W9-BMN-942

CURRENT
Diagnosis & Treatment
Cardiology

THIRD EDITION

Edited by

Michael H. Crawford, MD
Professor of Medicine
Lucy Stern Chair in Cardiology
Interim Chief of Cardiology
University of California, San Francisco

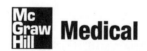

New York   Chicago   San Francisco   Lisbon   London   Madrid   Mexico City
Milan   New Delhi   San Juan   Seoul   Singapore   Sydney   Toronto

Current Diagnosis & Treatment: Cardiology, Third Edition

1 2 3 4 5 6 7 8 9 0   DOC/DOC   12 11 10 9

ISBN 978-0-07-144211-4; MHID 0-07-144211-1
ISSN 1079-1051

NOTICE

Medicine is an ever-changing science. As new research and clinical experience broaden our knowledge, changes in treatment and drug therapy are required. The authors and the publisher of this work have checked with sources believed to be reliable in their efforts to provide information that is complete and generally in accord with the standards accepted at the time of publication. However, in view of the possibility of human error or changes in medical sciences, neither the authors nor the publisher nor any other party who has been involved in the preparation or publication of this work warrants that the information contained herein is in every respect accurate or complete, and they disclaim all responsibility for any errors or omissions or for the results obtained from use of the information contained in this work. Readers are encouraged to confirm the information contained herein with other sources. For example and in particular, readers are advised to check the product information sheet included in the package of each drug they plan to administer to be certain that the information contained in this work is accurate and that changes have not been made in the recommended dose or in the contraindications for administration. This recommendation is of particular importance in connection with new or infrequently used drugs.

This book was set in Minion by Silverchair Science + Communications, Inc.
The editors were James Shanahan and Harriet Lebowitz.
The production supervisor was Catherine Saggese.
The cover designer was Mary McKeon.
The text was designed by Alan Barnett Design.
RR Donnelley was printer and binder.

Cover photos: Right, credit: Zsolt Nyulaszi; Top left, Doppler echocardiogram, credit: Chris Gallagher/Photo Researchers, Inc; Bottom left, credit: John Bavosi/Photo Researchers, Inc.

This book is printed on acid-free paper.

Contents

12. Infective Endocarditis 137

Bruce K. Shively, MD* & Michael H. Crawford, MD

13. Systemic Hypertension 153

William F. Graettinger, MD, FACC, FACP, FCCP

14. Hypertrophic Cardiomyopathies 164

Pravin M. Shah, MD, MACC

15. Restrictive Cardiomyopathies 172

John D. Carroll, MD & Michael H. Crawford, MD

16. Myocarditis 179

John B. O'Connell, MD & Michael H. Crawford, MD

21. Atrial Fibrillation 259

Melvin M. Scheinman, MD

22. Conduction Disorders & Cardiac Pacing 267

Richard H. Hongo, MD & Nora Goldschlager, MD

23. Ventricular Tachycardia 299

Nitish Badhwar, MD

30. Cardiac Tumors 432

Bill P.C. Hsieh, MD & Rita F. Redberg, MD, MSc, FACC, FAHA

31. Cardiovasular Disease in Pregnancy 446

Kirsten Tolstrup, MD, FACC, FASE

32. Endocrinology & the Heart 464

B. Sylvia Vela, MD & Michael H. Crawford, MD

33. Connective Tissue Diseases & the Heart 484

Carlos A. Roldan, MD

34. The Athlete's Heart   507

Cedela Abdulla, MD & J. V. (Ian) Nixon, MD, FACC, FAHA

Authors

Cedela Abdulla, MD
Department of Family Medicine, Memorial Hermann
    Hospital System, Houston, Texas
cedela_a@yahoo.com
The Athlete's Heart

Richard W. Asinger, MD
Director of Cardiology Division - HCMC, Professor of
    Medicine, University of Minnesota Medical School,
    Minneapolis, Minnesota
asing001@umn.edu
Long-Term Anticoagulation for Cardiac Conditions

Nitish Badhwar, MD
Assistant Clinical Professor of Medicine, University of
    California, San Francisco, California
badhwar@medicine.ucsf.edu
Ventricular Tachycardia

Andrew J. Boyle, MBBS, PhD
Assistant Clinical Professor of Medicine, University of
    California, San Francisco, California
aboyle@medicine.ucsf.edu
Acute Myocardial Infarction

Robert J. Bryg, MD
Professor of Medicine, David Geffen School of Medicine at
    UCLA, Los Angeles, California
nevsimbob@aol.com
Mitral Stenosis

Blase A. Carabello, MD
Professor, Baylor College of Medicine, Houston, Texas
blaseanthony.carabello@med.va.gov
Aortic Stenosis

Enrique V. Carbajal, MD
Assistant Clinical Professor of Medicine, University of
    California, San Francisco Medical Education Program;
    Assistant Chief, Cardiology Section, Veterans Affairs
    Central California Health Care System, Fresno,
    California
enrique.carbjal@med.va.gov
Congestive Heart Failure

John D. Carroll, MD
Professor of Medicine, Director Cardiac and Vascular
    Center; Chief, Interventional and Clinical Cardiology,
    University of Colorado Hospital, Denver, Colorado
john.carroll@uchsc.edu
Restrictive Cardiomyopathies

Kuang-Yuh Chyu, MD, PhD
Assistant Professor-in-Residence, Department of Medicine,
    University of California, Los Angeles, California
Kuang-Yuh.Chyu@cshs.org
Unstable Angina/Non-ST Evaluation Myocardial Infarction

Michael H. Crawford, MD
Professor of Medicine, Lucy Stern Chair in Cardiology;
    Interim Chief of Cardiology, University of California,
    San Francisco, California
crawfordm@medicine.ucsf.edu
*Approach to Cardiac Disease Diagnosis; Chronic Ischemic
    Heart Disease; Aortic Stenosis; Aortic Regurgitation; Mitral
    Regurgitation; Infective Endocarditis; Restrictive Cardio-
    myopathies; Myocarditis; Syncope; Endocrinology & the
    Heart*

Prakash C. Deedwania, MD
Chief, University of California, San Francisco School of
    Medicine, Cardiology Sections; Veterans Affairs Central
    California Health Care System, San Francisco, California
Congestive Heart Failure

Teresa De Marco, MD
Professor of Clinical Medicine and Surgery; Director, Heart
    Failure and Pulmonary Hypertension; Medical Director,
    Heart Transplantation, University of California, San
    Francisco, California
demarco@medicine.ucsf.edu
Pulmonary Hypertension

John P. DiMarco MD, PhD
Professor of Medicine; Director, Clinical Cardiac
    Electrophysiology Division of Cardiovacular Medicine
    University of Virginia Health System, Charlottesville,
    Virginia
jdimarco@virginia.edu
Sudden Cardiac Death

John A. Elefteriades, MD
Professor & Chief, Section of Cardiothoracic Surgery, Yale
    University School of Medicine, New Haven, Connecticut
john.elefteriades@yale.edu
Thoracic Aortic Aneurysms & Dissections

Elyse Foster, MD
Professor of Clinical Medicine and Anesthesia, University of
    California, San Francisco, California
foster@medicine.ucsf.edu
Congenital Heart Disease in Adults

Nora Goldschlager, MD

Professor of Clinical Medicine, University of California, San Francisco; Director, Coronary Care Unit, ECG Department and Pacemaker Clinic, San Francisco General Hospital, San Francisco, California

ngoldschlager@medsfgh.ucsf.edu

Conduction Disorders & Cardiac Pacing

William F. Graettinger, MD, FACC, FACP, FCCP

Professor & Vice-Chairman, Department of Internal Medicine, Chief, Division of Cardiology, University of Nevada School of Medicine, Reno; Chief, Cardiology Section, VA Sierra Nevada Healthcare System, Reno, Nevada

william.graettinger@med.va.gov

Systemic Hypertension

Ian S. Harris, MD

Assistant Professor of Medicine, Department of Internal Medicine, Division of Cardiology, Adult Congenital Heart Disease Service, University of California School of Medicine, San Francisco, California

harrisi@medicine.ucsf.edu

Congenital Heart Disease in Adults

Brian D. Hoit, MD

Professor of Medicine and Physiology and Biophysics, Case Western Reserve University; Director of Echocardiography, Case Medical Center, University Hospitals of Cleveland, Ohio

bdh6@cwru.edu

Tricuspid and Pulmonic Valve Disease

Richard H. Hongo, MD

California Pacific Medical Center, San Francisco, California

rhongo@cpcmg.com

Conduction Disorders & Cardiac Pacing

Bill P.C. Hsieh, MD

Instructor in Medicine, Albert Einstein College of Medicine, Montefiori Medical Center, New York, New York

Cardiac Tumors

Allan S. Jaffe, MD

Assistant Professor of Medicine & Consultant, Divisions of Cardiology and Laboratory Medicine, Mayo Clinic, Rochester, Minnesota

jaffe.allan@mayo.edu

Acute Myocardial Infarction

Peter R. Kowey, MD

Professor of Medicine, Jefferson Medical College; Chief, Division of Cardiovascular Diseases, Lankenau Hospital, Philadelphia, Pennsylvania

koweypr@mlhheart.org

Supraventricular Tachycardias

Byron K. Lee, MD

Assistant Professor of Medicine, Division of Cardiology, University of California, San Francisco, California

leeb@medicine.ucsf.edu

Supraventricular Tachycardias

Martin M. LeWinter, MD

Professor of Medicine & Molecular Physiology and Biophysics, University of Vermont College of Medicine, Attending Cardiologist and Director, Heart Failure Program, Fletcher Allen Health Care, Burlington, Vermont

martin.lewinter@vtmednet.org

Pericardial Disease

David D. McManus, MD

Instructor in Medicine, Cardiology Division, Department of Medicine, University of Massachusetts Medical Center, Worchester, Massachusetts

mcmanus.dave@gmail.com

Pulmonary Hypertension

Edward McNulty, MD

Assistant Clinical Professor of Medicine, University of San Francisco, San Francisco, California

edward.j.mcnulty@kp.org

Cardiogenic Shock

J. V. (Ian) Nixon, MD, FACC, FAHA

Professor of Internal Medicine & Cardiology, Virginia Commonwealth University School of Medicine Director, Noninvasive Cardiology Services, Pauley Heart Center, VCU Health System, Richmond, Virginia

jnixon@mcvh-vcu.edu

The Athlete's Heart

John B. O'Connell, MD

Professor & Chairman, Department of Internal Medicine, Wayne State University School of Medicine, Detroit, Michigan

joconnell@nmff.org

Myocarditis

Rajni K. Rao, MD

Assistant Clinical Professor of Medicine, University of California, San Francisco, California

rao@medicine.ucsf.edu

Pulmonary Embolic Disease

Rita F. Redberg, MD, MSc, FACC, FAHA

UCSF School of Medicine, Robert Wood Johnson
Foundation Health Policy Fellow, Professor of Medicine,
University of California, San Francisco Medical Center,
San Francisco, California
redberg@medicine.ucsf.edu
Cardiac Tumors

Carlos A. Roldan, MD

Associate Professor of Medicine, Cardiology Division,
Veterans Affairs Medical Center and University of New
Mexico, Albuquerque, New Mexico
carlosroldan2@med.va.gov
Connective Tissue Diseases & the Heart

Melvin M. Scheinman, MD

Professor of Medicine, Emeritus, Walter H., Shorenstein
Endowed Chair in Cardiology, University of California,
San Francisco, California
scheinman@medicine.ucsf.edu
Atrial Fibrillation

Pravin M. Shah, MD, MACC

Chair, Medical Director, Hoag Heart and Vascular Institute,
Newport Beach, California
pshah@hoaghospital.org
Hypertrophic Cardiomyopathies

Prediman K. Shah, MD

Shapell and Webb Chair & Director, Division of Cardiology
and Oppenheimer Atherosclerosis Research Center,
Cedar-Sinai Medical Center; Professor of Medicine,
University of California, Los Angeles, California
shahp@cshs.org
Unstable Angina/Non-ST Evaluation Myocardial Infarction

Sanjiv J. Shah, MD

Assistant Professor of Medicine, Division of Cardiology,
Department of Medicine; Director, Heart Failure with
Preserved Ejection Fraction, Bluhm Cardiovascular
Institute, Northwestern University Feinberg School of
Medicine, Chicago, Illinois
sanjiv.shah@northwestern.edu
*Heart Failure with Preserved Ejection Fraction; Evaluation &
Treatment of the Perioperative Patient*

Richard D. Taylor, MD

Director, Arrhythmia Management Program, Hennepin
County Medical Center; Assistant Professor of Medicine,
Minneapolis, Minnesota
rpkjtay@comcast.net
Long-Term Anticoagulation for Cardiac Conditions

Craig Timm, MD

Professor of Internal Medicine, Associate Dean of
Undergraduate Medical Education, University of New
Mexico Health Sciences Center, Albuquerque, New
Mexico
ctimm@salud.unm.edu
Cardiogenic Shock

Kristen Tolstrup, MD, FACC, FASE

Assistant Director, Cardiac Noninvasive Laboratory,
Cedars-Sinai Heart Institute; Associate Professor, UCLA
Geffen School of Medicine, Los Angeles, California
tolstrupk@cshs.org
Cardiovascular Disease in Pregnancy

Subha L. Varahan, MD

Fellow Division of Cardiovascular Medicine, University
Hospitals Case Medical Center, Division of
Cardiovascular Medicine, Department of Medicine,
Cleveland, Ohio
svarahan@gmail.com
Tricuspid and Pulmonic Valve Disease

B. Sylvia Vela, MD

Associate Professor of Clinical Medicine, University of
Arizona College of Medicine; Associate Chief of Staff,
Education, Phoenix VA Health Care System, Phoenix,
Arizona
sylvia.vela@med.va.gov
Endocrinology & the Heart

Christian Zellner, MD

Cardiology Fellow, University of California, San Francisco,
California
christian.zellner@ucsf.edu
Lipid Disorders

William A. Zoghbi, MD, FASE, FACC

William L. Winters Endowed Chair in CV Imaging;
Professor of Medicine, Weill Cornell Medical College;
Director, Cardiovascular Imaging Institute, The
Methodist DeBakey Heart & Vascular Center, Houston,
Texas
wzoghbi@tmhs.org
Aortic Regurgitation

Preface

Current Diagnosis & Treatment: Cardiology is designed to be a concise discussion of the essential knowledge needed to diagnose and manage cardiovascular diseases. *Current Diagnosis & Treatment: Cardiology* cannot be considered a condensed textbook because detailed pathophysiologic discussions are omitted; there are no chapters on diagnostic techniques; and rare or obscure entities are not included. Also, it is not a cardiac therapeutics text because diagnostic techniques, prevention strategies, and prognosis are fully discussed.

INTENDED AUDIENCE

Current Diagnosis & Treatment: Cardiology is designed to be a quick reference source in the clinic or on the ward for the experienced physician. Cardiology fellows will find that it is an excellent review for Board examinations. Also, students and residents will find it useful to review the essentials of specific conditions and to check the current references included in each section for further study. Nurses, technicians, and other health care workers who provide care for cardiology patients will find *Current Diagnosis & Treatment: Cardiology* a useful resource for all aspects of heart disease care.

COVERAGE

The 36 chapters in *Current Diagnosis & Treatment: Cardiology* cover the major disease entities and therapeutic challenges in cardiology. There are chapters on major management issues in cardiology such as pregnancy and heart disease, the use of anticoagulants in heart disease, and the perioperative evaluation of heart disease patients. Each section is written by experts in the particular area, but has been extensively edited to ensure a consistent approach throughout the book and the kind of readability found in single-author texts.

Since the second edition the book has changed somewhat. Each chapter has been thoroughly revised and the references updated, often by new authors. A new chapter has been added on heart failure with preserved ejection fraction and the chapters covering thoracic aortic diseases have been combined into one. My hope is that the book is found useful and improves patient care. Also, I hope it is an educational tool that improves knowledge of cardiac diseases. Finally, I hope it stimulates clinical research in areas where our knowledge is incomplete.

Michael H. Crawford, MD

Approach to Cardiac Disease Diagnosis

Michael H. Crawford, MD

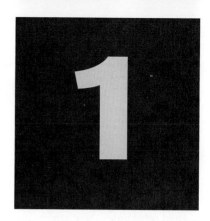

▶ General Considerations

The patient's history is a critical feature in the evaluation of suspected or overt heart disease. It includes information about the present illness, past illnesses, and the patient's family. From this information, a chronology of the patient's disease process should be constructed. Determining what information in the history is useful requires a detailed knowledge of the pathophysiology of cardiac disease. The effort spent on listening to the patient is time well invested because the cause of cardiac disease is often discernible from the history.

A. Common Symptoms

1. Chest pain—Chest pain is one of the cardinal symptoms (Table 1–1) of ischemic heart disease, but it can also occur with other forms of heart disease. The five characteristics of ischemic chest pain, or angina pectoris, are

- Anginal pain usually has a substernal location but may extend to the left or right chest, the shoulders, the neck, jaw, arms, epigastrium, and, occasionally, the upper back.
- The pain is deep, visceral, and intense; it makes the patient pay attention but is not excruciating. Many patients describe it as a pressure-like sensation or a tightness.
- The duration of the pain is minutes, not seconds.
- The pain tends to be precipitated by exercise or emotional stress.
- The pain is relieved by resting or taking sublingual nitroglycerin.

2. Dyspnea—A frequent complaint of patients with a variety of cardiac diseases, dyspnea is ordinarily one of four types. The most common is exertional dyspnea, which usually means that the underlying condition is mild because it requires the increased demand of exertion to precipitate symptoms. The next most common is paroxysmal nocturnal dyspnea, characterized by the patient awakening after being asleep or recumbent for an hour or more. This symptom is caused by the redistribution of body fluids from the lower extremities into the vascular space and back to the heart, resulting in volume overload; it suggests a more severe condition. Third is orthopnea, a dyspnea that occurs immediately on assuming the recumbent position. The mild increase in venous return (caused by lying down) before any fluid is mobilized from interstitial spaces in the lower extremities is responsible for the symptom, which suggests even more severe disease. Finally, dyspnea at rest suggests severe cardiac disease.

Dyspnea is not specific for heart disease, however. Exertional dyspnea, for example, can be due to pulmonary disease, anemia, or deconditioning. Orthopnea is a frequent complaint in patients with chronic obstructive pulmonary disease and postnasal drip. A history of "two-pillow orthopnea" is of little value unless the reason for the use of two pillows is discerned. Resting dyspnea is also a sign of pulmonary disease. Paroxysmal nocturnal dyspnea is perhaps the most specific for cardiac disease because few other conditions cause this symptom.

3. Syncope and presyncope—Lightheadedness, dizziness, presyncope, and syncope are important indications of a reduction in cerebral blood flow. These symptoms are nonspecific and can be due to primary central nervous system disease, metabolic conditions, dehydration, or inner-ear problems. Because bradyarrhythmias and tachyarrhythmias are important cardiac causes, a history of palpitations preceding the event is significant.

4. Transient central nervous system deficits—Deficits such as transient ischemic attacks (TIAs) suggest emboli from the heart or great vessels or, rarely, from the venous circulation through an intracardiac shunt. A TIA should prompt the search for cardiovascular disease. Any sudden loss of blood flow to a limb also suggests a cardioembolic event.

Table 1–1. Common Symptoms of Potential Cardiac Origin.

Chest pain or pressure
Dyspnea on exertion
Paroxysmal nocturnal dyspnea
Orthopnea
Syncope or near syncope
Transient neurologic defects
Edema
Palpitation
Cough

5. Fluid retention—These symptoms are not specific for heart disease but may be due to reduced cardiac function. Typical symptoms are peripheral edema, bloating, weight gain, and abdominal pain from an enlarged liver or spleen. Decreased appetite, diarrhea, jaundice, and nausea and vomiting can also occur from gut and hepatic dysfunction due to fluid engorgement.

6. Palpitation—Normal resting cardiac activity usually cannot be appreciated by the individual. Awareness of heart activity is often referred to by patients as palpitation. Among patients there is no standard definition for the type of sensation represented by palpitation, so the physician must explore the sensation further with the patient. It is frequently useful to have the patient tap the perceived heartbeat out by hand. Commonly, unusually forceful heart activity at a normal rate (60–100 bpm) is perceived as palpitation. More forceful contractions are usually the result of endogenous catecholamine excretion that does not elevate the heart rate out of the normal range. A common cause of this phenomenon is anxiety. Another common sensation is that of the heart stopping transiently or of the occurrence of isolated forceful beats or both. This sensation is usually caused by premature ventricular contractions, and the patient either feels the compensatory pause or the resultant more forceful subsequent beat or both. Occasionally, the individual feels the ectopic beat and refers to this phenomenon as "skipped" beats. The least common sensation reported by individuals, but the one most linked to the term "palpitation" is rapid heart rate that may be regular or irregular and is usually supraventricular in origin.

7. Cough—Although cough is usually associated with pulmonary disease processes, cardiac conditions that lead to pulmonary abnormalities may be the root cause of the cough. A cardiac cough is usually dry or nonproductive. Pulmonary fluid engorgement from conditions such as heart failure may present as cough. Pulmonary hypertension from any cause can result in cough. Finally, angiotensin-converting enzyme inhibitors, which are frequently used in cardiac conditions, can cause cough.

B. History

1. The present illness—This is a chronology of the events leading up to the patient's current complaints. Usually physicians start with the chief complaint and explore the patient's symptoms. It is especially important to determine the frequency, intensity, severity, and duration of all symptoms; their precipitating causes; what relieves them; and what aggravates them. Although information about previous related diseases and opinions from other physicians are often valuable, it is essential to explore the basis of any prior diagnosis and ask the patient about objective testing and the results of such testing. A history of prior treatment is often revealing because medications or surgery may indicate the nature of the original problem. A list should be made of all the patient's current medications, detailing the dosages, the frequency of administration, whether they are helping the patient, any side effects, and their cost.

2. Antecedent conditions—Several systemic diseases may have cardiac involvement. It is therefore useful to search for a history of rheumatic fever, which may manifest as Sydenham chorea, joint pain and swelling, or merely frequent sore throats. Other important diseases that affect the heart include metastatic cancer, thyroid disorders, diabetes mellitus, and inflammatory diseases such as rheumatoid arthritis and systemic lupus erythematosus. Certain events during childhood are suggestive of congenital or acquired heart disease; these include a history of cyanosis, reduced exercise tolerance, or long periods of restricted activities or school absence. Exposure to toxins, infectious agents, and other noxious substances may also be relevant.

3. Atherosclerotic risk factors—Atherosclerotic cardiovascular disease is the most common form of heart disease in industrialized nations. The presenting symptoms of this ubiquitous disorder may be unimpressive and minimal, or as impressive as sudden death. It is therefore important to determine from the history whether any risk factors for this disease are present. The most important are a family history of atherosclerotic disease, especially at a young age; diabetes mellitus; lipid disorders such as a high cholesterol level; hypertension; and smoking. Less important factors include a lack of exercise, high stress levels, the type-A personality, and truncal obesity.

4. Family history—A family history is important for determining the risk for not only atherosclerotic cardiovascular disease but for many other cardiac diseases as well. Congenital heart disease, for example, is more common in the offspring of parents with this condition, and a history of the disorder in the antecedent family or siblings is significant. Other genetic diseases, such as neuromuscular disorders or connective tissue disorders (eg, Marfan syndrome) can affect the heart. Acquired diseases, such as rheumatic valve disease, can cluster in families because of the spread of the streptococcal infection among family members. The lack of a history of hypertension in the family might prompt a more intensive search for a secondary cause. A history of atherosclerotic disease sequelae, such as limb loss, strokes, and heart attacks, may provide a clue to the aggressiveness of an atherosclerotic tendency in a particular family group.

▶ Physical Findings

A. Physical Examination

The physical examination is less important than the history in patients with ischemic heart disease, but it is of critical value in patients with congenital and valvular heart disease. In the latter two categories, the physician can often make specific anatomic and etiologic diagnoses based on the physical examination. Certain abnormal murmurs and heart sounds are specific for structural abnormalities of the heart. The physical examination is also important for confirming the diagnosis and establishing the severity of heart failure, and it is the only way to diagnose systemic hypertension because this diagnosis is based on elevated blood pressure recordings.

1. Blood pressure—Proper measurement of the **systemic arterial pressure** by cuff sphygmomanometry is one of the keystones of the cardiovascular physical examination. It is recommended that the brachial artery be palpated and the diaphragm of the stethoscope be placed over it, rather than merely sticking the stethoscope in the antecubital fossa. Current methodologic standards dictate that the onset and disappearance of the Korotkoff sounds define the systolic and diastolic pressures, respectively. Although this is the best approach in most cases, there are exceptions. For example, in patients in whom the diastolic pressure drops to near zero, the point of muffling of the sounds is usually recorded as the diastolic pressure. Because the diagnosis of systemic hypertension involves repeated measures under the same conditions, the operator should record the arm used and the position of the patient to allow reproducible measurements to be made on serial visits.

If the blood pressure is to be taken a second time, the patient should be in another position, such as standing, to determine any orthostatic changes in blood pressure. Orthostatic changes are a very important physical finding, especially in patients complaining of transient central nervous system symptoms, weakness, or unstable gait. The technique involves having the patient assume the upright position for at least 90 seconds before taking the pressure to be sure that the maximum orthostatic effect is measured. Although measuring the pressure in other extremities may be of value in certain vascular diseases, it provides little information in a routine examination beyond palpating pulses in all the extremities. Keep in mind, in general, that the pulse pressure (the difference between systolic and diastolic blood pressures) is a crude measure of left ventricular stroke volume. A widened pulse pressure suggests that the stroke volume is large; a narrowed pressure, that the stroke volume is small.

2. Peripheral pulses—When examining the peripheral pulses, the physician is really conducting three examinations. The first is an examination of the cardiac rate and rhythm, the second is an assessment of the characteristics of the pulse as a reflection of cardiac activity, and the third is an assessment of the adequacy of the arterial conduit being examined. The pulse rate and rhythm are usually determined in a convenient peripheral artery, such as the radial. If a pulse is irregular, it is better to auscultate the heart; some cardiac contractions during rhythm disturbances do not generate a stroke volume sufficient to cause a palpable peripheral pulse. In many ways, the heart rate reflects the health of the circulatory system. A rapid pulse suggests increased catecholamine levels, which may be due to cardiac disease, such as heart failure; a slow pulse represents an excess of vagal tone, which may be due to disease or athletic training.

To assess the characteristics of the cardiac contraction through the pulse, it is usually best to select an artery close to the heart, such as the carotid. Bounding high-amplitude carotid pulses suggest an increase in stroke volume and should be accompanied by a wide pulse pressure on the blood pressure measurement. A weak carotid pulse suggests a reduced stroke volume. Usually the strength of the pulse is graded on a scale of 1 to 4, where 2 is a normal pulse amplitude, 3 or 4 is a hyperdynamic pulse, and 1 is a weak pulse. A low-amplitude, slow-rising pulse, which may be associated with a palpable vibration (thrill), suggests aortic stenosis. A bifid pulse (beating twice in systole) can be a sign of hypertrophic obstructive cardiomyopathy, severe aortic regurgitation, or the combination of moderately severe aortic stenosis and regurgitation. A dicrotic pulse (an exaggerated, early, diastolic wave) is found in severe heart failure. Pulsus alternans (alternate strong and weak pulses) is also a sign of severe heart failure. When evaluating the adequacy of the arterial conduits, all palpable pulses can be assessed and graded on a scale of 0 to 4, where 4 is a fully normal conduit, and anything below that is reduced, including 0—which indicates an absent pulse. The major pulses routinely palpated on physical examination are the radial, brachial, carotid, femoral, dorsalis pedis, and posterior tibial. In special situations, the abdominal aorta and the ulnar, subclavian, popliteal, axillary, temporal, and intercostal arteries are palpated. In assessing the abdominal aorta, it is important to make note of the width of the aorta because an increase suggests an abdominal aortic aneurysm. It is particularly important to palpate the abdominal aorta in older individuals because abdominal aortic aneurysms are more prevalent in those older than 70. An audible bruit is a clue to significantly obstructed large arteries. During a routine examination, bruits are sought with the bell of the stethoscope placed over the carotids, abdominal aorta, and femorals at the groin. Other arteries may be auscultated under special circumstances, such as suspected temporal arteritis or vertebrobasilar insufficiency.

3. Jugular venous pulse—Assessment of the jugular venous pulse can provide information about the central venous pressure and right-heart function. Examination of the right internal jugular vein is ideal for assessing central venous pressure because it is attached directly to the superior vena cava without intervening valves. The patient is positioned into the semiupright posture that permits visualization of the top of the right internal jugular venous blood column. The height of this column of blood, vertically from the sternal angle, is added to 5 cm of blood (the presumed distance to the center of the right atrium from the sternal angle) to obtain an estimate of central venous pressure in centimeters of blood. This can be converted to millimeters of mercury (mm Hg) with the formula:

$$\text{mm Hg} = \text{cm blood} \times 0.736.$$

Examining the characteristics of the right internal jugular pulse is valuable for assessing right-heart function and rhythm disturbances. The normal jugular venous pulse has two distinct waves: *a* and *v*; the former coincides with atrial contraction and the latter with late ventricular systole. An absent *a* wave and an irregular pulse suggest atrial fibrillation. A large and early *v* wave suggests tricuspid regurgitation. The dips after the *a* and *v* waves are the *x* and *y* descents; the former coincide with atrial relaxation and the latter with early ventricular filling. In tricuspid stenosis the *y* descent is prolonged. Other applications of the jugular pulse examination are discussed in the chapters dealing with specific disorders.

4. Lungs—Evaluation of the lungs is an important part of the physical examination: Diseases of the lung can affect the heart, just as diseases of the heart can affect the lungs. The major finding of importance is rales at the pulmonary bases, indicating alveolar fluid collection. Although this is a significant finding in patients with congestive heart failure, it is not always possible to distinguish rales caused by heart failure from those caused by pulmonary disease. The presence of pleural fluid, although useful in the diagnosis of heart failure, can be due to other causes. Heart failure most commonly causes a right pleural effusion; it can cause effusions on both sides but is least likely to cause isolated left pleural effusion. The specific constellation of dullness at the left base with bronchial breath sounds suggests an increase in heart size from pericardial effusion (Ewart sign) or another cause of cardiac enlargement; it is thought to be due to compression by the heart of a left lower lobe bronchus.

When right-heart failure develops or venous return is restricted from entering the heart, venous pressure in the abdomen increases, leading to hepatosplenomegaly and eventually ascites. None of these physical findings is specific for heart disease; they do, however, help establish the diagnosis. Heart failure also leads to generalized fluid retention, usually manifested as lower extremity edema or, in severe heart failure, anasarca.

5. Cardiac auscultation—Heart sounds are caused by the acceleration and deceleration of blood and the subsequent vibration of the cardiac structures during the phases of the cardiac cycle. To hear cardiac sounds, use a stethoscope with a bell and a tight diaphragm. Low-frequency sounds are associated with ventricular filling and are heard best with the bell. Medium-frequency sounds are associated with valve opening and closing; they are heard best with the diaphragm. Cardiac murmurs are due to turbulent blood flow, are usually high-to-medium frequency, and are heard best with the diaphragm. Low-frequency atrioventricular valve inflow murmurs, such as that produced by mitral stenosis, are best heard with the bell, however. Auscultation should take place in areas that correspond to the location of the heart and great vessels. Such placement will, of course, need to be modified for patients with unusual body habitus or an unusual cardiac position. When no cardiac sounds can be heard over the precordium, they can often be heard in either the subxiphoid area or the right supraclavicular area.

Auscultation in various positions is recommended because low-frequency filling sounds are best heard with the patient in the left lateral decubitus position, and high-frequency murmurs, such as that of aortic regurgitation, are best heard with the patient sitting.

A. Heart sounds—The **first heart sound** is coincident with mitral and tricuspid valve closure and has two components in up to 40% of normal individuals. There is little change in the intensity of this sound with respiration or position. The major determinant of the intensity of the first heart sound is the electrocardiographic (ECG) PR interval, which determines the time delay between atrial and ventricular contraction and thus the position of the mitral valve when ventricular systole begins. With a short PR interval, the mitral valve is widely open when systole begins, and its closure increases the intensity of the first sound, as compared to a long PR-interval beat when the valve partially closes prior to the onset of ventricular systole. Certain disease states, such as mitral stenosis, also can increase the intensity of the first sound.

The **second heart sound** is coincident with closure of the aortic and pulmonic valves. Normally, this sound is single in expiration and split during inspiration, permitting the aortic and pulmonic components to be distinguished. The inspiratory split is due to a delay in the occurrence of the pulmonic component because of a decrease in pulmonary vascular resistance, which prolongs pulmonary flow beyond the end of right ventricular systole. Variations in this normal splitting of the second heart sound are useful in determining certain disease states. For example, in atrial septal defect, the second sound is usually split throughout the respiratory cycle because of the constant increase in pulmonary flow. In patients with left bundle branch block, a delay occurs in the aortic component of the second heart sound, which results in reversed respiratory splitting; single with inspiration, split with expiration.

A **third heart sound** occurs during early rapid filling of the left ventricle; it can be produced by any condition that causes left ventricular volume overload or dilatation. It can therefore be heard in such disparate conditions as congestive heart failure and normal pregnancy. A **fourth heart sound** is due to a vigorous atrial contraction into a stiffened left ventricle and can be heard in left ventricular hypertrophy of any cause or in diseases that reduce compliance of the left ventricle, such as myocardial infarction.

Although third and fourth heart sounds can occasionally occur in normal individuals, all other extra sounds are signs of cardiac disease. Early ejection sounds are due to abnormalities of the semilunar valves, from restriction of their motion, thickening, or both (eg, a bicuspid aortic valve, pulmonic or aortic stenosis). A midsystolic click is often due to mitral valve prolapse and is caused by sudden tensing in midsystole of the redundant prolapsing segment of the mitral leaflet. The opening of a thickened atrioventricular valve leaflet, as in mitral stenosis, will cause a loud opening sound (snap) in early diastole. A lower frequency (more of a knock) sound at the time of rapid filling may be an indication of constrictive pericarditis. These early diastolic sounds must be distinguished from a third heart sound.

B. MURMURS—**Systolic murmurs** are very common and do not always imply cardiac disease. They are usually rated on a scale of 1 to 6, where grade 1 is barely audible, grade 4 is associated with palpable vibrations (thrill), grade 5 can be heard with the edge of the stethoscope, and grade 6 can be heard without a stethoscope. Most murmurs fall in the 1–3 range, and murmurs in the 4–6 range are almost always due to pathologic conditions; severe disease can exist with grades 1–3 or no cardiac murmurs, however. The most common systolic murmur is the crescendo/decrescendo murmur that increases in intensity as blood flows early in systole and diminishes in intensity through the second half of systole. This murmur can be due to vigorous flow in a normal heart or to obstructions in flow, as occurs with aortic stenosis, pulmonic stenosis, or hypertrophic cardiomyopathy. The so-called innocent flow murmurs are usually grades 1–2 and occur very early in systole; they may have a vibratory quality and are usually less apparent when the patient is in the sitting position (when venous return is less). If an ejection sound is heard, there is usually some abnormality of the semilunar valves. Although louder murmurs may be due to pathologic cardiac conditions, this is not always so. Distinguishing benign from pathologic systolic flow murmurs is one of the major challenges of clinical cardiology. Benign flow murmurs can be heard in 80% of children; the incidence declines with age, but may be prominent during pregnancy or in adults who are thin or physically well trained. The murmur is usually benign in a patient with a soft flow murmur that diminishes in intensity in the sitting position and neither a history of cardiovascular disease nor other cardiac findings.

The **holosystolic,** or **pansystolic,** murmur is almost always associated with cardiac pathology. The most common cause of this murmur is atrioventricular valve regurgitation, but it can also be observed in conditions such as ventricular septal defect, in which an abnormal communication exists between two chambers of markedly different systolic pressures. Although it is relatively easy to determine that these murmurs represent an abnormality, it is more of a challenge to determine their origins. Keep in mind that such conditions as mitral regurgitation, which usually produce holosystolic murmurs, may produce crescendo/decrescendo murmurs, adding to the difficulty in differentiating benign from pathologic systolic flow murmurs.

Diastolic murmurs are always abnormal. The most frequently heard diastolic murmur is the high-frequency decrescendo early diastolic murmur of aortic regurgitation. This is usually heard best at the upper left sternal border or in the aortic area (upper right sternal border) and may radiate to the lower left sternal border and the apex. This murmur is usually very high frequency and may be difficult to hear. Although the murmur of pulmonic regurgitation may sound like that of aortic regurgitation when pulmonary artery pressures are high, it is usually best heard in the pulmonic area (left second intercostal space parasternally). If structural disease of the valve is present with normal pulmonary pressures, the murmur usually has a midrange frequency and begins with a slight delay after the pulmonic second heart sound. Mitral stenosis produces a low-frequency rumbling diastolic murmur that is decrescendo in early diastole, but may become crescendo up to the first heart sound with moderately severe mitral stenosis and sinus rhythm. The murmur is best heard at the apex in the left lateral decubitus position with the bell of the stethoscope. Similar findings are heard in tricuspid stenosis, but the murmur is loudest at the lower left sternal border.

A **continuous murmur** implies a connection between a high- and a low-pressure chamber throughout the cardiac cycle, such as occurs with a fistula between the aorta and the pulmonary artery. If the connection is a patent ductus arteriosus, the murmur is heard best under the left clavicle; it has a machine-like quality. Continuous murmurs must be distinguished from the combination of systolic and diastolic murmurs in patients with combined lesions (eg, aortic stenosis and regurgitation).

Traditionally, the origin of heart murmurs was based on five factors: (1) their timing in the cardiac cycle, (2) where on the chest they were heard, (3) their characteristics, (4) their intensity, and (5) their duration. Unfortunately, this traditional classification system is unreliable in predicting the underlying pathology. A more accurate method, **dynamic auscultation,** changes the intensity, duration, and characteristics of the murmur by bedside maneuvers that alter hemodynamics.

The simplest of these maneuvers is observation of any changes in murmur intensity with normal respiration because all right-sided cardiac murmurs should increase in intensity with normal inspiration. Although some exceptions exist, the method is very reliable for detecting such murmurs. Inspiration is associated with reductions in intrathoracic pressure that increase venous return from the abdomen and the head, leading to an increased flow through the right heart chambers. The consequent increase in pressure increases the intensity of right-sided murmurs. These changes are best observed in the sitting position, where venous return is smallest, and changes in intrathoracic pressure can produce their greatest effect on venous return. In a patient in the supine position, when venous return is near maximum, there may be little change observed with respiration. The ejection sound caused by pulmonic stenosis does not routinely increase in intensity with inspiration. The increased blood in the right heart accentuates atrial contraction, which increases late diastolic pressure in the right ventricle, partially opening the stenotic pulmonary valve and thus diminishing the opening sound of this valve with the subsequent systole.

Changes in position are an important part of normal auscultation; they can also be of great value in determining the origin of cardiac murmurs (Table 1–2). Murmurs dependent on venous return, such as innocent flow murmurs, are softer or absent in upright positions; others, such as the murmur associated with hypertrophic obstructive cardiomyopathy, are accentuated by reduced left ventricular volume associated with the upright position. In physically capable individuals, a rapid squat from the standing position is often diagnostically valuable because it suddenly increases venous return and left ventricular volume and accentuates flow murmurs but diminishes the murmur of hypertrophic obstructive cardiomyopathy. The stand-squat maneuver is also useful for altering the timing of the midsystolic click caused by mitral valve prolapse during systole. When the ventricle is small during standing, the prolapse occurs earlier in systole, moving the midsystolic click to early systole. During squatting, the ventricle dilates and the prolapse is delayed in systole, resulting in a late midsystolic click.

Valsalva maneuver is also frequently used. The patient bears down and expires against a closed glottis, increasing intrathoracic pressure and markedly reducing venous return to the heart. Although almost all cardiac murmurs decrease in intensity during this maneuver, there are two exceptions: (1) The murmur of hypertrophic obstructive cardiomyopathy may become louder because of the diminished left ventricular volume. (2) The murmur associated with mitral regurgitation from mitral valve prolapse may become longer and louder because of the earlier occurrence of prolapse during systole. When the maneuver is very vigorous and prolonged, even these two murmurs may eventually diminish in intensity. Therefore, the Valsalva maneuver should be held for only about 10 seconds, so as not to cause prolonged diminution of the cerebral and coronary blood flow.

Isometric hand grip exercises have been used to increase arterial and left ventricular pressure. These maneuvers increase the flow gradient for mitral regurgitation, ventricular septal defect, and aortic regurgitation; the murmurs should then increase in intensity. Increasing arterial and left ventricular pressure increases left ventricular volume, thereby decreasing the murmur of hypertrophic obstructive cardiomyopathy. If the patient is unable to perform isometric exercises, **transient arterial occlusion** of both upper extremities with sphygmomanometers can achieve the same increases in left-sided pressure.

Noting the changes in murmur intensity in the heart beat following a premature ventricular contraction, and comparing these to a beat that does not, can be extremely useful. The premature ventricular contraction interrupts the cardiac cycle, and during the subsequent compensatory pause, an extra-long diastole occurs, leading to increased left ventricular filling. Therefore, murmurs caused by the flow of blood out of the left ventricle (eg, aortic stenosis) increase in intensity. There is usually no change in the intensity of the murmur of typical mitral regurgitation because blood pressure falls during the long pause and increases the gradient

Table 1–2. Differentiation of Systolic Murmurs Based on Changes in Their Intensity from Physiologic Maneuvers.

Maneuver	Origin of Murmur					
	Flow	TR	AS	MR/VSD	MVP	HOCM
Inspiration	– or ↑	↑	–	–	–	–
Stand	↓	–	–	–	↑	↑
Squat	↑	–	–	–	↓	↓
Valsalva	↓	↓	↓	↓	↑	↑
Handgrip/TAO	↓	–	–	↑	↑	↓
Post-PVC	↑	–	↑	–	–	↑

AS, aortic stenosis; Flow, innocent flow murmur; HOCM, hypertrophic obstructive cardiomyopathy; MR, mitral regurgitation; MVP, mitral valve prolapse; PVC, premature ventricular contraction; TAO, transient arterial occlusion; TR, tricuspid regurgitation; VSD, ventricular septal defect; ↑ or ↓, change in intensity of murmur; –, no consistent change.

between the left ventricle and the aorta, allowing more forward flow. This results in the same amount of mitral regurgitant flow as on a normal beat with a higher aortic pressure and less forward flow. The increased volume during the long pause goes out of the aorta rather than back into the left atrium. Unfortunately, there is no reliable way of inducing a premature ventricular contraction in most patients; it is fortuitous when a physician is present for one. Atrial fibrillation with markedly varying cycle lengths produces the same phenomenon and can be very helpful in determining the origin of murmurs.

Various rapid-acting pharmacologic agents have been used to clarify the origin of cardiac murmurs. A once-popular bedside pharmacologic maneuver was the inhalation of amyl nitrite. Because this produces rapid vasodilatation and decreases in blood pressure, it diminishes the murmurs of aortic and mitral regurgitation and ventricular septal defect and increases systolic flow murmurs (eg, those caused by aortic stenosis and hypertrophic obstructive cardiomyopathy). Patients never liked the unpleasant odor of amyl nitrite and its popularity has since waned. Other pharmacologic maneuvers have occasionally been used to clarify the origin of a murmur. These include the infusion of synthetic catecholamines to increase blood pressure, isoproterenol to increase the heart rate, and intravenous β-blockers to decrease the heart rate. With the ready availability of echocardiography, these more invasive interventions have also diminished in popularity.

Brennan JM et al. A comparison by medicine residents of physical examination versus hand-carried ultrasound for estimation of right atrial pressure. Am J Cardiol. 2007 Jun 1;99(11):1614–6. [PMID: 17531592]

Marcus GM et al. Usefulness of the third heart sound in predicting an elevated level of B-type natriuretic peptide. Am J Cardiol. 2004 May 15;93(10):1312–3. [PMID: 15135714]

B. Diagnostic Studies

1. Electrocardiography—Electrocardiography is perhaps the least expensive of all cardiac diagnostic tests, providing considerable value for the money. Modern ECG-reading computers do an excellent job of measuring the various intervals between waveforms and calculating the heart rate and the left ventricular axis. These programs fall considerably short, however, when it comes to diagnosing complex ECG patterns and rhythm disturbances, and the test results must be read by a physician skilled at ECG interpretation.

Analysis of cardiac rhythm is perhaps the ECG's most widely used feature; it is used to clarify the mechanism of an irregular heart rhythm detected on physical examination or that of an extremely rapid or slow rhythm. The ECG is also used to monitor cardiac rate and rhythm; Holter monitoring and other continuous ECG monitoring devices allow assessment of cardiac rate and rhythm on an ambulatory basis. ECG radio telemetry is also often used on hospital wards and

between ambulances and emergency departments to assess and monitor rhythm disturbances. There are two types of ambulatory ECG recorders: continuous recorders that record all heart beats over 24 or more hours and intermittent recorders that can be attached to the patient or implanted subcutaneously for weeks or months and then activated to provide brief recordings of infrequent events. In addition to analysis of cardiac rhythm, ambulatory ECG recordings can be used to detect ST-wave transients indicative of myocardial ischemia and certain electrophysiologic parameters of diagnostic and prognostic value. The most common use of ambulatory ECG monitoring is the evaluation of symptoms such as syncope, near-syncope, or palpitation for which there is no obvious cause and cardiac rhythm disturbances are suspected.

The ECG is an important tool for rapidly assessing **metabolic and toxic disorders** of the heart. Characteristic changes in the ST-T waves indicate imbalances of potassium and calcium. Drugs such as tricyclic antidepressants have characteristic effects on the QT and QRS intervals at toxic levels. Such observations on the ECG can be life-saving in emergency situations with comatose patients or cardiac arrest victims.

Chamber enlargement can be assessed through the characteristic changes of left or right ventricular and atrial enlargement. Occasionally, isolated signs of left atrial enlargement on the ECG may be the only diagnostic clue to mitral stenosis. Evidence of chamber enlargement on the ECG usually signifies an advanced stage of disease with a poorer prognosis than that of patients with the same disease but no discernible enlargement.

The ECG is an important tool in managing **acute myocardial infarction.** In patients with chest pain that is compatible with myocardial ischemia, the characteristic ST-T-wave elevations that do not resolve with nitroglycerin (and are unlikely to be the result of an old infarction) become the basis for thrombolytic therapy or primary angioplasty. Rapid resolution of the ECG changes of myocardial infarction after reperfusion therapy has prognostic value and identifies patients with reperfused coronary arteries.

Evidence of **conduction abnormalities** may help explain the mechanism of bradyarrhythmias and the likelihood of the need for a pacemaker. Conduction abnormalities may also aid in determining the cause of heart disease. For example, right bundle branch block and left anterior fascicular block are often seen in Chagas cardiomyopathy, and left-axis deviation occurs in patients with a primum atrial septal defect.

A newer form of electrocardiography is the signal-averaged, or high-resolution, ECG. This device markedly accentuates the QRS complex so that low-amplitude afterpotentials, which correlate with a propensity toward ventricular arrhythmias and sudden death, can be detected. The signal-averaged ECG permits a more accurate measurement of QRS duration, which also has prognostic significance of established value in the stratification of risk of developing sustained ventricular arrhythmias in postmyocardial infarction patients, patients with coronary artery disease and unexplained syncope, and patients with nonischemic cardiomyopathy.

2. Echocardiography—Another frequently ordered cardiac diagnostic test, echocardiography is based on the use of ultrasound directed at the heart to create images of cardiac anatomy and display them in real time on a television screen. Two-dimensional echocardiography is usually accomplished by placing an ultrasound transducer in various positions on the anterior chest and obtaining cross-sectional images of the heart and great vessels in a variety of standard planes. In general, two-dimensional echocardiography is excellent for detecting any anatomic abnormality of the heart and great vessels. In addition, because the heart is seen in real time, this modality can assess the function of cardiac chambers and valves throughout the cardiac cycle.

Transesophageal echocardiography (TEE) involves the placement of smaller ultrasound probes on a gastroscopic device for placement in the esophagus behind the heart; it produces much higher resolution images of posterior cardiac structures. Transesophageal echocardiography has made it possible to detect left atrial thrombi, small mitral valve vegetations, and thoracic aortic dissection with a high degree of accuracy.

The older analog echocardiographic display referred to as M-mode, motion-mode, or time-motion mode, is currently used for its high axial and temporal resolution. It is superior to two-dimensional echocardiography for measuring the size of structures in its axial direction, and its 1/1000-s sampling rate allows for the resolution of complex cardiac motion patterns. Its many disadvantages, including poor lateral resolution and the inability to distinguish whole heart motion from the motion of individual cardiac structures, have relegated it to a supporting role.

Doppler ultrasound can be combined with two-dimensional imaging to investigate blood flow in the heart and great vessels. It is based on determining the change in frequency (caused by the movement of blood in the given structure) of the reflected ultrasound compared with the transmitted ultrasound, and converting this difference into flow velocity. Color-flow Doppler echocardiography is most frequently used. In this technique, frequency shifts in each pixel of a selected area of the two-dimensional image are measured and converted into a color, depending on the direction of flow, the velocity, and the presence or absence of turbulence. When these color images are superimposed on the two-dimensional echocardiographic image, a moving color image of blood flow in the heart is created in real time. This is extremely useful for detecting regurgitant blood flow across cardiac valves and any abnormal communications in the heart.

Tissue Doppler imaging is similar to color-flow Doppler except that myocardial tissue movement velocity is interrogated. This allows for the quantitation of the rate of tissue contraction and relaxation which is a measure of myocardial performance that can be applied to systole and diastole. Regional differences in myocardial performance can be assessed and used to guide biventricular pacemaker resynchronization therapy.

Because color-flow imaging cannot resolve very high velocities, another Doppler mode must be used to quantitate the exact velocity and estimate the pressure gradient of the flow when high velocities are suspected. Continuous wave Doppler, which almost continuously sends and receives ultrasound along a beam that can be aligned through the heart, is extremely accurate at resolving very high velocities such as those encountered with valvular aortic stenosis. The disadvantage of this technique is that the source of the high velocity within the beam cannot always be determined but must be assumed, based on the anatomy through which the beam passes. When there is ambiguity about the source of the high velocity, pulsed wave Doppler is more useful. This technique is range-gated such that specific areas along the beam (sample volumes) can be investigated. One or more sample volumes can be examined and determinations made concerning the exact location of areas of high-velocity flow.

Two-dimensional echocardiographic imaging of dynamic left ventricular cross-sectional anatomy and the superimposition of a Doppler color-flow map provide more information than the traditional left ventricular cine-angiogram can. Ventricular wall motion can be interrogated in multiple planes, and left ventricular wall thickening during systole (an important measure of myocardial viability) can be assessed. In addition to demonstrating segmental wall motion abnormalities, echocardiography can estimate left ventricular volumes and ejection fraction. In addition, valvular regurgitation can be assessed at all four valves with the accuracy of the estimated severity equivalent to contrast angiography.

Doppler echocardiography has now largely replaced cardiac catheterization for deriving hemodynamics to estimate the severity of valve stenosis. Recorded Doppler velocities across a valve can be converted to pressure gradients by use of the simplified Bernoulli equation (pressure gradient = $4 \times$ velocity^2). Cardiac output can be measured by Doppler from the velocity recorded at cardiac anatomic sites of known size visualized on the two-dimensional echocardiographic image. Cardiac output and pressure gradient data can be used to calculate the stenotic valve area with remarkable accuracy. A complete echocardiographic examination including two-dimensional and M-mode anatomic and functional visualization, and color, pulsed, and continuous wave Doppler examination of blood flow provides a considerable amount of information about cardiac structure and function. A full discussion of the usefulness of this technique is beyond the scope of this chapter, but individual uses of echocardiography will be discussed in later chapters.

Unfortunately, echocardiography is not without its technical difficulties and pitfalls. Like any noninvasive technique, it is not 100% accurate. Furthermore, it is impossible to obtain high-quality images or Doppler signals in as many as 5% of patients—especially those with emphysema, chest wall deformities, and obesity. Although TEE has made the examination of such patients easier, it does not solve all the problems of echocardiography. Despite these limitations, the technique is so powerful that it has moved out of the noninvasive laboratory and is now frequently being used in the operating room, the clinic, the emergency department, and even the cardiac catheterization laboratory, to help guide procedures without the use of fluoroscopy.

3. Nuclear cardiac imaging—Nuclear cardiac imaging involves the injection of tracer amounts of radioactive elements attached to larger molecules or to the patient's own blood cells. The tracer-labeled blood is concentrated in certain areas of the heart, and a gamma ray detection camera is used to detect the radioactive emissions and form an image of the deployment of the tracer in the particular area. The single-crystal gamma camera produces planar images of the heart, depending on the relationship of the camera to the body. Multiple-head gamma cameras, which rotate around the patient, can produce single-photon emission computed tomography (SPECT) images, displaying the cardiac anatomy in slices, each about 1-cm thick.

A. Myocardial perfusion imaging—The most common tracers used for imaging regional myocardial blood-flow distribution are thallium-201 and the technetium-99m-based agents, such as sestamibi. Thallium-201, a potassium analog that is efficiently extracted from the bloodstream by viable myocardial cells, is concentrated in the myocardium in areas of adequate blood flow and living myocardial cells. Thallium perfusion images show defects (a lower tracer concentration) in areas where blood flow is relatively reduced and in areas of damaged myocardial cells. If the damage is from frank necrosis or scar tissue formation, very little thallium will be taken up; ischemic cells may take up thallium more slowly or incompletely, producing relative defects in the image.

Myocardial perfusion problems are separated from nonviable myocardium by the fact that thallium eventually washes out of the myocardial cells and back into the circulation. If a defect detected on initial thallium imaging disappears over a period of 3–24 hours, the area is presumably viable. A persistent defect suggests a myocardial scar. In addition to detecting viable myocardium and assessing the extent of new and old myocardial infarctions, thallium-201 imaging can also be used to detect myocardial ischemia during stress testing (see section on Stress testing below) as well as marked enlargement of the heart or dysfunction. The major problem with thallium imaging is photon attenuation because of chest wall structures, which can give an artifactual appearance of defects in the myocardium.

The technetium-99m-based agents take advantage of the shorter half-life of technetium (6 hours; thallium 201's is 73

hours); this allows for use of a larger dose, which results in higher energy emissions and higher quality images. Technetium-99m's higher energy emissions scatter less and are attenuated less by chest wall structures, reducing the number of artifacts. Because sestamibi undergoes considerably less washout after the initial myocardial uptake than thallium does, the evaluation of perfusion versus tissue damage requires two separate injections.

In addition to detecting perfusion deficits, myocardial imaging with the SPECT system allows for a three-dimensional reconstruction of the heart, which can be displayed in any projection on a monitor screen. Such images can be formed at intervals during the cardiac cycle to create an image of the beating heart, which can be used to detect wall motion abnormalities and derive left ventricular volumes and ejection fraction. Matching wall motion abnormalities with perfusion defects provides additional confirmation that the perfusion defects visualized are true and not artifacts of photon attenuation. Also, extensive perfusion defects and wall motion abnormalities should be accompanied by decreases in ejection fraction.

B. Radionuclide angiography—Radionuclide angiography is based on visualizing radioactive tracers in the cavities of the heart over time. Radionuclide angiography is usually done with a single gamma camera in a single plane, and only one view of the heart is obtained. The most common technique is to record the amount of radioactivity received by the gamma camera over time. Although volume estimates by radionuclide angiography are not as accurate as those obtained by other methods, the ejection fraction is quite accurate. Wall motion can be assessed in the one plane imaged, but the technique is not as sensitive as other imaging modalities for detecting wall motion abnormalities.

4. Other cardiac imaging

A. Chest radiography—Chest radiography is used infrequently now for evaluating cardiac structural abnormalities because of the superiority of echocardiography in this regard. The chest radiograph, however, is a rapid, inexpensive way to assess pulmonary anatomy and is very useful for evaluating pulmonary venous congestion and hypoperfusion or hyperperfusion. In addition, abnormalities of the thoracic skeleton are found in certain cardiac disorders and radiographic corroboration may help with the diagnosis. Detection of intracardiac calcium deposits by the radiograph or fluoroscopy is of some value in finding coronary artery, valvular, or pericardial disease.

B. Computed tomographic scanning—Computed tomography (CT) has been applied to cardiac imaging by using ECG gating to account for the motion of the heart. The major application of this technology has been the detection of small amounts of coronary artery calcium as an indicator of atherosclerosis in the coronary arterial tree. With the development of multidetector CT and using intravenous contrast agents, noninvasive coronary angiography is possible and has a very high negative predictive value for detecting significant coronary artery lesions. Hybrid positron emission tomography (PET) or nuclear SPECT plus CT scanners are now available and can provide anatomic and perfusion data. CT scanning is also very useful for detecting thoracic aorta disease, such as dissection and pericardial disease.

C. MAGNETIC RESONANCE IMAGING—Magnetic resonance imaging (MRI) probably has considerable potential as a technique for evaluating cardiovascular disease. It is excellent for detecting aortic dissection and pericardial thickening and assessing left ventricular mass. Newer computer analysis techniques have solved the problem of myocardial motion and can be used to detect flow in the heart, much as color-flow Doppler is used. In addition, regional molecular disturbances can be created that place stripes of a different density in either the myocardium or the blood; these can then be followed through the cardiac cycle to determine structural deformation (eg, of the left ventricular wall) or the movement of the blood.

Gadolinium-based contrast agents can be injected intravenously to enhance MRI. In delayed images taken after contrast injection (approximately 10 minutes), hyperenhancement of the myocardium suggests irreversible scar formation. This determination can identify nonviable myocardium in patients with coronary artery disease. The major limitation of cardiac MRI is the length of the studies and the relative nonavailabilty of magnetic resonance systems to acute patient care areas compared with CT.

D. POSITRON EMISSION TOMOGRAPHY—Positron emission tomography (PET) is a technique using tracers that simultaneously emit two high-energy photons. A circular array of detectors around the patient can detect these simultaneous events and accurately identify their origin in the heart. This results in improved spatial resolution, compared with SPECT. It also allows for correction of tissue photon attenuation, resulting in the ability to accurately quantify radioactivity in the heart. Positron emission tomography can be used to assess myocardial perfusion and myocardial metabolic activity separately by using different tracers coupled to different molecules. Most of the tracers developed for clinical use require a cyclotron for their generation; the cyclotron must be in close proximity to the PET imager because of the short half-life of the agents. Agents in clinical use include oxygen-15 (half-life 2 minutes), nitrogen-13 (half-life 10 minutes), carbon-11 (half-life 20 minutes), and fluorene-18 (half-life 110 minutes). These tracers can be coupled to many physiologically active molecules for assessing various functions of the myocardium. Because rubidium-82, with a half-life of 75 seconds, does not require a cyclotron and can be generated on-site, it is frequently used with PET scanning, especially for perfusion images. Ammonia containing nitrogen-13 and water containing oxygen-15 are also used as perfusion agents. C-11-labeled fatty acids and ^{18}F fluorode-

oxyglucose are common metabolic tracers used to assess myocardial viability, and acetate containing carbon-11 is often used to assess oxidative metabolism.

The main clinical uses of PET scanning involve the evaluation of coronary artery disease. It is used in perfusion studies at rest and during pharmacologic stress (exercise studies are less feasible). In addition to a qualitative assessment of perfusion defects, PET allows for a calculation of absolute regional myocardial blood flow or blood-flow reserve. Positron emission tomography also assesses myocardial viability, using the metabolic tracers to detect metabolically active myocardium in areas of reduced perfusion. The presence of viability imply that returning perfusion to these areas would result in improved function of the ischemic myocardium. Although many authorities consider PET scanning the gold standard for determining myocardial viability, it has not been found to be 100% accurate. Thallium reuptake techniques and echocardiographic and MR imaging of delayed myocardial enhancement have proved equally valuable for detecting myocardial viability in clinical studies.

5. Stress testing—Stress testing in various forms is most frequently applied in cases of suspected or overt ischemic heart disease (Table 1–3). Because ischemia represents an imbalance between myocardial oxygen supply and demand, exercise or pharmacologic stress increases myocardial oxygen demand and reveals an inadequate oxygen supply (hypoperfusion) in diseased coronary arteries. Stress testing can thus induce detectable ischemia in patients with no evidence of ischemia at rest. It is also used to determine cardiac reserve in patients with valvular and myocardial disease. Deterioration of left ventricular performance during exercise or other stresses suggests a diminution in cardiac reserve that would have therapeutic and prognostic implications. Although most stress test studies use some technique (Table 1–4) for directly assessing the myocardium, it is important not to forget the symptoms of angina pectoris or extreme dyspnea: light-headedness or syncope can be equally important in evaluating patients. Physical findings such as the development of pulmonary rales, ventricular gallops, murmurs, peripheral cyanosis, hypotension, excessive increases in heart rate, or inappropriate decreases in heart rate also have diagnostic and prognostic value. It is therefore important that a symptom assessment and physical examination always be done before, during, and after stress testing.

Table 1–3. Indications for Stress Testing.

Evaluation of exertional chest pain
Assess significance of known coronary artery disease
Risk stratification of ischemic heart disease
Determine exercise capacity
Evaluate other exercise symptoms

Table 1–4. Methods of Detecting Myocardial Ischemia during Stress Testing.

Electrocardiography
Echocardiography
Myocardial perfusion imaging
Positron emission tomography
Magnetic resonance imaging

Electrocardiographic monitoring is the most common cardiac evaluation technique used during stress testing; it should be part of every stress test in order to assess heart rate and detect any arrhythmias. In patients with normal resting ECGs, diagnostic ST depression of myocardial ischemia has a fairly high sensitivity and specificity for detecting coronary artery disease in symptomatic patients if adequate stress is achieved (peak heart rate at least 85% of the patient's maximum predicted rate, based on age and sex). Exercise ECG testing is an excellent low-cost screening procedure for patients with chest pain consistent with coronary artery disease, normal resting ECGs, and the ability to exercise to maximal levels.

A **myocardial imaging** technique is usually added to the exercise evaluation in patients whose ECGs are abnormal or, for some reason, less accurate. It is also used for determining the location and extent of myocardial ischemia in patients with known coronary artery disease. Imaging techniques, in general, enhance the sensitivity and specificity of the tests but are still not perfect, with false-positives and false-negatives occurring 5–10% of the time.

Which adjunctive myocardial imaging technology to choose depends on the quality of the tests, their availability and cost, and the services provided by the laboratory. If these are all equal, the decision should be based on patient characteristics. For example, echocardiography might be appropriate when ischemia is suspected of developing during exercise and is profound enough to depress segmental left ventricular performance and worsen mitral regurgitation. On the other hand, perfusion scanning might be the best test to determine which coronary artery is producing the symptoms in a patient with known three-vessel coronary artery disease and recurrent angina after revascularization.

Choosing the appropriate form of stress is also important (Table 1–5). Exercise, the preferred stress for increasing myocardial oxygen demand, also simulates the patient's normal daily activities and is therefore highly relevant clinically. There are essentially only two reasons for not choosing exercise stress, however: the patient's inability to exercise adequately because of physical or psychological limitations; or the chosen test cannot be performed readily with exercise (eg, PET scanning). In these situations, pharmacologic stress is appropriate.

6. Cardiac catheterization—Cardiac catheterization is now mainly used for the assessment of coronary artery anatomy by coronary angiography. In fact, the cardiac catheterization laboratory has become more of a therapeutic than a diagnostic arena. Once significant coronary artery disease is identified, a variety of catheter-based interventions can be used to alleviate the obstruction to blood flow in the coronary arteries. At one time, hemodynamic measurements (pressure, flow, oxygen consumption) were necessary to accurately diagnose and quantitate the severity of valvular heart disease and intracardiac shunts. Currently, Doppler echocardiography has taken over this role almost completely, except in the few instances when Doppler studies are inadequate or believed to be inaccurate. Catheter-based hemodynamic assessments are still useful for differentiating cardiac constriction from restriction, despite advances in Doppler echocardiography. Currently, the catheterization laboratory is also more often used as a treatment arena for valvular and congenital heart disease. Certain stenotic valvular and arterial lesions can be treated successfully with catheter-delivered balloon expansion or the deployment of stents. Congenital shunts can also be closed by catheter-delivered devices.

Myocardial biopsy is necessary to treat patients with heart transplants and is occasionally used to diagnose selected cases of suspected acute myocarditis. For this purpose, a biotome is usually placed in the right heart and several small pieces of myocardium are removed. Although this technique is relatively safe, myocardial perforation occasionally results.

7. Electrophysiologic testing—Electrophysiologic testing uses catheter-delivered electrodes in the heart to induce rhythm disorders and detect their structural basis. Certain arrhythmia foci and structural abnormalities that facilitate rhythm disturbances can be treated by catheter-delivered radiofrequency energy (ablation) or by the placement of various electronic devices that monitor rhythm disturbances and treat them accordingly through either pacing or internally delivered defibrillation shocks. Electrophysiologic testing and treatment now dominate the management of arrhythmias; the test is more accurate than the surface ECG for diagnosing many arrhythmias and detecting their substrate, and catheter ablation and electronic devices have been

Table 1–5. Types of Stress Tests.

Exercise
Treadmill
Bicycle
Pharmacologic
Adenosine
Dipyridamole
Dobutamine
Isoproterenol
Other
Pacing

more successful than pharmacologic approaches at treating arrhythmias.

8. Test selection—In the current era of escalating health-care costs, ordering multiple tests is rarely justifiable, and the physician must pick the one test that will best define the patient's problem. Unfortunately, cardiology offers multiple competing technologies that often address the same issues, but in a different way. The following five principles should be followed when considering which test to order:

- What information is desired? If the test is not reasonably likely to provide the type of information needed to help the patient's problem, it should not be done, no matter how inexpensive and easy it is to obtain. At one time, for example, routine preoperative ECGs were done prior to major noncardiac surgery to detect which patients might be at risk for cardiac events in the perioperative period. Once it was determined that the resting ECG was not good at this, the practice was discontinued, despite its low cost and ready availability.

- What is the cost of the test? If two tests can provide the same information and one is much more expensive than the other, the less expensive test should be ordered. For example, to determine whether a patient's remote history of prolonged chest pain was a myocardial infarction, the physician has a choice of an ECG or one of several imaging tests, such as echocardiography, resting thallium-201 scintigraphy, and the like. Because the ECG is the least expensive test, it should be performed for this purpose in most situations.

- Is the test available? Sometimes the best test for the patient is not available in the given facility. If it is available at a nearby facility and the patient can go there without undue cost, the test should be obtained. If expensive travel is required, the costs and benefits of that test versus local alternatives need to be carefully considered.

- What is the level of expertise of the laboratory and the physicians who interpret the tests? For many of the high-technology imaging tests, the level of expertise considerably affects the value of the test. Myocardial perfusion imaging is a classic example of this. Some laboratories are superlative in producing tests of diagnostic accuracy. In others, the number of false-positive and false-negative results is so high that the tests are rendered almost worthless. Therefore, even though a given test may be available and inexpensive and could theoretically provide essential information, if the quality of the laboratory is not good, an alternative test should be sought.

- What quality of service is provided by the laboratory? Patients are customers, and they need to be satisfied. If a laboratory makes patients wait a long time, if it is tardy in getting the results to the physicians, or if great delays occur in accomplishing the test, choose an alternative laboratory (assuming, of course, that alternatives are available). Poor service cannot be tolerated.

Many other situations and considerations affect the choice of tests. For example, a young patient with incapacitating angina might have a high likelihood of having single-vessel disease that would be amenable to catheter-based revascularization. It might be prudent to take this patient directly to coronary arteriography with an eye toward diagnosing and treating the patient's disease in one setting for maximum cost-effectiveness. This approach, however, presents the risk of ordering an expensive catheterization rather than a less-expensive noninvasive test if the patient does not have significant coronary disease. If an assessment of left ventricular global performance is desirable in a patient known to need coronary arteriography, the assessment could be done by left ventricular cine-angiography at the time of cardiac catheterization. This would avoid the extra expense of echocardiography if it was not otherwise indicated. Physicians are frequently solicited to use the latest emerging technologies, which often have not been proved better than the standard techniques. It is generally unwise to begin using these usually more expensive methods until clinical trials have established their efficacy and cost-effectiveness.

Asch FM et al. Lack of sensitivity of the electrocardiogram for detection of old myocardial infarction: a cardiac magnetic resonance imaging study. Am Heart J. 2006 Oct;152(4):742–8. [PMID: 16996851]

Beanlands RS et al; PARR-2 Investigators. F-18-fluorodeoxyglucose positron emission tomography imaging-assisted management of patients with severe left ventricular dysfunction and suspected coronary disease; a randomized, controlled trial (PARR-2). J Am Coll Cardiol. 2007 Nov 13;50(20):2002–12. [PMID: 17996568]

Budoff MJ et al; American Heart Association Committee on Cardiovascular Imaging and Intervention; American Heart Association Council on Cardiovascular Radiology and Intervention; American Heart Association Committee on Cardiac Imaging, Council on Clinical Cardiology. Assessment of coronary artery disease by cardiac computed tomography: a scientific statement from the American Heart Association Committee on Cardiovascular Imaging and Intervention, Council on Cardiovascular Radiology and Intervention, and Committee on Cardiac Imaging, Council on Clinical Cardiology. Circulation. 2006 Oct 17;114(16):1761–91. [PMID: 17015792]

Cheitlin MD et al; American College of Cardiology; American Heart Association; American Society of Echocardiography. ACC/AHA/ASE 2003 guideline update for the clinical application of echocardiography: summary article: a report of the American College of Cardiology/American Heart Association Task Force on Practice Guidelines (ACC/AHA/ASE Committee to Update the 1997 Guidelines for the Clinical Application of Echocardiography). Circulation. 2003 Sep 2;108(9):1146–62. [PMID: 12952829]

Gibbons RJ et al; American College of Cardiology/American Heart Association Task Force on Practice Guidelines (Committee to Update the 1997 Exercise Testing Guidelines). ACC/AHA 2002 guideline update for exercise testing: summary article: a report of the American College of Cardiology/American Heart Association Task Force on the Practice Guidelines (Committee to Update the 1997 Exercise Testing Guidelines). Circulation. 2002 Oct 1;106(14):1883–92. [PMID: 12356646]

Klocke FJ et al; American College of Cardiology; American Heart Association Task Force on Practice Guidelines; American Society for Nuclear Cardiology. ACC/AHA/ASNC guidelines for the clinical use of cardiac radionuclide imaging executive summary: a report of the American College of Cardiology/American Heart Association Task Force on Practice Guidelines (ACC/AHA/ASNC Committee to Revise the 1995 Guidelines for the Clinical Use of Cardiac Radionuclide Imaging.) Circulation. 2003 Sep 16;108(11):1404–18. [PMID: 12975245]

Ommen SR et al. Clinical utility of Doppler echocardiography and tissue Doppler imaging in the estimation of left ventricular filling pressures: a comparative simultaneous Doppler-catheterization study. Circulation. 2000 Oct 10;102(15):1788–94. [PMID: 11023933]

Sampson UK et al. Diagnostic accuracy of rubidium-82 myocardial perfusion imaging with hybrid positron emission tomography/computed tomography in the detection of coronary artery disease. J Am Coll Cardiol. 2007 Mar 13;49(10):1052–8. [PMID: 17349884]

Sanz J et al. Detection of healed myocardial infarction with multidetector-row computed tomography and comparison with cardiac magnetic resonance delayed hyperenhancement. Am J Cardiol. 2006 Jul 15;98(2):149–55. [PMID: 16828583]

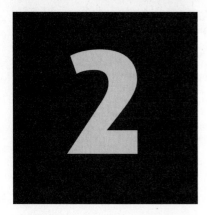

Lipid Disorders

Christian Zellner, MD

- ▶ Total serum cholesterol greater than 200 mg/dL.
- ▶ LDL cholesterol greater than 100 mg/dL.
- ▶ HDL cholesterol less than 40 mg/dL.
- ▶ Triglycerides greater than 150 mg/dL.
- ▶ Lipoprotein(a) less than 30 mg/dL.

▶ General Considerations

Over the last decade, lipid screening has been established as a cornerstone of cardiac prevention in guidelines in primary care, cardiology, and many other specialties. Statins, inhibitors of hydroxymethylglutaryl-coenzyme A (HMG-CoA) reductase have become indispensable in the treatment of coronary artery disease (CAD) as well as in prevention of vascular events in patients at high risk, such as those with diabetes mellitus.

Lipoproteins and Apolipoproteins

Esterified cholesterol and triglycerides are insoluble in blood and are transported in plasma by lipoproteins. These lipoproteins are known as high-density lipoprotein (HDL) cholesterol, low-density lipoprotein (LDL) cholesterol, very-low density lipoproteins (VLDL), intermediate-density lipoproteins (IDL), and chylomicrons (Figure 2–1). Lipoproteins carry characteristic apolipoproteins in their outer layer that have functional significance (apo A-I for HDL; apo B-100 for LDL, IDL, and VLDL; and apo B-48 for chylomicrons). For example, apo B-100 is recognized by the LDL receptor and is required for hepatic production and removal of LDL. Other apolipoproteins, such as apo E and apo CI-CIII, have long been known to play an important part in lipid metabolism, while the effects of many apolipoproteins remain incompletely understood.

1. Metabolism—Traditionally, the lipoprotein metabolism has been separated into exogenous (ie, uptake of cholesterol and fat from food) and endogenous pathways (ie, metabolic turnover in plasma, liver, and bile) (Figure 2–2). These pathways represent simultaneous events that are complementary. Key elements of dietary fat and cholesterol metabolism, and metabolism of major lipoprotein classes are discussed below.

2. Dietary fats—Dietary fats are processed by pancreatic lipase to fatty acids to allow absorption across the intestinal epithelium, where they are re-esterified to triglycerides. For further transport they form large chylomicrons, lipoproteins that also carry esterified cholesterol, apolipoprotein B-48, and apo CII (an apolipoprotein that acts as an activator of lipoprotein lipase). Chylomicrons are secreted into the lymphatic system, and eventually enter the bloodstream via the thoracic duct. After hydrolysis by lipoprotein lipase, an enzyme present in the endothelium of many tissues, chylomicrons release fatty acids into peripheral tissues to provide immediate energy for muscles or to be stored as fat in adipose tissue. Similar to the intestinal pathway of chylomicrons, VLDL serve as carriers to export triglycerides from the liver and are also targets of lipoprotein lipase. After chylomicrons and VLDL release most of their triglyceride content, these smaller particles (called chylomicron remnant, and VLDL remnant or IDL) contain a high core concentration of esterified cholesterol and are considered by many clinicians to be of high atherogenic potential. Chylomicron remnants and about half of VLDL remnants are then taken up by the liver in an apo E mediated process for subsequent cholesterol metabolism, while the remaining VLDL remnants act as the building block for LDL in plasma.

Turnover of chylomicrons and VLDL is rapid, with VLDL carrying less than 30% of overall plasma triglycerides. Fasting or zero-fat diets, therefore, lead to prompt improvement in acutely elevated triglycerides in hypertriglyceridemia.

3. Dietary cholesterol—Absorption of dietary or recirculated biliary cholesterol is largely by diffusion across the intes-

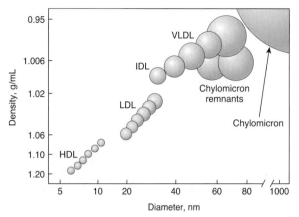

▲ **Figure 2–1.** The density and size-distribution of the major classes of lipoprotein particles. Lipoproteins are classified by density and size, which are inversely related. HDL, high-density lipoproteins; IDL, intermediate-density lipoproteins; LDL, low-density lipoproteins; VLDL, very low-density lipoproteins. (Reproduced, with permission, from Rader DJ et al. Disorders of Lipoprotein Metabolism. In: AS Fauci, E Braunwald, DL Kasper, SL Hauser, DL Longo, JL Jameson, J Loscaizo (eds). *Harrison's Principles of Internal Medicine,* 17th edition. New York: McGraw-Hill; 2008.)

tinal brush border in the jejunum. It is important to recognize that only half of the intestinal cholesterol is absorbed, mainly in the form of recirculated biliary cholesterol, while less than 30% comes from dietary cholesterol. Dietary plant sterols (phytosterols) or other sterols compete with cholesterol uptake in this process and lead to cholesterol lowering by way of reduced absorption. This explains why limiting the intake of dietary cholesterol often shows only modest improvement in cholesterol levels. After passive diffusion of cholesterol, the protein Nieman-Pick C1-like 1 (NPC1L1; inhibited by the drug ezetimibe) is critical in the uptake of sterols and cholesterol into intestinal enterocytes. In an active process involving the adenosine triphosphate–binding cassette (ABC)-Transporter ABCG5/G8, sterols and cholesterol are largely transported back into the gut, while a small amount of free cholesterol is esterified and transferred into chylomicrons for subsequent hepatic uptake. In the liver, cholesterol is either incorporated into VLDL or metabolized into bile acids. Cholesterol can also be synthesized from acetyl-CoA, a process that is regulated by HMG-CoA and inhibited by statins.

4. LDL and HDL—LDL and HDL are continuously remodeled in plasma, a complex process involving enzymes, transfer proteins, and receptors. This allows LDL to act as a transporter of cholesterol from the liver to target tissues, while HDL carries out the opposite function. Most enzymes or proteins affect both classes and include hepatic lipase (HL), cholesteryl-ester transfer protein (CETP), and phospholipids-transfer protein

(PLTP). LDL is taken up in the liver by the LDL receptor. The LDL receptor is down-regulated by feedback mechanisms such as high hepatic free cholesterol levels, likely one of the causes of increased LDL levels with high intake of saturated fats. Statins, HMG-CoA reductase inhibitors, act by lowering hepatic free cholesterol, leading to increased expression of LDL receptors and subsequent uptake of LDL in the liver.

5. Lipoprotein(a)—Lipoprotein(a) or Lp(a) is an LDL-like particle containing apo B-100 and apo (a), which has close structural homology with plasminogen. Lp(a) is not only an atherogenic lipoprotein, particularly in patients with elevated LDL, but it is also prothrombotic because it can displace plasminogen from its binding sites. Lp(a) can be elevated in patients with diabetes mellitus, chronic kidney disease, or nephrotic syndrome, but its levels are mainly determined by genetic factors. Lp(a) does not respond to statin therapy and is not included in routine lipid panels. Estimated levels by Vertical Auto Profile (VAP) are informative but need to be confirmed by enzyme-linked immunosorbent assay (ELISA).

6. Genetics—Abnormal lipid levels develop in most patients after weight gain, with sedentary lifestyle, or in the presence of other disorders, such as diabetes mellitus and renal or thyroid disease. While likely combinations of small genetic variants (ie, polygenic factors) are responsible for these lipid changes, only a few patients have known monogenic defects, the most common of which is familial hypercholesterolemia (FH), occurring in 1 in 500 patients. FH is caused by an LDL receptor gene mutation, resulting in elevated plasma cholesterol and premature CAD. The mutant receptor impairs clearance of LDL, but treatment with statins and other drugs typically remains effective because of clearance through normal receptors in heterozygous patients. Compound heterozygous states or homozygous mutations are infrequent, but always associated with severely increased plasma cholesterol, limited response to statins, and extensive tendon xanthomas. Because FH is diagnosed in most people after their first coronary event, family history of hypercholesterolemia, elevated LDL during childhood, and tendon xanthomas are important clues to FH and should trigger screening of family members. Early CAD is also common in familial combined hyperlipidemia (FCH), a familial disorder characterized by elevated triglycerides and LDL that occurs in 1–2% of the population. A single gene involved in this disease has not been found, and the disease is likely polygenic. Typically, patients are identified after their first cardiac event but do not have tendon xanthomas. Although these are examples of common genetic disorders associated with lipid abnormalities, current screening and treatment remains centered on lipid profiles until genetic testing becomes a clinical reality.

Brunzell JD. Clinical practice. Hypertriglyceridemia. N Engl J Med. 2007 Sep 6;357(10):1009–17. [PMID: 17804845]

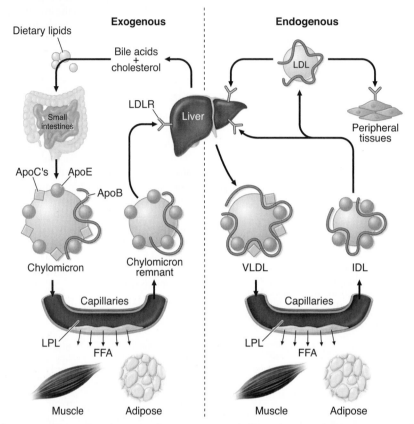

▲ **Figure 2-2.** The exogenous and endogenous lipoprotein metabolic pathways. The exogenous pathway transports dietary lipids to the periphery and the liver. The endogenous pathway transports hepatic lipids to the periphery. FFA, free fatty acids; IDL, intermediate-density lipoproteins; LDL, low-density lipoproteins; LDLR, low-density lipoprotein receptor; LPL, lipoprotein lipase; VLDL, very low-density lipoproteins. (Reproduced, with permission, from Rader DJ et al. In: AS Fauci, E Braunwald, DL Kasper, SL Hauser, DL Longo, JL Jameson, J Loscaizo (eds). *Harrison's Principles of Internal Medicine,* 17th edition. New York: McGraw-Hill; 2008.)

▶ Clinical Findings

A. History

History is a critical component of the initial visit, because by the time patients are referred to a cardiologist, many have already started taking lipid-lowering drugs. It is important to ask for lipid profiles obtained before medications were started, since lipid panels are now routinely included in screening of healthy adults by primary care physicians or are often offered at shopping malls or public events. When available, response to the initial drug and any adverse effects including myalgias and abnormal liver function tests should be noted. Family history of early coronary disease or dyslipidemia at a young age suggests a genetic component. A brief diet and exercise review, and recent weight gain or weight loss should also be recorded. It is important to screen for regular alcohol use as it a frequent cause of elevated triglycerides and weight gain.

In addition, a history or symptoms of other diseases associated with lipid abnormalities (eg, diabetes mellitus, hypothyroidism, end-stage renal disease, liver disease), other cardiovascular risk factors, a Framingham Risk Score, and dietary habits (grapefruit juice, red yeast rice) or medication interfering with lipid-lowering drugs should be included in the initial history.

B. Physical Examination

The physical examination should focus on the cardiovascular system but manifestations of metabolic diseases are often missed and include abdominal pain (enlarged liver or spleen, gallstones, pancreatitis), corneal changes, and tendon or eruptive xanthomas. The Achilles tendons are easily palpated while examining distal pulses and should resemble a "narrow string of steel." Broad tendons or tendon xanthomas are found in FH and are typically absent in FCH. Eruptive xanthomas are found in hypertriglyceridemia and dysbetalipoproteinemia. Other physical findings such as truncal obesity, lipodystrophy, acanthosis, reduced muscle bulk, muscle weakness, myalgia, or neuropathy are important clues to metabolic diseases or drug side effects.

C. Laboratory Assessment

The Third Report of the National Cholesterol Education Program (NCEP) Expert Panel on Detection, Evaluation, and Treatment of High Blood Cholesterol in Adults (Adult Treatment Panel (ATP) III) suggests that a fasting lipid profile should be obtained in all adults 20 years of age or older at least once every 5 years. Patients who are acutely ill; have significant weight change; are pregnant; or who recently had a significant illness, myocardial infarction, or stroke should be evaluated at a later time because cholesterol levels may be suppressed. Because of initial variability between laboratories, the NCEP has established guidelines for standardization of lipid and lipoprotein measurements. Compact chemical analyzers for routine office determinations should not be used for the initial diagnosis due to reported variability in results but can be useful for subsequent visits. In our practice, patients referred for dyslipidemia receive a detailed questionnaire and a laboratory request for a lipid panel prior to their first visit to facilitate management.

Lipid panels measure total cholesterol and triglycerides, as well as LDL, HDL, and VLDL after an overnight fast. Nonfasting samples primarily affect VLDL and triglycerides, while all other measurements (including LDL and HDL) remain interpretable but are less accurate. Routine lipid panels use precipitation of one fraction of cholesterol (ie, HDL) and measuring the remaining cholesterol while adjusting for cholesterol found in VLDL to estimate LDL. The so-called Friedman formula: LDL cholesterol = total cholesterol – HDL – triglycerides/5 is unreliable for triglycerides greater than 400 mg/dL. If direct measurement of LDL is not available, a repeat fasting sample should be ordered with instructions to fast for at least 12 hours. Newer technologies such as the Berkeley HeartLab Segmented Gradient Gel, the Atherotech VAP (Vertical Auto Profile), and the LipoScience Nuclear Magnetic Resonance assess lipid fractions independently. These tests are based on the initial discovery of lipoprotein classes in the 1950s using analytical ultracentrifugation and provide additional information of cholesterol subclasses, although not included in ATP III guidelines. Direct measurement of LDL and triglycerides using these techniques may be necessary when significant hypertriglyceridemia persists despite fasting.

Basic screening should also include thyroid function studies, liver function studies, fasting glucose, baseline creatine kinase, and urine analysis. Baseline uric acid levels may be needed before starting niacin therapy. A host of other screening tools exist to estimate cardiovascular risk, such as apo B, homocysteine, C-reactive protein (CRP), and lipoprotein-associated phospholipase A2 (Lp-PLA2). Vascular studies such as ankle-brachial-index (ABI), carotid intima-

medial thickness (IMT), coronary artery calcium scores (CACS), and coronary angiography by computed tomography (CTA) estimate subclinical vascular disease burden. These tests are not part of ATP III recommendations but may be useful in individual cases.

Expert Panel on Detection, Evaluation, and Treatment of High Blood Cholesterol in Adults. Executive Summary of the Third Report of The National Cholesterol Education Program (NCEP) Expert Panel on Detection, Evaluation, and Treatment of High Blood Cholesterol in Adults (Adult Treatment Panel III). JAMA. 2001 May 16;285(19):2486–97. [PMID: 11368702]
Kulkarni KR. Cholesterol profile measurement by vertical auto profile method. Clin Lab Med. 2006 Dec;26(4):787–802. [PMID: 17110240]

▶ Treatment

A. LDL Goals

Epidemiologic studies suggest that in middle-aged men, higher LDL (each 1 mg/dL increase is associated with a 1% risk increase) and lower HDL (each 1 mg/dL decrease is associated with a 2% risk increase) are important targets in cardiovascular prevention. In patients with established CAD, LDL lowering translates into up to 20% relative-risk reduction. To guide therapy, the NECP has established a classification of LDL, total cholesterol, and HDL levels (Table 2–1). The NCEP ATP III identifies LDL as the primary therapeutic target in addition to lifestyle changes and focuses on primary prevention in patients with increased risk as well as aggressive lipid lowering in patients with established vascular disease. Treatment with aspirin, β-blockers, angiotensin-converting-enzyme inhibitors in appropriate candidates, smoking cessa-

Table 2–1. ATP III Classification of LDL, Total, and HDL Cholesterol (mg/dL).

LDL Cholesterol	
< 100	Optimal
100–129	Near or above optimal
130–159	Borderline high
160–189	High
≥ 190	Very high
Total Cholesterol	
< 200	Desirable
200–239	Borderline high
≥ 240	High
HDL Cholesterol	
< 40	Low
≥ 60	High

ATP, adult treatment panel; HDL, high-density lipoprotein; LDL, low-density lipoprotein.

tion, moderation of alcohol use, increased exercise and weight loss, as well as incorporation of dietary intervention, as outlined in Table 2–2, are strongly advised.

Statin therapy is initiated immediately in patients with established CAD or at high risk; all others will be offered a trial of therapeutic lifestyle changes. When response to lifestyle changes and diet is inadequate, the NCEP recommends the addition of pharmacologic therapy after a few months (Figure 2–3). In patients without overt CAD, the Framingham Risk Score should be used to estimate 10-year CAD risk (Table 2–3). Framingham Risk Score calculators can be found online, as handheld applications, or as part of the ATP III guidelines. Because it is clear that *lifetime* risk of CAD remains very high in all individuals, many physicians have adopted a more aggressive approach to lipid lowering with LDL goals of less than 100 mg/dL in patients even considered low risk (10-year CAD risk of < 10%). The long-term risks, benefits, and costs of such an approach will likely be reevaluated in the next ATP revision.

Treatment decisions are guided by several large-scale clinical trials that established the role of LDL-lowering and statin therapy in primary and secondary prevention of cardiac events and stroke. The Heart Protection Study (HPS), Treat-to New Targets (TNT), PROVE-IT, and ASCOT-LLA trials showed that patients with very low LDL cholesterol and vascular disease benefited from statin therapy. These findings have only partially been included in the most recent update of the NCEP ATP III guidelines and are listed as an "optional" LDL goal of < 70 mg/dL in patients with high-risk features: (1) Optional

LDL goal: < 70 mg/dL for patients with CAD or high risk; (2) Optional LDL goal: < 100 mg/dL for patients with two risk factors and moderate risk (10-year CAD risk of 10–20%).

The optional LDL goal of < 70 mg/dL should be considered in all patients at high risk for subsequent events and include history of myocardial infarction, coronary artery or other bypass grafts, stroke, percutaneous coronary intervention, and stenting. Treatment with statins, irrespective of LDL goals, should be individualized for patients with aortic valve stenosis or prosthesis and chronic kidney disease until ATP guidelines are revised.

B. Non-HDL Goals and Hypertriglyceridemia

Because treating hypertriglyceridemia is not the primary lipid target in patients with CAD, it is frequently overlooked. Elevated triglycerides are common (more than 25% of population) and often associated with secondary causes (such as obesity; diabetes; renal disease; the metabolic syndrome; and a number of drugs, including protease inhibitors and estrogens). Most patients will show borderline high triglyceride levels of less than 200 mg/dL, and after achieving their LDL goal, lifestyle changes such as smoking cessation, abstinence from alcohol, increased exercise, weight loss, and reduced carbohydrate intake are primary treatment strategies in this group of patients. In patients with high triglycerides (> 200 mg/dL), LDL goals remain the primary treatment target, but lowering non-HDL cholesterol, comprising LDL, IDL, and VLDL, was introduced by ATP III as a secondary treatment goal in 2001. Non-HDL cholesterol has not been widely adopted as it is not always reported separately, but non-HDL cholesterol levels can be obtained easily by subtracting HDL from total cholesterol. This essentially aims to add atherogenic cholesterol in remnant particles to LDL goals in patients with elevated triglycerides. Therefore, the non-HDL goal is 30 mg/dL higher than the LDL goal. Very high triglyceride levels (> 500 mg/dL) are rare in the general population but are often associated with recurrent, acute pancreatitis and should be suspected with any history of abdominal pain (Table 2–4). Changes in lifestyle (weight loss, increased physical activity, restriction of alcohol, restriction of dietary fat to 10–20% of total caloric intake, reduction of high carbohydrate intake) and drug therapy are almost always required. In general, LDL cholesterol levels are low and statins are ineffective, but response to niacin or fibrates or in combination with omega-3 fatty acids is good. A significant number of patients, however, will not respond to drug therapy due to genetic mutations in lipoprotein lipase, apo CII or related pathways. A very low-fat diet is critical in these patients and hard to achieve without frequent visits with a dietitian.

Much of moderate hypertriglyceridemia (250–500 mg/dL) is due to various exogenous or secondary factors (Table 2–5), which include alcohol, diabetes mellitus, hypothyroidism, obesity, chronic renal disease, and drugs. Changes in lifestyle or treatment of the primary disease process may be sufficient to reduce triglyceride levels and high carbohydrate intake and

Table 2–2. Nutrient Composition of the Therapeutic Lifestyle Changes (TLC) Diet.

Nutrient	Recommended Intake
Saturated fat[1]	< 7% of total calories
Polyunsaturated fat	Up to 10% of total calories
Monounsaturated fat	Up to 20% of total calories
Total fat	25–35% of total calories
Carbohydrate[2]	50–60% of total calories
Fiber	20–30 g/day
Protein	Approximately 15% of total calories
Cholesterol	< 200 mg/day
Total calories[3]	Balance energy intake and expenditure to maintain desirable body weight and prevent weight gain.

[1]*Trans* fatty acids are another LDL-raising fat that should be kept at a low intake.

[2]Carbohydrates should be derived predominantly from foods rich in complex carbohydrates, including grains, especially whole grains, fruits, and vegetables.

[3]Daily energy expenditure should include at least moderate physical activity (contributing approximately 200 kcal/day).

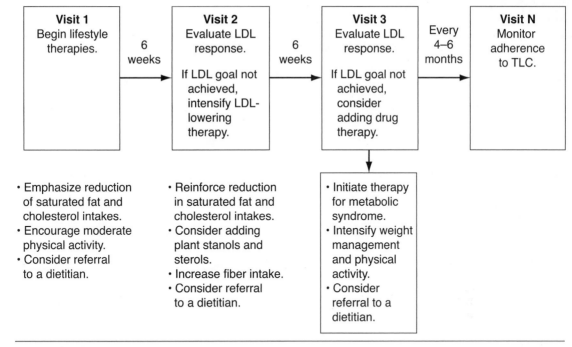

LDL, low-density lipoprotein.

▲ **Figure 2–3.** Model of steps in therapeutic lifestyle changes (TLC). (Source: Expert Panel on Detection, Evaluation and Treatment of High Blood Cholesterol in Adults: Executive summary of the Third Report of the NCEP Expert Panel on Detection, Evaluation and Treatment of High Blood Cholesterol in Adults (Adult Treatment Panel III). JAMA. 2001;285;2491.)

Table 2–3. Risk Factors That Modify LDL–Cholesterol Goals.[1]

Major Risk Factors (exclusive of LDL-cholesterol)
Cigarette smoking
Hypertension (blood pressure ≥ 140/90 mm Hg or on antihypertensive medication)
Low HDL-C (< 40 mg/dL)[2]
Family history of premature CAD (CAD in male first-degree relative < 55 years; CAD in female first-degree relative < 65 years)
Age (men ≥ 45 years; women ≥ 55 years)

Categories of Risk	LDL Goal (mg/dL)
CAD and CAD risk equivalents	< 100
Multiple (2+) risk factors	< 130
0–1 risk factor	< 160

[1]Diabetes is regarded as a CAD risk equivalent.
[2]HDL cholesterol ≥ 60 mg/dL counts as a "negative" risk factor; its presence removes one risk factor from the total count.
CAD, coronary artery disease; HDL, high-density lipoprotein; LDL, low-density lipoprotein.

alcohol use are frequently overlooked. Often, however, these patients not only need lifestyle changes, but also statin therapy in combination with other lipid-lowering drugs such as fibrates, niacin, or omega-3 fatty acids.

Hypertriglyceridemia in the presence of elevated LDL with or without low HDL remains a common lipid abnormality in patients with CAD, and both LDL and non-HDL cholesterol goals should be aggressively met to decrease the burden of CAD.

C. HDL and Lipoprotein(a)

Low HDL is a strong predictor of CAD and increased cardiovascular mortality. The major causes of reduced serum

Table 2–4. Categories of Triglyceride Levels.

Category	Triglyceride Levels
Optimal	< 150 mg dL
Borderline	150–199 mg/dL
High	200–499 mg/dL
Very high	≥ 500 mg/dL

Table 2–5. Some Acquired Causes of Hyperlipidemia.

Condition	Liproprotein Accumulating	Lipid Phenotype	HDL Level
Diabetes mellitus			
Type 1	Chylomicron, VLDL	↑ TG	↓
Type 2	VLDL	↑ TG	↓
Obesity	VLDL	↑ TG	– or ↓
Alcohol	VLDL	↑ TG	– or ↑
Oral contraceptives	VLDL	↑ TG	– or ↑
Hypothyroidism	LDL	↑ C	–
Nephrotic syndrome	VLDL, LDL	↑ TG, ↑ C	– or ↑
Renal failure	VLDL, LDL	↑ TG, ↑ C	– or ↓
Primary biliary cirrhosis	LDL	↑ C	
Acute hepatitis	VLDL	↑ TG	

C, cholesterol; HDL, high-density lipoprotein; LDL, low-density lipoprotein; TG, triglyceride; VLDL, very low-density lipoprotein.
↑, increase; ↓, decrease; –, no change.
Reproduced, with permission, from Frishman WH et al. Lipids and lipoproteins: Atherosclerotic risk and management. In Frishman WH, ed: Medical Management of Lipid Disorders: Focus on Prevention of Coronary Artery Disease. Armonk, NY: Futura, 1992.

HDL cholesterol are shown in Table 2–6. Low HDL is often part of the metabolic syndrome and associated with elevated triglycerides. Attempts should be made to raise low HDL cholesterol by nonpharmacologic means such as smoking cessation, weight loss, and increased exercise. Drug therapy should focus initially on LDL goals using statins. When low HDL is associated with increased VLDL, therapeutic modification of the latter should be considered, and should include fibrates, omega-3 fatty acids, and particularly niacin. Similar to low HDL, Lp(a) is independently associated with cardiovascular disease. Statins do not lower Lp(a) but appear to attenuate pro-atherogenic effects of Lp(a) in the setting of elevated LDL. ATP III, however, does not suggest a specific target for LDL cholesterol in patients with elevated Lp(a). Patients are often treated toward a low LDL goal (< 70 mg/dL) because of lack of effective drugs to lower Lp(a), as less than 30% of patients respond to niacin therapy.

D. Nonpharmacologic Approaches

1. Dietary modification—The NCEP recommends dietary modification as the first-line treatment for hyperlipidemia (see Table 2–2). It advises a diet that limits cholesterol intake to no more than 200 mg daily (typical US diet is over 400 mg/day) and fat intake of less than 30% of total calories, saturated fat constituting less than 7% of daily caloric intake (typical US diet is over 15% of daily caloric intake). ATP III also emphasizes the use of plant stanols and sterols and viscous (soluble) fiber as therapeutic dietary options to enhance lowering of LDL cholesterol.

Saturated fats typically raise cholesterol, while monounsaturated fats (eg, olive oil), and polyunsaturated fats can lower serum cholesterol. The favorable effects of polyunsaturated fat on serum cholesterol have been counterbalanced by evidence that high intake not only tends to lower HDL levels but may promote gallstone formation. In most outpatients, diet changes, even after seeing a dietitian, lead to only a 10% decrease in LDL, often with no long-term effects. Very low-fat diets such as the Dean Ornish Diet, the Pritikin Diet, and most vegetarian diets can even lower HDL cholesterol. In contrast,

Table 2–6. Major Causes of Reduced Serum HDL Cholesterol.

Cigarette smoking
Obesity
Lack of exercise
Androgenic and related steroids
  Androgens
  Progestational agents
Anabolic steroids
β-Adrenergic-blocking agents
Hypertriglyceridemia
Genetic factors
Primary hypoalphalipoproteinemia

Reproduced, with permission, from Frishman WH et al: Lipids and lipoproteins: Atherosclerotic risk and managment. In Frishman WH, ed: Medical Management of Lipid Disorders: Focus on Prevention of Coronary Artery Disease. Armonk, NY: Futura, 1992.

a diet rich in monounsaturated fats such as the Mediterranean or South Beach Diets may increase or maintain HDL levels.

Trans-fats are formed by commercial hydrogenation processes, which harden polyunsaturate-rich marine and vegetable oils. Lipid profiles are known to be adversely affected by a high trans-fat diet, which depresses HDL levels and elevates LDL levels. Trans-fats are listed on food labels as partially hydrogenized fats or oils and should be avoided.

Saturated fats, such as stearic acid, which contributes substantially to the fatty acid composition in beef and in plants such as cocoa, have been found to be as effective as oleic acid (monounsaturated fat) in lowering plasma cholesterol, by replacing other saturated fats. Lean beef, therefore, does not need to be excluded in a low-cholesterol diet.

2. Exercise—Physical inactivity is a modifiable risk factor, and daily exercise is recommended as an adjunct to dietary modification for the initial treatment of hyperlipidemia. More recently, the benefits of combined resistance and aerobic exercise have become apparent and should be encouraged in every patient. Walking of at least 5000 steps daily or a goal exercise of 1500 calories weekly should be recommended to all patients. Regular physical activity reduces VLDL and triglyceride levels in most, and, in some, lowers LDL and raises HDL. It also can lower blood pressure, reduce insulin resistance, and favorably influence cardiovascular function, but likely requires a modest degree of associated weight loss to achieve sustained benefits.

E. Pharmacologic Therapy

Table 2–7 summarizes the medications available to treat hyperlipidemia.

1. Omega-3 fatty acids (fish oil)—Omega-3 fatty acids are found in cold-water fish (salmon, Arctic char). Eicosapentaenoic acid (EPA) and docosahexaenoic acid (DHA) are the active compounds and sold as part of many dietary supplements. Purified EPA and DHA have recently become available by prescription to avoid concerns about contamination with mercury or other environmental toxins. The pathways by which DHA and EPA lower triglycerides are not completely understood and doses of at least 3–4 g per day are needed for significant triglyceride lowering. Omega-3 fatty acids can used in combination with statins, fibrates, and niacin without significant side effects, but frequently increase LDL in higher doses. Unpleasant aftertaste and soft stools often limit the compliance with higher doses, and liver function studies should be monitored. High-dose fish oil may affect platelet function when given in combination with aspirin and other platelet-antagonists, although no clear association with increased bleeding risk has been found.

2. Bile acid sequestrants—The bile acid-binding resins cholestyramine, colestipol, and colesevelam (WelChol) are used as second-line therapy and in combination with other agents to treat hypercholesterolemia without concurrent hypertriglyceridemia.

Resins interrupt the enterohepatic circulation of bile acids and lead to reduced uptake of biliary cholesterol. Resins have a synergistic effect when given in combination with statins but are now largely replaced by the cholesterol absorption inhibitor ezetimibe. Resins can cause a 5–20% increase in VLDL levels; hence, they should be restricted to patients with normal triglycerides. Cholestyramine and colestipol are powders that must be mixed with water or fruit juice before ingestion and are taken in two or three divided doses with or just after meals. Colestipol is also available in tablet form for greater ease of administration. Colesevelam is a newer bile acid resin, which may have fewer adverse effects and drug interactions than older resins due to its novel structure and higher affinity for bile acids. It should be noted that all bile acid sequestrants could decrease absorption of some antihypertensive agents, including thiazide diuretics and β-blockers. As a general recommendation, all other drugs should be administered either 1 hour before or 4 hours after the bile acid sequestrant. The response to therapy is variable in each individual, but a 15–30% reduction in LDL cholesterol may be seen with colestipol (20 g/day), cholestyramine (16 g/day), or colesevelam (3.8 g/day) treatment. The fall in LDL concentration becomes detectable 4–7 days after the start of treatment, and approaches 90% of maximal effect in 2 weeks. The initial dose should be 4 g of cholestyramine, 5 g of colestipol, or 1.88 g of colesevelam twice a day, and if there is an inadequate response, the dosage can be titrated upward accordingly. Using more than the maximum dosage does not increase the antihypercholesterolemic effect of the drug appreciably, but because it does increase side effects, it decreases compliance. Because resins are virtually identical in action, the choice is based on potential drug interactions and patient preference, specifically taste and the ability to tolerate the ingestion of bulky material.

3. Cholesterol absorption inhibitors—Ezetimibe, the first drug in this class, inhibits the absorption of cholesterol and phytosterols through the intestinal brush border and interrupts the enterohepatic recirculation of sterols from bile. Ezetimibe lowers LDL but does not affect triglycerides. When used with resins, its absorption is reduced, while use of fibrates increases its blood concentration. Ezetimibe should be avoided in pregnant or lactating women and in patients with liver disease, and used with caution in patients receiving cyclosporine. As a monotherapy of 10 mg daily, it reduces cholesterol by 15–20% and is synergistic with statin therapy. Although side effects are uncommon, when ezetimibe is given in combination with statins, liver function studies can become elevated. Rare cases of thrombocytopenia, pancreatitis, and arthralgias have been reported.

4. Fibrates—Fibrates are a class of drugs that activate the nuclear peroxisome proliferator activated receptor alpha. Fibrates inhibit the production of VLDL while enhancing VLDL clearance, as a result of the stimulation of lipoprotein

Table 2–7. Summary of the Major Drugs Used for the Treatment of Hyperlipidemia.

Drug	Major Indications	Starting Dose	Maximal Dose	Mechanism	Common Side Effects
HMG-CoA reductase inhibitors (statins)					
Lovastatin	Elevated LDL-C	20 mg/day	80 mg/day	↓ Cholesterol synthesis, ↑ hepatic LDL receptors, ↓ VLDL production	Myalgias, arthralgias, elevated transaminases, dyspepsia
Pravastatin		40 mg at bedtime	80 mg at bedtime		
Simvastatin		20 mg at bedtime	80 mg at bedtime		
Fluvastatin		20 mg at bedtime	80 mg at bedtime		
Atorvastatin		10 mg at bedtime	80 mg at bedtime		
Rosuvastatin		10 mg at bedtime	40 mg at bedtime		
Cholesterol absorption inhibitors					
Ezetimibe	Elevated LDL-C	10 mg/day	10 mg/day	↓ Intestinal cholesterol absorption	Elevated transaminases
Bile acid sequestrants					
Cholestyramine	Elevated LDL-C	4 g/day	32 g/day	↑ Bile acid excretion and ↑ LDL receptors	Bloating, constipation, elevated triglycerides
Colestipol		5 g/day	40 g/day		
Colesevelam		3750 mg/day	4375 mg/day		
Nicotinic acid					
Immediate-release	Elevated LDL-C, low HDL-C, elevated triglycerides	100 mg three times daily	1 g three times daily	↓ VLDL hepatic synthesis	Cutaneous flushing; GI upset; elevated glucose, uric acid, and liver function tests
Sustained-release		250 mg twice daily	1.5 g twice daily		
Extended-release		500 mg at bedtime	2 g at bedtime		
Fibric acid derivatives					
Gemfibrozil	Elevated triglycerides, elevated remnants	600 mg twice daily	600 mg twice daily	↑ LPL, ↓ VLDL synthesis	Dyspepsia, myalgia, gallstones, elevated transaminases
Fenofibrate		145 mg/daily	145 mg/daily		
Omega 3 fatty acids					
	Elevated triglycerides	3 g/day	6 g/day	↑ Triglyceride catabolism	Dyspepsia, diarrhea, fishy odor to breath

HDL-C, high-density lipoprotein cholesterol; LDL-C, low-density lipoprotein cholesterol; LPL, lipoprotein lipase; VLDL, very low-density lipoprotein.
Reproduced, with permission, from Radar DJ et al. Disorders of lipoprotein metabolism. In Fauci AS et al, eds: *Harrison's Principles of Internal Medicine*, 17th edition. New York: McGraw-Hill; 2008.

lipase activity. Fibrates reduce plasma triglycerides and concurrently raise HDL cholesterol levels. Their effects on LDL cholesterol are less marked and more variable.

Fibrates are first-line therapy to reduce the risk of pancreatitis in patients with very high levels of plasma triglycerides. The VA HIT study found that the fibrate gemfibrozil confers a significant risk reduction in major cardiovascular events in patients with established CAD and low HDL but normal LDL levels. The newer generation of fibric acid derivatives, such as fenofibrate, may decrease total cholesterol and LDL levels to a greater extent than gemfibrozil or clofibrate and is better tolerated. These drugs should not be used as first-line therapy for hypercholesterolemic patients unless hypertriglyceridemia is present. The combination of fibrates and statins is effective when triglycerides and cholesterol are elevated, but creatine kinase values must be closely monitored, as metabolism of statins may be affected. Side effects of fibrates include cholelithiasis, gastrointestinal disturbance, myositis, and liver function test abnormalities. The combination of cerivastatin and gemfibrozil was associated with significant increase in rhabdomyolysis, leading to withdrawal of cerivastatin from the market. While fenofibrate may have a lower incidence of rhabdomyolysis, close monitoring of combination therapy is required.

5. Niacin—Niacin, a water-soluble vitamin, has been shown to lower VLDL and LDL levels and to increase HDL levels when given in large doses. It is given either as a long-acting form once daily or as regular niacin in high doses three times daily. Its use is often limited by side effects and patient noncompliance.

The mode of action of niacin particularly on HDL is unknown and appears to be independent of the drug's role as a vitamin. One of its important actions is believed to be partial inhibition of free fatty acid release from adipose tissue, an effect mediated by the receptor HM74A. Niacin inhibits lipolysis, decreases the synthesis of VLDL and LDL by the liver, and increases the rate of triglyceride removal from the plasma as a result of increased lipoprotein lipase activity.

Through its beneficial effects on VLDL, LDL, and HDL levels, niacin is indicated for most forms of hyperlipidemia and for patients with low HDL. It is the most potent drug for raising HDL, and it is also particularly useful for patients who have elevated plasma VLDL-triglyceride levels as a part of their lipid profile.

Niaspan, a once daily prescription extended-release niacin, is available in doses up to of 2 g daily. If higher doses are needed, over-the-counter immediate-release crystalline niacin should be used and slowly uptitrated from 100 mg three times daily. The most common side effect is cutaneous flushing, often prevented by taking aspirin 30 minutes prior to each dose. Mild elevations in liver function studies occur in up to 15% of patients treated with any form of niacin. Changes in liver function studies rarely require discontinuation of niacin, but rapid drop in cholesterol levels, associated with abdominal pain and elevated liver function studies, should raise suspicion for acute niacin-induced hepatitis. Niacin also raises glucose and uric acid, which should be measured before and after dose increases, and it can worsen peptic ulcer disease. Successful therapy with niacin requires extensive patient motivation, but it is particularly useful in patients with combined hyperlipidemia and low plasma levels of HDL, and is effective in combination with statins.

6. Statins—Statins inhibit the conversion of HMG-CoA to mevalonic acid, a rate-limiting step in the synthesis of cholesterol. This, in turn, leads to increased hepatic LDL-receptor expression and clearance of circulating LDL. HMG-CoA reductase inhibitors produce substantial reduction in levels of LDL cholesterol and, to a lesser extent, triglyceride levels. In modest daily doses, statins reduce total and LDL cholesterol at a rate of 15–50% and may reduce triglycerides by 10–30%. Although effective as monotherapy, statin inhibitors can be combined with ezetimibe when LDL goals are not obtained, or with fibrates or niacin for an additive effect on triglycerides. Because cholesterol synthesis is maximal at night, it is recommended that some HMG-CoA reductase inhibitors be given at bedtime.

Statins have revolutionized the treatment of hyperlipidemia by their potency, efficacy, and tolerability and have evolved into first-line therapy for most forms of hyperlipidemia. Numerous studies with statins involving primary and secondary prevention of CAD have demonstrated a reduction in CAD events, CAD mortality, stroke, and mortality from all other causes. In addition, statins exhibit pleiotropic effects beyond the lowering of LDL cholesterol levels and are postulated to possess antiinflammatory properties, contribute to coronary plaque stabilization, and improve endothelial cell function, conditions that are increasingly recognized as emerging areas of therapy for the treatment of CAD. Statins may also play a role in the treatment of congestive heart failure, osteoporosis, sepsis, aortic stenosis, and chronic kidney disease.

Statins are contraindicated in pregnancy and lactation and can have significant drug interactions since they are metabolized by the cytochrome P-450 pathway. This affects the coadministration with immunosuppressive drugs, fibrates, niacin, macrolides, calcium channel blockers, and ketoconazoles that all may increase the risk of rhabdomyolysis. Although statins are well tolerated, 10% of patients experience some degree of side effects. Asymptomatic and transient elevation in liver function studies occur in up to 2% of patients. It is recommended that treatment be stopped if liver function studies increase to three times the upper limit of normal. Values usually revert to baseline after discontinuation of treatment.

Myositis, myalgia, and myopathy have been reported with increased creatine kinase levels in 5% of patients but can occur even with normal creatine kinase levels. Creatine kinase increase is more likely with the combined use of statins with fibrates or niacin, but rhabdomyolysis is rare, particularly with fenofibrate. The combination of cerivastatin and gemfibrozil has been discontinued from production because of a high incidence of rhabdomyolysis and death. Caution is advised for use of statins in the frail and elderly or in advanced renal disease, and patients should be closely monitored for symptoms, change in medications, and rise in creatine kinase levels.

7. Lipid effects of non-lipid-lowering drugs—Selective α_1-blockers have been shown to reduce triglycerides and increase HDL to a modest degree and are neutral with regard to glucose control. If clinically indicated for other reasons, they can add to the lipid management in these patients. Use of estrogens in postmenopausal women can lower LDL and total cholesterol with additional increases in HDL. Not infrequently, however, estrogens also increase triglycerides and are associated with increased risk of endometrial hyperplasia, possibly leading to endometrial cancer. The selective estrogen receptor modulator raloxifene also lowers total and LDL cholesterol, albeit with much lower risk of side effects. Because of an increase in thromboembolic and cardiovascular events with estrogens they should not be prescribed for cardiovascular prevention in postmenopausal women.

8. Combination drug therapy—When treating patients with most genetic dyslipidemias, such as heterozygous familial hypercholesterolemia or FCH, it is common for single-drug therapy to fail to achieve satisfactory lipid levels, even with high-dose statins. In this setting, combination drug therapy is often needed to control plasma lipid levels. In other cases, it may be beneficial to use a combination of low-dose therapeutic agents with complementary effects rather than high doses of either agent alone in order to minimize their individual dose-related toxicities.

In the past, resins have been used in combination therapy with statins but have now been replaced by the cholesterol uptake inhibitor ezetimibe. Ezetimibe is offered as a drug combination with simvastatin or can be used alone as an add-on to more potent statins. A combination of extended-release niacin with lovastatin is also available. Patients with resistant hypertriglyceridemia often require a combination of fibrates, niacin, and fish oil. Many patients on these drug combinations are stable without side effects, but challenging cases will require the combination of statin, ezetimibe, or fibrates and high-dose crystalline niacin with close monitoring for side effects. These patients are best managed by consulting with a lipid specialist and should be evaluated for alternative treatment options such as lipid-apheresis and genetic screening.

Armitage J. The safety of statins in clinical practice. Lancet. 2007 Nov 24;370(9601):1781–90. [PMID: 17559928]

Ashen MD et al. Clinical practice. Low HDL cholesterol levels. N Engl J Med. 2005 Sep 22;353(12):1252–60. [PMID: 16177251]

Grundy SM et al. Implications of recent clinical trials for the National Cholesterol Education Program Adult Treatment Panel III guidelines. Circulation. 2004 Jul 13;110(2):227–39. [PMID: 15249516]

Harper CR et al. The broad spectrum of statin myopathy: from myalgia to rhabdomyolysis. Curr Opin Lipidol. 2007 Aug;18(4):401–8. [PMID: 17620856]

Heart Protection Study Collaborative Group. MRC/BHF Heart Protection Study of cholesterol lowering with simvastatin in 20,536 high-risk individuals: a randomised placebo-controlled trial. Lancet. 2002 Jul 6;360(9326):7–22. [PMID: 12114036]

LaRosa JC et al; Treating to New Targets (TNT) Investigators. Intensive lipid lowering with atorvastatin in patients with stable coronary disease. N Engl J Med. 2005 Apr 7;352(14):1425–35. [PMID: 15755765]

Leeper NJ et al. Statin use in patients with extremely low low-density lipoprotein levels is associated with improved survival. Circulation. 2007 Aug 7;116(6):613–8. [PMID: 17664373]

Mozaffarian D et al. Trans fatty acids and cardiovascular disease. N Engl J Med. 2006 Apr 13;354(15):1601–13. [PMID: 16611951]

Pasternak RC et al; American College of Cardiology; American Heart Association; National Heart, Lung and Blood Institute. ACC/AHA/NHLBI clinical advisory on the use and safety of statins. J Am Coll Cardiol. 2002 Aug 7;40(3):567–72. [PMID: 12142128]

Rubins HB et al. Gemfibrozil for the secondary prevention of coronary heart disease in men with low levels of high-density lipoprotein cholesterol. Veterans Affairs High-Density Lipoprotein Cholesterol Intervention Trial Study Group. N Engl J Med. 1999 Aug 5;341(6):410–8. [PMID: 10438259]

Stampfer MJ et al. Primary prevention of coronary heart disease in women through diet and lifestyle. N Engl J Med. 2000 Jul 6;343(1):16–22. [PMID: 10882764]

Zarraga IG et al. Impact of dietary patterns and interventions on cardiovascular health. Circulation. 2006 Aug 29;114(9):961–73. [PMID: 16940205]

► When to Refer

Traditionally, endocrinologists have managed lipid clinics, but with the expanding use of statins in primary and secondary prevention of cardiovascular disease, this is changing. Today, management of lipid disorders is often multidisciplinary and requires collaboration with primary care physicians, vascular surgeons, rheumatologists, nephrologists, and infectious disease specialists (HIV). While over 90% of cases can easily be cared for by the general cardiologist, consultation with a lipid specialist should be considered for the following patients:

- Those with severe hypertriglyceridemia complicated by pancreatitis.
- Those with known or suspected complex genetic disorders (homozygous hypercholesterolemia, sitosterolemia, lipodystrophy, dysbetalipoproteinemia, Tangier disease).
- Those with recurrent statin myopathy or history of rhabdomyolyis.
- HIV-infected patients receiving highly active antiretroviral therapy with suboptimal lipid control.
- Patients who do not respond to statin therapy.
- Patients with poor lipid control after undergoing cardiac, renal, or liver transplantation.
- Patients considered for LDL-apheresis.

These patients require frequent dedicated visits with close monitoring of lipid responses, diet and medication review, and laboratory monitoring for side effects.

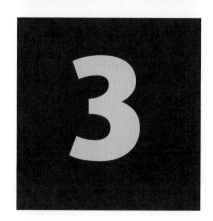

Chronic Ischemic Heart Disease

Michael H. Crawford, MD

ESSENTIALS OF DIAGNOSIS

- ▶ Typical exertional angina pectoris or its equivalents.
- ▶ Objective evidence of myocardial ischemia by electrocardiography, myocardial imaging, or myocardial perfusion scanning.
- ▶ Likely occlusive coronary artery disease because of history and objective evidence of prior myocardial infarction.
- ▶ Known coronary artery disease shown by coronary angiography.

▶ General Considerations

For clinical purposes, patients with chronic ischemic heart disease fall into two general categories: those with symptoms related to the disease, and those who are asymptomatic. Although the latter are probably more common than the former, physicians typically see symptomatic patients more frequently. The issue of asymptomatic patients becomes important clinically when physicians are faced with estimating the risk to a particular patient who is undergoing some stressful intervention, such as major noncardiac surgery. Another issue is the patient with known coronary artery disease who is currently asymptomatic. Such individuals, especially if they have objective evidence of myocardial ischemia, are known to have a higher incidence of future cardiovascular morbidity and mortality. There is, understandably, a strong temptation to treat such patients, despite the fact that it is difficult to make an asymptomatic patient feel better, and some of the treatment modalities have their own risks. In such cases, strong evidence that longevity will be positively influenced by the treatment must be present in order for its benefits to outweigh its risks.

▶ Pathophysiology & Etiology

In the industrialized nations, most patients with chronic ischemic heart disease have coronary atherosclerosis. Consequently, it is easy to become complacent and ignore the fact that other diseases can cause lesions in the coronary arteries (Table 3–1). In young people, coronary artery anomalies should be kept in mind; in older individuals, systemic vasculitides are not uncommon. Today, collagen vascular diseases are the most common vasculitides leading to coronary artery disease, but in the past, infections such as syphilis were a common cause of coronary vasculitis. Diseases of the ascending aorta, such as aortic dissection, can lead to coronary ostial occlusion. Coronary artery emboli may occur as a result of infectious endocarditis or of atrial fibrillation with left atrial thrombus formation. Infiltrative diseases of the heart, such as tumor metastases, may also compromise coronary flow. It is therefore essential to keep in mind diagnostic possibilities other than atherosclerosis when managing chronic ischemic heart disease.

Myocardial ischemia is the result of an imbalance between myocardial oxygen supply and demand. Coronary atherosclerosis and other diseases reduce the supply of oxygenated blood by obstructing the coronary arteries. Although the obstructions may not be enough to produce myocardial ischemia at rest, increases in myocardial oxygen demand during activities can precipitate myocardial ischemia. This is the basis for using stress testing to detect ischemic heart disease. Transient increases in the degree of coronary artery obstruction may develop as a result of platelet and thrombus formation or through increased coronary vasomotor tone. Although it is rare in the United States, pure coronary vasospasm in the absence of atherosclerosis can occur and cause myocardial ischemia and even infarction. In addition, in the presence of other cardiac diseases, especially those that cause a pressure load on the left ventricle, myocardial oxygen demand may outstrip the ability of normal coronary arteries to provide oxygenated blood,

Table 3–1. Nonatherosclerotic Causes of Epicardial Coronary Artery Obstruction.

Fixed	Congenital anomalies
	Myocardial bridges
	Vasculitides
	Aortic dissection
	Granulomas
	Tumors
	Scarring from trauma, radiation
Transient	Vasospasm
	Embolus
	Thrombus in situ

resulting in myocardial ischemia or infarction. A good example would be the patient with severe aortic stenosis, considerable left ventricular hypertrophy, and severely elevated left ventricular pressures who tries to exercise. The manifestations of chronic ischemic heart disease have their basis in a complex pathophysiology of multiple factors that affect myocardial oxygen supply and demand.

Vasan RS et al. Relative importance of borderline and elevated levels of coronary heart disease risk factors. Ann Intern Med. 2005 Mar 15;142(6):393–402. [PMID: 15767617]

Yusuf S et al. Effect of potentially modifiable risk factors associated with myocardial infarction in 52 countries (the INTERHEART study): case-controlled study. Lancet. 2004 Sep 11–17;364(9438): 937–52. [PMID: 15364185]

▶ Clinical Findings

A. Risk Factors

Coronary atherosclerosis is more likely to occur in patients with certain risk factors for this disease (Table 3–2). These include advanced age, male gender or the postmenopausal state in females, a family history of coronary atherosclerosis, diabetes mellitus, systemic hypertension, high serum cholesterol and other associated lipoprotein abnormalities, and tobacco smoking. Additional minor risk factors include a sedentary lifestyle, obesity, high psychological stress levels, and such phenotypic characteristics as earlobe creases, auricular hirsutism, and a mesomorphic body type. The presence of other systemic diseases—hypothyroidism, pseudoxanthoma elasticum, and acromegaly, for example—can accelerate a propensity to coronary atherosclerosis. In the case of nonatherosclerotic coronary artery disease, evidence of such systemic vasculitides as lupus erythematosus, rheumatoid arthritis, and polyarthritis nodosa should be sought. Although none of these risk factors is in itself diagnostic of coronary artery disease, the more of them that are present, the greater the likelihood of the diagnosis.

B. Symptoms

The major symptom of chronic ischemic heart disease is angina pectoris, with a clinical diagnosis based on five features:

- The character of the pain is a deep visceral pressure or squeezing sensation, rather than sharp or stabbing or pinprick-like pain.

- The pain almost always has some substernal component, although some patients complain of pain only on the right or left side of the chest, upper back, or epigastrium.

- The pain may radiate from the thorax to the jaw, neck, or arm. Arm pain in angina pectoris typically involves the ulnar surface of the left arm. Occasionally, the radiated pain may be more noticeable to the patient than the origin of the pain, resulting in complaints of only jaw or arm pain. These considerations have led some physicians to suggest that any pain between the umbilicus and the eyebrows should be considered angina pectoris until proven otherwise.

- Angina is usually precipitated by exertion, emotional upset, or other events that obviously increase myocardial oxygen demand, such as rapid tachyarrhythmias or extreme elevations in blood pressure.

- Angina pectoris is transient, lasting between 2 and 30 minutes. It is relieved by cessation of the precipitating event, such as exercise, or by the administration of treatment, such as sublingual nitroglycerin. Chest pain that lasts longer than 30 minutes is more consistent with myocardial infarction; pain of less than 2 minutes is unlikely to be due to myocardial ischemia.

For reasons that are unclear, some patients with chronic ischemic heart disease do not manifest typical symptoms of angina pectoris but have other symptoms that are brought on by the same precipitating factors and are relieved in the same

Table 3–2. Risk Factors for Coronary Heart Disease.

Major independent risk factors
Advancing age
Tobacco smoking
Diabetes mellitus
Elevated total and low-density lipoprotein cholesterol
Low high-density lipoprotein cholesterol
Hypertension
Conditional risk factors
Elevated serum homocysteine
Elevated serum lipoprotein(a)
Elevated serum triglycerides
Inflammatory markers (eg, C-reactive protein)
Prothrombic factors (eg, fibrinogen)
Small LDL particles
Predisposing risk factors
Abdominal obesity
Ethnic characteristics
Family history of premature coronary heart disease
Obesity
Physical inactivity
Psychosocial factors

way as angina. Because myocardial ischemia can lead to transient left ventricular dysfunction, resulting in increased left ventricular end-diastolic pressure and consequent pulmonary capillary pressure, the sensation of dyspnea can occur during episodes of myocardial supply-and-demand imbalance. Dyspnea may be the patient's only symptom during myocardial ischemia, or it may overshadow the chest pain in the patient's mind. Therefore, dyspnea out of proportion to the degree of exercise or activity can be considered an angina equivalent. Severe myocardial ischemia may lead to ventricular tachyarrhythmias manifesting as palpitations or even frank syncope. Severe episodes of myocardial ischemia may also lead to transient pulmonary edema, especially if the papillary muscles are involved in the ischemic myocardium and moderately severe mitral regurgitation is produced. The most dramatic result of myocardial ischemia is sudden cardiac death.

Patients with chronic myocardial ischemia can also have symptoms caused by the effects of repeated episodes of ischemia or infarction. Thus, patients may have manifestations of chronic cardiac rhythm disorders, especially ventricular arrhythmias. Patients may have chronic congestive heart failure or symptoms related to atherosclerosis of other vascular systems. Patients with vascular disease in other organs are more likely to have coronary atherosclerosis. Those with prior cerebral vascular accidents or symptoms of peripheral vascular disease may be so disabled by these diseases that their ability to either perceive angina or generate enough myocardial oxygen demand to produce angina may be severely limited.

C. Physical Examination

The physical examination is often not helpful in the diagnosis of chronic ischemic heart disease. This is because many patients with chronic ischemic heart disease have no physical findings related to the disease, or if they do, the findings are not specific for coronary artery disease. For example, a fourth heart sound can be detected in patients with chronic ischemic heart disease, especially if they have had a prior myocardial infarction; however, fourth heart sounds are very common in hypertensive heart disease, valvular heart disease, and primary myocardial disease. Palpation of a systolic precordial bulge can occur in patients with prior myocardial infarction, but this sign is not specific and can occur in patients with left ventricular enlargement from any cause. Other signs can also be found in cases of chronic ischemic heart disease, such as those associated with congestive heart failure or mitral regurgitation. Again, these are nonspecific and can be caused by other disease processes. Because coronary atherosclerosis is the most common heart disease in industrialized nations, any physical findings suggestive of heart disease should raise the suspicion of chronic ischemic heart disease.

D. Laboratory Findings

A complete blood count is useful to detect anemia, which will aggravate angina. Thyroid function tests are also impor-

tant since hyperthyroidism can aggravate angina and hypothyroidism can lead to atherosclerosis. High sensitivity C-reactive protein (CRP) has been used to detect the increased inflammation of active atherosclerosis. Values greater than 3 mg/L predict coronary events, but the additive value over standard risk factors is unclear. Mortality can be predicted by brain natriuretic peptide (BNP) levels in patients with coronary artery disease. Presumably, patients with high CRP or BNP levels should be treated more aggressively to reduce risk factors.

E. Diagnostic Studies

1. Stress tests—Because angina pectoris or other manifestations of myocardial ischemia often occur during the patient's normal activities, it would be ideal to detect evidence of ischemia at that time. This can be done with ambulatory electrocardiography (ECG). Under unusual circumstances, a patient may have spontaneous angina or ischemia in a medical facility, where it is possible to inject a radionuclide agent and immediately image the myocardium for perfusion defects. Detection of myocardial ischemia during a patient's normal activities, however, does not have as high a diagnostic yield as exercise stress testing does.

Of the various forms of exercise stress that can be used, the most popular is treadmill exercise, for several reasons: It involves walking, a familiar activity that often provokes symptoms. Because of the gravitational effects of being upright, walking requires higher levels or myocardial oxygen demand than do many other forms of exercise. In addition, walking can be performed on an inexpensive treadmill device, which makes evaluating the patient easy and cost-effective. Bicycling is an alternative form of exercise that is preferred by exercise physiologists because it is easier to quantitate the amount of work the person is performing on a bicycle than on a treadmill. Unfortunately, bicycle exercise does not require as high a level of myocardial oxygen demand as does treadmill walking. Thus, a patient may become fatigued on the bicycle before myocardial ischemia is induced, resulting in lower diagnostic yields. On the other hand, bicycle exercise can be performed in the supine position, which facilitates some myocardial ischemia detection methods such as echocardiography. In patients with peripheral vascular disease or lower limb amputations, arm and upper trunk rowing or cranking exercises can be substituted for leg exercise. Arm exercise has a particularly low diagnostic yield because exercising with the small muscle mass of the arms does not increase myocardial oxygen demand by much. Rowing exercises that involve the arms and the trunk muscles produce higher levels of myocardial oxygen demand that can equal those achieved with bicycle exercise—but not quite the levels seen with treadmill exercise. For these reasons, patients who cannot perform leg exercises are usually evaluated using pharmacologic stress testing.

There are two basic kinds of pharmacologic stress tests. One uses drugs, such as the synthetic catecholamine dobutamine, that mimic exercise; the other uses vasodilator drugs, such as dipyridamole and adenosine, that, by producing profound vasodilatation, increase heart rate and stroke volume, thereby raising myocardial oxygen demand. In addition, vasodilators may dilate normal coronary arteries more than diseased coronary arteries, augmenting any differences in regional perfusion of the myocardium, which can be detected by perfusion scanning. In general, vasodilator stress is preferred for myocardial perfusion imaging, and synthetic catecholamine stress is preferred for wall motion imaging.

2. Electrocardiography—ECG is the most frequently used method for detecting myocardial ischemia because of its ready availability, low cost, and ease of application. The usual criterion for diagnosing ischemia is horizontal or down-sloping ST segment depression, achieving at least 0.1 mV at 80 ms beyond the J point (junction of the QRS and the ST segment). This criterion provides the highest values of sensitivity and specificity. Sensitivity can be increased by using 0.5 mV, but at the expense of lower specificity; similarly, using 0.2 mV increases the specificity of the test at the expense of lower sensitivity. Furthermore, accuracy is highest when ECG changes are in the lateral precordial leads (V_4, V_5, V_6) instead of the inferior leads (II, III, aVF). In the usual middle-aged, predominantly male population of patients with chest pain syndromes, who have normal resting ECGs and can achieve more than 85% of their maximal predicted age-based heart rate during treadmill exercise, the preceding ECG criteria have a sensitivity and specificity of approximately 85%. If the resting ECG is abnormal, if the patient does not achieve 85% of maximum predicted heart rate, or if the patient is a woman, the sensitivity and specificity are lower and range from 70% to 80%. In an asymptomatic population with a low pretest likelihood of disease, sensitivity and specificity fall below 70%.

3. Myocardial perfusion scanning—This method detects differences in regional myocardial perfusion rather than ischemia per se; however, there is a high correlation between abnormal regional perfusion scans and the presence of significant **coronary artery occlusive lesions.** Thus, when coronary arteriography is used as the gold standard, the sensitivity and specificity of stress myocardial perfusion scanning in the typical middle-aged, predominantly male population with symptoms are approximately 85–95%. Testing an asymptomatic or predominantly female population would result in lower values. Failure to achieve more than 85% of the maximal predicted heart rate during exercise also results in lower diagnostic accuracy. Although treadmill exercise is the preferred stress modality for myocardial perfusion imaging, pharmacologically induced stress with dipyridamole or adenosine produces nearly as good results and is an acceptable alternative in the patient who cannot exercise. **Positron emission tomography** with vasodilator stress also can be used to detect regional perfusion differences indicative of coronary artery disease.

4. Assessing wall motion abnormalities—Reduced myocardial oxygen supply results in diminishment and, if severe enough, failure of myocardial contraction. Using methods to visualize the left ventricular wall, a reduction in inward endocardial movement and systolic myocardial thickening is observed with ischemia. **Echocardiography** is an ideal detection system for wall motion abnormalities because it can examine the left ventricle from several imaging planes, maximizing the ability to detect subtle changes in wall motion. When images are suboptimal (< 5% of cases), intravenous contrast agents can be given to fill the left ventricular cavity and improve endocardial definition. The results with either exercise or pharmacologic stress are comparable to those of myocardial perfusion imaging and superior to the ECG stress test detection of ischemia. The preferred pharmacologic detection method with wall motion imaging is dobutamine because it directly stimulates the myocardium to increase contractility, as well as raising heart rate and blood pressure, all of which increase myocardial oxygen demand. In some laboratories, if the heart rate increase is not comparable to that usually achieved with exercise testing, atropine is added to further increase myocardial oxygen demand. **Magnetic resonance imaging (MRI)** can also be used to assess left ventricular wall motion during pharmacologic stress testing, but there is relatively little experience with this technique.

5. Evaluating global left ventricular performance—Myocardial ischemia, if profound enough, results in a reduction in global left ventricular performance, which can be detected by either a decrease in left ventricular ejection fraction or a failure for it to increase during exercise. Therefore, techniques such as **radionuclide angiography,** single-photon emission computed tomography (SPECT) left ventricular reconstruction, and echocardiography have been used to detect changes in global left ventricular function. Because fairly profound ischemia is required to depress global left ventricular function, this method has not been as sensitive as other techniques. Furthermore, myocardial disease can lead to an abnormal exercise ejection fraction response, which lowers the specificity of the test. In addition, age and female gender blunt the ejection fraction response to exercise, making the test less reliable in the elderly and in women. As a result, there is currently little enthusiasm for the use of global left ventricular function tests alone for detecting ischemic heart disease.

6. Evaluating coronary anatomy

A. CORONARY ANGIOGRAPHY—Coronary angiography is the standard for evaluating the anatomy of the coronary artery tree. It is best at evaluating the large epicardial coronary vessels that are most frequently diseased in coronary atherosclerosis. Experimental studies suggest that lesions that reduce the lumen of the coronary artery by 70% or more in area (50% in diameter) significantly limit flow, especially during periods of increased myocardial oxygen demand. If such lesions are detected, they are considered compatible with symptoms or other signs of myocardial ischemia. This assessment is known to be imprecise for several reasons, however. First, the actual cross-sectional area of the coronary artery at the point of an atherosclerotic lesion must be estimated from two-dimensional diameter measurements in several planes. When compared with autopsy findings, stenosis severity is usually found to have been underestimated by the coronary angiography. Second, the technique does not take into consideration that lesions in series in a coronary artery may incrementally reduce the flow to distal beds by more than is accounted for by any single lesion. Thus, a series of apparently insignificant lesions may actually reduce myocardial blood flow significantly. Third, the cross-sectional area is not actually measured routinely. It is instead referenced to a supposed normal segment of artery in terms of a percentage of stenosis or percentage of reduction in the normal luminal diameter or cross-sectional area. The problem with this type of estimate is that it is often difficult to determine what a normal segment of artery is, especially in patients with diffuse coronary atherosclerosis.

Quantitative coronary angiogram measurements are an improvement over this visual inspection technique, but they are not commonly used except in research projects. **Epicardial coronary artery anatomy** is a static representation at the time of the study. It does not take into consideration potential changes in coronary vasomotor tone that may occur under certain circumstances and further reduce coronary blood flow. In addition, coronary angiography does not adequately evaluate disease in the intramyocardial blood vessels; this may be important in some patients, especially insulin-dependent diabetics. In patients with pure vasospastic angina, the coronary arteries are usually normal or minimally diseased. To establish increased vasomotion as the cause of the angina, provocative tests have been used to induce coronary vasospasm in the cardiac catheterization laboratory. The most popular of these is an **ergonovine infusion,** which is reputed to produce focal vasospasm only in naturally susceptible arteries and not in normal coronary arteries, which usually exhibit only a uniform reduction in vessel diameter. Ergonovine infusion has some risks, however, in that the resultant coronary vasospasm may be difficult to alleviate and can be quite profound. In addition, not all patients with vasospastic angina may respond to this agent. Thus, its use has diminished in favor of ECG monitoring during the patient's normal daily activities.

B. OTHER TECHNIQUES—ECG or imaging evidence of old myocardial infarction is often presumed to indicate that severe coronary artery stenoses are present in the involved vessel. Myocardial infarction, however, can occur as a result of thrombus on top of a minor plaque that has ruptured and occasionally from intense vasospasm or coronary emboli from the left heart. In these cases, coronary angiography would not detect significant (narrowing of more than 50% of the diameter) coronary lesions despite the evidence of an old myocardial infarction. Coronary artery imaging is therefore necessary because estimating the degree of stenosis from the presence of infarction is not accurate. The presence of inducible myocardial ischemia almost always correlates with significant coronary artery lesions. Under the right clinical circumstances, coronary angiography can often be avoided if noninvasive stress testing produces myocardial ischemia. Coronary angiography could then be reserved for patients who have not responded to medical therapy and were being considered for revascularization, where visualizing the coronary anatomy is necessary.

Other imaging techniques have also had some success. Echocardiography, especially transesophageal, can often visualize the first few centimeters of the major epicardial coronary arteries, and MRI has also shown promise. At present, neither of these noninvasive imaging techniques has reached the degree of accuracy needed to replace contrast coronary angiography; however, technical improvements may change this in the future.

Cardiac computed tomography (CT) is rapidly evolving. Noncontrast techniques can rapidly detect calcified coronary artery plaque. The amount of plaque can be quantitated, usually as the Agatston score, which is predictive of future coronary events in an incremental fashion beyond traditional risk factors. The major use of CT coronary calcium score may be to further stratify the risk of an event in intermediate-risk patients where the intensity of risk factor reduction could be altered accordingly. Contrast CT angiography can evaluate the lumen of the coronary arteries and is a useful alternative to stress testing for low to intermediate pretest risk of coronary artery disease patients. More recently, hybrid CT and either SPECT or positron emission tomography scanners are being used to visualize coronary lesions and assess their physiologic significance at one setting. Since most patients with a positive CT scan for either coronary calcium or lesions eventually get a stress test, this combination makes sense.

F. Choosing a Diagnostic Approach

Normally, noninvasive testing is performed first in the evaluation of suspected coronary atherosclerosis in symptomatic patients with an intermediate pretest likelihood of disease. There are several reasons for this: there is less risk with stress testing than with invasive coronary angiography and cardiac CT has almost no risks. Mortality rates for stress testing average 1 per 10,000 patients, compared with 1 per 1000 for coronary angiography. The physiologic demonstration of myocardial ischemia and its extent forms the basis for the therapeutic approach irrespective of coronary anatomy. Mildly symptomatic patients who show small areas of ischemia at intense exercise levels have an excellent prognosis and are usually treated medically. Knowledge of the coronary anatomy is not necessary to make this therapeutic decision. In general, therefore, a noninvasive technique should be used to detect myocardial ischemia and its extent before considering coronary angiography, which is both riskier and more costly. Asymptomatic patients with a low to intermediate pretest likelihood of coronary artery disease may be better served by a noninvasive coronary artery imaging technique, such as cardiac CT; symptomatic patients may be better served by undergoing the combination of cardiac CT and stress perfusion imaging.

Profound symptoms that occur with minimal exertion are almost certainly due to severe diffuse coronary atherosclerosis or left main obstruction, and it is prudent to proceed directly with coronary angiography. Patients with severe unstable angina should undergo coronary angiography because of the potential increased risk posed by stress testing. If this approach is not appropriate in a particular clinical setting, the clinician might medicate the patient and perform careful stress testing after demonstrating a lack of symptoms on medical therapy. Patients with angina or evidence of ischemia in the early period after myocardial infarction are categorized as having unstable angina and should be taken directly to coronary angiography. The post-infarction patient who is not having recurrent ischemia, however, can usually be evaluated by stress testing and then a decision can be made about the advisability of coronary angiography. If the clinical situation is such that it is likely that stress testing will be inaccurate or uninterpretable, CT or invasive coronary angiography should be performed. Left bundle branch block on the ECG, for example, not only renders the ECG useless for detecting myocardial ischemia but may also affect the results of myocardial perfusion imaging and wall motion studies. Noninvasive techniques have poor diagnostic accuracy in morbidly obese female patients who are unable to exercise. In general, patients whose medical conditions preclude accurate stress testing are candidates for direct coronary angiography.

Which type of noninvasive stress testing to select is based on several factors. The most important of these is the type of information desired; second, certain characteristics of the patient, which may make one test more applicable than another; and third, the pretest likelihood of disease. For example, cardiac CT may be most useful in low-risk patients; stress imaging in intermediate-risk patients; and invasive angiography in high-risk patients. Stress perfusion scanning is more likely than echocardiographic imaging to provide adequate technical quality in obese individuals or those with chronic obstructive pulmonary disease. Cost is also an important consideration, and the ECG stress test is the least expensive. In most patients with a low-to-medium clinical pretest likelihood of disease, using the ECG stress test makes sense, especially because good exercise performance with a negative ECG response for ischemia indicates an excellent prognosis even if coronary artery disease is present. In the patient who is highly likely to have coronary artery disease, however, it is useful to not only confirm the presence of the disease but to document its extent. For this purpose, myocardial imaging techniques are better at determining the extent of coronary artery disease than is the ECG. It is also believed that myocardial perfusion scanning is somewhat better at identifying the coronary arteries involved in the production of ischemia than are techniques for detecting wall motion abnormalities.

Budoff MJ et al; American Heart Association Committee on Cardiovascular Imaging and Intervention; American Heart Association Council on Cardiovascular Radiology and Intervention; American Heart Association Committee on Cardiac Imaging, Council on Clinical Cardiology. Assessment of coronary artery disease by cardiac computed tomography: a scientific statement from the American Heart Association Committee on Cardiovascular Imaging and Intervention, Council on Cardiovascular Radiology and Intervention, and Committee on Cardiac Imaging, Council on Clinical Cardiology. Circulation. 2006 Oct 17;114(16):1761–91. [PMID: 17015792]

Lee TH et al. Clinical practice. Noninvasive tests in patients with stable coronary artery disease. N Engl J Med. 2001 Jun 14;344(24):1840–5. [PMID: 11407346]

▶ Treatment

A. General Approach

Because myocardial ischemia is produced by an imbalance between myocardial oxygen supply and demand, in general, treatment consists of increasing supply or reducing demand—or both. Heart rate is a major determinant of myocardial oxygen demand, and attention to its control is imperative. Any treatment that accelerates heart rate is generally not going to be efficacious in preventing myocardial ischemia. Therefore, care must be taken with potent vasodilator drugs, such as hydralazine, which may lower blood pressure and induce reflex tachycardia. Furthermore, because most coronary blood flow occurs during diastole, the longer the diastole, the greater the coronary blood flow; and the faster the heart rate, the shorter the diastole.

Blood pressure is another important factor: Increases in blood pressure raise myocardial oxygen demand by elevating left ventricular wall tension, and blood pressure is the driving pressure for coronary perfusion. A critical blood pressure is required that does not excessively increase demand, yet keeps coronary perfusion pressure across stenotic lesions optimal. Unfortunately, determining what this level of blood pressure should be in any given patient is difficult, and a trial-and-error approach is often needed to achieve the right balance. Consequently, it is prudent to reduce blood pressure when it is very high, and it may be important to allow it to increase when it is very low. It is not uncommon to encounter patients whose myocardial ischemia has been so vigorously treated with a combination of pharmacologic agents that their blood pressure is too low to be compatible with adequate coronary perfusion. In such patients, withholding some of their medications may actually improve their symptoms. Although myocardial contractility and left ventricular volume also contribute to myocardial oxygen demand, they are less important than heart rate and blood pressure. Myocardial contractility usually parallels heart rate.

Attention should be paid to reducing left ventricular volume in anyone with a dilated heart, but not at the expense of excessive hypotension or tachycardia because these factors are more important than volume for determining myocardial oxygen demand.

It is important to eliminate any aggravating factors that could increase myocardial oxygen demand or reduce coronary artery flow (Table 3–3). Hypertension and tachyarrhythmias are obvious factors that need to be controlled. Thyrotoxicosis leads to tachycardia and increases in myocardial oxygen demand. Anemia is a common problem that increases myocardial oxygen demand because of reflex tachycardia; it reduces oxygen supply by decreasing the oxygen-carrying capacity of the blood. Similarly, hypoxia from pulmonary disease reduces oxygen delivery to the heart. Heart failure increases angina because it often results in left ventricular dilatation, which increases wall stress, and in excess catecholamine tone, which increases contractility and produces tachycardia.

The long-term outlook for patients with coronary atherosclerosis must be addressed by reducing their risk factors for the disease. Once a patient is known to have atherosclerosis, risk factor reduction should be fairly vigorous: If diet has not reduced serum cholesterol, strong consideration should be given to pharmacologic therapy because it has been shown to reduce cardiac events. Patients should be encouraged to exercise, lose weight, quit smoking, and try to reduce stress levels. Daily low-dose aspirin is important for preventing coronary thrombosis. The use of megadoses of vitamin E, β-carotene, and vitamin C should be discouraged in the patient with known coronary atherosclerosis because clinical trials have not demonstrated efficacy and some have shown harm.

B. Pharmacologic Therapy

1. Nitrates—Nitrates, which work on both sides of the supply-and-demand equation, are the oldest drugs used to treat angina pectoris (Table 3–4). These agents are now available in several formulations to fit the patient's lifestyle and disease characteristics. Almost all patients with known coronary atherosclerosis should carry rapid-acting nitroglycerin to abort acute attacks of angina pectoris. Nitrates work principally by providing more nitrous oxide to the vascular endothelium and the arterial smooth muscle, resulting in vasodilation. This tends to ameliorate any increased coronary vasomotor tone and dilate coronary obstructions. As long as blood pressure does not fall excessively, nitrates increase coronary blood flow. Nitrates also cause venodilation, reducing preload and decreasing left ventricular end-diastolic volume. The reduced left ventricular volume decreases wall tension and myocardial oxygen demand.

Sublingual nitroglycerin takes 30–60 seconds to dissolve completely and begin to produce beneficial effects, which can last up to 30 minutes. Although most commonly used to abort acute attacks of angina, the drug can be used prophylactically if the patient can anticipate its need 30 minutes prior to a precipitating event. Prophylactic therapy is best accomplished, however, with longer-acting nitrate preparations. Isosorbide dinitrate and mononitrate are available in oral formulations; each produces beneficial effects for several hours. Large doses of these agents must be taken orally to overcome nitrate reductases in the liver. Liver metabolism of the nitrates can also be avoided with cutaneous application. Nitroglycerin is available as a topical ointment that can be applied as a dressing; it is also available as a ready-made, self-adhesive patch that delivers accurate continuous dosing of the drug through a membrane. Although the paste and the patches produce similar effects, the patches are more convenient for patients to use.

Sublingual nitroglycerin tablets are extremely small and difficult for patients with arthritis to manipulate. A buccal preparation of nitroglycerin is available, which comes in a larger, more easily manipulable tablet that can be chewed and allowed to dissolve in the mouth, rather than being swallowed. This achieves nitrate effectiveness within 2–5 minutes and lasts about 30 minutes, as do the sublingual tablets. An oral nitroglycerin spray, which may be easier to manipulate and more convenient for some patients, is also available.

The major difficulty with all long-acting nitroglycerin preparations is the development of tolerance to their effects. The exact reason for tolerance development is not clearly understood, but it may involve liver enzyme induction or a lack of arterial responsiveness because of local adaptive factors. Regardless of the mechanism, however, round-the-clock nitrate administration will lead to progressively increasing tolerance to the drug after 24–48 hours. Because of this, nitroglycerin is usually taken over the 16-hour period each day that corresponds to the time period during which most of the ischemic episodes would be expected to occur. For most patients, this means not taking nitrate preparations before bed and allowing the ensuing 8 hours for the effects to

Table 3–3. Factors That Can Aggravate Myocardial Ischemia.

Increased myocardial oxygen demand	Tachycardia
	Hypertension
	Thyrotoxicosis
	Heart failure
	Valvular heart disease
	Catecholamine analogues
	   (eg, bronchodilators, tricyclic anti-
	   depressants)

Reduced myocardial oxygen supply	Anemia Hypoxia Carbon monoxide poisoning Hypotension Tachycardia

Table 3–4. Common Oral Antianginal Drugs.

Drug	Usual Dose	Comments; Adverse Effects
Nitrates		
Nitroglycerin	0.4–0.6 mg SL	Aborts acute attacks; headaches, hypotension
Nitroglycerin	1–3 mg buccal	Larger tablet for handicapped patients
Nitroglycerin	0.4 mg spray	More convenient than pills
Nitroglycerin	0.5–2 in of 2% ointment	Prophylactic therapy; tolerance a problem
Nitroglycerin	0.1–0.6 mg/h patches	Prophylactic therapy; tolerance a problem
Isosorbide dinitrate	10–60 mg three times daily	Need 8 h off q24h to avoid tolerance
Isosorbide mononitrate	20 mg twice daily	Take 7 h apart

Drug	Daily Dosage (mg)	Comments; Adverse Effects
β-Blockers		
Propranolol	160–320	CNS side effects—fatigue, impotence—common
Nadolol	80–240	Long half-life, noncardioselective
Timolol	10–45	Noncardioselective
Metaprolol	100–400	Cardioselective
Atenolol	50–200	Cardioselective
Acebutolol	400–1200	Cardioselective, some intrinsic sympathomimetic activity
Betaxolol	5–40	Cardioselective, long half-life
Bisoprolol	5–20	Cardioselective
Pindolol	5–40	Marked intrinsic sympathomimetic activity
Calcium Channel Blockers, Heart Rate Lowering		
Diltiazem	120–360	Heart-rate lowering; AV block, heart failure, edema
Verapamil	120–480	Heart-rate lowering; AV block, heart failure, constipation
Dihydroperidine Calcium Channel Blockers		
Amlodipine	5–10	Least myocardial depression
Nifedipine	30–60	Hypotension, tachycardia
Nicardipine	60–120	Potent coronary vasodilator
Felodipine	5–20	High vascular selectivity
Isradipine	2.5–10	Potent coronary vasodilator
Nisoldipine	10–40	Similar to nifedipine
Sodium Current Inhibitor		
Ranolazine	1000–2000 mg	May increase QT interval on ECG

wear off and responsiveness to the drug to be regained. This timing would have to be adjusted for patients with nocturnal angina. The difficulty with the 8-hour overnight hiatus in therapy, however, is that the patient has little protection during the critical early morning wakening period—when ischemic events are more likely to occur. Patients should therefore take the nitrate preparation as soon as they arise in the morning. For this reason, the nitroglycerin patches have a small amount of paste on the outside of the membrane that delivers a bolus of drug through the skin, which quickly elevates the patient's blood level of the drug. It is important that the patient be careful not to wipe this paste off the patch before applying it.

Nitrates, which are effective in preventing the development of angina as well as aborting acute attacks, are helpful in both patients with fixed coronary artery occlusions and those with vasospastic angina. Their potency, compared with other agents, is limited, however, and patients with severe angina often must turn to other agents. In such patients, nitrates can be excellent adjunctive therapy.

2. β-Blockers—β-Adrenergic blocking agents are highly effective in the prophylactic therapy of angina pectoris. They have been shown to reduce or eliminate angina attacks and prolong exercise endurance time in double-blind, placebo-controlled studies. They can be used around the clock because no tachyphylaxis to their effects has been found. β-Blockers mainly work by lowering myocardial oxygen demand through decreasing heart rate, blood pressure, and myocardial contractility. As mentioned earlier, however, they also increase myocardial oxygen supply by increasing the duration of diastole through heart rate reduction. Currently, several β-blocker preparations are available, with one or more features that may make them more—or less—attractive for a particular patient.

Among these features is the agent's pharmacologic half-life, which ranges from 4 to 18 hours. Various delivery systems have been developed to slow down the delivery of short-acting agents and prolong the duration of drug activity through sustained release or long-acting formulations. Note that the pharmacodynamic half-life of β-adrenergic blockers is often longer than their pharmacologic half-life, and drug effects can be detected for days after discontinuation of prolonged β-blocker therapy.

Ideally, β-blockers should be titrated against the heart rate response to exercise because blunting of the exercise heart rate response is the hallmark of their efficacy. Adverse effects of β-blockers include excessive bradycardia, heart block, and hypotension. Nonselective β-blockers can cause bronchospasm, but it occurs less often with the β₁-selective agents. Blocking β₂-peripheral vasodilatory actions may aggravate claudication in patients with severe peripheral vascular disease. β-Adrenergic stimulation is also important for the gluconeogenic response to hyperglycemia in severely insulin-dependent diabetic patients. Although β-blockers may impair this response, the major problem with their use in insulin-dependent diabetic patients is that the warning signals of hypoglycemia (sweating, tachycardia, piloerection) may be blocked. Because of their negative inotropic properties, β-blockers may also precipitate heart failure in patients with markedly reduced left ventricular performance or acute heart failure.

Other side effects of β-blockers are less predictably related to their anti-β-adrenergic effects. Adverse central nervous system effects are especially troublesome and include fatigue, mental slowness, and impotence. These side effects are somewhat less common with agents that are less lipophilic, such as atenolol and nadolol. Unfortunately, it is these side effects that make many patients unable to tolerate β-blockers.

3. Calcium channel antagonists—Calcium channel antagonists theoretically work on both sides of the supply-and-demand equation. By blocking calcium access to smooth muscle cells, they produce peripheral vasodilatation and are effective antihypertensive agents. In the myocardium, they block sinus node and atrioventricular node function and reduce the inotropic state. They dilate the coronary arteries and increase myocardial blood flow. The calcium channel blockers available today produce a variable spectrum of these basic pharmacologic effects. The biggest group is the dihydroperidine calcium channel blockers, which are potent arterial dilators and thereby cause reflex sympathetic activation, which overshadows their negative chronotropic and inotropic effects.

A second major group of calcium channel blockers are those that lower the heart rate. The two most commonly used drugs in this class are diltiazem and verapamil. Because these drugs have less peripheral vasodilatory action in individuals with normal blood pressure, they produce little reflex tachycardia. The average daily heart rate is usually reduced with these agents because their inherent negative chronotropic effects are not overridden; negative inotropic effects are also more common with these agents. Hypertensive and normotensive individuals seem to have a different vascular responsiveness to the rate-lowering calcium channel blockers. Interestingly, in hypertensive individuals, rate-lowering calcium channel blockers lower the blood pressure as well as the dihydroperidine agents. Diltiazem is more widely used because of its low side-effect profile. Verapamil, which is an excellent treatment for patients with supraventricular arrhythmias, has potent effects on the arteriovenous (A nnV) node; this can cause excessive bradycardia and heart block in patients with angina pectoris. Verapamil is also more likely than diltiazem to precipitate heart failure, and it often produces troublesome constipation, especially in elderly individuals. All the calcium channel blockers can produce peripheral edema. This is due not to their negative inotropic effects but rather to an imbalance between the efferent and afferent peripheral arteriolar tone, which increases capillary hydrostatic pressure. Other adverse effects of these drugs are idiosyncratic and include gastrointestinal and dermatologic effects.

Calcium channel blockers are titrated to the patient's symptoms because there is no physiologic marker of their effect, in contrast to the heart rate response to exercise with β-blockers. This makes choosing the appropriate dosage difficult, and many clinicians increase the dose until some side effect occurs and then they reduce it. The most common side effects are related to the pharmacologic effects of the drugs. With the dihydroperidines, vasodilatory side effects, such as orthostatic hypotension, flushing, and headache, occur. Hypotension is less common with the heart rate-lowering calcium channel blockers, and their side effects are more related to cardiac effects, such as excessive bradycardia. These drugs are very useful because they are excellent for preventing angina pectoris, lowering high blood pressure, and, in the case of the heart rate-lowering agents, controlling supraventricular arrhythmias.

4. Ranolazine—Ranolazine partially inhibits fatty acid oxidation and increases glucose oxidation which generates more ATP for each molecule of oxygen consumed. This shift in substrate selection may reduce myocardial oxygen demand without altering hemodynamics. Since all other antianginal agents reduce heart rate and blood pressure, this gives ranolazine an advantage. Studies have shown that ranolazine provides additive benefits to standard treatment described above and is useful as monotherapy. It has few adverse effects, but experience with this agent is limited.

5. Combination therapy—Although monotherapy is desirable for patient convenience and cost considerations, many patients, especially those with severe inoperable coronary artery disease, require more than one antianginal agent to control their symptoms. Because all antianginal agents have a synergistic effect in preventing angina, the initial choices should be for agents with complementary pharmacologic effects. For example, nitrates can be added to β-blocker therapy: Nitrates have an effect on dilating coronary arteries and increasing coronary blood flow, and their peripheral effects may increase reflex sympathetic tone and counteract some of the negative inotropic and chronotropic effects of the β-blockers. This has proved to be a highly effective combination. Similarly, combining a β-blocker with dihydroperidine drugs, when the β-blockers suppress the reflex tachycardia produced by the dihydroperidine, has also proved to be highly effective. Combinations of the heart rate-lowering calcium channel blockers and nitrates have also proved efficacious. Extremely refractory patients may respond to the combination of a dihydroperidine calcium channel blocker and a heart rate-lowering calcium channel blocker.

Combining a dihydroperidine calcium channel blocker and nitrates makes little sense, however, because of the high likelihood of producing potent vasodilatory side effects. This combination may excessively lower blood pressure to the point that coronary perfusion pressure is compromised and the patient's angina actually worsens. In fact, in as many as 10% of patients with moderately severe angina, both the nitrates and the dihydroperidine calcium channel blockers alone have been reported to aggravate angina. Although few corroborative data exist, this percentage is certainly higher with the combination of the two agents.

The most difficult cases often involve triple therapy, with a calcium channel blocker, a β-blocker, and a nitrate. Although there are few objective data on the benefits of this approach, it has proven efficacious in selected patients. The major problem with triple therapy is that side effects, such as hypotension, are increased, which often limits therapy. Ranolazine has no hemodynamic effects and can be used for those patients refractory to their current regimen but with heart rate or blood pressure levels as low as is tolerable. It has been successfully combined with atenolol, amlodipine, and diltiazem.

6. Adjunctive therapy—All patients with coronary artery disease should take aspirin (81–325 mg/d) and selected high-risk patients should also take clopidogrel. These drugs reduce platelet aggregation and retard the growth of atherothrombosis. Also important is correction of dyslipidemia, smoking cessation, exercise, weight loss, control of hyperten-sion, and management of stress. In patients with known coronary artery disease, it is important to decrease low-density lipoprotein (LDL) cholesterol and perhaps increase high-density lipoprotein (HDL) cholesterol to published targets (< 100 mg/dL, > 40 mg/dL, respectively). Angiotensin-converting enzyme (ACE) inhibitors may have a protective effect in patients with coronary artery disease, especially postmyocardial infarction. β-Blockers are also indicated postmyocardial infarction, but their use in chronic coronary artery disease without infarct or angina is controversial. However, both β-blockers and ACE inhibitors would be preferred agents for blood pressure control in patients with chronic coronary artery disease.

C. Revascularization

1. Catheter-based methods—The standard percutaneous coronary intervention (PCI) is balloon dilatation with placement of a metal stent. Such treatment is limited to the larger epicardial arteries and can be complicated by various types of acute vessel injury, which can result in myocardial infarction unless surgical revascularization is immediately performed. Smaller arteries may be amenable to plain old balloon angioplasty (POBA), and large arteries with complicated lesions may be candidates for other forms of PCI. PCI requires intense antiplatelet therapy usually with aspirin and clopidogrel to prevent stent thrombosis. After the stent has been covered with endothelium, this risk is much less.

In the absence of acute complications, initial success rates for significantly dilating the coronary artery are greater than 85%, and the technique can be of tremendous benefit to patients—without their undergoing the risk of cardiac surgery. The principal disadvantage to PCI is restenosis, which occurs in about one-third of patients treated with a bare metal stent during the first 6 months. Drug-eluting stents have reduced restenosis to 10% or less but have been associated with a small incidence of late thrombosis. Although many agents are under intense investigation, there is currently no systemic pharmacologic approach to preventing restenosis.

PCI is ideal for symptomatic patients with one or two discrete lesions in one or two arteries. In patients with more complex lesions or those with three or more vessels involved, bypass surgery is preferable for several reasons. First, the restenosis risk is the same for each lesion treated by PCI, so that if enough vessels are worked on the risk of restenosis in one of them will approach 100%. Second, the ability to completely revascularize patients with multivessel disease is less with PCI compared with bypass surgery. Finally, some clinical trials have shown that diabetic patients have better outcomes after bypass surgery relative to PCI.

2. Coronary artery bypass graft surgery—Controlled clinical trials have shown that coronary artery bypass graft (CABG) surgery can successfully alleviate angina symptoms in up to 80% of patients. These results compare very favorably with pharmacologic therapy and catheter-based techniques and can be accomplished in selected patients with less than 2% operative mortality rates. Although the initial cost of surgery is high, studies have shown it can be competitive with repeated angioplasty and lifelong pharmacologic therapy in selected patients.

The standard surgical approach is to use the saphenous veins, which are sewn to the ascending aorta and then, distal to the obstruction, in the coronary artery, effectively bypassing the obstruction with blood from the aorta. Although single end-to-side saphenous-vein-to-coronary-artery grafts are preferred, occasionally surgeons will do side-to-side anastomoses in one coronary artery (or more) and then terminate the graft in an end-to-side anastomosis in the final coronary artery. There is some evidence that although these skip grafts are easier and quicker to place than multiple single saphenous grafts, they may not last as long. The major problem with saphenous vein grafts is recurrent atherosclerosis in the grafts, which is often quite bulky and friable, and ostial stenosis, probably from cicatrization at the anastomotic sites. Although these problems can be approached with PCI and other interventional devices, the success rate of catheter-delivered devices to open obstructed saphenous vein grafts is not as high as that seen with native coronary artery obstructions, and many patients require repeat saphenous vein grafting after an average of about 8 years. It is believed that meticulous attention to a low-fat diet, cessation of smoking, and the ingestion of one aspirin a day (80–160 mg) will retard the development of saphenous vein atherosclerosis; some patients do well for 20 years or more after CABG.

There is now considerable evidence that arterial conduits make better bypass graft materials. The difficulty is finding large enough arteries that are not essential to other parts of the body. The most popular arteries used today are the internal thoracic arteries. Their attachment to the subclavian artery is left intact, and the distal end is used as an end-to-side anastomosis into a single coronary artery. If a patient requires more than two grafts, some surgeons, rather than using a saphenous vein, have used the radial artery or abdominal vessels, such as the gastroepiploic. There are less data on these alternative conduits, but theoretically they would have the same advantages as the internal thoracic arteries in terms of graft longevity. Efforts at preventing bypass graft failure are worthwhile because the risk of repeat surgery is usually higher than that of the initial surgery. There are several reasons for this, including the fact that the patient is older, the scar tissue from the first operation makes the second one more difficult, and finally, any progression of atherosclerosis in the coronary arteries makes finding good-quality insertion sites for the graft more difficult.

D. Selection of Therapy

Pharmacologic therapy is indicated when other conditions may be aggravating angina pectoris and can be successfully treated. For example, in the patient with coexistent hypertension and angina, it is often prudent to treat the hypertension and lower blood pressure to acceptable levels before pursuing revascularization for angina because lowering the blood pressure will often eliminate the angina. For this purpose, it is wise to use antihypertensive medications that are also antianginal (eg, β-blockers, calcium channel blockers) rather than other agents with no antianginal effects (eg, ACE inhibitors, centrally acting agents). The presence of heart failure can also produce or aggravate angina, and this should be treated. Care must be taken in choosing antianginal drugs that they do not aggravate heart failure. For this reason, nitrates are frequently used in heart failure and angina because these drugs may actually benefit both conditions. Rate-lowering calcium channel blockers should be avoided if the left ventricular ejection fraction is below 35%, unless it is clear that the heart failure is episodic and is being produced by ischemia. In this situation, however, revascularization may be a more effective strategy. β-Blockers can be effective, but they must be started at low doses and uptitrated carefully. Although β-blockers are now part of standard therapy for heart failure, there is little data on their use in patients with angina and reduced left ventricular performance. Finally, the presence of ventricular or supraventricular tachyarrhythmias may aggravate angina. Rhythm disorders also afford an opportunity for using dual-purpose drugs. The heart rate-lowering calcium channel blockers may effectively control supraventricular arrhythmias and also benefit angina. β-Blockers can often be effective treatment for ventricular arrhythmias in patients with coronary artery disease and should be tried before other, more potent antiarrhythmics or devices are contemplated. Keep in mind that digoxin blood levels may be increased by concomitant treatment with calcium channel blockers. In addition, the combination of digoxin and either heart rate-lowering calcium channel blockers or β-blockers may cause synergistic effects on the atrioventricular node and lead to excessive bradycardia or heart block.

The major indication for revascularization of chronic ischemic heart disease is the failure of medications to control the patient's symptoms. Drug-refractory angina pectoris is the major indication for revascularization. Note that myocardial ischemia should be established as the source of the patient's symptoms before embarking on revascularization, since symptoms may actually be due to gastroesophageal reflux. Consequently, some form of stress testing that verifies the relationship between demonstrable ischemia and symptoms is advisable before performing any revascularization procedure.

In some other instances—patient preference, for example—revascularization therapy might be considered before even trying pharmacologic therapy. Some patients do not like the prospect of lifelong drug therapy and would rather have open arteries. Although this is a valid reason to perform revascularization, the clinician must be careful that his or her own enthusiasm for revascularization as treatment does not pressure the patient into such a decision. Other candidates for direct revascularization are patients with high-risk occupations who cannot return to these occupations unless they are completely revascularized (eg, airline pilots).

Revascularization is preferred to medical therapy in managing certain types of coronary anatomy that are known (through clinical trials) to have a longer survival if treated with CABG rather than medically. Such lesions include left main obstructions of more than 50%, three-vessel disease, and two-vessel disease in which one of the vessels is the left anterior descending artery. Currently, left main stenoses are not effectively treated with catheter-based techniques, but two- and three-vessel coronary disease could potentially be treated by PCI. Clinical trials have shown equivalent long-term outcomes between PCI and CABG in patients with multivessel disease.

CABG is also recommended for patients with two- or three-vessel coronary artery disease and resultant heart failure from reduced left ventricular performance, especially if viable myocardium can be demonstrated. Because the tests for viable myocardium are not perfect, however, many clinicians believe that all these patients should be revascularized in the hope that some myocardial function will return. This seems a prudent approach, given that donor hearts for cardiac transplantation are difficult to obtain—and many patients with heart failure and coronary artery disease improve following bypass surgery.

Surgery is also recommended when the patient has a concomitant disease that requires surgical therapy, such as significant valvular heart disease, heart failure in the presence of a large left ventricular aneurysm, or mechanical complications of myocardial infarction, such as a ventricular septal defect. In the presence of hemodynamic indications for repairing these problems, any significant coronary artery disease that is found should be corrected with bypass surgery at the same time.

The risk of bypass surgery in a given individual must also be considered because several factors can increase the risk significantly and might make catheter-based techniques or medical therapy more desirable. Age is always a risk factor for any major surgery, and CABG is no exception. Also, female gender tends to increase the risk of CABG, possibly because women are, on the average, smaller and have smaller arteries than men. Some data indicate that if size is the only factor considered, gender disappears as a risk predictor with CABG. Other medical conditions that may complicate the perioperative period (eg, chronic kidney disease, obesity, lung disease, diabetes) also raise the risks of surgery. Another factor (discussed earlier) is whether this is a repeat bypass operation. The technical difficulties are especially troublesome when a prior internal thoracic artery graft has been placed because this artery lies right behind the sternum and can be easily compromised when reopening the chest.

The choice between catheter-based techniques and CABG surgery is based on several considerations: Is it technically feasible to perform either technique with a good anticipated result? What does the patient wish to do? The patient may have a strong preference for one technique over the other. Again, the clinician must be careful not to unduly influence the patient in this regard, lest it give the appearance of a conflict of interest. Consideration must also be given to factors that increase the risk of surgery. The most difficult decision involves the patient who is suitable for either surgery or a catheter-based technique. The few controlled, randomized clinical trials that have been done on such patients have shown equivalent clinical results with PCI and surgery in terms of mortality and symptom relief. Note that this is accomplished by PCI at the cost of repeated procedures in many patients. Despite the necessity for these repeated procedures, the overall cost of bypass surgery is higher over the short term. Unfortunately, the trials do not outline clear guidelines for choosing PCI or CABG in the patient who is a good candidate for either treatment; this continues to be a decision to be made by the clinician and the patient on a case-by-case basis. The availability of minimally invasive surgery has pushed the balance between CABG and PCI a little toward CABG but not all patients are suitable for a minimally invasive approach.

Bhatt DL et al; CHARISMA Investigators. Clopidogrel and aspirin versus aspirin alone for the prevention of atherothrombotic events. N Engl J Med. 2006 Apr 20;354(16):1706–17. [PMID: 16531616]

Boden WE et al; COURAGE Trial Research Group. Optimal medical therapy with or without PCI for stable coronary disease. N Engl J Med. 2007 Apr 12;356(15):1503–16. [PMID: 17387127]

Chaitman BR et al. Anti-ischemic effects and long-term survival during ranolazine monotherapy in patients with chronic severe angina. J Am Coll Cardiol. 2004 Apr 21;43(8):1375–82. [PMID: 15093870]

Chaitman BR et al; Combination Assessment of Ranolazine In Stable Angina (CARISA) Investigators. Effects of ranolazine with atenolol, amlodipine, or diltiazem on exercise tolerance and angina frequency in patients with severe chronic angina: a randomized controlled trial. JAMA. 2004 Jan 21;291(3):309–16. [PMID: 14734593]

Gibbons RJ et al; American College of Cardiology, American Heart Association Task Force on Practice Guidelines. Committee on the Management of Patients with Chronic Stable Angina. ACC/AHA 2002 guideline update for the management of patients with chronic stable angina—summary article: a report of the American College of Cardiology/American Heart Association Task Force on Practice Guidelines (Committee on the Management of Patients with Chronic Stable Angina). Circulation. 2003 Jan 7;107(1):149–58. [PMID: 12515758]

King SB 3rd et al. Eight-year mortality in the Emory Angioplasty versus Surgery Trial (EAST). J Am Coll Cardiol. 2000 Apr;35(5):1116–21. [PMID: 10758949]

Pocock SJ et al. Quality of life after coronary angioplasty or continued medical treatment for angina: three-year follow-up in the RITA-2 trial. Randomized Intervention Treatment of Angina. J Am Coll Cardiol. 2000 Mar 15;35(4):907–14. [PMID: 10732887]

Rodriguez A et al. Argentine randomized study: coronary angioplasty with stenting versus coronary bypass surgery in patients with multiple-vessel disease (ERACI II): 30-day and 1-year follow-up results. ERACI II Investigators. J Am Coll Cardiol. 2001 Jan;37(1):51–8. [PMID: 11153772]

Seven-year outcome in the Bypass Angioplasty Revascularization Investigation (BARI) by treatment and diabetic status. J Am Coll Cardiol. 2000 Apr;35(5):1122–9. [PMID: 10758950]

▶ Prognosis

There are two major determinants of prognosis in patients with chronic ischemic heart disease. The first is the clinical status of the patient, which can be semiquantitated by the Canadian Cardiovascular Society's angina functional class system. In this system, class I is asymptomatic, II is angina with heavy exertion, III is angina with mild-to-moderate exertion, and IV comprises patients who cannot perform their daily activities without getting angina or who are actually experiencing angina decubitus. The higher the Canadian class, the worse the prognosis. Clinical status can also be determined by exercise testing. If patients can exercise more than 9 minutes or into stage IV of the modified Bruce protocol, their prognosis is excellent. However, the presence of either angina or significant ischemic ST depression on the exercise test indicates a poorer prognosis. In addition, when using perfusion scanning, the more extensive the perfusion abnormalities with exercise, the worse the prognosis. Left ventricular dysfunction with exercise, as evidenced by a decrease or a failure to increase the ejection fraction on left ventricular imaging, or by significant lung uptake of thallium during stress perfusion imaging, also connotes a worse prognosis. Perhaps the most powerful predictor for future mortality is the resting left ventricular ejection fraction; values of less than 50% are associated with an exponential increase in mortality.

A second prognostic system is based solely on coronary anatomy. The more vessels involved, and the more severely they are involved, the worse the prognosis. This observation has formed the anatomic basis for revascularization in patients with coronary artery disease. Although this approach has some appeal, it has never been proven that revascularization in asymptomatic patients improves their prognosis. Even in patients with left main and severe three-vessel disease, proof is lacking that prophylactic revascularization is of any value if the patients are asymptomatic. Theoretical considerations suggest that ischemia—even in the absence of angina—that can be demonstrated by stress testing or ambulatory ECG recordings would support a decision to revascularize based on anatomy and the presence of ischemia. Although this seems like a much stronger case for revascularization in an asymptomatic patient, such treatment has not been proven efficacious in clinical trials.

The simplicity of the coronary anatomy approach to prognosis has resulted in considerable clinical data on the longevity of patients with chronic ischemic heart disease. Patients with one-vessel coronary artery disease have about a 3% per year mortality rate, less if the vessel is the right or circumflex coronary artery and somewhat more if it is the left anterior descending artery. Patients with two-vessel disease have a 5% or 6% mortality rate per year; in patients with three-vessel disease, this increases to 6–8% a year. Patients with left main disease, with or without other coronary occlusions, have about an 8–12% yearly mortality rate. Similar data do not exist for the clinical classification of patients because of the complexities of determining risk by this approach. A positive treadmill exercise test, at a low workload, for either angina or ischemic ST changes connotes a yearly mortality rate of 5%. This is less if the patient exercised a long time and had good left ventricular function and no previous myocardial infarction. It is worse if the patient exercised only a very short time on the treadmill and had evidence of left ventricular dysfunction or a prior myocardial infarction. How much modern pharmacologic and revascularization therapy can influence these prognostic figures is unclear at present.

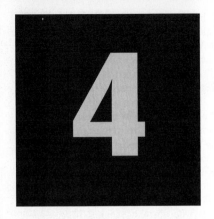

Unstable Angina/Non-ST Elevation Myocardial Infarction

Prediman K. Shah, MD & Kuang-Yuh Chyu, MD, PhD

ESSENTIALS OF DIAGNOSIS

▶ New or worsening symptoms (angina, pulmonary edema) or signs (electrocardiographic [ECG] changes) of myocardial ischemia.

▶ Absence or mild elevation of cardiac enzymes (creatine kinase and its MB fraction or troponin I or T) without prolonged ST segment elevation on ECG.

▶ Unstable angina and non-ST elevation myocardial infarction are closely related in pathogenesis and clinical presentation and are therefore discussed as one entity in this chapter.

▶ General Considerations

A. Background

Unstable angina and non-ST elevation myocardial infarction (USA/NSTEMI) are a part of the wide spectrum of acute coronary syndrome. They are closely related in pathogenesis but with different severity in presentation. Compared with ST elevation myocardial infarction (STEMI), the incidence of USA/NSTEMI has been increasing. In the current era, USA/NSTEMI is the admitting diagnosis for about 40–50% of all admissions to cardiac care units.

B. Clinical Spectrum

Atherosclerotic coronary artery disease comprises a spectrum of conditions that ranges from a totally asymptomatic state at one end to sudden cardiac death at the other (Table 4–1). It is clear that coronary artery disease, the primary cause of mortality and morbidity in much of the industrialized world, takes its toll through such acute complications (unstable coronary syndromes) as unstable angina, myocardial infarction, acute congestive heart failure, and sudden cardiac death. Also known as acute ischemic syndromes,

these are the first clinical expressions of atherosclerotic coronary artery disease in 40–60% of patients with coronary artery disease.

C. Pathophysiology

Angina pectoris is the symptomatic equivalent of transient myocardial ischemia, which results from a temporary imbalance in the myocardial oxygen demand and supply. Most episodes of myocardial ischemia are generally believed to result from an absolute reduction in regional myocardial blood flow below basal levels, with the subendocardium carrying a greater burden of flow deficit relative to the epicardium, whether triggered by a primary reduction in coronary blood flow or an increase in oxygen demand. As shown in Figure 4–1, the various acute coronary syndromes share a more-or-less common pathophysiologic substrate. The differences in clinical presentation result largely from the differences in the magnitude of coronary occlusion, the duration of the occlusion, the modifying influence of local and systemic blood flow, and the adequacy of coronary collaterals.

In patients with unstable angina, most episodes of resting ischemia occur without antecedent changes in myocardial oxygen demand but are triggered by primary and episodic reductions in coronary blood flow. Worsening of ischemic symptoms in patients with stable coronary artery disease may be triggered by such obvious extrinsic factors such as severe anemia, thyrotoxicosis, acute tachyarrhythmias, hypotension, and drugs capable of increasing myocardial oxygen demand or coronary steal; in most cases, however, no obvious external trigger can be identified. In these patients—who constitute the majority—the evolution of unstable angina and its clinical complications is the outcome of a complex interplay involving coronary atherosclerotic plaque and resultant stenosis, platelet-fibrin thrombus formation, and abnormal vascular tone.

1. Unstable plaque—Several studies have shown that the atherosclerotic plaque responsible for acute unstable coro-

Table 4–1. Clinical Spectrum of Atherosclerotic Coronary Artery Disease.

Subclinical symptoms or asymptomatic
Stable angina
Unstable angina[1]
Acute myocardial infarction[1]
Acute pulmonary edema[1]
Sudden death[1]

[1]Acute unstable ischemic syndromes.

nary syndromes is characterized by a fissure or rupture in its fibrous cap, most frequently at the shoulder region (junction of the normal part of the arterial wall and the plaque-bearing segment). These plaques tend to have relatively thin acellular fibrous caps infiltrated with foam cells or macrophages and eccentric pools of soft and necrotic lipid core. Many clinical and angiographic studies suggest that plaque fissure leading to unstable angina or acute MI may occur not only at sites of severe atherosclerotic stenosis, but even more commonly at minimal coronary stenoses. Serial angiographic observations have shown that development from stable to unstable angina is associated with progression of atherosclerotic disease in 60–75% of patients. This may reflect ongoing episodes of mural thrombosis and incorporation into the underlying plaque. These and other studies have shown that coronary lesions initially occluding less than 75% of the coronary artery area are likely to progress and lead to unstable angina or myocardial infarction; lesions occluding more than 75% are likely to lead to total occlusion. The latter are less likely to lead to myocardial infarction, probably because of the possibility of collateral blood vessel development in more severely stenotic arteries. Furthermore, outward positive remodeling (Glagov effect) of coronary artery segments containing large atherosclerotic plaques may minimize luminal compromise and yet enhance vulnerability for plaque disruption.

Although the precise mechanisms are not known, several hypotheses explain the propensity of plaques to rupture. These include circumferential hemodynamic stresses related to arterial pulse and pressure, intraplaque hemorrhage from small

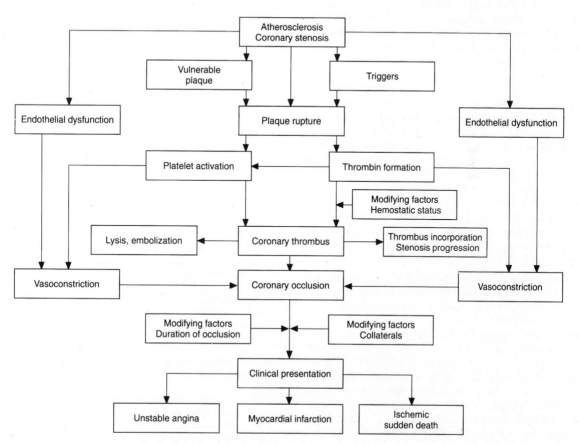

▲ **Figure 4–1.** Schematic summarizing the current view of the key pathophysiologic events in acute coronary syndromes.

intimal fissures, vasoconstriction, and the twisting and bending of arteries. Other possibilities are inflammatory processes that involve elaboration of matrix-degrading enzymes (collagenase, elastase, stromelysin, cathepsins) released by foam cells or macrophages and other mesenchymal cells in the plaques in response to undefined stimuli (including, but not limited to, oxidized low-density lipoprotein [LDL]). An excess of matrix-degrading enzymatic activity may contribute to loss of collagen in the protective fibrous cap of the plaque, predisposing it to disruption. Similarly reduced synthesis of collagen, resulting from increased death of matrix-synthesizing smooth muscle cells by apoptosis (programmed cell death), may also contribute to plaque disruption. Intracellular pathogens, such as *Chlamydophila pneumoniae*, *Helicobacter pylori*, cytomegalovirus (CMV), and immune activation have recently been shown to cause inflammatory responses in atherosclerotic plaques and are implicated as potential triggers for plaque rupture.

2. Dynamic obstruction

A. Thrombosis—Plaque fissure or rupture initiates the process of mural—and eventually luminal—thrombosis by exposing platelets to the thrombogenic components of plaque (eg, collagen, lipid gruel, and tissue factor). This leads to platelet attachment, aggregation, platelet thrombus formation, and the exposure of tissue factor, an abundant procoagulant in the plaque, which interacts with clotting factor VII. The ensuing cascade of events results in the formation of thrombin, which contributes to further platelet aggregation, fibrin formation, and vasoconstriction; it may also play a role as a smooth muscle cell mitogen and chemoattractant for inflammatory cells. The magnitude of the thrombotic response may be further modulated by such local rheologic factors as the shear rate, as well as the status of local and circulating coagulability, platelet aggregability, and fibrinolysis. The superimposition of thrombus on a fissured atherosclerotic plaque can abruptly worsen the local coronary stenosis and lead to a sudden decrease in blood flow. In about 20–40% of acute coronary syndromes seen during autopsy, however, neither plaque fissure nor rupture can be found underlying thrombosis (plaque erosion).

B. Vasoconstriction—It has become increasingly clear that atherosclerosis is generally associated with a reduced vasodilator response, an increased vasoconstrictor response, or a paradoxical vasoconstrictor response to a variety of stimuli: flow changes, exercise, vasoactive substances (eg, acetylcholine, platelet aggregates, thrombin). This abnormal vasomotor response has been observed well before the development of full-blown atherosclerosis; it has also been seen in patients with risk factors for coronary artery disease but no overt atherosclerosis. The response has generally been attributed to endothelial dysfunction with enhanced inactivation or a reduction in the release of nitric oxide or related nitrosovasodilators (eg, the relaxation factor produced by the normal endothelium). Some studies have also suggested other causes, such as enhanced sensitivity of the vascular smooth muscle, abnormal platelet function, and an increased release of endothelin (a vasoconstrictor peptide).

Braunwald E. Unstable angina, an etiologic approach to management. Circulation. 1998 Nov 24;98(21):2219–22. [PMID: 98226306]
Ross R. Atherosclerosis—an inflammatory disease. N Engl J Med. 1999 Jan 14;340(2):115–26. [PMID: 9887164]
Shah PK. Mechanisms of plaque vulnerability and rupture. J Am Coll Cardiol. 2003 Feb 19;41(4 Suppl S):15S–22S. [PMID: 12644336]

▶ Clinical Findings

A. Symptoms and Signs

Unstable angina is a clinical syndrome characterized by symptoms of ischemia, which may include classic retrosternal chest pain or such pain surrogates as a burning sensation, feeling of indigestion, or dyspnea (Table 4–2). Anginal symptoms may also be felt primarily or as radiation in the neck, jaw, teeth, arms, back, or epigastrium. In some patients, particularly the elderly, dyspnea, fatigue, diaphoresis, light-headedness, a feeling of indigestion and the desire to burp or defecate, or nausea and emesis may accompany other symptoms—or may be the only symptoms. The pain of unstable angina typically lasts 15–30 minutes; it can last longer in some patients. The clinical presentation of unstable angina can take any one of several forms.

There may be an onset of ischemic symptoms in a patient who had been previously free of angina, with or without a history of coronary artery disease. If symptoms are effort-induced, they are often rapidly progressive, with more frequent, easily provoked, and prolonged episodes. Rest pain may follow a period of crescendo effort angina—or exist from the beginning.

Symptoms may intensify or change in a patient with antecedent angina. Pain may be provoked by less effort and

---

Table 4–2. Clinical Presentation of Unstable Angina.

New onset of ischemic symptoms
At rest only
During exertion only
At rest and exertion
Intensification of previous ischemic symptoms
Increased frequency, severity, duration
Change in pattern (eg, symptoms at rest)
Recurrence of ischemic symptoms within 4–6 weeks after an acute myocardial infarction
Other
Recurrence of ischemia within 4–6 weeks following bypass surgery or coronary catheterization
Recurrent acute pulmonary edema
Prinzmetal (variant) angina

be more frequent and prolonged than before. The response to nitrates may decrease and their consumption increase. The appearance of new pain at rest or with minimal exertion is particularly ominous. On the other hand, recurrent long-standing ischemic symptoms at rest do not necessarily constitute an acute ischemic syndrome. Ischemic symptoms may recur shortly after (usually within 4 weeks) an acute myocardial infarction, coronary artery bypass surgery, or catheter-based coronary artery intervention. In some patients, an acute unstable coronary syndrome may manifest itself as acute pulmonary edema or sudden cardiac death.

B. Physical Examination

No physical finding is specific for unstable angina, and when the patient is free of pain the examination may be entirely normal. During episodes of ischemia, a dyskinetic left ventricular apical impulse, a third or fourth heart sound, or a transient murmur of ischemic mitral regurgitation may be detected. Similarly, during episodes of prolonged or severe ischemia there may be transient evidence of left ventricular failure, such as pulmonary congestion or edema, diaphoresis, or hypotension. Arrhythmias and conduction disturbances may occur during episodes of myocardial ischemia.

The findings from physical examination, especially as they relate to signs of heart failure, provide important prognostic information. An analysis of data from four randomized clinical trials (GUSTO IIb, PURSUIT, PARAGON A and B) revealed that Killip classification, a commonly used classification based on physical examination of patients at presentation of STEMI, is a strong independent predictor for short- and long-term mortality, with higher Killip class associated with higher mortality rate. This is also recently confirmed using data from the Canadian ACS Registries.

C. Diagnostic Studies

Unstable angina is a common reason for admission to the hospital, and the diagnosis, in general, rests entirely on clinical grounds. In a patient with typical effort-induced chest discomfort that is new or rapidly progressive, the diagnosis is relatively straightforward, particularly (but not necessarily) when there are associated ECG changes. Often, however, the symptoms are less clear-cut. The pain may be atypical in terms of its location, radiation, character, and so on, or the patient may have had a single, prolonged episode of pain—which may or may not have resolved by the time of presentation. The physician should strongly suspect unstable angina, particularly when coronary artery disease or its risk factors are present. When in doubt, it is safer to err on the side of caution and consider the diagnosis to be unstable angina until proven otherwise. Even though dynamic ST-T changes on the ECG make the diagnosis more certain, between 5% and 10% of patients with a compelling clinical history (especially middle-aged women) have no critical coronary stenosis on coronary angiography. In rare instances, especially in women, spontaneous coronary artery dissection, unrelated to coronary atherosclerosis, may be the basis for an acute coronary syndrome. In general, the more profound the changes in ECG, the greater the likelihood of an ischemic origin for the pain and the worse the prognosis.

1. ECG and Holter monitoring—ECG abnormalities are common in patients with unstable angina. In view of the episodic nature of ischemia, however, the changes may not be present if the ECG is recorded during an ischemia-free period or the ischemia involves the myocardial territories (eg, the circumflex coronary artery territory) that do not show well on the standard 12-lead ECG. Therefore, it is not surprising that 40–50% of patients admitted with a clinical diagnosis of unstable angina have no ECG abnormalities on initial presentation. The ECG abnormalities tend to be in the form of transient ST-segment depression or elevation and, less frequently, T wave inversion, flattening, peaking or pseudo-normalization (ie, the T wave becomes transiently upright from a baseline state of inversion). It must be emphasized, however, that a normal or unremarkable ECG should never be used to disregard the diagnosis of unstable angina in a patient with a compelling clinical history and an appropriate risk-factor profile.

Continuous Holter ambulatory ECG recording reveals a much higher prevalence of transient ST-T wave abnormalities, of which 70–80% are not accompanied by symptoms (silent ischemia). These episodes, which may be associated with transient ventricular dysfunction and reduced myocardial perfusion, are much more prevalent in patients with ST-T changes on their admission tracings (up to 80%) than in persons without such changes. Frequent and severe ECG changes on Holter monitoring, in general, indicate an increased risk of adverse clinical outcome.

2. Angiography—More than 90–95% of patients with a clinical syndrome of unstable angina have angiographically detectable atherosclerotic coronary artery disease of varying severity and extent. The prevalence of single-, two-, and three-vessel disease is roughly equal, especially in patients older than 55 and those with a past history of stable angina. In relatively younger patients and in those with no prior history of stable angina, the frequency of single-vessel disease is relatively higher (50–60%). Left mainstem disease is found in 10–15% of patients with unstable angina. A subset of patients (5–10%) with angiographically normal or near normal coronary arteries may have noncardiac symptoms masquerading as unstable angina, the clinical syndrome X (ischemic symptoms with angiographically normal arteries and possible microvascular dysfunction), or the rare primary vasospastic syndrome of Prinzmetal (variant) angina. It should be recognized, however, that most patients (even those with Prinzmetal angina) tend to have a significant atherosclerotic lesion on which the spasm is superimposed. In general, the extent (number of vessels involved, location of lesions) and severity (the percentage of diameter-narrowing, the minimal luminal diameter, or the length of the lesion) of coronary artery disease and the prevalence of collateral circulation, as judged by traditional angiographic criteria, do not differ between patients with unstable angina and those with stable coronary artery disease. The morphologic features of the culprit lesions do tend to differ, however. The culprit lesion in patients with unstable angina tends to be more eccentric and irregular, with overhanging margins and filling defects or lucencies. These findings (on autopsy or in vivo angioscopy) represent a fissured plaque, with or without a superimposed thrombus. Such unstable features in the culprit lesion are detected more frequently when angiography is performed early in the clinical course.

3. Noninvasive tests—Any form of provocative testing (exercise or pharmacologic stress) is clearly contraindicated in the acute phase of the disease because of the inherent risk of provoking a serious complication. Several studies of patients who had been pain-free and clinically stable for more than 3–5 days, however, have shown that such testing, using ECG, scintigraphic, or echocardiographic evaluation may be safe. Provocative testing is used primarily to stratify patients into low- and high-risk subsets. Aggressive diagnostic and therapeutic interventions can then be selectively applied to the high-risk patients; the low-risk patients are treated more conservatively. In general, these studies have shown that patients who have good exercise duration and ventricular function, without significant inducible ischemia or ECG changes on admission, are at a very low risk and can be managed conservatively. On the other hand, patients with ECG changes on admission, a history of prior myocardial infarction, evidence of inducible ischemia, and ventricular dysfunction tend to be at a higher risk for adverse cardiac events and therefore in greater need of further and more invasive evaluation.

4. Other laboratory findings—Blood levels of myocardial enzymes are, by definition, not elevated in unstable angina; if they are elevated without evolution of Q waves, the diagnosis is generally a non–Q wave myocardial infarction (or NSTEMI). This distinction is somewhat arbitrary, however.

There is evidence of elevated blood levels of biochemical inflammation markers (eg, C-reactive protein [CRP], serum amyloid A, fibrinogen) in patients presenting with USA/NSTEMI. An elevated blood level of CRP or serum amyloid A on admission is associated with a higher risk for early mortality, even in patients in whom classic myocardial damage marker (cardiac-specific troponins) is negative. Increased blood level of fibrinogen is also associated with increased rate of death or myocardial infarction. The presence of such markers may be useful in risk stratification for clinical outcomes; however, their current roles in diagnosing USA/NSTEMI have not been established. It is also unclear whether treatment strategies based on these biochemical markers would alter clinical outcomes.

Khot UN et al. Prognostic importance of physical examination for heart failure in non-ST-elevation acute coronary syndromes: the enduring value of Killip classification. JAMA. 2003 Oct 22;290(16):2174–81. [PMID: 14570953]

Morrow DA et al. C-reactive protein is a potent predictor of mortality independently of and in combination with troponin T in acute coronary syndromes: A TIMI 11A substudy. Thrombolysis in Myocardial Infarction. J Am Coll Cardiol. 1998 Jun;31(7):1460–5. [PMID: 9626820]

Morrow DA et al. Serum amyloid A predicts early mortality in acute coronary syndromes: a TIMI 11A substudy. J Am Coll Cardiol. 2000 Feb;35(2):358–62. [PMID: 10676681]

Segev A et al. Prognostic significance of admission heart failure in patients with non-ST-elevation acute coronary syndromes (from the Canadian Acute Coronary Syndrome Registries). Am J Cardiol. 2006 Aug 15;98(4):470–3. [PMID: 16893699]

Toss H et al. Prognostic influence of increased fibrinogen and C-reactive protein levels in unstable coronary artery disease. FRISC Study Group. Fragmin during Instability in Coronary Artery Disease. Circulation. 1997 Dec 16;96(12):4204–10. [PMID: 9416883]

▶ Differential Diagnosis

Conditions that simulate or masquerade as unstable angina include acute myocardial infarction, acute aortic dissection, acute pericarditis, pulmonary embolism, esophageal spasm, hiatal hernia, chest wall pain, and so on. Careful attention to the history, risk factors, and objective findings of ischemia (transient ST-T changes and mild elevations of troponins in particular) remain the cornerstones for the diagnosis.

A. Acute Myocardial Infarction

Although myocardial infarction often produces more prolonged pain, the clinical presentation can be indistinguishable from that of unstable angina. As stated earlier, this distinction should be considered somewhat arbitrary because abnormal myocardial technetium-99m pyrophosphate uptake, mild creatine kinase elevations detected on very frequent blood sampling, and increases in troponin-T and I levels (released from necrotic myocytes) are observed in some patients with otherwise classic symptoms of unstable angina.

B. Acute Aortic Dissection

The pain of aortic dissection is usually prolonged and severe. It frequently begins in or radiates to the back and tends to be relatively unrelenting and often tearing in nature; transient ST-T changes are rare. An abnormal chest radiograph showing a widened mediastinum, accompanied by asymmetry in arterial pulses and blood pressure, can provide clues to the diagnosis of aortic dissection, which can be verified by bedside echocardiography (transesophageal, with or without transthoracic echocardiography), MRI, CT scanning, or aortography.

C. Acute Pericarditis

Acute pericarditis may be difficult to differentiate from unstable angina. A history of a febrile or respiratory illness suggests the former. The pain of pericarditis is classically pleuritic in nature and worsens with breathing, coughing, deglutition, truncal movement, and supine posture. A pericardial friction rub is diagnostic, but it is often evanescent, and frequent auscultation may be needed. Prolonged, diffuse ST elevation that is not accompanied by reciprocal ST depression or myocardial necrosis is typical of pericarditis. Leukocytosis and an elevated erythrocyte sedimentation rate are common in pericarditis but not in unstable angina. Echocardiography may detect pericardial effusion in patients with pericarditis; diffuse ventricular hypokinesis may imply associated myocarditis. Regional dysfunction, especially if transient, is more likely to reflect myocardial ischemia.

D. Acute Pulmonary Embolism

Chest pain in acute pulmonary embolism is also pleuritic in nature and almost always accompanied by dyspnea. Arterial hypoxemia is common, and the ECG may show sinus tachycardia with a rightward axis shift. Precordial ST-T wave abnormalities may simulate patterns of anterior myocardial ischemia or infarction. A high index of suspicion, combined with a noninvasive assessment of pulmonary ventilation-perfusion mismatch, evidence of lower extremity deep venous thrombosis, CT angiography, and possibly pulmonary angiography, is necessary to exclude the diagnosis.

E. Gastrointestinal Causes of Pain

Various gastrointestinal pathologies can mimic unstable angina. These include esophageal spasm, peptic ulcer, hiatal hernia, cholecystitis, and acute pancreatitis. A history compatible with those conditions, the response to specific therapy, and appropriate biochemical tests and imaging procedures should help clarify the situation. It should be noted that these abdominal conditions may produce ECG changes that simulate acute myocardial ischemia.

F. Other Causes of Chest Pain

Many patients present with noncardiac chest pain that mimics unstable angina, and sometimes no specific diagnosis can be reached. The pain may be musculoskeletal or there may be nonspecific changes on the ECG that increase the diagnostic confusion. In these patients, a definite diagnosis often cannot be reached despite careful clinical observation. When the pain has abated and the patient is stable, a provocative test for myocardial ischemia may help rule out ischemic heart disease. Although coronary angiography may provide evidence of atherosclerotic coronary artery disease, anatomic evidence does not necessarily prove an ischemic cause for the symptoms. In some patients, acute myocarditis may also produce chest pain syndromes simulating unstable angina and acute myocardial infarction. Recreational drug use (cocaine and methamphetamine) may also produce clinical syndromes of chest pain, sometimes related to drug-induced

acute coronary syndrome precipitated by the vasoconstrictor and prothrombic effects of these drugs.

▶ Treatment

In treating unstable angina, the initial objective is to stratify patients for their short-term morbidity and mortality risks based on their clinical presentations (Figure 4–2). Following risk stratification, management objectives include eliminating episodes of ischemia and preventing acute myocardial infarction and death.

A. Initial Management

During this early in-hospital phase, therapy is primarily aimed at stabilizing the patient by stabilizing the culprit coronary lesion and thus preventing a recurrence of myocardial ischemia at rest and progression to myocardial infarction.

1. General measures—Patients whose history is compatible with a diagnosis of unstable angina should be promptly hospitalized—ideally, in an intensive or intermediate care unit. General supportive care includes bed rest with continuous monitoring of cardiac rate and rhythm and frequent evaluation of vital signs; relief of anxiety with appropriate reassurance and, if necessary, anxiolytic medication; treatment of associated precipitating or aggravating factors such as hypoxia, hypertension, dysrhythmias, heart failure, acute blood loss, and thyrotoxicosis. A 12-lead ECG should be repeated if it is initially unrevealing or if any significant change has occurred in symptoms or clinical stability. Serial cardiac enzyme evaluation should be performed to rule out an acute myocardial infarction.

2. Specific drug therapy

A. NITRATES—Nitrates are generally considered one of the cornerstones of therapy (Tables 4–3 and 4–4). They tend to relieve and prevent ischemia by improving subendocardial blood flow in the ischemic zone through their vasodilator actions, predominantly on the large epicardial vessels, including the stenotic segments and the coronary collaterals. Unlike acetylcholine and other endothelium-dependent vasodilators, nitrates produce their effects by directly stimulating cyclic guanosine monophosphate (GMP) in the vascular smooth muscle without requiring an intact or functional endothelium; hence their effects are generally well preserved in atherosclerosis. Reduction of left ventricular preload and afterload by peripheral vasodilator actions may contribute to the reduction of myocardial ischemia. Although nitrates may reduce the number of both symptomatic and asymptomatic episodes of myocardial ischemia in unstable angina, no effect has yet been demonstrated on the incidence of progression to myocardial infarction or death.

In the very acute phase, it is preferable to use intravenous nitroglycerin to ensure adequate bioavailability, a rapid onset and cessation of action, and easy dose titratability. Oral, sublingual, transdermal, and transmucosal preparations are better suited for subacute and chronic use. To minimize the

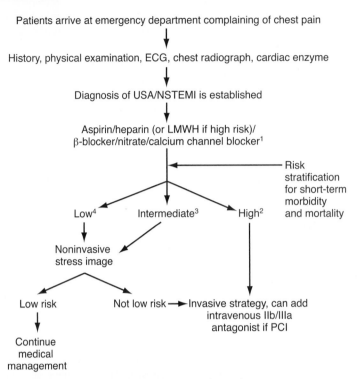

Patients arrive at emergency department complaining of chest pain

History, physical examination, ECG, chest radiograph, cardiac enzyme

Diagnosis of USA/NSTEMI is established

Aspirin/heparin (or LMWH if high risk)/
β-blocker/nitrate/calcium channel blocker[1]

Risk stratification for short-term morbidity and mortality

Low[4]   Intermediate[3]   High[2]

Noninvasive stress image

Low risk   Not low risk → Invasive strategy, can add intravenous IIb/IIIa antagonist if PCI

Continue medical management

▲ **Figure 4–2.** Algorithm in risk stratification and management of USA/NSTEMI.
[1]All patients should receive risk factor modification (lipid lowering, smoking cessation, blood pressure/diabetes mellitus control, dietary counseling, exercise program, weight control). [2]High risk features include accelerating ischemic symptoms in preceding 48 h, rest pain > 20 min, presence of clinical congestive heart failure, advanced age (> 75 years), new bundle-branch clock or rest angina with transient ST-segment changes > 0.5 mm, sustained ventricular tachycardia or marked elevation of cardiac enzyme. (ACC/AHA guidelines for unstable angina. J Am Coll Cardiol. 2000;36:970.) [3]Intermediate risk features include history of prior MI/PVD/CABG/CVA/aspirin use, resolved prolonged rest angina (> 20 min), rest angina (< 20 min) relieved with rest or sublingual nitroglycerin, age > 70 years, T-wave inversion > 2 mm, presence of pathologic Q wave, slightly elevated cardiac enzyme. (ACC/AHA guidelines for unstable angina. J Am Coll Cardiol. 2000;36:970.) [4]Low-risk features do not have the clinical features included in items 2 and 3 but have new-onset Canadian Cardiovascular Society (CCS) class III or IV angina in the past 2 weeks without prolonged (> 20 min) rest angina, normal or unchanged ECG, normal cardiac enzyme. (ACC/AHA guidelines for unstable angina. J Am Coll Cardiol. 2000;36:970.) CABG, coronary artery bypass grafting; CVA, cerebrovascular accident; ECG, electrocardiogram; LMWH, low-molecular-weight heparin; MI, myocardial infarction; PCI, percutaneous coronary intervention; PVD, peripheral vascular disease.

chances of abrupt hypotension, nitroglycerin infusion should be started at 10 mcg/min and the infusion rate titrated according to symptoms and blood pressure. The goal is to use the lowest dose that will relieve ischemic symptoms without incurring side effects. The side effects of nitrates include hypotension, which should be meticulously avoided; reflex tachycardia associated with hypotension; occasional profound bradycardia, presumably related to vagal stimulation; headaches; and facial flushing. Rare side effects include methemoglobinemia, alcohol intoxication, and an increase in intraocular and intracranial pressure. Some studies have shown a nitroglycerin-induced decrease in the anticoagulant effect of heparin; these results have not been confirmed by other

studies. More recent studies suggest that nitroglycerin may reduce the circulating levels of exogenously administered tissue plasminogen activator, possibly reducing its thrombolytic efficacy. Because the magnitude of reduced arterial pressure that a patient can tolerate without developing signs of organ hypoperfusion varies, it is difficult to define an absolute cut-off point. A reasonable approach in normotensive patients without heart failure is to maintain the arterial systolic blood pressure no lower than 100–110 mm Hg; in hypertensive patients, reduction below 120–130 mm Hg may be unwise.

Continuous and prolonged administration of intravenous nitroglycerin for more than 24 hours may lead to the attenuation of both its peripheral and coronary dilator

Table 4–3. Effects of Medical Therapy in Unstable Angina.

Therapy	Recurrent Ischemia	Progression to Acute Myocardial Infarction	Mortality
Nitrates	↓↓	?	?
Calcium channel blockers	↓↓	?*	?*
β-Blockers	↓↓	↓?	↓?
Aspirin/clopidogrel	↓?	↓↓	↓↓
UFH/LMWH	↓↓	↓↓↓	↓↓↓
Thrombolytics	?	?	?

↓, reduction in frequency; ?, benefit not clearly established; *, increased risk with nifedipine, decreased risk with diltiazem in non-Q wave infarction in two studies.
LMWH, low-molecular-weight heparin; UFH, unfractionated heparin.

actions. This effect is due to the development of tolerance in some patients, presumably from depletion of sulfhydryl groups. Some studies show that this attenuation diminishes when sulfhydryl donors such as *N*-acetylcysteine are administered. At the present time, however, there is no easy and practical way to avoid or overcome this problem other than

escalating the dose to maintain reduction in measurable end points (eg, the arterial blood pressure).

With the increasing use of phosphodiesterase-5 inhibitors (such as sildenafil) for erectile dysfunction among patients with coronary artery disease or the recreational use of such medication, it is important to obtain a history of whether the patient has taken such medication 24 hours prior to presentation of USA/NSTEMI. Nitrate-mediated vasodilation in the presence of phosphodiesterase-5 inhibition can lead to prolonged hypotension or even death.

B. ANTIPLATELET AND ANTICOAGULANT THERAPY—Coronary thrombosis has long been suspected as a culprit in the pathophysiology of unstable angina, and several observational studies published in the 1950s and 1960s reported on the beneficial effects of anticoagulation. The protective effects of aspirin (including the fact that taking a single aspirin had the same benefit as taking more than one) in coronary-prone patients were also described in the 1950s. The unequivocal benefits of antiplatelet and anticoagulant therapy in unstable angina were established only in the past 2 decades, however, when several placebo-controlled randomized trials were completed.

(1) Aspirin—Aspirin has been shown to reduce the risk of developing myocardial infarction by about 50% in at least four randomized trials. The protective effect of aspirin in unstable angina has been comparable, in the dosage range of 75–1200 mg/day. However, because of the potential for gastrointestinal side effects, low doses of aspirin (75–81 mg/day) are preferable. A lower dose should be preceded by a

Table 4–4. Mechanisms of Action and Adverse Effects of Drug Therapy in Unstable Angina.

Agent	Myocardial Blood Flow	Myocardial Oxygen Demand	Vasoconstriction	Platelet Fibrin Thrombus	Adverse Effects
Nitrates	↑↑	↓↓	↓↓	↓?	Hypotension, reflex tachycardia, rarely bradycardia, headaches, increased intracranial and intraocular pressure, methemoglobinemia, alcohol intoxication, tolerance, decreased heparin effect not established.
Calcium channel blockers	↑↑	↓↓	↓↓	—	Hypotension, excessive bradyarrhythmias (verapamil, dilitiazem), increased heart rate (nifedipine), worsening heart failure, worsening ischemia from coronary steal (nifedipine).
β-Blockers	↑	↓↓↓	?	?	Excessive bradyarrhythmias, worsening heart failure, increased bronchospasm.
Aspirin	↑↑↑*	?	?	↓↓↓	Gastritis or ulceration, bleeding, allergy.
Heparin	↑↑↑*	?	?	↓↓↓	Bleeding, thrombocytopenia, rarely increased thrombotic risk, osteoporosis, increased K⁺.

↑, increase; ↓, decrease; ?, not established; *, increase or maintenance of coronary flow is due to prevention of thrombotic occlusion rather than to any direct vasodilator action.

loading dose of 160–325 mg on the first day in order to initiate the antiplatelet effect more rapidly.

(2) Ticlopidine and clopidogrel—These two thienopyridine drugs are adenosine diphosphate (ADP) antagonists that are approved for antiplatelet therapy. They have been shown to be comparable to aspirin in reducing the risk of developing acute myocardial infarction in unstable angina. Both drugs have delayed onset of full antiplatelet effect, hence they are not suitable in acute cases. Because they are more expensive than aspirin and carry a 1% risk of agranulocytosis and, rarely, thrombotic thrombocytopenia purpura, ticlopidine and clopidogrel should be used only when a patient cannot tolerate aspirin due to hypersensitivity or major gastrointestinal side effects.

Due to a better safety profile and faster onset of action, clopidogrel is the preferred thienopyridine. Extrapolation based on the CURE trial suggested that the combination of aspirin and clopidogrel appears to modestly reduce the combined incidence of cardiovascular death, myocardial infarction, or stroke in USA/NSTEMI patients who are not undergoing revascularization procedures. However, this small additional benefit is at the expense of increased major or minor bleeding and cost. The optimal duration of such combination therapy has not been established either.

(3) Unfractionated heparin and low-molecular-weight heparin—The protective effect of intravenous unfractionated heparin (UFH) in treating unstable angina has been demonstrated in randomized trials. During short-term use, the risk of myocardial infarction in unstable angina is reduced by about 90%, and ischemic episodes are reduced by about 70%.

Two studies have compared the relative benefits of intravenous heparin with those of aspirin alone or combined with heparin. Although both agents offer protection against the development of acute myocardial infarction in unstable angina, the studies show that heparin may be somewhat more effective in reducing both the risk of infarct development and the number of ischemic episodes. Aspirin and heparin together may not be superior to heparin alone, but aspirin does offer protection against rebound reactivation of acute ischemic syndromes shortly after short-term heparin therapy ends—an argument for their combined use in unstable angina. Because combined therapy may increase the risk of bleeding, only low-dose aspirin should be used.

Recently, low-molecular-weight heparin (LMWH) was tested to examine its role as an alternative anticoagulation therapy to UFH in patients with USA/NSTEMI. LMWH has certain pharmacologically superior features to UFH: longer half-life, weaker binding to plasma protein, higher bioavailability with subcutaneous injection, more predictable dose response, and less incidence of heparin-induced thrombocytopenia. Dalteparin has been shown to be superior to placebo and equivalent to UFH for immediate, short-term treatment of USA/NSTEMI in reducing composite end points in the FRISC and FRIC trials, respectively. In the FRISC II trial, dalteparin also lowered the risk of death or myocardial infarction in patients receiving invasive procedures, especially in high-risk patients. In ESSENCE and thrombolysis in myocardial infarction (TIMI) 11B trials, enoxaparin (modestly but significantly) reduced the combined incidence of death, myocardial infarction, or recurrent angina over UFH. This reduction is mainly due to a decrease in recurrent angina. But in the SYNERGY trial, enoxaparin was not superior to UFH in reducing mortality or non-fatal myocardial infarction in high-risk patients undergoing early invasive therapy. Taken together, acute treatment with LMWH is likely as effective as UFH in USA/NSTEMI patients receiving aspirin. However, because LMWH is easier to use and does not require partial thromboplastin time monitoring, it is being increasingly preferred over UFH.

(4) Direct thrombin inhibitors—Medications in this class include hirudin, bivalirudin, argatroban, efegatran, and inogatran. Compared with heparin, direct thrombin inhibitors, as a class, appear to offer a small reduction in death or myocardial infarction in patients with USA/NSTEMI. However, hirudin is associated with an excess of major bleeding compared with heparin whereas argatroban, efegatran, and inogatran are associated with an increased risk of death or myocardial infarction.

Bivalirudin was recently tested in the ACUITY trial. Bivalirudin was shown to be noninferior to heparin in composite ischemia end points (death, myocardial infarction, or unplanned revascularization) in USA/NSTEMI patients with moderate- or high-risk features undergoing invasive therapy when it was used in conjuction with a glycoprotein IIb/IIIa (GP IIb/IIIa) inhibitor. Taken together, direct thrombin inhibitors have not been routinely used in the medical management of USA/NSTEMI; however, they are alternative antithrombotics for patients with heparin-induced thrombocytopenia.

(5) Glycoprotein IIb/IIIa receptor inhibitor—Activation of GP IIb/IIIa receptors leads to interaction of receptors with ligands such as fibrinogen followed by platelet aggregation. Several GP IIb/IIIa receptor antagonists have been developed to inhibit this agonist-induced platelet aggregation and tested in clinical trials. Currently available intravenous IIb/IIIa receptor inhibitors are abciximab, a monoclonal antibody against the receptor; nonpeptidic inhibitors, lamifiban and tirofiban; and a peptidic inhibitor, eptifibatide.

Four major randomized clinical trials (PRISM, PRISM-PLUS, PURSUIT, and PARAGON) evaluated the efficacy of intravenous GP IIb/IIIa receptor inhibitors in reducing clinical events (death, myocardial infarction, or refractory angina) in patients with USA/NSTEMI. Different inhibitors were tested in the trials (tirofiban in PRISM and PRISM-PLUS, eptifibatide in PURSUIT, and lamifiban in PARAGON). Although patient population, experimental designs, angiographic strategies, and end point measurement in these trials were different, these trials showed consistent, though small, reduction of short-term composite event rates in the management of the acute phase of USA/NSTEMI. However, the efficacy of these GP IIb/IIIa inhibitors in reducing short-term mortality is not as consistent if only death is considered as the clinical end point. Subgroup analysis of these trials indicated that patients with high-risk features would benefit more from the use of GP IIb/IIIa inhibitors.

The efficacy of intravenous abciximab on clinical outcome in patients with USA/NSTEMI without early intervention was tested in GUSTO-IV ACS trial. There was no survival benefit in patients receiving abciximab when compared with placebo at 30 days or at 1 year.

The efficacy of intravenous GP IIb/IIIa inhibitors in reducing clinical events in patients with USA/NSTEMI undergoing percutaneous coronary intervention (PCI) was also tested—abciximab in EPILOG and CAPTURE, tirofiban in RESTORE. These trials consistently showed a reduction of short-term clinical events (composite end point of death, myocardial infarction, urgent or repeat revascularization). The major benefit appears to be in nonfatal adverse events rather than mortality.

At the present time there is no clinical role for oral GP IIb/IIIa antagonists such as xemilofiban, orbofiban, and sibrafiban because of lack of proven clinical benefit and increased risk of bleeding.

Thus, overall data suggest that intravenous GP IIb/IIIa inhibitor used judiciously, along with aspirin and heparin, is beneficial in high-risk patients with USA/NSTEMI undergoing PCI. Table 4–5 summarizes the use of various antiplatelet, antithrombotic, and GP IIb/IIIa inhibitors in different USA/NSTEMI settings.

C. Thrombolytic drugs—A number of trials have examined the role of thrombolytic therapy in USA/NSTEMI. Despite improved angiographic appearance of the culprit vessel following thrombolytic therapy, no clear-cut benefit over and above antiplatelet and anticoagulant therapy alone has been demonstrated. The precise reasons for this are unclear, especially because there is general agreement about the important pathophysiologic contribution of thrombus to unstable angina. At this time, therefore, the routine use of thrombolytic therapy in unstable angina cannot be recommended.

D. β-Blockers—β-Blockers are commonly used in managing ischemic heart disease because they have been shown to reduce the frequency of both symptomatic and asymptomatic ischemic episodes in stable as well as unstable angina. The protective effects of β-blockers in ischemic heart disease are generally attributed to their negative chronotropic and inotropic effects, which reduce the imbalance of myocardial oxygen demand and supply. Their ability to reduce the risk of infarct development is less clear, but they do decrease reinfarction and mortality rates in postinfarction patients. The mechanism of their protective effect against reinfarction remains unexplained, although it has been speculated that they reduce the risk of plaque rupture by reducing mechanical stress on the vulnerable plaque. It is also unclear whether β-blockers offer any additional benefit in unstable angina in patients who are already receiving nitrates and antiplatelet-anticoagulant therapy. At present, the use of β-blockers in patients with unstable angina should be considered an adjunctive therapy.

E. Calcium channel blockers—Calcium channel blockers are also frequently used in managing ischemic heart

Table 4–5. Use of Antiplatelet, Antithrombotic, and GP IIb/IIIa Inhibitors in Different Subsets of Patients with USA/NSTEMI Based on AHA/ACC Guideline Recommendation.

	Aspirin	Clopidogrel	UFH or LMWH	GP IIb/IIIa inhibitors
Low risk[1]	✓	✓[2]	✓	No
Moderate risk[1]	✓	✓[2]	✓	No
High risk[1]				
No plan for early invasive therapy	✓	✓[3]	✓	✓[4,5]
Revascularization with PCI	✓	✓[6,7]	✓	✓[4,8]
Revascularization with CABG	✓	No[6]	✓	NA

[1]See Figure 4-2 for risk classification.
[2]Use in patients who are unable to take aspirin due to hypersensitivity or major gastrointestinal intolerance.
[3]Optimal duration of use has not been established; guideline recommends use for at least 1 month and for up to 9 months.
[4]Class IIa indication.
[5]Only tirofiban or eptifibatide (not abciximab) is indicated for this use.
[6]Hold clopidogrel until coronary anatomy is defined by angiography and the decision whether to use PCI or CABG is made.
[7]In the current "drug eluting stent" era, the use of such stent and optimal duration of treatment with clopidogrel after drug eluting stent has been under great debate due to the complication of late stent thrombosis.
[8]Administered prior to PCI.
CABG, coronary artery bypass grafting; GP, glycoprotein; LMWH, low-molecular-weight heparin; PCI, percutaneous coronary intervention; UFH, unfractionated heparin; USA/NSTEMI, unstable angina/non-ST elevation myocardial infarction.

disease. Their beneficial effects in myocardial ischemia are generally attributed to their ability to improve myocardial blood flow by reducing coronary vascular tone and dilation of large epicardial vessels and coronary stenoses through an endothelium-independent action. They also reduce myocardial workload through their negative chronotropic and inotropic and peripheral vasodilator effects. Because exaggerated vasoconstriction may play a role in unstable angina, calcium channel blockers have been used in its management. In general, although calcium channel blockers have been shown to reduce the frequency of ischemic episodes in unstable angina, their protective effect against the development of acute myocardial infarction has not been definitively demonstrated. In fact, the use of such calcium channel blockers as nifedipine tends to increase the risk of ischemic complications in unstable angina. Such adverse effects may well be due to reflex tachycardia or coronary steal caused by the arteriole-dilating actions of some calcium channel blockers. The protective effects of the heart rate-slowing calcium channel blocker diltiazem have been reported in patients with a non-Q wave myocardial infarction and preserved ventricular function. As in the case of β-blockers, the additive benefits of calcium channel blockers in patients with unstable angina who are receiving nitrates and antithrombotic therapy have not been defined, and their use should also be considered an adjunct to such drugs.

A comparison of aspirin plus tirofiban with aspirin plus heparin for unstable angina. The Platelet Receptor Inhibition in Ischemic Syndrome Management (PRISM) Study Investigators. N Engl J Med. 1998 May 21;338(21):1498–505. [PMID: 9599104]

Anderson JL et al; American College of Cardiology; American Heart Association Task Force on Practice Guidelines (Writing Committee to Revise the 2002 Guidelines for the Management of Patients with Unstable Angina/Non-ST-Elevation Myocardial Infarction); American College of Emergency Physicians; Society for Cardiovascular Angiography and Interventions; Society of Thoracic Surgeons; American Association of Cardiovascular and Pulmonary Rehabilitation; Society for Academic Emergency Medicine. ACC/AHA 2007 guidelines for the management of patients with unstable angina/non-ST-elevation myocardial infarction: a report of the American College of Cardiology/American Heart Association Task Force on Practice Guidelines (Writing Committee to Revise the 2002 Guidelines for the Management of Patients with Unstable Angina/Non-ST-Elevation Myocardial Infarction) developed in collaboration with the American College of Emergency Physicians, the Society for Cardiovascular Angiography and Interventions, and the Society of Thoracic Surgeons endorsed by the American Association of Cardiovascular and Pulmonary Rehabilitation and the Society for Academic Emergency Medicine. J Am Coll Cardiol. 2007 Aug 14;50(7):e1–e157. [PMID: 17692738]

Bertrand ME et al. Management of acute coronary syndromes: acute coronary syndromes without persistent ST segment elevation: recommendations of the Task Force of the European Society of Cardiology. Eur Heart J. 2000 Sep;21(17):1406–32. [PMID: 10952834]

Chew DP et al. Increased mortality with oral platelet glycoprotein IIb/IIIa antagonists: a meta-analysis of phase III multicenter randomized trials. Circulation. 2001 Jan 16;103(2):201–6. [PMID: 11208677]

Cohen M et al. A comparison of low-molecular-weight heparin with unfractionated heparin for unstable coronary artery disease. Efficacy and Safety of Subcutaneous Enoxaparin in Non-Q-Wave Coronary Events Study Group. N Engl J Med. 1997 Aug 14;337(7):447–52. [PMID: 9250846]

Direct Thrombin Inhibitor Trialists' Collaborative Group. Direct thrombin inhibitors in acute coronary syndromes: principal results of a meta-analysis based on individual patients' data. Lancet. 2002 Jan 26;359(9303):294–302. [PMID: 11830196]

Effects of platelet glycoprotein IIb/IIIa blockade with tirofiban on adverse cardiac events in patients with unstable angina or acute myocardial infarction undergoing coronary angioplasty. The RESTORE Investigators. Randomized Efficacy Study of Tirofiban for Outcomes and REstenosis. Circulation. 1997 Sep 2;96(5):1445–53. [PMID: 9315530]

Goodman SG et al. Randomized trial of low molecular weight heparin (enoxaparin) versus unfractionated heparin for unstable coronary artery disease: one-year results of the ESSENCE study. Efficacy and Safety of Subcutaneous Enoxaparin in Non-Q-Wave Coronary Events. J Am Coll Cardiol. 2000 Sep;36(3):693–8. [PMID: 10987586]

Inhibition of platelet glycoprotein IIb/IIIa with eptifibatide in patients with acute coronary syndromes. The PURSUIT Trial Investigators. Platelet Glycoprotein IIb/IIIa in Unstable Angina: Receptor Suppression Using Integrilin Therapy. N Engl J Med. 1998 Aug 13;339(7):436–43. [PMID: 9705684]

Inhibition of the platelet glycoprotein IIb/IIIa receptor with tirofiban in unstable angina and non-Q-wave myocardial infarction. The Platelet Receptor Inhibition in Ischemic Syndrome Management in Patients Limited by Unstable Signs and Symptoms (PRISM-PLUS) Study Investigators. N Engl J Med. 1998 May 21;338(21):1488–97. [PMID: 9599103]

International, randomized, controlled trial of lamifiban (a platelet glycoprotein IIb/IIIa inhibitor), heparin, or both in unstable angina. The PARAGON Investigators. Platelet IIb/IIIa Antagonism for the Reduction of Acute coronary syndrome events in a Global Organization Network. Circulation. 1998 Jun 23;97(24):2386–95. [PMID: 9641689]

Long-term low molecular mass heparin in unstable coronary artery disease: FRISC II prospective randomized multicenter study. FRagmin and Fast Revascularization during InStability in Coronary artery disease. Lancet. 1999 Aug 28;354(9180):701–7. [PMID: 10475180]

Low molecular weight heparin during instability in coronary artery disease, Fragmin during Instability in Coronary Artery Disease (FRISC) study group. Lancet. 1996 Mar 2;347(9001):561–8. [PMID: 8596317]

Kaul S et al. Low molecular weight heparin in acute coronary syndrome: evidence for superior or equivalent efficacy compared with unfractionated heparin? J Am Coll Cardiol. 2000 Jun;35(7):1699–712. [PMID: 10841215]

Klein W et al. Comparison of low molecular weight heparin with unfractionated heparin acutely and with placebo for 6 weeks in the management of unstable coronary artery disease. Fragmin in unstable coronary artery disease study (FRIC). Circulation. 1997 Jul 1;96(1):61–8. [PMID: 9236418]

Platelet glycoprotein IIb/IIIa receptor blockade and low-dose heparin during percutaneous coronary revascularization. The EPILOG investigators. N Engl J Med. 1997 Jun 12;336(24):1689–96. [PMID: 9182212]

Randomised placebo-controlled trial of abciximab before and during coronary intervention in refractory unstable angina: the CAPTURE study. Lancet. 1997 May 17;349(9063):1429–35. [PMID: 9164316]

Stone GW et al; ACUITY Investigators. Bivalirudin for patients with acute coronary syndromes. N Engl J Med. 2006 Nov 23;355(21):2203–16. [PMID: 17124018]

B. Definitive Management

1. Catheter-based interventions—Endovascular interventions such as percutaneous coronary angioplasty, atherectomy, and laser-assisted angioplasty are commonly performed in patients with unstable angina to reduce the critical stenosis in the culprit artery or in multiple coronary arteries. Although these interventions accomplish an acute reduction in the severity of stenosis (80–93%), in patients with unstable angina they carry a somewhat higher risk of acute complications, including death (0–2%), abrupt closure (0–17%), acute myocardial infarction (0–13%), and the need for urgent coronary artery bypass surgery (0–12%), than in patients with stable angina. The risk is especially great when the procedure is performed soon after the onset of symptoms, in the absence of prior treatment with heparin, or in the presence of an angiographically visible intracoronary thrombus. The 3- to 6-month restenosis rate with these interventions is 17–44%.

Several randomized clinical trials compared "early conservative" and "early invasive" strategies in treating patients with unstable angina. Earlier trials, such as TIMI IIIB and the Veterans Affairs non-Q wave infarction strategies in hospital (VANQWISH), did not show a beneficial role of early invasive strategy. In contrast, trials such as FRISC II, TACTICS-TIMI 18, and RITA-3 showed a reduction in nonfatal adverse events in USA/NSTEMI patients receiving early invasive treatment. Another recent trial (ICTUS) did not demonstrate superiority of early invasive strategy in reducing mortality compared with early conservative (selective invasive) strategy in high-risk USA/NSTEMI patients. Differences in patient characteristics, study designs, surgical mortality rates, and background antiischemic medications used may account for these conflicting results and thus it is difficult to reach a consensus recommendation when treating patients with USA/NSTEMI. A recent meta-analysis containing seven contemporary randomized trials suggested that early invasive therapy performed within 24 hours does not confer similar mortality benefit to the strategy to perform procedures more than 24 hours after randomization. Data from the CRUSADE registry also suggested that a delay of invasive procedure of 46 hours does not increase adverse events compared to a delay of 23 hours. Nevertheless, analysis from FRISC II, TACTICS-TIMI 18, and OPUS-TIMI 16 trials showed patients with high-risk features (such as older age, long-duration of ischemia, angina at rest, ST segment changes on ECG, positive cardiac enzymes, and high TIMI risk scores) benefit more from early invasive strategy with revascularization. Intentionally delaying invasive therapy should be cautioned against and not encouraged.

2. Coronary artery bypass surgery—Randomized trials and observational series have shown that surgical myocardial revascularization in patients with unstable angina is relatively superior to medical therapy for controlling symptoms and improving effort tolerance and ventricular function.

At the present time, surgical revascularization can be considered an appropriate option for patients with unstable angina who do not stabilize with aggressive medical therapy or for whom angioplasty is unsuccessful or is followed by acute complications not amenable to additional catheter-based intervention. It is also applicable to patients who have severe multivessel or left mainstem coronary artery disease, particularly when left ventricular function is also impaired. Although multivessel angioplasty is performed in many centers, the bypass angioplasty revascularization investigation (BARI) trial showed coronary artery bypass grafting offered a lower repeat revascularization rate and a reduced instance of clinical angina compared with multivessel percutaneous transluminal coronary angioplasty. The BARI trial also revealed that coronary artery bypass grafting has a better long-term survival benefit compared with multivessel percutaneous transluminal coronary angioplasty, especially in diabetic patients.

3. Intra-aortic balloon counterpulsation—Intra-aortic balloon counterpulsation is a useful adjunct in managing selected cases of unstable angina. It helps maintain or improve coronary artery blood flow and myocardial perfusion by augmenting diastolic aortic pressure; at the same time, systolic unloading contributes to a reduction in ventricular wall tension and myocardial oxygen demand and an improvement in ventricular function. These beneficial effects on myocardial oxygen supply and demand help stabilize patients with recurrent myocardial ischemia and those with serious intermittent or persistent hemodynamic or electrical instability. Cardiac catheterization and revascularization can then be carried out with relative safety.

Intra-aortic balloon counterpulsation (and the percutaneous method of insertion) carries a significant risk of vascular complications involving the lower extremities, especially in women, in patients older than 70 years, and in the presence of diabetes or aortoiliac disease. It should be viewed as a temporary stabilizing measure, pending definitive revascularization.

Bavry AA et al. Benefit of early invasive therapy in acute coronary syndromes; a meta-analysis of contemporary randomized clinical trials. J Am Coll Cardiol. 2006 Oct 3;48(7):1319–25. [PMID: 17010789]

Boden WE et al. Outcomes in patients with acute non-Q-wave myocardial infarction randomly assigned to an invasive as compared with a conservative management strategy. Veterans Affairs Non-Q-Wave Infarction Strategies in Hospital (VANQWISH) Trial Investigators. N Engl J Med. 1998 Jun 18;338(25):1785–92. [PMID: 9632444]

Cantor WJ et al. Early cardiac catheterization is associated with lower mortality only among high-risk patients with ST- and non-ST-elevation acute coronary syndromes: observations from the OPUS-TIMI 16 trial. Am Heart J. 2005 Feb;149(2):275–83. [PMID: 15846265] de Winter RJ et al; Invasive versus Conservative Treatment in Unstable Coronary Syndromes (ICTUS) Investigators. Early invasive versus selectively invasive management for acute coronary syndromes. N Engl J Med. 2005 Sep 15;353(11):1095–104. [PMID: 16162880]

Fox KA et al; Randomized Intervention Trial of Unstable Angina Investigators. Interventional versus conservative treatment for patients with unstable angina or non-ST-elevation myocardial infarction: the British Heart Foundation RITA 3 randomised trial. Randomized Intervention Trial of unstable Angina. Lancet. 2002 Sep 7;360(9335):743–51. [PMID: 12241831]

Ryan JW et al; CRUSADE Investigators. Optimal timing of intervention in non-ST-segment elevation acute coronary syndromes: insights from the CRUSADE (Can Rapid risk stratification of Unstable angina patients Suppress ADverse outcomes with Early implementation of the ACC/AHA guidelines) Registry. Circulation. 2005 Nov 15;112(20):3049–57. [PMID: 16275863]

Santa-Cruz RA et al. Aortic counterpulsation: a review of the hemodynamic effects and indications for use. Catheter Cardiovasc Interv. 2006 Jan;67(1):68–77. [PMID: 16342217]

Seven-year outcome in the Bypass Angioplasty Revascularization Investigation (BARI) by treatment and diabetic status. J Am Coll Cardiol. 2000 Apr;35(5):1122–9. [PMID: 10758950]

Table 4–6. ABCDE Approach for Long-Term Risk Reduction in Patients with USA/NSTEMI.

A:	Antiplatelet therapy (aspirin, clopidogrel)
B:	β-Blockers Blood pressure control
C:	Cholesterol-modifying medications (statins, fibrates, niacin) Converting enzyme inhibitors Cessation of smoking
D:	Dietary management (Mediterranean style diet, Ornish style low-fat diet)
E:	Exercise and weight control

USA/NSTEMI, unstable angina/non-ST elevation myocardial infarction.

Prognosis

With the advancement of treatment strategies, clinical event rates for refractory angina, myocardial infarction, and death have been reduced substantially. For example, in patients who were not treated with aspirin and heparin, the rate of refractory angina, myocardial infarction, and death was 23%, 12%, and 1.7%, respectively, within the first week of treatment and the rates became 10.7%, 1.6%, and 0%, respectively, if the patients were treated with aspirin and heparin. With the addition of a GP IIb/IIIa receptor inhibitor, the rate for refractory angina, myocardial infarction, or death was 10.6%, 8.3%, and 6.9%, respectively, at 6 months in the PRISM-PLUS trial. With the combination of early invasive strategy, GP IIb/IIIa inhibitor, heparin, and aspirin, the 6-month mortality rate decreased further to 3.3% in the TACTICS-TIMI 18 trial. Even with such decreases in the event rates, a substantial number of patients still continue to suffer from USA/NSTEMI and its complications due to the high prevalence of atherosclerosis. All patients should become acquainted with risk factor modification strategies, which include lipid lowering, smoking cessation, an exercise program, diabetes control, blood pressure control, dietary counseling, and weight control. Recently, the use of angiotensin-converting enzyme inhibitors has also been shown to reduce atherothrombotic events in patients with coronary artery disease especially in the presence of diabetes. With the advancement of therapies and risk factor modification, patients' short- and long-term outcomes can be further improved. A simple mnemonic—ABCDE (Table 4–6) summarizes the long-term risk-reducing approach for patients with unstable coronary artery disease.

Effects of ramipril on cardiovascular and microvascular outcomes in people with diabetes mellitus: results of the HOPE study and MICRO-HOPE substudy. Heart Outcomes Prevention Evaluation Study Investigators. Lancet. 2000 Jan 22;355(9200):253–9. [PMID: 10675071]

Acute Myocardial Infarction

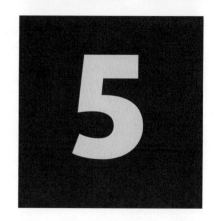

Andrew J. Boyle, MBBS, PhD & Allan S. Jaffe, MD

ESSENTIALS OF DIAGNOSIS

- ▶ Chest discomfort, usually described as "pressure," "dull," "squeezing," or "aching."
- ▶ Characteristic electrocardiographic changes.
- ▶ Elevated biomarkers, such as troponin.
- ▶ Imaging may show new regional wall motion abnormality with preserved wall thickness.
- ▶ The elderly, women, and diabetics may have atypical presentation.

▶ General Considerations

Acute myocardial infarction (MI) is a clinical syndrome that results from occlusion of a coronary artery, with resultant death of cardiac myocytes in the region supplied by that artery. Depending on the distribution of the affected coronary artery, acute MI can produce a wide range of clinical sequelae, varying from a small, clinically silent region of necrosis to a large overwhelming area of infarcted tissue resulting in cardiogenic shock and death. About 1.2 million people experience MI in the United States each year; every minute, one American will die of coronary artery disease.

The risk of having an acute MI increases with age, male gender, smoking, dyslipidemia, diabetes, hypertension, abdominal obesity, a lack of physical activity, low daily fruit and vegetable consumption, alcohol overconsumption, and psychosocial index. As much as 90% of the risk of acute MI has been attributed to the modifiable risk factors. The diagnostic criteria for acute MI are listed in Table 5–1.

▶ Pathophysiology & Etiology

A prolonged imbalance between myocardial oxygen supply and demand leads to the death of myocardial tissue. Coronary atherosclerosis is an essential part of the process in most patients. Ischemic heart disease seems to progress through stages of fatty-streak deposition in coronary arteries to development of fibro-fatty plaque, which then increases in size until it causes luminal obstruction, leading to exertional angina (see Chapter 3). However, at any stage in this process, the atherosclerotic lesion may erode, ulcerate, fissure, or rupture, thereby exposing subendothelial vessel wall substances to the circulating blood. Procoagulant factors (such as tissue factor) reside within the plaque itself and, in the absence of counterbalancing antithrombotic factors (eg, heparin, tissue-factor-inhibitor) and fibrinolytic activities (tissue plasminogen activator [t-PA] and single-chain urokinase-type plasminogen activator) within the endothelial cells of the coronary artery, can cause thrombosis. This potent procoagulant stimulus results in thrombus development in this region. In general, acute MI occurs when this thrombosis propagates and occludes flow within the artery, resulting in ischemia of cardiomyocytes distal to the obstruction. Recent work suggests that inflammation may play a pivotal role in the genesis of plaque rupture. Total thrombotic occlusion occurs most commonly in proximal coronary arteries; its presence has been documented during the first 4 hours after infarction in more than 85% of patients with ST-segment elevation (Figure 5–1).

A similar type of myocardial insult occurs occasionally despite angiographically normal coronary arteries and may be caused by emboli (eg, in patients with prosthetic valves or those with endocarditis), dissection of the coronary artery (most commonly in pregnant women), or coronary vasospasm (on rare occasions). It can also be caused by thrombosis in situ, the probable mechanism by which patients who have variant angina or who abuse cocaine can suffer acute infarction. In these cases, vasoconstriction secondary to endothelial dysfunction and a propensity to thrombosis is of sufficient magnitude and duration to cause thrombus formation. Oxygen consumption and possibly direct myocyte toxicity also increase with cocaine use. In addition, thrombosis in situ can apparently cause infarction among women who take estrogens

Table 5-1. ESC/ACC Definition of Myocardial Infarction.

Criteria for acute MI

1. Typical rise and gradual fall (troponin) or more rapid rise and fall (CK-MB) of biochemical markers of myocardial necrosis with at least one of the following:
   a. Ischemic symptoms
   b. Development of pathologic Q waves on the ECG
   c. ECG changes indicative of ischemia (ST segment elevation or depression)
   d. Coronary artery intervention (eg, coronary angioplasty)
2. Pathologic findings of an AMI

Criteria for established MI

Any one of the following criteria satisfies the diagnosis for established MI:

1. Development of new pathologic Q waves on serial ECGs. The patient may or may not remember previous symptoms. Biochemical markers of myocardial necrosis may have normalized, depending on the length of time that has passed since the infarct developed.
2. Pathologic findings of a healed or healing MI

MI, myocardial infarction; CK-MB, myocardial muscle kinase isoenzyme; ECG, electrocardiogram.
Adapted, with permission, from Beller GA et al. J Am Coll Cardiol. 2000;36:957.

(especially if they smoke). An increasingly recognized differential diagnosis of acute MI is stress cardiomyopathy (also known as apical ballooning syndrome or tako-tsubo cardiomyopathy). This entity can present with a variety of symptoms and electrocardiographic (ECG) changes, including ST elevation, and there is akinesis of the anterior and inferior walls and apex of the left ventricle in the absence of coronary artery disease. It is often accompanied by severe emotional stress. The diagnosis is one of exclusion, after angiography demonstrates patent coronary arteries. The prognosis is good, and recovery of ventricular function is the norm.

In addition to blockage of coronary arteries (reduced "supply"), acute MI may be seen when myocardial oxygen requirements are elevated (increased "demand"). This often occurs when other medical illnesses coexist with ischemic heart disease. Pulmonary embolism, pneumonia, arrhythmia, septic shock, severe anemia, or great emotional distress can increase myocardial oxygen demand, reduce coronary perfusion pressure, or evoke paradoxical coronary artery responses and lead to MI. However, these tend to be smaller infarctions with no ECG ST elevation that are diagnosed by elevated biomarkers.

Libby P et al. Inflammation and atherosclerosis. Circulation. 2002 Mar 5;105(9):1135–43. [PMID: 11877368]

Rosamond W et al; American Heart Association Statistics Committee and Stroke Statistics Subcommittee. Heart disease and stroke statistics—2007 update: a report from the American Heart Association Statistics Committee and Stroke Statistics Subcommittee. Circulation. 2007 Feb 6;115(5):e69–171. [PMID: 17194875]

Wittstein IS et al. Neurohumoral features of myocardial stunning due to sudden emotional stress. N Engl J Med. 2005 Feb 10;352(6):539–48. [PMID: 15703419]

▶ **Clinical Findings**

A. Symptoms and Signs

Chest discomfort is the most common symptom; it is usually described as "pressure," "dull," "squeezing," or "aching," although it may be described differently because of individual variability, differences in articulation or verbal abilities, or concomitant disease processes. The discomfort is usually in the center of the chest and commonly radiates to the left arm or the neck. However, it may also radiate to the right arm, epigastrium, jaw, teeth, or the back. The nature of the pain may lead patients to place a hand or fist over the sternum (Levine sign). These clinical signs and symptoms were originally defined in groups of males. It is now clear that women often have more atypical symptoms.

Associated symptoms may include dyspnea, nausea (particularly in inferior infarction), palpitations, and a sense of impending doom.

Patients, especially those with diabetes or hypertension, may have atypical presentations; for example, a diabetic person may have abdominal pain that mimics the discomfort commonly associated with gallstones. In elderly patients, heart failure is often the presenting symptom. By age 85, only 40% of patients will complain of chest discomfort as the initial symptom. The diagnosis of MI should be considered in patients in whom symptoms are atypical yet compatible with ischemia (paroxysms of dyspnea, for example) or in those with atypical chest discomfort. Patients can also have discomfort that is sharper or that radiates to the back. These patients can have pericarditis alone, pericarditis induced by infarction, or a dissecting aortic aneurysm—with or without concomitant infarction.

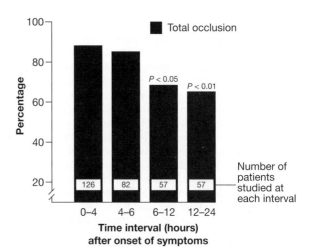

▲ **Figure 5–1.** Incidence of total occlusion in patients with acute myocardial infarction. (Reproduced, with permission, from DeWood MA et al. N Engl J Med. 1980;303:897.)

B. Physical Examination

The physical examination is a critical and underappreciated part of the initial assessment of patients with suspected acute MI. Findings may vary tremendously, from markedly abnormal, with signs of severe congestive heart failure (CHF), to totally normal.

On general inspection, most patients with a large MI appear pale or sweaty and may be agitated or restless. Heart rate should be measured for arrhythmia, heart block, or sinus tachycardia. This is crucial before administration of β-blockers. Assessment of blood pressure is important because severe hypertension (which may be due to the pain) is a contraindication to fibrinolytic treatment and must be treated emergently. Conversely, hypotension in the setting of acute MI may be due to cardiogenic shock, which alters treatment strategy. Fibrinolytic treatments are not effective in cardiogenic shock, and the patient should be considered for an urgent intra-aortic balloon pump (IABP) and primary percutaneous coronary intervention (PCI).

The jugular venous pulse should be carefully examined. Its elevation in the setting of inferior MI without left heart failure suggests right ventricular MI. Detection of right ventricular MI is vital because it portends a much worse prognosis than isolated inferior MI, and the management strategy is different than isolated inferior MI. Whereas elevated jugular venous pulse in left ventricular MI with left ventricular failure may respond to diuresis, right ventricular MI may require intravenous fluid therapy to maintain left ventricular filling.

Cardiac auscultation should be specifically targeted to complications of MI (see later in this chapter) and detection of important comorbidities. Acute MI may result in ischemic mitral regurgitation with a soft S_1 and a pansystolic murmur. Acquired ventricular septal defect (VSD) may also result in a pansystolic murmur, but it is usually loud and high-pitched and has a normal S_1 and usually occurs later (see Complications of Myocardial Infarction section below). Both ischemic mitral regurgitation and acquired VSD may result in heart failure. The presence of a pericardial friction rub may indicate established infarction which has happened days earlier. Heart failure due to large infarctions may result in a third heart sound. Signs of left heart failure, such as rales and pulmonary hypertension, should also be sought. Important comorbidities, such as concomitant severe aortic stenosis, should also be documented because they may change the initial reperfusion strategy from fibrinolysis or PCI to cardiac surgery with coronary artery bypass graft (CABG) and aortic valve replacement simultaneously.

Alternative diagnoses may also be suggested by clinical examination. The presence of atrial fibrillation or prosthetic valve may suggest that thromboembolism to the coronary artery is the cause of the coronary occlusion. Furthermore, a brief assessment of pulse equality and blood pressure in both arms should be performed. Inequalities in perfusion between arms may indicate aortic dissection, causing compromised blood flow in the branch vessels of the aortic arch. Aortic dissection may also be responsible for occlusion of the ostium of the coronary artery causing the acute MI. This is a surgical emergency and should not be treated with anticoagulation or fibrinolysis. Therefore, a focused clinical examination is an essential part of the initial patient assessment and can be invaluable in guiding therapy.

C. Diagnostic Studies

1. Electrocardiography—The most rapid and helpful test in assessing patients with suspected acute MI is the 12-lead ECG. It should be performed as soon as possible, preferably within 10 minutes, after the patient's arrival in the emergency department or clinician's office, since the presence or absence of ST elevation determines the preferred management strategy. For a diagnosis of ST elevation MI (STEMI), ST elevation must be present in at least two contiguous leads. For anterior MI, the precordial (V) leads demonstrate ST elevation (Figure 5–2), and if there is lateral wall involvement, I and aVL may also show ST elevation. In inferior MI, leads II, III, and aVF are affected.

In addition to standard ECG leads, right ventricular leads should be recorded in all patients with inferior MI. Inferior MI is usually caused by occlusion of the right coronary artery, which may also cause right ventricular infarction. Differentiating right ventricular infarction from left ventricular infarction is imperative because the management is different.

In posterior MI, usually due to circumflex artery occlusion, the only changes seen on a standard ECG may be reciprocal ST depression and R waves (reciprocal of Q waves) in the anterior leads. This ECG pattern should prompt the use of posterior ECG leads V7–9, which may show ST elevation. Even in the absence of ST elevation in posterior leads, true posterior infarction pattern on ECG in the presence of symptoms suggestive of MI should be treated like STEMI.

Non-ST elevation MI (NSTEMI) has a variable presentation on ECG. There may be no ECG changes, or patients may have ST depression, T wave flattening, or T wave inversion. Preexisting abnormalities like T wave inversion may also "pseudo-normalize" in NSTEMI, making it even more difficult to diagnose on ECG. Because determining whether ECG changes are new or old may be difficult, serial ECGs are necessary to diagnose dynamic changes. In patients with symptoms suggestive of MI and no evidence of ST elevation on ECG, the diagnosis of acute coronary syndrome is made. This encompasses unstable angina pectoris and NSTEMI. The distinction between these two entities is made on the presence or absence of elevated biomarkers of MI.

2. Cardiac biomarkers—The diagnosis of infarction requires increases in molecular markers of myocardial injury (Figure 5–3). Myoglobin release from injured myocardium occurs quite early and is very sensitive for detecting infarction. Unfortunately, it is not very specific because minor skeletal muscle trauma also releases myoglobin. Myoglobin is cleared

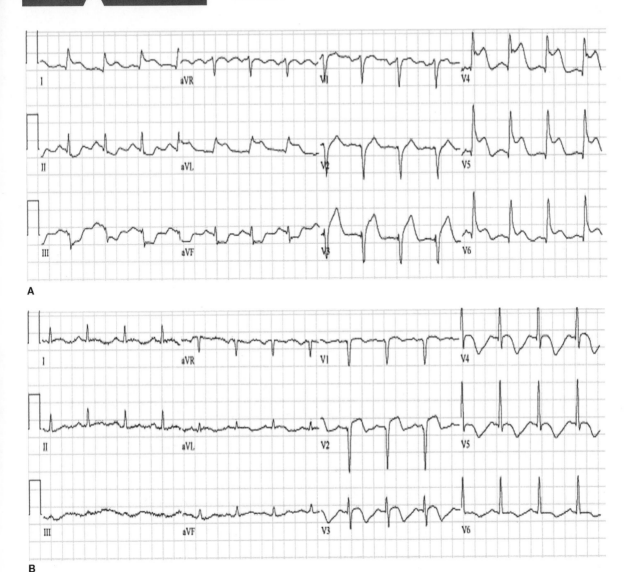

▲ **Figure 5-2.** ECG changes in anterolateral STEMI. **A:** Initial ECG on presentation shows ST segment elevation in the precordial leads, as well as I and aVL, indicative of acute anterolateral STEMI due to proximal left anterior descending (LAD) coronary artery occlusion. Note the reciprocal ST depression in the inferior leads. **B:** Following reperfusion, subsequent ECG 48 hours later demonstrates resolution of both the anterolateral ST elevation and the reciprocal changes. Note the Q wave in V2 and the development of T wave inversion.

renally, so even minor decreases in glomerular filtration rate lead to elevation. The other early marker advocated by some are isoforms of creatine kinase (CK). This marker has comparable early sensitivity and specificity to myoglobin. The marker of choice in past years was the MB isoenzyme of creatine kinase (CK-MB). A typical rising-and-falling pattern of CK and CK-MB (in the proper clinical setting) was sufficient for the diagnosis of acute infarction. In the typical

pattern of CK release after infarction, the enzyme marker level exceeds the upper bound of the reference range within 6–12 hours after the onset of infarction. Peak levels occur by 18–24 hours and generally return to baseline within no more than 48 hours. However, elevations can occur due to release of the enzyme from skeletal muscle. The lack of a rising-and-falling pattern should raise the suspicion that the release is from skeletal muscle, which is usually due to a chronic skeletal

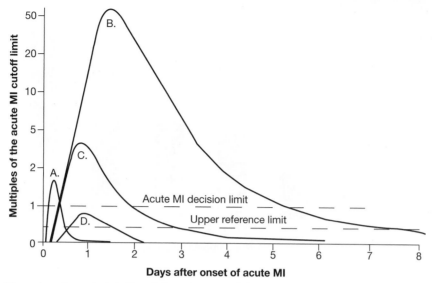

▲ **Figure 5–3.** Biomarkers in acute MI. Plot of the appearance of cardiac markers in blood versus time after onset of symptoms. Peak A, early release of myoglobin or CK-MB isoforms after acute MI. Peak B, cardiac troponin after acute MI. Peak C, CK-MB after acute MI. Peak D, cardiac troponin after unstable angina. Data are plotted on a relative scale, where 1.0 is set at the acute MI cutoff concentration. (Reprinted, with permission, from Wu AH et al. Clin Chem. 1999;45:1104.)

muscle myopathy. Elevations of CK in patients with hypothyroidism (where clearance of CK is slowed) and those with renal failure (where clearance is normal because CK is not cleared renally) are caused, in part, by myopathy.

Cardiac troponins I and T are proteins found in cardiac muscle cells and released into the circulation from damaged cardiac myocytes during acute MI. Troponin levels (either I or T) are significantly more sensitive and specific for myocardial damage than CK. Troponin becomes detectable in serum between 4 hours and 6 hours after onset of an acute MI, peaks and then falls to lower levels, and remains elevated at these low levels for 5–7 days (Figure 5–3). Thus, the late or retrospective diagnosis of acute MI can be made with this marker, making the use of lactate dehydrogenase isoenzymes superfluous. Therefore, because of its sensitivity and specificity for cardiac muscle damage as well as its early rise and continued low level detectability, troponin is the preferred biomarker for diagnosis of acute MI. Furthermore, it has been shown to correlate with prognosis even in the absence of CK or CK-MB elevation (Figure 5–4).

Coronary recanalization, whether spontaneous or induced pharmacologically or mechanically, alters the timing of all markers' appearance in the circulation. Because it increases the rapidity with which the marker is washed out from the heart, leading to rapid increases in plasma, the diagnosis of infarction can be made much earlier—generally within 2 hours of coronary recanalization. Although patency can be approximated from the marker rise, distinguishing between thrombolysis in myocardial infarction (TIMI) II and TIMI III flow is not highly accurate. It should also be

understood that peak elevations are accentuated, which must be taken into account if the clinician wants to use peak values as a surrogate for infarct size.

3. Imaging—In the emergency setting, most diagnoses of acute MI are made on history, physical examination, and ECG. However, when the history is atypical and the ECG is equivocal or uninterpretable, performance of a rapid bedside echocardiogram may demonstrate a new regional wall motion abnormality with preserved wall thickness, suggestive of acute MI. In most cases of STEMI, however, echocardiography is not warranted because it delays reperfusion therapy. Echocardiography is also helpful in diagnosing complications of MI, such as VSD, papillary muscle rupture or free wall rupture, and tamponade.

In NSTEMI that is diagnosed on elevated plasma levels of cardiac biomarkers, nuclear scintigraphy or echocardiography may help determine the region of the heart affected by the MI, but these are not standard diagnostic tools.

Alpert JS et al. Myocardial infarction redefined—a consensus document of the Joint European Society of Cardiology/American College of Cardiology Committee for the redefinition of myocardial infarction. J Am Coll Cardiol. 2000 Sep;36(3):959–69. [PMID: 10987628]

Menown IB et al. Early diagnosis of right ventricular or posterior infarction associated with inferior wall left ventricular acute myocardial infarction. Am J Cardiol. 2000 Apr 15;85(8):934–8. [PMID: 10760329]

Ottani F et al. Elevated cardiac troponin levels predict the risk of adverse outcome in patients with acute coronary syndromes. Am Heart J. 2000 Dec;140(6):917–27. [PMID: 11099996]

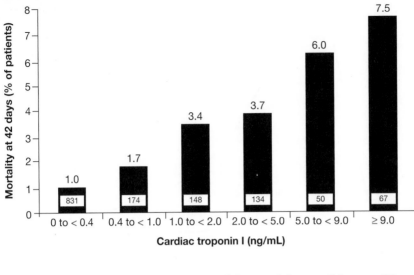

▲ **Figure 5-4.** Troponin I and mortality. Relationship between cardiac troponin levels and risk of mortality in patients with acute coronary syndromes. (Used with permission from Antman EM et al. N Engl J Med. 1996;335:1342.)

▶ Treatment

The goals of treatment in acute MI are stabilization of the patient and salvage of as much myocardium as possible. A number of general measures should be performed in all patients. In patients with ST elevation—who are at highest risk for complications and have ongoing cardiomyocyte necrosis—immediate reperfusion of the infarct artery should be attempted. The management of acute MI is summarized in Table 5–2.

Early recognition of symptoms of myocardial ischemia may lead to faster treatment and salvage of myocardium. Therefore, it is recommended that patients at risk for MI be educated about the symptoms suggestive of acute MI and call for emergency help immediately if they have these symptoms.

A. Pre-hospital Management

Aspirin, 162–325 mg, should be given immediately. Continuous cardiac monitoring, oxygen, and sublingual nitroglycerin should be administered to all patients with suspected acute MI. Communities usually have organized protocols for ambulance personnel regarding (1) whether or not they should obtain a 12-lead ECG, (2) whether there are designated hospitals that receive patients in whom an acute MI is suspected, or (3) whether the patient should be taken to the nearest emergency department. In some regions of the world, fibrinolytic treatment is initiated in the ambulance, based on a 12-lead ECG.

B. Emergency Department Therapy

On arrival, all patients with suspected acute MI should have a 12-lead ECG performed immediately. If aspirin has not been given, then 162–325 mg of aspirin should be administered immediately. All patients with suspected MI should have continuous cardiac ECG monitoring, and intravenous access (two separate intravenous lines) should be gained in all patients. Sublingual nitroglycerin and intravenous morphine should be administered if patients have active chest pain. Oxygen saturations should be monitored noninvasively, rather than by arterial blood gas measurement. Supplemental oxygen, 2–4 L/min, should be given to all patients, particularly if they are hypoxemic. A portable chest radiograph should be ordered but should not delay reperfusion, unless a diagnosis of aortic dissection is strongly considered. Echocardiography may be considered if the diagnosis of MI remains in doubt (eg, equivocal history, uninterpretable ECG). Oral β-blockers should be administered to all patients with acute MI, unless there is a contraindication, such as hypotension, bradycardia, or asthma. This has been shown to improve outcomes and limit the size of infarction. Intravenous β-blockers could be considered when there is hypertension or tachyarrhythmia, for example (Table 5–3). However, they should be avoided in patients with signs of heart failure, in those with contraindications to β-blockers, and in those at high risk for cardiogenic shock (age > 70 years, heart rate > 110/min or < 60/min, systolic blood pressure < 120 mm Hg, or prolonged time since the onset of symptoms).

Table 5–2. Overview of Management of Acute MI.

Pre-hospital management
    Aspirin
    Call 911
    Continuous cardiac monitoring
    Consider pre-hospital 12-lead ECG
Emergency department treatment
    Intravenous access
    Continuous cardiac monitoring
    12-lead ECG
    Aspirin
    Oxygen
    Nitroglycerin
    Morphine
    Heparin
    β-Blocker
Reperfusion strategies
    Primary PCI vs fibrinolysis for STEMI
    Glycoprotein IIb/IIIa for NSTEMI, followed by elective PCI
In-hospital management
    Initial bedrest
    Continuous cardiac monitoring
    Oxygen for hypoxemia
    Nitroglycerin for ongoing pain
    ACE inhibitor, β-blocker, aspirin, clopidogrel, statin
Post-discharge
    Prognostic indicators
    Cardiac rehabilitation
    Aggressive secondary prevention with smoking cessation, thera-
      peutic lifestyle changes, and medications

ACE, angiotensin-converting enzyme; ECG, electrocardiogram; NSTEMI, non-ST elevation myocardial infarction; PCI, percutaneous coronary intervention; STEMI, ST elevation myocardial infarction.

Heparin should be administered to all patients with acute MI, unless a contraindication exists. The choice between unfractionated heparin (UFH) infusion and low-molecular-weight heparin (LMWH) should be based on the likelihood of invasive therapy. Unfractionated heparin is preferred in most institutions for invasive therapy (primary PCI) because it has a short half-life, it can be turned off rapidly if there is a complication during invasive therapy, and because it can be monitored during procedures with a bedside activated clotting time test. In contrast, LMWHs have a long half-life, and there is no bedside test of their anticoagulant efficiency. In STEMI, patients undergoing fibrinolysis can have adjunctive UFH or LMWH, with both having evidence of benefit as adjunctive therapy.

C. Reperfusion Therapy

1. Patients with STEMI—All patients with STEMI who seek medical care within the first 12 hours after symptom onset should be considered for urgent reperfusion of the infarct-related artery, but the earlier therapy is begun, the greater the benefit. In addition, those patients who seek medical care within 12–24 hours of symptom onset may be considered for reperfusion, particularly if chest pain is ongoing or heart failure or shock has developed, but the benefit of reperfusion therapies after more than 12 hours is less well established. The definitive therapies for reperfusion in STEMI are fibrinolysis or PCI. Both these strategies improve patency of the infarct-related artery, reduce infarct size, and lower mortality rates. Therefore, one or the other method should be performed as quickly as possible. The goal of reperfusion therapies in the United States is a door-to-needle time of 30 minutes (for fibrinolysis) and a door-to-balloon inflation time of less than 90 minutes (for PCI). Percutaneous coronary intervention has been shown to be superior to fibrinolysis when it is performed without significant delay by experienced clinicians in experienced centers (Figure 5–5). However, significant delays in performing PCI reduce its benefit over fibrinolytic therapy. There are special cases where primary PCI is always preferred over fibrinolysis: cardiogenic shock, severe CHF or pulmonary edema (Killip class III), or if there are contraindications to fibrinolysis (Table 5–4). These patients may require insertion of an IABP and may benefit from mechanical reperfusion with primary PCI. The different management of patients with these high-risk clinical features underscores the need for careful clinical examination of all patients with chest pain.

Recent data suggest that all patients with STEMI, whether they undergo primary PCI or fibrinolytic therapy, benefit from early administration of clopidogrel. However, this may cause an increase in bleeding complications if the patient undergoes CABG surgery. Therefore, administration of a clopidogrel 300 mg loading dose followed by 75 mg daily should be considered in all STEMI patients, whether they receive fibrinolysis or primary PCI.

2. Patients with NSTEMI—These patients should not be treated with fibrinolytics. The definitive management of NSTEMI involves anticoagulation, platelet inhibition, and an early invasive strategy (ie, routine coronary angiography with or without PCI during the index hospitalization).

All patients should receive aspirin and general acute MI treatment as discussed above. Anticoagulation with heparin, either UFH or LMWH, should be given to all patients. Unless CABG surgery is anticipated, all patients should receive clopidogrel, since it reduces recurrent ischemia in NSTEMI. Clopidogrel should be continued for 9–12 months. In addition to aspirin, heparin, and clopidogrel, all NSTEMI patients should be treated with a glycoprotein IIb/IIIa inhibitor (eptifibatide, abciximab, or tirofiban) immediately after the diagnosis is made and continued until after coronary angiography with or without PCI. Most NSTEMI patients treated with all the above will experience recovery from their ischemic symptoms and therefore do not need to be taken to the cardiac catheterization laboratory emergently. However, if there is ongoing ischemia that cannot be controlled by the above measures, or if there is cardiogenic shock or pulmonary edema, the patient should be taken emergently to the cardiac catheterization laboratory for insertion of IABP and coronary angiography with or without PCI.

Table 5–3. Standard Intravenous Doses of Commonly Used Agents in Patients with Acute Myocardial Infarction.

Agents	Dosage	Comments
Antiarrhythmics		
Lidocaine	Initial bolus of 1 mg/kg and 2 mg/min infusion; additional bolus doses to 3 mg/kg may be necessary.	For symptomatic arrhythmias and sustained ventricular tachycardia and ventricular fibrillation, not arrest
Procainamide	20 mg/min–1 g, then 2–4 mg/min drip	May cause hypotension, QRS or QT lengthening, or toxicity
Magnesium	1–2 g over 1–2 min or infusion of 8 g over 24 h	Observe for changes in heart rate, blood pressure
Amiodarone	15 mg/min × 10 min, then 1 mg/min × 6 h and 0.5 mg/min × 24 h	For refractory ventricular tachycardia, ventricular fibrillation and arres
β-Blockers		
Esmolol	250 mcg/kg IV loading dose, then 25–50 mcg/kg/min to maximum dose of 300 mcg/kg/min	Very short half-life
Metoprolol	5 mg q 5 min IV × 3 then 25–50 mg q12h orally	Long duration of action; may exacerbate heart failure
Propranolol	0.1 mg/kg over 5 mm IV, followed by 20–40 mg q6h orally	Long duration of action; may exacerbate heart failure
Calcium channel blockers		
Diltiazem	20–25 mg IV test dose, then 10–15 mg/h as needed; 90–120 mg three times daily orally	May exacerbate heart failure
Inotropes and Pressors		
Amrinone	Initial bolus of 0.75 mg/kg, then 5–10 mg/kg/min	May exacerbate ischemia
Dobutamine	Begin at 2.5 mcg/kg/min and titrate to effect	Increases in heart rate > 10% may exacerbate ischemia
Dopamine	Start at 2 mcg/kg/min, titrate to effect	May exacerbate pulmonary congestion and ischemia
Norepinephrine	Start at 2 mcg/min, titrate to effect	Temporizing treatment only
Vasodilators		
Nitroglycerin	Begin at 10 mcg/min IV, titrate to effect	Avoid reducing blood pressure by > 10% if normotensive, > 30% if hypertensive
Nitroprusside	Begin at 0.1 mcg/kg/min, titrate to effect	Mean dose 50–80 mcg/kg/min
Nesiritide	2 mcg/kg bolus followed by 0.01 mcg/kg/min infusion, can increase by 0.005 to maximum infusion 0.03 mcg/kg/min	Hold diuretics and other vasodilators. Keep systolic blood pressure > 100 mm Hg
Anticoagulants		
Unfractionated heparin	5000 unit bolus followed by 1000 units/h adjusted by a PTT	Less efficacious than LMWH
Enoxaparin	1 mg/kg SQ q12h, can give immediate 30 mg bolus intravenously if necessary	Hard to reverse effects; avoid in patients with renal failure
Dalteparin	120 international units/kg q12h	Avoid in patients with renal failure
Abciximab	0.25 mg/kg followed by 0.125 mcg/kg/min × 12 h, maximum time-24 h	Care necessary if renal failure; thrombocytopenia greater with repeated use
Eptifibatide	180 mcg/kg bolus × 2 (30 min later) followed by 2 mcg/kg/min for as long as 96 h for ACS, 24 h post PCI	Care necessary if renal failure
Tirofiban	0.4 mcg/kg/min × 30 min followed by 0.1 mcg/kg/min for up to 108 h for ACS, 12–19 h for PCI	Care necessary if renal failure
Clopidogrel	300 mg loading dose, then 75 mg/day × at least 1 month	TTP possible

ACS, acute coronary syndromes; LMWH, low-molecular-weight heparin; PCI, percutaneous coronary intervention; PTT, partial thromboplastin time.

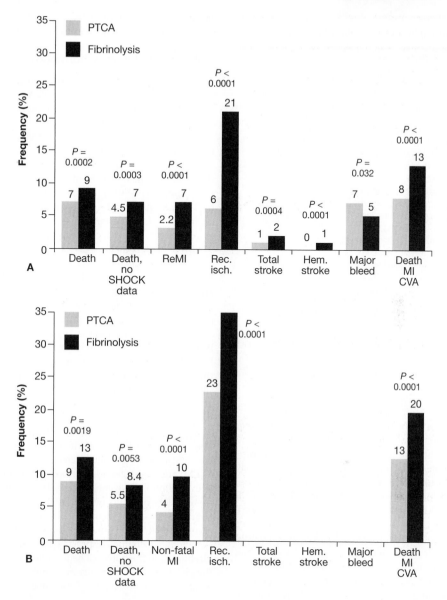

▲ **Figure 5–5.** PCI vs fibrinolysis for STEMI. Short-term (4 to 6 weeks; **A**) and long-term (**B**) outcomes for various end points shown are plotted for STEMI patients randomized to PCI or fibrinolysis for reperfusion in 23 trials (n = 7739). Primary angioplasty for acute STEMI improves both short- and long-term outcomes. (CVA, cerebrovascular accident; Hem. Stroke, hemorrhagic stroke; Rec. Isch, recurrent ischemia; ReMI, recurrent myocardial infarction; STEMI, ST elevation myocardial infarction.) (Modified, with permission, from Keeley et al. The Lancet. 2003;361:13 and Antman et al. J Am Coll Cardiol. 2004;44:671.)

D. In-hospital Management

All patients with acute MI should be admitted for continuous cardiac monitoring. Patients should have bed rest for the first 12–24 hours following MI and reperfusion, but in the absence of ongoing ischemia, should be mobilized after this time. All patients should receive the appropriate cardiac diet, adhering to the National Cholesterol Education Program (NCEP) Adult Treatment Panel III (ATP III) dietary guidelines, as well as education regarding the necessary dietary changes they should make after discharge.

Table 5–4. Contraindications for Fibrinolysis Use in STEMI.

Absolute contraindications
Any prior ICH
Known structural cerebral vascular lesion (eg, AVM)
Known malignant intracranial neoplasm (primary or metastatic)
Ischemic stroke within previous 3 months
Suspected aortic dissection
Active bleeding or bleeding diathesis (excluding menses)
Significant closed head or facial trauma within 3 months
Severe uncontrolled hypertension (SBP > 180 mm Hg and/or DBP > 110 mm Hg)

Relative contraindications
History of prior ischemic stroke greater than 3 months, dementia, or known intracranial pathology not covered in contraindications
Traumatic or prolonged (greater than 10 minutes) CPR or major surgery in previous 3 weeks
Recent internal bleeding (within 4 weeks)
Noncompressible vascular punctures
For streptokinase/anistreplase: prior exposure (more than 5 days ago) or prior allergic reaction to these agents
Pregnancy
Active peptic ulcer
Current use of anticoagulants: the higher the INR, the higher the risk of bleeding

AVM, arteriovenous malformation; CPR, cardiopulmonary resuscitation; DBP, diastolic blood pressure; ICH, intracranial hemorrhage; INR, international normalized ratio; SBP, systolic blood pressure; STEMI, ST elevation myocardial infarction.

Within the first 24 hours of presentation, the long-term medical management of patients with both STEMI and NSTEMI should be commenced (Table 5–5). Angiotensin-converting enzyme (ACE) inhibitors should be given on day 1, if the patient's blood pressure allows, particularly in those with anterior MI or impaired left ventricular function. ACE inhibitors reduce left ventricular remodeling and heart failure and should be continued long-term. β-Blockade should have already been started in the emergency department and should be continued orally in all patients, unless there are absolute contraindications, and should also be continued long-term. Aspirin, 162–325 mg daily, should be administered initially, then 81 mg daily for life. Clopidogrel, 75 mg daily, should be administered for at least 1 month in all patients, and longer-term therapy should be considered. Patients who receive bare metal stents should receive at least 1 month of aspirin 325 mg daily, and clopidogrel 75 mg daily, then aspirin 81 mg daily for life. Patients receiving drug-eluting stents should receive clopidogrel 75 mg daily for at least 1 year, and aspirin for life. Hydroxymethylglutaryl coenzyme A (HMG-CoA) reductase inhibitors (statin therapy) should be given soon after MI and should be continued at high dose long-term.

During hospitalization, all patients should be educated about adhering to therapeutic lifestyle changes, including dietary and lifestyle measures, smoking cessation, and medication compliance. Selected patients should be referred to a cardiac rehabilitation program to consolidate these messages and develop an appropriate exercise regimen.

E. Primary PCI versus Fibrinolysis

The goal of reperfusion is to rapidly restore blood flow to the myocardium to prevent ongoing ischemic cell death. Therefore, whichever means can achieve reperfusion most quickly should be used. Primary PCI results in improved patency rates of the infarct-related artery, as well as improved TIMI flow grade, compared with fibrinolysis. In general, the patency rate with primary PCI is 90% or higher, whereas with thrombolysis, the rate is about 65% and recurrent events are more common. With modern advances, coronary stenting has further improved long-term outcomes over balloon angioplasty alone. Percutaneous coronary intervention has therefore been widely accepted as the treatment of choice for STEMI in centers that can perform primary PCI rapidly and effectively (Figure 5–6). However, very early after the onset of symptoms, when the thrombus in the infarct-related artery is still soft, fibrinolysis may recanalize the artery as quickly as, if not more so than, primary PCI. This is true in the first hour and possibly the first 3 hours after symptom onset. Therefore, fibrinolysis is an acceptable treatment in these early time-points. However, after 3 hours, primary PCI has a clear benefit over fibrinolysis and should be considered the preferred therapy. It bears re-stating that primary PCI should only be performed in centers skilled in the treatment of STEMI that can achieve rapid reperfusion, with a goal door-to-balloon inflation time of 90 minutes.

In deciding whether elderly patients with acute STEMI should undergo PCI or fibrinolytic therapy, the risks and benefits must be weighed carefully. Elderly patients with STEMI are at high risk for increased morbidity and mortality with thrombolytic agents. Indeed, some studies suggest that these agents have no benefit in this group. On the other hand, PCI is clearly beneficial. However, if PCI cannot be accomplished, individual decisions concerning the risk (which is substantial, especially in regard to intracranial bleeding) and the potential benefits must be balanced. Given the high (20–30%) mortality rate from STEMI in the elderly, some increased risk may be reasonable.

F. Fibrinolytic Agents

There are a number of fibrinolytic agents that have been successfully used in acute MI. Table 5–6 shows the currently approved agents for use in the United States. A brief discussion of each is warranted before deciding on the most appropriate agent. Plasmin, the key ingredient in the fibrinolytic system, degrades fibrin, fibrinogen, prothrombin, and a variety of other factors in the clotting and complement systems. This effect inhibits clot formation and can lead to bleeding. Patients with acute MI and ST-segment elevation have little evidence of spontaneous or intrinsic fibrinolysis, despite the intense thrombotic stimulus present. This may be due in part

Table 5–5. Meta–Analysis of Randomized Trials of Drug Therapy Administered during and after Acute Myocardial Infarction.

Drug Class and Time Administered	Number of Trials	Number of Patients	Relative Risk of Death (95% CI)	P Value
β–Adrenergic antagonists				
During MI	29	28,970	0.87 (0.77–0.98)	0.02
After MI	26	24,298	0.77 (0.70–0.84)	< 0.001
ACE inhibitors				
During MI	15	100,963	0.94 (0.89–0.98)	0.006
After MI, patients with left ventricular dysfunction	3	5,986	0.78 (0.70–0.86)	< 0.001
Nitrates (during MI)	22	81,908	0.94 (0.90–0.99)	0.03
Calcium channel blockers (during and after MI)	24	20,342	1.04 (0.95–1.14)	0.41
Antiarrhythmic drugs				
Lidocaine (during MI)	14	9,155	1.38 (0.98–1.95)	> 0.05
Class I drugs (after MI)	18	6,300	1.21 (1.01–1.44)	0.04
Amiodarone (after MI)	9	1,557	0.71 (0.51–0.97)	0.03
Magnesium (during MI)	11	61,860	1.02 (0.96–1.08)	> 0.05

ACE, angiotensin-converting enzyme; MI, myocardial infarction.
Reproduced, with permission, from Hennekens CH et al. N Engl J Med. 1996;335:1660.

to increased levels of circulating plasminogen activator inhibitor (PAI-1) in plasma or PAI-1 that is elaborated locally from platelets. The pharmacologic administration of fibrinolytic agents (Table 5–6) to such patients seems reasonable. Plasminogen activators can be administered intravenously or directly into the coronary artery. Although more rapid patency occurs with local administration, and lower doses can be used, given the need for early treatment, plasminogen activators are generally administered intravenously.

In addition to invoking fibrinolysis and inhibiting clotting by degrading clotting factors, all plasminogen activators enhance clot formation. These effects seem greater with nonspecific plasminogen activators such as streptokinase and urokinase and could partly explain why fibrin-specific

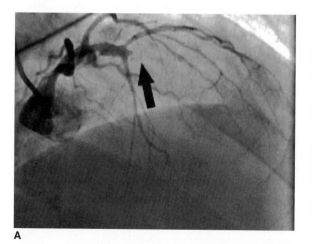
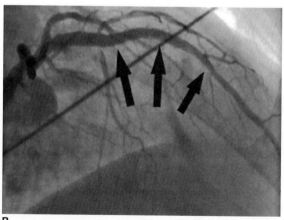

A   B

▲ **Figure 5–6.** Primary PCI for acute MI. **A:** Initial angiography of a patient presenting with acute anterior STEMI shows an occluded left anterior descending (LAD) coronary artery (arrow). **B:** Following angioplasty and stenting, patency of the LAD is restored.

Table 5–6. Fibrinolytic Agents.

Agent	Dosage	Adjunctive Treatments
Streptokinase	1,500,000 units over 1 h	Aspirin, ± heparin
Tissue plasminogen activator		
Standard	15 mg bolus, then 50 mg over 30 min and 35 mg over next 60 min	Aspirin, heparin, essential
Patients weighing less than 65 kg	1.25 mg/kg over 3 h, 10% of dose as initial bolus	
Urokinase	3,000,000 units over 1 h	Aspirin, ± heparin
Reteplase	10 mg initial bolus, second 10-mg bolus after 30 min	Aspirin, heparin, essential
Tenecteplase	< 60 kg: 30-mg bolus	
	60–70 kg: 35-mg bolus	
	71–80 kg: 40-mg bolus	
	81–90 kg: 45-mg bolus	
	> 90 kg: 50-mg bolus	Aspirin, heparin essential

activators such as t-PA open arteries more rapidly. The enhancement of coagulation by plasminogen activators suggests an important role for the concomitant use of antithrombotic agents.

All fibrinolytic agents increase the risk of bleeding and therefore patients at high risk for life-threatening bleeding should not be given fibrinolysis (Table 5–4).

1. Streptokinase—Streptokinase is derived from streptococcal bacteria and activates plasminogen indirectly, forming an activator complex with a slightly longer half-life than streptokinase alone (23 minutes versus 18 minutes after a bolus). Because it activates both circulating plasminogen and plasminogen bound to fibrin, both local and systemic effects occur; that is, circulating fibrinogen degrades substantially (fibrinogenolysis as well as fibrinolysis occurs).

Because antibodies to the streptococci exist in many patients, allergic reactions can occur; anaphylaxis is rare, however, and the use of corticosteroids to avoid allergic reactions is no longer recommended. When streptokinase is administered intravenously, a large dose is necessary to overcome antibody resistance. Because a dose of 250,000 units will suffice in 90% of patients, the recommended dose of 1.5 million units over a 1-hour period is generally more than adequate to overcome resistance. Patients who are known to have had a severe streptococcal infection or to have been treated with streptokinase within the preceding 5 or 6 months (or longer) should not receive the agent.

Rapid administration of streptokinase, even at the recommended dose, can cause a substantial reduction in blood pressure. Although this might be considered a potential benefit of the agent, it may also be detrimental. The rate of the infusion should therefore be reduced in response to significant hypotension, and the blood pressure should be monitored closely. Because streptokinase is more procoagu-

lant than other thrombolytic agents, it should not be surprising that patients benefit to a greater extent from the concomitant use of potent antithrombins such as hirudin. However, in combination with glycoprotein IIB/IIIA inhibitors, streptokinase seems to be associated with markedly increased bleeding rates.

2. Urokinase—Urokinase is a direct activator of plasminogen. It has a shorter half-life than streptokinase (14 ± 6 minutes) and is not antigenic. Its effects on both circulating and bound-to-fibrin plasminogen are similar to those from streptokinase. It is therefore difficult to understand why intravenous doses of urokinase (2.0 million units as bolus or 3 million over 90 minutes) seem to induce coronary artery patency more rapidly than does streptokinase. There is substantial synergism between urokinase and t-PA.

3. Tissue plasminogen activator—The initial human t-PA was made by recombinant DNA technology. The half-life in plasma was short (4 minutes) as a bolus but longer (46 minutes) with prolonged infusions. Despite the short half-life, lytic activity persisted for many hours after clearance of the activator. Although t-PAs are considered "fibrin-specific," no activator is totally fibrin-specific, and fibrin specificity is lost at higher doses. At clinical doses, however, less fibrinogen degradation took place than with nonspecific activators. Tissue plasminogen activator clearly opened coronary arteries more rapidly than nonspecific activators and this is likely why its use improved mortality rates. Bleeding was not less and there was a slight increase in the number of intracranial bleeds, which was in part due to the need for dosage adjustment for lighter-weight patients.

The original regimen for the use of t-PA was 100 mg over 3 hours: 10 mg as a bolus, followed by 50 mg over the first hour and 40 mg over the next 2 hours. Patients who weighed less than 65 kg received 1.25 mg/kg over 3 hours with 10% of the total dose given as a bolus. An alternative front-loaded regimen was found to be more effective and included an initial bolus of 15 mg, followed by 50 mg over 30 minutes and 35 mg over the next 60 minutes. Doses higher than 100 mg are associated with a higher incidence of intracranial bleeding.

4. Reteplase—Reteplase, a mutant form of t-PA, lacks several of the structural areas of the parent molecule (the finger domain, kringle 1, and the epidermal growth factor domain). It is less fibrin-specific (causes more systemic degradation of fibrinogen) than the parent molecule and has a longer half-life. Accordingly, it is used as a double bolus of 10 units initially followed by a second bolus 30 minutes later, and this requires no adjustment for patient weight. Although not shown to be superior to t-PA, many clinicians have elected to use reteplase because of the convenience of the double bolus administration.

5. Tenecteplase—Tenecteplase is also a mutant form of t-PA. It has substitutions in the kringle 1 and protease domains to increase its half-life, increase its fibrin specificity, and reduce its sensitivity to its native inhibitor (PAI-1). Although not shown to be superior to t-PA, tenecteplase is generally being used in preference to the parent molecule because of the convenience of a single bolus dose.

Regardless of the fibrinolytic agent used, all patients should receive aspirin and heparin (either UFH or LMWH) to counteract the procoagulant effect of the fibrinolytic agent.

Intravenous heparin, used with plasminogen activators, improves the rapidity with which patency is induced; it is essential for maintaining coronary patency, especially with t-PA type agents. Its use is less necessary after treatment with streptokinase, probably because of the anticoagulant effects of fibrinogen depletion and degradation products.

The standard dose of UFH is usually a bolus of 5000 units, followed by a 1000-unit-per-hour infusion until the partial thromboplastin time can be used to titrate a dose between 1.5 and 2 times the normal range. It has become clear that optimal titration of UFH is problematic and that if the activated partial thromboplastin time is either too high or too low, some benefit is lost. For this reason, the use of LMWH has been recommended. With the exception of patients with renal failure, a dose of 1 mg/kg of enoxaparin and 120 unit/kg of dalteparin provide consistent reduction in anti-Xa levels and thus consistent anticoagulation. This is probably the reason that recent studies suggest LMWH is more effective for the treatment of patients with acute MI. In addition, because LMWH inhibits Xa activity predominantly, there is some suggestion that discontinuing it may be less problematic than is the case for UFH, which has fewer effects on Xa and more direct effects (when combined with antithrombin 3) on thrombin itself. The ability to use LMWH intravenously in the catheterization laboratory has not been a problem in regions where this strategy has been embraced.

G. Adverse Effects of Fibrinolytic Therapy

The most serious complication of treatment with thrombolytic agents is bleeding, particularly intracranial hemorrhage; however, catheter-based interventions substantially reduce this complication. The mechanism of bleeding with thrombolytic agents is unclear but has been related to the efficacy of the agent; the concomitant use of antithrombotic agents, such as heparin and aspirin; and the degree of hemostatic perturbation induced by the plasminogen activators. In most studies, the incidence of stroke and intracranial bleeding has been slightly higher with t-PA type activators. This may be in keeping with the greater efficacy and rapidity of their effects. Although most bleeding occurs early during treatment, bleeding can occur 24–48 hours later, and vigilance even after the first few hours is important.

Intracranial bleeding is by far the most dangerous bleeding complication because it is often fatal. For most plasminogen activators, the incidence of intracranial hemorrhage is less than 1%, but it may be as high as 2–3% in elderly patients. Risk factors for intracranial bleeding include a history of cerebrovascular disease, hypertension, and age. These factors must be taken into account when determining whether a thrombolytic agent has an appropriate benefit-to-risk relationship. Changes in mental status require an immediate evaluation—clinical and computed tomography or magnetic resonance imaging. If bleeding is strongly suspected, heparin should be discontinued or neutralized with protamine.

There also is a substantial incidence of nonhemorrhagic, probably thrombotic, stroke that may be partly due to dissolution of thrombus within the heart, followed by migration. The exact mechanisms of this phenomenon are unclear. In some studies, the excess of strokes with t-PA has been found to be related to this phenomenon, and in other studies, it has been due to an apparent increase in intracranial bleeding.

Bleeding outside the brain can occur in any organ bed and should be prevented whenever possible. The puncture of noncompressible arterial or venous vessels is relatively contraindicated in all cardiovascular patients: those with unstable angina one day may be candidates for thrombolytic treatment on the next. Blood gas determinations should therefore be avoided if possible and oximeters used instead in cardiovascular patients. It should be understood that central lines placed in cardiovascular patients pose a substantial risk should there be a subsequent need for a lytic agent. Foley catheters and endotracheal (especially nasotracheal) intubation can also predispose to significant hemorrhage. Bleeding should be watched for assiduously. If severe bleeding occurs while heparin is in use, it should be antagonized with protamine. In general, this and supportive measures are all that can be done. In some studies, there appears to be a slightly higher incidence of extracranial bleeding with nonspecific activators than with t-PA; this finding has not been consistent. In an occasional patient, who begins to bleed shortly after receiving the plasminogen activator, aminocaproic acid, which changes the activation of plasminogen, may be useful. Otherwise, discontinuation of the drug and conservative local measures are all that can be done. If volume repletion is necessary, red blood cells are preferred to whole blood, and cryoprecipitate is preferred to fresh frozen plasma because it does not replenish plasminogen.

Allergic reactions related to the use of streptokinase are unusual but should be identified when they occur. Mild reactions, such as urticaria, can be treated with antihistamines; more severe reactions, such as bronchospasm, may require corticosteroids or epinephrine.

Bleeding after primary PCI can also be substantial, particularly if glycoprotein IIB/IIIA agents are administered. The use of newer closure devices are touted by some clinicians, but close observation is the key to minimizing bleeding from the catheter site. On occasion, platelet transfusions may be necessary.

Antman EM et al; American College of Cardiology; American Heart Association; Canadian Cardiovascular Society. ACC/AHA guidelines for the management of patients with ST-elevation myocardial infarction—executive summary. A report of the American College of Cardiology/American Heart Association Task Force on Practice Guidelines (Writing Committee to revise the 1999 guidelines for the management of patients with acute myocardial infarction). J Am Coll Cardiol. 2004 Aug 4;44(3):671–719. [PMID: 15358045]

Braunwald E et al; American College of Cardiology; American Heart Association. Committee on the Management of Patients with Unstable Angina. ACC/AHA 2002 guideline update for the management of patients with unstable angina and non–ST-segment elevation myocardial infarction—summary article: a report of the American College of Cardiology/American Heart Association task force on practice guidelines (Committee on the Management of Patients with Unstable Angina). J Am Coll Cardiol. 2002 Oct 2;40(7):1366–74. [PMID: 12383588]

Sabatine MS et al; CLARITY-TIMI 28 Investigators. Addition of clopidogrel to aspirin and fibrinolytic therapy for myocardial infarction with ST-segment elevation. N Engl J Med. 2005 Mar 24;352(12):1179–89. [PMID: 15758000]

Stone GW et al; Controlled Abciximab and Device Investigation to Lower Late Angioplasty Complications (CADILLAC) Investigators. Comparison of angioplasty with stenting, with or without abciximab, in acute myocardial infarction. N Engl J Med. 2002 Mar 28;346(13):957–66. [PMID: 11919304]

Yusuf S et al; Clopidogrel in Unstable Angina to Prevent Recurrent Events Trial Investigators. Effects of clopidogrel in addition to aspirin in patients with acute coronary syndromes without ST-segment elevation. N Engl J Med. 2001 Aug 16;345(7):494–502. [PMID: 11519503]

▶ Complications of Myocardial Infarction

The complications of acute MI are listed in Table 5–7.

A. Cardiogenic Shock

Cardiogenic shock is characterized by peripheral hypoperfusion and hypotension refractory to volume repletion. This occurs secondary to inadequate cardiac output resulting from severe left ventricular dysfunction.

Table 5–7. Complications of Acute MI.

Cardiogenic shock
Congestive heart failure (CHF)
Ischemic mitral regurgitation
Ventricular septal defect (VSD)
Free wall rupture
Recurrent ischemia
Pericarditis
Conduction disturbances
Arrhythmias
Mural thrombus
Aneurysm or pseudoaneurysm of the left ventricle
Right ventricular infarction

Goals of therapy for cardiogenic shock include hemodynamic stabilization to ensure adequate oxygenation of perfused tissue and prompt assessment for reversible causes of the cardiogenic shock. If reversible causes are not found, immediate reperfusion, especially with PCI, is indicated (see Chapter 6).

B. Congestive Heart Failure

In general, there is greater urgency in treating patients with CHF during the early phases of acute MI because such patients often have multivessel disease and are at increased risk for recurrent infarction and increased infarct size. A high degree of suspicion and close monitoring are key to anticipating this complication of acute MI.

Echocardiography has been the technique of choice in evaluating such patients from a perspective of both valvular and myocardial function. Swan-Ganz pulmonary artery catheterization can also be used to aid diagnosis and to assess ongoing management. Management strategies depend on the clinical history of the patient. Patients with new-onset acute CHF are typically euvolemic and benefit from nitrate therapy for ischemia. These patients in general should not receive diuretics initially because diuretic therapy often complicates the clinical course with the development of hypotension. In addition, reduced respiratory effort, reduced heart rate, and normalization of oxygen saturation are central to early clinical management.

Nitroglycerin is often the best agent to use for ischemia in patients with CHF. In some instances, the hemodynamic profile provided by nitroprusside may be desirable. However, nitroprusside may exacerbate ischemia by inducing a coronary steal phenomenon; in this setting, nitroprusside would be a second-line therapy.

Continuous positive airway pressure can reduce the work of breathing in patients with pulmonary edema and should be considered early in these patients.

Nesiritide (recombinant b-type natriuretic peptide) infusion has demonstrated hemodynamic and neurohormonal benefits in the management of acute heart failure.

Intravenous ACE inhibitor therapy should not be used in this setting until hemodynamic stability is achieved. Hypotension is a complicating factor because it reduces coronary perfusion and may lead to further ischemia. Low-dose dobutamine, starting at 2.5 mcg/kg/min, can be used to achieve hemodynamic benefit. Also, phosphodiesterase inhibitors can be considered although their vasodilating effects may limit their inotropic benefit in patients with significant hypotension.

The use of Swan-Ganz catheterization monitoring is controversial, and no randomized controlled data support their use as a first-line recommendation in the management of CHF with acute MI. However, Swan-Ganz monitoring can be beneficial in verifying diagnosis, and its use in the early phases of management may allow rapid titration of parenteral therapy.

Once hemodynamic stabilization has been achieved, which is generally within the first 6–12 hours, initiation of oral agents is appropriate. Drugs of choice in this setting are ACE inhibitors, which improve cardiac performance, have beneficial effects on ventricular remodeling, and have been demonstrated not only to reduce morbidity but also to reduce mortality rates in patients with CHF. Oral β-blocker therapy should also be initiated early in the treatment of these patients; however, this should be done in a stepwise fashion in relation to ACE inhibitor therapy to avoid hypotensive effects.

Aldosterone blockade with spironolactone or eplerenone should be given to patients with left ventricular impairment (left ventricular ejection fraction less than 40%) or clinical heart failure or both following MI. Aldosterone blockade should be started, in addition to ACE inhibitors, in patients who do not have significant renal impairment or hyperkalemia. The serum potassium level should be monitored closely, since both eplerenone and spironolactone can cause hyperkalemia.

C. Acute Mitral Valve Regurgitation

The development of acute severe mitral valve regurgitation occurs in approximately 1% of patients with acute MI and contributes to 5% of deaths. Mitral regurgitation occurs as a result of papillary muscle rupture most commonly involving the posterior medial papillary muscle because its singular blood vessel supply is derived from the posterior descending coronary artery. In contrast, the anterior lateral papillary muscle much less commonly ruptures because it has a dual blood supply derived from the left anterior descending and circumflex coronary arteries. Rupture of the papillary muscle may be complete or partial with the development of a flail mitral valve leaflet. Pulmonary edema usually ensues rapidly and occurs within 2–7 days after inferior infarction. The intensity of associated murmur varies depending on the extent of unobstructed flow back into the left atrium. If severe regurgitation is present, no murmur may be audible. As a result, a high degree of suspicion is needed to promptly diagnose acute mitral regurgitation. Two-dimensional echocardiography can be used to demonstrate the partial or completely ruptured papillary muscle head and the flail segment of the mitral valve. Typically, hyperdynamic left ventricular function is demonstrated, and its occurrence in severe CHF should prompt the diagnosis. The treatment of choice is to stabilize the patient hemodynamically with the use of intravenous vasodilators and possibly intra-aortic balloon counterpulsation. The basis of a successful outcome, however, is prompt emergency surgery. The operative mortality rate in this setting can be up to 10%, but this affords most opportunity for survival. Mitral valve repair with reimplantation of the severed papillary muscle is the preferred technique as an alternative to mitral valve replacement. The mortality rate is unacceptably high in the absence of prompt surgery.

Ischemic mitral regurgitation without papillary muscle rupture occurs in up to 50% of patients with acute inferior wall MI. In those patients in whom severe CHF symptoms develop, hemodynamic compensation needs to be undertaken and could include the use of IABP for adequate afterload reduction. Treatment of ischemia in this setting may include reperfusion therapy with PCI, intravenous vasodilator therapy, and mechanical support. Once the acute phase of the infarction is past, resolution of the severe mitral regurgitation may occur, which then avoids the need for surgery.

D. Acute Ventricular Septal Rupture

Rupture of the ventricular septum has been reported to occur in up to 3% of acute MIs and contributes to about 5% of deaths. Typically, half of VSDs occur in anterior wall MIs, often in patients with their first infarction, with peak incidence occurring 3–7 days after initial infarction. Findings associated with VSD can be confused with acute mitral regurgitation because both can result in hypotension, severe heart failure, and prominent murmur. However, the diagnosis of VSD should be suspected clinically when a new pansystolic murmur is noted. Generally, the murmur is most prominent along the left sternal border and may have an associated thrill. Prompt surgical intervention is recommended, which, if successful, can reduce the mortality rate from nearly 100% to below 50%.

Although percutaneous repair of postinfarction VSDs in the catheterization laboratory using septal occluding devices has been reported, surgical repair remains the gold standard.

E. Cardiac Rupture

Rupture of the free wall of the left ventricle occurs in approximately 1–3% of patients with acute infarction and accounts for up to 15% of peri-infarction deaths. Free wall rupture may occur as early as within the first 48 hours of infarction. Fifty percent of ruptures occur within the first 5 days of infarction and 90% within the first 2 weeks. Rupture may be due to expansion of the peri-infarct zone, with thinning of the infarcted wall occurring in response to increased stress. The paradoxical motion of the infarcted segment at the margin of the infarcted zone may also contribute stress, resulting in muscle rupture. Patients may complain of recurrence of chest pain, and an ECG may show persistent ST elevation with Q waves. Prompt intervention at that time may include echocardiography with pericardiocentesis, IABP placement, and urgent cardiac catheterization with anticipation of immediate surgery. Unfortunately, all too often signs of cardiac rupture are not present until acute hemodynamic decompensation occurs with cardiac arrest due to electromechanical dissociation. Successful treatment of cardiac rupture requires the clinician to have a high index of suspicion and undertake immediate intervention if there is to be any possibility of preventing death.

F. Recurrent Ischemia

Episodes of chest pain recur in up to 60% of patients after infarction. When chest discomfort recurs early (within 24 hours of MI), the discomfort usually reflects the process of completing the infarction. Chest discomfort may reflect the effects of ongoing ischemia or recurrent infarction. In this situation prompt reassessment and treatment is critical. Patients with hemodynamic compromise in association with new ECG changes in the distribution other than that of the infarct-related artery are at significant risk and require prompt attention, often including coronary angiography with catheter-based intervention.

In those patients who were treated initially with reperfusion therapy and have recurrent chest pain, prompt evaluation is needed to assess the adequacy of anticoagulation and the possibility of reocclusion of the culprit coronary artery. Adequacy of adjunctive therapy in the setting of recurrent chest pain is necessary, and often adjustments in drug doses are required. Occasionally short-term use of intravenous nitroglycerin and intravenous β-blockers are required to quiet the ischemic episode. In this setting, glycoprotein IIb/IIIa inhibitors should be considered if no contraindications are present. In patients who have had coronary angiography and PCI, correlation between angiographic findings and the 12-lead ECG should be made. Acute stent thrombosis will usually be seen on the ECG as recurrence of ST elevation. This requires emergent repeat catheterization. Conversely, patients with diffuse coronary artery disease may have ischemia due to narrowings in the non-culprit coronary arteries, precipitated by stress or tachycardia, for example. The treatment of this is anticoagulation, glycoprotein IIb/IIIa inhibitors, and β-blockers.

In patients with NSTEMI, recurrent chest pain is a marker of significant risk for reinfarction, especially if transient ST segment and T wave changes are noted or if persistent ST segment depression is associated with the initial presentation. Prompt coronary angiography and PCI is often required in this setting.

G. Pericarditis

Pericarditis is common in patients with acute MI, particularly in the course of transmural infarctions. In general, the larger the area of infarction, the more likely pericarditis will develop. Pericarditis may be clinically silent or may be associated with a pericardial rub, pleuritic chest pain, or pericardial effusion as suggested by chest radiograph or two-dimensional echocardiography. The associated chest discomfort, classically described as being relieved by sitting up, may also be associated with a description of shortness of breath and epigastric discomfort with inflammation of the contiguous diaphragm. Pericardial rubs are most commonly heard when the patient is seated with held inspiration. Late pericardial inflammation occurring 2 weeks to 3 months after MI is termed "Dressler syndrome" and most likely reflects an autoimmune mechanism. Dressler syndrome is often associated with large serosanguinous pleural and pericardial effusions, and tamponade develops in persons who die of this syndrome. The treatment of choice for Dressler syndrome is aspirin, or colchicine, and in some instances corticosteroids may be necessary. The use of corticosteroids, however, is not generally advocated because of the high frequency of relapse when corticosteroid therapy is discontinued. Echocardiographic assessment is appropriate as a follow-up tool in these patients to determine the extent of effusion if present and to exclude tamponade or the possibility of partial myocardial rupture. Nonsteroidal antiinflammatory drugs (NSAIDs) should be avoided in patients with ischemic heart disease, particularly those with evidence of acute infarction. Agents such as indomethacin inhibit new collagen deposition and, therefore, may impair the healing process necessary for stabilization of the infarcted region. This may, in a small number of patients, contribute to the development of myocardial rupture. When used in cases refractory to aspirin, NSAIDs should be used for the shortest time possible and tapered as rapidly as possible. In addition, recent data have linked the use of NSAIDs and cyclooxygenase-2 (COX-2) inhibitors to increased rates of cardiac events. Therefore, the use of NSAIDs and COX-2 inhibitors should be minimized or discouraged. Heparin use early in acute MI should not be stopped if pericarditis is present. However, the presence of Dressler syndrome is a contraindication to heparin use, because of its high incidence of hemorrhage into the pericardial fluid with resulting tamponade.

H. Conduction Disturbances

The presence of a conduction disturbance is associated with increased in-hospital and long-term mortality rates. The prognostic significance and management of these disturbances may vary with the location of the infarction, the type of conduction disturbance, associated clinical findings, and the extent of hemodynamic compromise. Patients whose conduction disturbances result in bradycardias and produce hemodynamic compromise generally require transvenous pacing. Bradycardias, especially those associated with inferior infarction, can often be treated with atropine. Recurrent episodes, however, warrant insertion of a pacemaker. Often ventricular pacing to provide a back-up rate is all that is required. A need for improved hemodynamics may be a reason to consider atrioventricular (AV) sequential pacing.

1. Anterior STEMI—The highest risk conduction disturbances occur in these patients. Abnormalities are present early after the onset of infarction and are usually the result of extensive infarction producing pump failure; treatment with a pacemaker may not improve the prognosis. Conduction disturbances in this circumstance are generally right bundle branch block (RBBB), with or without concomitant fascicular block. RBBB without fascicular block may have the same incidence of progression to complete heart block (20–40%) as does an RBBB with fascicular block. Patients with RBBB and a fascicular block with anterior MI should be considered for placement of temporary transvenous pacing and be observed for evidence of progression to complete heart block, warranting permanent transvenous pacing.

Left bundle branch block (LBBB) is most often a chronic manifestation of hypertension and myocardial dysfunction rather than an acute abnormality. In a setting of acute MI, however, it is often difficult to determine whether the LBBB is new. Recommendations have been to use pacemakers for patients with LBBB known to be new; this approach has also been advocated for patients with RBBB. Given the present availability of external pacemakers, these issues appear to be less critical.

In the absence of the signs and symptoms of hemodynamic instability or evidence of the progression to heart block, it is reasonable to observe patients with RBBBs or LBBBs and to use external pacing if conduction disturbances develop. Once such a disturbance develops, a transvenous pacemaker is indicated, and it is likely that AV sequential devices would be of benefit.

2. Inferior MI—Conduction disturbances with acute inferior MI are often less critical, but they do suggest a poorer prognosis. The conduction disturbances that commonly occur represent involvement of the AV node and usually include first-degree AV block, Mobitz I (Wenckebach) or Mobitz II second-degree AV block with narrow QRS complexes, and complete heart block with a junctional rhythm. Conduction disturbances are more common in patients with right ventricular infarction. If hemodynamic stability is maintained, patients with these conduction disturbances do not require pacemakers, and they often respond to the administration of atropine (0.5 mg intravenously). If hemodynamic compromise occurs in association with either Wenckebach block or a junctional rhythm, however, or if any arrhythmia requires treatment with more than one dose of atropine, a transvenous pacemaker is warranted. Large initial or total doses of atropine can lead to tachycardia with exacerbation of ischemia and, at times, ventricular tachycardia (VT) or ventricular fibrillation (VF). For patients with right ventricular infarction and hemodynamic compromise associated with the loss of atrial kick, an AV sequential pacemaker is recommended. In general, hemodynamically significant conduction disturbances occur in patients with inferior infarction early during the evolution of infarction; late conduction disturbances are usually well tolerated. Some of these conduction disturbances respond to an intravenous infusion of 250 mg of aminophylline.

3. Mobitz II second-degree AV block—Mobitz II second-degree AV block or complete heart block with a wide QRS complex are both absolute indications for transvenous pacemaker insertion. Such disturbances can occur from electrolyte abnormalities or conduction system disease, but they are most often associated with hemodynamic abnormalities caused by bradycardia. The use of temporary AV sequential pacing may benefit patients who have hemodynamic abnormalities; these patients are also likely to require permanent pacing (see the section, Prognosis, Risk Stratification, & Management).

I. Other Arrhythmias

1. Sinus tachycardia—Sinus tachycardia occurs in up to 25% of patients with acute MI. It is a marker of physiologic stress (pain, anxiety, hypovolemia) and often indicates the presence of CHF. In some patients, such as those with right ventricular infarction, it may represent relative or absolute volume depletion. In general, although tachycardia increases myocardial oxygen consumption and can exacerbate ischemia, it should not be treated as a discrete entity. The proper approach is to treat the underlying physiologic drive. It may be unwise to block a tachycardia that is compensating for the increased cardiac work required, for example, by sepsis. Accordingly, β-blockers should only be used once it is clear that no underlying abnormality is inducing the tachycardia or that the underlying abnormality (eg, hyperthyroidism) is amenable to such treatment. Making this determination may require hemodynamic monitoring.

2. Supraventricular tachycardia—Paroxysmal supraventricular tachycardia (PSVT), atrial flutter, and atrial fibrillation can all occur with acute MI. Atrial fibrillation is by far the most common arrhythmia and is often associated with the presence of high atrial filling pressures. The presence of supraventricular tachycardia should lead to consideration of CHF as a cause. A complete differential diagnosis, including conditions such as hyperthyroidism, pulmonary embolism, pericarditis, and drug-induced arrhythmias, is appropriate. Paroxysmal supraventricular tachycardia should be treated immediately because of the high likelihood in this setting that the tachycardia will induce ischemia. Adenosine in bolus doses of 6–12 mg intravenously is the initial approach of choice and often terminates the tachycardia. If it does not, cardioversion should be considered prior to other treatment, unless the PSVT terminates and restarts recurrently. Prolonged pharmacologic management before cardioversion may complicate the procedure, and the delay may induce toxicity if the heart rate is rapid, even in the absence of overt hemodynamic compromise. For recurrent or once-terminated PSVT (depending on the mechanisms of the tachycardia; see Chapter 20), small doses of digitalis, diltiazem, verapamil, or a class I antiarrhythmic agent are reasonable choices for maintenance, as long as the indications and contraindications for each of these agents are kept in mind.

Atrial flutter and atrial fibrillation are generally markers of CHF. Frequently the diagnosis of flutter or fibrillation is made after administration of adenosine; once diagnosed, control of the ventricular response is critical. This can generally be accomplished with digitalis, verapamil, or diltiazem in conventional doses (see Chapter 21) once the CHF is treated. Intravenous diltiazem is effective in an emergency situation, usually with an initial test dose of 20–25 mg. If the response is favorable, a titrated dose of 10–15 mg/h should be used. Intravenous diltiazem should be used cautiously in patients with acute MI and CHF. Cardioversion is indicated if a rapid ventricular response persists; the ventricular rate is difficult to control; or there are signs of hypotension, CHF, or recurrent ischemia. In general, PSVT and atrial flutter require 100 J as the initial shock energy; atrial fibrillation requires 200 J.

Arrhythmias that recur after transient reversion in response to pharmacologic maneuvers or cardioversion require additional treatment. Treatment of the underlying initiating stimulus is critical. β-Blockers can also be used to control the ventricular response acutely or for maintenance.

3. Ventricular arrhythmias—The incidence of postinfarct malignant ventricular arrhythmias in patients with acute MI appears to be diminishing, perhaps because of the use of reperfusion therapy. It also is conceivable that interventions such as intravenous β-blockers have also contributed to this decline. Because of the diminishing incidence of VT and fibrillation in patients with acute infarction, as well as an unfavorable benefit-risk ratio, the use of prophylactic lidocaine is not recommended. Although prophylactic lidocaine reduces the incidence of VF, it is associated in many series with an increase in cardiac death, possibly because it abolishes ventricular escape rhythms in patients who may also be prone to bradycardia. Because warning arrhythmias, once considered progenitors of VF, do not appear to be highly predictive, it is recommended that only symptomatic arrhythmias and VT be indications for treatment.

VT with hemodynamic compromise, angina or pulmonary edema, and VF should be treated with immediate electric shock. Sustained monomorphic VT without hemodynamic compromise, angina, or pulmonary edema can be treated with amiodarone. Amiodarone should be administered as an initial bolus of 150 mg over 10 minutes. If arrhythmias persist, additional boluses of 150 mg every 10–15 minutes can be given; however, the total dose should never exceed 2.2 g in 24 hours. Hypotension and CHF can be induced during the acute administration of amiodarone as a result of its negative inotropic effects. If amiodarone does not relieve the symptoms or the arrhythmias, patients can be treated with intravenous procainamide. The initial loading dose is 1 g, at no more than 50 mg/min, followed by a 2–6 mg/min drip. The infusion rate should be reduced if hypotension occurs; this effect is due to procainamide's α-adrenergic effects. If successful, the drug is continued until the patient is hemodynamically stable; it can then be tapered after initiation of treatment with secondary-prevention agents and an assessment made in terms of long-term risk stratification. On rare occasions, a pacemaker may need to be placed in the right ventricle to compete with or overdrive-suppress malignant ventricular arrhythmias. This is usually reserved for rhythms refractory to pharmacologic therapy and can, on occasion, be life-saving. The ventricular pacemaker is generally set at 90–110 bpm, or whatever rate is necessary to suppress the ventricular arrhythmias.

Accelerated idioventricular rhythm occurs in up to 40% of patients and can in some instances be a marker of reperfusion. This rhythm is generally thought to be benign and is usually not treated.

J. Mural Thrombi

Patients with acute MI are at risk for the development of endocardial thrombi for a variety of reasons. Left ventricular thrombus develops in up to 40% of patients with anterior wall infarction but uncommonly in inferior infarcts. Large areas of dyskinesis with poor flow are prone to develop clots. Because there may be a return in contractility in the borders of the infarcted zone during the remodeling process, it could paradoxically be that clots develop more readily in patients with larger infarctions, but those with somewhat smaller infarctions tend to have them result in emboli more frequently. It has been recommended that all patients with an anterior wall MI be considered for anticoagulation during hospitalization and for 3–6 months thereafter. If anticoagulation is not used routinely, echocardiographic evaluation for the presence of mural thrombi is recommended. Because short-term anticoagulation until the ventricle is remodeled might well be adequate for most patients, the value of long-term (3 months or more) anticoagulation is unclear. In the absence of contraindications, it is probably worthwhile to use heparin during hospitalization and subsequently to use warfarin for 3 months for patients with anterior infarction. Because it has not been established whether low doses of warfarin are as effective as larger doses in inhibiting left ventricular mural thrombi, only a full dose (an INR 2.0–2.5) is recommended. Anticoagulation may be valuable for some patients for other reasons, such as atrial fibrillation. Patients with inferior or non-Q wave infarctions do not require routine anticoagulation following MI but should receive warfarin if mural thrombi are detected by echocardiography. Some clinicians use echocardiographic criteria to select patients who should be treated; others would treat any thrombus detected.

In the current era of routine aspirin and clopidogrel use after MI, there is little data on which patients should receive warfarin. It is prudent to fully anticoagulate patients with established mural thrombi, and those with other reasons for warfarin therapy, such as atrial fibrillation or aspirin allergy. Other cases, including anterior MI, should be judged individually with the risk of thromboembolism from mural thrombus balanced against the risk of bleeding from warfarin.

Mural thrombi can form in the atrium as well as in the ventricle. Atrial fibrillation is common in patients with CHF; in the setting of atrial fibrillation, stagnation of blood in the atrial appendage leads to a high incidence of clots. This condition can be established only with transesophageal echocardiography, but it may explain the high incidence of emboli in patients with paroxysmal atrial fibrillation. Accordingly, patients with atrial fibrillation should receive anticoagulation, not only because of their increased incidence of thrombus but because it appears that emboli can be prevented in this group with reasonably modest doses of anticoagulants (goal INR 2.0–2.5). Anticoagulation is discussed in depth in Chapter 29.

Patients with CHF and acute MI are at increased risk for pulmonary emboli because of deep venous thrombosis in the calf and thigh. This may be prevented by the use of warfarin. An argument can be made to consider the use of warfarin in any patient with acute infarction who has had no contraindications for several months. Because aspirin was withheld in some studies, it is unclear whether it offers similar benefits, which would allow it to be substituted for warfarin. In the current era of aspirin and clopidogrel following MI, warfarin should be considered for MI with extensive wall motion abnormality, including anterior MI, and any MI with established mural thrombus on echocardiography. However, it is probably not necessary in other patients.

K. Aneurysm and Pseudo-aneurysms

Large areas of infarction tend to thin and bulge paradoxically. These large dyskinetic areas eventually form discrete aneurysms with defined borders. In general, treatment involves the same principles as those for patients with heart failure: vasodilatation and adequate control of filling pressures to reduce pulmonary congestion. Often patients with large dyskinetic areas will have a component of heart failure. If severe heart failure can be managed over time, an aneurysm may form that will then be amenable to surgical resection.

Occasionally, while aneurysms are forming, a myocardial rupture will occur. A small amount of rupture can become tamponaded by the pericardium, leading to what is known as a pseudo-aneurysm. Pseudo-aneurysms, which tend to have narrow necks and are not lined with endocardium, function like aneurysms in that they fill with blood during ejection, reducing systolic performance. In addition to reducing stroke volume and leading to increases in ventricular volume as a compensatory response with concomitant increases in pulmonary congestion, pseudo-aneurysms are prone to rupture. The larger the pseudo-aneurysm, the greater the possibility of rupture. Accordingly, the diagnosis of pseudo-aneurysm usually leads to relatively prompt surgery. Although pseudo-aneurysms can occur with both anterior and inferior MIs, true aneurysms are unusual in the inferior-posterior distribution. A large aneurysmal dilatation is therefore more apt to be a pseudo-aneurysm in an inferior-posterior location.

L. Right Ventricular Infarction

Right ventricular involvement in acute inferior wall MI is common. Hemodynamically significant right ventricular dysfunction, however, is uncommon, occurring in relatively few patients with right ventricular infarction. Substantial right ventricular infarction contributing to hemodynamic compromise occurs in up to 20% of patients with inferior and posterior infarction. These patients often clinically demonstrate hypotension and elevated jugular venous pressure but clear lung fields in the setting of acute inferior wall infarction. ST segment elevation in right-sided leads (V_3R or V_4R), right ventricular wall motion abnormalities on echocardiography help confirm the diagnosis of right ventricular involvement. With right ventricular infarction, the right ventricle becomes noncontractile, and cardiac output is maintained by increased excursion of the septum into the right ventricle and by elevated right-sided filling pressures. The incidence of high-grade AV block is also increased in patients with right ventricular infarction.

If reperfusion is not possible, the stunned right ventricle tends to resolve its dysfunction. Support entails intravenous fluid administration if left ventricular filling pressures are reduced, and occasionally the use of positive inotropic therapy or AV sequential pacing, or both are required. Early treatment with intravenous diuretics may lead to hypotension and confound patient presentation; therefore, focused clinical examination on presentation is paramount. Patients who display the development of shock despite supportive treatment may benefit from catheter-based intervention (angioplasty and stenting) of the occluded right coronary artery. The balance between the extent of right ventricular and left ventricular dysfunction, however, determines long-term outcome.

Crenshaw BS et al. Risk factors, angiographic patterns, and outcomes in patients with ventricular septal defect complicating acute myocardial infarction. GUSTO-I (Global Utilization of Streptokinase and TPA for Occluded Coronary Arteries) Trial Investigators. Circulation. 2000 Jan 4–11;101(1):27–32. [PMID: 10618300]

Hochman JS et al. Early revascularization in acute myocardial infarction complicated by cardiogenic shock. SHOCK Investigators. Should We Emergently Revascularize Occluded Coronaries for Cardiogenic Shock. N Engl J Med. 1999 Aug 26;341(9):625–32. [PMID: 10460813]

Welch PJ et al. Management of ventricular arrhythmias: a trial-based approach. J Am Coll Cardiol. 1999 Sep;34(3):621–30. [PMID: 10483940]

Yeo TC et al. Clinical characteristics and outcome in postinfarction pseudoaneurysm. Am J Cardiol. 1999 Sep 1;84(5):592–5, A8. [PMID: 10482162]

▶ Prognosis, Risk Stratification, & Management

A. Risk Predictors

1. Infarct size—Infarct size is an important determinant of long-term risk: the larger the infarction, the poorer the long-term prognosis. This association is easy to demonstrate in patients with first infarctions. In patients with multiple infarctions, the cumulative amount of damage is predictive. Measures that estimate cumulative infarct size (eg, ejection fraction; sestamibi scanning) provide important prognostic information. Nonetheless, the presence of an adverse prognosis does not, in and of itself, mandate a more aggressive therapeutic approach. However, ACE inhibitors and β-blockers are important adjunctive therapies.

2. Infarct type—Patients with NSTEMI are more prone to recurrent episodes of chest discomfort and infarction than are patients with STEMI. Patients with STEMI have an adverse short-term prognosis and should be considered for immediate reperfusion therapy; they often manifest arrhythmias that, especially in association with a low left ventricular ejection fraction, are an important marker of an adverse prognosis. Often these are the patients who have CHF during hospitalization for acute infarction. Their prognosis is worse than that of patients without heart failure, even if the left ventricular ejection fraction appears reasonably well preserved.

3. Malignant arrhythmias—Many patients who suffer malignant arrhythmias during evolution of the infarction are also at increased risk. The one exception appears to be patients with primary VF (ie, VF with no complication of infarction).

B. Risk Assessment

Advanced age (> 65 years), prior MI, anterior location of infarction, postinfarction angina, NSTEMI, mechanical complications of infarction, CHF, and the presence of diabetes all suggest higher risk for reinfarction or death in the 6 months following infarction. These patients require aggressive risk stratification prior to hospital discharge after infarction.

1. Myocardial ischemia—Patients with recurrent ischemia during hospitalization are generally considered unstable because of the adverse prognosis associated with recurrent angina following MI. For patients with multiple episodes of recurrent chest discomfort, or ischemia in a distribution distant from the current infarction, cardiac catheterization is recommended to permit consideration of PCI.

In patients without complications, who are not receiving reperfusion therapy, ECG treadmill stress tests provide additional prognostic information. Thallium or sestamibi scintigraphy add to the sensitivity and specificity of this analysis. Nuclear or echocardiographic imaging can be used in patients whose ECGs cannot be interpreted because of drug effects, resting ST-T wave changes, or conduction disturbances. Patients who are unable to exercise may benefit from pharmacologic stress tests, such as dobutamine echocardiography or dipyridamole or adenosine nuclear stress imaging. The inability to exercise is in itself a marker of poor prognosis.

Patients who have received thrombolytics or PCI and have not had recurrent episodes of chest discomfort constitute a very low-risk group for which the ability of any stress testing method to predict events is significantly reduced. Generally, however, patients who have been treated with thrombolytic agents and have evidence of ischemia undergo invasive investigation with cardiac catheterization.

The evidence that the prognosis of patients with NSTEMI is adequately determined by stress testing is controversial and in part depends on the nature of the stress procedure, perhaps including whether patients exercise rigorously enough. There is some suggestion that because most stress tests during acute hospitalization tend to be submaximal, a maximal stress test 6–8 weeks after the infarction is most appropriate for thorough risk stratification.

2. Ventricular function—Patients with complications of infarction or any findings of CHF should have a noninvasive evaluation of ventricular function during their acute hospitalization. Assuming the absence of intercurrent events, one evaluation of ventricular function generally suffices.

In the absence of such an assessment, a stress echocardiogram can provide information concerning both ischemia and ventricular performance. Advocates believe that the combination of these parameters is important; detractors argue that the evaluation of ischemia is less complete than can be accomplished with radionuclide scintigraphy.

The evaluation of some patients with poor ventricular function may also require determining the presence of viable but dysfunctional myocardium (stunned or hibernating regions). Sophisticated metabolic studies using positron emission tomography seem to have the most promise for delineating the regions apt to improve with revascularization; however, they are not widely available for routine use. The response of dysfunctional regions may also be evaluated with dobutamine echocardiography (improved function is thought to be predictive of viable myocardium) or delayed thallium imaging (delayed uptake suggests viability).

3. Arrhythmias—Patients who have VT or recurrent episodes of VF after the first day require further evaluation. Evaluation is mandatory for patients who have recurrent arrhythmias without easily remediable causes, especially sustained VT, which generally requires invasive electrophysiological studies. Although treadmill- and ambulatory ECG-guided therapy are equivalent in some studies, the use of invasive electrophysiological studies to select and titrate antiarrhythmic agents or choose a mechanical device provide one approach. Recent data suggest that if the ejection fraction is < 0.35 and VT is present that implantable cardioverter defibrillators (ICDs) save lives.

At present, it is unclear how to manage less severe arrhythmias, which may include frequent ectopy or nonsustained VT. Signal-averaged ECG can be used in such patients; although a negative study is reassuring, the sensitivity of the procedure for detecting risk is inadequate. Recent data suggest that prophylactic ICDs in the 6 weeks following MI for ejection fraction < 35% do not reduce mortality. Therefore, depressed ejection fraction alone, in the absence of life-threatening arrhythmias, following MI is not an indication for ICD therapy. Patients should have optimal medical therapy and left ventricular ejection fraction should be reassessed after 6 weeks.

Patients who have had bradycardias often require pacemakers. Long-term pacemakers improve the prognosis for patients in whom complete heart block has developed via a mechanism involving bundle branch block. Some clinicians advocate pacing for patients who had transient complete heart block without the development of bundle branch blocks (those with inferior MI and narrow QRS complexes), but supportive data are not conclusive. There also is controversy concerning the use of pacemakers in patients with conduction disturbance such as RBBB and anterior fascicular block, who may (or may not) have had transient Mobitz II second-degree AV block; the benefits of pacing have yet to be established.

C. Risk Management

Patients with recurrent ischemia, severe ventricular arrhythmias, reduced ejection fraction (< 0.40), or evidence of severe ischemia during stress testing require cardiac catheterization. Although, in general, treatment is guided by anatomic considerations and their relationship to a long-term prognosis, the ability to predict—from the anatomy—which vessels are apt to be involved in subsequent events is poor. Furthermore, it is unclear that mechanical interventions will reduce the incidence of infarction or death except in well-defined subsets of patients (eg, those with left main disease, proximal three-vessel disease, and a reduced ejection fraction).

1. Risk factor modification—Central to the patient's in-hospital treatment is the identification of factors that increase the risk for progression of coronary artery disease. These include the traditional risk factors for atherosclerosis: hypertension, diabetes, smoking, cholesterol abnormalities, family history, and a sedentary lifestyle. Attempts to modify the diet, stop smoking, and increase exercise should begin once the patient has left the intensive care unit. Although such efforts will vary with each patient, a structured program with active follow-up of patients to ensure some level of success may be helpful.

Recent statin therapy trials support aggressive reduction in cholesterol for the stabilization, and possibly regression, of atherosclerosis. Therefore, a very aggressive approach toward the reduction of LDL cholesterol and increases in high-density lipoprotein is justified early (within the first 24–48 hours) in postinfarction management. All post-MI patients should receive a statin, and aim to achieve an LDL of < 70 mg/dL.

2. Secondary prevention—β-Blockers should be given to all patients who have had acute ST and non–ST elevation MIs with or without reperfusion therapy. Patients with CHF tend to benefit most with gradual titration of dose.

Although secondary-prevention trials with aspirin have not indicated statistically significant benefits, most studies do show a trend toward improvement, and meta-analysis supports the concept that aspirin improves prognosis after acute infarction. Whether this benefit is synergistic with the effects of β-blockers is unclear. Nonetheless, it appears reasonable for patients to start taking low doses of aspirin (81–325 mg/day) after acute MI and to continue it long-term.

Long-term treatment with ACE inhibitors is recommended for patients at risk for ventricular remodeling and the sequelae associated with that process. In general, this includes patients with left ventricular ejection fractions of < 45%. Given the results of recent trials, even patients with a low normal ejection fraction after infarction should be considered for ACE inhibitor treatment, particularly with an anterior MI.

3. Rehabilitation—Studies of exercise rehabilitation have been confounded by the fact that individuals who participate in such programs generally have favorable risk factor and psychological profiles that lessen their risk of recurrent events. It has been argued that the improved prognosis of such patients is related to these initial characteristics—and not to the effects of exercise training. Nonetheless, exercise training clearly improves peripheral muscle efficiency, and intense long-term physical training (5 days a week for at least 9 months) has been shown to reduce the development of cardiac ischemia. Therefore, exercise rehabilitation programs are recommended whenever possible for postinfarction patients.

The amount of exercise prescribed must obviously be based on the patient's heart rate and blood pressure. These should be monitored as the patients start to walk during the convalescent phase in the hospital, and marked increases (eg, blood pressure more than 140/90 mm Hg) should be avoided. The patient's rehabilitation activity schedule should be reduced if this level of hypertension occurs. This may also indicate the need for treatment with β-blockers or ACE inhibitors to reduce the labile hypertensive response. In any event, the response of blood pressure and heart rate to exercise must be monitored. Phase II of the program begins at hospital dismissal and generally continues for 8–12 weeks. Objectives should include further patient education, risk factor modification, and gradual resumption of normal work and recreational activities.

4. Psychological factors—It is now clear that as many as 20–25% of patients with acute MI meet formal clinical criteria for depression. It also appears that this is an adverse prognostic feature and that such patients have increased morbidity and mortality rates. Although there is some argument that this is so because these patients have more severe disease, this hypothesis has not been supported by recent studies. It may well be that whatever leads to depression is negatively synergistic with underlying coronary artery disease, as suggested by the increase in catecholamines in such patients. Regardless of the mechanism, however, careful consideration of the presence or absence of depression in patients is recommended. Psychological consultation should be sought for patients in whom depression is suspected, and treatment should be initiated to improve both the quality of the individual's life and—to the extent that there is an interaction with ischemic heart disease—the prognosis. Because tricyclic antidepressants initially liberate catecholamines and may thereby induce adverse effects, drug treatment has previously been thought to be problematic in cardiovascular patients. On the other hand, these agents have membrane-stabilizing effects that may reduce the propensity to arrhythmias and it is believed that the potential for risk has been exaggerated. Newer agents that antagonize serotonin as their primary mode of action may be safer, but cognitive therapy has also been shown to be effective.

Ades PA. Cardiac rehabilitation and secondary prevention of coronary heart disease. N Engl J Med. 2001 Sep 20;345(12)892–902. [PMID: 11565523]

Antman EM et al. The TIMI risk score for unstable angina/non-ST elevation MI: a method for prognostication and therapeutic decision making. JAMA. 2000 Aug 16;284(7):835–42. [PMID: 10938172]

Hohnloser SH et al; DINAMIT Investigators. Prophylactic use of an implantable cardioverter-defibrillator after acute myocardial infarction. N Engl J Med. 2004 Dec 9;351(24):2481–88.

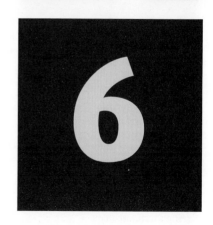

Cardiogenic Shock

Edward McNulty, MD & Craig Timm, MD

ESSENTIALS OF DIAGNOSIS

- Tissue hypoperfusion: Depressed mental status, cool extremities, decreased urinary output.
- Hypotension: Systolic blood pressure < 90 mm Hg.
- Reduced cardiac output: Cardiac index < 2.2 L/min/m².
- Adequate intravascular volume: Pulmonary artery wedge pressure > 15 mm Hg.

General Considerations

A diagnosis of cardiogenic shock has historically conferred a very high mortality. Despite recent advances in treating this condition, nearly 50% of patients with cardiogenic shock still do not survive to hospital discharge. In a strict sense, cardiogenic shock develops as a result of the failure of the heart in its function as a pump, resulting in inadequate cardiac output. This failure is most commonly caused by extensive myocardial damage from an acute myocardial infarction (MI), but other mechanical complications of an acute MI, valve lesions, arrhythmias, and end-stage cardiomyopathies can also lead to cardiogenic shock.

Definition

A number of definitions for cardiogenic shock have been proposed. Although these definitions differ in some ways, there is general agreement that both hemodynamic and clinical parameters should be included. There should be evidence of a reduced cardiac output without hypovolemia. Clinical signs of decreased peripheral perfusion should be present and include cool and clammy skin, weak distal pulses, altered mental status, and diminished urinary output (less than 30 mL/h). A commonly used set of hemodynamic criteria for cardiogenic shock are (1) a systolic blood pressure of less than 90 mm Hg for at least 30 minutes (or the

need for vasopressor or intra-aortic balloon pump support in order to maintain a systolic blood pressure ≥ 90 mm Hg), (2) a pulmonary capillary wedge pressure (PCWP) of greater than 15 mm Hg, and (3) a cardiac index less than 2.2 L/min/ m². Using a combination of clinical and hemodynamic criteria means that fewer patients are given an inappropriate diagnosis of shock.

Etiology

Acute MI accounts for most cases of cardiogenic shock. Acute MI results in cardiogenic shock in 5–10% of patients; however, it is likely that cardiogenic shock develops in many more patients following an acute MI, but they do not survive to receive medical attention. Cardiogenic shock may occur in a patient with a massive first infarction, or it may occur with a smaller infarction in a patient with an already substantially infarcted myocardium. "Mechanical" complications of acute MI can also cause shock, and these include ventricular septal rupture, acute mitral regurgitation as a result of papillary muscle rupture, and myocardial free wall rupture with tamponade. Right ventricular infarction in the absence of significant left ventricular infarction or dysfunction can lead to shock. Refractory tachyarrhythmias or bradyarrhythmias, usually in the setting of preexisting left ventricular dysfunction, are occasionally a cause of shock and can occur with either ventricular or supraventricular arrhythmias. Cardiogenic shock may occur in patients with end-stage cardiomyopathies (ischemic, valvular, hypertrophic, restrictive, or idiopathic in origin). Cardiogenic shock may also be the presenting manifestation of acute myocarditis (infectious, toxic, rheumatologic or idiopathic). A more recently recognized entity is **stress cardiomyopathy** (also known as apical ballooning syndrome or tako-tsubo cardiomyopathy) in which severe heart failure and sometimes cardiogenic shock result from extreme emotional distress. Finally, certain endocrine abnormalities may cause severe cardiac dysfunction and cardiogenic shock (Table 6–1).

Table 6-1. Causes of Cardiogenic Shock.

I. Acute myocardial infarction (MI)
  A. Pump failure
  B. Mechanical complications of acute MI
    1. Acute mitral regurgitation
    2. Ventricular septal defect
    3. Free wall rupture/tamponade
  C. Right ventricular MI
II. End-stage, severe cardiomyopathies secondary to
  A. Valvular disease
  B. Chronic ischemic disease
  C. Restrictive/infiltrative
  D. Idiopathic
III. Acute myocarditis: viral/infectious, toxic
IV. Stress cardiomyopathy
V. Endocrine disease (eg, hypothyroidism, pheochromocytoma)
  A. Bradyarrhythmias
  B. Tachyarrhythmias
VII. Secondary to medications
VIII. Post-traumatic

Babaev A et al. Trends in management and outcomes of patients with acute myocardial infarction complicated by cardiogenic shock. JAMA. 2005 Jul 27;294(4):448–54. [PMID: 16046651]

Hochman JS et al. Cardiogenic shock complicating acute myocardial infarction–etiologies, management and outcome: a report from the SHOCK Trial Registry. SHould we emergently revascularize Occluded Coronaries for cardiogenic shocK? J Am Coll Cardiol. 2000 Sep;36(3 Suppl A):1063–70. [PMID: 10985706]

Sharkey SW et al. Acute and reversible cardiomyopathy provoked by stress in women from the United States. Circulation. 2005 Feb 1;111(4):472–9. [PMID: 15687136]

▶ Pathogenesis

The principle feature of shock is hypotension with evidence of end-organ hypoperfusion. In cardiogenic shock, this occurs as a consequence of inadequate cardiac function. The usual response to low cardiac output is sympathetic stimulation to increase cardiac performance and maintain vascular tone. This results in tachycardia and increased myocardial contractility (β-adrenergic mediated effects) and peripheral vasoconstriction (an α-adrenergic mediated effect). The classic patient with cardiogenic shock has evidence of peripheral vasoconstriction (cool, clammy skin) and tachycardia. Corresponding classic hemodynamics are a reduced cardiac output and increased systemic vascular resistance (SVR), defined as:

$$(SVR) = \frac{(\text{mean arterial pressure} - \text{central venous pressure}) \times 80 (\text{dynes} \times s \times cm^{-5})}{\text{Cardiac output}}$$

Recent evidence suggests that many patients with cardiogenic shock do not have these classic hemodynamics and instead have a lower SVR much like patients in septic shock. In fact, it has been postulated that a systemic inflammatory response-like syndrome with a low SVR may be encountered in up to 25% of patients in cardiogenic shock. Furthermore, patients with severe septic shock often have depressed myocardial function, and patients with cardiogenic shock can have a component of hypovolemia. Thus, there can be considerable overlap in pathophysiologies.

A. Cardiogenic Shock after Acute MI

If at least 40% of the left ventricular myocardial muscle mass is lost, either acutely or as a result of prior damage, cardiogenic shock can result from pump failure (ie, there is not sufficient left ventricular muscle mass to maintain forward cardiac output). This usually occurs as a consequence of an MI. The initial event in an acute MI is obstruction of a coronary artery, commonly termed the "infarct-related artery." The acute obstruction decreases oxygen supply to a portion of the heart, resulting in myocardial ischemia and infarction, which in turn leads to diminished myocardial contractility. The ensuing drop in cardiac output and blood pressure leads to decreased perfusion pressures in other coronary beds. (Coronary perfusion becomes compromised when the aortic diastolic pressure falls below 50–55 mm Hg.) This results in further ischemia, especially if stenoses are present in these non–infarct-related vessels, and additional deterioration in left ventricular function occurs. Indeed, most patients with shock after acute MI have extensive coronary disease, and mortality correlates with the extent of coronary disease (Figure 6–1).

The process of ischemia and infarction leading to myocardial dysfunction leading to further ischemia and so on has been appropriately termed "a vicious cycle." Evidence for this vicious cycle is found in autopsy studies that show infarct extension at the edges of an infarct in addition to discrete, remote infarctions throughout the ventricle. This also explains the finding that cardiogenic shock can occur immediately, provided sufficient myocardium is dysfunctional, or occur hours after the initial infarct as a consequence of the vicious cycle. Tissue hypoperfusion also leads to accumulation of lactic acid. Acidemia is detrimental to left ventricular contractility, and this is another example of a vicious cycle contributing to the pathophysiology of cardiogenic shock.

B. Mechanical Complications of Acute MI

The pathophysiology of cardiogenic shock due to mechanical complications of acute MI is somewhat different. The three main mechanical problems are (1) acute mitral regurgitation as a consequence of papillary muscle rupture, (2) ventricular septal defect (VSD), and (3) myocardial free wall rupture leading to cardiac tamponade. These mechanical problems all occur in a bimodal distribution, with some occurring earlier in the presentation and others occurring later, and are a consequence of weakened, necrotic myocardium.

The papillary muscles anchor the the mitral valve apparatus to the left ventricle. Proper papillary muscle function is vital in ensuring that the two mitral valve leaflets close

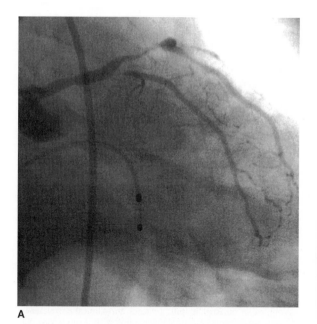

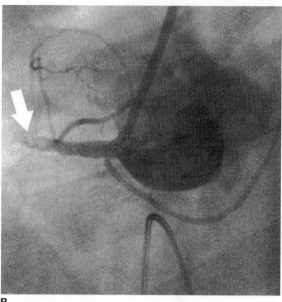

A   B

▲ **Figure 6–1.** Coronary angiogram of patient with an acute myocardial infarction and cardiogenic shock. Severe disease in left coronary system (**A**) and acute occlusion with thrombus in the right coronary artery (**B**).

completely to prevent leakage or regurgitation of blood backwards into the left atrium. Papillary muscle rupture is a term used somewhat erroneously; rupture and avulsion of the entire papillary muscle usually results in such severe regurgitation that it is rapidly fatal. If only a portion of the papillary muscle ruptures, then severe mitral regurgitation ensues, leading to pulmonary edema and a reduced forward cardiac output. This accounts for up to 7% of patients with cardiogenic shock after an acute MI. The sympathetic nervous system response to cardiac failure results in increased SVR (afterload) and a further increase in the regurgitant fraction, another example of a vicious cycle contributing to cardiogenic shock.

Rupture of the myocardial free wall results in bleeding into the relatively nondistendible pericardial space and leads rapidly to pericardial tamponade and cardiovascular collapse. Often this is immediately fatal, but occasionally patients survive and cardiogenic shock develops. The incidence of free wall rupture in patients with cardiogenic shock is as high as 3%.

Rupture of the intraventricular septum with the formation of a VSD has an incidence of approximately 0.3% in patients with acute MI and accounts for up to 6% of patients with cardiogenic shock after an acute MI. A large VSD causes significant shunting of blood from the left ventricle to the right ventricle, and results in right ventricular volume and pressure overload (Figure 6–2). Shock usually develops as a consequence of reduced forward cardiac output. As with acute mitral regurgitation, the sympathetic nervous system response results in increased afterload, thereby shunting an even larger fraction of the cardiac output across the interventricular septum.

C. Right Ventricular Infarction

Right ventricular infarctions occur in approximately 40% of patients with inferior MIs. Right ventricular infarctions may result in cardiogenic shock without significant left ventricular dysfunction. Failure of the right ventricle leads to diminished right ventricular stroke volume, which results in a decreased volume of blood returning to the left ventricle. This markedly diminished left ventricular preload, even with normal left ventricular contractility, causes a decreased systemic cardiac output. The right ventricle also becomes dilated, which results in displacement of the intraventricular septum to the left. If severe, this can actually impair left ventricular filling, with physiology similar to that seen in cardiac tamponade. Since left ventricular filling pressures are not elevated in pure right ventricular failure, pulmonary congestion will not be evident.

D. Arrhythmias

A variety of arrhythmias can contribute to the development of shock. A sustained arrhythmia, that is, one that does not culminate in ventricular fibrillation and sudden death, is generally a cause of shock only in the already compromised ventricle. Atrial and ventricular tachyarrhythmias can result in diminished time for ventricular filling in diastole as well as

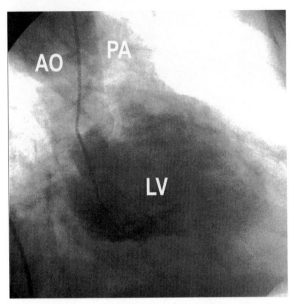

▲ **Figure 6-2.** Left ventriculogram of patient with ventricular septal defect. Note that contrast injected into the left ventricle (LV) opacifies both the aorta (AO) and the pulmonary artery (PA). (The right ventricle is superimposed upon the left in this projection and therefore is not visualized.)

the loss of the atrial contribution to ventricular diastolic filling. This results in a diminished preload, which in turn results in a decreased stroke volume. These factors may be enough to result in cardiogenic shock in patients with already impaired left ventricular function or with conditions such as severe aortic stenosis in which the left ventricle is especially sensitive to filling pressures. Bradyarrhythmias reduce cardiac output as a consequence of the slow heart rate. Because total cardiac output is a function of heart rate and stroke volume (cardiac output = stroke volume × heart rate), a markedly decreased heart rate, especially with concomitant left ventricular dysfunction may, result in shock.

E. Other Causes of Cardiogenic Shock

Many forms of heart disease can result in an end-stage dilated cardiomyopathy. These patients may be in such acutely decompensated states that they are in frank cardiogenic shock.

Birnbaum Y. Ventricular septal rupture after acute myocardial infarction. N Engl J Med. 2002 Oct 31;347(18):1426–32. [PMID: 12409546]

Bowers TR et al. Patterns of coronary compromise resulting in acute right ventricular ischemic dysfunction. Circulation. 2002 Aug 27;106(9):1104–9. [PMID: 12196336]

Crenshaw BS. Risk factors, angiographic patterns, and outcomes in patients with ventricular septal defect complicating acute

myocardial infarction. GUSTO-I (Global Utilization of Streptokinase and TPA for Occluded Arteries) Trial Investigators. Circulation. 2000 Jan 4–11;101(1):27–32. [PMID: 10618300]

Jacobs AK et al. Cardiogenic shock caused by right ventricular infarction: a report from the SHOCK registry. J Am Coll Cardiol. 2003 Apr 16;41(8):1273–9. [PMID: 12706920]

Kohsaka S et al. Systemic inflammatory response syndrome after acute myocardial infarction complicated by cardiogenic shock. Arch Intern Med. 2005 Jul 25;165(14):1643–50. [PMID: 16043684]

Menon V et al. Outcome and profile of ventricular septal rupture with cardiogenic shock after myocardial infarction: a report from the SHOCK trial registry. SHould we emergently revascularize Occluded Coronaries in cardiogenic shocK? J Am Coll Cardiol. 2000 Sep;36(3 Suppl A):1110–6. [PMID: 10985713]

Slater J et al. Cardiogenic shock due to cardiac free-wall rupture or tamponade after acute myocardial infarction: a report from the SHOCK trial registry. SHould we emergently revascularize Occluded Coronaries for cardiogenic shocK? J Am Coll Cardiol. 2000 Sep;36(3 Suppl A):1117–22. [PMID: 10985714]

Webb JG et al. Implications of the timing of onset of cardiogenic shock after acute myocardial infarction: a report from the SHOCK trial registry. SHould we emergently revascularize Occluded Coronaries in cardiogenic shocK? J Am Coll Cardiol. 2000 Sep;36(3 Suppl A):1084–90. [PMID: 10985709]

Wong SC et al. Angiographic findings and clinical correlates in patients with cardiogenic shock complicating acute myocardial infarction: a report from the SHOCK trial registry. SHould we emergently revascularize Occluded Coronaries for cardiogenic shocK? J Am Coll Cardiol. 2000 Sep;36(3 Suppl A):1077–83. [PMID: 10985708]

▶ Clinical Findings

A. History

The symptoms that precede the development of cardiogenic shock depend on the cause. Patients with acute MIs often have the typical history of acute onset of chest pain, possibly in the setting of known coronary artery disease. Often, however, patients seek medical care days later following unrecognized MIs once cardiogenic shock has developed. In such cases, there is no history of antecedent chest pain, but instead the insidious onset of dyspnea and weakness culminating in shock. Patients may be obtunded and lethargic as a result of decreased central nervous system perfusion. Mechanical complications of acute MI tend to occur several days to a week following the initial infarction but can occur earlier. They may be heralded by chest pain, but they more commonly present abruptly as acute dyspnea. Patients with arrhythmias may have a history of palpitations, presyncope, syncope, or a sensation of skipped beats. Regardless of the cause, however, by the time shock develops, the patient may be unable to give any useful history.

B. Physical Examination

The physical examination reveals signs consistent with hypoperfusion.

1. Vital signs—Hypotension is present (systolic blood pressure < 90 mm Hg). The heart rate is commonly elevated, and the respiratory rate is generally increased as a result of hypoxia from pulmonary congestion.

2. Neurologic—Patients may be confused, lethargic, or obtunded as a consequence of cerebral hypoperfusion.

3. Pulmonary—Patients may use accessory muscles of respiration and may have paradoxical respirations. The chest examination in most cases shows diffuse rales, often to the apices. Patients with isolated right ventricular infarction will not have pulmonary congestion.

4. Cardiovascular system—Jugular venous pulsations are commonly elevated. Peripheral pulses will be weak. The apical impulse is displaced in patients with dilated cardiomyopathies, and the intensity of heart sounds is diminished, especially in patients with pericardial effusions. A third or fourth heart sound suggesting significant left ventricular dysfunction and/or elevated filling pressures may be present. A mitral regurgitation murmur (holosystolic, usually at the apex) or a VSD murmur (harsh, holosystolic at the sternal border) can help in diagnosing these causes. Patients with a free wall rupture that is partially contained may have a pericardial friction rub. Patients with significant right heart failure may have signs on abdominal examination of liver enlargement with a pulsatile liver in the presence of significant tricuspid regurgitation.

5. Extremities—Peripheral edema may be present. Cyanosis and cool, clammy extremities are indicative of diminished tissue perfusion. Profound peripheral vasoconstriction can result in mottling of the skin (livedo reticularis).

C. Laboratory Findings

Patients with recent or acute MIs will have elevations in cardiac-specific enzymes (CPK-MB, troponin). Renal and hepatic hypoperfusion may result in elevations in serum creatinine and in transaminases (alanine transaminase [ALT] and aspartate transaminase [AST]). Coagulation abnormalities may be present in patients with hepatic congestion or hepatic hypoperfusion. An anion gap acidosis may be present and the serum lactate level may be elevated.

D. Diagnostic Studies

While further diagnostic studies are important in clarifying the diagnosis, it must be emphasized that rapid, definitive therapy should not be delayed once the diagnosis is apparent. In general, patients with cardiogenic shock and suspected acute MI should proceed to cardiac catheterization as quickly as possible.

1. Electrocardiography—The electrocardiogram (ECG) may be helpful in distinguishing between causes of cardiogenic shock. Patients with coronary disease and acute MI may show evidence of both old (Q waves) and new infarctions (ST segment elevation). Right-sided chest leads in patients with inferior MIs can detect the presence of a right ventricular infarction (ST elevation in V_4R). While ST elevations are often present on the ECGs of patients with cardiogenic shock, patients with non–ST-segment elevation MIs represent up to 50% of patients with cardiogenic shock. The ECG also readily aids in the diagnosis of arrhythmias contributing to cardiogenic shock.

2. Chest radiography—The chest radiograph may show an enlarged cardiac silhouette (cardiomegaly) and evidence of pulmonary congestion in patients with severe left ventricular failure. A VSD or severe mitral regurgitation associated with an acute infarction will lead to pulmonary congestion but not necessarily cardiomegaly. Findings of pulmonary congestion may be less prominent—or absent—in the case of predominantly right ventricular failure or in patients with superimposed hypovolemia.

3. Echocardiography—Given that it is noninvasive and able to be performed rapidly at the bedside, echocardiography is extremely useful in the diagnosis of cardiogenic shock. Furthermore, mechanical complications of an acute infarction can be readily diagnosed via echocardiography. Information obtained by echocardiography includes assessment of right and left ventricular size and function, valvular function (stenosis or regurgitation), right and left ventricular filling pressures, and the presence of pericardial fluid with tamponade.

4. Hemodynamic monitoring—Routine use of invasive pulmonary artery catheters in critically ill patients is controversial. However, this procedure is recommended in certain situations and can help in establishing the diagnosis and cause of cardiogenic shock. Catheters are usually placed from a central vein into the right heart and advanced into a pulmonary artery. By occluding flow temporarily in a branch of the pulmonary artery ("wedging" the catheter), an estimate of left atrial pressure can be obtained (the PCWP). The presence of a wedge pressure higher than 15 mm Hg in a patient with acute MI generally, but not always, indicates adequate intravascular volume. Patients with primarily right ventricular failure or significant superimposed hypovolemia may have cardiogenic shock with a normal or reduced PCWP. The presence of a large "v wave" on the PCWP tracing is consistent with significant mitral regurgitation, but may also be seen with a VSD or a very stiff left ventricle. A pulmonary artery catheter also allows calculation of the SVR. Hemodynamic criteria for cardiogenic shock vary and include a cardiac index of less than 2.2 L/min/m². (Cardiac index is preferred to cardiac output as a measure because it normalizes the cardiac output for body size.) It is important to note that some patients with chronic heart failure but not in cardiogenic shock have cardiac outputs in this range and are in fact ambulatory in a "compensated" state. Patients in cardiogenic shock usually have suffered an acute insult and cannot compensate.

5. Oxygen saturation—Invasive measurement of the mixed venous oxygen saturation can be obtained from pulmonary artery catheters and may be helpful in two ways. First, knowing the mixed venous oxygen saturation allows the arteriovenous difference in oxygen content to be calculated. The arteriovenous difference in oxygen content is inversely proportional to the cardiac output; it increases as more oxygen is extracted from the blood in the setting of low cardiac output. Serial determinations can be useful in monitoring a patient's course and response to therapy. Secondly, oxygen saturations obtained invasively with a pulmonary artery catheter may also be helpful in diagnosing a VSD. The shunting of oxygenated blood from the left ventricle to the right ventricle across the septal defect results in an abnormal "oxygen saturation step-up" when comparing oxygen saturations from the right atrium with those obtained from the right ventricle.

E. Left Heart (Cardiac) Catheterization

Left heart catheterization and invasive coronary angiography should be performed without delay in patients with ST-segment elevation MI, since survival and myocardial salvage depend on the time to reperfusion. This also applies to patients in cardiogenic shock with ST-segment elevation. In patients with cardiogenic shock without ST-segment elevation but with evidence of MI, cardiac catheterization should be expedited as well. In the cardiac catheterization laboratory, obstructions in coronary arteries or bypass grafts can be detected, appropriate treatments planned (either bypass surgery or percutaneous coronary intervention [PCI]) and an intra-aortic balloon pump (IABP) placed if necessary.

▶ Treatment

Although some general therapeutic considerations are applicable to all patients in cardiogenic shock, treatment is most effective when the cause is identified. In many situations, this identification allows rapid correction of the underlying problem. In fact, survival in most forms of shock requires a quick, accurate diagnosis. The patient is so critically ill that only prompt, directed therapy can reverse the process. The already high mortality rates in cardiogenic shock are even higher in patients for whom treatment is delayed. Therefore, although measures aimed at temporarily stabilizing the patient may provide enough time to start definitive therapy, potentially lifesaving treatment can be carried out only when the cause is known (Table 6–2).

A. Acute MI

In patients with cardiogenic shock caused by a large amount of infarcted or ischemic myocardium, the most effective treatment for decreasing mortality is prompt revascularization, with either PCI or coronary artery bypass grafting (CABG) surgery. A number of pharmacologic and nonpharmacologic measures may be helpful in stabilizing the patient prior to revascularization.

1. Ventilation-oxygenation—Because respiratory failure usually accompanies cardiogenic shock, every effort should

Table 6–2. Management of Cardiogenic Shock.

I. Diagnosis[1]
  A. Electrocardiogram
  B. Chest radiography
  C. Laboratory tests (complete blood count, coagulation profile, CK-MB, cardiac troponin, electrolytes + blood urea nitrogen/creatinine, arterial blood gases)
  D. Echocardiography
  E. Pulmonary artery catheterization (if diagnosis is in question, patient receiving inotropes/vasopressors, or patient is not responding to treatment)
  F. Cardiac catheterization
II. Treatment
  A. Oxygen supplementation; intubation, ventilation
  B. Vasopressors/inotropes; consider careful intravenous fluids, arterial line and pulmonary artery catheter insertion to guide management; correct underlying causes of acidemia
  C. Intra-aortic balloon pump, if needed
  D. For suspected acute MI: aspirin, heparin, urgent cardiac catheterization, revascularization (PCI, CABG); fibrinolysis if a delay in PCI is anticipated

[1]Patients with suspected acute MI should proceed directly to cardiac catheterization; this should generally not be delayed to facilitate additional diagnostic tests.
CABG, coronary artery bypass grafting; MI, myocardial infarction; PCI, percutaneous coronary intervention.

be made to ensure adequate ventilation and oxygenation. Adequate oxygenation is essential to avoid hypoxia and further deterioration of oxygen delivery to tissues. Patients with cardiogenic shock should receive supplemental oxygen and many require mechanical ventilation. Hypoventilation can lead to respiratory acidosis, which could exacerbate the metabolic acidosis already caused by tissue hypoperfusion. Acidosis worsens cardiac function and makes the heart less responsive to inotropic agents. A substantial proportion of the cardiac output in patients with cardiogenic shock is devoted to the "work of breathing," so mechanical ventilation is also advantageous in this regard.

2. Fluid resuscitation—Although hypovolemia is not the primary defect in cardiogenic shock, a number of patients may be relatively hypovolemic when shock develops following MI. The causes of decreased intravascular volume include increased hydrostatic pressure and increased permeability of blood vessels as well as patients simply being volume depleted for many hours. The physical examination may not always be helpful in determining the adequacy of the left ventricular filling pressure. In select patients, invasive monitoring with a pulmonary artery catheter can be helpful in determining the optimal volume status. Some patients with cardiogenic shock will actually have improved hemodynamics with slightly higher than normal filling pressures. Ventricular compliance is reduced in acute ischemia; the pressure–volume relationship changes such that cardiac output may be optimized at slightly higher filling pressures. In general, a PCWP of 18–22 mm Hg is considered adequate; further increases will lead to pulmonary congestion without a concomitant gain in cardiac output. Fluid administration, when indicated by low or normal PCWP, should be undertaken in 200–300 mL boluses of saline, followed by careful reassessment of hemodynamic parameters, especially cardiac output and PCWP, and generally should not be undertaken in patients with marginal oxygenation or in those not already mechanically ventilated.

3. Inotropic/vasopressor agents—A variety of drugs are available for intravenous administration to increase the contractility of the heart, the heart rate, and peripheral vascular tone. It is important to note that these agents also increase myocardial oxygen demand; improvements in hemodynamics and blood pressure therefore come at a cost, which can be deleterious in patients with ongoing ischemia. Furthermore, β-agonists can precipitate tachyarrhythmias and α-agonists can lead to dangerous vasoconstriction and ischemia in vital organ beds. When using these agents, attention should be given to the patient as a whole rather than focusing solely on a desired arterial pressure.

A. DIGOXIN—Although digoxin benefits patients with chronic congestive heart failure, it is of less benefit in cardiogenic shock because of its delayed onset of action and relatively mild potency (compared with other available agents).

B. β-ADRENERGIC AGONISTS—Dopamine is an endogenous catecholamine with qualitatively different effects at varying doses. At low doses (< 3 mcg/kg/min), it predominantly stimulates dopaminergic receptors that dilate various arterial beds, the most important being the renal vasculature. Although used frequently in low doses to improve renal perfusion, there is scant evidence to support the clinical usefulness of this strategy. Intermediate doses of 3–6 mcg/kg/min cause β_1-receptor stimulation and enhanced myocardial contractility. Further increases in dosage lead to predominant α-receptor stimulation (peripheral vasoconstriction) in addition to continued β_1 stimulation and tachycardia. Dopamine increases cardiac output, and its combination of cardiac stimulation and peripheral vasoconstriction may be beneficial as initial treatment of hypotensive patients in cardiogenic shock.

Dobutamine is a synthetic sympathomimetic agent that differs from dopamine in two important ways: It does not cause renal vasodilatation, and it has a much stronger β_2 (arteriolar vasodilatory) effect. The vasodilatory effect may be deleterious in hypotensive patients because a further drop in blood pressure may occur. On the other hand, many patients with cardiogenic shock experience excessive vasoconstriction with a resultant elevation in afterload (SVR) as a result of either the natural sympathetic discharge or the treatment with inotropic agents, such as dopamine, that also have prominent vasoconstrictor effects. In such patients, the combination of cardiac stimulation and decreased afterload with dobutamine may improve cardiac output without a loss of arterial pressure.

Other agents that are occasionally used include isoproterenol and norepinephrine. Isoproterenol is also a synthetic sympathomimetic agent. It has very strong chronotropic and inotropic effects, resulting in a disproportionate increase in oxygen consumption and ischemia. It is therefore not generally recommended for cardiogenic shock except occasionally for patients with bradyarrhythmias. Norepinephrine has even stronger α and β_1 effects than dopamine and may be beneficial when a patient continues to be hypotensive despite large doses of dopamine (more than 20 mcg/kg/min). Because of the intense peripheral vasoconstriction that occurs, perfusion of other vascular beds such as the kidney, extremities, and mesentery may be compromised. Therefore, norepinephrine should not be used for any extended time unless plans are made for definitive treatment.

4. Vasodilators—Vasodilation (especially of the arterioles to reduce SVR) can be effective in increasing cardiac output in patients with heart failure by countering the peripheral vasoconstriction caused by endogenous catecholamines. Although these agents have a role in treating acute, decompensated heart failure, they are rarely used in patients with cardiogenic shock given the risk of worsening hypotension. The IABP (see below) is generally more effective for reducing SVR without the risk of untoward hypotension.

5. Circulatory support devices—Among the mechanical devices developed to assist the left ventricle until more definitive therapy can be undertaken, the intra-aortic balloon pump (IABP) has been in use the longest and is the most well studied. The IABP is placed in the descending aorta, usually via the femoral artery. Its inflation and deflation are timed to the cardiac cycle (generally synchronized with the ECG). The balloon inflates in diastole immediately following aortic valve closure. The augmentation of diastolic pressure that occurs when the balloon inflates increases coronary perfusion as well as that of other organs. The balloon deflates at the end of diastole, immediately before left ventricular contraction, abruptly decreasing afterload and thereby enhancing left ventricular ejection. Unlike β-agonists, these benefits come without increases in myocardial demand.

Indications for use of the IABP include cardiogenic shock, especially when caused by ventricular septal rupture and acute mitral regurgitation. In both ventricular septal rupture and mitral regurgitation, the principle benefit is the decrease in afterload that occurs as the balloon deflates; this results in a larger fraction of the left ventricular volume being ejected forward into the aorta rather than into the left atrium (mitral regurgitation) or the right ventricle (ventricular septal rupture). An IABP should be placed as soon as possible in an effort to support these patients until emergency surgery can be performed. The most common side effects of the IABP are local vascular complications, but these have diminished substantially with the smaller caliber devices used currently. Nonrandomized data have shown that patients in cardiogenic shock treated with an IABP fare better than those not treated with an IABP.

A number of other circulatory support devices have been developed in recent years with the ability to provide even more circulatory support than the IABP. Devices can be implanted surgically (such as the left ventricular assist device or LVAD) or percutaneously, and are capable of creating flow rates of 3–5 L/min (close to a normal cardiac output). These devices can be used until cardiac transplantation can be facilitated, or occasionally to support patients who ultimately recover.

6. Revascularization—Revascularization, either by PCI or CABG surgery, decreases mortality in patients in whom cardiogenic shock develops following MI. The multicenter, randomized SHOCK trial (SHould we emergently revascularize Occluded Coronaries for cardiogenic shocK) showed a trend toward improved survival at 30 days in patients randomized to early revascularization (either PCI or CABG within 6 hours of enrollment). The survival benefit for early revascularization became significant at 6 months, a benefit that persisted to 6 years. Although the mortality of patients treated with a strategy of early revascularization was still high, the absolute reduction in mortality was substantial (13% at 1 year); stated alternatively, the "number needed to treat" with revascularization was approximately nine to prevent one death at 1 year, which is low and provides strong support for revascularization in these circumstances. Of note, patients 75 years of age and older did not benefit from revascularization at 1 year in the randomized trial but did benefit in the nonrandomized but much larger SHOCK registry. Many experts believe that the SHOCK trial was underpowered to show a mortality difference at 30 days and, based on the 6-month and now 6-year data, ACC/AHA guidelines recommend emergency revascularization for patients (especially those under the age of 75) with cardiogenic shock complicating acute MI.

A. PERCUTANEOUS CORONARY INTERVENTION—Patients undergoing PCI in the SHOCK trial had a similar benefit to those having bypass surgery. Mortality from cardiogenic shock has decreased over the past decade in parallel with increasing use of PCI for these patients. Although retrospective, other studies from large populations have shown that PCI use is associated with lower mortality in patients with cardiogenic shock.

B. CABG SURGERY—Despite the marked absolute reduction in mortality observed among patients treated with bypass surgery in the SHOCK trial, only a small proportion of patients with cardiogenic shock undergo urgent bypass surgery (approximately 3% in the National Registry of Myocardial Infarction 2004 database). Nevertheless, patients with multivessel disease in cardiogenic shock should be evaluated for bypass surgery, and for patients with mechanical complications of MI, surgery offers the best hope for survival at present.

7. Fibrinolytic therapy—Fibrinolytic therapy refers to treating patients with acute ST-segment elevation MIs with drugs that have fibrinolytic properties (that dissolve occlusive thrombus within coronary arteries or grafts). While PCI is superior therapy to fibrinolysis for ST-segment elevation MI, fibrinolysis is the recommended therapy if there will be a considerable delay in facilitating PCI. Most trials of fibrinolytic therapy excluded patients with cardiogenic shock. In earlier trials that included patients with cardiogenic shock, there was no benefit to fibrinolytic therapy over placebo. It has been suggested that the low flow state present in shock may contribute to the limited efficacy of fibrinolytic therapy. In contrast to these older studies, in the SHOCK trial and registry, patients treated medically with fibrinolytic therapy fared better than those medically treated without fibrinolytic therapy. Additional evidence comes from meta-analyses of more recent fibrinolytic trials that revealed improved survival among hypotensive patients treated with fibrinolytics. Current guidelines recommend fibrinolytic therapy for patients with an acute MI complicated by cardiogenic shock who cannot proceed directly to cardiac catheterization and PCI.

8. Other medical therapies—Aspirin and heparin are indicated in patients with MIs and cardiogenic shock, provided mechanical complications requiring surgery are not present. β-Blockers are contraindicated in patients in cardiogenic shock. Platelet IIb/IIIa inhibitors block the final pathway of platelet activation and aggregation and are beneficial in patients with acute coronary syndromes. Several clinical trials of IIb/IIIa inhibitors included patients with cardiogenic shock. Patients in cardiogenic shock treated with the IIb/IIIa inhibitor eptifibatide had improved survival in the PURSUIT trial, and patients in cardiogenic shock at presentation who undergo PCI and are treated with the IIb/IIIa inhibitor abciximab have improved survival. For patients who eventually stabilize and in whom hypotension is no longer a concern, most clinicians would recommend other medical therapies benefiting patients with heart failure including ACE inhibitors.

B. Mechanical Complications

Acute mitral regurgitation secondary to papillary muscle dysfunction, myocardial free wall rupture, and VSD are true emergencies. The definitive therapy for these catastrophes is surgical repair, although there are reports of using percutaneously placed devices to successfully repair VSDs. If the patient is to survive, all efforts must be made to get the patient to the operating room as soon as possible after the diagnosis is made. Pharmacologic agents and the IABP (see section on Circulatory Support Devices) are useful as temporizing measures.

C. Right Ventricular Infarction

Cardiogenic shock may occur with right ventricular MI and no or only minimal left ventricular dysfunction. Recent data have questioned the long-accepted notion that patients with shock from an islolated right ventricular MI have a better prognosis than those with primarily left ventricular dysfunction. In the SHOCK registry, patients with a right ventricular MI and shock fared similarly to those with primarily left ventricular dysfunction. Hemodynamic data suggesting right ventricular dysfunction out of proportion to left ventricular dysfunction and ST elevation in lead RV4 on a right-sided ECG are helpful in establishing the diagnosis, and assessment of right ventricular function on echocardiography can confirm the diagnosis. In cases of shock from right ventricular failure, initial treatment is aggressive fluid resuscitation to increase right ventricular preload and output. Significant amounts of fluid (1–2 L or more) may be required to develop an adequate preload for the failing right ventricle. Inotropic agents are usually necessary when the right ventricular failure is so profound that shock continues despite adequate volume administration, and the IABP may be helpful in this situation. Heart block is common in patients with right ventricular MIs. Patients with right ventricular infarction are relatively dependent on right atrial contraction. As a result, single-chamber right ventricular pacing may be inadequate in patients who require pacing, and atrioventricular sequential pacing may be required to improve cardiac output.

D. Arrhythmias

Arrhythmias contributing to cardiogenic shock are readily recognized with ECG monitoring and should be promptly treated. Tachyarrhythmias (ventricular tachycardia and supraventricular tachycardia) should be treated with electrical cardioversion in patients with hemodynamic compromise. Bradyarrhythmias may respond to pharmacologic agents (atropine, isoproterenol) in some circumstances, but external or transvenous pacing may be required.

Antoniucci D et al. Abciximab therapy improves survival in patients with acute myocardial infarction complicated by early cardiogenic shock undergoing coronary artery stent implantation. Am J Cardiol. 2002 Aug 15;90(4):353–7. [PMID: 12161221]

Barron HV et al. The use of intra-aortic balloon counterpulsation in patients with cardiogenic shock complicating acute myocardial infarction: data from the National Registry of Myocardial Infarction 2. Am Heart J. 2001 Jun;141(6):933–9. [PMID: 11376306]

Brodie BR et al. Comparison of late survival in patients with cardiogenic shock due to right ventricular infarction versus left ventricular pump failure following primary percutaneous coronary intervention for ST-elevation acute myocardial infarction. Am J Cardiol. 2007 Feb 15;99(4):431–5. [PMID: 17293178]

Dzavik V et al; SHOCK Investigators. Early revascularization is associated with improved survival in elderly patients with acute myocardial infarction complicated by cardiogenic shock: a report from the SHOCK trial registry. Eur Heart J. 2003 May;24(9):828–37. [PMID: 12727150]

Fang J et al. Trends in acute myocardial infarction complicated by cardiogenic shock, 1979–2003, United States. Am Heart J. 2006 Dec;152(6):1035–41. [PMID: 17161048]

Hasdai D et al. Platelet glycoprotein IIb/IIIa blockade and outcome of cardiogenic shock complicating acute coronary syndromes without persistent ST-segment elevation. J Am Coll Cardiol. 2000 Sep;36(3):685–92. [PMID: 10987585]

Hochman JS et al. Early revascularization and long-term survival in cardiogenic shock complicating acute myocardial infarction. JAMA. 2006 Jun 7;295(21):2511–5. [PMID: 16757723]

Hochman JS et al. One year survival following early revascularization for cardiogenic shock. JAMA. 2001 Jan 10;285(2):190–2. [PMID: 11176812]

Jacobs AK et al. Cardiogenic shock caused by right ventricular infarction: a report from the SHOCK registry. J Am Coll Cardiol. 2003 Apr 16;41(8):1273–9. [PMID: 12706920]

Martinez MW et al. Transcatheter closure of ischemic and post-traumatic ventricular septal ruptures. Catheter Cardiovasc Interv. 2007 Feb 15;69(3):403–7. [PMID: 17195200]

Sanborn TA et al. Impact of thrombolysis, intra-aortic balloon pump counterpulsation, and their combination in cardiogenic shock complicating acute myocardial infarction: a report from the SHOCK trial registry. SHould we emergently revascularize Occluded Coronaries for cardiogenic shocK? J Am Coll Cardiol. 2000 Sep;36(3 Suppl A):1123–9. [PMID: 10985715]

White HD et al. Comparison of percutaneous coronary intervention and coronary artery bypass grafting after acute myocardial infarction complicated by cardiogenic shock: results from the SHould we emergently revascularize Occluded Coronaries for cardiogenic shocK (SHOCK) trial. Circulation. 2005 Sep 27;112(13):1992–2001. [PMID: 16186436]

► Prognosis

Over the past 25 years, the prognosis of patients with cardiogenic shock has improved from over 80% in hospital mortality in the late 1970s to under 50% mortality in recent years. Revascularization (primarily PCI) appears to be the major contribution to improved outcomes. Demographic features associated with a better prognosis include younger age and male gender. Delayed time to revascularization predicts a worse outcome. Other clinical predictors of poorer outcome include a lower ejection fraction, extensive coronary disease, a left main or vein graft acute occlusion, higher heart rate, lower systolic blood pressure, and severe mitral regurgitation. Cardiac power (mean arterial pressure × cardiac output) was the strongest hemodynamic predictor of outcome in the SHOCK registry.

Fang J et al. Trends in acute myocardial infarction complicated by cardiogenic shock, 1979–2003, United States. Am Heart J. 2006;152(6):1035–41. [PMID: 17161048]

Fincke R et al. Cardiac power is the strongest hemodynamic correlate of mortality in cardiogenic shock: a report from the SHOCK trial registry. J Am Coll Cardiol. 2004 Jul 21;44(2):340–8. [PMID: 15261929]

Klein LW et al. Mortality after emergent percutaneous coronary intervention in cardiogenic shock secondary to acute myocardial infarction and usefulness of a mortality prediction model. Am J Cardiol. 2005 Jul 1;96(1):35–41. [PMID: 15979429]

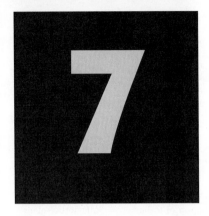

Aortic Stenosis

Blase A. Carabello, MD & Michael H. Crawford, MD

ESSENTIALS OF DIAGNOSIS

▶ Angina pectoris.

▶ Dyspnea (left ventricular heart failure).

▶ Effort syncope.

▶ Systolic ejection murmur radiating to the carotid arteries.

▶ Carotid upstroke delayed in reaching its peak and reduced in amplitude (parvus et tardus).

▶ Echocardiography shows thickened, immobile aortic valve leaflets.

▶ Doppler echocardiography quantifies increased transvalvular pressure gradient and reduced valve area.

▶ General Considerations & Etiology

Aortic stenosis is the narrowing of the aortic valve orifice, caused by failure of the valve leaflets to open normally. This reduction in orifice area produces an energy loss as laminar flow is converted to a less efficient turbulent flow, in turn increasing the pressure work that the left ventricle must perform in order to drive blood past the narrowed valve. The concentric left ventricular hypertrophy that develops as a major compensatory mechanism helps the left ventricle cope with the increased pressure work it must perform. These factors—turbulence, energy loss, and hypertrophy—constitute the pathophysiologic underpinnings for the patient's symptoms. The disease is confirmed through history and physical examination, Doppler echocardiography, and cardiac catheterization.

A. Bicuspid Aortic Valve

This is the most common congenital cardiac abnormality, occurring in approximately 2% of the population. It is believed that the bicuspid valve has hemodynamic disadvantages compared with the normal tricuspid valve, leading to

valvular degeneration by mechanisms that are still not fully understood. At least mild aortic stenosis develops in approximately 50% of all patients with bicuspid aortic valves, usually by age 50. Bicuspid aortic valve is associated with aortic dilatation and an increased risk of dissection and rupture, independent of any associated valve disease.

B. Tricuspid Aortic Valve Degeneration

Many patients born with normal tricuspid aortic valves eventually develop senile degeneration of the valve leaflets and leaflet calcification, thus producing valvular stenosis. Although hypercholesterolemia and diabetes have been defined as risk factors for this degeneration, these conditions account for only a small percentage of all cases. The mechanisms by which some valves degenerate and become stenotic while others remain relatively normal are unknown but are probably related to genetic polymorphisms.

C. Congenital Aortic Stenosis

Fusion of the valve leaflets before birth produces congenital aortic stenosis that is occasionally detected for the first time in adulthood. In many respects, however, congenital aortic stenosis appears to differ from acquired adult aortic stenosis. The hypertrophy in congenital aortic stenosis is more exuberant, yet heart failure symptoms. The first clinical manifestation of the disease can be sudden death without the development of premonitory symptoms in about 15% of patients.

D. Rheumatic Fever

Rheumatic fever still occasionally causes aortic stenosis in the United States, although this cause is more common in developing nations. Rheumatic heart disease almost never attacks the aortic valve in isolation, usually also affecting the mitral valve to some degree. A patient with aortic stenosis and a perfectly normal mitral valve is considered to have degenerative rather than rheumatic aortic stenosis.

E. Other Causes

Systemic lupus erythematosus, severe familial hypercholesterolemia, and ochronosis have occasionally been reported to cause valvular aortic stenosis.

Grotenhuis HB et al. Reduced aortic elasticity and dilatation are associated with aortic regurgitation and left ventricular hypertrophy in nonstenotic bicuspid aortic valve patients. J Am Coll Cardiol. 2007 Apr 17;49(15):1660–5. [PMID: 17433959]
O'Brien KD. Epidemiology and genetics of calcific aortic valve disease. J Investig Med. 2007 Sep;55(6):284–91. [PMID: 17963677]

▶ Clinical Findings

A. Symptoms and Signs

Angina, effort syncope, and congestive heart failure are the classic symptoms in patients with acquired aortic stenosis. Angina is the presenting symptom in approximately 35% of patients, effort syncope in 15%, and congestive heart failure in 50%. The onset of these symptoms heralds a dramatic increase in the mortality rate for these patients if aortic valve replacement is not performed. Symptoms are therefore the guidepost for intervention, and understanding them is key to understanding and managing the disease.

1. Angina—Angina occurs in response to myocardial ischemia, which develops when left ventricular oxygen demand exceeds supply. It should be noted that although epicardial coronary artery disease may coexist with aortic stenosis, angina frequently occurs in aortic stenosis in the absence of coronary artery disease.

As noted earlier, concentric left ventricular hypertrophy develops as a compensatory response to the pressure overload of aortic stenosis. The load on individual myocardial fibers can best be described as left ventricular wall stress and defined by the Laplace equation:

$$\text{Stress} = \frac{\text{pressure} \times \text{radius}}{2 \times \text{thickness}}$$

As left ventricular pressure increases, a parallel increase in left ventricular wall thickness (concentric hypertrophy) helps offset the pressure overload and maintain stress in the normal range. The left ventricular myocardium must produce stress in order to shorten; maintaining normal stress facilitates shortening. This compensatory mechanism is attended by negative pathophysiologic sequelae, however. Despite normal epicardial coronary arteries, the coronary blood flow is reduced; although the flow may be normal at rest, the reserve needed to offset increased oxygen demands during stress or exercise is inadequate, and thus ischemia develops. The exact mechanism by which the coronary blood flow reserve is reduced in aortic stenosis is uncertain, but low capillary density per unit of muscle is at least one operative factor.

Oxygen demand is best estimated clinically by the product of heart rate and wall stress. As noted earlier, the hypertrophy initially maintains wall stress in the normal range, and despite the pressure overload, myocardial oxygen demand is not increased. Eventually, however, the hypertrophy cannot keep pace with the pressure demands of the ventricle, and wall stress increases. This increases oxygen demand and is another factor contributing to ischemia and the symptoms of angina.

2. Effort syncope—In general, syncope results from inadequate cerebral perfusion. The syncope of aortic stenosis usually occurs during exercise. One theory for exertional syncope in aortic stenosis is that during exercise total peripheral resistance decreases, but cardiac output cannot increase as it normally does because the narrowed aortic valve restricts the output. Blood pressure is the product of peripheral resistance and cardiac output, so this imbalance causes a drop in blood pressure, leading to syncope.

Another theory is that the very high left ventricular pressure that develops during exercise triggers a reflexive vasodepressor response, leading to a fall in blood pressure. In addition, exercise can cause both ventricular and supraventricular arrhythmias, which in aortic stenosis lead to a fall in effective output and consequently a decrease in blood pressure.

3. Congestive heart failure—Both left ventricular systolic and diastolic failure occur in aortic stenosis and produce the symptoms of dyspnea on exertion as well as orthopnea and paroxysmal nocturnal dyspnea. In some patients, the attendant high left-sided filling pressure leads to pulmonary hypertension, which overloads the right ventricle and thereby produces right ventricular failure and the symptoms of edema and ascites.

Impaired diastolic left ventricular filling in aortic stenosis is primarily due to the increased wall thickness caused by concentric hypertrophy. Because the increased thickness makes the ventricle harder to fill, producing any left ventricular volume requires increased filling pressure. The increased diastolic filling pressure is referred to the left atrium and to the pulmonary veins, where pulmonary venous congestion develops, leading to increased lung water, increased lung stiffness, and dyspnea. The wall composition also changes. Collagen content increases (Figure 7–1), creating a compensatory mechanism that helps translate the increased force generated by the myocardium into chamber contraction. Unfortunately, the increase in collagen further increases ventricular stiffness.

Systole is governed by two mechanical properties: contractility and afterload. Contractility is the ability of the myocardium to generate force; afterload is the force the ventricle must overcome to contract. Either property can impair ventricular systole, and both are operative in aortic stenosis. Although the initial concentric hypertrophy normalizes wall stress (afterload), as the disease progresses, the hypertrophy may not keep pace with the increase in pressure and wall stress increases. As stress increases, ejection fraction (EF) decreases:

$$\text{EF} = \frac{\text{stroke volume}}{\text{end-diastolic volume}}$$

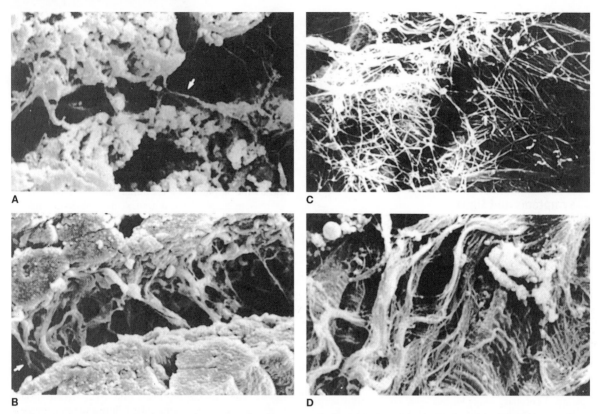

▲ **Figure 7–1.** Scanning electron microscopy of normal myocardium (**A** and **C**) and pressure-overloaded hypertrophied myocardium (**B** and **D**). **B** shows denser perimysial collagen connections in the hypertrophied myocardium (compared with **A, D** shows the thickened tendons in the hypertrophied myocardium (compare with normal myocardium in **C**). (Adapted, with permission, from Weber KT. J Am Coll Cardiol. 1989;13:1637.)

Reduced ejection fraction is more common in men than women. Inexplicably, women tend to generate more hypertrophy, keeping wall stress low and thus maintaining normal or even supernormal ejection fraction.

Ejection fraction may also decline if contractility falls; however, the exact mechanism of reduced contractility in aortic stenosis is unclear. In the simplest sense, reduced contractility is the result of prolonged overload on the heart. Loss of contractile elements and ischemia from abnormal coronary blood flow are two of the mechanisms that have been postulated to explain the reduction.

B. Physical Examination

1. Systolic ejection murmur—The classic murmur of aortic stenosis is a medium-pitched and often harsh systolic ejection murmur, heard best in the aortic area and radiating to the carotid arteries. In mild disease, the murmur peaks early in systole. As the disease worsens, the murmur peaks later, increases in intensity, and may be associated with a thrill palpated in the aortic area. With further progression of aortic

stenosis, the murmur peaks very late in systole. It may decrease in intensity as cardiac output begins to fall, and the thrill may disappear. In advanced but still correctable disease, the murmur may become very unimpressive and be reduced to a grade II/VI or even a grade I/VI murmur, sometimes misleading the examiner into believing that severe disease is not present.

Sometimes the murmur is heard well over the aortic area, fades over the midsternum, and reappears over the apex (Gallavardin phenomenon). The diagnostician may be misled into believing that two separate murmurs—one of aortic stenosis and one of mitral regurgitation—are present. Distinguishing between Gallavardin phenomenon and two separate murmurs is difficult but important: The appearance of even mild mitral regurgitation in aortic stenosis is an ominous prognostic sign. If the diagnosis cannot be settled at the bedside, color-flow Doppler examination of the mitral valve will resolve the issue.

2. Carotid upstroke—Carotid upstroke in aortic stenosis is typically low in volume and delayed in reaching the peak amplitude (Figure 7–2). Palpation of this **parvus et tardus**

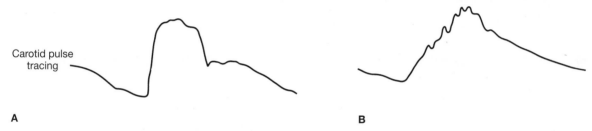

▲ **Figure 7–2. A:** A carotid pulse tracing from a normal subject. **B:** A tracing from a patient with aortic stenosis. The upstroke in **B** is quite delayed and demonstrates a shudder.

pulse is probably the single best way to estimate the severity of aortic stenosis at the bedside. The examiner should palpate his or her own carotid artery with one hand while palpating the patient's carotid artery with the other, thus gauging the difference between normal and abnormal. A palpable shuddering sensation of the carotid pulse may also be noted. In elderly patients, increased stiffness of the carotid arteries may falsely normalize the upstroke, making it feel relatively brisk in nature. Even in this circumstance, however, the upstroke is rarely completely normal in character.

3. Second heart sound—Paradoxic splitting of the second heart sound is due to the prolonged ejection time required to expel stroke volume through the stenotic valve, which delays the closure of the aortic valve (A_2) past closure of the pulmonic valve (P_2). Although paradoxic splitting is emphasized in many texts, a more common finding is that the reduced movement of the aortic valve renders A_2 inaudible and only a soft, single second sound (P_2) is heard.

4. Apical impulse—Because in aortic stenosis the left ventricle is usually concentrically hypertrophied and its volume is not increased, the point of maximum impulse is usually felt in its normal position. The apex beat, however, is abnormally forceful and sustained in nature. The left atrial contribution to left ventricular filling may be both visible and palpable; it corresponds to the fourth heart sound and is usually present in aortic stenosis as a result of increased left ventricular stiffness.

5. Other findings—In far-advanced disease with congestive heart failure, a third heart sound is often heard. Pulmonary hypertension may develop, increasing the intensity of the pulmonic component of the second sound. At their initial visit, patients with aortic stenosis may also have right ventricular failure manifested as edema and ascites.

C. Diagnostic Studies

1. Electrocardiography—The concentric left ventricular hypertrophy that develops in aortic stenosis is often reflected in the electrocardiogram (ECG) as increased QRS voltage, left atrial abnormality, and ST and T wave abnormalities. The ECG, however, does not always demonstrate left ventric-

ular hypertrophy even though the heart is actually hypertrophied. No ECG findings are, therefore, either sensitive or specific for aortic stenosis.

2. Chest radiography—Patients with aortic stenosis usually show a normal-sized heart on a chest radiograph. The left heart border may develop a rounded appearance consistent with concentric left ventricular hypertrophy; the aortic shadow may become enlarged because of post-stenotic dilation. Occasionally, calcification of the aortic valve can be seen on the lateral view.

3. Echocardiography—Echocardiographic examination of the heart combined with Doppler investigation of the aortic valve usually can confirm the diagnosis of aortic stenosis; a technically adequate study can accurately quantify its severity. Echocardiography shows thickening of the aortic valve, reduced leaflet mobility, and concentric left ventricular hypertrophy, demonstrating the presence of aortic stenosis but not quantifying its severity.

The Doppler study can be used to determine the gradient across the aortic valve and to calculate aortic valve area. Doppler quantification of aortic stenosis is based on the ability to measure blood velocity. Flow through an orifice is equal to cross-sectional orifice area times velocity. As shown in Figure 7–3, velocity must increase when a moving stream of a given flow reaches a narrowed area if the flow is to remain constant when it reaches the constriction. That is, the product of the velocity times area at the first orifice must be equal to that at the second orifice.

Measuring the area of the aortic outflow tract (A_1), the velocity of flow there (V_1), and the velocity at the stenosis (V_2), the aortic valve area (A_2) can be calculated as follows:

$$A_2 = \frac{A_1 \times V_1}{V_2}$$

The velocity of flow at the stenosis can also be used to calculate the aortic pressure gradient using the modified Bernoulli equation:

$$\text{Gradient} = 4V^2$$

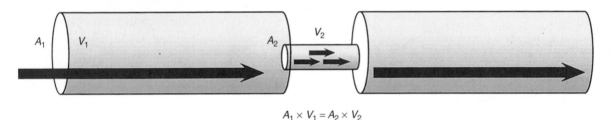

$$A_1 \times V_1 = A_2 \times V_2$$

▲ **Figure 7–3.** Constant flow through a tube of different diameters. As the flow reaches the narrowed orifice A_2, velocity must increase in order for the flow to remain constant.

Figure 7–4 shows the velocity profile from Doppler examination of a patient with aortic stenosis. The velocity of 4 m/s thus translates to a gradient of 64 mm Hg.

This technique is remarkably accurate compared with gradients measured invasively by catheter. In general, a mean gradient greater than 50 mm Hg or an aortic valve area less than 0.8 cm² indicates that the aortic stenosis is severe enough to cause the patient's symptoms. Many exceptions to this rule exist, however. Some patients remain asymptomatic despite higher gradients and smaller valve areas, and others become symptomatic with lower gradients and larger valve areas.

4. Cardiac catheterization—Although Doppler echocardiography is an accurate means of determining the severity of aortic stenosis in most patients, other noninvasive techniques are generally not recommended. Stress testing, for example, can be dangerous, and left-ventricular hypertrophy makes cardiac perfusion imaging and the interpretation of ECGs problematic. Cardiac catheterization (whose main purpose is coronary angiography) is indicated when symptoms such as angina pectoris could be caused by coronary disease or aortic stenosis or when valve replacement surgery is planned. The presence and severity of coronary disease will influence the course of therapy, tipping the balance toward surgery when the aortic stenosis is of borderline severity.

During cardiac catheterization, cardiac output and aortic valve gradient are measured; these data are used to assess stenosis severity by calculation of aortic valve area. Great care must be used in assessing both parameters because errors in estimating the stenosis will be proportional to any measurement errors. The cardiac output is measured using the Fick principle or the indicator-dilution principle (usually thermodilution). The gradient is obtained by placing one catheter in the left ventricle (by retrograde or transseptal technique) and a second catheter in the proximal aorta on the other side of the stenotic valve. The pressure difference (gradient) is measured by recording the two pressures simultaneously. Recent studies discredit the use of a femoral artery sheath to record the downstream pressure. Left ven-

tricular and femoral artery pressure waves occur at different times, so the tracings are aligned to compensate for this. This practice, however, may underestimate the true gradient by as much as 50%.

The cardiac output and gradient are then used to calculate the aortic valve area using the Gorlin formula:

$$AVA = \frac{CO(cm^3/min)/SEP \times HR}{44.3\sqrt{G}}$$

where AVA = aortic valve area, CO = cardiac output, G = mean aortic valve gradient, SEP = systolic ejection period (in seconds), and HR = heart rate. A valve area of less than 0.7–0.8 cm² usually indicates critical aortic stenosis, a severity of disease capable of causing symptoms, morbidity, and death. A symptomatic patient with a valve area of less than 0.8 cm² will usually require aortic valve replacement because the presence of symptoms connotes a poor prognosis and the constricted valve area suggests that the aortic stenosis is causing those symptoms. A caveat: Although the Gorlin formula is reasonably accurate in predicting the orifice area in severe disease, it was validated in patients with mitral—not aortic—stenosis. When used to calculate the aortic valve area, the Gorlin formula is flow-dependent; that is, the valve area varies directly with the flow. This dependence can be the result of the increased flow physically increasing the orifice; the increased calculated area and flow can also represent a problem with the formula. In either case, the calculated area depends on the patient's cardiac output at the moment. This is not a factor in severe disease with a large transvalvular gradient for which the formula almost always correctly predicts a critically narrowed valve. In some patients with very low cardiac outputs and low transvalvular gradients, however, the formula calculates a severely narrowed aortic valve area when no severe aortic stenosis is actually present. In such cases, increasing the cardiac output by infusion of dobutamine allows for recalculation of the valve area at a higher output. If the aortic valve area then exceeds 1.0 cm² or the gradient fails to increase markedly despite an increase in output, the stenosis is probably relatively mild and not the cause of the patient's symptoms

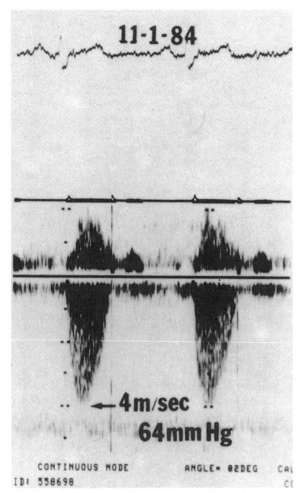

▲ Figure 7–4. The Doppler wave form; flow across a stenotic aortic valve. Flow accelerates to 4 m/s, which translates to a gradient of 64 mm Hg. (Adapted, with permission, from Assey et al. The patient with valvular heart disease. In: Pepine CJ, Hill JA, Lambert CR, eds. *Diagnostic and Therapeutic Cardiac Catheterization.* Philadelphia: Williams & Wilkins, 1998.)

or cardiac failure. Dobutamine infusion can be used with echocardiography or cardiac catheterization.

Valve resistance, which is simply the gradient divided by flow, is gaining credibility as another measure of stenosis severity. A resistance greater than 250 dynes × s × cm^{-5} probably indicates severe stenosis. Valve resistance (VR) is calculated using the following formula:

$$AR = \frac{Gradient \times HR \times SEP \ (in \ seconds) \times 1.33}{CO \ L/min}$$

and is expressed as dynes × s × cm^{-5}.

PATIENT EXAMPLES OF AORTIC STENOSIS—The following cases are examples of patients with varying degrees of aortic stenosis (PCW = pulmonary capillary wedge):

Case 1

Symptoms: angina, dyspnea
PCW: 16 mm Hg
CO: 4.5 L/min
HR: 70 bpm
SEP: 0.33 s
G: 72 mm Hg
EF: 55%

$$AVA = \frac{4500/(0.33 \times 70)}{44.37\sqrt{2}} = 0.52 \ cm^2$$

$$VR = \frac{70 \times 0.33 \times 72}{4.5} \times 1.33 = 492 \ dynes \cdot s \cdot cm^{-5}$$

Both calculations indicated severe aortic stenosis; the gradient was large and the patient symptomatic. Surgery was therefore mandatory because this patient undoubtedly suffered from severe symptomatic aortic stenosis.

Case 2

Symptoms: dyspnea, orthopnea
PCW: 26 mm Hg
CO: 3.3 L/min
HR: 70 bpm
SEP: 0.28 s
G: 30 mm Hg
EF: 30%

$$AVA = \frac{3300/(0.28 \times 70)}{44.3\sqrt{30}} = 0.70 \ cm^2$$

$$VR = \frac{70 \times 0.28 \times 30}{3.3} \times 1.33 = 237 \ dynes \cdot s \cdot cm^{-5}$$

In this case, the calculated aortic valve area indicated moderately severe aortic stenosis that required surgery; the valve resistance was borderline, suggesting the stenosis might be less severe. To evaluate the patient further, nitroprusside was cautiously infused and titrated. The repeat hemodynamics showed the following:

PCW: 16 mm Hg
CO: 4.5 L/min
HR: 80 bpm
SEP: 0.25 s
G: 30 mm Hg
AVA: 0.93 cm^2
VR: 177 dynes × s × cm^{-5}

Both indexes now indicated moderate—but not critical—aortic stenosis. That the disease was only moderate is further suggested by the lack of an increase in gradient when the cardiac output increased. It was also indicated by improvement in the hemodynamics with infusion of a vasodilator (which, in true aortic stenosis, could be expected to cause deterioration rather than improvement). In this case, an independent cardiomyopathy was probably responsible for the reduced ejection performance. The moderate aortic stenosis played a detrimental role but was not responsible for the patient's condition. He subsequently improved with long-term administration of an angiotensin-converting enzyme (ACE) inhibitor, a result that would not have been anticipated in severe outflow tract obstruction.

5. Cardiac computed tomography (CT)—The progression of aortic sclerosis (calcium deposits in the aortic valve) can be monitored by cardiac CT, and it can be used to quantify the amount of calcium in the aortic valve. However, there is poor correlation between valve calcium and the hemodynamic severity of aortic stenosis. One study has found that the severity of calcification of the valve in aortic stenosis is associated with worse clinical outcomes.

Attenhofer Jost CH et al. Echocardiography in the evaluation of systolic murmurs of unknown cause. Am J Med. 2000 Jun 1;108(8):614–20. [PMID: 10856408]

Freeman RV et al. Spectrum of calcific aortic valve disease: pathogenesis, disease progression, and treatment strategies. Circulation. 2005 Jun 21;111(24):3316–26. [PMID: 15967862]

Monin JL et al. Low-gradient aortic stenosis: operative risk stratification and predictors for long-term outcome: a multicenter study using dobutamine stress hemodynamics. Circulation. 2003 Jul 22;108(3):319–24. [PMID: 12835219]

Nishimura RA et al. Low-output, low-gradient aortic stenosis in patients with depressed left ventricular systolic function: the clinical utility of the dobutamine challenge in the catheterization laboratory. Circulation. 2002 Aug 13;106(7):809–13. [PMID: 12176952]

Phoon CK. Estimation of pressure gradients by auscultation: an innovative and accurate physical examination technique. Am Heart J. 2001 Mar;141(3):500–6. [PMID: 11231450]

Popovic AD et al. Echocardiographic evaluation of valvular stenosis: the gold standard for the next millennium? Echocardiography. 2001 Jan;18(1):59–63. [PMID: 11182784]

Rifkin RD. Physiological basis of flow dependence of Gorlin formula valve area in aortic stenosis: analysis using an hydraulic model of pulsatile flow. J Heart Valve Dis. 2000 Nov;9(6):740–51. [PMID: 11128779]

Rosenhek R et al. Predictors of outcome in severe, asymptomatic aortic stenosis. N Engl J Med. 2000 Aug 31;343(9):611–7. [PMID: 10965007]

▶ Treatment

The only effective therapy for severe aortic stenosis is relief of the mechanical obstruction posed by the stenotic valve. Figure 7–5 shows the natural course of aortic stenosis: Survivorship is excellent until the classic symptoms of angina, syncope, or congestive heart failure develop. At that point, survival declines sharply. Treatment includes such modalities as aortic balloon valvotomy, valve débridement, and valve replacement.

A. Pharmacologic Therapy

There is no effective pharmacologic treatment for severe aortic stenosis, and in some instances medication may be harmful. Although digitalis and diuretics may temporarily help improve congestive heart failure, unless the aortic valve is replaced, the heart failure will worsen and lead to death. It should also be noted that although ACE inhibitors prolong life in most cases of congestive heart failure, they are contraindicated in severe aortic stenosis. Vasodilators decrease total peripheral resistance, usually increasing cardiac output and providing a beneficial effect in other cardiac diseases. In severe aortic stenosis, however, because cardiac output across the stenotic valve cannot increase, the fall in total peripheral resistance leads to hypotension—which can be fatal. In milder disease (such as Case 2 [described earlier]) that is associated with other causes of heart failure, vasodilators can be used to treat the underlying independent cardiomyopathy. Nitrates can be used cautiously in severe disease to treat angina until surgery is performed. β-Adrenergic blocking agents must be used with great caution or avoided entirely: They may unmask the left ventricle's dependence on adrenergic support for pressure generation and thereby cause shock or heart failure.

Because patients with aortic stenosis share some risk factors with patients with atherosclerosis, there has been enthusiasm for using cholesterol lowering drugs to decrease the progression of aortic stenosis. Studies to date have shown mixed results. Clearly, if patients with aortic stenosis have elevated low-density lipoprotein (LDL) cholesterol levels, they should be treated.

The latest guidelines have eliminated the need for antibiotic prophylaxis in patients with aortic stenosis to prevent infective endocarditis except for prosthetic valves.

B. Aortic Balloon Valvuloplasty

This procedure involves a percutaneous catheterization in which a large-bore balloon is placed retrograde across the stenotic aortic valve. Inflating the balloon fractures calcium deposits in the leaflets and stretches the aortic annulus, increasing the valve area. Although the procedure is of some benefit in cases of congenital aortic stenosis, in which the leaflets are not calcified, the results in adults have been disappointing. The procedure produces no regression in left ventricular hypertrophy, the gradient is reduced acutely by only about 50%, and the valve area remains in the critical stenosis range. Six months after the procedure, 50% of the patients have completely lost even that modest benefit. The periprocedural mortality rate is 2–5%, and the ultimate mortality rate is the same as that of the natural course of the disease without intervention.

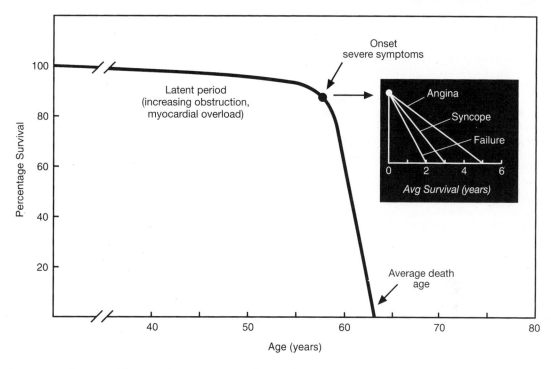

▲ **Figure 7–5.** The natural history of aortic stenosis. There is little change in survival until the symptoms of angina, syncope, or heart failure develop. Then the decline is precipitous. (Adapted, with permission, from Ross J Jr et al. Circulation. 1968;38(Suppl V):V-61.)

It is important that patients understand that balloon valvuloplasty is not an alternative to aortic valve replacement. Because the procedure produces only transient mild hemodynamic benefits at high risk and does not reduce the high mortality rate of untreated aortic stenosis, it should be considered only a palliative measure for patients whose other severe systemic illnesses preclude surgery. Occasionally, it may provide a bridge to surgery for severely symptomatic patients who need time to recover from another illness prior to aortic valve surgery.

C. Surgical Therapy

1. Aortic valve replacement

A. INDICATIONS—As noted earlier, survival in aortic stenosis drops sharply when the classic symptoms of angina, effort syncope, or congestive heart failure appear. Fifty percent of the patients with aortic stenosis in whom angina pectoris develops are dead within 5 years of its onset if aortic valve replacement is not undertaken. Half the patients with syncope will be dead within 3 years, and 50% of the patients with congestive heart failure will be dead within 2 years without surgical correction. The exact pathophysiologic changes that produce the onset of

symptoms and begin this rapid downhill course are unknown. It is known that in some cases the stenosis can worsen relatively rapidly, going from mild to severe in a year or two. Worsening stenosis increases the pressure overload on the left ventricle, which presumably reaches a point of decompensation manifested as the onset of symptoms.

Recent studies confirm the benignity of the asymptomatic state in aortic stenosis. In asymptomatic patients with proven peak Doppler gradients equal to or greater than 50 mm Hg, the incidence of sudden death is less than 1% per year. Therefore, surgery is generally not indicated for asymptomatic patients with aortic stenosis. The surgical mortality is at least 2–3%, and even this low figure cannot be justified in the absence of symptoms. However, outcomes in asymptomatic patients vary widely. Some evidence suggests that those with severe valve calcification or rapidly increasing valvular velocity on repeated Doppler studies have a poor prognosis and perhaps should be considered for surgery despite a lack of symptoms.

It must be made clear, however, that benignity of the asymptomatic condition pertains only to adult-acquired aortic stenosis. Children in whom the disease has been present from birth respond differently, and sudden death in the absence of symptoms is common. Asymptomatic children with aortic stenosis should probably undergo surgery once a peak gradient of 75 mm Hg develops, and sooner if symptoms are present.

The mortality rate in adults rapidly increases to about 5% within 3 months of the onset of symptoms and is a remarkable 75% in 3 years if surgical correction is not undertaken. Adults with aortic stenosis should be operated on shortly after the development of symptoms. A reasonable strategy for patients with asymptomatic aortic stenosis is to obtain an initial Doppler echocardiographic study. If the mean gradient is more than 30 mm Hg, the patient should undergo a history and physical examination every 6 months—with instructions to alert the physician immediately if symptoms occur. When close questioning reveals that symptoms have developed, the Doppler echocardiographic study can be repeated to confirm that the aortic stenosis has worsened. If the patient is in the coronary-disease-prone age range, cardiac catheterization to confirm the hemodynamics and to define coronary anatomy should be performed at that time, with an eye toward aortic valve replacement in the near future.

B. In advanced disease—Because aortic valve replacement instantaneously reduces afterload by removing or substantially reducing the pressure gradient, left ventricular performance improves immediately. Thus, patients with far-advanced disease and severe congestive heart failure may respond to aortic valve replacement with a dramatically rapid improvement following surgery. Even patients with ejection fractions of less than 20% may experience a doubling in both ejection fraction and forward output, with a reduction in filling pressures and pulmonary edema early after aortic valve replacement. Over time, left ventricular hypertrophy regresses, contractile function may improve, and ejection fraction may return completely to normal—even though it was profoundly depressed before surgery (Figure 7–6). Therefore, even when the disease is far advanced and is attended by severe congestive heart failure, it is almost never too late to perform aortic valve replacement for patients with aortic stenosis except, of course, when it is inappropriate.

C. Contraindications—The amount of afterload reduction that can be effected by removing the aortic valve obstruction is proportional to the gradient. In patients with a low mean transvalvular gradient, the increase in ejection fraction and cardiac output that occurs after surgery is limited because afterload reduction is limited. In fact, most patients with a low transvalvular gradient (< 30 mm Hg) and far-advanced heart failure do not improve following aortic valve replacement. It is also clear, however, that some patients do improve—even dramatically—despite a low gradient. Why some patients improve and most do not is currently unknown. Unfortunately, at this time, the outcome for the patient with a low gradient and far-advanced heart failure cannot be predicted. What is known is that such patients are at high risk when undergoing aortic valve

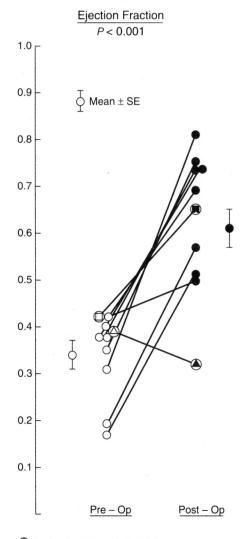

▲ **Figure 7–6.** The effect of aortic valve replacement on preoperatively depressed ejection fraction. With the exception of one patient who suffered an intraoperative myocardial infarction, all patients demonstrated improved ejection fraction as afterload was reduced following surgery. (Adapted, with permission, from Smith N et al. Circulation. 1978;58:255.)

replacement, and such patients need to be advised of the precarious nature of the surgery if it is undertaken.

D. Effects of age—Age should not be considered a major factor when deciding if surgery should be undertaken. Although advanced age increases the risks of surgical mortality and postsurgical morbidity, it must be recognized that age is a risk factor in even apparently healthy patients without aortic stenosis. Once age is corrected for, the mortality rate following aortic valve replacement surgery for aortic stenosis approaches that of the normal population for that age range. In fact, aortic valve replacement for aortic stenosis in patients older than age 65 is one of the few conditions where cardiac surgery returns the patient to the expected longevity of the general population of that age range.

E. BENEFITS—Replacement of the aortic valve removes or greatly reduces the pressure overload placed on the left ventricle by aortic stenosis. Left ventricular systolic pressure and afterload are significantly reduced, leading to improved ejection performance and cardiac output and reduced left ventricular filling pressure. Subsequently, the left ventricular hypertrophy regresses, most of it in the first year following surgery; full regression, however, may not occur for as long as a decade. The abnormal coronary blood flow and blood flow reserve caused by aortic stenosis also improve as the hypertrophy regresses. Although diastolic function improves as the wall thins, it may not completely return to normal because the increased collagen content (see Figure 7–1) that developed in response to the pressure overload does not regress fully. A persistently increased collagen content causes the left ventricular stiffness to be greater than normal.

F. TECHNIQUES—Aortic valve replacement can be accomplished using the patient's own pulmonic valve, a bioprosthesis, or a mechanical prosthesis. Each has its own inherent risks and benefits.

(1) Pulmonic valve transplantation (Ross procedure)— In this procedure, the patient's native pulmonic valve (autograft) is removed and sewn into the aortic position. A prosthetic valve or a pulmonic homograft is then sewn into the pulmonic position. This maneuver improves the patient's condition because the native, viable pulmonic valve with its excellent hemodynamic characteristics and durability is sewn into the high-pressure, high-stress, left-sided circuit where prostheses can fail. The bioprosthesis or homograft placed in the pulmonic position is under low pressure and low stress; it is more durable here than it would be in the aortic position.

The major disadvantage of the pulmonic autograph is the amount of surgery involved. It is a technically very demanding procedure and, although excellent results have been reported from a few centers, it may not be applicable to every hospital's surgical program.

(2) Bioprostheses—Two general types of bioprostheses are available: heterografts and homografts. Heterografts are constructed from either porcine aortic valve leaflets or bovine pericardium (both preserved with glutaraldehyde). Heterografts have had a wide application, and much is known about their advantages and disadvantages. The major advantage of this bioprosthesis is its low thromboembolic potential. In the absence of atrial fibrillation, the risk of

thromboembolism following aortic valve bioprosthetic implantation is less than 1 event per 100 patient years, and anticoagulation is not required. Atrial fibrillation substantially increases thromboembolic risk, as it does in patients with native valves. In the absence of a contraindication, anticoagulation is therefore probably advisable in patients with atrial fibrillation. Anticoagulation is unnecessary in patients with normal sinus rhythm.

The major disadvantage of heterografts is their limited durability. Primary valve failure occurs in only 10% of patients 10 years following implantation of a bioprosthesis in the aortic position, but valve failure rapidly accelerates after that period; approximately 50% of valves have failed within 15 years. Calcification and degeneration of the valves leads to tears in the cusps or stenosis of the valve or flail leaflets. Degeneration is greatly accelerated in younger patients, and heterograft bioprostheses should not be used in patients younger than 35 years of age—except for young women who wish to become pregnant. Because anticoagulation with warfarin produces an unacceptable rate of fetal mortality, valve replacement with a bioprosthesis that does not require anticoagulation may be preferable. The patient must understand, however, that a second valve replacement will probably be required.

A second disadvantage to bioprosthesis is a modest obstruction to outflow and a residual pressure gradient in patients requiring implantation of small valves.

The ideal patient for heterograft bioprosthesis implantation is the elderly patient whose life expectancy is less than the durability span of the valve or the patient for whom anticoagulation poses a significant risk.

Cryopreserved homografts, which are harvested from human donors, have an excellent hemodynamic profile. They are ideal for use in patients with a small aortic root where other types of prostheses might cause a transvalvular gradient. They are also relatively resistant to bacterial endocarditis. Although homografts may be more durable than heterograft valves, long-term follow-up data on large numbers of cryopreserved homografts are currently unavailable. In addition, the use of homograft valves is limited by availability. Because many potential donors for homograft valves are also whole-heart donors, the number of available homografts is small.

(3) Mechanical valves—Compared with bioprostheses, mechanical valves, such as the bileaflet valve, have superior durability. All mechanical valves require anticoagulation, however. Thromboembolic complications possible in the absence of anticoagulation include stroke and fixation of the valve in either the open or closed position. With proper anticoagulation, these events are reduced to 1 event per 100 patient years; the risk of anticoagulant hemorrhage is approximately 0.5%/year. Anticoagulation therapy should be targeted to maintain the prothrombin time at 1.5 times control (international normalized ratio [INR] 2.5–3.5). Mechanical valves are typically implanted in younger patients for whom long-term durability is important and in whom anticoagula-

tion can be accomplished at lower risk than in elderly patients. Although caged-ball and tilting-disk valves were popular in the twentieth century, the bileaflet valves are most commonly used today.

2. Aortic valve débridement—Both mechanical and ultrasonic débridement of the aortic valve to remove calcium deposits and increase leaflet mobility have met with limited success in calcific aortic stenosis. Surgical débridement usually results in significant residual stenosis that worsens in time. Ultrasonic débridement, using sound waves to pulverize the calcium deposits, dramatically reduces the aortic valve gradient and produces excellent results 6 months after surgery. Unfortunately, aortic insufficiency develops in many patients shortly thereafter as the integrity of the leaflets is impaired. Most current data suggest either mechanical or ultrasonic débridement is a poor alternative to aortic valve replacement.

The development of new techniques for engaging the patient with the heart–lung pump and stabilizing the heart during surgery have allowed for heart operations through limited thoracic incisions. Although results similar to conventional sternotomy have been reported for aortic valve surgery in some centers, total surgical time, pump time, and aorta cross-clamp time are significantly increased. On the other hand, patients appreciate the smaller incisions. Whether these minimally invasive approaches will replace conventional techniques is not clear at this time.

Recently, a collapsible bioprosthetic valve mounted in a large stent has been deployed percutaneously for aortic stenosis. Although often successful, some have failed to stay put and damage to the left-sided conduction system can occur. Currently, such devices are experimental, but improvements with experience will eventually result in a percutaneous alternative to aortic valve surgery.

Aikawa K et al. Timing of surgery in aortic stenosis. Prog Cardiovasc Dis. 2001 May–Jun;43(6):477–93. [PMID: 11431802]

Connolly HM et al. Severe aortic stenosis with low transvalvular gradient and severe left ventricular dysfunction: result of aortic valve replacement in 52 patients. Circulation. 2000 Apr 25;101(16):1940–6. [PMID: 10779460]

Cowell SJ et al; Scottish Aortic Stenosis and Lipid Lowering Trial Impact on Regression (SALTIRE) Investigators. A randomized trial of intensive lipid-lowering therapy in calcific aortic stenosis. N Engl J Med. 2005 Jun 9;352(23):2389–97. [PMID: 15944423]

Cribier A et al. Early experience with percutaneous transcatheter implantation of heart valve prosthesis for the treatment of end-stage inoperable patients with calcific aortic stenosis. J Am Coll Cardiol. 2004 Feb 18;43(4):698–703. [PMID: 14975485]

Moura LM et al. Rosuvastatin affecting aortic valve endothelium to slow the progression of aortic stenosis. J Am Coll Cardiol. 2007 Feb 6;49(5):554–61. [PMID: 17276178]

Oswalt JD et al. Highlights of a 10-year experience with the Ross procedure. Ann Thorac Surg. 2001 May;71(5 Suppl):S332–5. [PMID: 11388217]

Pereira JJ et al. Survival after aortic valve replacement for severe aortic stenosis with low transvalvular gradients and severe left ventricular dysfunction. J Am Coll Cardiol. 2002 Apr 17;39(8):1356–63. [PMID: 11955855]

Pessotto R et al. Midterm results of the Ross procedure. Ann Thorac Surg. 2001 May;71(5 Suppl):S336–9. [PMID: 11388218]

Pierri H et al. Clinical predictors of prognosis in severe aortic stenosis in unoperated patients > or = 75 years of age. Am J Cardiol. 2000 Oct 1;86(7):801–4. [PMID: 11018208]

Rosenhek R et al. Predictors of outcome in severe, asymptomatic aortic stenosis. N Engl J Med. 2000 Aug 31;343(9):611–7. [PMID: 10965007]

Sundt TM et al. Quality of life after aortic valve replacement at the age of > 80 years. Circulation. 2000 Nov 7;102(19 Suppl 3):III70–4. [PMID: 11082365]

▶ **Prognosis**

As noted earlier, the natural course and thus the prognosis of unoperated aortic stenosis are widely known. Once symptoms develop, aortic stenosis becomes a lethal disease with a 3-year mortality rate of 75%. Figure 7–7 compares the mortality rate of two groups of patients with symptomatic aortic stenosis: those who refused surgery, and patients who underwent it. The difference is dramatic. Overall, the 10-year

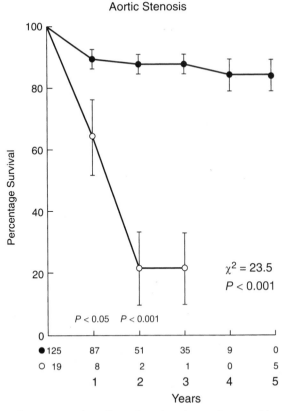

▲ **Figure 7–7.** The effect of aortic valve replacement in patients with symptomatic severe aortic stenosis (solid circle) compared with the survivorship of similar patients who refused surgery (open circle). (Adapted, with permission, from Schwarz F et al. Circulation. 1982;66:1105.)

survival rate following aortic valve replacement for pure aortic stenosis is 75%. The age-adjusted survivorship after surgery remains excellent even in octogenarians free of other cardiac or systemic diseases.

Asymptomatic patients generally have a good prognosis; however, symptoms will develop within 5 years in most patients with hemodynamically significant aortic stenosis, and the risk of sudden death will be 1% per year. Certain factors, such as reduced left ventricular ejection fraction, an enlarged left ventricle, and severe valve calcification, are known to reduce patient's survival. Also, patients with hypercholesterolemia, hypercalcemia, or elevated serum creatinine tend to progress more rapidly and should be monitored closely. Whether progressive stenosis can be delayed or halted by altering cholesterol levels or other biologic factors is unknown.

A. Coincident Disease

Coronary artery disease is the single most important coincident disease that affects the prognosis of aortic stenosis. Figure 7–8 shows that the prognosis for patients with aortic stenosis and coronary disease worsens almost immediately following surgery, compared with the prognosis of corrected isolated aortic stenosis. Coronary bypass surgery may improve this prognosis, but this point is controversial. What is not controversial is that even with complete revascularization the prognosis of combined aortic stenosis and coronary disease does not equal that of isolated aortic stenosis. Some experts have advocated correcting only the aortic stenosis in patients with combined disease because the addition of coronary bypass grafting has not been clearly shown to prolong survival. These results, however, were acquired before the more recent extensive use of artery grafts, which are superior to vein grafts. Modern results may be better.

Therefore, because there is no definitive answer regarding the efficacy of combined coronary bypass grafting and aortic valve replacement, grafting seems prudent when angina is one of the patient's symptoms or when left-main or three-vessel disease is present.

Acquired von Willebrand syndrome (type 2A) is observed in most patients with severe aortic stenosis and is associated with increased skin or mucosal bleeding in about 20%. Hemostatic abnormalities often disappear the first day after valve replacement surgery suggesting that they are related to high shear stress. These abnormalities can recur if there is a mismatch between patient and prosthesis size. Patients with severe aortic stenosis are at risk for bleeding before and during surgery, especially if they have Heyde syndrome with gastrointestinal angiodysplasia.

B. Follow-up

Implantation of a prosthetic heart valve is not curative. The severe risks of native valve aortic stenosis have instead been exchanged for the lesser risks inherent to prosthetic valves. Lifelong regular follow-up of patients with prostheses is therefore required. If anticoagulation therapy is used, periodic surveillance of the prothrombin time is needed, and alterations in dosage must be made to maintain it at 1.5 times control. The prothrombin time should be tested at least once a month and more frequently if a stable dose of warfarin and the degree of anticoagulation have not yet been obtained. Many avoidable complications of prostheses result from improper anticoagulation.

Endocarditis prophylaxis is more important in the presence of a prosthetic valve than in the presence of an abnormal native valve. Infection of a prosthesis is often fatal, and even when the infection is cured, the valve almost always requires re-replacement. Prevention of prosthetic valve endocarditis

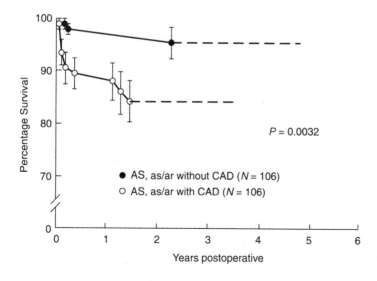

▲ **Figure 7–8.** The effects of coronary disease (open circle) on survivorship of patients with aortic stenosis (AS) or aortic stenosis and regurgitation (as/ar) following surgery shown and compared with that of isolated AS or as/ar (solid circle). CAD, coronary artery disease. (Adapted, with permission, from Miller DC et al. Am J Cardiol. 1979;43:494.)

by antibiotic administration before and after dental and other surgery is therefore advised.

Implantation of a prosthesis makes the Doppler echocardiographic evaluation of valve function difficult. Although acoustic shadowing around the prosthesis hinders echocardiographic and Doppler interpretation, each valve has a characteristic Doppler profile that should be recorded early following surgery. If subsequent symptoms of congestive heart failure or syncope develop, another ultrasound study can be made for comparison. A significant deviation from the initial study may indicate that prosthetic stenosis or regurgitation is now present and responsible for the recurrence of the patient's symptoms. Transesophageal echocardiography is usually better able to visualize morphologic details of a prosthetic valve than transthoracic echocardiography and is indicated for suspected valve failure, thrombosis, or endocarditis. Cinefluoroscopy is also useful for assessing valve motion and diagnosing leaflet or ball-motion abnormalities. The suspicion of valve dysfunction is usually confirmed by cardiac catheterization. It should be noted, however, that when prosthetic stenosis is suspected, the gradient across the valve may be difficult to obtain invasively. Retrograde passage of the catheter across a tilting disk valve may result in catheter entrapment, a potentially fatal complication. Retrograde passage of a catheter across a bileaflet valve may damage the leaflets; this practice should be avoided. Transseptal catheterization is often the safest way to obtain a transvalvular gradient if prosthetic aortic valve stenosis is suspected.

Palta S et al. New insights into the progression of aortic stenosis: implications for secondary prevention. Circulation. 2000 May 30;101(21):2497–502. [PMID: 10831524]

Pellikka PA et al. Outcome of 622 adults with asymptomatic hemodynamically significant aortic stenosis during prolonged follow-up. Circulation. 2005 Jun 21;111(24):3290–5. [PMID: 15956131]

Rossi A et al. Echocardiographic prediction of clinical outcome in medically treated patients with aortic stenosis. Am Heart J. 2000 Nov;140(5):766–71. [PMID: 11054623]

Veyradier A et al. Abnormal von Willebrand factor in bleeding angiodysplasias of the digestive tract. Gastroenterology. 2001 Feb;120(2):346–53. [PMID: 11159874]

Vincentelli A et al. Acquired von Willebrand syndrome in aortic stenosis. N Engl J Med. 2003 Jul 24;349(4):343–9. [PMID: 12878741]

Aortic Regurgitation

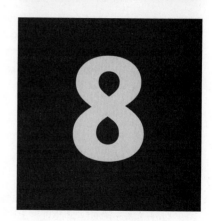

William A. Zoghbi, MD, FASE, FACC
& Michael H. Crawford, MD

ESSENTIALS OF DIAGNOSIS

- Following a long asymptomatic period, presentation with heart failure or angina.
- Wide pulse pressure with associated peripheral signs.
- Diastolic decrescendo murmur at the left sternal border.
- Left ventricular dilation and hypertrophy with preserved function.
- Presentation and findings dependent on the rapidity of onset of regurgitation.
- Diagnosis confirmed and severity estimated by Doppler echocardiography, aortography, magnetic resonance imaging, or computed tomography angiography.

Etiology

Normally, the integrity of the aortic orifice during diastole is maintained by an intact aortic root and firm apposition of the free margins of the three aortic valve cusps. Aortic regurgitation (AR) may therefore be caused by a variety of disorders affecting the valve cusps or the aortic root (or both) (Table 8–1). With rheumatic heart disease becoming less common, nonrheumatic causes currently account for most of the underlying causes of aortic insufficiency, including congenitally malformed aortic valves, infective endocarditis, and connective tissue diseases. Disorders affecting the aortic root also account for a large number of patients with AR. These conditions include cystic medial necrosis, Marfan syndrome, aortic dissection, and inflammatory diseases. Even in the absence of any obvious abnormality of the aortic valve or root, severe systemic hypertension has been reported to cause significant AR.

Roberts WC et al. Causes of pure aortic regurgitation in patients having isolated aortic valve replacement at a single US tertiary hospital (1993 to 2005). Circulation. 2006 Aug 1;114(5):422–9. [PMID: 16864725]

Pathophysiology

The presentation and findings in patients with AR depend on its severity and rapidity of onset. The hemodynamic effects of acute severe AR are entirely different from the chronic type and the two will be discussed separately.

A. Chronic Aortic Regurgitation

In response to the left ventricular volume overload associated with AR, progressive left ventricular dilation occurs. This results in a higher wall stress, which stimulates ventricular hypertrophy and which, in turn, tends to normalize wall stress. Patients with severe AR may have the largest end-diastolic volumes produced by any other heart disease and yet, their end-diastolic pressures are not uniformly elevated. In keeping with the Frank-Starling mechanism, the stroke volume is also increased. Thus, despite the presence of regurgitation, a normal effective forward cardiac output can be maintained. This state persists for several years. Gradually, left ventricular diastolic properties and contractile function start to decline. The adaptive dilation and hypertrophy can no longer match the loading conditions. The left ventricular end-diastolic pressure begins to rise and the ejection fraction drops with a decline in effective forward output and development of heart failure.

B. Acute Aortic Regurgitation

In contrast to chronic AR, when sudden severe regurgitation occurs, the left ventricle has no time to adapt. The acute ventricular volume overload therefore results in a small increase in end-diastolic volume and severe elevation of end-diastolic pressure, which is transmitted to the left atrium and pulmonary veins, culminating in acute pulmonary edema. Because the ventricular end-diastolic volume is normal, the total stroke volume is not increased and the effective forward cardiac output drops. To compensate for the low output state, sympathetic stimulation occurs, which produces tachycardia and peripheral vasoconstriction, the latter further worsening AR.

Table 8–1. Causes of Aortic Regurgitation.

Aortic cusp abnormalities
  Infectious: Bacterial endocarditis, rheumatic fever
  Congenital: Bicuspid aortic valve, Marfan syndrome
  Inflammatory: Systemic lupus erythematosus, rheumatoid arthritis,
    Beçhet syndrome
  Degenerative: Myxomatous (floppy) valve, calcific aortic valve
  Trauma
  Postaortic valvuloplasty
  Diet drug valvulopathy
Aortic root abnormalities
  Aortic root dilatation: Marfan syndrome, syphilis, ankylosing
    spondylitis, relapsing polychondritis, idiopathic aortitis, annu-
    loaortic ectasia, cystic medial necrosis, Ehlers-Danlos syndrome
  Loss of commissural support: Aortic dissection, trauma, ventricular
    septal defect
Increased afterload
  Systemic hypertension
  Supravalvular aortic stenosis

▶ Clinical Findings

A. Symptoms and Signs

1. Chronic aortic regurgitation—Patients with chronic AR remain asymptomatic for a long time. Palpitations are common and may be due to either awareness of forceful left ventricular contractions or occurrence of premature atrial or ventricular beats. Angina may occur either from concomitant coronary disease or from a combination of low diastolic pressure and increased oxygen demand from ventricular hypertrophy. When left ventricular dysfunction supervenes, patients initially experience exertional dyspnea and fatigue. At a later stage, resting heart failure symptoms occur with orthopnea and paroxysmal nocturnal dyspnea.

On physical examination, visible cardiac pulsations are common. The area of the apical impulse is increased on palpation and is displaced caudally and laterally. The first heart sound is usually normal. The aortic component of the second heart sound may be decreased in conditions where cusp excursion is reduced, such as with valve calcification. An S_4 is often present due to underlying hypertrophy, and an S_3 is audible when ventricular failure occurs. On auscultation, the characteristic sound of AR is a soft, high-pitched diastolic decrescendo murmur best heard in the third intercostal space along the left sternal border at end expiration, with the patient sitting and leaning forward. In the presence of aortic root disease, the murmur may be best heard to the right of the sternum. A systolic ejection murmur may be present at the aortic area due to the high flow state. Occasionally, a diastolic rumble may be heard at the apex, referred to as the Austin Flint murmur. The mechanism underlying this murmur remains unclear. A number of different causes have been proposed, the most recent being

the aortic jet encountering the mitral inflow resulting in turbulence.

The systolic arterial pressure is increased due to a large stroke volume, whereas the diastolic pressure is decreased due to runoff from the aorta into both the ventricle and peripheral arteries. This is the underlying reason for a wide pulse pressure and for a variety of associated peripheral signs in chronic significant AR (Table 8–2). However, it must be remembered that these signs are not specific for AR and may occur in any high flow state such as occurs in anemia, thyrotoxicosis, and arteriovenous malformations. With the development of heart failure, the pulse pressure narrows and the peripheral signs of AR are attenuated.

2. Acute aortic regurgitation—In contrast to chronic AR, most patients with acute severe AR are symptomatic. Initial presentation may vary depending on the underlying cause, which most commonly is aortic dissection, infective endocarditis, or trauma. In the presence of associated acute AR, clinical manifestations of severe dyspnea, orthopnea, and weakness often develop. The onset of symptoms is sudden, with rapid progression to hemodynamic collapse if left untreated.

In acute AR, the left ventricle has had no time to adapt to the volume overload state. The peripheral signs associated with chronic AR are therefore absent. Pulse pressure is usually normal, and hypotension may be present in severe cases. Bilateral rales are usually present on examination of the lungs and reflect underlying pulmonary edema. On precordial palpation, the apical impulse is not shifted. The first heart sound may be soft or absent due to the premature closure of the mitral valve. An S_3 is often present, but an S_4 is usually absent because there is little or no atrial contribution to ventricular filling due to high left ventricular end-diastolic pressure. The typical diastolic murmur of AR is shortened in duration, often difficult to hear, and easily missed.

Table 8–2. Peripheral Signs of Aortic Regurgitation.

Name of Sign	Description
Corrigan pulse	Rapid and forceful distention of arterial pulse with quick collapse
De-Musset sign	To and fro head bobbing
Müller sign	Visible pulsation of uvula
Quincke sign	Capillary pulsations seen on light compression of nail bed
Traube sign	Systolic and diastolic sounds (pistol shots) over the femoral artery
Duroziez sign	Bruits heard over femoral artery on light compression by stethoscope
Hill sign	Popliteal cuff pressure exceeding brachial pressure by 60 mm Hg or greater

B. Laboratory Findings

Laboratory findings depend on the underlying cause of AR. Elevated white blood cell count and erythrocyte sedimentation rate are seen in inflammatory conditions, such as infection and aortitis. Abnormal antinuclear antigen and rheumatoid factor titers may be seen in patients with rheumatologic disorders. When syphilis is suspected, serologic tests may be indicated.

C. Diagnostic Studies

1. Electrocardiography—No specific electrocardiographic abnormalities are characteristic of AR. Signs of left atrial enlargement, left ventricular hypertrophy, and a "strain pattern" (ST depression with T-wave inversion in lateral leads) are often seen in chronic significant AR. Arrhythmias, including ventricular ectopy and ventricular tachycardia, may occur in advanced cases with left ventricular dysfunction. In acute AR, sinus tachycardia may be the only abnormality. In cases of infective endocarditis, inflammation or abscess formation may spread to the atrioventricular node, resulting in prolongation of the PR interval or development of atrioventricular block.

2. Chest radiography—Chest radiographic findings are not specific for AR and reflect an estimate of cardiac size and pulmonary vascular changes. In chronic significant AR, an increase in the size of the cardiac silhouette is seen. In acute AR, the cardiac size is normal; the lung fields show increased markings due to pulmonary edema. When AR is due to aortic dissection, the chest film may show an enlarged ascending aorta. If calcification of the aortic knob is present,

a helpful sign of dissection is increased separation between the outer margin of the aorta and the calcific density.

3. Echocardiography and Doppler techniques—With recent technologic advances, particularly the introduction of color-flow Doppler, echocardiography has become the method of choice for evaluating patients with AR. Two-dimensional echocardiography in combination with various Doppler modalities and, in selected cases, transesophageal imaging has provided a noninvasive means for not only diagnosing AR with a high sensitivity and specificity but also for assessing its etiology and severity. Furthermore, important information can be obtained on the hemodynamic impact of the regurgitant lesion, prognosis, and effectiveness of therapy.

A. DETECTION OF AORTIC REGURGITATION—Currently, the best noninvasive method for detecting AR is Doppler echocardiography. Doppler techniques are extremely sensitive and specific in the detection of AR, manifested as a diastolic flow abnormality arising from the aortic valve, directed toward the left ventricle. Even trivial regurgitation can be detected, which commonly is not audible on physical examination. Although most cases of moderate-to-severe chronic AR have typical findings on physical examination, moderate lesions may occasionally be missed on examination because of the subtlety of auscultatory findings. Doppler echocardiography is also extremely valuable in patients with acute AR when the typical clinical findings of chronic AR are absent and the murmur can often be missed. Among the available Doppler techniques (including color Doppler, pulsed and continuous wave Doppler), color Doppler echocardiography has proven to be extremely helpful in the evaluation of AR (Figure 8–1).

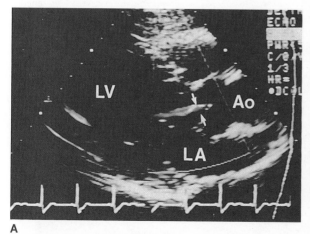

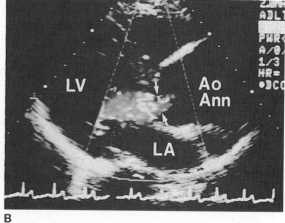

A   B

▲ **Figure 8–1.** Color Doppler echocardiographic frames in diastole from the parasternal long axis view in (**A**) a patient with mild aortic regurgitation and another with (**B**) severe regurgitation. The patient with severe aortic regurgitation (**B**) has a large ascending aortic aneurysm (Ao Ann). The width of the aortic regurgitation jet in the left ventricular outflow (between arrows) provides a good estimate of the severity of aortic regurgitation by color Doppler echocardiography. Ao, aorta; Ao Ann, aortic aneurysm; LA, left atrium; LV, left ventricle.

Its major advantage over conventional Doppler is that it provides a spatial orientation of the regurgitant jet arising from the aortic root. A completely negative color Doppler examination in multiple planes virtually excludes the presence of AR. Although pulsed and continuous wave Doppler are almost equally sensitive in the detection of AR, eccentric aortic insufficiency jets can be missed with these techniques and are better delineated with color-flow imaging.

Echocardiographic imaging with M-mode and two-dimensional examinations cannot detect the presence of AR but can provide indirect clues to its presence. These include diastolic fluttering of the anterior mitral leaflet or septum depending on the impingement of the regurgitant flow on these structures. These signs, although specific, are not sensitive for the detection of AR and do not relate to the severity of regurgitation.

B. Assessment of cause—Because two-dimensional echocardiography can image cardiac structures, it provides valuable information on the cause of the AR. Structural abnormalities of the aortic valve, including calcifications or thickening, congenital deformities, vegetations, rupture, or prolapse, can be identified. Dilatation of the aortic root, calcifications, or dissection can also be evaluated. Although most of these conditions can be assessed with transthoracic echocardiography, transesophageal echocardiography has provided high-resolution images that allow for improved detection of such abnormalities, especially in technically difficult cases or in conditions such as infective endocarditis. Transesophageal echocardiography is also routinely performed when an aortic abnormality, such as aneurysm or dissection, is suspected (Figure 8–2). In patients with AR due to aortic disease, precisely defining the morphology of the valve and involvement of the aortic root is important in determining the surgical approach and deciding whether the valve can be preserved or requires replacement.

C. Assessment of severity—In addition to the detection of AR, Doppler echocardiography combined with two-dimensional echocardiographic imaging has recently allowed an assessment of the severity of the lesion. Several methods have been proposed, including color Doppler assessment of regurgitant jet size, continuous wave Doppler using the pressure half-time method, measurements of regurgitant volume and

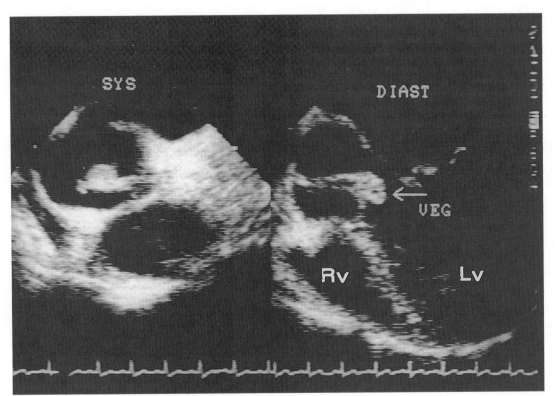

▲ **Figure 8–2.** Transesophageal echocardiographic frames in systole (SYS) and diastole (DIAST), showing a vegetation attached to the aortic valve that prolapses into the left ventricular outflow tract during diastole. In this patient, transthoracic echocardiographic imaging was difficult and failed to demonstrate the large vegetation.

Table 8-3. Grading the Severity of Aortic Regurgitation Using Doppler Techniques Combined with Echocardiography.

Severity of AR	Color-Flow Doppler JH/LVOH (%)	Continuous Wave Doppler PHT (ms)	Pulsed Doppler Regurgitant Fraction (%)
Mild	< 24	> 500	< 20
Moderate	25–45	500–349	20–35
Moderately severe	46–64	349–200	36–50
Severe	> 65	< 200	> 50

AR, aortic regurgitation; JH/LVOH, Ratio of aortic regurgitant jet height to left ventricular outflow height in the parasternal long axis view, PHT, pressure half-time.

effective regurgitant orifice area derived from two-dimensional echocardiography and pulsed Doppler techniques.

With color-flow Doppler, the AR jet can be spatially oriented in the two-dimensional plane arising from the aortic valve and directed toward the left ventricle. The ratio of the AR jet diameter just below the leaflets to that of the left ventricular outflow diameter has been shown to correlate well with the severity of regurgitation when compared with the angiographic standard (Table 8–3, see Figure 8–1). Similarly, a good estimation of AR severity has been found by relating the cross-sectional area of the jet at its origin to the left ventricular outflow area. Recently, measurement of the width of the AR jet at the level of the leaflets (vena contracta) has been used to quantitatively approximate AR severity. A vena contracta of > 0.6 cm is considered a sign of severe AR. On the other hand, it is important to note that the length of the AR jet does not correlate well with AR severity. This is in part because color Doppler flow mapping is also highly dependent on the velocity of regurgitation, or the driving pressure, in addition to the regurgitant volume.

Another index of AR severity that has been useful clinically is the pressure half-time derived from continuous wave Doppler recordings of the AR jet velocity. The velocity of the regurgitant jet is related to the instantaneous pressure difference between the aorta and left ventricle in diastole by the modified Bernoulli equation: $\Delta = 4V^2$, where ΔP is the pressure gradient in millimeters of mercury and V is the blood velocity in meters per second. The pressure half-time index is the time it takes for the initial maximal pressure gradient in diastole to fall by 50%. In patients with mild regurgitation, there is a gradual small drop in the pressure difference in diastole, whereas with severe AR, a more precipitous drop occurs (Figure 8–3). A pressure half-time greater than 500 ms is seen in mild AR, but more significant regurgitation is usually associated with a shorter pressure half-time (see Table 8–3, Figure 8–3). The severity of AR using this index may be overestimated in patients who have elevated left ventricular end-diastolic pressure.

The severity of AR can also be assessed using regurgitant volume and regurgitant fraction derived from two-dimensional and pulsed Doppler echocardiography. This method is based on the continuity equation, which states that, in the absence of regurgitation, blood flow is equal across all valves.

Stroke volume at the level of a valve annulus is calculated as the product of the cross-sectional area obtained by two-dimensional echocardiography and the time velocity integral of flow recorded by pulsed Doppler. In the presence of AR, stroke volume at the left ventricular outflow tract is higher than that across another valve without regurgitation. Therefore, AR volume can be calculated as the difference between stroke volume at the left ventricular outflow and that derived at another valve site. Dividing the regurgitant volume by stroke volume across the aortic valve gives an estimate of regurgitant fraction. A regurgitant fraction of less than 30% is usually mild, whereas regurgitant fraction greater than 50% denotes severe AR (see Table 8–3). A similar approach to estimating severity of AR can be achieved using pulsed Doppler echocardiography in the proximal descending aorta. In patients with significant AR, a large reversal of flow is observed in diastole toward the aortic arch and ascending aorta. This simple method should be used routinely to qualitatively grade the severity of regurgitation and can also be used quantitatively to derive a regurgitant fraction.

Proximal flow convergence is more difficult to identify in AR, but when it is present, the proximal isovelocity surface area method can be used to determine the effective regurgitant orifice area. This method is less accurate in eccentric jets and aortic root dilatation.

Although color-flow Doppler allows a good estimation of the severity of AR in most patients, its accuracy depends on optimization of the color Doppler examination, including gainsettings, frame rate, and interrogation of multiple tomographic planes. The availability of other independent Doppler indices of AR severity further allows the corroboration of color Doppler findings. This is particularly helpful in patients with eccentric AR jets, for which severity may be difficult to assess by color-flow Doppler alone. A detailed transthoracic examination usually provides all the necessary information. When the transthoracic approach is inadequate or inconclusive, transesophageal echocardiography can be performed in this setting for the diagnosis and assessment of severity of the lesion.

Another important caveat in classifying the severity of AR is that it is in part dependent on hemodynamic status, including preload and, more importantly, afterload. Raising blood pressure may significantly increase AR severity.

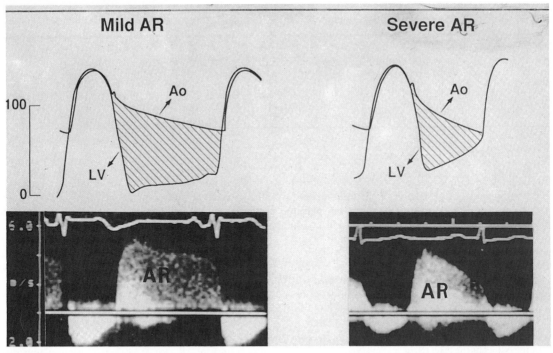

▲ **Figure 8-3.** Schematic of aortic and left ventricular pressure tracings in (*left*) a patient with mild and (*right*) another with severe aortic regurgitation and corresponding examples of continuous wave Doppler recording of aortic jet velocity in such patients. In mild aortic regurgitation, a gradual, small drop in the difference between aortic and ventricular pressures occurs in diastole, reflected by the small decrease in the velocity of the aortic regurgitation jet. In contrast, in severe aortic regurgitation, a more precipitous drop occurs in the pressure gradient and in the corresponding jet velocity. AR, aortic regurgitation; Ao, aorta; LV, left ventricle.

D. Assessment of hemodynamic effects—The hemodynamic effects of AR are assessed with both echocardiographic imaging and Doppler echocardiography. Two-dimensional echocardiography provides quantitation of ventricular size and function, in addition to the degree of left ventricular hypertrophy and ventricular mass. End-diastolic and end-systolic left ventricular dimensions and volumes as well as left ventricular ejection fraction provide important measures of the hemodynamic effects of AR and help identify patients at higher risk. In patients with acute AR, premature closure of the mitral valve can be demonstrated by both two-dimensional and M-mode imaging. In these situations, diastolic mitral regurgitation can also be detected by Doppler echocardiography, reflecting the rapid rise of left ventricular pressure in diastole, exceeding that of left atrial pressure. These findings indicate severe AR. In patients with chronic AR, assessment of the ventricular and atrial filling dynamics at the mitral and pulmonary venous inflow, respectively, allows for noninvasive estimation of ventricular diastolic pressure, further adding to the overall evaluation of the hemodynamic effect of AR on ventricular function. Newer modalities such as Doppler tissue imaging further enhance the accuracy of noninvasive assessment of ventricular diastolic function. Thus, in patients with chronic AR, two-dimensional echocardiography with Doppler provides serial assessment of left ventricular volumes, hypertrophy, and function and helps assess the progression of the disease and optimum timing of surgical intervention.

4. Cardiac catheterization and angiography—Prior to the introduction of Doppler echocardiography, the evaluation of the severity of AR invariably required invasive testing by cardiac catheterization. With the improvement in the accuracy of noninvasive tests, routine cardiac catheterization is no longer necessary in most patients. At catheterization, the detection of AR is achieved with the injection of radiopaque contrast into the aortic root and the appearance of dye in the left ventricle (Figure 8–4). In addition, aortography allows evaluation of the ascending aorta for dilatation or dissection. Some of the structural abnormalities of the aortic valve may also be identified. The severity of AR is quantitatively approximated using a grading system that takes into account the intensity of contrast dye in the left ventricle and its clearance (Table 8–4). This grading system has been

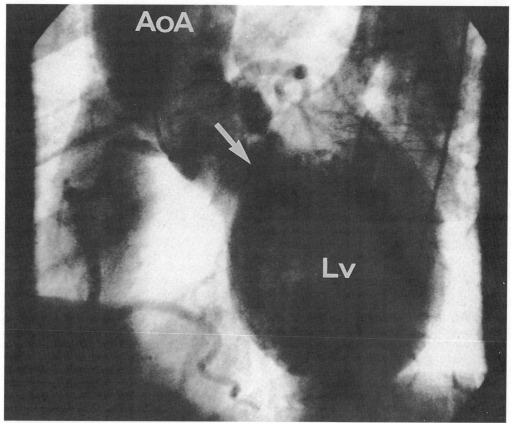

▲ **Figure 8–4.** Aortic root contrast injection in the left anterior oblique projection in a patient with severe aortic regurgitation, showing significant opacification of the left ventricle. The aortography also shows an ascending aortic aneurysm. AoA, aortic aneurysm; Lv, left ventricle.

helpful clinically in the assessment of AR severity. However, it is important to emphasize that, similar to other diagnostic techniques, a number of technical factors may also affect interpretation. Positioning the catheter too close to the valve may itself cause regurgitation. The volume and rapidity of contrast injection, ventricular function, and type of catheter used are important factors that may affect the interpretation of AR severity.

At catheterization, the severity of AR can also be assessed by the determination of regurgitant volume and regurgitant fraction. In the absence of regurgitation or shunts, the left ventricular stroke volume derived from contrast ventricu-

Table 8–4. Angiographic Grading of the Severity of Aortic Regurgitation.

Grade	Degree of LV Opacification	Intensity of Dye	Clearance of Dye from LV
I (mild)	Incomplete	Ao > LV	Completely cleared on each beat
II (moderate)	Complete but faint	Ao > LV	Incomplete clearance
III (moderately severe)	Complete opacification in several beats	Ao = LV	Slow
IV (severe)	Complete on first beat	Ao < LV	Slow

Ao, aorta; LV, left ventricle.

lography is equal to right ventricular stroke volume obtained by the Fick method or thermodilution. When isolated AR is present, subtracting left ventricular from right ventricular stroke volume gives the regurgitation volume. Regurgitant fraction is derived as the regurgitant volume divided by left ventricular stroke volume. In the presence of concomitant mitral regurgitation, a total regurgitant volume or fraction can only be assessed using this method. Because of inherent variability in the determination of stroke volume, a 10–15% error in these measurements is not infrequent and is similar to those obtained with Doppler echocardiography.

Cardiac catheterization provides an accurate assessment of the hemodynamic effect of AR. Using contrast ventriculography, preferably in biplanar projections, accurate determination of left ventricular volumes and ejection fraction can be performed. Furthermore, direct measurements of pressures in the various cardiac chambers can be recorded. In compensated chronic AR, the only abnormality that may be observed is a widened pulse pressure on the aortic pressure tracing. As decompensation occurs, left ventricular end-diastolic pressure rises. In severe, particularly acute AR, aortic and left ventricular pressures may equalize at end-diastole.

With the improvement in noninvasive testing, routine cardiac catheterization is no longer necessary in most patients for the sole assessment of the lesion. Currently, cardiac catheterization is indicated in the assessment of AR severity when noninvasive testing is equivocal or discordant with the clinical presentation and, more commonly, in the assessment of coronary artery disease prior to aortic valve surgery. Preoperative coronary angiography should be performed prior to elective surgery for AR in men older than 35 years of age, premenopausal women over 35 who have risk factors for coronary artery disease, postmenopausal women, and any patients with clinical suspicion of coronary artery disease.

5. Electrocardiographically gated 64-slice computed tomography angiography (CTA)—This test allows rapid diastolic frame rates from which the regurgitant orifice can be planimetered. Studies have shown excellent agreement with echo Doppler measures in the same patients. In addition, the size of the aorta and left ventricle can be determined as well as ejection fraction. CTA can also be used to detect significant coronary artery disease in patients with chest pain or who are being considered for surgery.

6. Magnetic resonance imaging—Advances in magnetic resonance imaging (MRI) have recently allowed for evaluation of patients with AR. At present, three basic approaches are available: spin echo imaging, gradient echo imaging (cine-MRI), and phase velocity mapping. Spin echo imaging provides an excellent approach for depicting cardiac morphology and detecting aortic root disease. However, aortic valve visualization is poor. Using cine-MRI, AR is detected as a decrease in the signal intensity in the left ventricular outflow during diastole. In preliminary studies, the ratio of area of low-intensity signal to the area of the left ventricular outflow has provided an

accurate estimate of AR severity. Regurgitant fractions have been determined by comparing right and left ventricular volumes and stroke volumes. Furthermore, using phase velocity mapping, flow in a region of interest can be assessed. Regurgitant fraction with this method can be derived by comparing flows in the ascending aorta and pulmonary artery.

The use of MRI is promising in the assessment of AR. It is particularly helpful in defining the severity and extent of AR. Imaging can be performed in any plane, without attenuation from lung or bone. However, this modality cannot be used in patients carrying metallic objects such as defibrillators or pacemakers. Its current drawbacks are lack of availability of cardiac MRI and high cost. It is an alternative to echocardiography and for centers with expertise in cardiac MRI.

7. Exercise stress testing—Exercise stress testing can be used to evaluate patients with equivocal symptoms or to guide patients who wish to participate in athletic activities. Early studies using exercise radionuclide angiography to assess ejection fraction suggested that a failure to rise or a fall in ejection fraction correlated with poor outcomes and was a criteria for considering surgery. However, when resting ejection fraction and end-diastolic left ventricular volume were considered, this exercise response in asymptomatic patients had no independent predictive value. Thus, radionuclide imaging with exercise in patients has been largely abandoned. In patients with inadequate echocardiograms, radionuclide imaging can be used to assess left ventricular size and function, but MRI or CT are probably superior.

Alkadhi H et al. Aortic regurgitation: assessment with 64-section CT. Radiology. 2007 Oct;245(1):111–21. [PMID: 17717329]

Bekeredjian R et al. Valvular heart disease: aortic regurgitation. Circulation. 2005 Jul 5;112(1):125–134. [PMID: 15998697]

Debl K et al. Assessment of the anatomic regurgitant orifice in aortic regurgitation: a clinical magnetic resonance imaging study. Heart. 2008 Mar;94(3):e8. [PMID: 17686805]

Scheffel H et al. Accuracy of 64-slice computed tomography for the preoperative detection of coronary artery disease in patients with chronic aortic regurgitation. Am J Cardiol. 2007 Aug 15;100(4):701–6. [PMID: 17697832]

Willett DL et al. Assessment of aortic regurgitation by transesophageal color Doppler imaging of the vena contracta: validation against an intraoperative aortic flow probe. J Am Coll Cardiol. 2001 Apr;37(5):1450–5. [PMID: 11300460]

▶ Treatment

The treatment of AR depends on its underlying cause, severity, cardiac function, and the presence or absence of symptoms. Mild-to-moderate AR may not require any specific treatment, whereas severe acute AR due to aortic dissection is a medical and surgical emergency.

A. Acute Aortic Regurgitation

Severe acute AR carries a high mortality rate if left untreated. It requires aggressive supportive measures, a rapid assessment of cause, and institution of definitive therapy. Because early death due to left ventricular failure and hemodynamic collapse is frequent in these patients despite intensive medical therapy, prompt surgical intervention is indicated. While the patient is being prepared for surgery, pharmacologic therapy can be initiated. Vasodilator therapy with sodium nitroprusside is the treatment of choice in acute AR because of its afterload and preload reduction. The dose is titrated to optimize forward cardiac output and pulmonary capillary wedge pressure. Positive inotropic agents such as dobutamine can be used if the patient remains hypotensive with a low systemic cardiac output.

When acute AR is associated with hemodynamic instability, the only definitive therapy is surgical correction. The timing of surgery depends on the cause and degree of hemodynamic derangement. In infective endocarditis with severe AR, it is preferable to give several days of appropriate antibiotics prior to aortic valve replacement (AVR), provided the patient is hemodynamically stable. Indications for urgent surgery are New York Heart Association (NYHA) class III–IV congestive heart failure, systemic embolization, persistent bacteremia, fungal endocarditis, or abscess formation. When AR results from aortic dissection with disruption of commissural support, urgent surgical repair is indicated.

B. Chronic Aortic Regurgitation

1. Mild-to-moderate aortic regurgitation—Patients who have mild or moderate AR and are asymptomatic and who have normal or minimally increased cardiac size, require no therapy for the AR. They should be followed with clinical evaluation yearly and echocardiography at 2–3 year intervals. In patients with a history of rheumatic fever, prophylaxis using either penicillin or erythromycin is indicated until the age of 25 years and 5 years after the last episode. If rheumatic carditis has already occurred, lifelong prophylaxis is recommended, even following valve replacement. Any occurrence of systemic hypertension should be treated because it aggravates the degree of regurgitation. Patients with AR secondary to syphilis should receive a full course of penicillin therapy. Patients with moderate AR should avoid isometric exercise, competitive sports, and heavy physical exertion. If symptoms present in such patients, an alternative cause for the symptoms should be considered.

2. Moderate-to-severe aortic regurgitation with symptoms and normal left ventricular function—Patients with chronic significant AR and normal left ventricular ejection fraction (LVEF) (> 50%) who have NYHA class III or IV symptoms or Canadian Cardiovascular Society class II–IV angina should undergo AVR. Patients with NYHA class II symptoms should be evaluated on a case-by-case basis. If the cause or severity of symptoms is unclear, an exercise test should be done. If exercise capacity is normal, treatment should be given as for asymptomatic patients as outlined in the following section. If new, even mild symptoms appear in

a patient with chronic significant AR—particularly if left ventricular size is increased or the ejection fraction is on the low side of normal—then AVR should be considered.

Medical therapy is attempted in symptomatic patients who are awaiting surgery or are not surgical candidates due to refusal, terminal medical illness, or advanced age. The aim of therapy in these patients is primarily relief of symptoms and improvement of exercise capacity. Medical therapy includes digitalis, diuretics, and vasodilator drugs. Oral vasodilators, such as hydralazine, and angiotensin-converting enzyme (ACE) inhibitors reduce afterload, allowing for greater forward cardiac output which may improve exercise tolerance. Preload reduction with diuretics and nitrates is also helpful in reducing pulmonary congestion.

3. Moderate-to-severe aortic regurgitation with symptoms and abnormal left ventricular function—Symptomatic patients with mild-to-moderate left ventricular dysfunction (LVEF = 25–50%) should undergo AVR. Treatment decisions for patients with more advanced left ventricular dysfunction (LVEF < 25% or left ventricular end-systolic dimension > 60 mm) is difficult. The operative risk is high, and not all patients benefit from AVR. On the other hand, outcome with medical therapy is poor as well. Patients with class II–III symptoms and recent onset of left ventricular dysfunction should be considered for surgical treatment. In patients not considered surgical candidates, aggressive medical therapy is useful in controlling symptoms. Diuretics and vasodilators are the mainstay of medical treatment. If symptoms persist, short-term inotropic support using dobutamine along with intravenous nitroprusside and diuretics may provide relief.

4. Moderate-to-severe aortic regurgitation without symptoms—The optimal timing of AVR in asymptomatic patients remains a challenging clinical decision. Clearly, patients with normal left ventricular function and good exercise capacity can live for several years without symptoms or left ventricular dysfunction, and surgery is clearly not indicated for such patients. These patients are candidates for long-term oral vasodilator therapy. It has been shown that the use of oral hydralazine in patients with AR produces a number of beneficial hemodynamic effects, including a reduction in regurgitant volume, end-diastolic and end-systolic volumes, and improvement in ejection fraction and effective cardiac output. Similar results have been shown with nifedipine and ACE inhibitors. Vasodilator therapy has also been shown to delay onset of symptoms, occurrence of left ventricular dysfunction, and the need for AVR. However, not all studies have demonstrated a benefit from vasodilator drugs.

When the evidence of left ventricular dysfunction (ejection fraction < 50%) is clear, despite the absence of symptoms, AVR is recommended to prevent further left ventricular dysfunction and improve prognosis. However, once the ejection fraction is decreased, surgical risk is higher and left ventricular dysfunction may become irreversible. The ideal time to intervene is late enough in the course of the disease to justify the surgical risk and postoperative sequelae such as anticoagulation, but early enough to prevent irreversible left ventricular contractile dysfunction. To determine the optimal time for surgery in chronic asymptomatic AR, it is important to identify preoperative variables that predict postoperative left ventricular function. A number of parameters have been investigated in the hope of identifying the ideal predictor. Regurgitant volume or fraction are not predictors of postoperative outcome because they are significantly influenced by loading conditions. End-diastolic volume has modest correlation with surgical outcome. The cutoff used varies from 150 to 250 mL/m². An end-diastolic minor dimension of greater than 70 mm has also been associated with a poor postoperative outcome. A major limitation of end-diastolic indices is their dependence on preload and thus may not reflect intrinsic myocardial contractile function. Left ventricular ejection fraction has been shown to be an important predictor of postoperative survival. An LVEF of less than 0.50 is associated with significantly reduced 3-year survival rate (64 ± 10%)

compared with an LVEF greater than 0.50 (91 ± 28%). Although LVEF has high sensitivity for identifying patients with worse postoperative outcome, it is less specific. This is understandable because LVEF reflects loading conditions in addition to the inotropic state of the myocardium. Similarly, LVEF response to exercise may be modulated by multiple factors, including peripheral resistance, preload heart rate, sympathetic tone, and type of exercise. Therefore, although a decrease in ejection fraction during exercise was previously considered to predict a poor outcome in chronic AR, recent data suggest that this is a nonspecific response. However, exercise capacity by itself is an important predictor of survival in AR.

End-systolic indices are less load-dependent and have been used to predict left ventricular function following surgery for AR. An end-systolic minor dimension greater than 55 mm or end-systolic volume greater than 60 mL/m² identifies patients with persistent left ventricular dysfunction and a poor survival rate following AVR. Recently, the ratio of left ventricular end-systolic dimension in millimeters and body surface area in square meters that exceeds 25 has been advocated as a marker

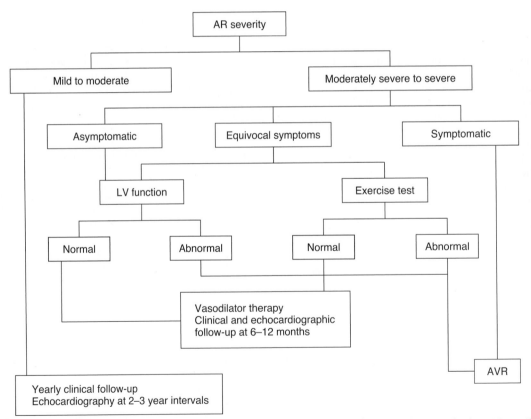

▲ **Figure 8–5.** Schematic of proposed treatment of patients with chronic significant aortic regurgitation. AR, aortic regurgitation; AVR, aortic valve replacement; LV, left ventricle.

of occult left ventricular dysfunction. If, in addition to an increased end-systolic ventricular size, the ejection fraction is also reduced, the survival rate drops further. Even though they are preload-independent, end-systolic indices are still affected by afterload. The ratio of end-systolic pressure or wall stress to end-systolic volume has been advocated as an index of contractility, which is less dependent on loading conditions. In patients with chronic severe AR, abnormalities of the end-systolic pressure-volume relationship have been shown, despite a normal LVEF, reflecting depressed myocardial contractility. Such patients are more likely to have symptoms and a need for earlier valve replacement.

For asymptomatic patients with moderate-to-severe AR, a noninvasive evaluation of left ventricular size and function is recommended as well as an exercise test if functional capacity is unclear (Figure 8–5). If exercise capacity is poor or LVEF is less than 50%, surgical treatment is recommended. Those with good exercise tolerance and normal left ventricular function should be followed at 6- to 12-month intervals. Oral vasodilators may be considered in these patients. In patients who remain asymptomatic, AVR should be considered when serial testing shows decreased exercise tolerance, progressive left ventricular enlargement, or worsening left ventricular function.

▶ Prognosis

Asymptomatic patients with chronic AR have a stable course for many years. The mean rate of progression to surgery is approximately 4% per year. Symptoms are the major determinant of outcome in AR. The mortality rate for patients with NYHA class II–IV symptoms is over 20% per year. Even for patients with class II symptoms, the mortality rate is 6% per year compared with 3% for patients with class I symptoms. In general, good results have been observed with AVR for AR, with an average operative mortality rate of 3–4% and a 5-year survival rate of 85%. These results depend on several factors, including preoperative ventricular function, concomitant coronary artery disease, and the underlying cause of AR. Aortic valve replacement is necessary in most patients. In some cases of AR secondary to loss of commissural support, aortic valve repair can be performed. The feasibility of aortic valve repair can be determined by a transesophageal echocardiogram. In patients with excessive aortic root dilatation or aneurysm, a composite aortic graft with reimplantation of the coronary arteries is performed more frequently. Most patients show resolution of symptoms following surgery to correct AR. The end-diastolic volume is reduced immediately, with some further reduction occurring over several days after surgery. The LVEF continues to improve up to 1–2 years after surgery. There is also a gradual decline in left ventricular mass. About 20–30% of patients will have incomplete symptomatic relief and persistent left ventricular dysfunction. These findings are associated with the presence of preoperative left ventricular dysfunction, particularly if the duration of dysfunction is prolonged (> 18 months). Even though the outcome is less than optimal in patients with moderate left ventricular dysfunction, with recent surgical advances, many of them still do better with surgery than with medical management. Surgery should be considered in all symptomatic patients unless left ventricular dysfunction is very severe.

Bhudia SK et al. Improved outcomes after aortic valve surgery for chronic aortic regurgitation with severe left ventricular dysfunction. J Am Coll Cardiol. 2007 Apr 3;49(13):1465–71. [PMID: 17397676]

de Waroux JB et al. Functional anatomy of aortic regurgitation: accuracy, prediction of surgical repairability, and outcome implications of transesophageal echocardiography. Circulation. 2007 Sep 11;116(11 Suppl):I264–9. [PMID: 17846315]

Enriquez-Sarano M et al. Clinical practice. Aortic regurgitation. N Engl J Med. 2004 Oct 7;351(15):1539–46. [PMID: 15470217]

Evangelista A et al. Long-term vasodilator therapy in patients with severe aortic regurgitation. N Engl J Med. 2005 Sep 29;353(13):1342–9. [PMID: 16192479]

Tornos P et al. Long-term outcome of surgically treated aortic regurgitation: influence of guideline adherence toward early surgery. J Am Coll Cardiol. 2006 Mar 7;47(5):1012–7. [PMID: 16516086]

St John Sutton M. Predictors of long-term survival after valve replacement for chronic aortic regurgitation. Eur Heart J. 2001 May;22(10):808–10. [PMID: 11350089]

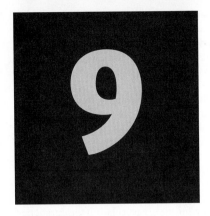

Mitral Stenosis

Robert J. Bryg, MD

ESSENTIALS OF DIAGNOSIS

- Exertional dyspnea, paroxysmal nocturnal dyspnea, orthopnea, or fatigue (later stages).

- Opening snap, loud S_1 (closing snap), diastolic rumbling murmur; with pulmonary hypertension, a parasternal lift with a loud P_2.

- ECG evidence of left atrial enlargement or atrial fibrillation; right ventricular hypertrophy in later stages.

- Chest radiographic signs of left atrial enlargement and normal left ventricular size.

- Thickened mitral valve leaflets with restricted valve motion and reduced orifice area demonstrated on two-dimensional echocardiography.

- An elevated transmitral pressure gradient and prolonged pressure half-time by Doppler echocardiography.

General Considerations

The normal mitral apparatus is a complex structure whose components must permit a large volume of blood to pass from the left atrium to the left ventricle. The cross-sectional area of a normal mitral valve ranges from 4 cm² to 6 cm² in an adult and a transmitral pressure gradient develops when the valve is narrowed to < 2.5 cm². Left atrial pressures begin to rise and are transmitted to the pulmonary vasculature and right side of the heart. Several congenital and acquired conditions result in impaired filling of the left ventricle and may be confused with mitral stenosis (Table 9–1).

The predominant cause of mitral stenosis in adults is rheumatic involvement of the mitral valve and approximately two-thirds of all patients with rheumatic mitral stenosis are female. However, a large proportion of patients with rheumatic valve disease—nearly 50%—have no history of rheumatic fever. Other causes of mitral stenosis are extremely rare. These figures will most likely change due to the impressive reduction of rheumatic fever in developed countries, although rheumatic fever remains a problem in developing countries and most likely reflects the reduced availability of antibiotics and the virulence of the strains of *Streptococcus*.

Acute rheumatic fever may produce a pancarditis involving the endocardium, myocardium, and pericardium. Aschoff bodies in the myocardium are very specific for a history of rheumatic carditis. Involvement of the mitral valve apparatus is the rule and may produce fusion and thickening of the commissures, cusps, and chordae tendineae. In addition, the fibrosis and calcification of the leaflets may extend to the valve ring. It is still debatable if the progression of mitral stenosis is due to a smoldering rheumatic process and recurrent infections or the constant trauma of turbulent flow produced by a deformed valve.

As the stenosis progresses, a transmitral pressure gradient develops to facilitate flow across the stenotic valve in diastole. Furthermore, the atrial contraction may augment this diastolic pressure gradient (assuming the heart is in normal sinus rhythm). Both the mitral valvular gradient (MVG) and mitral valvular flow (MVF) are required to assess the mitral valve area (MVA) as expressed by the Gorlin formula:

$$MVA\ (cm^2) = \frac{MVF}{37.7\sqrt{MVG}}$$

The mitral valvular flow is a function of cardiac output and heart rate. An increase in cardiac output or heart rate will increase the transmitral flow. As expressed by the Gorlin formula, the increased mitral valvular flow (produced by an increased cardiac output or tachycardia) elevates the mitral valvular gradient exponentially assuming the mitral valve area remains constant. The increased mitral valvular gradient produces an elevated left atrial pressure. This is an important concept for the development of symptoms.

Table 9–1. Conditions Causing
Left Ventricular Inflow Obstruction.

Congenital
Valvular mitral stenosis
Subvalvular ring
Cor triatriatum
Pulmonary vein stenosis
Acquired
Valvular mitral stenosis
Atrial myxoma
Thrombus
Neoplasm
Large fungal or bacterial vegetation
Prosthetic valve dysfunction

Essop MR et al. Rheumatic and nonrheumatic valvular heart disease: epidemiology, management and prevention in Africa. Circulation. 2005 Dec 6;112(23):3584–91. [PMID: 16330700]

▶ Clinical Findings

A. Symptoms and Signs

Early in the disease, patients may be asymptomatic. However, conditions that increase cardiac output or heart rate will increase the mitral valvular gradient and left atrial pressure as described earlier. The elevated left atrial pressure is subsequently transmitted into the pulmonary circulation, leading to dyspnea, and may facilitate the early diagnosis of mitral stenosis. Common conditions that increase cardiac output or heart rate are exercise, hyperthyroidism, pregnancy, atrial fibrillation, and fever. In addition, venous return is augmented in the supine position and may produce orthopnea and paroxysmal nocturnal dyspnea in patients with moderate disease.

As the disease progresses, the pulmonary artery pressure increases proportionally to the pulmonary capillary pressure. The proportional increase is termed "passive pulmonary hypertension" because the increased pressure produced by the right ventricle is required to drive blood across the pulmonary vascular bed into the left atrium. In some patients with severe mitral stenosis, the pulmonary artery pressure is increased disproportionally to the pulmonary capillary pressure. The disproportional increase is termed "reactive pulmonary hypertension." The reactive pulmonary hypertension is secondary to pulmonary artery constriction and organic obliterative changes in the pulmonary vascular bed. These changes typically produce symptoms of right-heart failure and may not be completely reversible.

The mitral valve stenosis and atrial inflammation secondary to rheumatic fever may produce dilatation and postinflammatory changes of the left atrium. These changes predispose the patient to palpitations and atrial fibrillation. In addition, there is an increased risk of systemic embolization resulting in a stroke, myocardial infarction (coronary embolism), splenic or renal infarction, and peripheral artery occlusion. For patients in sinus rhythm, age, the presence of a left atrial thrombus, mitral valve area, and the presence of significant aortic regurgitation are positively associated with embolism. In cases of atrial fibrillation, previous embolism is positively associated with embolism; percutaneous balloon mitral commissurotomy is a negative predictor. Spontaneous echo contrast (also known as smoke) detected by transesophageal echocardiography is associated with systemic embolism. Most emboli appear to originate from the left atrium, especially the left atrial appendage.

Increased pulmonary pressures and vascular congestion produce hemoptysis. Hemoptysis may present as a sudden hemorrhage (termed "pulmonary apoplexy"; this condition is rarely life-threatening), pink frothy sputum resulting from pulmonary edema, blood-tinged sputum associated with dyspnea or bronchitis, and pulmonary infarction due to a pulmonary embolism. Chest pain may develop and resembles angina. The chest pain is most likely the result of pulmonary hypertension and right ventricle hypertrophy and is typically relieved with correction of the mitral stenosis, although concomitant coronary artery disease should be evaluated with the development of chest pain. Endocarditis is primarily associated with mild mitral stenosis and is quite unusual with calcification in severe mitral stenosis.

B. Physical Examination

The general appearance of patients with mitral stenosis is usually unremarkable. Older studies reported mitral facies, which is characterized by pinkish-purple patches on the cheeks produced by low cardiac output, systemic vasoconstriction, and right-sided heart failure. This sign is now extremely rare. Right-sided heart failure also produces an elevated jugular venous pulse with a prominent *a* wave (assuming the heart is in normal sinus rhythm) and *v* wave (produced by tricuspid regurgitation).

The apical impulse is generally normal or decreased, representing normal left ventricular function and decreased left ventricular volume. Palpation of the S_1 over the precordium is a pathognomonic finding and suggests that the anterior mitral valve leaflet is pliable. When the patient is in the left lateral decubitus position, a diastolic thrill may be appreciated. When pulmonary hypertension is present, a parasternal right ventricular heave develops along with a palpable P_2.

Auscultation of the heart sounds may reveal an accentuated S_1 early in the disease. Accentuation of S_1 occurs when the left ventricular pressure rises rapidly in early systole, and the flexible mitral valve leaflets transgress a wide closing excursion. As the severity of mitral stenosis increases with calcification and fibrosis of the leaflets, the amplitude of S_1 subsequently diminishes. When pulmonary hypertension is present, the splitting of the second heart sound may narrow and become a single accentuated S_2. An S_3 originating from the left ventricle is absent in patients with mitral stenosis unless there is concomitant coronary artery disease, mitral regurgitation, or aortic regurgitation. An S_4, if present, originates from the right ventricle when it is hypertrophied and dilated secondary to pulmonary hypertension.

The opening snap is due to sudden tensing of the valve leaflets after they have completed their opening excursion. The vigorous opening of the leaflets is secondary to high left atrial pressures accompanied by a fall in left ventricular pressures in early diastole. The opening snap is audible (high frequency) at the apex, using the diaphragm of the stethoscope.

It is imperative to examine the patient in the left lateral decubitus position for a diastolic murmur. In addition, the murmur may be accentuated by having the patient exercise prior to auscultation. The murmur is described as a rumble (low frequency) and is audible at the apex, using the bell of the stethoscope. The diastolic murmur of mitral stenosis reflects the mitral valvular gradient and the duration of blood flow across the valve. In mild mitral stenosis, the early diastolic decrescendo murmur is brief and is accompanied by a presystolic murmur. The presystolic murmur is secondary to the gradient produced by the atrial contraction. However, the presystolic murmur may be produced in atrial fibrillation and is due to the narrowing of the mitral orifice produced by ventricular systole prior to S_1. A murmur of pulmonary regurgitation (Graham Steell murmur) may be present and difficult to distinguish from the murmur of aortic regurgitation.

Reliable indicators of the severity of mitral stenosis are the A_2–OS interval and the length (rather than intensity) of the diastolic murmur. As the severity of mitral stenosis increases, the A_2–OS interval decreases and the length of the murmur increases. The decreased interval is the result of increased left atrial pressures, producing a mitral valvular gradient at the very onset of diastole. The gradient leads to an early excursion of the valve leaflets (early OS) and continues throughout all of diastole (pandiastolic murmur). The opening snap and murmur may become inaudible when mitral stenosis is very severe and the valve leaflets are rigid.

C. Diagnostic Studies

1. Electrocardiography—Early in the disease, the electrocardiogram (ECG) typically reveals a normal sinus rhythm and is very insensitive. As the disease progresses, left atrial enlargement leads to changes in the P wave. The P wave in lead II becomes broad and notched (termed "P-mitrale") along with a prominent terminal component of the P wave in lead V_1. The P wave axis migrates between +45 and –30 degrees. Atrial fibrillation subsequently develops in many patients, and the previously described findings are lost. As the pulmonary hypertension becomes severe (70–100 mm Hg), right axis deviation develops in addition to an R wave greater than the S wave in lead V_1. In pure mitral stenosis, left ventricular hypertrophy is absent.

2. Chest radiography—Radiologic examination of the cardiac silhouette is quite advantageous. Left atrial enlargement may produce a "double-density," straightening of the left heart border, along with elevation of the left mainstem bronchus (PA view), and impingement on the esophagus due to posterior extension (lateral view). Right ventricular enlargement may occupy the retrosternal space (lateral view). The left ventricular silhouette is normal in pure mitral stenosis, and calcification of the mitral valve is difficult to see on routine chest radiograph. Radiologic examination of the lung fields reveals elevated pulmonary pressures. The pulmonary arteries are prominent, and blood flow is redistributed to the upper lobes (cephalization). Transudation of fluid into the interstitium occurs, resulting in Kerley A lines, Kerley B lines, and pulmonary edema.

3. Echocardiography—The echocardiographic examination is now the keystone of the diagnostic assessment of mitral stenosis. Valuable information is provided with the following echocardiographic techniques: M-mode, two-dimensional, three-dimensional, Doppler, stress, and transesophageal echocardiography (TEE).

A. M-MODE—As mitral stenosis progresses, the usual M-shaped configuration of the anterior mitral leaflet is altered. The diastolic posterior motion of the anterior leaflet is reduced, producing a reduced E-F slope. In patients in sinus rhythm, the A wave, which is normally seen with an atrial contraction, may be reduced or absent. Fusion of the commissures produces a concordant motion of the anterior and posterior mitral leaflets. Although this mode of echocardiography can provide a qualitative diagnosis, it is the least reliable means of quantifying the severity of obstruction.

B. TWO-DIMENSIONAL ECHOCARDIOGRAPHY—This method provides a more complete view of the mitral valve apparatus. The parasternal long axis may reveal diastolic "doming" of the mitral valve and a "hockey stick" configuration of the anterior leaflet. Pliable leaflets with restricted mobility of the leaflet tips produce this configuration. The parasternal short axis can image the orifice of the mitral valve that demonstrates the typical "fish mouth" configuration. After visualization, the orifice is planimetered in diastole to obtain an accurate measurement of the mitral valve area. This measurement is very reliable but may be operator-dependent and prone to error. The inaccuracy is further evident after commissurotomy due to the distortion produced by commissural splitting. With the advent of percutaneous mitral balloon valvotomy (PMBV), the mitral apparatus morphology determined by two-dimensional echocardiography plays an extremely important role for selection criteria.

C. THREE-DIMENSIONAL ECHOCARDIOGRAPHY—Three-dimensional echocardiography can be used to assess mitral valve area via planimetry. The three-dimensional nature helps optimize the plane of the mitral valve. This technique has been demonstrated to be as accurate as other methods for determining mitral valve area. It is limited in the ability of the transducer to obtain adequate images.

D. TRANSESOPHAGEAL ECHOCARDIOGRAPHY—TEE is useful in assessing the left atrium prior to PMBV. It assists with the detection of left atrial thrombi and spontaneous echocardiographic contrast (smoke). It is extremely useful in assessing mitral valve commissural morphology to help guide optimal management in patients undergoing evaluation for balloon mitral valvotomy. Its use, especially with three-dimensional echocardiography, in assessing mitral valve area is less clear. Planimetry of the proper mitral valve plane for mitral stenosis is more difficult with this technique.

E. Doppler echocardiography—Doppler accurately assesses the hemodynamic effects of the mitral valve stenosis; the indicators are mitral valvular gradient, mitral valve area, and pulmonary artery pressures. The mitral valvular gradient is measured by obtaining the velocity of mitral inflow. The velocity (V) is converted to the pressure gradient between the atrium and ventricle using the modified Bernoulli equation:

$$\text{Gradient (mm Hg)} = 4(V^2)$$

The mitral valve area can be estimated using the pressure half-time method, the proximal isovelocity surface area (PISA), or the continuity of flow method. The pressure half-time is currently the most widely used technique for estimating the mitral valve area from Doppler-derived data. The pressure half-time is the time required for the peak pressure gradient between the left atrium and the left ventricle to decline to one-half of its original value. Doppler velocity is converted into a pressure gradient by dividing the initial flow velocity by the square root of 2. Empirically, a pressure half-time of 220 ms correlates with a mitral valve area of 1 cm^2.

$$\text{MVA (cm}^2) = \frac{220}{\text{pressure half-time}}$$

As the mitral valve area decreases, the pressure half-time increases. However, the pressure half-time may be inaccurate in patients with abnormalities of left atrial or left ventricular compliance, those with associated aortic regurgitation, and those with a previous mitral valvotomy. In addition, the presence of severe mitral regurgitation appears to underestimate mitral valve area by pressure half-time. The PISA and the continuity of flow method provide more accurate estimates of mitral valve area in these circumstances but are rarely used in clinical practice.

Pulmonary artery pressures are determined using continuous wave Doppler. The velocity of tricuspid regurgitation produced by pulmonary hypertension is measured, yielding a gradient between the right atrium and right ventricle with the use of the modified Bernoulli equation described previously. The right ventricular systolic pressure is obtained by adding the estimated right atrial pressure to the gradient.

Use of tissue Doppler imaging can also be used in monitoring mitral stenosis. Specifically, measurements of the isovolumetric relaxation time (IVRT), mitral inflow velocity (E), and annular early diastolic velocity (Ea) can be followed annually, especially after PMBV, to assess left ventricular filling pressure. This is especially useful in tracking patients after valve intervention.

F. Stress echocardiography—Dobutamine stress echocardiography (DSE) and exercise echocardiography are also used to assess valve function. With DSE, development of a mean mitral valve gradient of greater than 18 mm Hg demonstrates high-risk patients. Exercise echocardiography can be used to demonstrate increased pulmonary artery pressures with exercise to help determine who would benefit from early intervention, such as valvotomy or valve replacement.

Each method has several limitations, and it is imperative to achieve cross validation. In most instances, measurements of the mitral valvular gradient, mitral valve area, and pulmonary artery pressures correlate well with one another with the use of a transthoracic echocardiogram. If correlation does not occur, a cardiac catheterization, TEE, three-dimensional echocardiogram, or exercise with simultaneous Doppler estimation of the transmitral and pulmonary pressures should be sought to clarify inconsistencies. In addition, a TEE can assess the presence or absence of left atrial thrombus in patients being considered for PMBV or cardioversion.

4. Cardiac catheterization—Direct measurements of left atrial and left ventricular pressures require a transseptal catheterization and predispose the patient to unnecessary risks. Conventional cardiac catheterization uses the pulmonary capillary wedge pressure for indirect measurement of left atrial pressures. Although the pulmonary capillary wedge accurately reflects the mean left atrial pressure, it overestimates the transmitral gradient. Presently, cardiac catheterization has a very limited role in determining the severity of mitral stenosis due to the recent advances in echocardiography.

5. Magnetic resonance imaging—MRI has been shown to be accurate in determining mitral valve area. Two different methods of MRI can be used. Three-dimensional reconstruction can accurately determine mitral valve area compared with echocardiography and Doppler pressure half-time. In addition, velocity encoded cardiovascular magnetic resonance (VE-CMR) compares favorably with Doppler in determining pressure half-time and calculating mitral valve area.

Binder TM et al. Improved assessment of mitral valve stenosis by volumetric real-time three-dimensional echocardiography. J Am Coll Cardiol. 2000 Oct;36(4):1355–61. [PMID: 11028494]

Diwan A et al. Doppler estimation of left ventricular filling pressures in patients with mitral valve disease. Circulation. 2005 Jun 21;111(24):3281–9. [PMID: 15956127]

Djavidani B et al. Planimetry of mitral valve stenosis by magnetic resonance imaging. J Am Coll Cardiol. 2005 Jun 21;45(12):2048–53. [PMID: 15963408]

Fabricius AM et al. Three-dimensional echocardiography for planning of mitral valve surgery: current applicability? Ann Thorac Surg. 2004 Aug;78(12):575–8. [PMID: 15276524]

Hildick-Smith DJ et al. Pulmonary capillary wedge pressure in mitral stenosis accurately reflects mean left atrial pressure but overestimates transmitral gradient. Am J Cardiol. 2000 Feb 15;85(4):512–5. [PMID: 10728964]

Lin SJ et al. Quantification of stenotic mitral valve area with magnetic resonance imaging and comparison with Doppler ultrasound. J Am Coll Cardiol. 2004 Jul7;44(1):133–7. [PMID: 15234421]

Mohan JC et al. Does chronic mitral regurgitation influence Doppler pressure half-time-derived calculation of the mitral valve area in patients with mitral stenosis? Am Heart J. 2004 Oct;148(4):703–9. [PMID: 15459604]

Mohan JC et al. Is the mitral valve area flow-dependent in mitral stenosis? A dobutamine stress echocardiographic study. J Am Coll Cardiol. 2002 Nov 20;40(10):1809–15. [PMID: 12446065]

Reis G et al. Dobutamine stress echocardiography for noninvasive assessment and risk stratification of patients with rheumatic mitral stenosis. J Am Coll Cardiol. 2004 Feb 4;43(3):393–401. [PMID: 15013120]

Sutaria N et al. Transoesophageal echocardiographic assessment of mitral valve commissural morphology predicts outcome after balloon valvotomy. Heart. 2006 Jan;92(1):52–7. [PMID: 16365352]

Xie MX et al. Comparison of accuracy of mitral valve area in mitral stenosis by real-time, three-dimensional echocardiography versus two-dimensional echocardiography versus Doppler pressure half-time. Am J Cardiol. 2005 Jun 15;95(12):1496–9. [PMID: 15950582]

Zamorana J et al. Real-time three-dimensional echocardiography for rheumatic mitral valve stenosis evaluation: an accurate and novel approach. J Am Coll Cardiol. 2004 Jun 2;43(11):2091–6. [PMID: 15172418]

▶ Treatment

A. Medical Therapy

Primary prophylaxis consists of an early diagnosis of group A streptococcal pharyngitis. Treatment started within 7–9 days after onset of illness may prevent rheumatic fever. Secondary prophylaxis may be individually tailored, but there are no firm guidelines. Recurrence of rheumatic fever is more common in young patients and in patients in whom carditis developed during the initial episode. Therefore, with carditis, secondary prevention continues for 10 years or until age 25. Without carditis, secondary prevention continues for 5 years or until age 18. The prevention of repeated attacks may delay the progression of mitral stenosis.

Patients with mitral stenosis are considered to be at moderate risk for bacterial endocarditis. Therefore, endocarditis prophylaxis was recommended for certain procedures specified by older guidelines. However, there is a recent debate concerning whether dental procedures predispose to endocarditis and whether antibiotic prophylaxis is of any value; current guidelines do not recommend antibiotic prophylaxis for mitral stenosis. The choice of antibiotics to treat endocarditis may be further complicated if the patient is receiving penicillin for prophylaxis against rheumatic fever. Resistance to penicillin and cephalosporins may develop in this scenario, and an alternative antibiotic should be given for prophylaxis against endocarditis.

Medical management of mitral stenosis with normal sinus rhythm is limited. A benefit is derived from salt restriction and diuretics when there is evidence of pulmonary vascular congestion. Digitalis does not benefit patients in sinus rhythm unless an associated left ventricular dysfunction is present. β-Blockers can significantly decrease heart rate and cardiac output. The decreased heart rate and cardiac output subsequently lead to a decrease in the transmitral gradient. Although there appears to be a physiologic advantage with the use of β-blockers, the data are conflicting. β-Blockers may be reserved for patients who have exertional symptoms if the symptoms occur at high heart rates. Anticoagulation is beneficial for cases with normal sinus rhythm with a prior embolic event or a left atrial dimension > 55 mm Hg by echocardiography.

Medical management of mitral stenosis and atrial fibrillation can alleviate a variety of complications. Atrial fibrillation in patients with mitral stenosis is poorly tolerated due to a loss of atrial contraction and an associated rapid ventricular rate. The rate control is achieved by using a β-blocker, calcium channel blocker, or digitalis. Electrical or chemical cardioversion should be performed with appropriate anticoagulation. Class IA, IC, and III agents can be used to terminate acute-onset atrial fibrillation and prevent recurrences of atrial fibrillation. Most antiarrhythmics increase the likelihood of maintaining normal sinus rhythm to approximately 50–70% of patients per year after cardioversion. Amiodarone appears to be more effective than sotalol or propafenone, although the antiarrhythmic should be tailored to the patient because of the risks of side effects with each agent. Heart rate control is most commonly achieved with a combination of nondihydropine calcium channel blockers, β-blockers, and digoxin. Anticoagulation is recommended for all patients who are unable to maintain normal sinus rhythm.

In pregnancy, the heart rate and cardiac output are increased substantially along with an increase in maternal blood volume. Nevertheless, most healthy pregnant women with mild to moderate mitral stenosis can be treated medically. Diuretics and β-blockers appear to be safe for use in pregnancy. Quinidine or procainamide are the drugs of choice if an antiarrhythmic drug is needed to maintain normal sinus rhythm. If anticoagulation is necessary, warfarin should be avoided and the patient should be treated appropriately with heparin.

B. Percutaneous Mitral Balloon Valvotomy

PMBV involves a transseptal puncture during cardiac catheterization. The transseptal approach offers direct access to the mitral orifice, after which a single- or double-balloon commissurotomy is performed. The mechanism of action is primarily commissural splitting and fracture of calcium deposits that improve valvular function. The Inoue and double-balloon techniques produce similar long-term results.

Two newer approaches are gaining acceptance. The retrograde nontransseptal balloon mitral valvuloplasty is based on an externally steerable cardiac catheter that enters the left atrium retrograde via the left ventricle. This technique avoids the need for a transseptal puncture and dilatation of the interatrial septum. Balloon valvuloplasty is recommended in patients who are symptomatic, have moderate to severe mitral stenosis, have pliable leaflets, and do not have a left atrial thrombus or significant mitral regurgitation. Patients who are either asymptomatic but have severe mitral stenosis or are symptomatic but have high surgical risks are considered acceptable candidates for balloon valvuloplasty. It is not recommended in cases of mild mitral stenosis. Important baseline variables include operator experience, age, New York Heart Association (NYHA) functional class, atrial fibrillation, cardiothoracic index, echocardiographic score, mean pulmonary artery pressure, and mitral regurgitation. The underlying mitral valve morphology is the most important factor in determining outcome, and echocardiographic scoring systems have been developed for assessing the morphology.

Balloon valvotomy is especially useful in the younger population. Children do extremely well with this technique and avoid surgical replacement of the valve indefinitely. Repeat balloon valvotomy is well tolerated and provides good immediate results, but the long-term results are inferior to initial balloon valvotomy. There is increased restenosis, mitral regurgitation, and atrial fibrillation in this population.

Balloon valvotomy during pregnancy is extremely well tolerated. Women with severe symptomatic mitral stenosis safely undergo valvotomy with marked increases in mitral valve area. Fetal development is normal for most women undergoing this procedure.

Mitral balloon valvotomy does not prevent the development of atrial fibrillation. Patients may require the maze procedure in order to lessen the risk or the development of atrial fibrillation.

C. Surgical Therapy

Three surgical approaches are used to treat mitral stenosis: closed commissurotomy, open commissurotomy, and mitral valve replacement. A closed commissurotomy is performed without the aid of a cardiopulmonary bypass. The surgeon enters the heart using either a transatrial or a transventricular approach. A dilator is subsequently introduced across the mitral valve without direct visualization. The lack of direct visualization is an obvious limitation, and patients are selected in a manner similar to that used for PMBV. Without cardiopulmonary bypass, the closed approach allows for a substantial reduction in cost compared with open commissurotomy and PMBV. Due to the substantial reduction of cost, closed commissurotomy is the procedure of choice in developing nations.

Open commissurotomy has several advantages over the closed procedure. Under direct visualization, the surgeon can incise commissures, débride calcium deposits, and separate fused chordae tendineae and the underlying papillary muscle. In addition, thrombi are removed from the left atrium, and many surgeons will amputate the left atrial appendage to remove a potential source of postoperative emboli. Open commissurotomy is usually preferred in patients with a left atrial thrombus or severe subvalvular and calcific disease; however, it is costly with the use of cardiopulmonary bypass.

Mitral valve replacement is primarily indicated for patients with moderate or severe mitral stenosis (mitral valve area < 1.5 cm^2) and NYHA III–IV symptoms who are not considered candidates for PMBV or mitral repair. The choice of a mechanical valve versus a bioprosthetic should be individualized. A recent study suggested that there is no difference between the St. Jude and Medtronic Hall prosthesis with respect to late clinical performance or hemodynamic results. Therefore, the choice of mechanical valve should be based on the surgeon's experience and preference. Mechanical valves offer durability and a larger effective orifice area than bioprosthetics; however, mechanical valves are more thrombogenic and require continuous anticoagulation. Although there is a lower frequency of embolic complications with bioprosthetics, the rate of structural deterioration over 10 years is substantial in younger patients. Stentless bioprosthetic valves are available and have similar long-term outcomes as stented bioprosthetic valves. Homograft mitral valves, in contrast with homograft aortic valves, do not fair well long term.

Minimally invasive surgery with port systems can be used for mitral valve repair or replacement. To date, there is not a significant clinical advantage to this approach. Robotic surgery is also used, although this remains rare even in developed countries and is nonexistent in the developing world.

Desai DK et al. Mitral stenosis in pregnancy: a four-year experience at King Edward VIII Hospital, Durban, South Africa. BJOG. 2000 Aug;107(8):953–8. [PMID: 10955424]

deSouza JA et al. Percutaneous balloon mitral valvuloplasty in comparison with open mitral valve commissurotomy for mitral stenosis during pregnancy. J Am Coll Cardiol. 2001 Mar 1;37(3):900–3. [PMID: 11693768]

Dogan S et al. Minimally invasive port access versus conventional mitral valve surgery: prospective randomized study. Ann Thorac Surg. 2005 Feb;79(2):492–8. [PMID: 15680822]

Esteves CA et al. Immediate and long-term follow-up of percutaneous balloon valvuloplasty in pregnant patients with rheumatic mitral stenosis. Am J Cardiol. 2006 Sep 15;98(6):812–6. [PMID: 16950192]

Fawzy ME et al. Immediate and long-term results of mitral balloon valvotomy for restenosis following previous surgical or balloon mitral commissurotomy. Am J Cardiol. 2005 Oct 1;96(7):971–5. [PMID: 16188526]

Fawzy ME et al. Long term clinical and echocardiographic results of mitral balloon valvotomy in children and adolescents. Heart. 2005 Jun;91(6):743–8. [PMID: 15894766]

Krasuski RA et al. Usefulness of percutaneous balloon mitral commissurotomy in preventing the development of atrial fibrillation in patients with mitral stenosis. Am J Cardiol. 2004 Apr 1;93(7):936–9. [PMID: 15050505]

Kypson AP et al. Robotic mitral valve surgery. Am J Surg. 2004 Oct;188(4A Suppl):83S–88S. [PMID: 15476657]

McElhinney DB et al. Current management of severe congenital mitral stenosis: outcomes of transcatheter and surgical therapy in 108 infants and children. Circulation. 2005 Aug 2;112(5):707–14. [PMID: 16043648]

Mohr FW et al. Clinical experience with stentless mitral valve replacement. Ann Thorac Surg. 2005 Mar;79(3):772–5. [PMID: 15734374]

Nakajima H et al. Consequence of atrial fibrillation and the risk of embolism after percutaneous mitral commissurotomy: the necessity of the maze procedure. Ann Thorac Surg. 2004 Sep;78(3):800–5. [PMID: 15336994]

Saunders PC et al. Minimally invasive technology for mitral valve surgery via left thoracotomy: experience with forty cases. J Thorac Cardiovasc Surg. 2004 Apr;127(4):1026–31. [PMID: 15052199]

Singer DE et al. Antithrombotic therapy in atrial fibrillation: the Seventh ACCP Conference on Antithrombotic and Thrombolytic Therapy. Chest. 2004 Sep;126(3 Suppl):429S–456S. [PMID: 15383480]

Sivadasanpillai H et al. Long-term outcome of patients undergoing balloon mitral valvotomy in pregnancy. Am J Cardiol. 2005 Jun 15;95(12):1504–6. [PMID: 15950584]

Turgeman Y et al. Feasibility, safety, and morphologic predictors of outcome of repeat percutaneous balloon mitral commissurotomy. Am J Cardiol. 2005 Apr 15;95(8):989–91. [PMID: 15820172]

Wang A et al. Serial echocardiographic evaluation of restenosis after successful percutaneous mitral commissurotomy. J Am Coll Cardiol. 2002 Jan 16;39(2):328–34. [PMID: 11788227]

Wilson W et al; American Heart Association Rheumatic Fever, Endocarditis, and Kawasaki Disease Committee; American Heart Association Council on Cardiovascular Disease in the Young; American Heart Association Council on Clinical Cardiology; American Heart Association Council on Cardiovascular Surgery and Anesthesia; Quality of Care and Outcomes Research Interdisciplinary Working Group. Prevention of infective endocarditis: guidelines from the American Heart Association Rheumatic Fever, Endocarditis and Kawasaki Disease Committee, Council on Cardiovascular Disease in the Young, and the Council on Clinical Cardiology, Council on Cardiovascular Surgery and Anesthesia, and the Quality of Care and Outcomes Research Interdisciplinary Working Group. Circulation. 2007 Oct 9;116(15):1736–54. [PMID: 17446442]

▶ Prognosis

The natural history of mitral stenosis has been profoundly influenced by the advancement of cardiovascular interventions. In most patients, rheumatic mitral stenosis is a progressive disease. In a large referral population without intervention, the mitral valve area decreased at a mean rate of 0.09 cm^2/year; however, the rate of mitral valve narrowing in individual patients is variable and cannot be predicted by the initial mitral valve area, mitral valve score, or transmitral gradient, alone or in combination. The mean interval between rheumatic fever and the appearance of symptoms was 16.3 ± 5.2 years. In 84.3% of these patients, death was cardiac-related and due to right-heart failure (27.7%), lung edema resistant to medical therapy (14.5%), thromboembolic (10.8%) or hemorrhagic complications (7.2%), myocardial infarction (9.3%), or infective endocarditis (3.6%); 14.5% of the patients had a sudden death. Progression from mild symptoms to severe disability is typically accelerated and the prognosis dramatically worsens.

In addition to lower rates of restenosis, PMBV and open commissurotomy provided lower rates of reintervention than closed commissurotomy. These results appear consistent with earlier studies. The excellent results, lower cost, and obviation of a thoracotomy and cardiopulmonary bypass advocate PMBV for all patients with favorable mitral valve morphology.

The perioperative mortality rate for mitral valve replacement is less than 5% in young healthy individuals; however, the mortality rate may exceed 20% in older patients who are in NYHA Class IV. Therefore, the procedure should be performed prior to the development of significant left ventricular dysfunction. Despite the increased risk of perioperative mortality, a tangible benefit is derived from mitral valve replacement.

Carabello BA. Is it ever too late to operate on the patient with valvular heart disease? J Am Coll Cardiol. 2004 Jul 21;44(2):376–83. [PMID: 15261934]

Choudhary SK et al. Open mitral commissurotomy in the current era: indications, technique and results. Ann Thorac Surg. 2003 Jan;75(1):41–6. [PMID: 12537190]

Hellgren L et al. Survival after mitral valve replacement: rationale for surgery before occurrence of severe symptoms. Ann Thorac Surg. 2004 Oct;78(4):1241–7. [PMID: 15464479]

Nowicki ER et al. Mitral valve repair and replacement in northern New England. Am Heart J. 2003 Jun;145(6):1058–62. [PMID: 12796763]

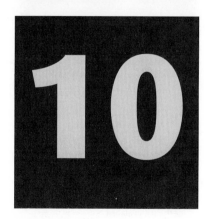

Mitral Regurgitation

Michael H. Crawford, MD

ESSENTIALS OF DIAGNOSIS

► Dyspnea or orthopnea.

► Characteristic apical systolic murmur.

► Color-flow Doppler echocardiographic evidence of systolic regurgitation into the left atrium.

General Considerations

The mitral apparatus consists of the left ventricular walls that support the papillary muscles, the chordae tendineae, mitral leaflets, annulus, and adjacent left atrial walls. Because defects in any of these components can lead to systolic regurgitation, the list of diseases that can cause mitral regurgitation includes many types of heart disease. Anything that causes left ventricular dilatation may disrupt the alignment of the papillary muscles, impairing their function and dilating the annulus, resulting in mitral regurgitation. Myocardial infarction involving the papillary muscles or the left ventricular walls that support them can impair the function of the mitral apparatus. Mitral chordae can rupture, especially in patients with hypertension or mitral valve prolapse. The most common diseases affecting the mitral leaflets are rheumatic heart disease and the myxomatous changes of mitral valve prolapse. In addition, infectious endocarditis can destroy the mitral leaflets, and mitral annular calcification can impair the normal systolic contraction of the annulus, leading to mitral regurgitation. Finally, left atrial dilatation from any cause can disrupt annular function and cause mitral regurgitation. Some patients have combinations of these defects, making mitral regurgitation both more likely and more severe.

For clinical purposes, mitral regurgitation can be divided into two broad categories: organic and functional. The former refers to diseases that involve the valve leaflets and their immediate supporting apparatus, ie, chordae and annu-lus. The latter refers to diseases that affect the left ventricle and atrium, leaving the valve apparatus intact (Table 10–1). Most clinical studies involve patients with organic mitral regurgitation, so, unless otherwise specified, the following discussion focuses on organic mitral regurgitation.

Among the many causes of chronic organic mitral regurgitation, mitral valve prolapse is a unique entity in many ways. An increase in the middle connective tissue layer of the mitral valve causes an increase in leaflet size and elongated chordae. The resultant systolic prolapse of the valve into the left atrium may or may not be accompanied by regurgitation. In some patients, regurgitation depends on left ventricular volume. Large volumes tend to reduce prolapse and hence regurgitation; small volumes have the opposite effect.

Consequently, the presence or absence of regurgitation and its severity and timing in systole (the ventricle becomes progressively smaller during systole) are determined by a complex interplay of left ventricular volume, pressure, and contractile state. Patients with mitral valve prolapse are also unique because the condition can be hereditary connective tissue disease (eg, Marfan syndrome) or acquired (inflammation of the valve). Some patients exhibit abnormalities of connective tissue in other organs (eg, thoracic skeleton) and have demonstrable abnormalities in the autonomic nervous system. Thus, the clinical presentation of mitral valve prolapse varies from one that is similar to other forms of mitral regurgitation to a unique presentation that is dominated by extracardiac manifestations.

In **chronic mitral regurgitation,** the more common of the two general clinical presentations, the mitral regurgitation progressively worsens as the underlying heart disease worsens. In this situation, the heart has time to adapt to the mitral leak. The increased pressure in the left atrium during systole causes left atrial dilatation. If this is not adequate to decompress the left atrial pressure, the pulmonary arterial tone increases to protect the pulmonary capillaries from increased hydrostatic pressure, resulting in pulmonary hypertension. Because the regurgitated blood returns to the

Table 10–1. Etiologic Classification of Mitral Regurgitation.

Organic Mitral Regurgitation
  Myxomatous changes (mitral valve prolapse)
  Rheumatic heart disease
  Infectious endocarditis
  Spontaneous chordal rupture
  Collagen vascular disease
  Trauma: penetrating and nonpenetrating
Functional Mitral Regurgitation
  Coronary artery disease
  Hypertrophic cardiomyopathy
  Dilated cardiomyopathy
  Left atrial dilatation

left ventricle in diastole, along with the normal atrial stroke volume, the volume load on the left ventricle results in left ventricular dilatation and eccentric hypertrophy.

Initially, the loading conditions in mitral regurgitation enhance left ventricular performance because preload is increased and afterload is normal. Preload is increased by the augmentation of left ventricular diastolic volume, which increases left ventricular systolic function via the Frank-Starling mechanism. Afterload, or the left ventricular wall tension after the aortic valve opens in systole, is not increased, despite increased left ventricular volume, because much of the increased volume is regurgitated into the left atrium in early systole before the aortic valve opens and because the continued regurgitation during systole reduces forward stroke volume and blood pressure. As the severity of mitral regurgitation increases over time, the ability of the dilated left ventricle to augment systolic function reaches its limits, left ventricular systolic function falls, and heart failure ensues.

Acute mitral regurgitation presents differently because there is insufficient time for these compensatory mechanisms to develop. Sudden rupture of the chordae tendineae, for example, may result in severe acute mitral regurgitation, which markedly increases left atrial pressure. Because the left atrium has no time to dilate, the pulmonary capillary pressure rises markedly, and pulmonary edema usually ensues. The left ventricle also does not dilate adequately to handle the tremendous volume load, and forward failure occurs because of an impaired left ventricular stroke volume. Acute mitral regurgitation (caused by the abrupt failure of a component of the mitral apparatus) can precipitate or aggravate symptoms in a patient with chronic mitral regurgitation.

Nesta F et al. New locus for autosomal dominant mitral valve prolapse on chromosome 13: clinical insights from genetic studies. Circulation. 2005 Sep 27;112(13):2022–30. [PMID: 16172273]

▶ Clinical Findings

A. Symptoms and Signs

1. Chronic mitral regurgitation—The medical history of patients with chronic mitral regurgitation may suggest its cause. Look for a possible history of acute rheumatic fever, coronary artery disease, or a cardiomyopathy. The most common symptom in patients with chronic mitral regurgitation is progressive dyspnea, beginning with dyspnea on exertion and progressing to paroxysmal nocturnal dyspnea and finally orthopnea. Patients may also complain of fatigue and other symptoms associated with congestive heart failure, such as edema. Chronic mitral regurgitation can lead to atrial fibrillation, and palpitations or other symptoms related to this rhythm disturbance may present in patients. Some patients with mitral valve prolapse may have atypical chest pain or inappropriate sympathetic nervous system activation (eg, tachycardia, orthostatic hypotension).

2. Acute mitral regurgitation—The patient with acute mitral regurgitation is usually markedly symptomatic, with severe orthopnea or frank pulmonary edema. Although sudden pulmonary edema in itself may suggest the diagnosis, other features of the history may point to the cause of mitral apparatus failure, such as a history of acute myocardial infarction, uncontrolled hypertension, or symptoms of infectious endocarditis.

B. Physical Examination

1. Chronic mitral regurgitation—In chronic mitral regurgitation, the heart rate may be increased because of atrial fibrillation or heart failure. The carotid pulse is usually brief and of low amplitude, and blood pressure examination shows a narrow pulse pressure. These findings reflect the reduced forward stroke volume. In the presence of heart failure, the respiratory rate may be increased and rales, pleural effusion, edema, increased jugular venous pressure, or ascites may be present. Left ventricular enlargement may result in an enlarged apical impulse. The first and second heart sounds are usually normal, and the pulmonic component of the second heart sound may be increased if pulmonary hypertension is evident. A third heart sound is common because of the left ventricular volume overload, but it does not necessarily indicate heart failure. A fourth heart sound is unusual unless associated coronary artery disease or hypertension is present. The characteristic murmur of chronic mitral regurgitation is usually holosystolic and heard best at the apex, with radiation to the axilla. Occasionally, in patients with posterior leaflet defects, the direction of the regurgitant jet may be anterior, and the murmur is heard in the aortic area. With anterior leaflet defects, the direction of the mitral jet may be posterior and transmitted to the back, where it can be heard up and down the spine. Some reports even note hearing this murmur with the stethoscope on the top of the head. In patients with mitral valve prolapse, the murmur can be crescendo and late systolic. This type of murmur, in fact, almost always represents mitral regurgitation. Often, the late systolic crescendo murmur of mitral valve prolapse is preceded by a midsystolic click from the sudden tensing of the prolapsing leaflets when the end of chordal tethering is reached. Some patients may manifest only a midsystolic click. Occasionally, mitral murmurs will be honking or musical in quality, presumably from a prolapsing leaflet that vibrates in the regurgitant stream. Some patients occasionally have other murmur configurations, whereas others with echocardiographically documented mitral regurgitation have no audible murmur, especially if the regurgitation is mild.

Because murmur configuration and radiation vary in mitral regurgitation, dynamic auscultation is of a great deal of value at the bedside for differentiating this murmur from other heart murmurs. Handgrip exercise is the favored bedside maneuver because it frequently increases the intensity of a mitral regurgitation murmur. In patients with poor grip strength, transient arterial occlusion with two blood pressure cuffs, one on each arm, is useful for producing the same effect (Table 10–2, and Chapter 1). The murmur of mitral valve prolapse behaves like that of mitral regurgitation from any cause, but it has a few unique features. Any maneuver that increases left ventricular volume will (as noted earlier) decrease the amount of mitral valve prolapse and decrease the amount of mitral regurgitation, thereby lessening the intensity of the murmur. Thus, rapid squatting will diminish the murmur of mitral valve prolapse and move the timing of the click-murmur complex later in systole (Figure 10–1). Conversely, maneuvers that decrease left ventricular volume increase the intensity and duration of the murmur of mitral valve prolapse. Thus, standing rapidly from a squatting position will make the murmur louder and move the click-murmur complex toward early systole. Extreme left ventricular volume increases can eliminate the click-murmur and mitral regurgitation, and extreme decrease can result in a

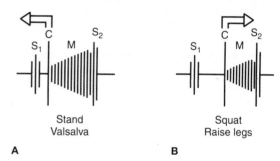

Stand
Valsalva

A

Squat
Raise legs

B

▲ **Figure 10–1.** Change in the position of the click (C)-murmur (M) complex during systole and the intensity of the murmur as a result of bedside maneuvers. **A:** Maneuvers that lengthen the murmur and increase intensity. **B:** Maneuvers that shorten the murmur and reduce its intensity. Note that the position of the midsystolic click also changes with these maneuvers.

pansystolic murmur without a click. Consequently, the auscultatory findings in mitral valve prolapse vary greatly, which can make accurate clinical diagnosis difficult.

2. Acute mitral regurgitation—In acute mitral regurgitation the physical findings are different. The marked increase in left atrial pressure, caused by regurgitation into a noncompliant left atrium, may raise left atrial pressure in late systole to the point that there is no longer any gradient for regurgitant flow. The murmur thus becomes an early systolic murmur rather than the holosystolic murmur characteristic of patients with chronic mitral regurgitation. In fact, when the acute mitral regurgitation is very severe, the murmur may not be audible. In mild-to-moderate acute mitral regurgitation, the murmur responds like the murmur of chronic mitral regurgitation with dynamic auscultation. More severe acute regurgitation is associated with high catecholamine tone and a lack of responsiveness to bedside maneuvers. Other charac-

Table 10–2. Differentiation of Systolic Murmurs Based on Changes in Their Intensity from Physiologic Maneuvers.

	Origin of Murmur					
Maneuver	**Flow**	**TR**	**AS**	**MR/VSD**	**MVP**	**HOCM**
Inspiration	– or ↑	↑	–	–	–	–
Stand	↓	–	–	–	↑	↑
Squat	↑	–	–	–	↓	↓
Valsalva maneuver	↓	↓	↓	↓	↑	↑
Handgrip/TAO	↓	–	–	↑	↑	↓
Post-PVC	↑	–	↑	–	–	↑

AS, aortic stenosis; Flow, benign flow murmur; HOCM, hypertrophic obstructive cardiomyopathy; MR, mitral regurgitation; MVP, mitral valve prolapse; PVC, premature ventricular contraction; TAO, transient arterial occlusion; TR, tricuspid regurgitation; VSD, ventricular septal defect; ↑, increase in murmur intensity; ↓, decrease in murmur intensity; –, no predictable change.

teristic features of acute mitral regurgitation include a fourth heart sound caused by vigorous atrial contraction following exaggerated expansion during ventricular systole (atrial diastole). In the presence of pulmonary hypertension, the pulmonary second sound increases, and murmurs of pulmonic and tricuspid regurgitation may be present. As mentioned earlier, acute mitral regurgitation invariably results in pulmonary edema. Consequently, the patient will have an increased respiratory rate, diffuse rales, evidence of plural effusion, increased heart rate, a narrow pulse pressure with low systolic blood pressure, and signs of acute right-heart failure, such as increased jugular venous pressure.

3. Mixed valvular disease—Patients with rheumatic valvular disease often have mixed mitral disease, which is defined as at least 2+ (on a scale of 1–4; see following section on Echocardiography) mitral regurgitation, with a mean mitral valve diastolic gradient of more than 10 mm Hg. The clinical course of mixed mitral valve disease is similar to that of mitral regurgitation, and such patients should be treated similarly. Aortic regurgitation frequently occurs with mitral regurgitation, either because of left ventricular dilatation or because the same disease process affects the aortic valve (eg, Marfan syndrome). This places an additional volume load on the left ventricle and usually accelerates the patient's clinical deterioration.

When aortic stenosis and mitral regurgitation occur together, it is sometimes difficult to ascertain whether the same disease process (eg, rheumatic disease) involved both valves or whether the pressure load of significant aortic stenosis altered left ventricular geometry, performance, or both, resulting in functional mitral regurgitation. Diagnostic imaging studies usually resolve this issue and help direct therapy.

C. Diagnostic Studies

1. Electrocardiography—Patients with chronic mitral regurgitation may have evidence of left ventricular hypertrophy, left atrial abnormality and, sometimes, right ventricular enlargement. Patients with coronary artery disease might have evidence of myocardial infarction or ischemia. Electrocardiographic (ECG) exercise testing is usually done only to confirm the patient's physical limitations, because ECG changes in the face of a left ventricular volume load are not likely to be accurate for the diagnosis of coronary artery disease. Ambulatory ECG monitoring is occasionally done in patients with palpitations to document atrial fibrillation or other intermittent rhythm disorders.

2. Chest radiography—In cases of chronic mitral regurgitation, an enlarged left ventricle and left atrium would be expected. In severe regurgitation, right-heart enlargement and pulmonary hypertension may be evident. Patients in heart failure will show pulmonary congestion and pleural effusions. In acute mitral regurgitation, there are often signs of pulmonary congestion without enlargement of the heart.

3. Echocardiography—The color-flow Doppler identification of a systolic regurgitant jet across the mitral valve into the left atrium is diagnostic of mitral regurgitation. There are several ways of estimating the severity of mitral regurgitation by analyzing the characteristics of the regurgitant jet on color-flow Doppler. The first method is the depth of penetration of the jet into the left atrium. A penetration of 1 cm or less is considered mild; 2–3 cm, moderate; and 4 cm or more, severe. If the jet is very narrow, the actual volume of regurgitant flow may not be as great as occurs with a more voluminous flow disturbance that penetrates to the same depth. Some investigators have therefore suggested also taking the area of the jet into consideration. One problem with this assessment system, however, is that if the jet impinges on a wall of the left atrium, it appears to penetrate less and be of a smaller area than if it is free in the atrial cavity. There is thus a tendency to underestimate the severity of mitral regurgitation when the jet hits the atrial wall. In addition, a regurgitant jet of any size occurring in a large left atrium will not appear as impressive as the same size jet in a small left atrium. The size of the leak in the mitral valve can be determined by evaluating the jet in a cross-sectional plane at the level of the mitral valve. This method gives an estimate of the size of the hole through which the jet is originating. These qualitative criteria for mitral regurgitation severity can be highly subjective.

For these reasons, there has been interest in more quantitative methods for estimating the severity of mitral regurgitation. The proximal isovelocity surface area observed where flow acceleration and convergence occur on the left ventricular side of the mitral leaflets allows the estimates of regurgitant volume and effective regurgitant orifice area. Fluid dynamics theory states that flow through an isovelocity surface is equal to the velocity times the surface area, which yields instantaneous regurgitant flow. This technique uses the color-flow Doppler color change interfaces observed with accelerating velocity through the orifice to estimate isovelocity surface area. Pulsed Doppler echocardiography can be used to quantitate regurgitant volume. The principle used is that of flow continuity. Systolic flow out the left ventricular outflow tract represents the forward stroke volume. This can be determined by multiplying the outflow tract area (measured on the two-dimensional echocardiographic image) times the outflow tract systolic velocity–time integral. Flow across the mitral valve in diastole represents the total stroke volume (forward plus regurgitant flow) and can be determined by multiplying mitral annulus area times the diastolic velocity–time integral. Regurgitant volume is the difference between total and forward stroke volume. Typically, the regurgitant volume is reported as the regurgitant fraction, which is the regurgitant stroke volume divided by the total stroke volume. Unfortunately, the calculation of regurgitant stroke volume has many possible sources of error, the largest of which is measuring the flow areas—mitral annular and outflow tract. Thus, individuals without valvular regurgitation can have regurgitant fractions of up to 20%. Also, the calculation of regurgitant flow is time-consuming and requires considerable skill. Effective regurgitant orifice area can be estimated as the ratio of regurgitant volume to the regurgitant jet velocity–time integral by pulsed Doppler.

Assessment of pulmonary venous flow velocity by pulsed Doppler echocardiography can also be of value in estimating the severity of mitral regurgitation. Normal pulmonary venous flow velocity is biphasic, with a predominant systolic forward velocity and a lesser diastolic forward velocity in older adults. Systolic forward velocity is reduced in patients with mitral regurgitation, and often the diastolic velocity predominates. In severe mitral regurgitation, the systolic flow in the pulmonary vein signal may reverse. Systolic flow reversal is highly specific for severe regurgitation but sensitivity is low. Unfortunately, pulmonary venous flow velocity patterns vary considerably in patients with mitral regurgitation, and the predictive value for regurgitation severity is low. In many laboratories, all these factors are integrated to produce a composite estimate of the severity of regurgitation, usually on a scale of 1 to 4, with 4 being severe mitral regurgitation. Table 10–3 exhibits the criteria for grading the severity of mitral regurgitation.

Echocardiography can be used to evaluate the anatomy of the mitral apparatus to determine where the defect lies and what its cause may be. For example, patients with rheumatic mitral valve disease have thickening of the mitral leaflets, especially at the tips, with rolled edges and regurgitation along the commissural fissure lines. Patients with mitral valve prolapse have voluminous mitral leaflets that prolapse into the left atrium in the latter part of systole. Patients with coronary artery disease have wall motion abnormalities near the papillary muscle attachments. Ruptured and flail chordae tendineae are readily detected by echocardiography, as is mitral annular calcification.

The echocardiogram is also useful for assessing the compensatory changes in the cardiovascular system resulting from mitral regurgitation. The degree of left ventricular and left atrial enlargement are related to the severity of the mitral regurgitation and its chronicity. Left ventricular systolic performance is an important determinant of prognosis in mitral regurgitation (see Prognosis). Doppler estimation of pulmonary artery pressures from pulmonic or tricuspid regurgitant jets is valuable for estimating the effect of mitral regurgitation on the pulmonary circulation. An assessment of right-heart chamber sizes and function is additional useful information. Echocardiography is also used for differentiating other conditions, such as ventricular septal defect (VSD), aortic stenosis, and hypertrophic obstructive cardiomyopathy (HOCM), that might be confused on history and physical examination with mitral regurgitation.

Table 10–3. Echocardiographic Grading of Mitral Regurgitation Severity.

Grading System	Mild	Mild to Moderate	Moderate to Severe	Severe
Angiographic grade	1+	2+	3+	4+
Specific signs	Jet area < 4 cm² Jet area to LA area < 20% Visual orifice width < 0.3 cm No or minimal flow convergence			Jet area > 40% of LA area Visual orifice width > 0.7 cm Flow reversed in pulmonary veins Major flail segment of leaflet Papillary muscle rupture
Supportive signs	Systolic dominant PV flow to A wave dominant mitral inflow Low density continuous wave Doppler MR signal Normal LV and LA size			Dense continuous wave Doppler signal E wave dominant mitral inflow, E > 1.2 m/s Enlarged LV and LA Normal LV function
Quantitative measurements				
Regurgitant volume, mL/beat	< 30	30–44	45–59	≥ 60
Regurgitant fraction, %	< 30	30–39	40–49	≥ 50
Effective orifice area, cm²	< 0.2	0.2–0.29	0.3–0.39	≥ 40

Modified, with permission, from Zoghbi WA et al. J Am Soc Echocardiogr. 2003;16:777.
LA, left atrium; LV, left ventricle; MR, mitral regurgitation; PV, pulmonary vein.

Color-flow Doppler echocardiography can detect trivial or mild mitral regurgitation in up to half of otherwise healthy adults. The incidence increases with age and with the rigor with which the operator interrogates the valve. In the absence of anatomic abnormalities, small degrees of regurgitation are probably benign effects of aging. In most cases, mild mitral regurgitation found by echocardiography is not associated with a murmur on physical examination.

Transesophageal echocardiography (TEE) can provide the anatomic details of leaflet anatomy needed to plan surgical repair. The probe is rotated progressively to identify the scallops of the two mitral valve leaflets in midesophageal long axis views. The rotation of the color-flow jet helps confirm the incompetent scallops. In addition, annular size can be determined and the subvalvular apparatus interrogated. TEE during surgery can be of value to the surgeon. Also, three-dimensional transthoracic echocardiography is useful for identifying the culprit scallops and may replace TEE.

4. Cardiac catheterization—Cardiac catheterization is rarely needed to diagnose mitral regurgitation, nor is it usually needed to assess the severity of the regurgitation, left ventricular size and function, or any resultant pulmonary hypertension. Coronary angiography is useful, however, for establishing artery disease as the likely cause of mitral regurgitation as well as the risk from surgical correction of mitral regurgitation from any cause.

Hemodynamic evaluation at the time of cardiac catheterization in patients with moderate-to-severe mitral regurgitation will show an increase in pulmonary artery pressures, increases in the pulmonary capillary wedge pressure (PCWP), and possibly a reduction in forward cardiac output. The PCWP tracing often displays a large v wave, which is more than 50% greater than the height of the a wave. Although much has been made of the diagnostic value of large v waves in the PCWP tracing (especially in the ICU setting) it must be remembered that any cause of left atrial pressure elevation will elevate the height of the v wave. It is only when the v wave is elevated out of proportion to the a wave that the diagnosis of mitral regurgitation is likely ($> 150\%$ of the a wave).

Left ventricular angiography is graded with a 1–4+ system, where 1+ is mild and 4+ is severe, indicating regurgitation of the angiographic dye into the pulmonary veins (see Table 10–3). This assessment method correlates well with the color-flow Doppler system. In addition, left ventricular angiography is useful for estimating left ventricular volume and ejection fraction. Cardiac catheterization can exclude the presence of other diseases, such as VSD, HOCM, and aortic stenosis, that might be confused with mitral regurgitation. Certain aspects of the patient's hemodynamics, such as the presence of pulmonary hypertension, are of prognostic value in mitral regurgitation.

Gutierrez-Chico JL et al. Accuracy of real-time 3-dimensional echocardiography in the assessment of mitral prolapse. Is transesophageal echocardiography still mandatory? Am Heart J. 2008 Apr;155(4):694–8. [PMID: 18371478]

O'Gara P et al. The role of imaging in chronic degenerative mitral regurgitation. J Am Coll Cardiol Img. 2008;1:221–37.

Pepi M et al. Head-to-toe comparison of two- and three-dimensional transthoracic and transesophageal echocardiography in the localization of mitral valve prolapse. J Am Coll Cardiol. 2006 Dec 19;48(12):2524–30. [PMID: 17174193]

Pu M et al. Comparison of quantitative and semiquantitative methods for assessing mitral regurgitation by transesophageal echocardiography. Am J Cardiol. 2001 Jan 1;87(1):66–70. [PMID: 11137836]

Supino PG et al. Prognostic value of exercise tolerance testing asymptomatic chronic nonischemic mitral regurgitation. Am J Cardiol. 2007 Oct 15;100(8):1274–81. [PMID: 17920370]

▶ Differential Diagnosis

Because the symptoms seen in chronic mitral regurgitation are not specific for this condition, the physical examination is crucial for the differential diagnosis. The murmur of tricuspid regurgitation, for example, can occasionally be heard at the apex, especially if the right ventricle is enlarged and displaced leftward. Differentiating features include the increase in the intensity of the murmur with inspiration, the large v waves in the jugular pulse, a right ventricular lift, and a pulsatile liver. It should be noted that tricuspid regurgitation can result from pulmonary hypertension caused by mitral regurgitation, so some patients have both murmurs. In this situation, the murmur of tricuspid regurgitation is best assessed at the left or right sternal border, and those of mitral regurgitation at the apex. It may be difficult, however, to distinguish between the two murmurs in patients where both are moderately severe.

The murmur of **aortic stenosis** is often confused with mitral regurgitation, especially when the mitral regurgitant murmur is atypical or radiates to the aortic area. The murmur of aortic stenosis is usually lower in pitch than that of mitral regurgitation; it radiates to the neck and is often accompanied by an S_4 sound. In aortic stenosis, the left ventricular apical impulse amplitude often increases but not necessarily in size, as is found in patients with mitral regurgitation. On dynamic auscultation, there is no change in the murmur of aortic stenosis with handgrip exercise, but the murmur does increase in the beat following a premature ventricular contraction. Perhaps the best bedside maneuver for distinguishing between these two murmurs is the inhalation of amyl nitrite. This potent vasodilator causes the murmur of aortic stenosis to become louder and that of mitral regurgitation softer.

A **VSD**, especially a muscular defect low in the septum, may mimic the murmur of mitral regurgitation. Because dynamic auscultation will not distinguish between these two left ventricular regurgitant murmurs, other signs must be used. The patient with VSD usually has a large right ventricle, and a vibration (thrill) over the anterior chest may be palpable. The murmur of **HOCM** can also be confused with mitral regurgitation. The major differential features are that the murmur of HOCM increases with the Valsalva maneuver, whereas the murmur of mitral regurgitation decreases; the murmur of HOCM decreases with handgrip, and the murmur of mitral regurgitation increases. In addition, the patient with HOCM usually has a prominent fourth heart sound. However, because many patients with HOCM also have mitral regurgitation, the ability to distinguish it from mitral regurgitation is difficult in some patients.

The murmur of **mitral valve prolapse** can be difficult to distinguish from the murmur of HOCM because both murmurs change in intensity and in a similar direction with the stand and squat and Valsalva maneuvers.

In this situation, other features of each disease, such as the midsystolic click with mitral valve prolapse and the left ventricular hypertrophy evident on palpation of the chest, or the fourth heart sound in the patient with HOCM, are useful for differentiating the two conditions by physical examination. The major differential diagnosis of acute mitral regurgitation is acute VSD because both may occur in the setting of acute myocardial infarction. A palpable vibration is more common, and the right ventricle is usually more prominent with VSD, but perhaps the best differentiation is that the patient with acute VSD has much less dyspnea than does the patient with acute mitral regurgitation. The response to dynamic auscultation is the same in these two conditions.

▶ Treatment

A. Pharmacologic Therapy

Vasodilators are useful in acute mitral regurgitation to decrease aortic pressure and impedance, favoring forward over regurgitant flow during systole. This decreases left ventricular size and left ventricular and atrial pressures, improves forward cardiac output, and decreases the amount of regurgitation. Studies of acute regurgitation with vasodilators, such as hydralazine, nifedipine, and nitroprusside, have demonstrated this effect in the hemodynamics laboratory and, thus, their usefulness for managing acute mitral regurgitation. Studies on the pharmacologic treatment of patients with chronic mitral regurgitation are scant, and the available data are not particularly encouraging. Because afterload is not increased in patients with well-compensated chronic mitral regurgitation, lowering it further may not improve forward flow and would more likely reduce it. Many patients experience vasodilator side effects, and if forward cardiac output is not improved, the patient's overall hemodynamic status is actually worsened. Thus, until further data are obtained, there is no evidence to support vasodilator therapy for asymptomatic patients with mitral regurgitation. In mildly symptomatic patients who presumably have left ventricular dilation and dysfunction, but who want to avoid surgery, vasodilators could be tried. Markedly symptomatic patients, however, are better treated surgically.

1. Digoxin—Digoxin is useful in atrial fibrillation for controlling the heart rate. Whether it is of any value for improving forward output with mitral regurgitation in patients with normal sinus rhythm is unknown. If there are other indications for using the drug, however, it is not known to be harmful to the overall hemodynamic status of patients with mitral regurgitation.

2. Oral anticoagulation—Oral anticoagulation is indicated for patients in atrial fibrillation and those with concomitant mitral stenosis. Whether patients with moderate-to-severe mitral regurgitation, with large left ventricles and large left atria, who are in normal sinus rhythm and have normal left ventricular function would benefit from anticoagulants is controversial. Eccentric regurgitant jets may produce areas of stasis in the left atrium, according to color-flow Doppler studies. Furthermore, patients with moderate-to-severe mitral regurgitation are always at risk for developing atrial fibrillation. Although an argument can be made for longterm anticoagulation in such patients, no clinical trials support this approach.

3. Antibiotic prophylaxis—Only patients with prosthetic heart valves now require antibiotics to prevent the development of bacterial endocarditis. Patients in whom rheumatic heart disease is the likely cause of mitral regurgitation should also have rheumatic fever antibiotic prophylaxis.

B. Surgical Treatment

Patients with acute, severe, or decompensated chronic severe mitral regurgitation will need urgent surgical therapy—if it is appropriate to their general medical condition. Such patients can usually be stabilized with intravenous vasodilators, such as hydralazine or nitroprusside, and other therapies for heart failure, such as diuretics. If there is no response to pharmacologic therapy, an intra-aortic balloon pump is indicated. This mechanical approach will reduce arterial and left ventricular pressure in systole, favoring forward flow rather than regurgitant and increased diastolic aortic pressure, and may improve left ventricular contractility. Most patients will stabilize on this therapy, allowing for an appropriate evaluation (eg, coronary angiography), thereby maximizing the benefits of surgery.

Patients with either acute or chronic moderately severe mitral regurgitation will eventually need surgical therapy. The issue is the appropriate timing of surgery. If the physician waits until the symptoms are marked because of left heart failure with depressed left ventricular systolic function and severe pulmonary hypertension, not much symptomatic improvement is achieved after surgery, and left ventricular function remains depressed. On the other hand, if surgery is performed earlier, the patient may become relatively asymptomatic, with normal left ventricular function. Considerable effort has been directed at determining prognostic indicators for avoiding a poor response to surgical therapy. Prospective studies have shown that the following are all markers of a poor prognosis following surgery: an ejection fraction of 60% or less, an end-systolic volume index of 50 mL/m^2 or more, an end-diastolic dimension on echocardiography of 45 mm or more, significant pulmonary hypertension, and atrial fibrillation. Although it seems logical that surgery should therefore be performed before these indicators are obtained in a patient, even one who is asymptomatic, this decision analysis has never been tested in clinical trials (Table 10–4).

In patients with aortic and mitral regurgitation, if the mitral valve is not obviously diseased and the mitral regurgitation is mild to moderate (1–2+), replacing the aortic valve will often diminish left ventricular size enough to reduce or eliminate the mitral regurgitation. Sometimes a mitral annular ring will be required to reduce mitral annular size. In cases where the mitral valve leaflets and chordae are diseased or the regurgitation is severe, valve repair or replacement will be necessary—at the cost of a higher likelihood of operative mortality or postoperative morbidity. Severe aortic stenosis is often accompanied by mild-to-moderate mitral regurgitation. In this situation, the reduction in left ventricular pressure produced by aortic valve replacement usually reduces the mitral regurgitation, and further mitral surgery can be avoided.

The pulmonary hypertension that often accompanies mitral regurgitation may lead to tricuspid and pulmonic regurgitation. The latter usually resolves when the pulmonary pressure is reduced by mitral valve surgery, and pulmonary valve replacement is rarely necessary. Tricuspid regurgitation, if mild-to-moderate and associated with moderately severe pulmonary hypertension, will usually resolve after successful mitral surgery. If the tricuspid regurgitation is moderately severe, but the leaflets are not diseased, a tricuspid ring may be effective; if tricuspid valve disease is present, repair or replacement will be necessary. One clinical guideline for the need for tricuspid valve repair or replacement is a mean right atrial pressure of more than 15 mm Hg; however, the decision for this is often made during surgery, after the mitral procedure has been completed.

The onset of heart failure symptoms should prompt consideration of surgical treatment. Symptoms such as dyspnea, fatigue, and edema develop in some patients before the clinical and hemodynamic signs and symptoms of mitral regurgitation develop. The importance of other symptoms, such as a history of arrhythmias or recurrent systemic emboli, is less certain. If the hemodynamic indicators are absent, other therapies for these conditions should be attempted first, before surgery.

Other factors to be taken into account when deciding when to perform surgery are the type of operation—valve repair or replacement—and the type of prosthetic valve, should one be needed. It is now possible in many patients with mitral regurgitation to repair rather than replace the mitral valve. Patients with mitral valve prolapse, ruptured chordae tendineae, or a ruptured papillary muscle are especially likely to respond to reparative surgery, whereas patients with markedly deformed valves and fused chordae from rheumatic heart disease, patients with infective endocarditis, or patients with left ventricular disease are less likely to be

Table 10–4. General Indications for Considering Mitral Valve Surgery in Patients with Chronic Severe Organic Mitral Regurgitation.

Symptoms such as dyspnea
Left ventricular ejection fraction $\leq 60\%$
Left ventricular end-systolic dimension ≥ 45 mm
Left ventricular end-systolic volume index ≥ 50 mL/m^2
Atrial fibrillation
Pulmonary artery systolic pressure > 50 mm Hg

helped by mitral valve repair and often require valve replacement. Repair is preferable, especially for the patient with normal sinus rhythm because there is no need for long-term anticoagulation therapy following surgery. In addition, mitral valve repair is generally associated with better preservation of left ventricular systolic function following surgery and is therefore highly advantageous for patients with a low left ventricular ejection fraction and a repairable mitral valve. Also, mitral valve repair can be done with minimally invasive approaches, often involving robotic surgical and endoscopic devices. Thus, if it is likely that mitral valve repair can be done, there is less reluctance about operating in asymptomatic patients that otherwise meet criteria for surgery.

If valve replacement is necessary, ventricular function can be preserved by leaving the chordae intact; chordal tethering of the papillary muscles is presumed to improve left ventricular performance. With valve replacement, the choice between a mechanical and a bioprosthetic valve may influence the timing of surgery.

In general, mechanical prosthetic valves are preferred because of their better long-term reliability. Bioprosthetic valves can be chosen when valve longevity is not an issue or when patients want to try to avoid anticoagulation therapy. The latter would apply mainly to young women with normal sinus rhythm who want to become pregnant. They will be much easier to treat without anticoagulation therapy—a feasible goal with a bioprosthetic valve. These patients must realize, however, that this valve will need to be replaced in approximately 10–15 years, as a result of deterioration. This should give these patients time for several pregnancies, if they so desire.

Generally, patients with a mechanical valve and no contraindications to anticoagulation therapy should be treated with such agents. The incidence of systemic emboli is higher with mitral than with aortic prosthetic valves. Without anticoagulation, there is a 1–3% per year chance of systemic emboli with a bioprosthetic valve in the mitral position, so aspirin therapy is recommended for patients with bioprosthetic valves. The use of warfarin for 3 months after bioprosthetic mitral valve replacement is sometimes done until the endothelium grows over the sewing ring reducing the risk of thrombus development. Patients with other risks for thrombus formation, such as atrial fibrillation, should also receive warfarin. Percutaneous approaches to mitral valve repair and replacement are under development. One approach is to put a clip at the tip of the mitral leaflets creating a double orifice valve similar to the surgical Alfieri technique. Another is to deliver an annuloplasty ring into the coronary sinus, reducing the annulus size. Finally, stent-mounted tissue valves can be used in the mitral area. At this time, these devices have not been released for routine use, but they hold great promise for the future.

Feldman T et al. Percutaneous mitral valve repair using the edge-to-edge technique: six-month results of the EVEREST PHASE I Clinical Trial. J Am Coll Cardiol. 2005 Dec 6;46(11):2134–40. [PMID: 16325053]

Harris KM et al. Effects of angiotensin-converting enzyme inhibition on mitral regurgitation severity, left ventricular size, and functional capacity. Am Heart J. 2005 Nov;150(5):1106. [PMID: 16291006]

Nifong LW et al. Robotic mitral valve surgery: a United States multicenter trial. J Thorac Cardiovasc Surg. 2005 Jun;129(6):1395–404. [PMID: 15942584]

Webb JG et al. Percutaneous transvenous mitral annuloplasty: initial human experience with device implantation in the coronary sinus. Circulation. 2006 Feb 14;113(6):851–5. [PMID: 16461812]

▶ Prognosis

Patients with chronic mitral regurgitation have an average survival curve similar to that of patients with chronic aortic regurgitation and chronic mitral stenosis. The cause of the chronic mitral regurgitation in individual patients influences the prognosis. In general, patients with coronary artery disease as the cause have a poor prognosis, those with the myxomatous changes of mitral valve prolapse have the best prognosis, and those with rheumatic heart disease have an intermediate prognosis. The onset of infectious endocarditis can markedly alter the prognosis. In addition, any sudden deterioration of mitral valve function that leads to acute worsening of the mitral regurgitation lessens the prognosis.

The prognosis in acute mitral regurgitation, when it is associated with acute pulmonary edema and severe symptoms, is guarded; it also depends on the cause. For example, patients with acute severe mitral regurgitation from acute myocardial infarction have a much worse prognosis than do otherwise healthy individuals who rupture a chorda. In general, most patients with acute mitral regurgitation require immediate surgical attention, and their prognosis is not as good as that for patients with chronic mitral regurgitation.

American College of Cardiology/American Heart Association Task Force on Practice Guidelines; Society of Cardiovascular Anesthesiologists; Society for Cardiovascular Angiography and Interventions; Society of Thoracic Surgeons, Bonow RO et al. ACC/AHA 2006 guidelines for the management of patients with valvular heart disease: a report of the American College of Cardiology/American Heart Association Task Force on Practice Guidelines (writing committee to revise the 1998 Guidelines for the Management of Patients with Valvular Heart Disease): developed in collaboration with the Society of Cardiovascular Anesthesiologists: endorsed by the Society for Cardiovascular Angiography and Interventions and the Society of Thoracic Surgeons. Circulation. 2006 Aug 1;114(5):e84–231. [PMID: 16880336]

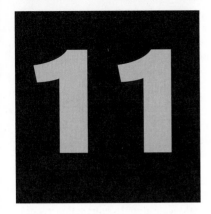

Tricuspid & Pulmonic Valve Disease

Brian D. Hoit, MD & Subha L. Varahan, MD

TRICUSPID VALVE DISEASE

ESSENTIALS OF DIAGNOSIS

Tricuspid regurgitation

▶ Prominent *v* wave in jugular venous pulse.

▶ Systolic murmur at left lower sternal border that increases with inspiration.

▶ Characteristic Doppler echocardiographic findings, including right ventricular (RV) volume overload (RV enlargement, paradoxical septal motion, and diastolic flattening of the interventricular septum), right atrial enlargement, and systolic turbulence in the right atrium.

Tricuspid stenosis

▶ Prominent *a* wave and reduced *y* descent in jugular venous pulse.

▶ Diastolic murmur at left lower sternal border that increases with inspiration.

▶ Characteristic Doppler echocardiographic findings, including a thickened and domed valve with restricted motion, right atrial enlargement, and increased diastolic velocity across the tricuspid valve.

▶ General Considerations

Clinical interest in tricuspid valve disorders has increased because of several distinct but interrelated events in clinical cardiology. First, high-resolution, noninvasive imaging techniques have been developed and validated, allowing clinicians to easily assess the morphology and function of the tricuspid valve. Second, the frequency of tricuspid valve endocarditis has increased significantly, owing largely to an increasing population of injection drug users, patients with

implanted cardiac devices or long-term central venous catheters, and, to a lesser extent, a growing number of immunocompromised patients. Third, several reparative percutaneous and surgical techniques with acceptable morbidity and mortality rates now exist. In addition, investigations in both animals and humans have demonstrated the influence of right-heart disease on cardiovascular performance vis-à-vis series and parallel interactions with the left ventricle.

▶ Pathophysiology & Etiology

The tricuspid valve has three leaflets that are unequal in size (anterior > septal > posterior). The papillary muscles are not as well defined as those of the left ventricle and are subject to considerable variation in both their size and leaflet support. Like the mitral valve, the leaflets, annulus, chordae, papillary muscles, and contiguous myocardium contribute individually to normal valve function and can be altered by pathophysiologic processes (Table 11–1).

A. Tricuspid Regurgitation

Tricuspid regurgitation most frequently occurs with a structurally normal tricuspid valve (functional tricuspid regurgitation), which is the result of a dilated right ventricle and tricuspid annulus and papillary muscle dysfunction.

Functional tricuspid regurgitation is usually observed in patients with disease of the left heart (eg, left ventricular [LV] dysfunction, mitral valve disease), pulmonary vascular and parenchymal disease, right ventricular (RV) infarction, arrhythmogenic RV dysplasia, and congenital heart disease.

By contrast, primary tricuspid regurgitation occurs when the intrinsic structure of the valve is anatomically abnormal.

Rheumatic tricuspid regurgitation almost always coexists with mitral valve involvement. Although two-thirds of patients with rheumatic mitral valve disease have pathologic evidence of tricuspid valve involvement, clinically significant tricuspid disease, which generally affects young and middle-

Table 11–1. Causes of Tricuspid Valve Disease.

Tricuspid Regurgitation	Tricuspid Stenosis
Functional (structurally normal tricuspid valve)	Rheumatic
Rheumatic	Carcinoid heart disease
Infective endocarditis	Tumors
Congenital (eg, tricuspid valve prolapse, Ebstein anomaly)	Congenital (eg, Ebstein anomaly)
Carcinoid heart disease	Regional cardiac tamponade
Systemic lupus erythematosus	Systemic lupus erythematosus
Catheter-induced	Whipple disease
Trauma	Fabry disease
Tumors	Infective endocarditis
Orthotopic heart transplantation	Endomyocardial fibrosis
Endomyocardial fibrosis	Endocardial fibroelastosis
Antiphospholipid syndrome	Methysergide therapy
	Antiphospholipid syndrome

aged women, is much less common. Rheumatic tricuspid involvement is usually mild and generally is shown clinically as pure regurgitation or mixed insufficiency and stenosis, caused by the fibrosis of the valve leaflets and chordae tendineae; contracture of the leaflets and commissural fusion produce regurgitation and stenosis, respectively.

Tricuspid valve endocarditis, which occurs primarily in injection drug users and patients with chronic intravascular hardware, may complicate left-to-right shunts, burns, and immunocompromised states. Infective endocarditis is more common in injecting drug users who are HIV-positive than in those who are HIV-negative. Infective endocarditis is typically caused by virulent pathogens that infect structurally normal valves. *Staphylococcus aureus* is the most common organism; the next most common pathogens are streptococci and enterococci. *Pseudomonas* and *Candida* species also predominate, and polymicrobial infections are not uncommon. Geographic location should also be considered when attempting to identify the responsible pathogens. Fungal endocarditis should be considered when vegetations are large; they occasionally cause obstruction. Abscesses may involve the annulus and septum, and chordal rupture or valve perforations may cause tricuspid regurgitation.

Carcinoid tumors are a rare cause of both tricuspid and pulmonic valve disease. The vasoactive substances (principally serotonin) produced by these tumors are believed to be causal, and patients with carcinoid valvular disease have higher serum levels of serotonin and increased urinary excretion of its metabolite, 5-hydroxyindoleacetic acid (5-HIAA), than those without cardiac disease. Left-sided valve involvement is unusual due to inactivation of these vasoactive molecules by monoamine oxidase in the lungs but can be seen in patients with right-to-left shunts or bronchial tumors. The valve exhibits pathognomonic plaque-like deposits of fibrous tissue (which may also deposit on the endocardium); leaflet distortion leads to regurgitation, ste-

nosis, or both. Tricuspid regurgitation is the most common lesion and is detected by echocardiography in virtually all patients with carcinoid tricuspid valve disease. Cardiac involvement is progressive and causes significant morbidity and mortality in such patients but early detection and surgical management may prolong survival. Long-term survival has been reported after tricuspid valve replacement, but carcinoid plaques may deposit on the bioprosthetic leaflets.

Tricuspid valve prolapse, owing to myxomatous degeneration, is seen almost exclusively in patients with mitral valve prolapse and occurs in as many as 50% of cases. Isolated involvement has been confirmed, however, by both echocardiography and necropsy. Anterior leaflet prolapse is most common, followed by septal and posterior leaflet prolapse. The associated tricuspid regurgitation is usually mild. Although tricuspid valve prolapse may be a marker of generalized connective tissue disease and a poor prognostic indicator in patients with mitral valve prolapse, its clinical significance remains undefined. Like mitral valve prolapse, the precise incidence of tricuspid valve prolapse is difficult to determine because of inconsistent clinical, echocardiographic, and angiographic definitions.

Tricuspid regurgitation is a frequent component of **Ebstein anomaly** of the tricuspid valve because of the apical displacement of septal and posterior tricuspid leaflets. This results in "atrialization" of a variable portion of the right ventricle and a range of abnormalities involving the anterior leaflet and atrial septum. The downward displacement of the tricuspid valve frequently causes a tricuspid regurgitant murmur (heard best in the apical area). This uncommon congenital abnormality is associated with right-to-left intra-atrial shunting, RV dysfunction, supraventricular arrhythmias, and sudden death.

Tricuspid regurgitation of at least moderate severity may complicate as many as 25% of cases of **systemic lupus erythematosus**; significant tricuspid regurgitation is usually due to the pulmonary hypertension produced by lupus pulmonary disease. Libman-Sacks endocarditis that involves the tricuspid valve is far less common. However, Libman-Sacks endocarditis has been associated with antiphospholipid antibodies, which have been shown to cause valvular thickening, isolated tricuspid involvement, and the development of nonbacterial vegetations. The cause of the valve disease is poorly understood, but intravalvular capillary thrombosis is believed to be a factor. Most patients present with combined tricuspid regurgitation and stenosis, and the regurgitation is typically moderate or severe. Pulmonary hypertension is usually present, and contributes to the valvular dysfunction.

Although **catheter-induced** tricuspid regurgitation occurs in approximately 50% of cases with catheters across the valve, the regurgitation is quantitatively small, clinically unimportant, and usually disappears when the catheter is removed. Tricuspid regurgitation can occur as a late complication of successful mitral valve replacement (MVR). In one series,

Doppler-detected moderate-to-severe regurgitation occurred in two-thirds of patients at a mean of over 11 years following MVR; over one-third of these patients had clinically evident tricuspid regurgitation. Other causes include blunt and penetrating trauma (rupture of papillary muscles, chordal disruption or detachment, leaflet rupture, complete valve destruction), primary or secondary cardiac tumors, orthotopic heart transplantation, and endomyocardial fibrosis.

B. Tricuspid Stenosis

Tricuspid stenosis is an uncommon lesion that is usually rheumatic in origin and almost exclusively accompanies mitral stenosis. Isolated rheumatic tricuspid stenosis is rare, and subvalvular disease is usually less severe in tricuspid than in mitral stenosis. Isolated carcinoid tricuspid stenosis is also rare; tricuspid regurgitation is more frequent and often occurs with pulmonic stenosis. Right atrial (RA) myxomas and obstructing metastatic tumors may produce hemodynamic changes that are indistinguishable from tricuspid stenosis. Tricuspid stenosis may be congenital and is infrequently predominant in Ebstein anomaly. Extrinsic compression of the tricuspid valve by a loculated pericardial effusion is an uncommon cause of tricuspid stenosis. Other unusual causes include systemic lupus erythematosus, Whipple disease, Fabry disease, antiphospholipid syndrome, infective endocarditis, endocardial fibroelastosis, and as a sequela to methysergide therapy. It should be noted that prosthetic tricuspid valves, like all prosthetic valves, are inherently stenotic.

Perez-Villa F et al. Severe valvular regurgitation and antiphospholipid antibodies in systemic lupus erythematosus: a prospective, long-term, followup study. Arthritis Rheum. 2005 Jun 15;53(3):460–7. [PMID: 15934103]
Raman SV et al. Tricuspid valve disease: tricuspid valve complex perspective. Curr Probl Cardiol. 2002 Mar;27(3):103–42. [PMID: 11979238]
Wilson LE et al. Prospective study of infective endocarditis among injection drug users. J Infect Dis. 2002 Jun 15;185(12):1761–6. [PMID: 12085322]

▶ Clinical Findings

A. Symptoms and Signs

Tricuspid valve disease can be difficult to recognize clinically. The symptoms may be overshadowed by associated illness, such as systemic lupus erythematosus, infective endocarditis, trauma, or neoplasia. The dominant presenting features may be symptoms that are usually not considered cardiac in origin: abdominal discomfort, jaundice, wasting, and inanition. In addition, patients with associated cardiovascular disease may have nonspecific symptoms (exertional dyspnea and fatigue in mitral stenosis) that obfuscate the diagnosis and deflect the suspicion of tricuspid valve disease. In patients with mitral stenosis, for example, tricuspid valve disease protects the pulmonary circulation and exertional dyspnea, pulmonary edema, and hemoptysis are less commonly reported, although a history of excessive fatigue may be elicited. Most often, however, the history is insufficient to diagnose tricuspid valve disease, and only a careful physical examination provides the necessary clues.

B. Physical Examination

1. Jugular venous pulse—Because the internal jugular veins lack effective valves, they should be inspected for an estimate of RA pressure (Figure 11–1 shows a normal jugular venous pulse). There are three waves (a, c, and v) and two descents, x and y (which correspond to the a and v waves, respectively). The a wave and the initial descent are produced by atrial contraction and relaxation, respectively. The x descent is interrupted by a c wave that is caused by isovolumetric contraction of the right ventricle and resultant bowing of the tricuspid valve toward the right atrium. The continuation of the x descent (sometimes called x') is caused by the descent of the arteriovenous (AV) ring toward the apex during RV ejection. The right atrium fills and, because the tricuspid valve is closed, RA pressure rises, causing the v wave. The rapid fall in volume and pressure when the valve opens produces the y descent. Except for a small but variable delay, the jugular venous pulse and RA pressure contours are similar.

When inspecting the jugular venous pulse, the examiner should pay careful attention to the magnitude of the central venous (mean RA) pressure, the dominant wave (a or v), and changes in pulse contour with respiration. Tricuspid valve disease is typically associated with increased central venous pressure.

A. Tricuspid regurgitation—The x descent of the jugular venous pulse is interrupted by an early v wave (c-v wave) with a rapid y descent (Figure 11–2). These findings are characteristically augmented during inspiration. The neck veins are distended, and the earlobes may pulsate. Because venous distention may obscure the jugular pulse contour, it is important to elevate the patient's head. RV volume overload leads to prominent pulsations over the left lower sternal border.

B. Tricuspid stenosis—In tricuspid stenosis (Figure 11–3), inspection of the jugular veins reveals a dominant a wave (assuming sinus rhythm), which increases with inspiration, and a slow and shallow y descent due to resistance to early RV diastolic filling.

2. Cardiac auscultation

A. Tricuspid regurgitation—Tricuspid regurgitation is classically associated with a holosystolic murmur that is best heard at the right or left midsternal border, but when the right ventricle is markedly dilated, the location of the murmur may move toward the left and suggest mitral regurgitation. The auscultatory hallmark of tricuspid regurgitation is an inspiratory augmentation from increased systemic venous return and tricuspid valve flow (Figure 11–4). Under such circumstances as severe tricuspid regurgitation, markedly increased RA pressures, and RV systolic failure, the murmur

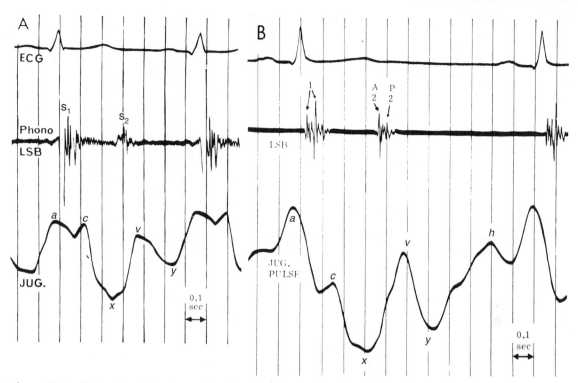

▲ **Figure 11–1.** Normal jugular venous pulse tracings at fast (**A**) and slow (**B**) heart rates. The *a* wave is the dominant reflection. At slow heart rates, an *h* wave signifying the end of right ventricular filling can be seen. LSB, left sternal border. (Reproduced, with permission, from Tavel ME. *Clinical Phonocardiograpy and External Pulse Recoding.* Yearbook Medical Publishers, 1978.)

may not increase with inspiration. Although usually described as holosystolic, the timing of the murmur may be early, mid, or late systolic. The murmur may be decrescendo when tricuspid regurgitation is severe and acute, and its character reflects the presence of a giant *c-v* wave; there may be a middiastolic flow rumble that resembles tricuspid stenosis. The murmur of tricuspid regurgitation is usually not accompanied by a thrill, and there is little radiation of the murmur. When the tricuspid valve is wide open in systole, there may be no murmur. An S_3, which can vary in intensity and with inspiration, is often associated with an extremely dilated right ventricle. An S_4 may also be heard if there is significant RV hypertrophy.

B. Tricuspid Stenosis—The tricuspid opening snap is difficult to distinguish from the mitral opening snap and auscultatory findings may be difficult to distinguish from existing mitral stenosis. Unlike mitral stenosis, however, the diastolic rumble of tricuspid stenosis has a higher pitch, increases with inspiration, is usually loudest at the lower left sternal border, and follows the opening snap of mitral stenosis. The tricuspid stenosis murmur is often scratchy, ends before the first heart sound, and has no pre-systolic

crescendo in patients with normal sinus rhythm. A diastolic murmur from relative tricuspid stenosis may be heard with large atrial septal defects and severe tricuspid regurgitation. In patients with normal sinus rhythm, a pre-systolic hepatic pulsation may be felt; this is due to reflux from atrial contraction against the stenotic valve. Both tricuspid stenosis and regurgitation can, if chronic, lead to ascites, jaundice, wasting, and muscle loss. Tricuspid valve disease, which is often diagnosed or suspected at the bedside, can almost always be confirmed with echocardiography.

C. Diagnostic Studies

The diagnostic evaluation of suspected tricuspid valve disease includes electrocardiography (ECG), plain chest film, two-dimensional and Doppler echocardiography, and cardiac catheterization. Limited experience with cine magnetic resonance imaging (MRI) and computed tomography (CT) suggests that, except in certain instances (such as the evaluation of carcinoid heart disease), the technique offers no clear advantage over Doppler echocardiography. Except for RV volume and ejection fraction determinations, nuclear studies are generally not clinically useful in tricuspid valve disease.

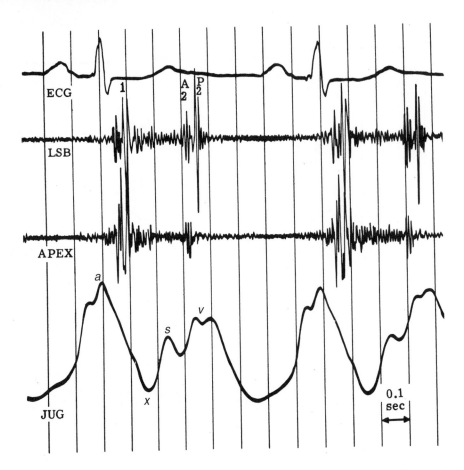

▲ **Figure 11-2.** Jugular venous pulse tracing from a patient with mitral stenosis and tricuspid regurgitation secondary to pulmonary hypertension. Note the shallow *x* descent, the midsystolic *s* wave, and the respiratory increase in the *v* wave. (Reproduced, with permission, from Tavel ME. *Clinical Phonocardiography and External Pulse Recording.* Yearbook Medical Publishers, 1978.)

1. Electrocardiography—P waves characteristic of RA enlargement with no evidence of RV hypertrophy suggest isolated tricuspid stenosis. Most often, however, the rhythm is atrial fibrillation. When pulmonary hypertension is the cause of tricuspid regurgitation, the ECG may show evidence of RV hypertrophy with right axis deviation and tall R waves in V_1 to V_2 and RA enlargement (Figure 11–5A). Atrial fibrillation is also common and incomplete right bundle branch block and Q waves in V_1 are occasionally seen. Preexcitation frequently accompanies Ebstein anomaly (Figure 11–5B).

2. Chest radiography—In tricuspid stenosis, the chest film is characterized by cardiomegaly, with a prominent right-heart border caused by RA enlargement, and a dilated superior vena cava and azygous vein. Pulmonary vascular markings may be notably absent. The chest film in tricus-

pid regurgitation shows cardiomegaly from RA and RV enlargement; pleural effusions and elevated diaphragms from ascites may be seen. In general, a dilated heart in the absence of pulmonary congestion or pulmonary hypertension should suggest either tricuspid valve disease or pericardial effusion. Massive RA enlargement suggests Ebstein anomaly.

3. Echocardiography—Echocardiography is the most useful noninvasive diagnostic test for evaluating tricuspid valve disease. Two-dimensional and Doppler echocardiographic examinations can identify associated disease of the left ventricle and other cardiac valves (eg, mitral stenosis), show the anatomic sequelae of chronic tricuspid valve disease (eg, dilated right heart chambers), and detect structural abnormalities of the tricuspid valve (eg, a thickened tricuspid

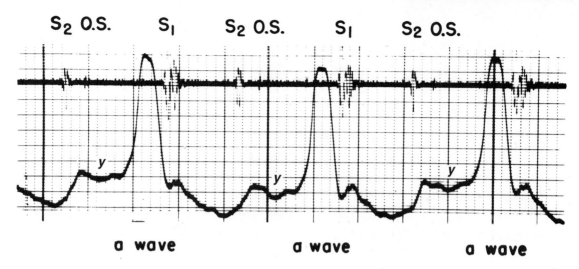

▲ Figure 11–3. Jugular venous pulse tracing and phonocardiogram from a patient with rheumatic tricuspid stenosis. Note the striking *a* waves and the shallow *y* descents. A loud S, and opening snap (O.S.) are evident on the accompanying phonocardiogram. (Courtesy of Fowler NO.)

valve with decreased mobility, compression of the tricuspid annulus, or involvement by tumor or prolapsing or displaced leaflets and vegetations; Figure 11–6). Multiplane transesophageal echocardiography may be helpful when diagnostic images cannot be obtained from transthoracic views or when associated disease of the interatrial septum, atria, and mitral valve is suspected. Agreement between transesophageal echocardiographic and intraoperative surgical findings in patients with infective endocarditis is excellent.

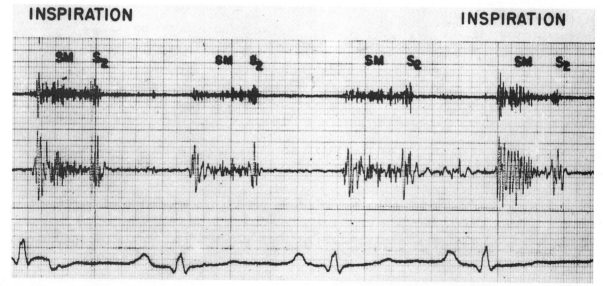

▲ Figure 11–4. Phonocardiogram from a patient with tricuspid regurgitation secondary to heart failure. The systolic murmur increases with inspiration, seen most clearly on the lower phonocardiographic tracing. Note that the murmur does not extend to the second heart sound. (Courtesy of Fowler NO.)

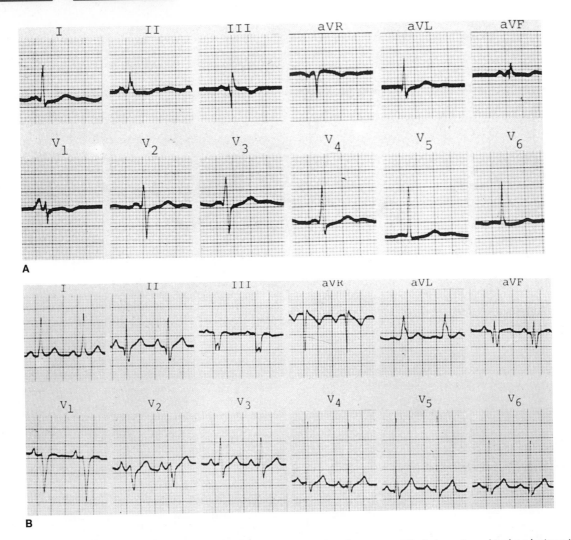

▲ **Figure 11–5.** Electrocardiograms from patients with tricuspid valve disease. **A:** Mitral stenosis and isolated tricuspid stenosis. The tall initial P-wave forces in lead V indicate right atrial enlargement. There is no electrocardiographic evidence of right ventricular hypertrophy. (Reproduced, with permission, from Chou TE. *Electrocardiography in Clinical Practice,* 3rd ed. Philadelphia: WB Saunders, 1991.) **B:** Patient with Ebstein anomaly and preexcitation. Delta waves create a pseudoinfarct pattern. P-wave amplitude in leads II and V_2 is consistent with right atrial enlargement. (Courtesy of Chou TE.)

A. TRICUSPID REGURGITATION—In tricuspid regurgitation, the echocardiographic findings usually show RV volume overload with a dilated right ventricle, paradoxical septal motion, and diastolic flattening of the interventricular septum. Contrast or color-flow Doppler echocardiography can visualize the tricuspid regurgitant jet. Turbulence can be detected by pulsed wave Doppler, the tricuspid valve diastolic gradient can be quantified using continuous wave Doppler, and pulmonary arterial pressure can be estimated from the pulmonary artery acceleration time or the peak velocity of the tricuspid regurgitant jet. Two-dimensional echocardiography distinguishes between primary disease of the left heart and RV disease, both of which cause functional tricuspid regurgitation and organic disease of the tricuspid valve. Contrast found in the inferior vena cava and hepatic veins following injection of agitated saline into an arm vein implies significant tricuspid regurgitation. On the other hand, a tricuspid valve annulus less than 3.4 cm in diameter

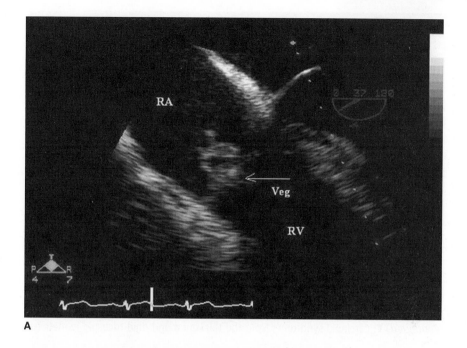

A

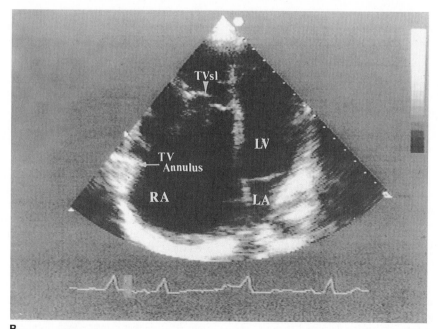

B

▲ **Figure 11–6.** Two-dimensional echocardiograms illustrating abnormalities of the tricuspid valve leaflets. **A:** Infective endocarditis. RA, right atrium; RV, right ventricle; Veg, tricuspid valve vegetation. **B:** Ebstein anomaly. Note the displacement of the septal leaflet (TVsl) relative to the tricuspid valve annulus. LV, left ventricle; RA, right atrium. (*continued*)

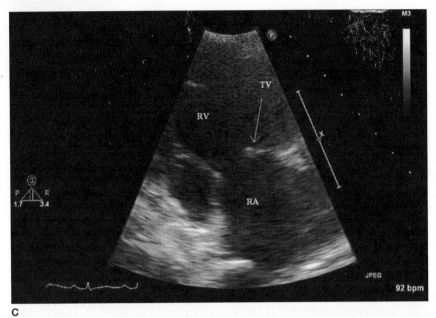

c

▲ **Figure 11–6.** (*Continued*) **C:** Carcinoid syndrome. Note the thickened and rigid tricuspid leaflets (*arrow*).

during diastole virtually excludes significant tricuspid regurgitation. The temporal and spatial distribution of systolic turbulence in the right atrium, using either color-flow mapping or pulsed wave Doppler, can be a means of estimating the severity of the regurgitation. Systolic reversal of the Doppler signal in the hepatic veins indicates significant tricuspid regurgitation. Newer Doppler techniques that quantitatively estimate effective regurgitant orifice, regurgitant volume, and regurgitant fraction have been developed and validated. It should be recognized that Doppler-detected tricuspid regurgitation occurs commonly in normal individuals. In such cases, the Doppler signal tends not to be holosystolic, and systolic turbulence occupies only a small area of the right atrium.

B. Tricuspid stenosis—As shown in Figure 11–7, the stenotic tricuspid valve is thickened and domed and has restricted motion. The echocardiographic appearance alone may be misleading because many patients with two-dimensional echocardiographic findings that suggest tricuspid stenosis have normal tricuspid valve diastolic pressure gradients. Although the right atrium is usually dilated, the right ventricle is not enlarged in isolated tricuspid stenosis. The severity of the stenosis is determined with continuous wave Doppler. Accurate peak instantaneous and mean gradients across the stenotic tricuspid valve are readily calculated using the modified **Bernoulli equation,** which relates a pressure drop (dP) to the velocity (V) across a stenosis ($dP = 4V^2$). The pressure half-time method for calculating valve orifice area, used successfully for the mitral valve, has not been

validated for the tricuspid valve. A tricuspid valve area less than 1.0 cm^2 indicates severe tricuspid stenosis.

4. Cardiac catheterization

A. Tricuspid regurgitation—Opacification of the right atrium following injection of radiographic contrast into the right ventricle detects and estimates the severity of the regurgitation. Although right ventriculography requires a catheter across the tricuspid valve, there is no significant contrast leak into the right atrium under normal circumstances. Right atrial and ventricular pressures are elevated, and the RA pressure may become "ventricularized" as a result of a large *c-v* wave and an absent *x* descent (Figure 11–8A). **Kussmaul sign** (increased RA pressure with inspiration or the absence of a normal fall in RA pressure) may be seen when the regurgitation is severe.

B. Tricuspid stenosis—In tricuspid stenosis, the mean RA pressure is increased; characteristically, the *a* wave is prominent and the *y* descent is slow. The hallmark of tricuspid stenosis is a diastolic gradient between the right atrium and right ventricle that increases with inspiration (Figure 11–8B). The gradients are frequently small, however, their detection is enhanced by recording RA and RV pressures simultaneously with two optimally damped catheters and equally sensitive transducers. Because of the low gradient, calculation of the valve area is unreliable. Injection or rapid volume infusion of atropine to increase the heart rate can increase the diastolic gradient and facilitate the diagnosis.

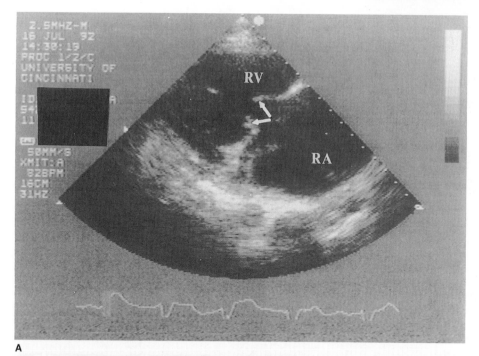

▲ **Figure 11-7. A:** Two-dimensional echocardiogram from a patient with rheumatic tricuspid valve disease, showing a thickened and domed tricuspid valve (*arrows*). The right atrium (RA) is considerably dilated and the right ventricle (RV) is enlarged. **B:** Continuous wave Doppler study from the same patient confirms tricuspid stenosis and regurgitation. The high-velocity signal above the baseline during diastole represents right ventricular inflow; the signal below the baseline during systole represents tricuspid regurgitation.

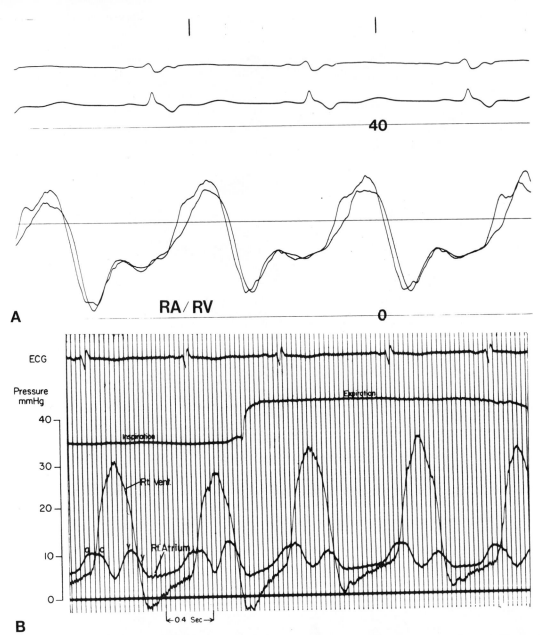

40

RA / RV

A

0

ECG

Pressure
mmHg

40 —

30 —

Expiration

Inspiration

Rt Vent.

20 —

10 —

a c
          v
Rt Atrium

0 —

←0 4 Sec→

B

▲ **Figure 11–8.** Hemodynamic recordings from patients with tricuspid valve disease. **A:** Severe tricuspid regurgitation. There is "ventricularization" of the right atrial (RA) pressures, which are indistinguishable from right ventricular (RV) pressures. **B:** Simultaneous and equally sensitive recordings of RA and RV pressures from a patient with rheumatic tricuspid stenosis. Note the RA-RV gradient throughout diastole, which increases with inspiration. (Reproduced, with permission, from Fowler et al. *Diagnosis of Heart Disease*. New York: Springer-Verlag, 1991.)

American College of Cardiology; American Heart Association Task Force on Practice Guidelines (Writing Committee to revise the 1998 guidelines for the management of patients with valvular heart disease); Society of Cardiovascular Anesthesiologists; Bonow RO et al. ACC/AHA 2006 guidelines for the management of patients with valvular heart disease: a report of the American College of Cardiology/American Heart Association Task Force on Practice Guidelines (writing Committee to Revise the 1998 guidelines for the management of patients with valvular heart disease) developed in collaboration with the

Society of Cardiovascular Anesthesiologists endorsed by the Society for Cardiovascular Angiography and Interventions and the Society of Thoracic Surgeons. J Am Coll Cardiol. 2006 Aug 1;48(3):e1–148. [PMID: 16875962]

Bonow RO et al. Task Force 3: valvular heart disease. J Am Coll Cardiol. 2005 Apr 19;45(8):1334–40. [PMID: 15837283]

Zoghbi WA et al; American Society of Echocardiography. Recommendations for evaluation of the severity of native valvular regurgitation with two-dimensional and Doppler echocardiography. J Am Soc Echocardiogr. 2003 Jul;16(7):777–802. [PMID: 12835667]

▶ Treatment

A. Medical

Tricuspid regurgitation is well tolerated in the absence of pulmonary hypertension. When pulmonary arterial pressures increase, cardiac output falls, leading to symptoms of right-heart failure (edema, fatigue, dyspnea). Restriction of sodium and the use of potent loop diuretics, angiotensin-converting enzyme (ACE) inhibitors, or angiotensin receptor antagonists decrease RA pressure. Medical therapy is also aimed at the cause of pulmonary hypertension, which is usually treated with nitric oxide donors, phosphodiesterase inhibitors, endothelin antagonists, and prostacyclin analogues (alone or in combination), depending on the specific cause. Treatment of associated systemic diseases is a critically important aspect of the therapeutic paradigm; it is, however, beyond the scope of this discussion. Symptomatic tricuspid stenosis is treated surgically.

B. Surgical

Surgery on the tricuspid valve may involve repair, reconstruction, excision, or replacement with a prosthetic valve. The decision to operate on the stenotic tricuspid valve is a straightforward one; the decision to operate on a regurgitant valve is more challenging. The surgeon must determine whether the regurgitation is functional or organic (ie, associated with a structurally normal or abnormal tricuspid valve), and if it is functional, the response of the pulmonary arterial pressure to the primary procedure should be anticipated. For example, repair may be unnecessary for functional tricuspid regurgitation if there is a high likelihood of a postoperative fall in pulmonary arterial pressure. In addition, repair of the functionally regurgitant tricuspid valve in patients with severe right ventricular dysfunction is unlikely to improve their status. However, the response of tricuspid regurgitation to reduced pulmonary artery pressure can be difficult to predict, and, as mentioned previously, significant tricuspid regurgitation often complicates successful MVR despite reduced pulmonary artery pressures. Given the high morbidity and mortality associated with reoperation to correct tricuspid regurgitation following MVR, the presence of any degree of preoperative tricuspid regurgitation, especially organic regurgitation, warrants consideration of concurrent tricuspid valve repair. Moreover, because "functional" tricuspid regurgitation may be due to unrecognized annular involvement and because annular dilation may be progressive, "prophylactic" tricuspid annuloplasty has been recommended when the annular diameter exceeds 21 mm/m^2. Interestingly, in patients with chronic pulmonary thromboembolic disease, pulmonary thromboendarterectomy dramatically reduces functional tricuspid regurgitation without a change in tricuspid annular diameter.

The decision whether to repair or replace the tricuspid valve with a prosthesis depends on the suitability of valve repair, the associated surgical procedures, and the underlying disease. Thrombosis is a more frequent problem with tricuspid than with mitral prostheses. Thus, primary valve repair, when possible, is the preferred procedure. Repair of the stenotic tricuspid valve involves identifying and separating the fan chordae (the chords that support the leaflets in the area of the commissure), leaflet decalcification, and chordal or papillary muscle division.

Annuloplasty procedures correct dilatation of the tricuspid valve annulus. The dilatation, which is not symmetric, typically involves the annulus around the anterior and posterior leaflets (posterior more than anterior). The procedure involves sizing and selectively plicating the anterior and posterior annuli. Although the routine use of an annuloplasty ring is considered superior to non-ring methods and is recommended by some groups, this position is not universally accepted.

When the tricuspid valve cannot be repaired and replacement is necessary, a porcine prosthesis is often used because of the lower risk of thrombosis, although recent changes in valve design have significantly lowered the risk of thrombosis with mechanical prostheses. Bioprosthetic valves are also more prone to late failure than mechanical prostheses. If anticoagulation is necessary for other reasons, a St. Jude prothesis is preferred by some surgeons—especially for younger patients. A recent meta-analysis indicates that long-term outcomes (mortality, thrombosis, structural deterioration) for bioprosthetic and mechanical valves are similar.

The primary indications for surgery in patients with tricuspid valve endocarditis are uncontrollable infection, septic emboli, or refractory congestive heart failure. Because virulent organisms are the rule, they are not, per se, an indication for surgery. Total excision of the tricuspid valve is an attractive option in injection drug users, considering both recidivism and the threat of prosthetic valve endocarditis. As noted earlier, tricuspid regurgitation without pulmonary hypertension is well tolerated; however, 20% of these patients ultimately may require valve replacement for right-heart failure. Debridement and valve repair have been suggested as alternative procedures to valve excision.

Successful percutaneous balloon valvuloplasty has been reported for native valve tricuspid stenosis and stenotic bioprosthetic tricuspid valves but experience is limited. There are no published studies to compare percutaneous balloon valvotomy with surgical valvuloplasty, and only limited long-term results have been published.

C. Postoperative Management

Postoperative management is dictated largely by the surgical procedures involved. Catheters are not left across prosthetic tricuspid valves, although this does not pose a difficulty with either valve repairs or annuloplasty procedures. Cardioversion to sinus rhythm is generally not successful if preoperative atrial fibrillation was present.

Antunes MJ et al. Management of tricuspid valve regurgitation. Heart. 2007 Feb;93(2):271–6. [PMID: 17228081]

Chang BC et al. Long-term clinical results of tricuspid valve replacement. Ann Thorac Surg. 2006 Apr;81(4):1317–23. [PMID: 16564264]

Dreyfus G et al. Secondary tricuspid regurgitation or dilatation: which should be the criteria for surgical repair? Ann Thorac Surg. 2005 Jan;79(1):127–32. [PMID: 15620928]

Fukuda S et al. Determinants of recurrent or residual functional tricuspid regurgitation after tricuspid annuloplasty. Circulation. 2006 Jul 4;114(1 Suppl):I582–7. [PMID: 16820642]

Jassal DS et al. Surgical management of infective endocarditis. J Heart Valve Dis. 2006 Jan;15(1):115–21. [PMID: 16480022]

Rizzoli G et al. Biological or mechanical prostheses in tricuspid position? A meta-analysis of intra-institutional results. Ann Thorac Surg. 2004 May;77(5):1607–14. [PMID: 15111151]

Sadeghi HM et al. Does lowering pulmonary arterial pressure eliminate severe functional tricuspid regurgitation? Insights from pulmonary thromboendarterectomy. J Am Coll Cardiol. 2004 Jul 7;44(1):126–32. [PMID: 15234420]

Sastry BK. Pharmacologic treatment for pulmonary arterial hypertension. Curr Opin Cardiol 2006 Nov;21(6):561–8. [PMID: 17053404]

Tang GH et al. Tricuspid valve repair with an annuloplasty ring results in improved long-term outcomes. Circulation. 2006 Jul 4;114(1 Suppl):I577–81. [PMID: 16820641]

▶ Prognosis

The natural history of tricuspid valve disease is a function of the associated valvular lesions and the primary disease (eg, rheumatic fever, carcinoid syndrome, Ebstein anomaly). Isolated lesions are rare, and their natural history is unknown.

Regardless of etiology, tricuspid regurgitation is associated with decreased survival. In a study of 5223 patients who underwent echocardiography between 1998 and 2002, patients were stratified according to whether they had no, mild, moderate, or severe tricuspid regurgitation (11%, 73%, 12%, and 4% of the study group, respectively). The survival rates at 1 year for patients in these four groups were 92%, 90%, 79%, and 64%, respectively. In general, the results of tricuspid valve surgery depend on the types of valve lesions, the corrective procedures, the degree and reversibility of LV and RV function, and the pulmonary vascular resistance. Residual tricuspid regurgitation usually occurs when the pulmonary vascular resistance remains elevated. Many patients have small-to-moderate tricuspid valve gradients after tricuspid valve replacement; like residual tricuspid valve leaks, these are usually not clinically important.

Although most surgeons favor repair over replacement, the superiority of this approach is difficult to prove. The hemodynamics are comparable, with a greater gradient after prosthetic valve replacement and more tricuspid regurgitation following repair. Because the problem of thromboemboli is reduced, complications should be less of a problem after repair. Data suggest that long-term survival in patients may be better after repair than valve replacement, but a randomized trial has never been performed.

Nath J et al. Impact of tricuspid regurgitation on long-term survival. J Am Coll Cardiol. 2004 Feb 4;43(3):405–9. [PMID: 15013122]

PULMONIC VALVE DISEASE

 ESSENTIALS OF DIAGNOSIS

Pulmonic regurgitation

▶ Diastolic murmur at the left upper sternal border that increases with inspiration.

▶ Split S_2 with a loud P_2.

▶ Characteristic Doppler echocardiographic findings, including valvular abnormalities (depending on etiology), right ventricular enlargement, and diastolic turbulence in the right ventricular outflow tract.

Pulmonic stenosis

▶ Systolic murmur at the left second intercostal space preceded by a systolic click.

▶ Split S_2 with a soft P_2.

▶ Characteristic Doppler echocardiographic findings, including thickened and domed leaflets, and increased systolic velocities across the pulmonic valve.

▶ General Considerations

The technologic advances made in the fields of noninvasive cardiac imaging, interventional cardiology, and cardiac surgery over the past few decades have had a noticeable effect on the diagnosis and management of pulmonic valve disease.

▶ Pathophysiology & Etiology

The normal pulmonic valve is a semilunar valve with anterior, left, and right leaflets. The function and texture of the valve leaflets, as well as the size of the valve annulus can be adversely affected in a variety of diseases.

A. Pulmonic Regurgitation

Pulmonic regurgitation most commonly occurs in the setting of pulmonary hypertension. The regurgitation is caused by dilatation of the pulmonic valve ring, and any cause of pulmonary hypertension can precipitate pulmonic regurgitation. **Idiopathic dilation** of the pulmonary trunk and **Marfan syndrome** also cause pulmonic regurgitation via a similar distortion of the valve ring. **Infective endocarditis** is the most frequently encountered cause of acquired pulmonic regurgitation, with vegetations causing dysfunction of the leaflets themselves. Although the pulmonic valve is the least likely to be seeded in endocarditis, the rising number of injecting drug users, immunocompromised persons, and patients with subclinical pulmonic stenosis represent a growing population at risk. Pulmonic regurgitation can also occur as a consequence of surgical treatment for **tetralogy of Fallot, congenital pulmonic stenosis,** or balloon valvuloplasty. The pulmonic regurgitation is generally mild and hemodynamically insignificant, but in rare cases it can progress to RV dilation, necessitating pulmonic valve replacement. **Rheumatic heart disease** is an infrequent cause of pulmonic regurgitation, and it invariably occurs in the setting of multiple valve disease. Other rare causes of pulmonic regurgitation include chest trauma, carcinoid tumors, syphilis, and catheter-related valve dysfunction. It should be noted that trivial pulmonic regurgitation is frequently encountered on routine echocardiography and is considered a normal variant.

B. Pulmonic Stenosis

Pulmonic stenosis is a congenital disorder in over 95% of cases. Congenital pulmonic stenosis is usually caused by a valvular lesion although subvalvular (infundibular hypertrophy) and supravalvular (rare intracardiac tumors, congenital rubella syndrome) lesions do occur. Valvular pulmonic stenosis is most often due to fibrosis of the valve with thickening of the leaflets. The leaflets dome into the pulmonary trunk during systole, producing a narrow central aperture. Less commonly, the valve leaflets are dysplastic and rubbery with a small valve annulus. Bicuspid pulmonic valves also occur. The pathologic distinctions made earlier do have some clinical relevance, as dysplastic valves are less responsive to balloon dilatation than dome-shaped valves. **Isolated congenital pulmonic stenosis** is the most commonly encountered congenital pulmonic valve disease in adulthood, and it typically causes valvular pulmonic stenosis. **Tetralogy of Fallot** also causes pulmonic stenosis with a bicuspid valve, and **Noonan syndrome** can be associated with dysplastic pulmonic stenosis. Other congenital syndromes associated with pulmonic stenosis include double-outlet right ventricle, atrioventricular canal defect, and univentricular atrioventricular connection.

The most common acquired form of pulmonic stenosis occurs with **carcinoid heart disease.** The proposed mechanism for carcinoid valve disease has been discussed earlier in this chapter. The whitish carcinoid plaques adhere to the valve leaflets and can cause both pulmonic stenosis and pulmonic regurgitation. Rheumatic heart disease is a rare cause of pulmonic stenosis and when present is generally seen with multiple valve disease. Large vegetations on an infected pulmonic valve can rarely cause pulmonic stenosis.

Moller JE et al. Factors associated with the progression of carcinoid heart disease. N Engl J Med. 2003 Mar 13;348(11):1005–15. [PMID: 12637610]

▶ Clinical Findings

A. Symptoms and Signs

As with tricuspid disease the symptoms of pulmonic valve disease can be subtle and overshadowed by coexisting illnesses. Patients with pulmonic regurgitation are often asymptomatic unless symptoms of pulmonary hypertension and RV failure eventuate. Patients with pulmonic stenosis are also frequently asymptomatic. Symptoms can appear gradually as the pulmonic valve pressure gradient increases and include exertional dyspnea, chest pain, and fatigue.

B. Physical Examination

1. Jugular venous waveform—The presence of pulmonic stenosis is suggested by a prominent jugular venous *a* wave in the setting of a relatively normal central venous pressure.

2. Cardiac auscultation

A. PULMONIC REGURGITATION—The pulmonic component of S_2 is usually loud because most patients have pulmonary hypertension, and the second heart sound is often split due to prolonged RV emptying. RV S_3 and S_4 gallops are sometimes heard in the left parasternal area. In the absence of pulmonary hypertension, the murmur of pulmonic regurgitation is a low-pitched, crescendo–decrescendo diastolic murmur that is best heard near the left third or fourth intercostal space. The murmur is augmented during inspiration. However, in patients with significant pulmonary hypertension the murmur assumes a different quality. The dilatation of the pulmonic valve annulus allows for a more forceful regurgitant jet, resulting in a high-pitched, decrescendo murmur that is best heard at the left parasternal border near the second or third intercostal space, otherwise known as the **Graham Steell murmur.**

B. PULMONIC STENOSIS—The second heart sound is also split with pulmonic stenosis, and this splitting is proportional to the degree of stenosis. Unlike in pulmonic regurgitation, the pulmonic component of S_2 is soft in pulmonic stenosis, and an S_4 can frequently be appreciated over the lower left sternal border. A high-frequency systolic click can be heard near the left upper sternal border that precedes the late-peaking crescendo–decrescendo systolic murmur that typifies pulmonic stenosis. Unlike the murmur, the click becomes softer during inspiration due to enhanced late diastolic pulmonic valve opening with the increased RV filling. The murmur can be associated with a thrill, and an RV impulse is frequently palpable.

C. Diagnostic Studies

The diagnostic evaluation of pulmonic valve disease should include an ECG, chest film, and a transthoracic echocardiographic study with Doppler imaging. Cardiac catheterization is generally unnecessary given the high degree of agreement between echocardiographic and catheterization data in pulmonic valve disease.

1. Electrocardiography—Pulmonic regurgitation and pulmonic stenosis can both demonstrate the effects of RV strain and pulmonary hypertension on surface tracings. Typical findings include right bundle branch block, right axis deviation, and RV hypertrophy. Mild or moderate pulmonic stenosis frequently presents with a normal ECG.

2. Chest radiography—Nonspecific enlargement of the right ventricle and pulmonary arteries can be seen with pulmonic regurgitation. Characteristically, pulmonic stenosis is associated with dilatation of the main pulmonary artery.

3. Echocardiography—In pulmonic regurgitation, the pulsed Doppler technique is used to accurately detect the presence and severity of pulmonic regurgitation. In addition, the presence of pulmonary hypertension, RV hypertrophy and dilation, and coexistent valve disease can be detected. Transesophageal echocardiography has a role in the evaluation of suspected pulmonic valve endocarditis.

Echocardiography determines the nature, location, and severity of the stenosis. Pulmonary stenosis is diagnosed almost exclusively by Doppler echocardiography, and, as with pulmonic regurgitation, data regarding the status of the ventricles and other valves can also be obtained. Transesophageal studies may be useful when the location of the stenosis is unclear from the surface study.

4. Cardiac catheterization—According to the 2006 AHA/ACC Guidelines, cardiac catheterization is recommended in adolescents and young adults with congenital pulmonic stenosis for evaluation of the valvular gradient if the Doppler peak jet velocity is greater than 3 m per second and balloon valvotomy is feasible.

▶ Treatment

Pulmonic regurgitation rarely requires specific treatment. Treatment of predisposing cardiac conditions, such as pulmonary hypertension, endocarditis, or left-sided valve disease, often improves the pulmonic regurgitation. As mentioned previously, certain patients may progress to right-heart failure from pulmonic regurgitation following repair of tetralogy of Fallot. These patients may require valve replacement, often with a porcine valve or pulmonary allograft.

Pulmonic stenosis has been managed with great success by balloon valvuloplasty. Treatment is based on severity of disease: balloon valvotomy is recommended if the RV–to–pulmonary artery peak-to-peak gradient is greater than 30 mm Hg at catheterization in the symptomatic patient, and greater than 40 mm Hg in the asymptomatic patient. Patients with dysplastic valves may not respond to balloon valvuloplasty and may require valve replacement with a porcine valve or pulmonary homograft. Percutaneous stented pulmonary valve implantation is being evaluated as an alternative to surgical repair of pulmonic stenosis and regurgitation in selected patients; initial results suggest significant early symptomatic improvement and low procedural morbidity.

▶ Prognosis

The prognosis of pulmonic valve disease is generally excellent. With pulmonic regurgitation, clinicians must consider the comorbidities involved (particularly pulmonary hypertension) that may influence prognosis. Patients with congenital pulmonic stenosis can expect a life expectancy comparable to that of the general population.

American College of Cardiology; American Heart Association Task Force on Practice Guidelines (Writing Committee to revise the 1998 guidelines for the management of patients with valvular heart disease); Society of Cardiovascular Anesthesiologists; Bonow RO et al. ACC/AHA 2006 guidelines for the management of patients with valvular heart disease: a report of the American College of Cardiology/American Heart Association Task Force on Practice Guidelines (writing Committee to Revise the 1998 guidelines for the management of patients with valvular heart disease) developed in collaboration with the Society of Cardiovascular Anesthesiologists endorsed by the Society for Cardiovascular Angiography and Interventions and the Society of Thoracic Surgeons. J Am Coll Cardiol. 2006 Aug 1;48(3):e1–148. [PMID: 16875962]

Nordmeyer J et al. Current experience with percutaneous pulmonary valve implantation. Semin Thorac Cardiovasc Surg. 2006 Summer;18(2):122–5. [PMID: 17157232]

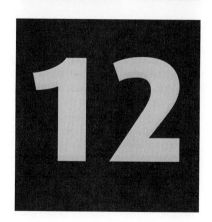

Infective Endocarditis

Bruce K. Shively, MD* & Michael H. Crawford, MD

Bruce K. Shively, MD* & Michael H. Crawford, MD

ESSENTIALS OF DIAGNOSIS

▶ Fever.

▶ Blood cultures positive for bacteria or fungi.

▶ Cardiac lesions on echocardiography.

General Considerations

Infective endocarditis is one of several infections in which endothelium is the initial site of infection. Healthy endothelium possesses an effective system of defense against both hemostasis and infection. Infection of the endothelium of blood vessels occurs only at sites markedly altered by disease or surgery, such as the severely atherosclerotic aorta or the suture lines of vascular grafts. By contrast, infection of the cardiac valve leaflet endothelium (endocardium) is not rare and occurs even in the absence of identifiable preexisting valve disease.

Pathophysiology & Etiology

A. Cardiac Infection—Vegetations

1. Precursor lesion and bacteremia—Valve infection probably begins when minor trauma, with or without accompanying valve disease, impairs the antihemostatic function of valve endocardium. Infection usually first appears along the coapting surface of the leaflets, suggesting a role for valve opening and closing. This hypothesis is supported by the observation that the ranking of valves in order of frequency of infection corresponds to the ranking of valves according to the force acting to close the valve (mitral > aortic > tricuspid > pulmonic).

This minor trauma may cause the formation of a microscopic thrombus on the leaflet surface. A small noninfected thrombus on the leaflet is called **nonbacterial thrombotic endocarditis (NBTE).** The next step is infection of the fibrin matrix of the thrombus by blood-borne organisms, which appear briefly in blood under many circumstances, such as brushing one's teeth. When transient bacteremia coincides with the presence of an NBTE lesion, organisms may adhere to the valve leaflet and begin to proliferate.

This theory for the pathogenesis of endocarditis is supported by observations regarding the circumstances under which endocarditis occurs and the particular organisms involved. Patients with endocarditis often tell of a preceding event that likely resulted in transient bacteremia. The common infecting organisms are those that gain entry to the blood because they colonize body surfaces and are adapted for attachment and proliferation in the NBTE lesion (see Clinical Syndromes).

2. Growth of vegetations—Vegetations begin near the coaptation line of the leaflet on the side that contacts the opposite leaflet during valve closure. Mitral valve vegetations are typically attached within 1–2 cm of the leaflet tip on the left atrial side and prolapse into the left atrium during systole. Aortic valve vegetations usually occur on the left ventricular (LV) side of the mid- or distal portions of the aortic cusps and prolapse into the LV outflow tract during diastole. A similar distribution of lesions occurs on the tricuspid and pulmonic valves.

Although the course of cardiac lesions in endocarditis varies, in a typical sequence of events (without treatment), the infection progresses by enlargement of the vegetation and extension of its region of attachment toward the base of the leaflet. Valve regurgitation almost always develops, as a result of either destruction of the leaflet tip or scarring and retraction of the leaflet. Erosion of the leaflet may lead to perforation (usually associated with clinically significant regurgitation). Weakening of the leaflet's spongiosum layer may result in a deformity called a leaflet aneurysm. Mitral or tricuspid chordal involvement may cause rupture and acute severe regurgitation. In rare cases (primarily in mitral bioprosthetic endocarditis; see Management of High-Risk

---

*Deceased.

Endocarditis), a large vegetation may cause hemodynamically significant valve obstruction.

3. Metastatic vegetations—These vegetations may form when the regurgitant jet of blood from an infected valve strikes an endocardial surface in the receiving chamber (wall or chordae), producing a small area of denuded endothelium. The thrombus that forms at this site also becomes infected, constituting a secondary vegetation. Such metastatic vegetations most often appear on the ventricular side of the anterior mitral leaflet where it is struck by a regurgitant jet from aortic valve endocarditis. Another common location is on the mitral chordae, also from aortic regurgitation. Metastatic lesions on the mural endocardium of the cardiac chambers can occur as well.

4. Abscess and fistula formation—Organisms eventually invade the valve annulus and adjacent myocardium. Abscess formation can take multiple forms and may occur with or without fistula formation. Aortic annular abscess is an infective mass that burrows into or around the outside of the annulus. The abscess may extend upward to the sinus of Valsalva or ascending aorta (a type of mycotic aneurysm). This extension may lead to a fistulous communication between the aorta and the left atrium or (rarely) the right atrium. In other patients, the abscess extends down through the fibrous trigone and forms a fistula to the LV outflow tract.

A band of fibrous tissue at the base of the anterior mitral leaflet (the intervalvular fibrosa) separates the aortic annulus from the left atrial wall. Infection extending down from the posterior aortic annulus may produce an aneurysm in this area, which may in turn fistulize to the left atrium, aortic root, or into the pericardial space. Infection extending down from the anterior aortic annulus may invade the septal myocardium, causing a block in the conduction system.

When mitral valve infection extends to the base of the anterior leaflet, abscess formation involving the fibrous trigone may track upward and become fistulous. Infection from the posterior leaflet may extend to form a myocardial abscess in the LV posterior wall or a fistula around or through the mitral annulus between the left atrium and left ventricle. Infection may even penetrate through to the pericardial space, producing purulent pericarditis.

B. Extracardiac Disease

At any time during cardiac infection, extracardiac complications may supervene and dominate the clinical picture. Although these manifestations are emphasized in the medical literature, it should be kept in mind that many patients with endocarditis do not have them, especially at the time of presentation. The extracardiac disease in endocarditis results from immunologic phenomena and the shedding of bacteria and fragments of infected thrombus from the valve vegetations.

1. Immune disease—The bacteremia accompanying endocarditis persists over long periods of time and represents a prolonged antigenic challenge to the immune system. Various antibodies and immune complexes appear in the blood—more so with longer duration of illness. Rheumatoid factors (anti-IgG or IgM antibody) and the antibodies yielding a false-positive Venereal Disease Research Laboratory (VDRL) test are rarely of interest for their diagnostic value. Other antibodies, such as those that form circulating immune complexes and activate complement, are of major importance because they cause microvascular damage, most frequently glomerulonephritis and vasculitic skin lesions.

2. Systemic and pulmonary emboli—The embolization of fragments of vegetation is a frequent and potentially catastrophic complication of endocarditis. The clinical consequences are highly variable and depend on many factors, including the size of the embolus, the site at which it lodges in the vasculature, the type and quantity of organisms carried, the point during treatment at which embolism occurs, and the host response. Small emboli are likely to present as metastatic infection; the most dreaded of these is brain abscess. Septic embolization may also lead to abscesses in the kidney, liver, bone, and (from the right heart) lung.

Large emboli present with signs and symptoms of major vascular obstruction. For endocarditis of the left heart, the most frequent and serious extracardiac complication is embolism to the brain; these strokes tend to be large, complicating subsequent management and often causing death. Emboli may also cause infarction of the spleen, liver, kidney, and the myocardium. Embolism to large arteries of the extremities is unusual and occurs primarily in fungal endocarditis.

3. Mycotic aneurysms—When infection of the arterial wall results in localized dilatation and progresses to abscess formation, mycotic aneurysms can occur. The cause is thought to be embolization of vegetation that does not obstruct blood flow enough to present clinically as embolism. These lesions frequently occur at vessel branch points. The mycotic aneurysm may produce signs and symptoms many weeks after the diagnosis of endocarditis, and recognition may be difficult. Their effects are especially devastating in the central nervous system. Aneurysms may act as a protected site of infection and cause persistent fever or bacteremia despite appropriate antibiotic therapy. Alternatively, if antibiotic therapy has sterilized the aneurysm, it may present months or years later as unexplained hemorrhage.

C. Clinical Syndromes

Endocarditis can assume any of a wide variety of forms because of the many possible combinations of infecting organisms, portals of entry, and other factors such as the patient's immune status and the presence of concomitant diseases. Although the list of organisms capable of causing endocarditis is very long (and the list of possible combinations of organisms and other factors is even longer), there are several common and distinctive clinical syndromes.

A distinction between the acute and subacute forms of endocarditis has been found to be of some clinical value. The differing characteristics of patients with these two forms are shown in Table 12–1. Many patients with endocarditis cannot be easily placed into one or the other of these two categories.

1. Viridans streptococcal endocarditis—The bacterial species classified as viridans streptococci account for approximately 25% of cases of endocarditis. These organisms can be divided into three groups: normal human oral flora (*Streptococcus mitis, Streptococcus sanguinis, Streptococcus anginosus, Streptococcus mutans, Streptococcus salivarius,* and other nutritionally variant species), inhabitants of the lower gastrointestinal and genitourinary tracts (nonenterococcal group D organisms, of which *Streptococcus bovis* is important), and *Streptococcus pneumoniae,* or pneumococcus, which infrequently causes endocarditis—and causes a syndrome very different from the other viridans streptococci. The first two groups of streptococci cause almost no other disease in humans, except for endocarditis. This predilection appears to stem from bacterial cell wall proteins that bind to fibronectin, platelets, laminin, and other components of blood clots.

Viridans streptococci usually grow slowly, and the patient typically has a febrile illness of at least 10 days' duration and modest intensity; many cases fit the clinical syndrome of subacute bacterial endocarditis. Although valve destruction may be extensive, it is gradual, and abscess formation in the heart or elsewhere is uncommon. Infection of a normal valve by viridans streptococci is probably unusual. The renal disease accompanying endocarditis caused by these organisms is usually mild and rarely causes significant renal insufficiency. Viridans streptococcal endocarditis is therefore often treatable medically and has a relatively good prognosis if antibiotic treatment is begun before complications occur.

Endocarditis from *S bovis* is strongly associated with underlying colorectal disease, especially malignancy. Colonization of the gastrointestinal tract by this organism increases with age and with malignancy for reasons that are not well understood. After initial endocarditis treatment, a patient with this disease should undergo colonoscopy.

Extra vigilance for complications is needed when treating patients with endocarditis from certain other streptococci. *Streptococcus anginosus* and *Streptococcus milleri* tend to cause abscesses in the brain and other major organs, and nutritionally variant streptococci are associated with higher morbidity and mortality rates than are the other viridans organisms—again for reasons that are not understood.

Complications from viridans streptococcal endocarditis are almost never due to failure to sterilize vegetations. Nevertheless, the sensitivity of these organisms to penicillin is not uniform, and testing for resistance is essential for establishing an appropriate antibiotic regimen.

2. *Staphylococcus aureus* endocarditis—*S aureus* is a relatively common cause of endocarditis, accounting for approximately 33% of all cases. In hospitals serving a large

Table 12–1. Characteristics of Acute and Subacute Endocarditis.[1]

Acute	Subacute
Symptom onset to diagnosis: 1 week	Symptom onset to diagnosis: 4 weeks
Acute malaise	Weight loss
Shaking chills	Fatigue
	Night sweats
Fever (may be high)	Low or no fever
Leukocytosis	Normal white cell count or leukopenia
Normal gamma globulins	Elevated gamma globulins
Rheumatoid factor +	Rheumatoid factor +

[1]Elevated erythrocyte sedimentation rate and anemia common to both syndromes.

population of injecting drug users, this may be the most common cause of endocarditis. Although *S aureus* frequently enters the circulation from the skin or nares, a culprit lesion may not be apparent on examination of these areas. Less than 25% of episodes of *S aureus* bacteremia in hospitalized patients are caused by endocarditis.

Unlike patients with streptococcal endocarditis, those with endocarditis caused by *S aureus* are likely to seek medical attention soon after the onset of bacteremia, which generally produces a febrile illness with marked constitutional symptoms and often rigors. This picture is especially common in injecting drug users. *S aureus* tends to cause valve destruction more rapidly than do other organisms; approximately 30% of cases result in extensive left-heart valve involvement complicated by abscess or fistula formation or pericarditis. *S aureus* endocarditis of the aortic valve is the most common cause of aortic annular abscess, often signaled by the appearance of PR interval prolongation. Mitral annular and myocardial abscesses are also associated with this organism.

Central nervous system involvement is present in 20% or more of cases and manifests as cerebral embolization, intracranial hemorrhage from mycotic aneurysm rupture, and microscopic or macroscopic brain abscesses. Other significant complications include septic arthritis, osteomyelitis, and major organ abscesses. Renal involvement, as indicated by an active urine sediment, is present in almost all cases, and frank renal impairment occurs in approximately 20%. The renal dysfunction caused by *S aureus* rarely progresses to dialysis or permanent renal failure.

S aureus is the most lethal of the organisms commonly causing endocarditis, with mortality rates of approximately 30% in non–injecting drug users and greater than 50% in patients with prosthetic valves. Injecting drug users have a much lower mortality rate (approximately 5%).

3. Enterococcal endocarditis—This form accounts for approximately 5% of cases of endocarditis—almost all from *Enterococcus faecalis*. Enterococcal endocarditis tends to occur in elderly men undergoing diagnostic manipulation or surgery involving areas colonized by this organism, such as the gastrointestinal and genitourinary tracts, in injecting drug users, or in women following obstetric procedures. An acute or insidious syndrome may be present in patients with enterococcal endocarditis, although the findings typical of subacute bacterial endocarditis are unusual.

Enterococcal endocarditis is especially difficult to treat because of antibiotic resistance (discussed later). It is markedly different from and far more serious than streptococcal endocarditis. Overall mortality is only slightly less than that for staphylococcal endocarditis, and the incidence of major complications and need for valve replacement is approximately 30–40%.

4. Endocarditis from gram-negative bacteria—Gram-negative bacteria rarely cause endocarditis, with the exception of three groups of organisms: *Pseudomonas aeruginosa*, the HACEK organisms (*Haemophilus* spp., *Actinobacillus*, *Cardiobacterium*, *Eikenella*, *Kingella*) and the enteric organisms (*Escherichia coli*, *Proteus*, *Klebsiella*, and *Serratia marcescens*). *Pseudomonas* and *Serratia* are occasional causes of endocarditis in injecting drug users.

The HACEK organisms are relatively slow growing and usually cause a subacute clinical syndrome. Organisms such as *Haemophilus* and *Cardiobacterium* are thought to account for cases of culture-negative endocarditis. Despite the often mild symptoms and signs of endocarditis caused by these organisms, valve destruction may be extensive by the time of diagnosis. The HACEK organisms are associated with endocarditis that causes major vessel embolism from large vegetations. Enteric organisms tend to produce an acute clinical syndrome similar to that caused by *Pseudomonas*.

5. Fungal endocarditis—Fungal endocarditis is associated with settings of immune compromise and procedures that give the organism access to the bloodstream, such as surgery, intravenous catheter placement, and injecting drug use. *Candida* species (especially *C albicans*), *Histoplasma capsulatum*, and *Aspergillus* account for approximately 80% of cases of fungal endocarditis. Other less common causative organisms include *Mucor* and *Cryptococcus*. Clinicians must recognize when patients are at risk for fungal endocarditis because the signs and symptoms of the disease often escape notice or lead to misdiagnosis. Risk factors are listed in Table 12–2. In most patients with fungal endocarditis of a native valve, the infection is related to a fundamental immune system impairment. Fungal superinfection should be considered when a patient with bacterial endocarditis relapses either late in the antibiotic course or after completing treatment. This observation is especially true for bacterial infection of a prosthetic valve. *Candida* species infection is usually hospital-acquired, whereas histoplasmosis may be a community-acquired infec-

Table 12–2. Risk Factors for Fungal Endocarditis.

History of an implanted cardiac device (eg, prosthetic valve, pacemaker, AICD)
Indwelling vascular catheter and prolonged hospitalization
Prolonged treatment with broad-spectrum antibiotics
Immunosuppression (eg, steroid or cytotoxic drugs, radiation, malnutrition, untreated malignancy)
Injecting drug use

AICD, automatic implantable cardioverter-defibrillator.

tion. Fungal endocarditis in injecting drug users is almost always due to non-*albicans* species of *Candida*.

The clinical syndrome of fungal endocarditis is more difficult to recognize than that of bacterial endocarditis. This may be due partly to the postsurgical state or multisystem disease common in these patients. It has also been suggested that fever and murmurs develop later in the course of fungal disease than in bacterial endocarditis and that leukocytosis and such peripheral manifestations as petechiae are less frequent. The development of symptoms is often insidious, extending over weeks or months. Cardiac involvement is generally limited to the development of vegetations; invasion of the myocardium occurs with a lower frequency than in bacterial endocarditis. The vegetations usually lead to leaflet destruction and valve regurgitation; they may be large and may occasionally cause valve orifice obstruction. The most likely complication of fungal infective endocarditis is embolism, including occlusion of large peripheral arteries from embolization. Table 12–3 lists the approximate frequency of causative organisms in native valve endocarditis.

6. Prosthetic valve endocarditis—The risk of developing endocarditis is higher with prosthetic heart valves than with severely diseased native valves, approximately 0.5% per patient-year. Despite some overlap, there is a clear difference between the causes of disease that develops within 2 months

Table 12–3. Native Valve Endocarditis: Causative Organisms.

Organism	% of cases
Viridans streptococci	28
Other streptococci	23
Enterococci	4
Staphylococcus aureus	28
Coagulase-negative staphylococcus	7
Gram-negative bacteria	4
Other	5
No growth	5

of implantation and the causes of disease that occurs later (Table 12–4). The difference is probably due to infection occurring during surgery in early prosthetic endocarditis, with organisms from the skin of the patient and operating room personnel (*Staphylococcus epidermidis* and *S aureus*) accounting for more than half the cases. The incidence of early prosthetic endocarditis has been greatly reduced by the routine use of prophylactic antibiotics for several days after operation. Prosthetic infection after 2 months usually involves the same mechanism as does native valve endocarditis, except that the causative organisms are those adapted to nonbiologic material.

Infection of a bioprosthesis involves primarily the sewing ring. Vegetations similar to those of native valve endocarditis can occur when the prosthesis is biologic, but infection more often begins in the area of attachment of the sewing ring to the annulus. Vegetations may form in this area, but—most important—early in the disease abscesses often form along the suture line, resulting in fistulization, paravalvular regurgitation, and partial or complete detachment (dehiscence) of the prosthesis.

Infection of a mechanical prosthesis centers on the sewing ring. The inward growth of an infective mass from the ring frequently causes the occluder to become stuck in a partially open or closed position. The lesions caused by sewing ring infection of mechanical prostheses are otherwise similar to those of bioprostheses.

Two important differences distinguish prosthetic valve endocarditis from native valve infection. Prosthetic valve infection may be extensive without the clinical signs, such as a murmur of regurgitation, heart failure, or embolism, usually seen in advanced native valve infection. When prosthetic valve dysfunction does occur (especially in a mechanical prosthesis), it tends to be abrupt and severe, as when the occluder becomes fixed in a half-open position. (Other differences are discussed later in this chapter.)

7. Endocarditis in the injection drug user—The patient usually has an intense febrile illness of several days' duration, starting within 24–48 hours of the last injection. The mode of infection is a needle contaminated by skin flora, and an intravenous injection site may show an abscess or thrombophlebitis. The most likely causative organism is *S aureus* which, overall, causes 70% of endocarditis in injecting drug users, and which in this setting has a benign prognosis with only a 2–5% mortality rate. Many other organisms can cause endocarditis in injection drug users, including gram-negative bacilli, especially *P aeruginosa, C albicans,* enterococci, and *S marcescens;* as well as viridans streptococci. The prevalence of specific causative organisms varies widely in different urban areas. Endocarditis from these organisms tends to be less acute than that caused by *S aureus,* but only rarely is it truly subacute.

Infection of the tricuspid valve is almost unique to injecting drug users and occurs in approximately 60% of cases of endocarditis in this population. Significant tricuspid regurgitation may not be clinically apparent. In as many as 40% of cases, the left heart valves alone are infected. Despite its proximity to the portal of entry in injecting drug users, the pulmonic valve is rarely involved, probably because of the low pressure gradient and low wear and tear of this valve. Chest pain and dyspnea should prompt consideration of septic pulmonary emboli, which occur in 30% of tricuspid valve endocarditis. This complication usually presents as chest pain accompanied by scattered fluffy pulmonary infiltrates. On serial chest films, these lesions may appear migratory because of simultaneous resolution of older infiltrates and appearance of new ones. Infiltrates may also progress to cavitation.

8. Endocarditis and HIV—HIV infection and AIDS do not increase the risk of infective endocarditis. The increased frequency of endocarditis in patients with HIV is due to the prevalence of injecting drug use in this population. HIV/AIDS patients appear to have an increased susceptibility to *Salmonella* endocarditis, a relatively antibiotic-responsive infection. Otherwise, the types of causative organisms seen is not altered by HIV status. The clinical syndrome and natural history of the disease in HIV-positive patients is also unchanged, except that patients with advanced AIDS (CD4 count < 200 cells/mcL) tend to have a more fulminant course and increased mortality rates.

Table 12–4. Prosthetic Valve Endocarditis: Causative Organisms.

Early (< 60 days postsurgery)	%	Late (> 60 days postsurgery)	%
Staphylococcus epidermidis	33	Streptococci	30
Gram-negative bacteria	19	*Staphylococcus epidermidis*	26
Staphylococcus aureus	17	*S aureus*	12
Diptheroids	10	Gram-negative bacteria	12
Candida albicans	8	Enterococci	6
Streptococci	7	Diptheroids	4
Enterococci	2	*Candida albicans*	3
Aspergillus	1		

9. Hospital-acquired endocarditis—Hospital-acquired endocarditis is uncommon; overall approximately 5% of positive blood cultures in hospitalized patients are due to infective endocarditis (exceptions include streptococcal viridans and nutritionally variant streptococci). Prosthetic valves are at far greater risk than native valves: endocarditis develops in 15–20% of patients with prosthetic valves who become bacteremic. Hospital-acquired endocarditis is marked by an increased likelihood of the presence of unusual or antibiotic-resistant organisms and an infected indwelling catheter as the likely portal of entry. Endocarditis occurs only rarely in postsurgical patients, usually after prolonged sepsis.

The usual causative organisms are coagulase-negative staphylococcus; *S aureus; Enterococcus;* and enteric gram-negative organisms, such as *Pseudomonas* and *Serratia.* Fungi, especially *Candida,* and fastidious organisms should also be suspected when endocarditis occurs in debilitated, leukopenic patients and those previously treated with long courses of antibiotics. Hospital-acquired endocarditis should be suspected when fever develops in a hospitalized patient who has positive blood cultures without an apparent source. Potential culprit catheters should be removed and cultured, followed by transesophageal echocardiography (TEE) if an additional risk factor for endocarditis exists. Examples of risk factors in this setting include a prosthetic valve, native valve disease predisposing to infection, or *S aureus* bacteremia. If the findings of TEE are normal, and other sources of infection have been ruled out, a short (2-week) course of antibiotics is usually appropriate. Surveillance blood cultures during and after treatment and a repeat TEE should be considered if uncertainty regarding the response to treatment persists. In the case of exposure of a prosthetic valve to bacteremia, blood culture surveillance should be extended for at least 2 months.

10. Pacemaker endocarditis—Pacemaker endocarditis is infection of the lead or of parts of the heart in contact with the lead (tricuspid valve, right ventricular endocardium). Mortality is high, up to 25%, and the diagnosis is often missed due to the indolent nature of the infection. Most cases are due to contamination at the time of implant; hematogenous infection of a lead is rare. Most cases have evidence of present or prior infection at the implant site. The delay from the most recent pacemaker procedure to the diagnosis of endocarditis may be as long as 2 years or as little as 6 weeks. In addition to fever and positive blood cultures, infection causes septic pulmonary emboli in about one-third of cases. Transesophageal echocardiography is the diagnostic test of choice, with a sensitivity of over 90%. The findings on transthoracic echocardiography (TTE) are often falsely normal.

Staphylococci are the usual infecting organisms, with *S epidermidis* accounting for 70% of cases and *S aureus* for most of the rest. As with prosthetic valve endocarditis, *S aureus* is the most likely culprit when endocarditis develops soon after implant, whereas *S epidermidis* is more likely when endocarditis develops later. *Staphylococcus* species produce a slime-like

"sleeve" along the lead that protects bacteria from the patient's immunologic defense as well as from antibiotic therapy. Treatment requires removal of the lead, and usually the entire system. Lead removal can be accomplished percutaneously with reasonable safety if the masses attached to the lead are small (< 1 cm). Surgery is indicated if the lead is fixed, if a large mass (> 1 cm) is present (with dislodgement likely to result in severe pulmonary embolism), or if tricuspid valve involvement is extensive. Lead removal is followed by 6 weeks of antibiotic therapy. The pacemaker-dependent patient is given an epicardial lead; reimplant of a transvenous system can be considered after 2 months with negative surveillance blood cultures.

▶ Clinical Findings

A. Diagnostic Criteria

In the current era, with the availability of sensitive blood culture techniques and TEE, the clinician will rarely need to rely on a formal schema for the diagnosis of endocarditis. The most useful schema is the Duke criteria which involves two "major" criteria (definite echocardiographic evidence of endocarditis, positive blood cultures) and six "minor" criteria (predisposing cardiac condition, fever, vascular phenomena, immunologic phenomena, suggestive echocardiogram, ambiguous blood cultures) to reach a probable diagnosis. This approach was useful because of the low sensitivity and specificity of clinical features by themselves. Now TEE and blood cultures independently have a diagnostic sensitivity of greater than 90%, and TEE has a specificity of greater than 90%. Diagnostic uncertainty may arise when the result of TEE is ambiguous or when adequate blood cultures are not obtained before starting antibiotics. In many such situations, a diagnosis can be reached by gathering more data. For example, if the TEE fails to show endocarditis-specific valve disease and the patient is doing well, discontinuing antibiotics in order to repeat cultures should be considered. Many of the common features of endocarditis—fever, a cardiac murmur, and a set of positive blood cultures—occur frequently in other diseases and are occasionally absent in patients with endocarditis. Other diseases frequently mimicked by endocarditis include malignancy, autoimmune disease, and septicemia. In addition, patients with endocarditis may come to the physician because of a complication of endocarditis so dramatic as to distract attention from the underlying infection. Typical settings in which this error occurs include heart failure, stroke, and myocardial infarction.

The recognition of possible **prosthetic valve endocarditis** may be difficult because the signs of infection may be very subtle. In early prosthetic endocarditis, the symptoms and signs may be incorrectly ascribed to other diseases. Fever and bacteremia during the first few weeks after prosthetic implantation should be considered to indicate prosthetic valve endocarditis until proven otherwise. This is especially important because early prosthetic valve endocarditis appears to follow a more fulminant course than either late prosthetic or native valve endocarditis. These patients often have other potential causes of bacteremia, however, and an effort to prove infection from another site should be pursued vigorously. Transesophageal echocardiography probably has a sensitivity of approximately 80% for prosthetic valve endocarditis and should be performed whenever an alternative explanation for fever or bacteremia is not readily apparent. If the TEE findings are normal but bacteremia persists (especially if the organism is a frequent cause of prosthetic endocarditis), prosthetic infection should be presumptively treated. Fluoroscopy to rule out dehiscence has been replaced by TEE.

Fungal endocarditis is also often difficult to diagnose. Blood cultures are negative in approximately half of cases caused by *C albicans,* the majority of histoplasmosis cases, and almost all cases caused by *Aspergillus*. Histologic examination and culture should be performed whenever possible on specimens of embolic material, oropharyngeal lesions (especially for histoplasmosis), skin lesions (for *Candida* species and *Aspergillus*), liver, bone marrow, and urine (for histoplasmosis). In addition, a careful eye examination should be performed in patients with suspected fungal endocarditis because of the high frequency of anterior uveitis and chorioretinitis.

Tricuspid valve endocarditis (as seen in injecting drug users) produces a distinctive picture because of the frequent occurrence of septic pulmonary emboli. Scattered fluffy infiltrates seen on chest film are accompanied by pleuritic chest pain. Less often, the presentation may mimic pneumonia or include pleural effusion. The murmur of tricuspid regurgitation may be inaudible or soft because right-heart pressures are normally low, even when tricuspid infection is extensive. A loud holosystolic murmur at the left lower sternal border that increases with inspiration, *v* waves in jugular veins, and a pulsatile liver indicate the development of severe tricuspid regurgitation and pulmonary hypertension.

B. Symptoms and Signs

Constellations of certain symptoms should arouse suspicion of endocarditis. One combination of symptoms often seen is constitutional symptoms (eg, fatigue, malaise, headache, arthralgias or myalgias, nausea, anorexia, weight loss) and fever, which can range from mild feverish feelings and night sweats to shaking chills. When these symptoms are chronic or mild, other diagnoses are often considered, such as malignancy and autoimmune disease.

A high suspicion of endocarditis is warranted when this picture is associated with any symptom pointing to the circulatory system, such as complaints associated with left- or right-heart failure (dyspnea, orthopnea, cough, peripheral edema), vascular occlusion (stroke, systemic embolism), and chest pain (Table 12–5).

C. Physical Examination

The physical examination is not essential for the diagnosis of endocarditis. Most of the physical findings caused by endo-

Table 12–5. Frequency of Symptoms and Signs in Endocarditis.

Frequency	Symptom	Sign
High (> 40% of patients)	Fever	Fever
	Chills	Murmur
	Weakness	Skin lesions or emboli
	Dyspnea	Petechiae
Moderate (10–40% of patients)	Sweats	Osler or Janeway lesions
	Anorexia/weight loss	Splinter hemorrhages
	Cough	Splenomegaly
	Stroke	Major complication: stroke, heart failure, pneumonia, meningitis
	Rash	
	Nausea/vomiting	
	Headache	
	Chest pain	
	Myalgias/arthralgias	
Low (< 10% of patients)	Abdominal pain	New or changing murmur
	Delirium/coma	Retinal lesions
	Hemoptysis	Renal failure
	Back pain	

carditis are not specific for this diagnosis and should be interpreted in the context of the overall examination and the patient's history. There are also no physical findings that, when absent, are useful for ruling out the diagnosis. A prominent murmur or skin lesion may arouse a clinical suspicion of endocarditis, but a murmur of valve regurgitation may be absent in patients with endocarditis. Vegetations may be present but may cause only slight regurgitation.

The examination is absolutely essential, however, to the treatment of endocarditis. The initial examination assists the clinician in assessing the severity of the illness. During treatment (or observation for more definite evidence of endocarditis), serial physical examinations are vital for identifying important changes in the patient's status because physical findings may signal the need for surgery.

1. Fever—Fever is usually present when the patient seeks medical attention, although it may be intermittent or already resolved through inappropriate antibiotic treatment. It may be infrequently masked by severe comorbid conditions, such as alcoholic cirrhosis, leukopenia, or malnutrition. The diversity of endocarditis does not permit generalizations about the temporal pattern or degree of fever. Fever may be low grade (37.5–38.5 °C) and accompanied by only malaise and anorexia, or it may be hectic with rigors, sweats, and temperature higher than 40 °C. Recurrence of fever during treatment of endocarditis is a very important problem (see section on Failure of antibiotic therapy).

2. Cardiac examination—The cardiac examination in the patient with suspected or known endocarditis focuses on identifying which heart valves are infected, the hemodynamic severity of the resultant regurgitation (or stenosis), and the adequacy of the patient's circulatory state.

At the time of initial evaluation of a patient with suspected endocarditis, the value of a detected murmur may be low because there may be no reliable information about the patient's prior cardiac condition. Systolic murmurs, for example, are common in the general population and very frequent in older or hospitalized patients; they are usually due to LV outflow or degenerative sclerosis of the aortic valve. Because endocarditis rarely causes valve stenosis, a systolic murmur related to endocarditis is almost always regurgitant.

Specific auscultatory features occasionally may be useful for determining how a valve has been damaged by infection. In mitral valve endocarditis, the examination may help identify which mitral leaflet has become partially flail. If the mitral regurgitant murmur radiates to the patient's back, the jet is likely to be directed posteriorly as a result of anterior leaflet prolapse into the left atrium. If the murmur radiates to the upper parasternal area (mimicking aortic stenosis), the posterior leaflet is likely to have lost its support.

It is essential that the examiner carefully note and document the cardiac findings as soon as the diagnosis of endocarditis is suspected. In addition to murmurs, the clinician should pay close attention to those aspects of the examination related to hemodynamic consequences of valvular dysfunction. Signs of pulmonary edema, dysfunction of either ventricle, and a low output state should be sought.

3. Skin and extremities—Assessment of the severity of extracardiac disease in endocarditis begins with a careful examination of the skin and peripheral circulation for evidence of vasculitis and emboli. Although these findings are not specific for the diagnosis of endocarditis, in the context of probable endocarditis, they strongly support that diagnosis. Their appearance during antibiotic therapy may signal the need for a change in the treatment plan.

A. PETECHIAE—Examine the soft palate, buccal mucosa, conjunctiva, and the skin of the extremities for petechiae, which are often transient, appearing in crops and fading in 2–3 days.

B. SPLINTER HEMORRHAGES—These brown streaks are 1–2 mm in length and found under the fingernails and toenails. Lesions in the proximal nail bed are moderately specific for endocarditis, whereas similar lesions under the distal nails are commonly found in healthy persons who work with their hands.

C. ROTH SPOTS—Vasculitis affecting small arteries of the retina may, on rare occasions, produce retinal infarction. The resulting funduscopic lesion, usually seen near the optic disc, is a pale retinal patch surrounded by a darker ring of hemorrhage.

D. OSLER NODES—These painful indurated nodules are 2–15 mm in diameter and appear on the palms and soles and often involve the distal phalanges. They are usually multiple and, like petechiae, tend to occur in crops and fade over 2–3 days. Osler nodes are thought to be caused by either vasculitis or septic embolization.

E. JANEWAY LESIONS—These painless, flat red macules are similar in size and location to Osler nodes that usually persist longer than a few days. Their pathogenesis is uncertain but is suspected to be vasculitis.

F. BLUE-TOES SYNDROME—Embolization of small vegetation fragments may cause ischemia in the distal arterial distribution of an upper or lower extremity. The affected finger or toe is tender, mottled, and cyanotic; over a period of days to weeks, the area becomes black and develops dry gangrene. Management is usually conservative (see Embolism section, later in this chapter). Acute arterial occlusive ischemia of a larger portion of an extremity raises the possibility of fungal endocarditis and is usually managed by embolectomy.

4. Neurologic examination—Cerebral embolization in endocarditis signals a poor prognosis and has a major impact on the overall management approach. The neurologic examination is an integral part of the evaluation of any patient with known or suspected endocarditis. During antibiotic treatment, symptoms that may be of neurologic origin justify careful repeat examination, often with CT.

5. Abdominal examination—Splenomegaly occurs in patients with endocarditis as part of generalized hyperplasia of the reticuloendothelial system. Its presence usually indicates endocarditis of at least 10 days' duration. Marked splenomegaly may be accompanied by abdominal pain from splenic infarction.

D. Diagnostic Studies

1. Detection of blood-borne infection—Bacteremia or fungemia invariably occurs at some point during endocarditis (a role for viruses is unproven). The presence of the organism in the blood is generally of low grade and continuous because of the vegetations in the circulating bloodstream. Bacteremia may be intermittent or of variable intensity, however, especially if abscess formation has occurred or if the patient is under treatment.

The method of obtaining blood cultures depends on the severity of the patient's illness, as judged from the clinical syndrome and results of TEE. The preferred method in cases of suspected endocarditis is to obtain two or three sets of aerobic and anaerobic cultures, each from a separate venipuncture site, over 12 or more hours. This approach should be used if the suspicion of endocarditis is low, the patient appears well enough to tolerate a 12-hour delay of antibiotic therapy, or the TEE is normal or inconclusive.

Initiation of antibiotic therapy, however, should not be delayed if the suspicion of endocarditis is high and the patient is acutely ill, with a temperature more than 40 °C, tachycardia, discomfort, or hypotension; the TEE is abnormal; or complications of endocarditis, such as embolism or congestive heart failure, have already occurred. Under these conditions, the cultures should be obtained over 30 minutes, followed immediately by antibiotic therapy.

Blood cultures have been found positive for an infecting organism in 70–95% of cases of endocarditis reported in studies since 1970. Proper technique and timing of blood cultures can improve the positive yield. Potential causes of negative blood cultures in patients with endocarditis are shown in Table 12–6. When blood cultures remain negative at 24–48 hours in a patient with probable endocarditis, the most important concern is infection from unusual organisms, such as the fungi, HACEK organisms, *Coxiella burnetii* (Q fever), *Chlamydophila psittaci*, *Bartonella* and *Abiotrophia* species (nutritionally variant streptococci). The laboratory should be notified of the suspected diagnosis, and infectious disease consultation obtained.

If antibiotics have already been started for another diagnosis, modification of the blood culture technique can increase the positive yield. The importance of recovering the causative organism may warrant stopping all antibiotics. (The use of antibiotic removal devices or specialized media have not been proven to be useful for increasing the yield from blood cultures in this situation.) Blood cultures then should be drawn according to the routine outlined earlier, usually with an additional two blood cultures drawn at 24 hours.

If the suspicion of endocarditis remains moderate or high after the initial blood culture sets are drawn, empiric antibiotic therapy should also begin. The antibiotics should be changed according to the blood culture results as soon as these become available. If the initial blood cultures are negative after 24 hours but endocarditis is still suspected, three more sets should be obtained and processed under the guidance of an infectious disease specialist. Hypertonic and nutri-

tionally supplemented media are useful for detecting cell wall-deficient and nutritionally variant organisms, respectively. The lysis-centrifugation method of blood culture preparation also should be used in an attempt to detect fungi, and the microbiology laboratory should be notified to hold the cultures for 4 weeks. Serologic testing should be considered.

2. Serologic testing—Serologic testing can be helpful for identifying certain causes of endocarditis when blood cultures are negative. Histoplasmosis antigen is highly specific for systemic infection by this organism. Positive antibody titers for Q fever (*C burnetii*) or *Brucella* in a patient with culture-negative endocarditis identify these organisms as the cause. The usefulness of other serologic tests, such as that for *C albicans*, is highly dependent on the clinical situation.

Although not essential to the diagnosis of endocarditis, serologic testing is supportive and can be useful in certain situations. A positive rheumatoid factor, commonly found in patients with endocarditis of longer than 2 weeks' duration, and a false-positive VDRL, which is less common, signal the presence of high titers of antibodies (stimulated by the prolonged antigenemia occurring in endocarditis). These two laboratory abnormalities are not specific for endocarditis, however, and are found in other diseases that may imitate endocarditis, such as systemic lupus erythematosus. When blood cultures are positive but other evidence of endocarditis is lacking or equivocal, a positive rheumatoid factor or VDRL should prompt careful follow-up and retesting (eg, repeat TEE) for further evidence of endocarditis. Under some circumstances, these positive serologic tests may even warrant extension of antibiotic therapy to treat presumed endocarditis.

3. Echocardiography

A. Transesophageal echocardiography—Patients with suspected endocarditis should undergo TEE as soon as possible. With its detailed images of the heart valves and related structures, TEE is highly sensitive and specific for the diagnosis of endocarditis and is essential to defining the extent of disease. A TEE that shows a mass with the characteristics of a vegetation has a specificity of more than 90% for endocarditis (in the absence of a history of endocarditis, since it is difficult to distinguish between old and new vegetations). A normal TEE does not rule out endocarditis, but it has a negative predictive accuracy of at least 90%. Because false-normal TEE studies can occur, however, a patient with a normal study but a high clinical suspicion of endocarditis should be either observed carefully or treated, depending on the clinical severity of the illness. The TEE should be repeated if needed.

(1) Classification—Transesophageal echocardiographic studies in patients with suspected endocarditis may be classified according to the probability of the disease. A useful scheme is based on four categories: normal, possible, probable, and almost certain. In the **normal** category, no substrate for endocarditis or other abnormalities is present.

Table 12–6. Causes of Negative Blood Cultures in Endocarditis.

Failure to obtain more than one set of blood cultures
Failure to hold blood cultures for longer than 1 week
Prior antibiotic prescription (normally within 2–3 days of culture)
Organism grows slowly in standard culture (eg, HACEK organisms, nutritionally variant streptococci)
Organism fails to grow in standard culture (eg, fungi, rickettsiae, Q fever, psittacosis, nutritionally variant streptococci)
Intermittent bacteremia or fungemia (rare)

The TEE findings are classified as **possible endocarditis** in the presence of valve disease, such as a prosthetic heart valve, rheumatic or degenerative valvular sclerosis, or valve regurgitation likely to be pathologic, that predispose the patient to endocarditis—but without evidence of lesions. The classification of **probable endocarditis** is used when less specific lesions are found. Examples of such abnormalities include localized leaflet thickening or an nonmobile leaflet-related mass (especially if the lesion has the reflectance of soft rather than sclerotic tissue), mitral or aortic valve prolapse, chordal rupture, intracardiac thrombi, and paravalvular regurgitation in patients with prosthetic valves.

Patients with no history of endocarditis who have a lesion very strongly associated with infective endocarditis fall into the **almost-certain** category. In such cases, TEE shows an intracardiac mass with typical vegetation characteristics—a pedunculated mass attached near the leaflet tip and prolapsing during valve closure into the lower pressure chamber. Vegetations have soft-tissue reflectance (like myocardium) and vibratory or rotatory motion independent of the motion of the leaflet. Vegetations apparent on TEE vary in length from 1 mm or 2 mm to several centimeters.

Other lesions considered almost certain for endocarditis would be an abscess or fistula, a metastatic vegetation, and an aneurysm of the intervalvular fibrosa. An abscess appears on TEE as an echolucent space adjacent to a valve annulus or prosthetic sewing ring. The abscess often appears to be separated from adjacent structures by thin septa, and jets of blood flowing into the abscess during systole or diastole (depending on abscess location) may be shown by Doppler interrogation. The abscess is considered a fistula when there is communication with two or more adjacent cardiac chambers or blood vessels. Metastatic vegetations appear on echocardiography as vibratory or rotatory masses attached to an endocardial surface at a site with a regurgitant jet.

It should be noted that this TEE classification scheme is appropriate only in patients with other reasons to suspect endocarditis (eg, unexplained fever, positive blood cultures) and no prior history of endocarditis.

(2) Diagnostic accuracy—Possible causes of false TEE results are shown in Table 12–7. Of particular importance is the possibility that TEE findings may be normal because endothelial infection may be in the vasculature rather than in the heart. Because vascular infection is rare in the absence of prior vascular surgery, the diagnosis is usually suspected based on the patient's history. Nevertheless, the TEE examination in patients with suspected endocarditis routinely includes the thoracic aorta. Transesophageal echocardiography may identify severe atherosclerosis with mobile atheroma or thrombi. Although these abnormalities are not nearly as specific for infection as are intracardiac vegetations, the clinical picture may justify antibiotic treatment.

In general, less than 10% of TEE results are falsely abnormal. By causing thickened, prolapsing leaflets and ruptured chordae, a myxomatous mitral valve can closely

Table 12–7. Causes of False Results of Transesophageal Echocardiography.

False-Abnormal
Myxomatous mitral valve disease
Papillary fibroelastomas
Partially flail leaflet
Healed vegetations
Mitral valve strands
Nodules of Arantii (aortic valve)
Lambl excrescences (mitral valve)
False-Normal
Aortic valve prosthesis
Mitral valve mechanical prosthesis (includes shadowing of aortic valve by a mitral prosthesis)
Calcified aortic root shadowing tricuspid or pulmonic valves
Mitral annular calcification
Aortic atheroma or aneurysm infection
Study done too early in disease course

mimic endocarditis. A benign leaflet tumor, called a **papillary fibroelastoma,** may give the appearance of a vegetation. Several other abnormalities seen by TEE have lower specificity for the diagnosis of endocarditis than do typical vegetations; examples include para-aortic cavities (potentially representing either an abscess or an aneurysm of the sinus of Valsalva) and paraprosthetic regurgitation. Clinical context is often crucial to the interpretation of these findings. The paraneoplastic syndrome of myxomas may mimic endocarditis, although usually location and morphologic features of myxomas distinguish them from thrombi or vegetations. Intracardiac thrombi may be innocent bystanders in a patient with a clinical syndrome suggesting endocarditis, or they may be secondarily infected.

Lambl excrescences are thin, strand-like structures extending 1–10 mm from the mitral leaflet margins. Because they prolapse a few millimeters into the left atrium and exhibit hypermobility, Lambl excrescences can be mistaken for small vegetations. Nodules of Arantii are similar extensions, not more than a few millimeters in length, from the center of the aortic cusp margin. When the aortic valve is closed, a TEE may show these nodules prolapsing from the center of the valve.

In addition to detecting vegetations, TEE usually provides a detailed picture of the extent of cardiac infection; it is very accurate at assessing the exact size and location of vegetations. Several complicated forms of cardiac involvement are usually identifiable by TEE. Because many of these complex lesions require surgery, TEE should be performed as soon as possible in a patient with a moderate or high suspicion of endocarditis.

Blood cultures should be drawn either before or 15 minutes after TEE to avoid the transient bacteremia that infrequently occurs during the procedure. Prophylaxis for endocarditis is not indicated prior to TEE.

B. TRANSTHORACIC ECHOCARDIOGRAPHY—The initial diagnostic value of TTE is limited in patients with possible endocarditis because of its low sensitivity: a large number of false-abnormal results occur, particularly in patients with prosthetic valves. On the other hand, a TTE showing typical vegetations is at least 90% specific for the diagnosis of endocarditis. Transthoracic echocardiography, however, cannot provide the detailed information regarding the anatomic extent of infection available from TEE.

Despite these limitations, TTE has a valuable ancillary role in patients with known endocarditis. It is well suited to assessing cardiac chamber dilatation, left and right ventricular dysfunction, and the patient's hemodynamic status. Presystolic closure of the mitral valve on TTE is a sign of elevated LV end-diastolic pressure and is an indication that the patient with aortic insufficiency should be considered for surgery. Similarly, right atrial and pulmonary artery pressures can be estimated by transthoracic Doppler examination. Additional Doppler data are essential to assessing the severity and hemodynamic sequelae of mitral regurgitation, including elevated left atrial pressure. Changes in the patient's clinical status during treatment often can be readily diagnosed by comparison of serial TTE studies. For these reasons, it is advisable to perform transthoracic study at the same time as the initial TEE. One useful strategy is to discuss the results of TTE with the referring physician while the patient is still in the laboratory, and then proceed to TEE if appropriate.

4. Electrocardiography and chest radiography—The electrocardiogram (ECG) is occasionally useful in alerting the clinician to the severity of endocarditis. In patients with known or suspected aortic valve endocarditis, the PR interval should be monitored closely for prolongation, an indication of aortic annular abscess formation. Less frequently, the ECG may show increased QRS voltage and a precordial strain pattern in patients with either severe aortic or mitral regurgitation and marked LV enlargement. The chest radiograph is primarily useful in evaluating the patient with suspected endocarditis to assess the presence and severity of pulmonary edema and to detect septic pulmonary emboli in patients with possible right-heart endocarditis.

Cecchi E et al. Are the Duke criteria really useful for the early bedside diagnosis of infective endocarditis? Results of a prospective multicenter trial. Ital Heart J. 2005 Jan;6(1):41–8. [PMID: 15773272]

Crawford MH et al. Clinical presentation of infective endocarditis. Cardiol Clin. 2003 May;21(2):159–66. [PMID: 12874890]

Li JS et al. Proposed modifications to the Duke criteria for the diagnosis of infective endocarditis. Clin Infect Dis. 2000 Apr;30(4):633–8. [PMID: 10770721]

Sachdev M et al. Imaging techniques for diagnosis of infective endocarditis. Cardiol Clin. 2003 May;21(2):185–95. [PMID: 12874892]

Thuny F et al. Risk of embolism and death in infective endocarditis: prognostic value of echocardiography: a prospective multicenter study. Circulation. 2005 Jul 5;112(1):69–75. [PMID: 15983252]

► Management

A. Initial Decisions

Management of newly diagnosed endocarditis requires the physician to make two decisions promptly. The first is whether to initiate empiric antibiotic therapy based on available clinical information or to await the exact identity and antibiotic sensitivities of the infecting organism and then to select the optimal regimen. The second decision is whether valve surgery is indicated immediately or can be deferred to allow assessment of the patient's response to antibiotic therapy.

Both decisions depend on the extent of cardiac infection (usually characterized by TEE), the severity of the patient's symptoms and signs of infection, the patient's circulatory status, the seriousness of extracardiac complications, and the available data about the organism.

Once initial treatment is underway, the physician must maintain a high level of vigilance for evidence of an inadequate response to treatment or the development of complications that will require additional medical or surgical intervention.

B. Antibiotic Therapy

The goal of antibiotic therapy is to sterilize vegetations. For most causative organisms, this is an achievable goal and will cure the patient if cardiac abscess and metastatic infection to other organs have not occurred. Vegetations, however, provide proliferating organisms with an environment that is protected against both the patient's immune system and antibiotics. Organisms grow under the surface of the vegetation where phagocytes cannot penetrate, and bacterial metabolism is slowed within the nutrient-poor vegetation, contributing to antibiotic resistance. For these reasons, antibiotic treatment is directed toward achieving bactericidal concentrations of drug within the vegetation over an extended period. It must be noted that certain important aspects of antibiotic dosing, especially in seriously ill patients, are beyond the scope of this text, and infectious disease consultation is advised.

1. Principles of antibiotic therapy

A. IN VITRO SENSITIVITY TESTING—For organisms with variable antibiotic sensitivity (eg, streptococci), the choice of drug and the dosage depend on in vitro sensitivity testing of the strain infecting the patient. An organism's sensitivity to an antibiotic is quantified by the minimum inhibitory concentration (MIC) and minimum bactericidal concentration (MBC). The MIC is defined as the minimum concentration of antibiotic that prevents proliferation of the organism in a standardized culture system. The MBC is the minimum concentration that kills 99.9% of the bacteria at 24 hours in a similarly standardized system. These tests are widely used to guide treatment of endocarditis.

MIC and MBC data are also used to identify organisms with antibiotic tolerance, which is defined as an MBC more than ten times higher than the MIC. In such cases, although the infecting organism is susceptible to the antibiotic, the rate of killing is not increased at higher antibiotic concentrations, as would be expected. The tolerance of *Enterococcus* for penicillin, for example, probably explains the substantial failure rate of medical therapy in diseases caused by this organism despite the use of a high-dose multidrug regimen. In all patients with enterococcal endocarditis, the organism's MIC for penicillin and vancomycin should guide the choice of which antibiotic to pair with an aminoglycoside. Resistance to gentamicin should be determined as well. *S aureus* is among the other potentially tolerant organisms that may require an alteration in the antibiotic regimen. Methicillin resistance, if present, requires pairing of vancomycin with an aminoglycoside.

B. Drug combinations—Combinations of drugs with additive, or synergistic, killing power are used frequently for treating endocarditis. A common combination is a β-lactam antibiotic (the penicillins and cephalosporins) with an aminoglycoside. This combination is synergistic because the β-lactam drug damages the bacterial cell wall, which allows more rapid penetration of the aminoglycoside into the cell.

C. Parenteral treatment—Antibiotic treatment must be given parenterally to ensure high and consistent serum drug levels and compliance. Outpatient intravenous drug therapy can be undertaken only under specific conditions (see section on Outpatient Treatment), and oral therapy is almost never sufficient.

D. Prolonged treatment—The duration of antibiotic administration is almost always for a month or more. Prolonged exposure of the patient to antibiotics can lead to frequent side effects and serious toxicity (monitoring antibiotic therapy is discussed in the following section).

2. Empiric antibiotic therapy—Empiric antibiotic therapy is the initiation of antibiotics for the purpose of treating endocarditis without identifying the causative organism. Ideally, empiric therapy is needed only briefly until culture and sensitivity data are available. It requires treating the patient for the worst-case organism and can subject the patient to the additional risk of receiving multiple antibiotics over a prolonged period. This approach should be avoided whenever the patient's clinical status allows waiting for blood culture results, and the physician should make every effort to draw blood cultures consistent with a tolerable delay in the initiation of appropriate therapy.

Empiric therapy may be necessary if the patient has the syndrome of acute endocarditis, appears with symptoms of significant toxicity, or shows signs of septic shock; if the patient shows signs and symptoms of left-heart failure and is likely to need surgery in the near future; or if the patient's echocardiogram (preferably TEE) shows evidence of extensive cardiac involvement. Although data on the prognostic implications of specific TEE findings are still incomplete, extensive involvement probably includes a vegetation longer than 2–3 cm, valve dysfunction likely to be hemodynamically significant, more than one infected valve, leaflet perforation, annular abscess, and pericarditis. The choice of antibiotic for empiric therapy may be guided by considering the most likely infecting organisms based on the clinical presentation.

3. Outpatient treatment—Outpatient parenteral antibiotic therapy, now widely used, can provide an excellent outcome. Careful patient selection and management are mandatory. The first 2 weeks of treatment should almost always be as an inpatient because complications are most likely during this time. If the patient has a low-virulence organism, if valve involvement is limited to vegetations attached to leaflets and vegetations are not large (< 15 cm), and the first 2 weeks have been uncomplicated, then outpatient treatment should be considered. Endocarditis due to viridans streptococci and the HACEK group can be treated as an outpatient. At present, it is less certain that infection with *S aureus,* especially of the aortic valve, can be safely treated this way, due to the frequency of abscess and subvalve extension.

In addition to a specialized team of nurses managing the infusion and assessing the patient daily, a physician experienced in the treatment of endocarditis should be available for a same-day visit in the event of evidence of complications (discussed further under the Management of Complications section below). The patient should live close to a hospital and have drug levels, blood cultures, and other blood work monitored as with an inpatient.

4. Monitoring antibiotic therapy

A. Drug levels—Monitoring the levels and effects of antibiotics is important in managing endocarditis because the patient's prolonged exposure to high doses of antibiotics increases the frequency of adverse drug effects. The use of aminoglycosides requires monitoring of serum levels at peak (1–2 hours after infusion is started) and trough (immediately before the next dose). A peak level for gentamicin or vancomycin of less than 5 mcg/mL is associated with treatment failure for many organisms and may warrant adjustment of the dose or the dosing interval. At a trough level of more than 2 mcg/mL, gentamicin carries an increased risk of nephrotoxicity, and the dose should be reduced. Monitoring these levels assumes even greater importance in the setting of renal insufficiency, especially if renal function is changing. Although vancomycin and flucytosine levels should always be monitored for the same reasons, levels for β-lactam antibiotics are available but rarely needed.

B. Adverse effects—The most common adverse effects are a pruritic maculopapular rash and low-grade fever seen with β-lactam antibiotics. The rash may signify delayed hypersensitivity and may be accompanied by hepatic or renal dysfunction. Liver biochemical tests (aspartate aminotransferase and alkaline phosphatase) and creatinine should be checked in this situation. If these tests are abnormal, substitution of another drug is required. If not, it is preferable to continue the antibiotic and treat the symptoms. Patients taking β-lactam antibiotics should have a routine complete blood count every 3 or 4 days during therapy to detect anemia, thrombocytopenia, and leukopenia. The sodium content of β-lactam antibiotics may require diuretic therapy in patients with heart failure.

Patients taking aminoglycosides should have the serum creatinine checked routinely at 3- to 4-day intervals. Equally useful for detection of renal dysfunction is the periodic examination of urine for white cell or granular casts. Ototoxicity is an idiosyncratic reaction unrelated to aminoglycoside levels that occurs in 10–20% of cases.

Diarrhea may occur during antibiotic therapy; this is usually due to overgrowth of gut organisms competing with those sensitive to the antibiotic (eg, *Clostridium difficile* colitis).

C. Management of Complications

1. Failure of antibiotic therapy—Changes in the cardiac examination during antibiotic treatment are particularly important in detecting failure of medical therapy. Changes in a regurgitant murmur almost always indicate valve dysfunction, and the appearance of a new murmur may signal metastatic infection of another valve. Such new findings almost always warrant repeat echocardiography (usually TEE) and blood cultures. There may also be an increase in the resting sinus rate and the appearance of heart failure.

Failure of antibiotic therapy is usually heralded by persistent or recurrent fever. Persistent fever is defined as continuing for more than a week during antibiotic treatment. Recurrent fever develops after an afebrile period of several days and occurs at least a week after initiation of antibiotics. Persistent infection is only one cause of fever in this setting; others include hypersensitivity to antibiotics and other drugs, phlebitis, silent emboli (especially pulmonary and splenic), intercurrent urinary or upper respiratory tract infection, or simply a delayed response to antibiotic therapy. Blood cultures should be obtained and efforts made to rule out these possibilities. If blood cultures are negative, and the patient shows no other evidence of deterioration, watchful waiting is appropriate.

Positive blood cultures after more than 1 week of antibiotic therapy strongly suggest persistent infection. The cause may be either antibiotic resistance or a protected site of infection. The site may be an intracardiac annular or myocardial abscess or an extracardiac site of metastatic infection, septic embolization, or mycotic aneurysm. Repeat TEE is strongly indicated. Careful comparison to the studies obtained at the time of initial diagnosis may detect intracardiac suppurative complications; there is a sensitivity range of 80–90%. If TEE findings are abnormal, urgent surgery is indicated. If they are normal, a careful history and physical examination coupled with CT or a technetium, gallium, or indium scan will often reveal an infective focus.

2. Worsening valve dysfunction and heart failure—At any time during the course of endocarditis, heart failure signs and symptoms may appear as a result of worsening regurgitation and failure of ventricular compensatory mechanisms. In fact, heart failure may appear despite effective antibiotic therapy—and even after bacteriologic cure. The onset of heart failure may be insidious and difficult to recognize, or it may be abrupt and catastrophic. Frequent appraisal of the patient's status by history and physical examination is the best way to ensure early detection of heart failure. Any change in the patient's regurgitant murmur during antibiotic therapy usually signifies progression of valvular dysfunction and the likely need for surgery. A persistent tachycardia or slowly increasing heart rate is a useful sign of impending heart failure prior to the appearance of the typical signs such as rales, S_3, and pulmonary vascular redistribution on chest radiograph. In patients with aortic valve endocarditis, the appearance of a widened pulse pressure usually indicates increased valve regurgitation.

Serial TTE or TEE is useful in confirming a suspected change in the patient's hemodynamic status; it may even identify the cause. Worsening of the mitral regurgitant lesion is suggested by an increase in size of the color-flow Doppler jet or an increase in the radius of the flow convergence region on the LV side of the regurgitant orifice. A rise in transmitral early filling velocity (E wave) and a fall in forward systolic pulmonary venous flow (S wave) may indicate a rise in mean left atrial pressure.

In the case of aortic regurgitation, jet enlargement over time is also a useful indicator of worsening regurgitation. Additional indications of severe aortic regurgitation include closure of the mitral valve on M-mode echocardiography prior to the onset of the QRS and shortening of the pressure half-time of the aortic insufficiency velocity, both from a rapid rise of LV pressure to a high level in late diastole. For either mitral or aortic regurgitation, the presence or development of a hyperdynamic left ventricle (increased ejection fraction, stroke volume, or both) and progressive LV dilatation on two-dimensional echocardiography are useful indirect indications of an excessive regurgitant burden. The appearance of pulmonary or right atrial hypertension, as estimated from tricuspid jet velocity and inferior vena caval dynamics, is another sign of hemodynamic decompensation. Transesophageal echocardiography has the additional major advantage of being able to detect the intracardiac complications accounting for the change in the patient's hemodynamic status.

If heart failure is mild, surgery should be deferred while diuretics, digoxin, and afterload-reducing drugs are given to optimize the patient's hemodynamic status. If the patient responds readily to therapy, surgery might be optional. In most cases, however, surgery should be undertaken as soon as feasible because it is almost certain that valve repair or replacement will be required eventually (for the hemodynamic lesion, if not for infection), and the patient's surgical risk is lowest at this early stage. One clear exception to surgery for mild heart failure is sodium overload (related to antibiotic therapy) and suspected valve dysfunction not confirmed by echocardiography.

If heart failure is moderate or severe, valve surgery should be undertaken immediately while drug therapy is used to stabilize the patient. Because of the difficulty in predicting the rate of progression of valve dysfunction, delaying surgery for hemodynamic optimization is ill-advised. Rapid development of heart failure may signal the occurrence of a major intracardiac complication, such as leaflet perforation, chordal rupture, or fistula formation. Preoperative or intraoperative TEE is usually helpful in guiding surgical planning in this setting.

3. Embolism—Embolism most often occurs early in the course of antibiotic therapy but can occur at any time, even after biologic cure. Suspected cerebral embolism should be evaluated immediately by CT; if necessary, cerebral angiography should be performed in order to rule out an intracranial mycotic aneurysm. Nonhemorrhagic infarcts may warrant measures to reduce cerebral edema.

If the patient is already receiving anticoagulant therapy prior to development of endocarditis, anticoagulation is usually continued. After cerebral embolism in a patient with endocarditis, however, anticoagulation therapy is usually discontinued (if possible) for 7–14 days to reduce the likelihood of massive intracerebral bleeding. If stroke occurs in mechanical prosthetic valve endocarditis, the balance of risks and benefits of continuing anticoagulation is unknown. In patients with stroke from endocarditis, serial neurologic examinations and (if a change is suspected) repeated CT scans are indicated to permit early detection of brain abscess.

Because no clinically useful means (including echocardiography) has been found to identify patients at high risk for embolism, valve surgery in endocarditis is not indicated to prevent embolism. Even the probability of embolism recurring after one episode is not necessarily high enough to warrant surgery for prevention. On the other hand, surgery may be advised if the patient has had more than one episode and has a persistent vegetation.

Peripheral embolization is managed conservatively and without anticoagulation whenever possible. Vascular surgery to restore the circulation may be indicated if major organ embolization becomes life-threatening. Embolectomy is generally indicated in culture-negative endocarditis in order to make a causative diagnosis; likely organisms include *Aspergillus, Candida,* and the HACEK group. Embolectomy is necessary, strictly for treatment, in fungal endocarditis in order to remove as much infection as possible from the circulation.

4. Mycotic aneurysm—A complaint of severe headache or visual disturbance (especially homonymous hemianopsia) in a patient with endocarditis should prompt an urgent CT scan for the possibility of an expanding intracranial mycotic aneurysm. This catastrophic complication may also present as a subarachnoid or intracerebral hemorrhage, usually massive. If the scan is negative, cerebral angiography is often necessary to confirm or rule out the diagnosis. Treatment is surgical removal as soon as the patient's condition will allow.

5. Myocardial infarction—Chest pain in the course of infective endocarditis is most likely due to myocardial infarction, pericarditis, or septic pulmonary embolization. Myocardial infarction during infective endocarditis is almost always caused by coronary embolization, although it may occasionally complicate purulent pericarditis or myocardial abscess. In the latter setting, inflammatory thrombosis of the artery probably occurs. Treatment is noninterventional. Anticoagulation is probably not indicated because its benefits for reducing myocardial ischemia in this setting are unknown and the risks of potential cerebral embolization are significant.

6. Pericarditis—The possibility of purulent pericarditis complicating infective endocarditis should be evaluated by TTE. If pericardial fluid is seen, prompt pericardiocentesis is needed. A transudate may be present; in this infrequent case, management can be conservative. Usually a purulent exudate will be found, necessitating surgical drainage or pericardiectomy. Most important, purulent pericarditis may signal the presence of an intracardiac abscess. Transesophageal echocardiography is indicated, and if an abscess is found, surgical drainage and valve surgery should be performed. Fortunately, the treatment of these related problems can be performed in a single operation. If an underlying myocardial abscess is not found, a pericardial window may be sufficient therapy. Continued observation is indicated because of the risk of subsequent additional cardiac or pericardial suppurative complications.

D. Management of High-Risk Endocarditis

1. Prosthetic valve endocarditis—Far higher morbidity and mortality rates are associated with prosthetic valve endocarditis than with native valve endocarditis. Infection of a prosthesis by fungi carries a mortality rate of more than 90%, whereas prosthetic infection from streptococci has a mortality rate of approximately 30%. In addition, the mortality rate from prosthetic valve endocarditis early after implantation is around twice that of late infection (after 2 months). Survival is improved by early operation in most cases, when the patient's surgical risk is acceptable. Surgical replacement is necessary in 85% of cases of biologic valve endocarditis and in almost all cases of mechanical prosthetic infection. Indications for surgery in prosthetic valve endocarditis are summarized in Table 12–8.

Medical treatment can be attempted in mechanical valve endocarditis when the surgical risk is high and the only evidence of valve involvement (using TEE) is a vegetation in the area of the sewing ring. In such cases, frequent serial TEE may be useful to monitor valve function and the response of the infected mass to treatment. Initial medical treatment of bioprosthetic endocarditis may be attempted when infection is due to a low-risk organism (such as *Streptococcus*) and involvement is limited to a vegetation on either the prosthetic leaflets or sewing ring. Repeated TEE is very useful if the

Table 12-8. Indications for Surgery in Prosthetic Valve Endocarditis.

Mechanical prosthesis (almost all cases)
Bioprosthesis if:
New paravalvular regurgitation or fistula
Sewing-ring abscess or dehiscence
Infection from *Staphylococcus epidermidis* or *aureus*, *Enterococcus*,
gram-negative bacteria, fungi
Blood cultures still positive after 1 week of antibiotics
Embolism or other major complication

patient does not respond to antibiotics. Blood cultures should be obtained every 4–7 days during treatment and weekly for a month following apparently successful treatment.

2. Fungal endocarditis—Overall mortality rates for fungal endocarditis are more than 80%; they are especially high in cases caused by *Aspergillus* and *Candida* species. Treatment requires the close collaboration of the primary physician, cardiologist, surgeon, and infectious disease specialist. Treatment is almost always a combination of valve replacement and a full course of an antifungal agent. Late relapses are common and require prolonged surveillance for years following successful completion of antifungal therapy. In addition to serologic tests and blood cultures, TEE is useful in monitoring the patient during and after treatment. Some clinicians have advocated long-term suppressive therapy with an oral azole agent for patients who survive the surgical and medical therapies for the acute infection.

3. Endocarditis from gram-negative bacteria—*Pseudomonas* endocarditis carries a mortality rate of almost 80% because of the frequent inability to sterilize vegetations by medical treatment. Among the causes for this inability is the frequent emergence of antibiotic-resistant bacterial strains during therapy. Surgery is usually performed as soon as possible after the diagnosis of *Pseudomonas* endocarditis of the left-sided valves. Surgery is also frequently indicated for endocarditis caused by the HACEK organisms, but here the reason is extensive valvular destruction by the time of diagnosis. In contrast to *Pseudomonas*, infection from HACEK organisms is readily cured by antibiotics. The treatment of endocarditis from enteric gram-negative bacteria is similar to that for *Pseudomonas* in that antibiotic therapy may fail, leading to a need for valve replacement. In vitro antibiotic sensitivity testing is crucial to antibiotic therapy of gram-negative bacteria.

E. Surgery

The indications for valve replacement or repair during infective endocarditis (discussed in the preceding section) are summarized in Table 12–9. The indications and timing of valve surgery are guided by several important principles.

Surgical morbidity and mortality rates are much higher if the patient is in even mild heart failure, is hypotensive, or has a low cardiac output when sent to the operating room. Similarly, uncontrolled infection, with its attendant systemic stress and peripheral dilatation, confers a higher surgical risk. In the absence of these factors, surgical risk is generally low despite active infective endocarditis. Surgery should not be delayed with the intention of prolonging preoperative antibiotic therapy. It has never been shown that either the risk of reinfection of the new prosthetic valve or surgical complications are reduced by longer preoperative antibiotic treatment.

The anatomic location and extent of valve involvement and other factors may allow valve debridement and repair rather than replacement. The advantages of valve repair are that future anticoagulation is not needed, and subsequent valve replacement carries a lower risk. The disadvantages of valve repair are the greater possibility of residual infected tissue and significant valve regurgitation. Valve repair is not considered in the presence of abscess or fistula near the valve or when significant leaflet erosion has occurred. As part of a repair, however, leaflet perforation can be patched and chordal support reconstructed. In general, valve repair is feasible when excision of the infected leaflet with a 2-mm margin of normal tissue will still leave enough normal leaflet to preserve valvular competence. Preoperative or intraoperative TEE is usually indicated for surgical planning and guidance.

F. Follow-up after Endocarditis

Long-term survival of the patient following an episode of endocarditis is much lower than that of the general population. Overall survival following native valve endocarditis is approximately 80% at 5 years and 50% at 10 years. Survival is considerably lower after prosthetic valve endocarditis. The patient remains at risk for three consequences of the disease: relapse of the original infection, noninfective sequelae of the infection, and recurrent endocarditis.

Failure to eradicate infection completely is usually apparent within 15 days after antibiotics are discontinued, although

Table 12-9. Indications for Valve Surgery in Native Valve Endocarditis.

Absolute Indications
Intracardiac abscess or fistula
Left heart failure from severe regurgitation or (rarely) obstruction
Endocarditis caused by fungi and resistant gram-negative organisms
Relative Indications
Mild heart failure in otherwise uncomplicated case
Recurrent embolization with persistent vegetation
Purulent pericarditis
Bacteremia despite optimal antibiotic therapy
Recurrent life-threatening septic pulmonary emboli
Severe tricuspid regurgitation with a low output state

relapse has been reported up to 6 months after apparently successful treatment. Relapse rates tend to be low with viridans streptococci (< 5%), intermediate with enterococci (8–20%), and high with *Pseudomonas* and fungi (> 20%). Relapse of *S aureus* endocarditis is not common (5%) but should prompt a search for an extracardiac source. Treatment of a relapse includes a reassessment of the extent of cardiac infection, and surgery warrants careful consideration. If a trial of antibiotic therapy is given, the patient should be carefully monitored during therapy to determine the need for surgery.

After successful treatment of infection, the patient remains at risk for the development of heart failure, stroke, and rupture of a mycotic aneurysm. A new baseline TTE should be obtained after treatment completion. If the patient had moderate or severe valve regurgitation or an episode of heart failure prior to hospital discharge, the probability of late heart failure is greatly increased. The risk of embolic stroke is very low after the first 4 weeks of antibiotic treatment but may persist for an unknown length of time. Rupture of a mycotic aneurysm after treatment is also rare but should be considered when a patient with stroke has a history of prior endocarditis.

Although estimates vary, recurrent endocarditis, defined as a repeat episode after more than 6 months, occurs in approximately 5–8% of cases. Controversy exists regarding the tendency for the infecting organism and the involved valve to be similar to those of the original episode. The recurrent episode probably carries a higher mortality rate than the original one. Risk factors for recurrent endocarditis include injecting drug use, congenital heart disease, rheumatic and myxomatous disease, and periodontitis. Any new febrile illness requires three sets of blood cultures before starting antibiotic therapy.

Andrews MM et al. Patient selection criteria and management guidelines for outpatient parenteral antibiotic therapy for native valve infective endocarditis. Clin Infect Dis. 2001 Jul 15;33(2):203–9. [PMID: 11418880]

Baddour LM et al; Committee on Rheumatic Fever, Endocarditis, and Kawasaki Disease; Council on Cardiovascular Disease in the Young; Councils on Clinical Cardiology, Stroke and Cardiovascular Surgery and Anesthesia; American Heart Association; Infectious Diseases Society of America. Infective endocarditis: diagnosis, antimicrobial therapy, and management of complications: a statement for healthcare professionals from the Committee on Rheumatic Fever, Endocarditis, and Kawasaki Disease, Council on Cardiovascular Disease in the Young, and the Councils on Clinical Cardiology, Stroke and Cardiovascular Surgery and Anesthesia, American Heart Association: endorsed by the Infectious Diseases Society of America. Circulation. 2005 Jun 14;111(23):e394–434. [PMID: 15956145]

Cabell CH et al; International Collaboration on Endocarditis Merged Database (ICE-MD) Study Group Investigators. Use of surgery in patients with native valve infective endocarditis: results from the International Collaboration on Endocarditis Merged Database. Am Heart J. 2005 Nov;150(5):1092–8. [PMID: 16291004]

Delahaye F et al. Indications and optimal timing for surgery in infective endocarditis. Heart. 2004 Jun;90(6):618–20. [PMID: 15145858]

Moreillon P et al. Infective endocarditis. Lancet. 2004 Jan 10;363(9403):139–49. [PMID: 14726169]

Mylonakis E et al. Infective endocarditis in adults. N Engl J Med. 2001 Nov 1;345(18):1318–30. [PMID: 11794152]

Olaison L et al. Current best practices and guidelines. Indications for surgical intervention in infective endocarditis. Cardiol Clin. 2003 May;21(2):235–51. [PMID: 12874896]

Systemic Hypertension

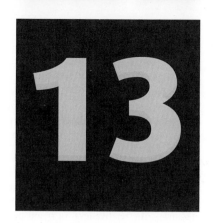

William F. Graettinger, MD, FACC, FACP, FCCP

ESSENTIALS OF DIAGNOSIS

- ► Prehypertension: systolic pressure of 120–139 mm Hg or diastolic pressure of 80–90 mm Hg.
- ► Stage 1 hypertension: systolic pressure of 140–159 mm Hg or diastolic pressure of 90–99 mm Hg.
- ► Stage 2 hypertension: systolic pressure of ≥ 160 mm Hg or diastolic pressure of ≥ 100 mm Hg.
- ► Measure on three separate occasions.
- ► In diabetic patients, diastolic pressure > 80 mm Hg, systolic pressure > 130 mm Hg, or both, on three separate occasions.

▶ General Considerations

Hypertension is a major modifiable risk factor for cardiovascular disease that can, if untreated, result in serious morbidity and mortality from cardiac, cerebrovascular, vascular, and renal disease. In excess of 62 million persons in the United States are estimated to have hypertension, and only about 70% of these individuals are aware of their diagnosis. Of those, only a third are at their therapeutic goal. The potential for death and disability is therefore quite high and represents a serious public health issue. Once the diagnosis of hypertension is made and therapy instituted, elevated blood pressure can be lowered, reducing the risk of cardiovascular disease in most patients. Major antihypertensive trials, in large populations, have conclusively demonstrated that there is a direct continuous relationship between the level of blood pressure and cardiovascular morbidity and mortality. These studies have shown that treating all levels of hypertension significantly decreases fatal and nonfatal stroke, coronary events, heart failure, and chronic kidney disease and renal failure. The wide array of antihypertensive agents is very effective in reducing blood pressure. Despite similar blood pressure and

overall mortality reductions, the reductions in incidence of stroke, coronary ischemic events, heart failure, and renal failure are not the same for all classes of antihypertensive agents. The reasons for these differences have not been totally explained and are the topic of much speculation.

A growing body of direct and inferential evidence suggests that reduction of blood pressure should not be the only goal of antihypertensive therapy. Therapy should also be directed toward controlling all of the patient's modifiable cardiovascular risk factors, including dyslipidemia, smoking, obesity, physical inactivity, microalbuminuria, and diabetes mellitus.

▶ Pathophysiology & Etiology

Until recently, high blood pressure was synonymous with hypertension; now, however, data suggest that there is considerably more to hypertension than increased blood pressure. Several metabolic and functional abnormalities have even been observed in the children of hypertensive patients prior to blood pressure elevation that are similar to, but of a lesser magnitude than, those found in their parents. Hypertension is also associated with insulin resistance and glucose intolerance. Insulin levels are consistently higher in hypertensive patients than in normotensive persons. Hyperinsulinemia is worsened by thiazide diuretics, especially in the presence of β-blocker therapy. Hyperinsulinemia produces a proliferation of vascular smooth muscle and fibrous tissue and adversely affects the serum lipid profile.

Renin and angiotensin levels are also important factors in determining both the response to therapy and the prognosis. Hypertensive patients with high renin levels have a greater incidence of myocardial infarction than do similar patients with lower levels. Normotensive young adults with a family history of hypertension have been found to have thicker left ventricular (LV) walls and alterations of LV diastolic filling in comparison with control subjects. Although not frankly abnormal, these latter two findings are similar to but less severe than those observed in hypertensive patients. Renal reserve also appears diminished in the children of hypertensive parents. LV hypertrophy, a direct result of hypertension, is twice as prevalent in patients with prehypertension than in normotensive persons, demonstrating target organ effects of blood pressures that were previously thought to be normal. Hypertension, therefore, is a multisystem disorder with involvement of the cardiovascular, neuroendocrine, and renal systems with a strong genetic component.

A. Natural History

Blood pressure gradually increases throughout childhood and adolescence. The best predictor of the level of future blood pressure is the relative level of blood pressure of a child in relation to his or her peers. During childhood and adolescence, body weight is a major determinant of blood pressure, with heavier children having higher blood pressures. High blood pressure is uncommon under the age of 20; if present, it is usually associated with renal insufficiency, renal artery stenosis, or coarctation of the aorta. The initial presentation of high blood pressure usually occurs in the third to the sixth decade, and blood pressure may fluctuate significantly during the early course of the disease. The prevalence of hypertension increases with age and is greater in men than women. In the elderly population, the gender distribution reverses, and more women than men have high blood pressure. More than 50% of the US population age 60–69 years and 75% of those 70 years or older have hypertension.

Large epidemiologic and intervention trials have clearly defined the risks of elevations of blood pressure and the benefits of treatment. Evidence of target organ damage has been demonstrated at lower levels of blood pressure than was previously known. As a result, the definition of hypertension has been revised. The new definition includes a new classification of prehypertension, which is thought to identify individuals at increased risk for hypertension and therefore require closer follow-up. Everyone should be screened for the presence of high blood pressure; testing should be done routinely in the physician's office or at one of the larger community screening activities.

These activities are typically targeted at those at greater risk for high blood pressure: older individuals, individuals with previously high-normal blood pressures (prehypertension), blacks, sedentary individuals, and those with a family history of hypertension.

B. Ethnic and Socioeconomic Factors

Blacks have both an earlier onset and a greater prevalence of high blood pressure than do whites, Asians, and Native Americans at all ages. Over the age of 50 years, hypertension is prevalent in more than 40% of black males, compared with approximately 27% in white males. Severe high blood pressure (diastolic blood pressure at least 115 mm Hg) is five times more common in black men than in white men and seven

times more common in black women than in white women. Blacks therefore tend to have more serious complications, especially strokes, from high blood pressure. Other factors also affect the prevalence of high blood pressure. Among all ethnic groups, less-educated individuals have a greater prevalence of high blood pressure than do more highly educated individuals, especially in lower socioeconomic groups.

The level of blood pressure elevation is directly related to total cardiovascular risk, and the presence of other cardiovascular disease risk factors, especially diabetes or dyslipidemia, is synergistic with high blood pressure.

▶ Clinical Findings

Blood pressure is a continuous variable with a reasonably normal, or bell-shaped-curve, distribution across the general population. The higher the blood pressure, the greater the risk of a cardiovascular event; conversely, the lower the blood pressure, the lower the cardiovascular risk. It is important to stress that isolated systolic hypertension, a systolic pressure of greater than 140 mm Hg with a diastolic pressure of less than 90 mm Hg, is abnormal and requires attention.

The diagnosis of hypertension should not be based on measurements taken at a single office visit. Elevated readings should be confirmed at a second or third visit to establish the diagnosis, and any factors that might elevate blood pressure should be excluded. The patient should refrain from smoking for at least 30 minutes prior to blood pressure measurement. The blood pressure should be measured, with a cuff of the appropriate size, after at least 5 minutes of rest in a seated or supine position. The cuff should cover approximately one-third of the length of the upper arm and should completely or almost completely encircle the arm. Too small a cuff may overestimate the true blood pressure because it may only partially compress the artery, requiring a higher pressure for total occlusion. The measurements should be made twice in both arms, for a total of four measures. The average of the two measurements in the arm with the higher values is used as the baseline value of blood pressure. Systolic blood pressure is indicated by the phase 1 Korotkoff sound (onset) and diastolic pressure by phase 5, or disappearance, in adults. In children, phase 4, or muffling, has been suggested as the best indicator of diastolic pressure.

The blood pressure obtained in the physician's office, however, does not always accurately represent that experienced by the patient during routine daily living. About 20–30% of patients with mildly elevated office blood pressure may have a hyperadrenergic response to having their blood pressure measured. This hyperreactivity is called white-coat, pseudo-, or office hypertension and may be related to anxiety from merely being in the physician's office or clinic. If the blood pressure is measured in a non-threatening situation by a friend or relative or with an automated device, the blood pressure in these individuals may be normal. Blood pressure hyperreactivity should be suspected in patients who have persistently elevated blood pressure in the office and normal pressure measurements out of the office or in patients who have hypotensive symptoms but remain hypertensive in the office despite therapy. It has not been clearly established whether the blood pressure in these individuals is truly normal or whether they have an early or different form of hypertension. Several studies have found alterations in cardiac structure and function that are somewhere between those found in normotensive subjects and those found in hypertensive patients. No large outcome studies are available.

The best way to evaluate a patient with suspected white-coat hypertension is to use an automated ambulatory blood pressure device that measures the blood pressure periodically throughout the day and night. The patient quickly becomes accustomed to the small, light-weight, portable device, and a representative series of recordings can be obtained. The accuracy of these devices allows separation of those patients with true elevations of blood pressure from those who are hyperreactors. The devices are also useful in evaluating patients with episodic hypertension and those with borderline blood pressure elevations who already have evidence of involvement of the heart, kidneys, or vasculature. Automated blood pressure monitoring can be used to evaluate the duration and effectiveness of antihypertensive medication; correlate blood pressure with damage to the heart, kidneys, or blood vessels; and determine the prognosis. Its value in routine evaluation of hypertensive patients has not been clearly established, however.

A. Initial Evaluation

The initial evaluation should be focused on excluding secondary or reversible causes of hypertension and looking for the presence and severity of organ damage caused by hypertension. A reversible cause for high blood pressure is found in less than 5% of adult patients. The causes of secondary hypertension include renovascular, chronic kidney disease, coarctation of the aorta, pheochromocytoma, obstructive uropathy, primary hyperaldosteronism, Cushing syndrome, obstructive sleep apnea, and thyroid or parathyroid disease. Signs of a secondary cause are frequently present and should be looked for in the patient's history, the screening physical examination, blood chemistries, and urinalysis. A more exhaustive evaluation for a secondary cause is needed for patients whose blood pressure is difficult to control medically, who have malignant hypertension, or who have a sudden onset of high blood pressure.

Most patients with mild-to-moderate hypertension are asymptomatic. A careful history should be obtained, including first-degree relatives (siblings, parents, children, aunts, uncles) with high blood pressure, stroke, coronary artery disease, or diabetes; any knowledge or personal history of high blood pressure; smoking; alcohol consumption; and history of headache, sweats, palpitations, and pallor. Alcohol consumption can cause acute elevations of blood pressure; long-term consumption can cause sustained elevations. A complete evaluation of all prescription and nonprescription medications the patient is taking should be done to exclude

any possible contribution to the elevation or any interaction that might limit a given drug's antihypertensive effects. In particular, the clinician should ask about use of estrogens, nonsteroidal antiinflammatory agents, and decongestants. Approximately 5% of women taking oral contraceptives have elevations of blood pressure; these usually resolve when the medication is discontinued. This side effect of oral contraceptives is more common in women over the age of 35 and in the presence of obesity; the use of low-dose estrogen oral contraceptives greatly reduces the incidence. Nonsteroidal antiinflammatory agents may cause hypertension or antagonize the antihypertensive effects of medications, especially angiotensin-converting enzyme inhibitors (ACEIs) and angiotensin receptor blockers (ARBs). Any previous antihypertensive medication use should be documented as well as the blood pressure response and side effects.

B. Physical Examination

The physical findings suggestive of secondary or potentially reversible high blood pressure include abdominal or flank bruits suggestive of renovascular hypertension; absent or diminished femoral pulses suggestive of aortic coarctation; and flank or abdominal masses suggestive of polycystic renal disease or abdominal aortic aneurysm. Careful evaluation for target organ damage from hypertension should include funduscopic examination for arteriovenous nicking, arteriolar narrowing, hemorrhages, exudates, or papilledema; and cardiac examination for signs of heart failure (S_3 or a laterally displaced LV apical impulse), LV hypertrophy (S_4 or a sustained LV apical impulse). The patient should also be examined for any neurologic deficit compatible with stroke.

C. Diagnostic Studies

Clinical laboratory tests should be performed to screen for occult renal or cardiac disease that might contribute to the elevation of blood pressure and to assess overall cardiovascular risk. The complete blood count might demonstrate the presence of anemia, suggesting chronic renal disease. Urinalysis is a good screening tool for occult renal disease, diabetes, renal protein loss, or abnormal sediment. All hypertensive diabetic patients and patients with moderate to severe hypertension should be tested for microalbuminuria. Levels of serum electrolytes; blood urea nitrogen; creatinine; fasting blood glucose; hemoglobin A_{1c}; total, high-density lipoprotein (HDL), and low-density lipoprotein (LDL) cholesterol; triglycerides; calcium; uric acid; and magnesium provide information on other potential cardiovascular risk factors and also establish a baseline for the effects of drug therapy.

1. Electrocardiography—Although not a particularly sensitive tool, an electrocardiogram (ECG) should be obtained to look for LV hypertrophy, which, if present, is an independent risk factor for cardiovascular morbidity and mortality. In hypertensive patients, this is a significant predictor of poor cardiovascular outcomes.

2. Chest radiography—Chest radiography is not a routine part of the screening process for the uncomplicated cases of hypertension.

3. Echocardiography—This imaging method, which is much more sensitive for the presence of LV hypertrophy, should be done in selected individuals. Although the role of echocardiography as a screening tool has not been established, it is excellent for assessing the degree of LV hypertrophy and systolic functional status in hypertensive patients. Cardiac Doppler allows the assessment of LV diastolic dysfunction, which may be associated with signs and symptoms of heart failure. Borderline hypertensive patients whose echocardiograms show LV hypertrophy should probably be treated.

D. Organ Involvement

The main organs (target or end organs) that suffer the ravages of high blood pressure are the heart, brain, kidneys, and blood vessels. High blood pressure is an independent risk factor for coronary artery disease, and cardiac involvement is responsible for the largest portion of the increase in morbidity and mortality observed in patients with high blood pressure. Up to one-third of untreated patients with mild-to-moderate elevations of blood pressure have LV hypertrophy. Increasing LV mass is generally associated with increasing blood pressure, although patients vary greatly in the extent of hypertrophy for any given level of blood pressure. Increased LV mass also can be present in the absence of elevated blood pressure, however, and may be related to metabolic differences in hypertensive patients. The prognosis is significantly worse when LV hypertrophy is present with any amount of blood pressure elevation. Effective antihypertensive therapy will cause regression of LV hypertrophy, but it is apparent that simple reduction of blood pressure is not always sufficient to cause regression. The anticipated beneficial effects of LV mass reduction with antihypertensive therapy have yet to be convincingly demonstrated.

1. Atherosclerotic complications—The most common causes of death in patients with high blood pressure are complications from atherosclerosis. These are unstable coronary syndromes characterized by angina, acute myocardial infarction, and sudden cardiac death. Large blood pressure reduction trials have shown disappointingly small decrease in the incidence of these atherosclerotic complications. When therapy is directed at reducing both blood pressure and cholesterol, the results are somewhat more encouraging—although not consistent. The addition of any of the "statins" or hydroxymethylglutaryl coenzyme A (HMG-CoA) reductase inhibitors is particularly effective in reducing acute coronary ischemic events.

2. Cardiac dysfunction—Other sequelae of long-standing high blood pressure are systolic and diastolic dysfunction. Reduced systolic function may result from myocardial ischemia, infarction, fibrosis, or cardiomyopathy. Diastolic dysfunction results directly from LV hypertrophy and, even in the absence of systolic dysfunction, can cause symptoms of heart failure. It is estimated that 40–50% of patients admitted to a hospital for heart failure have preserved systolic cardiac function. This is especially prevalent in the older (> 65-years-old) population. Cardiac dysrhythmias and sudden cardiac death are also more prevalent in the presence of LV hypertrophy.

3. Stroke—Hypertension is the major risk factor for hemorrhagic stroke and, to a lesser extent, cerebral infarction. The level of systolic pressure is more closely related to stroke incidence than is diastolic pressure. The incidence of hemorrhagic stroke, at any raised level of systolic pressure, is significantly higher among blacks than among other groups; when stroke occurs, it also tends to be more extensive. Effective antihypertensive therapy reduces the risk of stroke to almost normotensive levels.

4. Hypertensive renal disease—Renal disease due to hypertension is characterized by nephrosclerosis with chronic renal insufficiency and ultimately renal failure. Microalbuminuria is a marker of asymptomatic renal dysfunction in hypertensive patients with renal dysfunction. The renal complications of high blood pressure can be virtually eliminated by effective antihypertensive therapy. All agents have been shown to be equally effective in their renal protective effects in nondiabetic patients. The combination of hypertension and diabetes mellitus is particularly damaging to the kidneys and causes earlier onset and more rapid progression of renal insufficiency and renal failure if untreated (see section on Diabetes mellitus).

5. Aorta and peripheral blood vessels—The aorta and peripheral blood vessels are involved in the genesis of high blood pressure and in its consequences. High blood pressure is a contributing and exacerbating factor in ascending aortic dissection and contributes to abdominal aortic aneurysm by virtue of the expansile effect of increased distending pressure. Changes in the elastic properties of the peripheral vasculature are manifest early in the course of hypertension as a decrease in arterial compliance that is related to the increase in blood pressure.

6. Eyes—The eyes suffer vascular damage as a result of untreated hypertension. The characteristic ocular findings of hypertensive retinopathy include arteriolar narrowing, arteriovenous nicking, flame hemorrhages, hard exudates, and papilledema-progressive changes related to increasing severity and duration of hypertension.

Chobanian AV et al; Joint National Committee on Prevention, Detection, Evaluation, and Treatment of High Blood Pressure. National Heart, Lung, and Blood Institute; National High Blood Pressure Education Program Coordinating Committee. Seventh report of the Joint National Committee on Prevention, Detection, Evaluation, and Treatment of High Blood Pressure. Hypertension. 2003 Dec;42(6):1206–52. [PMID: 14656957]

▶ Treatment

The treatment of hypertension has evolved over the past four decades as knowledge of the natural history, pathophysiology, and risk factors for hypertension as well as the effects of therapy and the interactions of these factors has accumulated. The goal of treating high blood pressure is to reduce blood pressure and thereby prevent or reverse end-organ damage without causing significant side effects or requiring unacceptable changes in lifestyle. Many classes of antihypertensive agents that effectively lower blood pressure, either alone or in conjunction with an agent from another class of drugs, are available. Because of the potentially detrimental metabolic changes caused by some agents, their failure to reduce the incidence of myocardial infarction, and the multisystem involvement of hypertension, it is essential to choose a regimen that effectively lowers blood pressure without causing abnormalities. The following recommendations incorporate data from large long-term trials and experimental evidence from human and animal studies.

Nonpharmacologic therapy and coronary risk factor reduction should be initiated in all patients once the diagnosis of sustained hypertension is made. Individuals with stage 1 hypertension can be treated with nonpharmacologic therapy for 3–6 months. If this fails to reduce blood pressure to below 140/90 mm Hg within that time, pharmacologic therapy should be initiated. If end-organ damage is already present at diagnosis, or if other major coronary risk factors such as diabetes or dyslipidemia are present, pharmacologic therapy should be initiated once the diagnosis has been made. Individuals with severe hypertension (systolic blood pressure higher than 160 mm Hg; diastolic higher than 100 mm Hg) should have both nonpharmacologic and drug therapy initiated once the diagnosis is confirmed.

A. Nonpharmacologic Therapy

Nonpharmacologic therapy should be encouraged in all hypertensive patients. The approaches of proven benefit are weight reduction especially in obese patients; moderate aerobic exercise in sedentary patients; a reduction in alcohol consumption in all patients who drink; and a reduction of salt intake in some patients.

1. Obesity—Obesity (more than 10% over ideal weight) is associated with hypertension, diabetes, hyperlipidemia, and excess coronary mortality. In obese patients, a decrease of as much as 2 mm Hg of diastolic blood pressure can be achieved for every 3 lbs of weight loss. The benefits of weight reduction start early in the course, with a loss of as little as 10–15 lb. Although all obese patients should be encouraged to lose weight, the process is usually difficult and frequently requires extensive support and sometimes a financial investment. The use of all "stimulant" type weight reduction therapies should be strictly avoided because they tend to elevate blood pressure. The fat substitutes or avoidance therapies do not raise blood pressure but have their own side effects.

2. Exercise—Regular exercise in a previously sedentary individual may reduce diastolic blood pressure as much as 10 mm Hg. The level of exercise should be that required to raise the heart rate to 50–60% of the maximal predicted heart rate. Walking briskly for 45 minutes three to five times per week should suffice for most previously sedentary individuals. Increasing the amount of exercise in a previously active individual, however, seldom decreases blood pressure.

3. Alcohol consumption—Alcohol consumption causes acute increases in blood pressure and can cause sustained hypertension in a significant proportion of individuals. Hypertensive patients should be encouraged to limit their alcohol consumption to 1 oz of ethanol per day, the equivalent of 2 oz of 100-proof hard liquor, 8 oz of wine, or 24 oz of beer. Even this level of alcohol consumption is associated with increased overall mortality. Alcohol decreases cardiovascular mortality and appears to decrease the onset of diabetes by improving insulin resistance. The best data for these benefits are for wine. Beer with its even higher carbohydrate load should be avoided in diabetic patients.

4. Sodium reduction—Reducing sodium in the diet has been shown to reduce blood pressure in most people to a modest degree. Hypertensive patients, older individuals, and blacks tend to be more salt-sensitive, and achieve larger reductions in blood pressure with salt restriction. Hypertensive patients should be encouraged to keep sodium chloride consumption to less than 4–6 g/d.

5. Stress—Stress has long been known to raise blood pressure acutely and has been implicated in the genesis of sustained hypertension, even though no clear relationship has been demonstrated. Reducing stress would seem to be a reasonable form of nonpharmacologic therapy, but no controlled studies have demonstrated significant improvement in blood pressure with stress avoidance or relaxation therapy.

B. Pharmacologic Therapy

Table 13–1 lists the available antihypertensive medications. Although all of these classes of agents have been shown to be roughly equal in their ability to lower blood pressure in large population studies, they are not equally effective in all demographic groups or in preventing all complications. The initial choice for a given patient should take age, race, metabolic side effects, other cardiac risk factors and, most importantly, concomitant diseases into consideration. The report of the Joint National Committee on Detection, Evaluation and Treatment of High Blood Pressure recommends monotherapy with diuretics or β-blockers as initial therapy. Calcium channel blockers, ACEIs, and ARBs, are alternative first-line agents. The report does recognize special populations, such as diabetic patients and patients with coronary disease, which need special consideration.

Until the most recent JNC7 recommendations, the traditional initial approach, known as monotherapy, was

Table 13-1. Common Oral Antihypertensive Agents.

Drug	Total Daily Dose[1] (mg)	Frequency	Drug	Total Daily Dose[1] (mg)	Frequency
Adrenergic inhibitors			**Calcium channel blockers**		
α-Blockers			Diltiazem (SR)	120–160	Twice daily
Doxasosin	1–16	Once daily	(CD, XR)	120–160	Once daily
Prazosin	1–20	Two or three times daily	Verapamil	80–480	Two or three times daily
Terazosin	1–20	Once daily	(long-acting)	120–480	Once or twice daily
β-Blockers			Dihydropyridines		
Atenolol	25–100	Once daily	Amlodipine	2.5–10	Once daily
Betaxolol	5–40	Once daily	Felodipine	5–20	Once daily
Bisoprolol	5–20	Once daily	Isradipine	2.5–10	Twice daily
Carvedilol	3.125–25	Twice daily	Nifedipine (GITS)	30–120	Once daily
Metoprolol	25–200	Twice daily			
Nadolol	20–240	Twice daily	**Diuretics**		
Propranolol (long-acting)	60–240	Once daily	Thiazide-type		
			Bendroflumethiazide	2.5–5	Once daily
Timolol	20–40	Once daily	Benzthiazide	12.5–50	Once daily
β-Blockers with ISA			Chlorthalidone	12.5–50	Once daily
Acebutolol	200–1200	Once daily	Chlorthiazide	12.5–50	Once daily
Carteolol	2.5–10	Once daily	Hydroclorthiazide	12.5–50	Once daily
Penbutolol	20–80	Once daily	Indapamide	2.5–5	Once daily
Pindolol	10–60	Twice daily	Metolazone	1.25–5	Once daily
α-β-Blockers			Methyclothiazide	2.5–5	Once daily
Labetalol	200–1200	Once or twice daily	Polythiazide	1.0–4	Once daily
ACE inhibitors			Trichlormethiazide	1.0–4	Once daily
Benazepril	10–40	Once or twice daily	Loop diuretics		
Captopril	25–50	Three times daily	Bumetanide	0.5–5	Twice daily
Enalapril	10–40	Once or twice daily	Furosemide	10–300	Twice daily
Fosinopril	10–40	Once or twice daily	Torsemide	2.5–10	Once daily
Lisinopril	10–40	Once or twice daily	Potassium-sparing agents		
Moexipril	7.5–30	Once or twice daily	Amiloride	5–10	Once or twice daily
Perindopril	4–16	Once daily	Spironolactone	25–100	Two or three times daily
Quinapril	10–80	Once or twice daily	Triamterene	50–150	Once or twice daily
Ramipril	2.5–20	Once or twice daily			
Trandolapril	1–8	Once daily	**Centrally acting agents**		
			Clonidine	0.1–1.2	Once or twice daily
Angiotensin receptor blockers			Transdermal	0.1–0.3	Once a week
Candesartan	2–32	Once daily	Guanabenz	4–64	Twice daily
Eprosartan	600–800	Once or twice daily	Methyldopa	250–2000	Twice daily
Irbesartan	75–300	Once daily			
Losartan	25–100	Once or twice daily	**Peripheral vasodilators**		
Telmisartan	20–80	Once daily	Hydralazine	50–200	Once or twice daily
Valsartan	80–320	Once daily	Minoxidil	2.5–80	Once or twice daily

[1]The total daily dose should be given in divided doses at the frequency specified. The initial dose should be the smallest listed.
ISA, intrinsic sympathomimetic activity.

to start with one drug and titrate it to blood pressure control or limiting side effects. The main advantage of starting with a diuretic or β-blocker (JNC6 recommendations) is that it is both moderately effective and reasonably inexpensive. The main drawback of monotherapy is that blood pressure is controlled to recommended levels in only a small number of patients; most patients require two or more medications.

Initial therapy should take concomitant diseases and ethnicity into consideration. Individual patient responsiveness is also very important. Blood pressure should be checked at home in the morning and at night and reported to the physician, since antihypertensive medications may lose efficacy late in the day, resulting in high morning pre-dose hypertension. An additional evening dose may be required for some "once daily" medications.

The use of β-blockers as initial therapy has been called into question by several large clinical trials, and the UK's National Institute of Health and Clinical Excellence (NICE) revised its guidelines to move β-blockers to fourth-line initial therapy. Their initial recommendation is to start with calcium channel blockers in all hypertensive patients older than 55 years and in all black patients.

Table 13–2 lists the generalized response to antihypertensive therapy based on demographic groups. It is important to note that gender does not appear to affect the response in any group. Such data can serve as a starting point in picking initial antihypertensive agents, but they provide only an indication of the likelihood of response in an individual patient. Concomitant diseases should be a major influence in the decision-making process. Demographics cannot predict individual responses and therefore should not be used to exclude consideration of any class of agents in a given patient (eg, ACEI for a black patient). Because pharmaceutical agents are quite costly, the economic burden must also factor into the decision-making process. If a patient cannot afford to buy his or her medications, it is unlikely that the patient will purchase it and hence that medication will be ineffective.

Concomitant diseases—Other diseases occurring along with hypertension clearly must influence the choice of initial and subsequent antihypertensive agents. In patients with diabetes, inhibitors of the renin-angiotensin-aldosterone system (RAAS) decrease hypertension-related nephropathy and should be used as initial antihypertensive agents unless contraindicated. In such patients, diuretics may exacerbate glucose intolerance and should be added to RAAS blockers only if they are needed to reach target levels or to manage fluid accumulation.

Because thiazide diuretics raise plasma triglycerides and LDL cholesterol, they worsen the already present dyslipidemias prevalent in diabetics. The current recommendations are to only use low-dose diuretics, which will avoid some of the deleterious side effects but tend to be less effective when used as monotherapy.

β-Blockers may exacerbate heart block and reactive airway disease. They may also increase plasma triglyceride levels and decrease HDL cholesterol, thereby potentially increasing atherosclerosis (see section on β-Adrenergic blocking agents). Nonetheless, β-blockers are a good choice for patients with hypertension and angina and are recommended for all patients with known coronary artery disease. They effectively treat both conditions and can simplify patient care without sacrificing efficacy. β-Blockers decrease mortality following myocardial infarction and should therefore not be withheld in such patients because of fears of increased atherogenesis or heart failure. Calcium channel blockers are also very effective in patients with combined hypertension and angina. RAAS blockers have been shown to improve survival in patients with dilated cardiomyopathy from any cause and with post-myocardial infarction systolic dysfunction.

1. Diuretics—When used as monotherapy, diuretics are effective in approximately 30–40% of patients and are espe-

Table 13–2. Response by Demographic Group.

Group	Effective Agents	Ineffective Agents
Young white	ACEI, calcium channel blocker, β-blocker	Diuretics
Older white	Calcium channel blocker, diuretic	
Young black	Calcium channel blocker	ACEI, β-blocker
Other black	Calcium channel blocker, diuretic	ACEI, β-blocker
Isolated systolic hypertension	Diuretic, calcium channel blocker	ACEI

ACEI, angiotensin-converting enzyme inhibitor.

cially effective in lowering systolic blood pressure. They are extremely inexpensive. Several studies and meta-analyses have shown diuretic therapy to significantly decrease cardiac and stroke mortality rates. Diuretics are particularly effective antihypertensive agents in the elderly.

The adverse side effects of diuretics are urinary frequency and metabolic disturbances. They cause loss of potassium, which can precipitate cardiac dysrhythmias, renal insufficiency, and resistance to antihypertensive agents. Thiazide diuretics may induce gout in gout-prone individuals. Low doses (eg, 12.5–25 mg/day of hydrochlorothiazide) usually prevent hypokalemia and may reduce the metabolic alterations in glucose and lipids.

The shorter acting loop diuretics, such as furosemide, are poor antihypertensive agents and should be used for managing fluid overload. No outcome data are available for these agents in hypertension.

Spironolactone inhibits aldosterone and is a weak diuretic. It may be used in conjunction with a thiazide or loop diuretic to conserve potassium if hypokalemia occurs. Serum potassium should be monitored especially carefully when spironolactone is used with other potassium-sparing agents such as RAAS blockers. Aldosterone blockers are also indicated in patients with New York Heart Association (NYHA) class III and IV heart failure and are useful in addition to ACEI and ARBs and β-blockers in patients with hypertension and heart failure.

2. Angiotensin-converting enzyme inhibitors—These agents block the conversion of inactive angiotensin I to the potent vasoconstrictor substance angiotensin II. The use of this group of agents is rapidly increasing as first-line therapy, especially in the young white population, due to the low incidence of associated side effects. The success rate is 40–50% as monotherapy and when used in combination with a low-dose diuretic, β-blocker, or calcium channel blocker, ACEIs are highly effective in controlling blood pressure in more than 80% of patients. Some of the additional benefits thought to be achieved with ACEIs are related to the reduction of the potent vasoconstrictor and mitogen effects of angiotensin II on cardiac and vascular tissue. They produce no adverse effect on glucose metabolism or lipid profile and have a potent renal-protective effect in diabetic patients. ACEIs preserve renal function and avoid or delay the onset of microalbuminuria and slow or prevent the progression to proteinuria and end-stage renal disease. ACEIs work by inhibiting the renin-angiotensin-aldosterone system and may cause mild elevations of serum potassium. If supplemental potassium is concomitantly administered, life-threatening hyperkalemia may result. Renal function and potassium levels should be monitored during initiation and titration of ACEI therapy in all patients, especially those with preexisting renal insufficiency. Of special note, ACEI may cause life-threatening fetal abnormalities and should be avoided in pregnant women. A chronic nonproductive cough develops in 5–15% of patients treated with an ACEI and may be bothersome enough to cause discontinuation of the agent. Recently, a rare potentially fatal side effect of angioedema has been described with ACEI use. This side effect should be aggressively treated, and the patient should not be rechallenged with an ACEI.

The antihypertensive efficacy of ACEI may be attenuated by concomitant administration of nonsteroidal antiinflammatory agents (including aspirin and over-the-counter ibuprofen, naproxen, etc), which should therefore be avoided.

3. Angiotensin receptor blockers—These agents selectively block the vascular angiotensin II (AT_1) receptors, causing vasodilation similar to the ACEI. They are as effective and very well tolerated with a side-effect profile similar to that of ACEI. ARBs appear to have the same renal protective effects in diabetic patients as ACEI. No large head-to-head trials of ACEIs and ARBs in diabetic patients are available. Due to the much higher cost of ARBs and the proven efficacy of ACEIs, diabetic patients should start on an ACEI, and patients intolerant of ACEI should use ARBs. The incidence of cough with ARBs is less than that observed with ACEI (< 5%) but is much higher in those patients who have already had an ACEI-associated cough. Angioedema has also been described with ARB use although it is significantly less frequent than with ACEI. If a patient has had angioedema with an agent in either of the two classes, the other class should be avoided.

4. β-Adrenergic blocking agents—β-Blockers are effective monotherapy in 50–60% of patients, especially those with an activated renin-angiotensin system. They lower blood pressure by decreasing both heart rate and cardiac contractility and thus cardiac output. All β-blockers are similar in antihypertensive efficacy, regardless of whether they are cardioselective ($β_1$-specific) or nonselective ($β_1$ and $β_2$) receptor blockers; possess intrinsic sympathomimetic activity (ISA); or are lipid-soluble. The side-effect profile does differ, however, and is based on these properties. $β_1$-Selective agents cause less

bronchial constriction at lower doses but are similar to nonselective β-blockers at high doses. Agents with ISA produce less resting bradycardia than do those without. Lipid solubility determines whether the agent will cross into the brain. Lipid-soluble β-blockers, which cross the blood-brain barrier, may cause more central nervous system disturbances, including nightmares and confusion. All β-blockers depress LV systolic function, tend to reduce cardiac output, and may cause impotence. Fatigue is a frequent side effect and may limit use in young active patients. β-Blockers also cause the alterations in lipid profile mentioned earlier; the HDL depression is less significant with cardioselective β-blockers at low doses (eg, metoprolol, 25–50 mg twice daily) and insignificant with the ISA β-blockers. The clinical significance of these abnormalities has not been established and the concomitant use of appropriate lipid therapy probably makes this a moot point.

5. Calcium channel blockers—Calcium channel blockers are very well tolerated and effective as monotherapy in 50–60% of patients in all demographic groups. The mechanism of antihypertensive action is vasodilatation with all such agents and a decrease in heart rate and cardiac output with the nondihydropyridines agents (verapamil and diltiazem). Because of the negative inotropic effects in all but the newest dihydropyridines agents, calcium channel blockers should not be used in patients with cardiac failure. All calcium channel blockers are now available in formulations that can be taken once or twice daily, a regimen that greatly improves compliance. Immediate-release preparations of short-acting agents have no place in the antihypertensive armamentarium. Combinations of calcium channel blockers and a β-blocker, an ACEI, or ARB are very effective in lowering blood pressure. Concomitant use of a β-blocker and a calcium channel blocker with significant sinus and atrioventricular node-slowing properties (eg, diltiazem, verapamil) should be done with caution to avoid profound bradycardia or heart block. Other side effects include peripheral edema (dihydropyridines) and constipation (verapamil).

In several large meta-analyses, calcium channel blockers have been shown to be highly effective in lowering blood pressure but have a 25% excess incidence of acute myocardial infarction and heart failure. The mechanisms are as yet to be delineated. Until this is resolved, use of calcium channel blockers as monotherapy for hypertension is not encouraged in patients with known coronary artery disease.

6. α-Receptor blockers—α-Blockers act at vascular postsynaptic α-receptors to produce arterial and venous dilatation. Because the α-blockers do not reduce cardiac output, they do not adversely affect exercise tolerance. The major side effect of this group is postural hypotension, especially after the first dose, a problem that can be minimized by taking the first dose at bedtime. α-Blockers increase HDL cholesterol and reduce LDL cholesterol and may thereby decrease coronary risk. The LDL-cholesterol-lowering effect of doxazosin is similar in magnitude to that of 10 mg of lovastatin. It is therefore surprising that the α-blocker arm of the ALLHAT trial, a large randomized trial comparing the major antihypertensive classes, was stopped early due to a 25% higher incidence of major cardiac events in hypertensive patients treated primarily with α-blockers compared with diuretics. The reasons for these unexpected results are unclear. α-Blockers should therefore not be used as initial therapy and should be relegated to the status of add-on therapy until more data clarify the reasons for this increased risk.

7. Centrally acting agents—The group of agents with central sympatholytic action includes methyldopa, clonidine, and guanabenz. This class of drugs acts by stimulating central α_1-adrenergic receptors, which exert an inhibitory effect on peripheral sympathetic outflow and is moderately effective as monotherapy in lowering blood pressure. The predominant side effects of this class are sedation, postural hypotension, dry mouth, and fatigue. Rebound hypertension may be a significant problem if the agent is withdrawn suddenly following high-dose therapy, especially with clonidine. Gradual reduction of the dose will avoid the rebound effect. This class of agents is now used infrequently because of its significant and often limiting side effects. The transcutaneous patch formulation of clonidine, which is applied once a week, is useful in enhancing compliance in selected patients or in patients unable to take oral therapy.

8. Direct arteriolar dilators—Agents such as hydralazine and minoxidil that lower blood pressure by relaxing vascular smooth muscle do so by direct arteriolar dilation. The resulting decrease in peripheral resistance induces a reflex tachycardia and inotropic cardiac stimulation. Because fluid retention develops almost universally, diuretics must usually be used concomitantly. Vasodilators should be avoided in patients with coronary artery disease because the reflex tachycardia may induce angina. These agents are used almost exclusively as additional agents in patients whose blood pressure is extremely difficult to control with more commonly used agents.

9. Combination therapy—Combining antihypertensive medications from different classes may be even more effective than expected from their individual responses. Many experts now recommend combination therapy to enhance efficacy and reduce side effects. This synergistic result frequently allows lower doses of each agent to be used with fewer side effects. A low-dose thiazide diuretic, for example, will significantly augment the antihypertensive efficacy of an ACEI, an ARB, an α-blocker, a β-blocker, or a vasodilator. β-Blockers will enhance the blood pressure-lowering effects of a vasodilator and reduce any reflex increase in heart rate. The use of lower dose combinations is highly effective and is likely to produce fewer side effects.

Pharmaceutical companies have made fixed-dose combinations of two medications in the same pill. The combinations may or may not work for a given patient, so it is recommended that blood pressure be controlled initially with appropriate doses of two or more agents and then a fixed-dose combination that approximates the effective therapy be substituted. This strategy will improve compliance.

10. Direct renin inhibitors—Aliskiren (Tekturna), the first member of this new class of antihypertensive agents, was recently approved by the FDA. The drug inhibits the ability of renin to form angiotensin I and reduces plasma renin activity. Aliskiren appears to be safe and does not produce rebound hypertension on withdrawal. It appears to be effective in all patient groups but as with all RAAS inhibitors, is less effective in blacks. Second-generation renin inhibitors are under development.

C. Management of Complicated Hypertension

The goals of antihypertensive therapy, to lower the blood pressure to a safe level, reduce LV hypertrophy, and improve other cardiovascular risk factors without adversely affecting other organ systems or risk factors, become more difficult to attain in the presence of concomitant disease of the heart, lungs, or kidneys. In tailoring antihypertensive therapy to the individual patient, it is best to simplify therapy by using medications that will improve the hypertension as well as (or at least not exacerbate) any coexisting condition (Table 13–3).

1. Coronary artery disease—In hypertensive patients with concomitant coronary artery disease manifested by angina, lowering blood pressure alone may improve anginal symptoms by decreasing myocardial oxygen demand. Beneficial agents include the non-ISA β-blockers, ACEI, ARBs, and calcium channel blockers. Care should be taken to avoid sudden drops in blood pressure to hypotensive levels. Patients with an acute coronary syndrome, unstable angina or non–ST-segment elevation myocardial infarction and hypertension should receive standard therapy for acute coronary

Table 13–3. Recommended Initial Agent in Patients with Concomitant Disease.

Disease	Initial Agent	Additional Agent
CAD	β-Blocker	ACEI, ARB, calcium channel blocker, diuretic
CHF	ACEI	β-Blockers, ARB, diuretic
CRI	Calcium channel blocker, β-blockers	Diuretic[1]
Diabetes	ACEI	β-Blocker, ARB, diuretic

[1]If CRI is due to decreased cardiac output, ACEI/ARB may be used with caution.
ACEI, angiotensin-converting enzyme inhibitor; ARB, angiotensin receptor blocker; CAD, coronary artery disease; CHF, congestive heart failure; CRI, chronic renal insufficiency.

syndrome (ie, intravenous heparin or low-molecular-weight heparin and nitroglycerin, aspirin, and β-blockers). This will usually lower blood pressure to a safe level. In patients with acute ST-segment elevation myocardial infarction complicated by hypertension, β-blockers are the mainstay of therapy. Blood pressure should be reduced to < 140/90 mm Hg. Drastic reductions should be avoided because coronary perfusion pressure is directly related to mean arterial pressure; coronary vascular reserve is exhausted in the peri-infarction area, and further ischemia or infarction could result. β-Blockers have been clearly demonstrated to decrease postmyocardial infarction mortality and ischemic event rates. In several large meta-analyses, calcium channel blockers have been shown to be highly effective in lowering blood pressure but have a 25% excess incidence of acute myocardial infarction and heart failure in patients with acute coronary syndromes. The mechanisms are as yet to be delineated.

2. Heart failure—In patients with reduced LV systolic function (from any cause), elevated blood pressure may contribute to further signs and symptoms of heart failure. Even normal levels of blood pressure may be too high in patients with moderate-to-severe LV systolic dysfunction. The goal of therapy should be to lower systolic blood pressure as low as possible without symptoms (< 110 mm Hg and lower if tolerated). ACEIs have proved very useful in reducing blood pressure and symptoms of heart failure and improving survival rates in such patients (see Table 13–3). Diuretics augment the antihypertensive effects of ACEI and are useful additions for the hypertensive patient with or without congestive heart failure. When starting an ACEI in a patient who is already taking a diuretic, the dose of the ACEI should be reduced and the diuretic should be withheld or given at a reduced dose that day to avoid hypotension. ARBs may be substituted in ACEI-intolerant patients.

β-Blockade has been definitively shown to improve symptoms, LV systolic function, and longevity in patients with heart failure when added to ACEI or alone. Metoprolol, bisoprolol, and carvedilol are the agents that have been used in the major heart failure trials.

It is not yet clear as to the most beneficial way to treat patients with preserved systolic function heart failure. The cornerstone of therapy is to reduce the invariably present hypertension to the usual target levels. These patients respond similarly to other hypertensive patients. Clinicians should be careful to not reduce preload too much with diuretics.

3. Cerebrovascular disease—Patients with symptomatic or otherwise evident cerebrovascular disease coexistent with hypertension should receive antihypertensive therapy. Such patients tend to be older and therefore respond similarly to other older patients (see Table 13–2). Acute cerebrovascular accidents are frequently accompanied by hypertension, which is sometimes severe. Rapid reduction of blood pressure in patients with acute stroke is associated with increased morbidity and mortality and should be avoided during the acute phase. In fact, unless the diastolic blood pressure is greater than 115 mm Hg, treatment should either be withheld or instituted slowly and with great caution until the patient has stabilized. Because cerebrovascular disease and coronary artery disease frequently coexist, antihypertensive therapy should be instituted judiciously in patients with stroke and evidence of ischemia or heart failure.

4. Renal insufficiency—Effective antihypertensive therapy will halt or slow the progression of renal insufficiency in most hypertensive patients (see Table 13–3). In patients with established renal insufficiency, ACEI therapy may be very effective and improve renal function but should be used carefully, with frequent monitoring of renal function and serum potassium during initiation and titration of therapy. Patients with renovascular hypertension may have rapid worsening of renal function when treated with ACEI. Such patients must be monitored carefully during initiation of antihypertensive therapy for worsening of renal function or the development of hyperkalemia. Potassium supplementation or potassium-sparing diuretics should be avoided in patients with even moderate renal insufficiency. Even a modest decrease in renal function could cause serious or fatal hyperkalemia. Most patients with renal insufficiency and hypertension respond well to all types of antihypertensive therapy, however. Such patients tend to have volume-dependent hypertension and respond well to loop diuretics, although higher doses must be used as renal function deteriorates.

5. Diabetes mellitus—Diabetic patients are known for their almost universal incidence of vascular disease and increased susceptibility to cardiovascular complications. The coexistence of diabetes and hypertension markedly increases the risk of coronary artery disease, stroke, and renal failure. If dyslipidemia is also present, the risk is even greater. Hypertension should be treated aggressively in diabetic patients, using agents that are renal-protective and do not further aggravate glucose intolerance or adversely affect lipids (see Table 13–3). ACEI, β-blockers, and ARBs are extremely useful in both controlling blood pressure and preventing or slowing the onset of proteinuria and renal failure in diabetic patients. The Hypertension Optimal Treatment Trial (HOT) established that lowering diastolic blood pressure in diabetic patients to levels below 80 mm Hg decreases the risk of major cardiovascular events and mortality compared with lowering diastolic blood pressure to "normal" (< 90 mm Hg) levels. The goal for systolic blood pressure is < 130 mm Hg. α-Blockers, ACEI, and ARBs, which are effective in diabetic patients, are glucose- and lipid-beneficial or neutral. It is recommended that an ACEI be used as the first agent in all diabetic patients. ARBs appear to have the same renal protective effects in diabetic patients as ACEI. No clear-cut superiority of ACEI compared with ARBs in diabetic patients has been demonstrated. Due to the much higher cost of ARBs and the proven efficacy of ACEI, diabetic patients should start on an ACEI and ACEI-intolerant patients should use ARBs.

Table 13–4. Antihypertensive Therapy for Hypertensive Emergencies.

Drug	Dose	Comments
Nitroprusside	0.25–10 mcg/kg/min	Treatment of choice
Fenoldopam	0.1 mcg/kg/min, increased by 0.05 mcg/kg/min	Does not require thiocyanate monitoring
Labetalol	20–40 mg IV q10 min to 300 mg	Commonly used after surgery
Esmolol	500 mcg/kg over 1 min, then 25–200 mcg/kg/min	Can aggravate heart failure
Clonidine	0.1–0.2 mg PO, 0.05–0.1 mg qh until 0.8 mg	Sedation possible
Captopril	6.25–50 mg PO q 6–8 h	Excessive hypotension possible

6. Hypertensive emergencies—Patients with severe hypertension (> 220/120 mm Hg) and signs and symptoms of encephalopathy, acute myocardial ischemic syndromes, stroke, pulmonary edema, or aortic dissection should be treated emergently to achieve rapid reduction of their blood pressure (Table 13–4). Because of its rapid onset and short duration of therapy, which allow for smoother titration of blood pressure, intravenous sodium nitroprusside is the treatment of choice. Patients should be admitted to the intensive care unit and monitored closely during therapy. The aim is to reduce blood pressure very quickly within the first hour or two after presentation but to avoid hypotension. Patients must be monitored for thiocyanate toxicity if therapy is prolonged. An alternative is intravenous fenoldopam, a selective dopamine-1 receptor agonist. It has a similar antihypertensive profile to nitroprusside with a rapid predictable onset of action, short half-life (9.8 min), and few side effects at effective doses. There is a linear correlation between fenoldopam infusion rate and blood pressure lowering. Its use still requires monitoring in the intensive care unit.

If aortic dissection is present, a short-acting β-blocker such as esmolol should be added to decrease shear forces in the aorta. Intravenous labetalol is highly effective and can also be used. Oral immediate-release clonidine and ACEI are effective in rapidly reducing blood pressure and can be added orally. Oral immediate-release nifedipine may cause unpredictable hypotension and should not be used.

Hypertensive urgencies (defined as patients who have severe hypertension but with minimal or no symptoms) may be treated more slowly, achieving a significant reduction in blood pressure within the first 24 hours. Intravenous labetalol is particularly useful in these patients.

Hansson L et al. Effects of intensive blood-pressure lowering and low-dose aspirin in patients with hypertension: principal results of the Hypertension Optimal Treatment (HOT) randomised trial. HOT Study Group. Lancet. 1998 Jun 13;351(9118):1755–62. [PMID: 9635947]

Major cardiovascular events in hypertensive patients randomized to doxazosin vs chlorthalidone: the antihypertensive and lipid-lowering treatment to prevent heart attack trial (ALLHAT). ALLHAT Collaborative Research Group. JAMA. 2000 Apr 19;283(15):1967–75. [PMID: 10789664]

National Collaborating Centre for Chronic Conditions. *Hypertension: management of hypertension in adults in primary care: partial update.* London: Royal College of Physicians, 2006.

Oh B-H et al. Aliskiren, an oral renin inhibitor, provides dose-dependent efficacy and sustained 24-hour blood pressure control in patients with hypertension. J Am Coll Cardiol. 2007 Mar 20;49(11):1157–63. [PMID: 17367658]

▶ **Prognosis**

Significant reductions in blood pressure definitely reduce the incidence of stroke, renal and cardiac failure, and acute coronary syndromes. To prevent cardiac and vascular disease, all the relevant risk factors and concomitant diseases, not just blood pressure alone, must be taken into account. Because coronary artery disease is the most common adverse outcome of hypertension, antihypertensive drugs must be chosen not only for their blood pressure-lowering properties but also for their effects on other critical cardiovascular, metabolic, and renal end points. Aggressive control of all of the cardiac risk factors is essential for optimal outcomes in hypertensive patients.

National Collaborating Centre for Chronic Conditions. *Hypertension: management of hypertension in adults in primary care: partial update.* London: Royal College of Physicians, 2006.

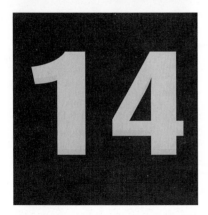

Hypertrophic Cardiomyopathies

Pravin M. Shah, MD, MACC

ESSENTIALS OF DIAGNOSIS

▶ Dyspnea.
▶ Systolic ejection murmur with characteristic changes during bedside maneuvers.
▶ Marked asymmetric left ventricular hypertrophy on echocardiogram.
▶ Normal or hyperkinetic left ventricular systolic function.

General Considerations

The term "hypertrophic cardiomyopathy (HCM)" can best be defined as a condition characterized by idiopathic or unexplained myocardial hypertrophy that is associated with small or normal ventricular cavity size, hyperdynamic ventricular function, and diastolic dysfunction. The qualifier *unexplained* is used to suggest that this condition may coexist with hypertension or aortic valve disease, although the extent and distribution of hypertrophy are disproportionate to these associated disorders. Therefore, mild-to-moderate hypertension and mild or moderate aortic valve disease cannot be implicated in massive asymmetric hypertrophy with hyperdynamic ventricular function. (The definition also requires hyperdynamic systolic function, a feature that is rarely absent even in the late stages of HCM.)

Although the condition has also been called idiopathic hypertrophic subaortic stenosis, which connotes a condition characterized by myocardial hypertrophy without underlying cause, HCM is a more accurate term because it describes the major feature of idiopathic hypertrophy, especially in patients with no evidence of subaortic stenosis or intraventricular obstruction.

HCM can be classified as nonobstructive or obstructive, based on the presence and the location (midventricle or outflow tract) of intraventricular obstruction. Other classifications may relate to the distribution of the hypertrophy: asymmetric septal hypertrophy, disproportionate upper septal thickening, apical asymmetric hypertrophy, and the like. Such approaches are generally not fruitful except when apical hypertrophy is localized.

Pathophysiology & Etiology

The underlying cause and pathogenesis of this disease are largely unknown. The asymmetric type of HCM is commonly transmitted genetically, but sporadic cases are also recognized. An abnormal response of the myocardium to normal catecholamines has been postulated as a pathogenetic mechanism. The clinical association between HCM and pheochromocytoma, neurofibromatosis, and lentiginosis suggests a genetic disorder of neural crest tissue. More recent studies have linked familial HCM to the cardiac myosin heavy-chain genes on chromosome 14 in some—but not all—families, indicating genetic heterogeneity. The presence of different disease genes or mutations within a given gene may account for differences in the clinical expression of familial HCM.

The pathologic findings at autopsy are remarkably uniform and include massive and generally asymmetric hypertrophy. Both the atria and the ventricles are affected, with the left ventricle most commonly involved. The interventricular septum is generally far more massively hypertrophied than the free wall, a peculiar asymmetric septal hypertrophy that may provide the necessary hemodynamic conditions to cause a dynamic outflow obstruction. In this situation, the condition is referred to as hypertrophic obstructive cardiomyopathy (HOCM). Localization of such hypertrophy in the midlateral wall may result in midventricular obstruction and distribution of the hypertrophy in the right ventricular infundibulum in subpulmonic stenosis. Asymmetric localization of hypertrophy can involve virtually any segment of the left ventricle, except for the posterobasal region.

In some patients, the hypertrophy involves primarily the apical portion of the left ventricle (asymmetric apical hypertrophy) rather than the outflow tract. Such patients exhibit none of the clinical features of intraventricular obstruction.

Striking pathologic features common to most patients with left ventricular outflow obstruction include fibrous thickening of the anterior mitral leaflet and plaques in the upper interventricular septum. The thickening of the anterior mitral leaflet is thought to represent the result of frequent contact with the interventricular septum. The endocardial plaques in the septum may be the result of jet lesions distal to the obstruction. The epicardial coronary arteries are large and patent.

Microscopically, a bizarre and disorderly array of muscle fibers is a striking feature associated with increased connective tissue that interrupts and crisscrosses the muscle bundles.

At times, the hypertrophied septum assumes a peculiar catenoid shape—convex to the left in the apex-to-base plane, but concave on its left ventricular surface in the cross sections. This bizarre and characteristic shape is thought to be responsible for the adynamic nature of the septum. It is hypothesized that fiber disarray and local hypertrophy could result from isometric contraction of a catenoid septum.

A. Systolic Function

The integrity of overall systolic function is rather well preserved even in advanced cases; indeed, hypercontractility is a hallmark of the disorder. The cardiac output is generally normal or mildly increased; the ejection fraction is often supernormal. Although global function is well preserved, regional abnormalities may occur; the upper interventricular septum is often hypodynamic and shows reduced thickening during systole. The free walls are generally hyperdynamic.

Left ventricular outflow obstruction is dynamic and variable. The variability can be observed within the same cardiac cycle, from one beat to the next and from one physiologic state to another. When present, the outflow obstruction begins sometime after the onset of early uninterrupted ejection. The obstruction is caused by a sharp systolic anterior motion (SAM) of the anterior mitral leaflet, which obliterates the outflow space. The actual mechanism is not clear, although it is likely to be the result of a Venturi effect from the rapid ejection of a jet of blood through an anatomically narrowed outflow space. The degree of left ventricular outflow obstruction can be accentuated by factors that reduce preload (end-diastolic volume), diminish afterload (arterial pressure), or increase contractility or heart rate. Echocardiographic recordings have demonstrated that a sharp systolic anterior motion of the mitral valve is both accentuated and prolonged by interventions that exacerbate the outflow obstruction, and vice versa (ie, it is diminished and shortened by interventions that reduce the outflow obstruction). Some investigators interpret intraventricular pressure gradients as not indicative of true obstruction because left ventricular emptying is normal or exaggerated and because early emptying is unimpeded. These gradients have been attributed to cavity obliteration. Echocardiographic techniques have elucidated differences between true gradients resulting from obstruction and those from cavity obliteration.

Mitral regurgitation is shown by color-flow Doppler echocardiography in more than 90% of patients with HOCM and is related to the dynamic outflow obstruction in most of them. Mitral regurgitation is more severe when a more persistent and prominent SAM accentuates outflow obstruction. The factors that decrease outflow obstruction tend to reduce the degree of mitral regurgitation.

Severe right ventricular infundibular stenosis is rare and may be either independent of or concurrent with left ventricular outflow obstruction. The mechanism of right ventricular outflow obstruction is different from that on the left side because the infundibulum is circumferentially bound by muscle. Excessive muscle contraction in this disorder results in outflow obstruction, and the factors resulting in increased contractility tend to accentuate obstruction. The tricuspid valve does not play any important role in the right-sided outflow obstruction.

B. Diastolic Function

Distensibility and compliance of the hypertrophied ventricles are reduced, with resulting elevation in end-diastolic pressure without an increase in volume. The prolongation of early diastolic relaxation coupled with increased wall stiffness tends to influence the pattern of diastolic filling. Early, rapid, passive filling is notably impaired, requiring a stronger atrial contraction to deliver diastolic inflow into a relatively nondistensible left ventricle. This dependence on atrial contraction to maintain efficient flow is exemplified by a sudden drop in cardiac output when atrial fibrillation supervenes. Although this abnormality of diastolic compliance has important hemodynamic consequences (eg, elevations of left atrial and pulmonary venous pressures causing pulmonary congestion and edema), actual inflow obstruction is rare.

▶ Clinical Findings
A. Symptoms and Signs

Effort dyspnea and paroxysmal nocturnal dyspnea constitute the most common symptoms (Table 14–1) and provide evidence of pulmonary congestion. Because elevations in pulmonary venous and left atrial pressures occur in the presence of a hyperdynamic, hypercontractile left ventricle, they must be attributed to increased stiffness of the hypertrophic ventricles. In some patients, especially in those with volume overload, frank pulmonary edema may be noted.

Frank syncope and presyncope (dizziness short of loss of consciousness) are common. These symptoms may be effort-related, although not predictably so, and the frequency of the episodes is highly variable. The exact mechanism is obscure; however, it is probably related to reflex vasodilatation and hypotension induced by stretching the left ventricular baroreceptors. On the other hand, arrhythmia may play a role by producing a decrease in cardiac output.

Typical effort angina simulating symptomatic coronary artery disease is frequent, although episodes of chest pain

Table 14–1. Characteristic Clinical Features of Hypertrophic Cardiomyopathy.

Symptoms
  Dyspnea: Effort-induced, paroxysmal nocturnal, or orthopnea
  Angina: Stable or unstable
  Syncope: Generally following exertion
  Dizziness (presyncope)
  No symptoms
Signs
  Sustained bifid apical impulse
  Palpable atrial impulse (S_4)
  Brisk carotid upstroke
  Bisferious pulse with normal pulse pressure (with LVOT obstruction)
  Gallop sounds: S_4 common, S_3 uncommon
  Ejection systolic murmur along left systolic border
  Longer, higher-pitched apical systolic murmur
  Effects of Valsalva maneuver: increased murmur intensity during peak strain phase (II) and decrease in later strain-release phase (IV)

LVOT, left ventricular outflow tract.

may be prolonged and may occur spontaneously at rest. Sublingual nitroglycerin typically (but not always) fails to provide prompt relief. When the epicardial coronary arteries are large and patent, the ischemia may be due to compression of the intramyocardial coronary arteries and increased myocardial tension and muscle mass, with oxygen requirements outstripping oxygen delivery.

Palpitations may merely be the result of the patient's awareness of forcible heartbeats, especially in the left lateral decubitus position. Atrial and ventricular arrhythmias are more commonly responsible. Tachyarrhythmias are poorly tolerated and are often associated with symptoms of low output and hypotension. Isolated or short runs of ventricular and supraventricular premature depolarizations often occur without symptoms.

The physical signs also tend to vary considerably—from minimal or nonspecific to highly characteristic. The characteristic signs include evidence of left ventricular hypertrophy, obstruction of left ventricular outflow, and resistance to left ventricular inflow.

B. Physical Examination

A powerful systolic thrust of the left ventricle on palpitation indicates an increase in muscle mass; although less frequent, the characteristic bifid apex in systole is virtually diagnostic of this condition. A prominent atrial contraction imparts a strong presystolic impulse that is palpable at the apex. A trifid impulse composed of a prominent *a* wave and bifid systolic peaks is rarely palpable but can often be recorded on apex cardiogram. Such a finding is highly characteristic of this disease. S_4 is commonly observed in the presence of sinus rhythm.

A jerky arterial pulse with sharp upstroke is typical, although not diagnostic. Occasionally, a bifid pulse may be felt, especially in the carotid artery. A bifid arterial pulse in association with a normal pulse pressure is characteristic of HOCM. The pulse contour is influenced by the presence and severity of outflow obstruction. In the absence of resting obstruction, the arterial pulse is essentially normal, although with a brisk upstroke.

A systolic murmur of variable intensity is present along the left sternal border and apex. It is poorly transmitted to the aortic area and neck vessels. It is medium- or high-pitched, with onset after the S_1. The murmur resembles a long ejection murmur along the left sternal border and attains a regurgitant quality (high-pitched, blowing) toward the apex. The apical murmur may be well transmitted to the axilla. The S_2 is clearly audible, and both components are well preserved. Reverse splitting with a delayed aortic component, when present, is diagnostic of severe outflow obstruction in the absence of left bundle branch block. The signs of outflow obstruction, including intensity of the systolic murmur, are accentuated by maneuvers that augment the severity of obstruction (Table 14–2).

The blowing apical murmur of mitral regurgitation also generally varies in intensity with dynamic outflow obstruction. In a few patients, associated severe mitral valve regurgitation, independent of outflow obstruction, may be present. Its presence can be determined by raising the blood pressure with methoxamine or angiotensin, which—although relieving outflow obstruction—will not diminish the murmur's intensity if the regurgitation is unrelated to obstruction. Because these patients may be candidates for mitral valve surgery, this differentiation is clinically important.

Although a prominent atrial sound (S_4) is a common feature of a noncompliant hypertrophied left ventricle, a

Table 14–2. Effects of Maneuvers on Murmur Intensity and Obstruction Severity in Hypertrophic Obstructive Cardiomyopathy.

Maneuvers	Left Ventricular Outflow Obstruction	Severity of Mitral Regurgitation	Murmur Intensity
Upright posture	↑	↑	↑
Squatting	↓	↓	↓
Valsalva			
Phase 2–3	↑	↑	↑
Phase 4	↓	↓	↓
Exercise	↑	↑	↑
Amyl nitrite inhalation	↑	↑	↑
Methoxamine	↓	↓	↓

↑, increased; ↓, decreased.

mitral diastolic murmur simulating mitral stenosis may occasionally lead to consideration of rheumatic mitral disease. The absence of an opening snap and the presence of severe, unexplained left ventricular hypertrophy should point to a correct diagnosis.

A systolic murmur of infundibular pulmonic stenosis is often prominent at the left sternal edge. The ejection sound is absent, and the pulmonary closure sound is delayed. When infundibular obstruction accompanies left ventricular outflow obstruction, the clinical signs of the latter dominate. However, isolated right ventricular outflow obstruction may be difficult to differentiate from congenital infundibular pulmonic stenosis until evidence for unexplained left ventricular hypertrophy is demonstrable.

C. Diagnostic Studies

1. Electrocardiography—A routine 12-lead electrocardiogram (ECG) often discloses evidence of left ventricular hypertrophy with increased QRS voltage or ST-T wave changes in the lateral precordial leads (V_4–V_6). Because no signs of left ventricular hypertrophy may be present in some patients despite the massive increase in cardiac muscle mass, a normal ECG does not exclude the diagnosis of HCM. Occasionally, large, abnormal Q waves that simulate myocardial infarction are noted as a result of septal depolarization. These changes of pseudo-infarction are uncommon. Other features include a short PR interval, Wolff-Parkinson-White syndrome, left-axis deviation from left anterior hemiblock, and complete left or right bundle branch block. Atrial and ventricular premature depolarizations are common, but sometimes can be detected only with ambulatory ECG recording. Complete heart block is rare.

Deep symmetric inversion of the T waves in the precordial leads has been described with apical HCM but may also be seen in other types. These changes in a patient with chest pain are often mistaken for subendocardial infarction.

2. Chest radiography—Posteroanterior and lateral chest radiographs are often normal. Evidence of left ventricular enlargement may be subtle because the cavity size is not increased. Left atrial size is either normal or only slightly increased, except in a stage of advanced decompensation. Pulmonary venous engorgement may be seen, but frank pulmonary edema and signs of pulmonary arterial hypertension are infrequent.

3. Echocardiography—Echocardiography is the most important method for diagnosing HCM (Table 14–3). This technique is useful for evaluating the thickness of the interventricular septum and left ventricular posterior wall and their movements in systole; the end-diastolic and end-systolic dimensions of the left ventricular cavity along its minor axis; the left ventricular outflow size (the space between the anterior mitral leaflet and the interventricular septum); and the functional aspects of mitral and aortic valve motion. It also permits differentiation of concentric and asymmetric hypertrophy.

Table 14–3. Echocardiographic Clues in Diagnosis of Hypertrophic Cardiomyopathy.

Two-dimensional echocardiography
Massive hypertrophy
Asymmetric wall thickness
Sparkling or granular appearance of walls
Normal cavity size
Dilated left atrium
Hyperdynamic LV function (EF > 70)
Systolic anterior motion of anterior (or posterior) mitral leaflet (obstructive cases)
Thickened, elongated anterior leaflet
Endocardiac thickening of LVOT
Hypodynamic basal septum
Doppler echocardiography
Mitral regurgitation
Mitral inflow: diastolic dysfunction pattern with impaired relaxation
Pulsed wave Doppler
High velocities in LVOT
Color-flow Doppler
High velocities and turbulent flow in LVOT
Continuous wave Doppler
Dagger-shaped velocity waveform in LVOT

EF, ejection fraction; LV, left ventricle; LVOT, left ventricular outflow tract.

The presence of dynamic left ventricular outflow obstruction is diagnosed by analyzing the systolic motion of the mitral valve. Abnormal motion of the anterior mitral leaflet against the interventricular septum localizes the site of outflow obstruction in HOCM. It begins sometime after completion of early ejection and is terminated in end-systole before aortic valve closure.

The dynamic nature of the obstruction can be interpreted from variations in the extent of the systolic anterior motion with maneuvers designed to alter the obstruction. Patients without a resting obstruction usually have small and incomplete SAM, whereas those with high resting gradients tend to have a large and complete SAM that is consistently noted from one beat to the next. Systolic anterior motion has also been noted in hyperkinetic circulatory states, in aortic regurgitation, during infusion of dopamine in a patient in shock, and following mitral valve repair for myxomatous mitral valve prolapse. As a result of the dynamic midsystolic obstruction to outflow, the aortic valve cusps may show premature closure with late systolic reopening.

A combination of narrow left ventricular outflow space, thickened interventricular septum, and the typical SAM of the anterior mitral leaflet is virtually diagnostic of HOCM. When the interventricular septal wall/posterior wall thickness ratio exceeds 1.5:1.0, asymmetric hypertrophy can be diagnosed confidently. With some exceptions, patients with HCM demonstrate asymmetric septal hypertrophy. Two-dimensional echocardiography may show that the asymmetric hypertrophy involves the lateral free wall, the apex, the distal septum and, rarely, the posteroinferior wall. Additional findings include midsystolic preclosure of one or more aortic valve cusps, a hypodynamic interventricular septum with diminished systolic motion, and reduced early diastolic slope of the anterior mitral leaflet. Two-dimensional echocardiography generally permits differentiation of SAM involving the mitral leaflet and that involving the chordae tendineae. The leaflet SAM is more characteristically associated with HOCM; the chordal motion may represent passive buckling of the chordae tendineae in a rapidly emptying left ventricle. When multiple criteria are sought, the diagnosis can be made from the echocardiographic examination alone.

Doppler echocardiography makes it possible to obtain information on flow and pressure dynamics, using pulsed and continuous wave modes. Pulsed wave Doppler can localize the site of obstruction by showing high velocities in the subaortic region when the obstruction is localized in the left ventricular outflow tract; the measurement of high velocities by continuous wave Doppler can be used to estimate the pressure drop across the subvalvular obstruction. The contour of the outflow tract velocity profile mirrors the profile of the pressure drop from the left ventricular cavity to the outflow tract and assumes a characteristic dagger shape (Figure 14–1). As ventricular ejection begins, the early velocity is in the range of 1.0–1.5 m/s, commensurate with the rapid early ejection. Subsequently, the velocity progressively increases to reach a peak in mid-to-late

systole and return to baseline at the end of ejection. This profile differs sharply from that seen in fixed obstruction (eg, valvular aortic stenosis), where a smooth contour of increasing velocity is observed, even when it peaks in midsystole. The presence and severity of mitral regurgitation can also be assessed. A similar Doppler velocity contour may also be observed to evaluate right ventricular infundibular obstruction.

Doppler techniques also provide information regarding left ventricular diastolic function. The heterogenous ventricular wall relaxation is associated with flow signals that are generally directed toward the apex and suggest earlier relaxation of the apical than the basal segments. These findings are also seen in other forms of hypertrophy, however, and lack diagnostic value. The overall rate of relaxation is prolonged, resulting in a small mitral-flow, early-filling wave. The subsequent atrial contraction accounts for the major proportion of ventricular filling and results in a prominent mitral inflow *a* wave. These features of mitral inflow velocity pattern can be readily evaluated by pulsed wave Doppler techniques and provide useful information. The pulmonary venous flow pattern detected by pulsed wave Doppler provides supplementary information. A more forceful atrial contraction results in a more prominent retrograde flow wave into the pulmonary veins (*ar*, or *a* reversal, wave). An important limitation of these Doppler methods, however, is their dependence on loading conditions and heart rate.

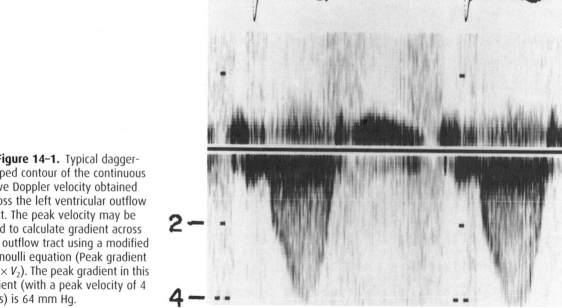

▲ **Figure 14–1.** Typical dagger-shaped contour of the continuous wave Doppler velocity obtained across the left ventricular outflow tract. The peak velocity may be used to calculate gradient across the outflow tract using a modified Bernoulli equation (Peak gradient $= 4 \times V_2$). The peak gradient in this patient (with a peak velocity of 4 m/s) is 64 mm Hg.

4. Cardiac catheterization and angiography—Before the advent of echocardiography, final confirmation of the diagnosis rested on cardiac catheterization and selective cardiac angiography, specifically the demonstration of dynamic left ventricular outflow obstruction. When catheterization is necessary, special care must be taken to avoid recording an artifactual gradient caused by entrapment of the catheter. Analysis of the recorded arterial pressure and pressure gradient during a postectopic beat often provides an important clue. Typically, the arterial pulse pressure is narrower in the postectopic than in the sinus beat, in contrast to both the normal and the fixed forms of left ventricular outflow obstruction (eg, valvular aortic stenosis), when the pulse pressure is wider in the postectopic beat. Accentuation of the outflow gradient with the Valsalva maneuver, amyl nitrite inhalation, or isoproterenol infusion provides added confirmation.

Selective left ventricular cine-angiography demonstrates the characteristic anatomic and functional features of HCM. Ventricular geometry is altered, with the cavity assuming a sausage shape in the right anterior oblique projection. In a few patients, simultaneous left and right ventricular angiograms have demonstrated a massively thickened interventricular septum, especially in its midportion. Such techniques, however, are no longer routinely used because echocardiography provides a reliable, noninvasive diagnostic tool. Therefore, catheterization-angiography studies should be reserved for selected patients and used on rare occasions for diagnostic confirmation.

▶ Treatment

Both medical and surgical management are palliative (Table 14–4), since the cause of this bizarre cardiomyopathy is unknown. The major objectives of therapy include improvement of symptoms, amelioration of outflow obstruction, improvement of left ventricular compliance, suppression of arrhythmias, and the prevention and treatment of major complications such as bacterial endocarditis, thromboembolism, and sudden death.

A. Medical Management

The cardiac drugs commonly used for symptomatic relief of dyspnea or angina in other cardiac disorders are either contraindicated or must be used with caution. Digitalis must be avoided except to treat rapid atrial fibrillation when β-adrenergic blockade and calcium channel blockers are unsuccessful or poorly tolerated. Nitrates are generally contraindicated and are often ineffective in relieving angina. Diuretics must be used with caution so as not to produce hypovolemia.

β-Adrenergic blocking agents are used extensively. Slowing the heart rate and decreasing contractility are generally beneficial. Although exercise and β-adrenergic stimulation have been shown to ameliorate obstruction, resting gradients are reduced only in some patients with labile obstruction. Symptomatic improvement is striking in some patients and

Table 14–4. Management Strategies in Hypertrophic Cardiomyopathy.

Medical therapy
β-Blockers
Calcium channel blockers
Disopyramide
Cautious combination of β-blockers and calcium channel blockers
Judicious use of diuretics for symptom relief
Antiarrhythmics as needed
Antibiotic prophylaxis against endocarditis
Anticoagulation for atrial fibrillation
Surgical therapy
Myectomy to relieve LVOT obstruction
Mitral valve replacement and myectomy with severe mitral regurgitation unrelated to LVOT obstruction
Other procedures
Permanent pacemaker insertion (currently experimental)
Appropriate AV delay to minimize LVOT gradient
Alcohol septal ablation

AV, atrioventricular; LVOT, left ventricular outflow tract.

may last several years. Increasing doses are often needed, however, and other patients do not experience sustained improvement. Although a daily dose of as high as 480 mg may be required for some patients, it is doubtful that left ventricular compliance is improved with β-adrenergic blockade. These agents have not been shown to decrease the incidence of ventricular arrhythmias or sudden death. The dose should be increased gradually and the effects monitored, especially in patients without a major component of outflow obstruction.

Calcium channel blockers (eg, verapamil, long-acting nifedipine) have provided beneficial effects, and amelioration of symptoms is frequently observed. The resting and exercise pressure gradients are reduced, and there seems to be improved compliance. The use of these agents should be carefully monitored, however. In some patients with undue hypotensive effect, severe deterioration or death may occur. Although disopyramide has been used for its negative inotropism to provide symptomatic improvement in some patients with HOCM, the frequency of side effects limits its widespread use.

In some patients with refractory symptoms, combined use of a β-blocker and a calcium channel blocker has proved successful; this regimen should be attempted under close observation, however.

Disopyramide, another negative inotropic agent, provides symptomatic improvement. Side effects include anticholinergic actions such as dry mouth and eyes, constipation, difficulty in micturition. Patients in atrial fibrillation may experience rapid ventricular rate and may require addition of β-blockers. Because of disopyramide's class IA antiarrhythmic properties, patients taking this agent should be closely monitored for proarrhythmias. Similarly, QT interval should be monitored for prolongation.

Sudden cardiac death is overwhelmingly the most common cause of demise among patients with HCM, probably from arrhythmias (their causal role has not yet been definitely established); effective antiarrhythmic agents may therefore be important. Atrial and ventricular arrhythmias are common in patients with HCM, regardless of their symptomatic or hemodynamic state. Although supraventricular tachycardias may worsen symptoms, they have not been associated with sudden death. Ventricular tachycardia and other high-grade ventricular arrhythmias have been found in at least 30% of patients monitored by 72-h ambulatory ECG recordings. Asymptomatic family members screened and found to have HCM also have a high incidence of asymptomatic ventricular arrhythmias. Although aggressive treatment of ventricular tachycardia is currently recommended, ventricular arrhythmias are generally refractory to conventional agents alone or in combination with β-adrenergic blockade. Amiodarone, a class III antiarrhythmic, has been reported (in an uncontrolled clinical trial) to prevent sudden cardiac death in this disorder, and sotalol, with its β-blocking and class III antiarrhythmic effects, may prove ideal, although systematic studies are not available.

Bacterial endocarditis is a common complication, and the use of prophylactic antibiotics at times of risk is recommended. Thromboembolism is another complication, especially in the presence of intermittent or sustained atrial fibrillation. Anticoagulation with warfarin sodium is advised in such cases, particularly if an embolic episode has been diagnosed.

B. Surgical Myectomy

Considerable experience has been reported with trans-aortic ventriculomyectomy in patients with HOCM. Creation of a small tunnel in the left ventricular outflow tract (by removing a small amount of muscle with a deep incision) provides postoperative relief of outflow obstruction and associated mitral regurgitation. Symptomatic improvement is often dramatic, along with reduction or abolition of the systolic murmur and other features of left ventricular outflow obstruction. Replacement of the mitral valve to relieve outflow obstruction is not indicated, unless severe independent mitral regurgitation can be demonstrated.

Surgical relief of right ventricular outflow obstruction can be carried out successfully (as it can in infundibular pulmonary stenosis). The current surgical approach to myectomy is considerably aided by intraoperative echocardiography. Multiplanar transesophageal echocardiography accurately localizes the hypertrophy and permits visualization of the resected muscle, showing the abolition of systolic anterior motion and the improvement of mitral regurgitation. The current operative risk for uncomplicated myectomy should not exceed 5%, and the obstruction should be relieved in more than 95% of cases. The surgical risk at several large centers is reported to be less than 2%.

C. Chemical Myectomy

This technique uses alcohol to partially ablate the septum. During this procedure a special catheter is threaded into the septal perforator branch of the left anterior descending coronary artery to enable the injection of absolute alcohol, which produces a controlled myocardial infarction in the proximal interventricular septum. The desired end result is thinning of the upper interventricular septum and dyskinesia, thereby enlarging the left ventricular outflow tract and subsequently reducing systolic gradients. Experience at several centers has demonstrated a high level of success with hemodynamic and symptomatic improvement in most patients. The procedure-related mortality rate has been in the range of 1–2%. Additional procedure-related complications include ventricular arrhythmias, atrioventricular (AV) block often requiring permanent pacemaker implantation and large anteroseptal infarction, and coronary artery dissection. Although alcohol septal ablation is an attractive alternative to surgical myectomy, this procedure should be considered experimental and its use limited to few centers with significant experience in a sufficient number of patients. The criteria for patients who may derive most benefit are evolving, but it is clear that not all patients with outflow obstruction are suitable candidates.

D. Pacemaker Implantation

An AV sequential permanent pacemaker has been used to ameliorate obstruction of the left ventricular outflow tract. The AV delay and ventricular activation are synchronized to provide a minimum outflow tract gradient, and the pacing continues for months or years. Long-term follow-up studies have reported substantial symptomatic and objective benefits. Further independent investigations are needed to confirm these findings. It appears that improvement with this approach, as with drugs, does not last long and may only delay rather than avoid a consideration of myectomy in symptomatic patients. This approach is therefore not recommended for general use.

E. Cardioverter Defibrillator Implantation

A subset of patients with a high risk of sudden death may benefit from implantation of a cardiac defibrillator. The risk factors for sudden death include genetic predisposition with known genotypes, sustained ventricular tachycardia or prior cardiac arrest, recurrent syncope, hypotension with exercise, and extreme hypertrophy with maximal wall thickness of 30 mm or more, particularly in adolescents and young adults.

▶ Prognosis

The natural history of HCM is quite variable, probably because of the complexity of disease expression. In general, the earlier the onset of clinical findings, the worse the prognosis. The major problem is sudden death, which is often the first manifestation of the disease in teenagers or young adults. Sudden death rates in hospital-based populations have ranged from 2% to 6% a year; in community-based patients, the rate is probably 1%/year. Patients who survive past 35 years of age usually have a better long-term prognosis. The only factors that seem to predispose to sudden death are a history of syncope and a family history of sudden death. Although some studies have shown a link with marked wall thickness on echocardiography and nonsustained ventricular tachycardia on ambulatory ECG monitoring, these two factors have a low predictive accuracy for sudden death.

Patients who live to old age (older than 65 years) may reach the heart failure stage, characterized by a dilated, thinned left ventricle with reduced systolic function. Outflow obstruction is minimal or absent at this stage, and digoxin, vasodilators, and diuretics may be indicated to reduce congestive heart failure symptoms and signs.

▶ Future Prospects

The genetic research on HCM has provided significant clues in the mutations in any of the ten genes of interest, each encoding proteins of the cardiac sarcomere. It promises to enable preclinical diagnosis of individuals affected by a mutant gene and characterize those likely to experience a malignant or rapidly progressive course. This could result in triage of patients with this diagnosis for selection of appropriate treatment options. A more readily available gene typical for this disorder is likely to revolutionize its management and progress.

Elliott PM et al. Sudden death in hypertrophic cardiomyopathy: identification of high risk patients. J Am Coll Cardiol. 2000 Dec;36(7):2212–8. [PMID: 11127463]

Elliott PM et al. Relation between severity of left-ventricular hypertrophy and prognosis in patients with hypertrophic cardiomyopathy. Lancet. 2001 Feb 10;357(9254):420–4.

Flores-Ramirez R et al. Echocardiographic insights into the mechanisms of relief of left ventricular outflow tract obstruction after nonsurgical septal reduction therapy in patients with hypertrophic obstructive cardiomyopathy. J Am Coll Cardiol. 2001 Jan;37(1):208–14. [PMID: 11153740]

Lim DS et al. Expression profiling of cardiac genes in human hypertrophic cardiomyopathy: insight into the pathogenesis of phenotypes. J Am Coll Cardiol. 2001 Oct;38(4):1175–80. [PMID: 11583900]

Maron BJ. Role of alcohol septal ablation in treatment of obstructive hypertrophic cardiomyopathy. Lancet. 2000 Feb 5;355(9202):425–6. [PMID: 10841119]

Maron BJ et al. Efficacy of implantable cardioverter-defibrillators for the prevention of sudden death in patients with hypertrophic cardiomyopathy. N Engl J Med. 2000 Feb 10;342(6):365–73. [PMID: 10666426]

Yu EH et al. Mitral regurgitation in hypertrophic obstructive cardiomyopathy: relationship to obstruction and relief with myectomy. J Am Coll Cardiol. 2000 Dec;36(7):2219–25. [PMID: 11127464]

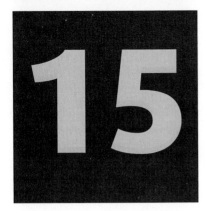

Restrictive Cardiomyopathies

John D. Carroll, MD & Michael H. Crawford, MD

ESSENTIALS OF DIAGNOSIS

▶ Symptoms and signs of heart failure with predominant right-sided findings.

▶ Normal left and right ventricular size and systolic function with dilated atria.

▶ Diastolic ventricular functional abnormalities suggestive of reduced ventricular compliance.

▶ Increased ventricular filling pressure (left > right) and reduced cardiac output.

▶ General Considerations

A. Definitions and Terminology

1. Restrictive cardiomyopathy—The World Health Organization defines cardiomyopathies as heart muscle diseases of unknown cause; restrictive cardiomyopathy is one of three forms (the others are dilated cardiomyopathy and hypertrophic cardiomyopathy). Restrictive cardiomyopathies are classified as primary (endocardial fibrosis and eosinophilic endomyocardial disease) or secondary to cardiac infiltrative diseases. Diseases with a defined cause that produce a dilated cardiomyopathy with restrictive characteristics are specifically excluded from this classification of cardiomyopathies.

For the clinician, restrictive cardiomyopathy is usually due to infiltrative diseases, such as the cardiomyopathy that occurs in systemic amyloidosis, hemochromatosis, sarcoidosis, and glycogen storage diseases (Table 15–1). These secondary cardiomyopathies are included because the cardiac involvement typically displays features of restrictive physiology that are pivotal in the diagnosis. Restrictive cardiomyopathies represent less than 1% of cases of congestive heart failure, and most of these are of the secondary form.

2. Restrictive physiology—Also known as **diastolic dysfunction** and **diastolic heart failure**, restrictive physiology requires a precise definition, even though clinical methods often yield only indirect evidence of this functional abnormality. It is characterized by elevated filling pressures and impaired ventricular filling from myocardial or endocardial abnormalities in a nondilated ventricle with no significant impairment of systolic performance. Numerous common cardiac diseases can produce the functional abnormalities of the restrictive or diastolic type, but the diseases are not classified as a restrictive cardiomyopathy.

3. Infiltrative cardiomyopathy—An alternative term applied to many of these diseases, infiltrative cardiomyopathy emphasizes that the endocardial, interstitial, or intracellular infiltration of a variety of materials (eg, extensive collagen bundles, amyloid protein) is the central histologic and pathophysiologic feature. The infiltration of material with tissue less compliant than normal myocardium and the increase in the wall thickness of the cardiac chambers reduce chamber compliance.

4. Obliterative cardiomyopathy—This term is sometimes used to describe the reduction in left ventricular chamber volume as the consequence of endocardial fibrosis and extensive mural thrombus formation.

B. Pathophysiology

1. Abnormalities in diastolic function—Although there are several causes of abnormal diastolic function in restrictive cardiomyopathy, loss of ventricular chamber compliance is the most common. Fibrosis and the presence of amyloid and hemosiderin all change the intrinsic mechanical properties of the chamber wall. Furthermore, the rate and extent of myocardial relaxation and elastic recoil are reduced in restrictive cardiomyopathy, causing increased diastolic pressures, an increased rate of early diastolic filling, and a reduced rate of atrial filling. Myocardial ischemia may further compromise diastolic function. In cardiac amyloidosis particularly, the coronary arteries may be infiltrated, reducing myocardial blood supply.

Table 15–1. Classification of Restrictive Cardiomyopathy.

Primary	Secondary
Idiopathic	Infiltrative disease
Familial ± skeletal myopathy	Amyloidosis
Löffler cardiomyopathy (endocarditis parientalis fibroplastica)	Glycogen storage diseases Hemochromatosis
Tropical endomyocardial fibrosis	Sarcoidosis
	Interstitial disease
	Radiation-induced fibrosis
	Chronic allograft rejection

2. Restrictive physiology—Restrictive physiology is best quantified by an assessment of the passive properties of the ventricles, usually of left ventricular compliance. No routine clinical methods measure chamber compliance, but a variety of tests are available to assess the consequences of altered chamber compliance. Specifically, alterations in the pattern of ventricular filling, absolute filling pressures, and pressure waveforms may be routinely determined by noninvasive and invasive techniques.

C. Etiology

1. Idiopathic restrictive cardiomyopathy—Patients with this condition have hemodynamic findings consistent with restrictive cardiomyopathy and endomyocardial biopsies that show fibrosis or variable degrees of cellular hypertrophy. The thickness of the ventricular wall need not be increased.

The average age of these patients at presentation is 20–30 years old. Most patients are women. The clinical course is variable, with many patients being symptomatically stable for years whereas others die quickly without cardiac transplantation to treat severe heart failure.

An idiopathic restrictive cardiomyopathy has also been described in children—predominantly girls—with a mean age of 4 years. Most were dead within several years of presentation, suggesting that idiopathic restrictive cardiomyopathy in childhood has a worse prognosis than in adults.

2. Familial cardiomyopathy—Sporadic case reports describe restrictive cardiomyopathy in multiple members of families. The coexistence of a skeletal myopathy has been seen in a family with a dominantly inherited restrictive cardiomyopathy.

3. Löffler cardiomyopathy—In 1936, Löffler described a cardiomyopathy associated with eosinophilia. It is now established that the degree and duration of eosinophilia quantitatively relate to the extent of endomyocardial disease. Males are more commonly affected. The disease has different stages and presentations; the most common is multiorgan involvement, evidence of a systemic inflammatory response, and thromboembolic events. Occasionally, it presents as a classic restrictive cardiomyopathy.

4. Tropical endocardial fibrosis—This form of restrictive cardiomyopathy is rarely seen in the industrialized societies of the West but is quite common in subtropical and tropical regions. Although overt eosinophilia is not the rule, the gross and microscopic features of the disease resemble those of Löffler cardiomyopathy. Overt manifestations of heart failure with ascites and edema frequently emerge in late childhood and early adulthood. The scarring process usually involves both ventricles, producing restrictive hemodynamics, although isolated right and left ventricular involvement occasionally occurs. The early stages of the disease have not been well characterized.

Management is unlike that for other causes of restrictive cardiomyopathy, and endocardiectomy may produce significant clinical improvement.

5. Amyloidosis—Cardiac amyloidosis occurs in several forms of this systemic disease; a description of each is beyond the scope of this chapter. In general, however, patients with evidence of cardiac amyloidosis should undergo an evaluation of other organ involvement, the nature of any serum gammopathy, and the nature of any plasma cell dyscrasia in the bone marrow.

Patients with heart failure symptoms caused by cardiac amyloidosis are typically dead in 6 months. The severity of the restrictive hemodynamics and the independent problems of low systemic arterial pressure and renal insufficiency make treatment of these patients difficult.

6. Inborn metabolic errors—Biochemical defects, typically genetically determined, may alter a variety of metabolic pathways and lead to direct or secondary effects on cardiac function. Restrictive-cardiomyopathy-like features have been described in glycogen storage disease, Fabry disease, Gaucher disease, and the mucopolysaccharidoses. The result is generally an infiltrative process, although other cardiac manifestations can occur for each of these complex entities (discussion of these is beyond the scope of this chapter).

7. Hemochromatosis and hemosiderosis—These conditions can produce a restrictive cardiomyopathy. This is an unusual manifestation; most cases of cardiac involvement are associated with a dilated cardiomyopathy.

8. Sarcoidosis—Restrictive cardiomyopathy from sarcoidosis is rare. Cardiac involvement is most commonly manifested by arrhythmias and conduction abnormalities. When congestive heart failure occurs, systolic function may be reduced, and a ventricular aneurysm is occasionally produced.

9. Radiation-induced fibrosis—Radiation more often causes constrictive pericarditis, but it can produce restrictive cardiomyopathy, and the pericardial and myocardial fibrotic pictures may be combined.

10. Other causes—Other diseases have been reported (generally as case reports) with a restrictive-cardiomyopathy-type of presentation. These include pseudoxanthoma elasticum, coronary arteritis, myocardial tuberculosis, fatty infiltration of the myocardium, carnitine deficiency, neoplastic disease, and carcinoid heart disease.

Kuperstein R et al. Prevalence, etiology, and outcome of patients with restrictive left ventricular filling and relatively preserved systolic function. Am J Cardiol. 2003 Jun 15;91(12):1517–9. [PMID: 12804751]

▶ Clinical Findings

A. Symptoms and Signs

The clinical presentation (Table 15–2) of most patients with restrictive cardiomyopathy is based on the hemodynamic abnormalities that produce symptoms of congestive heart failure. The symptoms are, therefore, not specific for restrictive cardiomyopathy but include dyspnea, paroxysmal nocturnal dyspnea, orthopnea, peripheral edema, ascites, and more general complaints of fatigue and weakness in everyday activities.

Anginal symptoms are not typical except in the setting of amyloidosis, where true coronary artery narrowing may be caused by vessel infiltration. Cardiac amyloidosis commonly presents as classic restrictive cardiomyopathy, although other presentations have been noted. Syncope, lightheadedness, and palpitations should suggest coexisting conduction system involvement and atrial or ventricular arrhythmias.

Table 15–2. Characteristic Findings in Restrictive Cardiomyopathy.

Anatomic
Nondilated left ventricle
Dilated atria
Thick chamber walls
AV valve regurgitation
Physiologic
Elevated filling pressures
Restricted filling pattern
Minimally altered systolic function
Reduced stroke volume
Clinical
Heart failure symptoms, including unexplained right heart failure
Unexplained diastolic dysfunction on Doppler echocardiography or cardiac catheterization
Arrhythmias
Conduction abnormalities
Thromboembolic events
Suspected chronic constrictive pericarditis
Cardiac abnormalities with systemic disorder known to cause restrictive cardiomyopathy

AV, artioventricular.

B. Physical Examination

Depending on the stage of the disease, the physical examination may be only slightly abnormal or may show severe congestive heart failure with extensive peripheral edema, ascites, and low cardiac output manifested by cold extremities, hypotension, and lethargy.

The arterial pressure is usually normal. Hypotension is not uncommon as the disease progresses, particularly in systemic amyloidosis, in which arterial infiltration and autonomic neuropathy may complicate the clinical picture.

The jugular venous waveform is an important aspect of the physical examination in restrictive cardiomyopathy. The absolute degree of elevation is an immediate indication of the severity of the hemodynamic impairment. The waveform also contains additional details helpful in categorizing the hemodynamic profile. The a wave will be absent in the presence of atrial fibrillation and a large regurgitant v wave will be present when tricuspid regurgitation complicates the restrictive cardiomyopathy. Rapid x and y descents should be expected in most patients with restrictive cardiomyopathy in sinus rhythm. Kussmaul sign (lack of inspiratory decrease in pressure or increase) may be present.

The carotid pulse is often of low volume and may become very weak in the later stages of the disease characterized by a low cardiac output state.

Precordial palpitation often reveals a right ventricular heave that accompanies a moderate degree of pulmonary hypertension. Left ventricular heaves are not pronounced, and the apical impulse is usually only slightly displaced laterally.

The presence of left- and right-sided S_3 gallops is common. The intensity of the first heart sound is usually not markedly diminished, as it is with significant systolic dysfunction; an exception is a diminished S_1 intensity caused by first-degree heart block. The second heart sound often reveals an increased P_2. The splitting of the second heart sound may be increased when a right bundle branch block is present, or it may be reversed in the presence of a left bundle branch block. The S_4 gallop may be present earlier in the course of the disease and then disappear because of the development of atrial fibrillation or true atrial systolic failure (as occurs in advanced amyloidosis).

Peripheral edema and ascites are present in many cases. Hepatomegaly with a pulsatile sensation on palpation is frequently present as a result of severe tricuspid regurgitation.

C. Diagnostic Studies

The initial diagnostic studies necessary in cases of suspected restrictive cardiomyopathy include an electrocardiogram, a chest radiograph, and an echocardiogram. Based on this preliminary evaluation, further testing is often needed to more completely define the hemodynamics (with cardiac catheterization), exclude confounding coronary artery disease (using coronary arteriography), examine pericardial thickness to exclude constrictive pericarditis (with cardiac imaging), and make a tissue diagnosis (using endomyocardial biopsy). Brain natriuretic peptide levels may be of some value if they are low (< 150 ng/L), which favors constrictive pericarditis, or high (> 650 ng/L), which favors restrictive cardiomyopathy. Intermediate values are of less diagnostic usefulness.

1. Electrocardiography—Electrocardiography is used to delineate rhythm (atrial fibrillation is quite common) and assess conduction abnormalities and variations in QRS voltage and ST-T wave morphology from either hypertrophy or infiltration.

2. Chest radiography—The chest radiograph often shows pulmonary venous congestion and pleural effusions. It also can give additional information useful in the diagnosis of sarcoidosis, neoplastic disease, scleroderma, radiation-induced disease, and other causes of restrictive cardiomyopathy.

3. Echocardiography—The central role of cardiac echocardiography in the diagnosis and management of restrictive cardiomyopathy should be emphasized. Serial echocardiographic studies are frequently useful in making the initial diagnosis and in subsequent management of this generally progressive group of diseases.

The normal-to-small-sized left ventricle with fairly well-preserved systolic performance is usually seen. Apical cavity obliteration is a feature on echocardiography that is fairly peculiar to tropical endocardial fibrosis. The dilated atria are visualized, and left atrial thrombi may be suggested by transthoracic studies and should lead to transesophageal echocardiography. Wall thickness is measured, and tissue characteristics of the myocardium are noted. Cardiac amyloidosis has unique echocardiographic features. The differential echogenicity of amyloid frequently produces a sparkling appearance of the myocardium in two-dimensional images. In addition, the relationship between electrocardiographic QRS voltage and echocardiographically determined left ventricular mass or wall thickness is characteristically altered. The reduction in QRS voltage is associated with an increased mass due to amyloid infiltration and is easily distinguished from the reduced voltage and unaltered or reduced mass in constrictive pericarditis and from the increased voltage and increased mass in left ventricular myocardial hypertrophy.

Doppler echocardiography adds another dimension to assessing tricuspid and mitral valve regurgitation, an estimation of pulmonary artery systolic pressures, and a profile of the inflow velocities of the left and right ventricle. The mitral and tricuspid inflow velocity profile is related—but not identical—to the filling volume profile. A characteristic restrictive pattern of left ventricular filling has been described as a reduced rate of early diastolic filling with an increased atrial contribution. The diagnostic value of this approach has been severely curtailed by several factors, however. Filling velocity profiles can be normalized by elevating left atrial pressure from simple intravascular volume expansion. The inflow velocity profile is also influenced by changes in the annular dimensions of the mitral and tricus-

pid valves. In addition, restrictive cardiomyopathies are frequently complicated by atrial fibrillation, atrioventricular (AV) valve regurgitation, and atrial pump failure, which all independently alter the dynamics of ventricular filling. Because of these factors, a single, diagnostic restrictive filling pattern cannot be defined. However, restrictive cardiomyopathy characteristically exhibits an increased mitral Doppler inflow early velocity (E > 1.0 m/s) due to increased left atrial pressure, a decrease in the atrial inflow velocity (A < 0.5 m/s), an E/A ratio > 1.5, a reduction in mitral E deceleration time to < 125 m/s; and a reduction in isovolumic relaxation time. Pulmonary venous Doppler shows a reduction in systolic and an increase in diastolic forward velocity, as well as an increase in the atrial contraction associated backward velocity. Tricuspid E deceleration time is also reduced (< 160 ms). Hepatic vein flow velocity shows diastolic predominance and flow velocity may be reversed during inspiration.

4. Radionuclide angiography—This method can be used to assess diastolic filling characteristics. It has the advantage of quantifying volume change in the ventricle during diastole. The characteristic reduction in early diastolic filling and the rate of filling with a corresponding increase in late diastolic filling is readily determined by the multiple-gated acquisition technique. The diagnostic value of this characteristic restrictive pattern suffers from the same limitations as the Doppler technique (discussed earlier) and has an added drawback in that the sampling rate of most nuclear imaging systems may not adequately represent volume filling rates. The diagnostic image of large atria and normal-to-small-sized ventricles can be observed on radionuclide imaging, but they are better defined by echocardiography.

Tissue Doppler echocardiography has been used to differentiate restrictive cardiomyopathy from constrictive pericarditis. In persons with restrictive disease, posterior wall myocardial isovolumic relaxation velocity is reversed, unlike in healthy persons or in persons with constrictive disease. During rapid ventricular filling, myocardial velocity is slower in restriction, but during atrial contraction, myocardial velocity is the same in restriction and constriction. Tissue Doppler interrogation of the mitral annulus shows that a velocity of longitudinal expansion in early diastole of > 8 m/s favors constriction over restriction.

5. Cardiac catheterization—Many adult patients with restrictive cardiomyopathy do not need a complete cardiac catheterization; the decision depends on the quality of the noninvasive hemodynamic data, the certainty of the diagnosis, and whether the symptoms or other clinical findings suggest confounding cardiac problems, such as coronary artery disease. Right- and left-heart catheterization are frequently needed to confirm the restrictive physiology and to assess the severity of the elevation of filling pressures and the reduction of cardiac output. Ventriculography may be useful in assessing the degree of mitral or tricuspid valve regurgitation. A major manifestation of a reduction in chamber compliance is elevation of filling pressures, both diastolic pressures in the ventricle and mean pressure in the atrium. The absence of elevated filling pressures in the euvolemic patient is strong evidence against a functionally important restrictive cardiomyopathy. The continued absence of elevated filling pressures after intravascular volume infusion or during exercise is definitive evidence against the presence of a restrictive cardiomyopathy. On the other hand, elevated filling pressures are so commonly found in cardiac disorders of all types that they have limited specific diagnostic value for restrictive cardiomyopathy.

The pressure waveforms recorded in the ventricles and atria may have characteristic shapes in restrictive cardiomyopathy. The right and left ventricular pressure recordings have a square-root sign (early diastolic dip followed by a plateau), and the prominent x and y descents in the right atrium produce an M or W configuration. Also, right atrial pressure usually does not change with respiration. Right ventricular systolic pressure may be elevated, but end-diastolic pressure is usually less than a third of the systolic pressure. Left ventricular end diastolic pressure is characteristically 5 mm Hg or more greater than right ventricular end diastolic pressure, but they may be nearly equal in some patients.

Perhaps the most accurate hemodynamic parameter for distinguishing between constrictive and restrictive disease is the response of left and right ventricular pressures to respiration. This is best assessed by having catheters in both ventricles and observing the changes in pressure with normal respiration. In restrictive cardiomyopathy, the ventricular pressures are concordant; they rise and fall together with respiration. Whereas, in constrictive pericarditis they are discordant; when right ventricular pressure rises with inspiration left ventricular pressure decreases and vice versa during expiration.

6. Endomyocardial biopsy—Endomyocardial biopsy is an essential test in the diagnosis of several specific diseases that lead to a restrictive cardiomyopathy, such as hemochromatosis and sarcoidosis (see Table 15–1). It is necessary to exclude these specific diseases when the final diagnosis is idiopathic restrictive cardiomyopathy. Furthermore, a negative biopsy is important information when considering thoracotomy to diagnose and surgically treat presumed constrictive pericarditis.

Endomyocardial biopsy is most commonly performed on the right ventricular aspect of the interventricular septum. The right internal jugular vein is the entry port of first choice although the femoral vein can be used, especially if the biopsy accompanies a full cardiac catheterization. Although left ventricular biopsy is not routinely done at most tertiary centers, it should be considered when selective left ventricular involvement is strongly suspected and a skilled physician is available.

The myocardial biopsy specimen is quite small, approximately 1–3 mm in diameter. Because many of the diseases in question are scattered in the wall of the septum rather than homogeneously present, at least five specimens should be taken.

7. Pericardial imaging—Computed tomography (CT), specifically fast CT, is extremely important in excluding constrictive pericarditis in many patients presumed to have restrictive cardiomyopathy. Echocardiography is frequently inadequate because the gain settings of the instrument factiously modify the true pericardial thickness. Cardiac magnetic resonance imaging is an alternative method that visualizes the pericardium as a lucent, low-intensity line bordered by opaque pericardial and subepicardial fat. Many clinicians believe magnetic resonance imaging is superior to conventional CT for defining pericardial thickness.

▶ Differential Diagnosis

The major differential diagnosis in cases of suspected restrictive cardiomyopathy is constrictive pericarditis. Table 15–3 outlines some of the distinguishing features of each disorder. The diagnostic approach includes echocardiography, a hemodynamic profile, pericardial imaging, and endomyocardial biopsy. The Doppler echocardiographic features that distinguish between restrictive cardiomyopathy and constrictive pericarditis are shown in Table 15–4. Because hemodynamic studies cannot always correctly distinguish between these two disorders, pericardial imaging and endocardial biopsy play an important role in establishing the diagnosis in some patients.

Babuin L et al. Brain natriuretic peptide levels in constrictive pericarditis and restrictive cardiomyopathy. J Am Coll Cardiol. 2006 Apr 4;47(7):1489–91. [PMID: 16580543]

Hassan WM et al. Pitfalls in diagnosis and clinical, echocardiographic, and hemodynamic findings in endomyocardial fibrosis: a 25-year experience. Chest. 2005 Dec;128(6):3985–92. [PMID: 16354870]

Ha JW et al. Differentiation of constrictive pericarditis from restrictive cardiomyopathy using mitral annular velocity by tissue Doppler echocardiography. Am J Cardiol. 2004 Aug 1;94(3):316–9. [PMID: 15276095]

Rajagopalan N et al. Comparison of new Doppler echocardiographic methods to differentiate constrictive pericardial heart disease and restrictive cardiomyopathy. Am J Cardiol. 2001 Jan 1;87(1):86–94. [PMID: 11137840]

Palka P et al. Differentiation between restrictive cardiomyopathy and constrictive pericarditis by early diastolic doppler myocardial velocity gradient at the posterior wall. Circulation. 2000 Aug 8;102(6):655–62. [PMID: 10931806]

▶ Treatment

The therapeutic plan for treating restrictive cardiomyopathy has three directions: management of the diastolic dysfunction; treatment of rhythm, conduction system, and thromboembolic complications; and treatment of the underlying disorder, if possible.

A. Diastolic Dysfunction

Most patients with restrictive cardiomyopathy require diuresis to treat venous congestion in the pulmonary and

Table 15–3. Differentiating between Restrictive Cardiomyopathy and Constrictive Pericarditis.

	Restrictive Cardiomyopathy	Constrictive Pericarditis
At the bedside	S₃ gallop	Pericardial knock
	Increased apical impulse	Reduced apical impulse
	Regurgitant murmurs	No murmurs
Electrocardiography	Usually low voltage	Low voltage
	Atrial fibrillation common	Atrial fibrillation common
Echocardiography	Increased wall thickness	Normal-to-reduced wall thickness
Cardiac catheterization	Square root sign	Square root sign
	Increased atrial pressure with M or W configuration	Increased atrial pressure with M or W configuration
	Kussmaul sign usually absent	Kussmaul sign usually present
	Pulsus paradoxus occasionally present	Pulsus paradoxus occasionally present
	LV diastolic pressure usually > RV	LV and RV diastolic pressures equal
	RV systolic pressure variable	RV systolic pressure usually < 50 mm Hg
	RV-LV pressure concordance	RV-LV pressure discordance
Ventriculography	Slow early diastolic LV filling	Rapid early diastolic LV filling
CT scan	Normal pericardium	Thickened pericardium

LV, left ventricular; RV, right ventricular.

systemic circulation. Unfortunately, the nature of restrictive cardiomyopathy complicates this goal in that normalization of right- and left-sided filling pressures may lead to a clinically significant reduction in preload. During diuretic therapy, attention must be directed toward detecting such symptoms of excessively reduced preload and cardiac output as fatigue and light-headedness. There may be direct signs of hypotension and hypoperfusion and such laboratory evidence as rising blood urea nitrogen. In severe restrictive cardiomyopathy, a very narrow intravascular volume status may prevent overt congestion without excessively reducing preload. No such window exists in the terminal phases of the disease.

Conventional medications used to treat other heart failure states are of no proven value in restrictive cardiomyopathy. Angiotensin-converting enzyme inhibitors may be limited by a low systemic arterial pressure; they have caused complications in children with restrictive cardiomyopathy. Digitalis preparations have no proven benefit in diastolic dysfunction and may pose a risk of toxicity.

Calcium antagonists have been advocated in diastolic dysfunction found in the setting of coronary artery disease, hypertensive heart disease, and hypertrophic cardiomyopathy. Their value in restrictive cardiomyopathy is uncertain, and their use should be approached with caution because they may further lower blood pressure.

Table 15–4. Differentiation of Constrictive Pericarditis from Restrictive Cardiomyopathy by Doppler Echocardiography.

Parameter	Normal	Constriction	Restriction
MVE respiratory variation	< 10%	≥ 25%	None
MVEDT	> 160 ms	< 160 ms	< 160 ms
TVE respiratory variation	< 15%	> 40%	None
TVEDT	> 160 ms	< 160 ms	< 160 ms
HV velocity	Systole > diastole	Variable	Systole < diastole
HV respiratory reversal	Expiratory	More marked expiratory	Inspiratory
Mitral annular velocity in early diastole	> 8 m/s	> 8 m/s	< 8 m/s

DT, deceleration time; HV, hepatic vein; MVE, mitral valve E wave velocity; TV, tricuspid valve; TVE, tricuspid valve E wave velocity.

B. Cardiac Complications

1. Rhythm disturbances

A. ATRIAL FIBRILLATION—The most frequent rhythm complication in the management of restrictive cardiomyopathy is atrial fibrillation. Not only is this rhythm disturbance common in restrictive cardiomyopathy, but loss of atrial contraction may worsen diastolic dysfunction because a higher mean atrial pressure is needed to achieve an adequate preload. In addition, a rapid ventricular response in atrial fibrillation further compromises pump function. Maintenance of normal sinus rhythm is therefore a reasonable goal, and such medications as flecainide, propafenone, and amiodarone may be necessary. Atrial fibrillation cannot be successfully prevented in some patients, however.

Digoxin may also be used to control the ventricular rate if fibrillation persists, although careful attention to serum drug levels and monitoring for digitalis-induced rhythm disturbances are mandatory. β-Blockers are less useful for rate control because they can lower blood pressure further. In an occasional patient, especially one with restrictive cardiomyopathy from amyloidosis, atrial contractile function may be minimal. If this can be discerned by Doppler echocardiographic studies, the need to maintain normal sinus rhythm would not be as urgent as in someone in whom ventricular filling is highly dependent on atrial contraction.

B. BRADYCARDIA—Restrictive cardiomyopathy may be complicated by advanced conduction system disease leading to complete heart block or by severe sinus node dysfunction leading to hemodynamically compromising bradycardia. Atrioventricular pacing at a reasonable rate can be achieved after pacemaker placement.

C. VENTRICULAR ARRHYTHMIAS—Ventricular arrhythmias may also complicate the course of the patient with restrictive cardiomyopathy. Management revolves around the issues of whether the arrhythmias are symptomatic, hemodynamically compromising, or sustained or whether they deteriorate into a life-threatening state. There are no special issues in managing these arrhythmias in the context of restrictive cardiomyopathy.

2. Thromboembolic complications—These complications of restrictive cardiomyopathy are similar to those of dilated cardiomyopathy. Thrombus formation in the atrial appendage or the left ventricle may occur and subsequently embolize to the central nervous system or elsewhere in the circulation. Patients with restrictive cardiomyopathy with atrial fibrillation, AV valve regurgitation, and low cardiac output are at particular risk, and prophylactic anticoagulation with warfarin should be considered. Patients with endocardial fibrosis should be particularly considered for long-term anticoagulation because of their higher thromboembolic risk and the possible progressive obliteration of the left ventricle from thrombus formation. Systemic venous thrombosis with pulmonary embolism is also a risk, especially in the bedridden, edematous patient. Heparin prophylaxis is recommended for all patients in an inpatient setting.

C. Underlying Disease

Certain treatment strategies are applied to specific causes of restrictive cardiomyopathy. Although details of these approaches are beyond the scope of this chapter, they include chemotherapy for underlying plasma cell dyscrasia in amyloidosis, treatment of underlying inflammation in sarcoidosis, treatment of underlying inflammation and hypereosinophilia in Löffler endocardial fibrosis, and the use of iron chelation therapy in hemochromatosis.

Cardiac transplantation should be considered in patients with restrictive cardiomyopathy with intractable symptoms. This therapy is pertinent to those with idiopathic and familial restrictive cardiomyopathy and chronic allograft rejection. Although transplantation has been performed in systemic disorders such as amyloidosis, reoccurrence of the disease in the transplanted heart and the progression of disease in other organ systems argue against the use of this approach in these diseases.

The latter stage of Löffler cardiomyopathy shows a restrictive cardiomyopathy with gross and microscopic anatomic features virtually identical to those of tropical endocardial fibrosis. Treatment of the underlying eosinophilic disorder and management of the restrictive cardiomyopathy are usually necessary. Occasionally, surgical stripping of the endocardial scar (endocardiectomy) and replacement of an AV valve (if severely regurgitant) are beneficial. When endomyocardial fibrosis progresses to cause severe chamber obliteration, surgical resection should be considered.

▶ Prognosis

As the causes of restrictive cardiomyopathy vary, so do the prognoses, depending essentially on the course of the underlying disease. Survival rates for patients with amyloidosis, for example, drop sharply within the first year, generally declining to zero within 4 years. After 10 years, patients with idiopathic restrictive cardiomyopathy have a survival rate of about 50%; those with hypertrophic cardiomyopathy, about 70%; and those with dilated cardiomyopathy, between 30% and 40%.

Ammash NM et al. Clinical profile and outcome of idiopathic restrictive cardiomyopathy. Circulation. 2000 May 30;101(21): 2490–6. [PMID: 10831523]

Myocarditis

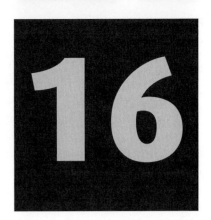

16

John B. O'Connell, MD & Michael H. Crawford, MD

- ► New congestive heart failure with a history of an antecedent viral syndrome.
- ► Elevated erythrocyte sedimentation rate, or cardiac markers.
- ► ECG shows sinus tachycardia, nonspecific ST-T changes, atrial or ventricular arrhythmias, or conduction abnormalities.
- ► Echocardiogram demonstrates chamber enlargement, wall motion abnormalities, systolic or diastolic dysfunction, or mural thrombi.
- ► Endomyocardial biopsy reveals an inflammatory infiltrate with adjacent myocyte injury.

► General Considerations

Myocarditis is defined simply as an inflammatory process with necrosis that involves the myocardium. In the past, the myocardial injury was believed to be a direct result of the cytotoxic effects of the relevant organisms. Even as early as 1806, however, it was thought that a persistent inflammatory process following such an infection (eg, diphtheria) of the myocardium led to progressive cardiac damage and dysfunction. When the term "myocarditis" was first introduced in 1837 as inflammation or degeneration of the heart, the diagnosis could be made only postmortem. Fortunately, endomyocardial biopsy now allows the sampling of human myocardial tissue during life and thus the accurate antemortem diagnosis of myocarditis.

► Pathophysiology

The histologic hallmark of myocarditis is a focal patchy or diffuse inflammatory infiltrate with adjacent myocyte injury. The inflammation may not be restricted to the myocardium but may also involve the adjacent endocardium, pericardium, and valvular structures.

Myocarditis is most commonly initiated by viral infection (Table 16–1). Initiation of the pathophysiologic abnormalities, however, may result from a variety of insults, including drugs, toxins, hypersensitivity reactions, collagen vascular diseases, and autoimmune reactions. The most common viruses associated with myocarditis in the United States and Western Europe in immunocompetent persons are adenoviruses, coxsackievirus B (enterovirus), parvovirus B19, herpes simplex, influenza A, and cytomegalovirus (CMV). Other viruses, bacteria, rickettsiae, spirochetes, fungi, protozoans, or metazoans can also produce myocarditis; such causes are uncommon, however (see Table 16–1). Successful identification of the most common offending pathogens depends on knowledge of the geographic region's relevant endemic and epidemic infectious diseases, the person's immunization status and immunocompetence, and the sophistication and availability of public health services.

Several mechanisms of myocardial damage have been proposed. (1) Direct injury of myocytes by the infectious agent. (2) Myocyte injury caused by a toxin such as that from *Corynebacterium diphtheriae.* (3) Myocyte injury as a result of infection-induced immune reaction or autoimmunity.

The autoimmunity hypothesis is the most widely accepted theory. It is believed that the viral infection triggers a cell-mediated immunologic response that ultimately causes myocardial injury; the myocardial injury persists despite viral clearance.

In the murine model, coxsackievirus B3 causes an infectious phase, which lasts 7–10 days, and is characterized by active viral replication. During this phase, initial myocyte injury takes place, causing the release of antigenic intracellular components (such as myosin) into the bloodstream. Subsequently, after viral clearance, a second phase of myocyte damage will start. This phase is immune-mediated by CD8 lymphocytes and autoantibodies against various myocyte components. Antimyosin antibodies were isolated from mice that developed

Table 16–1. Important Causes of Myocarditis.

Infectious	
Viral	**Bacterial**
Coxsackie A and B	β-Hemolytic streptococci
Influenza A and B	*Corynebacterium diphtheriae*
Echovirus	*Neisseria meningitides*
Arbovirus	*Staphylococcus aureus*
Cytomegalovirus	*Mycoplasma pneumoniae*
HIV	*Salmonella typhi*
Hepatitis	*Mycobacterium tuberculosis*
Epstein-Barr virus	*Borrelia burgdorferi*
Mumps	*Rickettsia rickettsii*
Poliomyelitis	*Campylobacter jejuni*
Herpes simplex	*Chlamydia trachomatis*
Herpes zoster	*Listeria monocytogenes*
Human herpes virus 6	*Legionella pneumophila*
Parvovirus B19	*Coxiella burnetii*
Rabies	
Rubella	
Rebeola	
Vaccinia	
Protozoal	**Metazoal**
Trypanosoma cruzi	*Echinococcus*
Toxoplasma gondii	*Trichinella spiralis*
Fungal	
Noninfectious	
Toxic	**Hypersensitivity**
Anthracyclines	?
Catecholamines	**Autoimmune**
Interleukins	?
Alpha-2 interferon	
Trastuzumab	

?, No dominant organisms.

myocarditis following coxsackievirus B infection, as well as from patients with myocarditis. Antigenic mimicry, the cross reactivity of antibodies to both virus and myocardial proteins, occurs when an infectious agent shares an identical antigen with the normal myocyte. This mechanism is documented in animal models, and it may play a role in humans. Myocyte injury may be a direct result of CD8 lymphocyte infiltration. The local release of cytokines, such as interleukin-1, interleukin-2, interleukin-6, tumor necrosis factor (TNF), and nitric oxide may play a role in determining the T-cell reaction and the

subsequent degree of autoimmune perpetuation. These cytokines may also cause reversible depression of myocardial contractility without causing cell death.

The popularity of the autoimmune hypothesis deemphasizes the role of the virus. Animal studies show, however, that viral proliferation itself might cause myocarditis. Some studies demonstrate the persistence of viral genomic fragments in myocardial cells of patients with active myocarditis and in some patients with dilated cardiomyopathy. Although these fragments may not be infectious, viral RNA may still serve as a persistent antigen to drive the immunologic response.

Exposure to cardiotropic viruses, presumably followed by a viral infection of the myocardium, is common. Based on the detection of serum antibodies to cardiotropic viruses, approximately 70% of the adult population has had prior exposure. Nonetheless, resultant abnormalities in cardiac function or symptomatic heart failure are unusual. The host factors predisposing to these deleterious immune responses are as yet undefined. Immunocompromised patients, such as pregnant women and patients with AIDS, are predisposed to myocarditis. The susceptibility to viral myocarditis may also be age-related or, based on familial occurrence, genetically predetermined.

Liu PP et al. Advances in the understanding of myocarditis. Circulation. 2001 Aug 28;104(9):1076–82. [PMID: 11524405]
Mahrholdt H et al. Presentation, patterns of myocardial damage, and clinical course of viral myocarditis. Circulation. 2006 Oct 10;114(5):1581–90. [PMID: 17015795]

▶ **Clinical Findings**

A. Symptoms and Signs

Myocarditis is most commonly asymptomatic, with no evidence of left ventricular dysfunction. The clinical manifestations of myocarditis are protean, when they are present. Myocardial involvement may be overshadowed or completely masked by the constitutional symptoms of the illness or other organ dysfunction. Cardiac symptoms may result from systolic or diastolic left ventricular dysfunction or from tachyarrhythmias or bradyarrhythmias. Patients frequently seek medical attention days to weeks after an acute febrile illness, particularly a flu-like syndrome. Common constitutional symptoms include fever, malaise, fatigue, arthralgias, myalgias, and skin rash.

Chest discomfort is a common symptom and is typically pericardial in nature; ischemic or atypical pain may also occur. Occasionally, patients have the syndrome of acute myocardial infarction with ischemic chest pain, electrocardiographic (ECG) abnormalities, elevated cardiac isoenzymes, or evidence of left ventricular wall motion abnormalities. Viral coronary arteritis and vasospasm have been implicated as the cause of this syndrome, but the epicardial coronary arteries are usually widely patent.

The acute onset of symptoms of congestive heart failure in a young person or in a patient without known coronary artery disease often suggests the diagnosis of myocarditis. Classic symptoms of congestive heart failure, including dyspnea, fatigue, decreased exercise tolerance, palpitations, and right heart failure, may be present. This constellation of signs and symptoms may be indistinguishable from dilated cardiomyopathy. It should be noted that because the metabolic demands on the heart associated with fever or a viral illness may initiate the first episode of congestive heart failure in patients with asymptomatic left ventricular dysfunction or reduced cardiac reserve, heart failure following a viral syndrome does not necessarily imply myocarditis.

Patients may also present with other symptoms that have been described in myocarditis: dizziness, syncope, or palpitations caused by atrial and ventricular arrhythmias and conduction disturbances. Myocarditis may present as sudden death, as a result of malignant ventricular arrhythmias or complete heart block; systemic and pulmonary thromboemboli have also been noted.

B. Physical Examination

The findings on physical examination vary widely. The patient may appear ill because the other manifestations of a viral illness dominate the clinical picture, and myocardial involvement may become evident only later in the course of the illness. Preexisting heart disease can also obscure the findings of myocarditis on examination.

Tachycardia, hypotension, and fever are associated with myocarditis. The tachycardia may be disproportionate to the degree of fever, and the heart rate is frequently elevated both at rest and with effort. Bradycardia is seen rarely, and a narrow pulse pressure is occasionally detected. Murmurs of mitral or tricuspid regurgitation are common, but diastolic murmurs are rare. The intensity of S_1 may be decreased and the intensity of pulmonic closure increased, and S_3 and S_4 gallops may also be heard.

In more severe cases, congestive heart failure with distended neck veins, pulmonary rales, wheezes, gallops, and peripheral edema may be detected. Pleural and pericardial rubs are common in acute viral myocarditis, and a rhythm disturbance or conduction delay may be evident. Circulatory collapse and shock may occur, but these are rare.

C. Diagnostic Studies

1. Electrocardiography—Electrocardiographic abnormalities are common in patients with myocarditis. These ECG changes are often nonspecific and transient, usually appearing only in the first 2 weeks of the illness. The most common abnormality is sinus tachycardia. While the presence of ST segment and T wave changes suggest the diagnosis of myocarditis during a viral syndrome, subtle ECG changes may be caused solely by fever, hypoxia, hyperkalemia, and other metabolic abnormalities associated with the syndrome. Atrioventricular (AV) and intraventricular conduction delays are also common. Left bundle branch block occurs in approxi-

mately 20% of patients with active myocarditis. Complete AV block is not an uncommon finding and is often diagnosed after the patient presents with syncope. Heart block is usually transient but may occasionally require a temporary pacemaker. Supraventricular tachycardia is common, particularly with associated congestive heart failure or pericarditis. Ventricular ectopy may be the only clinical finding that suggests myocarditis. Other reported abnormalities include axis shifts and repolarization abnormalities.

2. Chest radiography—The chest radiograph may be normal, or it may demonstrate mild to moderate cardiomegaly from dilatation of the left or right ventricular cavity (or both). The cardiac silhouette may also be globular when a pericardial effusion is present, however. Evidence of venous congestion and pulmonary edema may be seen in more severe cases, and pulmonary infiltrates from concomitant pneumonia may be present.

3. Echocardiography—Two-dimensional echocardiography is a convenient and noninvasive method of evaluating chamber sizes, valvular function, and myocardial contractility. Left ventricular systolic dysfunction is commonly seen in patients with congestive heart failure. Regional wall motion abnormalities mimicking a myocardial infarction are surprisingly common; however, global hypokinesis may also occur. The left ventricular cavity may be normal in size or minimally enlarged; it may be markedly enlarged in those with fulminant disease. Mitral or tricuspid regurgitation may be present. Interestingly, an increase in wall thickness mimicking hypertrophic cardiomyopathy may be seen early in the course of the disease, presumably secondary to edematous inflammation. Mural thrombi occur in approximately 15% of cases. Echocardiography is also helpful in demonstrating abnormalities of diastolic filling that mimic restrictive cardiomyopathy and in distinguishing ventricular dilatation from pericardial effusion. Echocardiograms are commonly obtained serially to monitor the course of the illness and to evaluate therapy. Echocardiographic changes may persist, improve, or even worsen after clinical resolution of acute myocarditis.

4. Magnetic resonance imaging—Acute myocarditis can be detected by gadolinium-enhanced cardiovascular magnetic resonance imaging (MRI). Focal areas of contrast enhancement are characteristic and are present in 75–90% of patients with acute myocarditis. In more chronic myocarditis, MRI has reduced sensitivity. Specificity is similar (70–95%) and is higher in more acute cases. MRI may help localize the areas where biopsy specimens should be taken. MRI is most often positive when biopsy specimens shows definite myocarditis. Borderline biopsy criteria cases are less likely to be detected by MRI. No MRI parameter predicts the presense of viral genomics by polymerase chain reaction (PCR).

5. Cardiac catheterization—Cardiac catheterization is not routinely performed in all cases of myocarditis; however, it may help in the diagnosis when the presentation mimics myocardial infarction. Characteristic hemodynamic findings of myocarditis include an elevated left ventricular end-diastolic pressure, a depressed cardiac output, and increased ventricular volumes. Ventriculography may also confirm abnormalities seen on echocardiography or MRI. Coronary angiogram typically demonstrates normal coronary arteries.

6. Endomyocardial biopsy—Myocardial biopsy is considered the gold standard for the diagnosis of myocarditis. It is an invasive procedure, although it only involves minimal morbidity and discomfort. The Stanford-Caves reusable bioptome is typically introduced to the right ventricular cavity. Newer, single-use bioptomes and sheaths can be introduced through right and left jugular, subclavian, or femoral veins and femoral arteries. Four to six tissue fragments are obtained, usually from the right side of the intraventricular septum, but cardiovascular MRI can be used to direct the bioptome to areas of focal disease. The major risk of myocardial biopsy is cardiac puncture. It occurs in less than 1% of cases but is often fatal. Computed tomography or three-dimensional echocardiography guidance can reduce the risk of right ventricular free wall puncture.

The histologic criteria for the diagnosis of myocarditis are defined as an inflammatory infiltrate of the myocardium with injury to the adjacent myocytes not typical for the ischemic damage associated with coronary artery disease. The diagnosis of borderline myocarditis is made when the infiltrate is not accompanied by myocyte injury. In large trials, only about 10% of patients with unexplained congestive heart failure met the criteria for active myocarditis. Many patients with negative biopsies have the classic clinical presentation of myocarditis. One explanation for the low yield of endomyocardial biopsy is that the inflammation may be focal or patchy. Another reason might be that some patients have purely humoral or cytokine-mediated forms of myocarditis with little or no cellular infiltrate. Furthermore, the histologic changes may be transient with rapid resolution. It should be noted that endomyocardial biopsy may rule in but never rule out active myocarditis.

In recent years, the role of endomyocardial biopsy has changed. It is no longer mandatory and essential in the evaluation of unexplained heart failure because the information it provides will rarely determine specific therapy. This became particularly evident after publication of the results of the Myocarditis Treatment Trial, which failed to show any benefit of the immunosuppressive therapy. It remains important to consider biopsy in some special cases of myocarditis, particularly in patients who do not respond to conventional therapy. Some patients in this group may have giant cell myocarditis, which requires a more aggressive approach with immunosuppressive therapy and consideration for early transplantation. Current guidelines suggest that biopsy may be appropriate in cases of unexplained new-onset (< 2 weeks) heart failure. After 2 weeks, no response to treatment or suspicion of special diagnoses, such as eosinophillic myocarditis, are considered valid indications for biopsy.

7. Other tests—An elevated erythrocyte sedimentation rate (ESR) is detected in approximately 60% of patients with active myocarditis. If the ESR is elevated, it may help monitor the course of the illness and effectiveness of therapy. The accuracy of this test may be affected by coexisting hepatic congestion or hepatitis; these conditions decrease the synthesis of fibrinogen and lower the ESR.

Mild to moderate leukocytosis occurs in approximately 25% of patients, along with neutrophilia or lymphocytosis and occasionally eosinophilia, particularly in parasitic illnesses. The percentage of eosinophils may also increase in the recovery phase of myocarditis.

The creatine phosphokinase-myocardial band (CK-MB) fraction is elevated in approximately 6% of patients, with the degree of elevation being proportional to the degree of myocyte injury. Cardiac troponin-I (Tn I) is a sensitive and specific marker for myocyte injury and is increased in about one-third of patients with myocarditis.

Measurement of serum antibody titers to various cardiotropic viruses is useful for establishing exposure to these agents. The titers may be neutralizing antibodies, complement-fixing antibodies, or hemagglutination-inhibiting antibodies. Because a fourfold rise in titer over a 4–6 week period is required to document an acute infection, serial blood samples must be obtained. It must be kept in mind that an elevated antibody titer or rise in dilution only implies infection with the offending organism. Proof of active myocarditis also requires a positive biopsy result. Cultures of throat washings, urine, and feces may help identify a viral pathogen. Unfortunately, viral cultures are usually negative, and serologic studies are often nondiagnostic. In addition, viral recovery is usually possible only during the acute phase of the illness when active replication is occurring. Because this phase is not associated with viral injury, the diagnostic yield of culture of myocardial samples obtained by endomyocardial biopsy is minimal. Other laboratory analyses that may be useful include a Mono-spot test, Epstein-Barr virus titers, hepatitis serology, and urine and serum for CMV.

The detection of viral genomic material in endomyocardial biopsies using recombinant DNA techniques is a promising diagnostic tool. Two methods are used: PCR and in situ hybridization. Plus-strand RNA indicates persistent viral state, and minus-strand RNA indicates active viral replication. Unfortunately, studies have been inconsistent, with viral detection ranging between 10% and 60% of patients with dilated cardiomyopathy and myocarditis, compared with almost no viral detection in the control groups. Some studies have noted a relationship between viral persistence and progressive myocardial dysfunction. At the present time, routine viral study of endomyocardial biopsy is not recommended and remains investigational with the possibility of clinical application in the future.

Abdel-Aty H et al. Diagnostic performance of cardiovascular magnetic resonance in patients with suspected acute myocarditis: comparison of different approaches. J Am Coll Cardiol. 2005 Jun 7;45(11):1815–22. [PMID: 15936612]

Bowles NE et al. Detection of viruses in myocardial tissues by polymerase chain reaction. Evidence of adenovirus as a common cause of myocarditis in children and adults. J Am Coll Cardiol. 2003 Aug 6;42(3):466–72. [PMID: 12906974]

Cooper LT et al; American Heart Association, American College of Cardiology; European Society of Cardiology; Heart Failure Society of America; Heart Failure Association of the European Society of Cardiology. The role of endomyocardial biopsy in the management of cardiovascular disease: a scientific statement from the American Heart Association, the American College of Cardiology, and the European Society of Cardiology. Endorsed by the Heart Failure Society of America and the Heart Failure Association of the European Society of Cardiology. J Am Coll Cardiol. 2007 Nov 6;50(19):1914–31. [PMID: 17980265]

De Cobelli F et al. Delayed gadolinium-enhanced cardiac magnetic resonance in patients with chronic myocarditis presenting with heart failure or recurrent arrhythmias. J Am Coll Cardiol. 2006 Apr 18;47(18):1649–54. [PMID: 16631005]

Feldman AM et al. Myocarditis. N Engl J Med. 2000 Nov 9;343(19):1388–98. [PMID: 11070105]

Gutberlet M et al. Suspected chronic myocarditis at cardiac MR: diagnostic accuracy and association with immunohistologically detected inflammation and viral persistence. Radiology. 2008 Feb;246(2):401–9. [PMID: 18180335]

Kühl U et al. High prevalence of viral genomes and multiple viral infections in the myocardium of adults with "idiopathic" left ventricular dysfunction. Circulation. 2005 Feb 22;111(7):887–93. [PMID: 15699250]

Kühl U et al. Viral persistence in the myocardium is associated with progressive cardiac dysfunction. Circulation. 2005 Sep 27;112(13):1965–70. [PMID: 16172268]

Mahrholdt H et al. Cardiovascular magnetic resonance assessment of human myocarditis: a comparison to histology and molecular pathology. Circulation. 2004 Mar 16;109(10):1250–8. [PMID: 14993139]

▶ Treatment

Patients with suspected acute myocarditis should be hospitalized and monitored closely for evidence of worsening congestive heart failure, arrhythmias, conduction disturbances, or emboli. Bed rest is essential, and activities that increase cardiac workload should be strongly discouraged. In the animal model, exercise has been shown to both intensify the inflammatory process in the myocardium and increase morbidity and mortality. Activities should be restricted until clinical improvement occurs or a follow-up biopsy documents the resolution of inflammation.

Antipyretics, other than nonsteroidal antiinflammatory drugs (NSAIDs), should be given to febrile patients, and analgesics are helpful in dealing with pleuropericardial chest pain. Hypoxia, decrease in cardiac output, and tachycardia warrant the administration of supplemental oxygen. If anemia is present, correcting it may improve cardiopulmonary function. The use of tobacco and alcohol should be strongly discouraged.

Patients with congestive heart failure should be treated by restricting sodium and fluids and by administering diuretics, angiotensin-converting enzyme (ACE) inhibitors or angiotensin-receptor blockers, β-blockers, and spironolactone. Patients with fulminant disease manifesting as cardiogenic shock will require more aggressive therapy with intravenous vasodilators and inotropic agents such as dobutamine or milrinone. Occasionally, cases may be refractory to conservative measures and require mechanical circulatory support. Favorable reports have used extracorporeal membrane oxygenation, intra-aortic balloon, and ventricular assist devices. Recent reports have demonstrated that early aggressive approach with mechanical circulatory support might help as a "bridge to recovery." As a last resort, cardiac transplantation may be considered in patients with acute myocarditis if all other measures have failed and the patient's condition is rapidly deteriorating. Unfortunately, an increased morbidity and mortality in transplant rejection results from the activated immunologic system that the donor heart encounters.

Antiarrhythmic agents are warranted in patients with tachyarrhythmias or ventricular arrhythmias. It is best to avoid agents with strong negative inotropic effects. Occasionally, amiodarone or an implantable cardioverter defibrillator may be used after all other attempts at controlling arrhythmia have failed. These measures must be used only as a last resort, however, because myocarditis frequently resolves spontaneously. Patients with symptomatic bradyarrhythmias or high-grade conduction blocks will benefit from the implantation of a pacemaker.

Anticoagulation therapy is indicated in patients with systemic or pulmonary emboli or mural thrombi detected by echocardiography or ventriculography. Patients with active myocarditis and even mild left ventricular dysfunction should probably receive anticoagulation (animal models have demonstrated a propensity toward mural thrombi). Anticoagulation may be contraindicated in patients with coexisting pericarditis.

Immunosuppressive therapy has been reported in few studies with disappointing results. Controlled trials of prednisone plus cyclosporine or azathioprine did not show significant differences in left ventricular ejection fraction (LVEF) or left ventricular diastolic diameter at 1 year. Also, no significant difference in survival occurred during the follow-up period.

Intravenous immune globulin was suggested to be useful by some reports. In those with persistent viral genome interferon-beta has been reported to eliminate viruses and improve left ventricular function, although immunosuppressive therapy is generally not indicated except in special cases.

The prognosis in giant cell myocarditis is very poor, and immunosuppressive therapy may be helpful. Another situation where immunosuppressive therapy may be indicated is myocarditis associated with underlying immune diseases, such as systemic lupus erythematosus (SLE). In a small percentage of myocarditis patients, the disease may recur after initial resolution; in these patients, immunosuppressive therapy may help in decreasing the recurrences.

Chandra D et al. Usefulness of percutaneous left ventricular assist device as a bridge to recovery from myocarditis. Am J Cardiol. 2007 Jun 15;99(12):1755–6. [PMID: 17560889]

Gojo S et al. Successful LVAS and RVAS-ECMO support in a patient with fulminant myocarditis who failed to recover from ventricular fibrillation with PCPS and IABP. J Thorac Cardiovasc Surg. 2003 Sep;126(3):885–6. [PMID: 14502181]

Kuhl U et al. Interferon-beta treatment eliminates cardiotropic viruses and improves left ventricular function in patients with myocardial persistence of viral genomes and left ventricular dysfunction. Circulation. 2003 Jun 10;107(22):2793–8. [PMID: 12771005]

McNamara DM et al. Controlled trial of intravenous immune globulin in recent-onset dilated cardiomyopathy. Circulation. 2001 May 8;103(18):2254–9. [PMID: 11342473]

Parrillo JE. Inflammatory cardiomyopathy (myocarditis): which patients should be treated with anti-inflammatory therapy? Circulation. 2001 Jul 3;104(1):4–6. [PMID: 11435327]

Wojnicz R et al. Randomized, placebo-controlled study for immunosuppressive treatment of inflammatory dilated cardiomyopathy: two-year follow-up results. Circulation. 2001 Jul 3;104(1):39–45. [PMID: 11435335]

▶ Prognosis

Most patients with myocarditis have self-limited, asymptomatic disease without residual cardiac dysfunction. Symptomatic patients have a poorer prognosis. Patients may spontaneously recover at any point during the illness, the degree of ventricular dysfunction may stabilize, or it may progress to dilated cardiomyopathy and heart failure, especially in the face of such causes as AIDS or giant cell myocarditis. Unfortunately, a small percentage of patients will die suddenly and unexpectedly, regardless of therapy. The overall prognosis is poor, with an estimated cumulative mortality rate at 5 years of about 50%. Progressive heart failure is the predominant cause of death. Interestingly, patients with fulminant myocarditis have a better long-term prognosis than patients with mild acute or chronic presentations. These patients should therefore be supported aggressively with vasopressor therapy and mechanical circulatory support, if necessary, to give them the best chance of surviving the initial critical phase, since the likelihood of long-term recovery is high.

Magnani JW et al. Survival in biopsy-proven myocarditis: a long-term retrospective analysis of the histopathologic, clinical, and hemodynamic predictors. Am Heart J. 2006 Feb;151(2):463–70. [PMID: 16442915]

McCarthy RE 3rd et al. Long-term outcome of fulminant myocarditis as compared with acute (nonfulminant) myocarditis. N Engl J Med. 2000 Mar 9;342(10):690–5. [PMID: 10706898]

Pulerwitz TC et al. Mortality in primary and secondary myocarditis. Am Heart J. 2004 Apr;147(4):746–50. [PMID: 15077094]

▶ Specific Forms of Myocarditis

A. Chagas Disease, or American Trypanosomiasis

Chagas disease is endemic in the rural areas of Central and South America.

A few cases have been reported in the Southwestern United States among immigrants from endemic areas. It is estimated that 18–20 million people are infected with the protozoan *Trypanosoma cruzi*, the organism that causes Chagas disease; of those infected, 50,000 die each year. *T cruzi* is transmitted by reduviid insects (Triatominae family). The insect becomes infected when it bites an animal or human carrier. Humans acquire the trypanosomes when the insects bite them during sleep. Alternatively, the insect might deposit its feces on the skin; trypanosomes then gain access to the bloodstream by the person rubbing the abraded skin or the conjunctivae.

Acute Chagas disease will develop in approximately 1% of the people bitten by reduviid bugs. Myocarditis may develop in this phase; however, patients usually recover within several weeks to several months. The patient may have an erythematous, pruritic skin lesion (chagoma) at the inoculation site. Unilateral, painless, palpebral edema with local lymphadenopathy (Romaña sign) is particularly common in children. After resolution of the acute phase, many patients enter a latent period during which a subclinical cardiomyopathy may develop. Approximately 30% of these patients progress to chronic Chagas disease, manifested as visceral organ enlargement (megaesophagus and megacolon) and cardiac disease, which is characterized by unrelenting congestive heart failure, malignant arrhythmias, heart block, thromboembolic phenomena, and sudden death. Cellular and humoral immune responses to *T cruzi*-altered host's cells appear to be responsible for myocardial injury. Characteristic ECG changes include right bundle branch block, with or without a left anterior fascicular block, and variable degrees of AV block. Echocardiography may demonstrate dilated ventricles, wall motion abnormalities, and specifically apical aneurysms. Active myocarditis can be demonstrated by endomyocardial biopsy using the Dallas criteria. Complement fixation test (Machado-Guerreiro test), and indirect immunofluorescent antibody assay is helpful in the diagnosis of chronic Chagas disease.

Treatment of Chagas disease is difficult, and primarily symptomatic. Heart failure is treated in the usual manner, and the use of anticoagulants and antiarrhythmic agents (amiodarone) may be warranted. Heart block may necessitate pacemaker placement. For life-threatening ventricular arrhythmia implantable cardioverter-defibrillator (ICD) implantation is indicated. Antiparasitic agents such as nifurtimox, benzimidazole, or itraconazole may be beneficial in both acute and untreated chronic Chagas disease. Cardiac transplantation may be an option in some cases; however, parasitemia is a common result of immunosuppression, and nifurtimox prophylaxis should be considered.

B. HIV

Infection with HIV is one of the leading causes of acquired heart diseases. The cardiac complications tend to occur late in the disease, and with lower CD4 counts. The HIV-related cardiac manifestations are likely to become more prevalent as therapy and longevity improve. Evidence of cardiac involvement is found at autopsy in more than 50% of patients dying with AIDS. There is a wide spectrum of cardiac manifestations in HIV patients, including pericardial, myocardial, and valvular involvement. Myocarditis in HIV patients is common. Causes may be a direct effect of HIV on the myocardium, or an autoimmune process induced by HIV alone or in conjunction with other viruses. About 20% of HIV-related myocarditis is caused by multiple infectious organisms, such as coxsackievirus group B, Epstein-Barr virus, CMV, adenovirus, *Toxoplasma gondii*, and *Histoplasma capsulatum*. HIV itself is responsible for the remaining 80% of cases. HIV cardiomyopathy is probably more related to HIV than to opportunistic infections.

Clinical presentation may be asymptomatic left ventricular systolic dysfunction or congestive heart failure. Echocardiography shows increased left ventricular dimensions, and decreased function. Myocardial biopsy reveals patchy lymphocytic infiltrate, the lymphocytes consist of T cells—mostly CD8, CD2, CD3, and rarely CD4.

Prognosis in HIV cardiomyopathy is grim, and the mortality rate is high independent of CD4 count. Rapid-onset congestive heart failure carries a worse prognosis, with 50% mortality in 6–12 months. Treatment is similar to that for other forms of cardiomyopathy. Intravenous immunoglobulins have been used with some success in acute congestive heart failure and in myocarditis in HIV-infected patients.

C. Toxoplasmosis

Active myocarditis may result from acute infection by the intracellular protozoan *T gondii*. This form is primarily diagnosed in immunocompromised persons, such as HIV patients, but may also occur following cardiac transplantation. The infection can be transmitted by the donor heart. Endomyocardial biopsy reveals edema, organisms within the myocytes in areas of focal myocyte necrosis, and a mixed inflammatory infiltrate containing eosinophils. Toxoplasmic cysts may also be seen, and a rise in antibody titer may be detected. The infection is usually asymptomatic, although heart failure, arrhythmias, and conduction abnormalities may occur. If detected early, pyrimethamine and sulfadiazine may be curative.

D. Cytomegalovirus

Symptomatic myocarditis caused by CMV infection usually occurs only in immunosuppressed patients, such as those with neoplasms, HIV disease, or transplanted organs. Asymptomatic myocarditis is known to occur in the general population but is usually self-limited. Endomyocardial biopsy may demonstrate viral inclusions within myocytes, and viral DNA can be found within the myocardium. A focal lymphocytic infiltration with fibrosis is characteristic. Treatment is with intravenous ganciclovir.

E. Lyme Myocarditis

Infection with the tick-borne spirochete *Borrelia burgdorferi* causes Lyme disease, which manifests primarily with myal-gias, arthralgias, headache, fever, adenopathy, and erythema chronicum migrans. Symptomatic, but usually transient, cardiac involvement develops in approximately 10% of infected patients. Conduction abnormalities or fluctuating degrees of AV block may be present. Syncope secondary to complete heart block is common and may require temporary transvenous pacing. Left ventricular dysfunction is rare. Endomyocardial biopsy may reveal active myocarditis. Spirochetes have been isolated from the myocardium in some patients. It is unclear whether the myocarditis of Lyme disease is a direct result of spirochetal infection or the immunologic response to it. The course of the disease is usually benign, and complete recovery is the rule.

Treatment with penicillin or doxycycline is recommended, but it is unknown if this treatment alters the course of the cardiac disease.

F. Giant Cell Myocarditis

Giant cell myocarditis is a rare form of myocarditis characterized by multinucleated giant cells within the myocardium, particularly at the margins of necrosis. The precise cause is as yet unknown although it has been associated with several autoimmune diseases, such as ulcerative colitis, Crohn disease, and myasthenia gravis. This form of myocarditis is rapid in onset and usually associated with fever and widespread ECG changes. Conduction abnormalities, including high-grade AV block and ventricular tachyarrhythmias, are more commonly seen in giant cell myocarditis than in viral myocarditis. The disease course is characterized by a progressive downhill trend regardless of medical therapy. Early recognition of this form of myocarditis is important, as the prognosis is far worse than viral myocarditis. It should be suspected in young patients with rapidly progressive heart failure that is refractory to conventional therapy. Myocardial biopsy is usually diagnostic.

Immunosuppressive therapy with a combination of cyclosporine, azathioprine, and corticosteroids appears to be beneficial, possibly prolonging the time to transplant or death. Cardiac transplantation should be considered early despite the possibility of disease recurrence in the transplanted heart.

G. Sarcoidosis

This systemic granulomatous disease is of unknown origin. The pathologic hallmark of this disease is noncaseating granuloma. The granuloma consists of activated helper-inducer T lymphocytes, macrophages, and multinucleated giant cells. The granulomas trigger a fibrotic response, resulting in organ damage.

The disease may be widespread or limited to a single organ. The lymphoid, pulmonary, cardiovascular, hepatobiliary, and hematologic systems are most commonly involved, with the lungs being affected in over 90% of patients. Cardiac sarcoidosis is more common than previously recognized and is less likely to be diagnosed antemortem than pulmonary sarcoidosis. Frequently, the initial presentation is sudden death. In myocardial sarcoidosis, portions of the myocardial wall are replaced by sarcoid granulomas. Based on the degree of myocardial involvement, the presenting signs and symptoms vary from first-degree AV block to fulminant heart failure. About 25% of deaths due to cardiac sarcoidosis are from heart failure, whereas sudden death accounts for about a third of the deaths. The diagnosis of cardiac sarcoidosis can be challenging, so evidence of other organ involvement should be sought. Chest radiography, ECG, and echocardiography are helpful diagnostic tools. Myocardial perfusion scintigraphy may demonstrate small diffusely scattered perfusion defects consistent with the granulomas (swiss cheese heart). Due to the scattered nature of the granulomas, endomyocardial biopsy lacks sensitivity and seldom aids the diagnosis despite high specificity. Treatment of sarcoidosis has not been studied by controlled trials; however, corticosteroids can improve cardiac symptoms and reverse ECG changes in over half of the treated patients. Antiarrhythmic drugs and automatic internal defibrillator placement may be indicated to decrease the risk of sudden death.

Pericardial Diseases

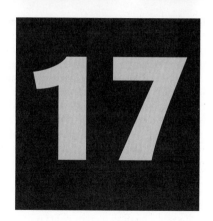

Martin M. LeWinter, MD

► General Considerations

A. Normal Pericardial Anatomy and Physiology

The pericardium consists of two layers: a serous visceral layer, which is intimately adherent to the heart and epicardial fat, and a fibrous parietal layer. The pericardium encloses the greater part of the surface of the heart, the juxtacardial portions of the pulmonary and systemic veins, and the proximal segments of the great vessels. A significant portion of the left atrium, however, is not enclosed within the pericardium. The pericardium is attached by ligaments to the manubrium sterni, the xiphoid process, the vertebral column, and the central tendon of the diaphragm. The pericardium is not essential for sustaining life or health, as evidenced by preservation of cardiac function even if the pericardium is congenitally absent or surgically removed. The pericardium does play a role in normal cardiovascular function, however, and can be involved in a number of important disease states. The normal functions of the pericardium include maintaining an optimal cardiac shape, promoting cardiac chamber interaction, preventing the overfilling of the heart, reducing friction between the beating heart and adjacent structures, providing a physical barrier to infection, and limiting displacement during the cardiac cycle.

B. Pericardial Pressure and Normal Function

The true pressure in the normal pericardial space is a matter of some controversy. When measured with fluid-filled catheters, pericardial pressure is very similar to intrapleural pressure: from −1 to −2 mm Hg on average, falling to about −5 mm Hg with normal inspiration. There is considerable evidence, however, that the pressure in the normal pericardial space is best considered as a contact force between visceral and parietal pericardium and therefore is more appropriately measured by specially-designed flat balloons. When measured in this way, the pericardial pressure is clearly higher than the intrapleural pressure, although its true magnitude

remains somewhat uncertain. The bulk of current evidence indicates that with normal cardiac volumes, the effective pericardial pressure ranges from 0–1 mm Hg to (at most) 3–4 mm Hg. The pericardial space between the parietal and visceral layers normally contains 15–50 mL of fluid, and the reserve volume of the pericardium is relatively small. Once this modest reserve is exceeded, intrapericardial pressure rises significantly. This can occur if the cardiac volume increases rapidly, for example, due to acute right ventricular myocardial infarction, or if additional fluid accumulates. With significant fluid in the pericardial space, fluid-filled catheters do provide accurate intrapericardial pressure measurements.

► Pathogenesis

A. Infectious Pathogens

1. Viral pericarditis—The most common clinical manifestation of viral involvement is acute pericarditis. An unidentified virus almost certainly underlies most cases of acute idiopathic pericarditis. The possibility of a viral cause is suggested when pericarditis occurs in the absence of other factors; it is supported by a more than fourfold rise in serial viral antibody titers during the initial weeks of illness. (Such measurement, however, is not a routine part of the management of viral pericarditis.) Frequently, a prodromal syndrome consistent with a viral infection is present.

The viral pathogens most commonly associated with pericarditis include coxsackievirus B (most common), coxsackievirus A, echovirus 8, and HIV. Although a wide range of viral agents have been implicated, no specific antiviral therapy has been shown to be effective; management and outcome are described in the section on acute pericarditis.

2. Bacterial pericarditis—Bacterial infection of the pericardium can occur following thoracic surgery, as a result of a contiguous pleural, mediastinal, or pulmonary infection, as a complication of bacterial endocarditis, or as a result of systemic bacteremia. Direct extension from pneumonia or empyema with staphylococci, pneumococci, and strepto-cocci accounts for most cases. The incidence of hospital-acquired penicillin-resistant staphylococcal pericarditis after thoracic surgery has increased during the past decade. Preexisting pericardial effusions and immunosuppressed states are important predisposing factors.

Common clinical manifestations include fever, chills, night sweats, and dyspnea; pleuritic chest pain and pericardial friction rubs are present in only a minority of patients. Leukocytosis with a shift to the left is generally present, and chest radiography usually reveals an increase in the cardiac silhouette. Although electrocardiograms (ECGs) are frequently normal, they can show typical changes of acute pericarditis.

Although high intrapericardial antibiotic levels are achievable, medical therapy alone is usually insufficient, and prompt percutaneous or surgical drainage is essential. Cardiac tamponade may occur very rapidly with hemodynamic deterioration that can be confused with septic shock. In view of the continuing high mortality rates of 65–77%, bacterial pericarditis should be considered a medical emergency.

3. Tuberculous pericarditis—Although several decades of effective antituberculous therapy and public health measures have brought about a declining rate of tuberculous pericarditis, this condition remains a major problem in immunocompromised persons and in the non-industrialized world. Thus, HIV-associated tuberculosis is a common cause of symptomatic pericardial effusion.

Tuberculous pericarditis typically occurs with no demonstrable pulmonary or extrapulmonary tuberculosis. Symptoms may be insidious and nonspecific. Findings are predominantly systemic, and pericardial friction rubs are unusual. Large effusions (Figure 17–1) and resulting tamponade are common, and constriction occurs as a late complication. Demonstration of tubercle bacillus by stain or culture is possible in only one-third to one-half of the patients, and the diagnosis is often presumptively established through a history of contact or a positive purified protein derivative (PPD) skin test. Alternatively, finding characteristic granulomata on pericardial biopsy specimens confirms the diagnosis, but even these are often falsely negative. High levels of adenosine deaminase (ADA), an enzyme produced by white blood cells in pericardial fluid, is a sensitive and specific test for tuberculous pericarditis. Increased interferon-gamma in pericardial fluid is an additional marker. Combined with ADA it provides even greater diagnostic accuracy. Most recently, polymerase chain reaction (PCR) to detect *Mycobacterium tuberculosis* DNA has been used and can be performed in minute amounts of pericardial fluid. Use of one or more of these modern tests should be routine whenever tuberculous pericarditis is suspected. Often the diagnosis of tuberculous pericarditis is made retrospectively in patients with constrictive pericarditis and a history of tuberculosis. Such cases are managed like any case of constrictive pericarditis.

Untreated tuberculous pericarditis is associated with mortality rates in excess of 80%. Management consists of

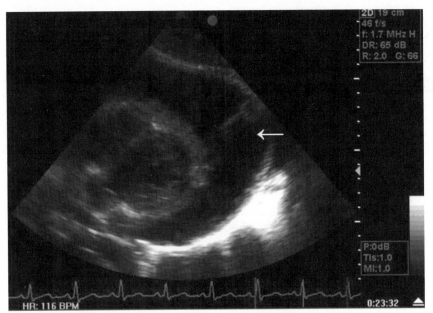

▲ **Figure 17–1.** Subcostal echocardiographic view of the heart demonstrating a large pericardial effusion (*arrow*) in a case of tuberculous pericarditis. The surface of the heart has a shaggy appearance, with frond-like structures extending to the parietal pericardium. This is typical of a tuberculous pericardial effusion. (Modified from Mayosi BM et al. Circulation. 2005;112:3608. Reprinted by permission of the American Heart Association.)

triple-drug antituberculous therapy for at least 9 months. Some authorities advocate the use of corticosteroids to prevent the development of constrictive pericarditis, but data to support this approach are inconclusive. Pericardiocentesis is indicated for patients with large or compromising effusions. As much as one-third of patients will require pericardial resection despite antibiotic therapy.

4. AIDS—The most common pericardial abnormality encountered in AIDS is an asymptomatic pericardial effusion. Small effusions can occur in HIV-positive individuals who do not have full-blown AIDS, although they often herald the transition to AIDS. Pericardial effusion can be considered part of a generalized effusive process that can involve the peritoneum and pleura as well. Asymptomatic effusions do not mandate invasive diagnostic studies or treatment, and many will resolve spontaneously without specific treatment.

In AIDS patients, symptomatic pericardial effusion with or without chest pain, friction rub, and ECG changes is caused by a variety of opportunistic infections and neoplasms. The most common infectious pathogens identified in symptomatic pericardial effusion are *M tuberculosis,* and *Mycobacterium avium-intracellulare.* The HIV virus itself can cause an effusion. Lymphomas and Kaposi sarcoma are the most common neoplasms associated with effusion. Pericarditis or symptomatic pericardial effusion in a patient with AIDS should therefore prompt an immediate search for infection or neoplasm. Pericardial effusion in HIV disease usually occurs in the context of full-blown AIDS and is strongly associated with a shortened survival time independent of the CD4 count. The mortality rate at 6 months for patients with effusion was nine times greater than for patients without effusion. There is no published information describing the effects of modern, highly active antiretroviral therapy on HIV-associated pericardial disease.

B. Iatrogenic Causes

1. Surgery-related syndromes—Several distinct pericardial syndromes may occur after heart surgery.

Cardiac tamponade may occur during in-hospital recuperation, most commonly in the first 24 hours. It is identified by the hemodynamic perturbations typical of tamponade. The sudden cessation of previously brisk bleeding from drains should alert the physician to the possibility of clogging. Therapy consists of prompt surgical exploration and evacuation. Cardiac tamponade is less common after the first 24 hours, with fewer typical clinical manifestations, and symptoms may consist largely of nonspecific generalized complaints. Two-dimensional echocardiography establishes the presence of a significant effusion and may delineate its anatomic distribution. Pericardial effusions in this setting are often loculated and may compress only one cardiac chamber. The approach to drainage is largely dictated by the location of the effusion.

Early pericarditis, consisting of fever, chest pain, pericardial friction rubs, and typical ECG features, is common. In most cases, the syndrome resolves spontaneously, and nonsteroidal antiinflammatory drugs (NSAIDs) are effective treatment.

Postpericardiotomy syndrome is reported in as many as 30–40% of patients. This syndrome, which usually occurs during the first several postoperative weeks, consists of fever, pleuritis, and pericarditis. Diagnosis proceeds by exclusion, and treatment consists of administering NSAIDs; the need for corticosteroids is rare.

Constrictive pericarditis occurs rarely as a complication of cardiac surgery. Its incidence is estimated to only be 0.2–0.3% of cardiac operations. However, cardiac surgery is emerging as an important cause of constrictive pericarditis because so many cardiac surgeries are performed in the United States annually.

Constrictive pericarditis has been reported to occur at times ranging from 2 weeks to 21 years after the surgery. Because of the relative rarity of this complication, it has been difficult to identify specific predisposing procedural factors. In the cases of constriction reported in the literature, 95% have been associated with an open pericardium, which may serve as a reservoir for the collection of blood. Occasionally, constrictive pericarditis appears within days or weeks after surgery. These cases appear to respond well to a course of corticosteroids. With this exception, the mainstay of therapy for postsurgical constrictive pericarditis is pericardiectomy.

2. Trauma—Traumatic hemorrhagic pericardial effusions, which can result from blunt or penetrating injuries of the chest, can also be caused by a variety of iatrogenic causes such as cardiac catheterization and coronary interventional procedures, pacemaker insertion, arrhythmia ablation procedures, endoscopy, and closed chest cardiac massage. The rapidity with which pericardial fluid can accumulate can quickly cause hemodynamic compromise. Hypotension in this setting should prompt both an immediate echocardiographic search for pericardial fluid and swift evacuation of any significant effusions. Delayed manifestations may include recurrent pericardial effusions and, in rare cases, constrictive pericarditis.

3. Radiation therapy—The incidence of pericardial injury from therapeutic radiation is related to dose, duration, and technical features. Pericardial damage from radiation may appear during the course of therapy or following it. The syndrome that appears during radiation therapy is acute pericarditis. The onset of clinical manifestations in the delayed form is usually within 12 months but may take many years. The clinical features of the late form range from asymptomatic pericardial effusions to acute pericarditis or constrictive pericarditis. Radiation therapy is now one of the leading causes of constrictive pericarditis. Diagnosis and management are discussed later in the sections on pericardial effusion and constrictive pericarditis.

C. Connective Tissue Disorders

1. Rheumatoid arthritis—Pericarditis has been found during postmortem examination in up to 50% of patients with rheumatoid arthritis. The clinical recognition of pericarditis during life, however, is far less frequent. Tamponade may occur rarely as a complication of pericardial effusion in rheumatoid arthritis and should be treated appropriately. Patients with nodular rheumatoid arthritis are much more likely to develop pericarditis than are those without nodules, and pericarditis commonly occurs in association with arthritis and pleuritis. Symptomatic pericarditis can be treated with NSAIDs. There is no evidence to support a role for corticosteroids in preventing constrictive pericarditis; as in other conditions, the presence of constrictive pericarditis warrants pericardiectomy.

2. Systemic lupus erythematosus—Pericarditis is the most common cardiac manifestation of systemic lupus erythematosus (SLE) and tends to occur during periods of active disease. Clinical and ECG features tend to be typical of acute pericarditis. Although tamponade can complicate pericarditis, progression to constrictive pericarditis is rare. Pericarditis generally subsides as systemic manifestations improve in response to corticosteroid or immunosuppressive therapy.

3. Progressive systemic sclerosis—As in rheumatoid arthritis, pericarditis is found during autopsy more frequently than during life. Asymptomatic pericardial effusions can be found in up to 40% of patients. Patients with scleroderma may have typical symptoms of pericarditis and nonspecific ECG changes, and tamponade may occur. The prognosis is generally poor for patients with scleroderma in whom pericarditis develops. Pericardial involvement can also occur in association with myocardial involvement and differentiating constrictive pericarditis from restrictive cardiomyopathy may be difficult.

D. Other Causes

1. Myocardial infarction—Clinical evidence of pericarditis can be found in 7–20% of patients within the first week after myocardial infarction, although autopsy series suggest a significantly higher incidence of clinically silent, localized fibrinous pericarditis. The incidence is greatest with large, ST-segment elevation myocardial infarctions. Anticoagulant therapy and antiplatelet therapy administered in conjunction with percutaneous revascularization procedures do not appear to increase the incidence of pericardial effusions after myocardial infarction. While it is theoretically possible that these drugs may increase the chance of hemorrhage into the pericardial space if an effusion does occur, they are not generally considered to be contraindicated in the setting of early postmyocardial infarction pericarditis. Thrombolytic therapy has been associated with a decreased incidence of pericarditis in placebo-controlled studies. Because these agents can contribute to the development of tamponade, however, their use may be relatively contraindicated when concurrent pericarditis is identified.

Dressler syndrome (postmyocardial infarction syndrome) occurs from 1 to 6 weeks after myocardial infarction and consists of fever, pleuropericardial pain, malaise, and evidence of pleural and pericardial effusions. The syndrome is a contraindication to anticoagulant therapy because pericardial hemorrhage can occur, increasing the likelihood of tamponade. The incidence of this syndrome has been decreasing in recent years. It is believed to have an autoimmune cause due to sensitization to myocardial cells at the time of necrosis. Antimyocardial antibodies have been demonstrated in patients with Dressler syndrome. Management is as outlined in the section on pericarditis.

2. Malignancy—A variety of hematologic and solid malignancies can cause pericardial metastases that are more frequently revealed during autopsy than during life. Typically, the diagnosis of malignancy has already been established in the patient with a malignant pericardial effusion, and other sites of metastatic spread are evident. On rare occasions, tamponade from the malignant effusion is the first manifestation of tumor. It is important to distinguish malignant effusions from other causes of effusion, such as radiation, infection, and uremia, because the management and prognosis of malignant and nonmalignant effusions in cancer patients differ substantially. The diagnosis is established through echocardiography and cytologic examination; the fluid will be positive in approximately 80% of malignant effusions, with the balance usually positively identified through surgical biopsy of the pericardium. There may be a role for routine measurement of selected tumor markers as a general screen for malignant effusion and an adjunct to direct detection of malignant cells.

Patients may survive for a number of months or occasionally longer after a diagnosis of malignant effusion; therapy to alleviate symptoms and prevent reaccumulation of the effusion is therefore indicated (treatment of nonmalignant effusions is discussed in the section on Pericardial Effusion). Pericardiocentesis usually provides immediate relief. Subsequent management to control the effusion may include radiation or chemotherapy for tumors, such as breast cancer, lymphoma, and leukemia, that are sensitive to these modalities. Instillation of chemicals, most commonly tetracycline, into the pericardium is effective in most cases but can be associated with unpleasant side effects such as pain and fever. Surgical approaches include subxiphoid pericardiotomy or thoracotomy with either pleuropericardiotomy or pericardiectomy. The subxiphoid approach, which can frequently be carried out under local anesthetic, has the advantage of high success rates and low morbidity and mortality. Malignancies, most commonly lymphomas, can also involve the pericardium through enlargement of anterior mediastinal lymph nodes and obstruction of lymphatic drainage. Shrinking the lymph nodes by chemotherapy or radiation therapy may dramatically improve the resulting effusions.

3. Renal failure—Pericardial involvement in patients with renal failure can take several forms. Pericardial effusions can be found on an echocardiogram in many patients with chronic kidney disease who are asymptomatic. These effusions, which are typically small, are related more closely to the patient's volume status than other variables and usually warrant no intervention beyond clinical vigilance.

The incidence of uremic pericarditis has been decreasing for years, a trend attributable to earlier and more intensive dialysis. Uremic pericarditis typically occurs before the initiation of long-term dialysis; its development is related, in part, to the elevation of absolute levels of blood urea nitrogen (BUN) and serum creatinine, and it almost always responds to dialysis. Patients in this setting can have symptoms and signs typical of acute pericarditis, or they may have few symptoms despite large pericardial effusions, with or without a pericardial rub. Although uremic pericarditis can lead to tamponade, it is more commonly associated with the slow accumulation of large, low-pressure pericardial effusions. As in any clinical setting, tamponade warrants prompt evacuation of the pericardial fluid.

Classic ECG changes of acute pericarditis are present in less than half the patients; abnormalities are more often nonspecific and may include atrial fibrillation. Complications from pericardiocentesis in this patient population may be more frequent than in other groups of patients with pericardial effusions.

Pericardial involvement can also occur in patients who are already undergoing dialysis. The development of dialysis-related pericardial disease is not strongly related to serum BUN or creatinine levels. Chest pain, typically pleuritic, is the most common symptom. Pericarditis in a patient undergoing dialysis presents complicated management issues. In a significant fraction of these patients, the pericarditis may have an identifiable, remediable cause that should be promptly identified. Although most patients in whom pericarditis develops while undergoing dialysis respond to intensification of the dialysis regimen, a significant subset do not improve. Clinical predictors of failure include fever higher than 102 °F, evidence of heart failure, a white blood cell count greater than 15,000/mcL, a large effusion observed echocardiographically, and the use of peritoneal dialysis as a sole treatment modality. NSAIDs may be tried, but a randomized, prospective study found indomethacin effective only in ameliorating fever. It did not affect the duration of chest pain and pericardial rub or the subsequent development of tamponade. When intensive dialysis and NSAIDs have failed to remedy symptomatic pericarditis, colchicine therapy (see below) should be considered. Effusions resulting in tamponade should be treated in the usual fashion. If tamponade recurs following an initial episode, creation of a pericardial window is recommended.

4. Drug-related causes—A number of pharmacologic agents have been implicated in pericardial disease. Pericarditis can occur as a feature of drug-induced SLE syndrome caused by procainamide, hydralazine, diphenylhydantoin, reserpine, methyldopa, and isoniazid. In addition to their propensity for causing myocardial inflammation, anthracycline antineoplastic agents can cause acute pericarditis. Methysergide can cause pericardial constriction as part of the syndrome of mediastinal fibrosis, and pericarditis can be part of a hypersensitivity reaction to penicillin. Minoxidil has been reported to cause pericarditis and tamponade; the mechanism is unknown.

5. Hypothyroidism—Pericardial effusion can be found in one-third of patients with myxedema. The frequency of pericardial involvement is related to both the severity and duration of hypothyroidism. The accumulation of pericardial fluid in this condition appears to be a result of a combination of increased capillary permeability and retarded lymphatic drainage. Because the pericardial fluid accumulates slowly, tamponade is rare. The ECG demonstrates low QRS. If pericardiocentesis is required before the diagnosis of hypothyroidism is made, the diagnosis can be suspected if the fluid is yellow and contains a high level of cholesterol. Pericardial disease in hypothyroidism reliably responds to thyroid hormone replacement therapy.

Alpert MA et al. Pericardial involvement in end-stage renal disease. Am J Med Sci. 2003 Apr;325(4):228–36. [PMID: 12695728]

Barbaro G. Pathogenesis of HIV-associated cardiovascular disease. Adv Cardiol. 2003;40:49–70. [PMID: 14533546]

Ben-Horin S et al. Large symptomatic pericardial effusion as the presentation of unrecognized cancer: a study in 173 consecutive patients undergoing pericardiocentesis. Medicine (Baltimore). 2006 Jan;85(1):49–53. [PMID: 16523053]

Fasseas P et al. Incidence, correlates, management, and clinical outcome of coronary perforation: analysis of 16,298 procedures. Am Heart J. 2004 Jan;147(1):140–5. [PMID: 14691432]

Frankel KM. Treating malignancy-related effusions. Chest. 2003 May;123(5):1775. [PMID: 12740308]

Gowda RM et al. Cardiac tamponade in patients with human immunodeficiency virus disease. Angiology. 2003 Jul–Aug;54(4):469–74. [PMID: 12934767]

Hoit BD. Management of effusive and constrictive pericardial heart disease. Circulation. 2002 Jun 25;105(25):2939–42. [PMID: 12081983]

Hsu LF et al. Incidence and prevention of cardiac tamponade complicating ablation for atrial fibrillation. Pacing Clin Electrophysiol. 2005 Jan;28 Suppl 1:S106–9. [PMID: 15683473]

Imazio M et al. Relation of acute pericardial disease to malignancy. Am J Cardiol. 2005 Jun 1;95(11):1393–4. [PMID: 15904655]

Maisch B et al. Guidelines on the diagnosis and management of pericardial diseases executive summary; The Task force on the diagnosis and management of pericardial diseases of the European society of cardiology. Eur Heart J. 2004 Apr;25(7):587–610. [PMID: 15120056]

Maisch B et al. Intrapericardial treatment of autoreactive pericardial effusion with triamcinolone; the way to avoid side effects of systemic corticosteroid therapy. Eur Heart J. 2002 Oct;23(19):1503–8. [PMID: 12242070]

Maisch B et al. Practical aspects of the management of pericardial disease. Heart. 2003 Sep;89(9):1096–103. [PMID: 12923044]

Mayosi BM et al. Tuberculous pericarditis. Circulation. 2005 Dec 6;112(23):3608–16. [PMID: 16330703]

Silva-Cardoso J et al. Pericardial involvement in human immunodeficiency virus infection. Chest. 1999 Feb;115(2):418–22. [PMID: 10027441]

Weich HS et al. Large pericardial effusions due to systemic lupus erythematosus: a report of eight cases. Lupus. 2005;14(6):450–7. [PMID: 16038109]

Witzke CF et al. The changing pattern of coronary perforation during percutaneous coronary intervention in the new device era. J Invasive Cardiol. 2004 Jun;16(6):257–301. [PMID: 15155997]

ACUTE PERICARDITIS

 ESSENTIALS OF DIAGNOSIS

▶ Central chest pain aggravated by coughing, inspiration, or recumbency.

▶ Pericardial friction rub on auscultation.

▶ Characteristic ECG changes.

▶ General Considerations

Acute pericarditis is an inflammatory condition of the pericardium that can be caused by virtually any of the conditions just discussed. As discussed above, a viral infection is the most common cause.

▶ Clinical Findings

A. Symptoms and Signs

The primary symptom of acute pericarditis is chest pain whose location, intensity, and nature are variable. The pain may be described as sharp or dull. Most often it is precordial or retrosternal in location and may be referred to the trapezius ridge, which is almost pathognomonic for pericarditis. It is characteristically aggravated by inspiration, coughing, or recumbency and lessened by sitting upright and leaning forward. Although it typically takes an hour or two to develop fully, the pain can sometimes appear remarkably abruptly. Many patients relate prodromal symptoms suggestive of a viral infection.

B. Physical Examination

Patients with pericarditis may be febrile and tachycardiac. The pericardial friction rub—the characteristic auscultatory finding—is typically scratchy and has three components corresponding to atrial contraction, ventricular systole, and early diastole. It is not unusual for only one or two components to be audible; the systolic component is most consistently present. Exercise may facilitate the identification of all three components. Because the friction rub may be evanescent, varying widely in intensity even in the course of a single day, repeated auscultation is important. Furthermore, because posture can affect the pericardial rub, auscultation

with the patient in several positions, (supine, sitting, etc) is often helpful. When the intensity of the rub is modulated significantly by respiration, it is termed a "pleuropericardial friction rub."

C. Diagnostic Studies

Evaluation of a patient with suspected pericarditis should routinely include an ECG, complete blood count, chest radiograph, creatine kinase with MB fraction, troponin I, and an echocardiogram. Additional diagnostic laboratory tests should be tailored to the clinical presentation. Echocardiography is a sensitive test for detecting pericardial effusion; however, pericardial effusion can occur in the absence of pericardial inflammation.

1. Electrocardiography—Serial ECGs are valuable in diagnosing pericarditis. Four stages of ECG changes have been described (Table 17–1). In stage I, the changes accompany the onset of chest pain and consist of widespread ST-segment elevation (Figure 17–2). The ST segment is concave upward (in distinction to the elevation in myocardial infarction). ST-segment elevation is typically present in all leads except aVR and V_1, where ST-segment depression is often present. The T waves are upright in the leads with ST elevation. The stage I pattern of pericarditis may be difficult to distinguish from the normal variant of early repolarization. A differentiating point that may be useful is the ST:T ratio in V_6. A T-wave apex four times (or greater) higher than the height of the ST segment is more likely to indicate early repolarization; if this ratio is less than 4, pericarditis is more likely. In addition, pericarditis causes changes in the ECG that distinguish it from early repolarization. In stage II, typically occurring several days later, the ST segments return to baseline, and the initially upright T waves flatten. In stage III, the T waves invert, and the ST segments may become depressed—changes that may persist indefinitely. Finally, in stage IV, which may occur weeks or months later, the T waves revert to normal. All four stages can be serially identified in about 50% of patients.

2. Other tests—Laboratory evidence of inflammation, such as mild leukocytosis and a modestly elevated erythrocyte sedimentation rate, is common in viral or idiopathic pericarditis. These findings are less consistent in pericarditis

Table 17–1. Serial Electrocardiographic Changes in Pericarditis.

Stage	ST Segment	T Waves
I	Elevated	Upright
II	Isoelectric	Upright → flat
III	Isoelectric	Inverted
IV	Isoelectric	Upright

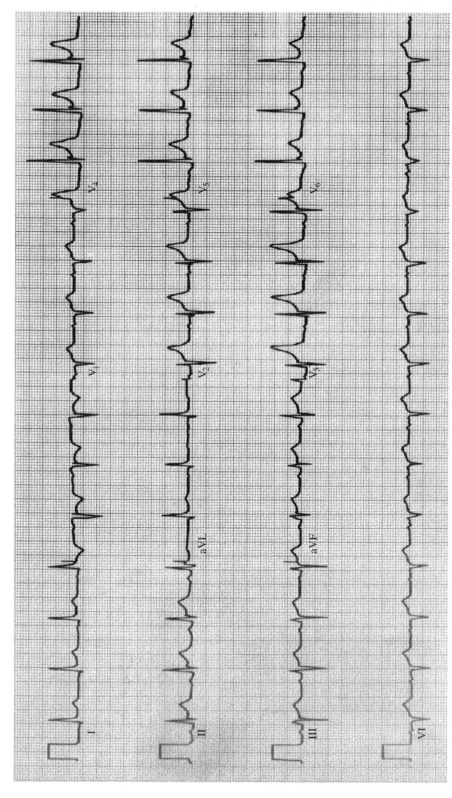

▲ **Figure 17–2.** Electrocardiogram of the first stage of pericarditis demonstrating diffuse ST-segment elevation and upright T waves.

associated with uremia or connective tissue disorders. Cardiac enzymes may be slightly elevated when the inflammatory process involves subepicardial myocardium. Alternatively, some cases occur in conjunction with a true viral myocarditis with more substantial elevations in creatine kinase and troponin I. Although the chest radiograph most often reveals no abnormalities in uncomplicated pericarditis, it may occasionally show evidence of pericardial effusion (discussed in the following section).

Treatment

The management of pericarditis associated with an identifiable etiology is directed primarily to the underlying cause. In the usual case of idiopathic acute pericarditis, treatment with any of the NSAIDs usually suppresses the clinical manifestations within 24 hours—and frequently more rapidly. Because of its excellent side-effect profile, ibuprofen, 800 mg orally three times a day for 10–14 days, is recommended. Colchicine, which has an excellent track record in the prophylaxis of recurrent pericarditis (see below), may be added if there is a slow or inadequate response to initial NSAID treatment. A 2–3 mg loading dose followed by 1 mg daily is recommended. A short course of corticosteroids is very effective in ameliorating the pain of acute pericarditis. However, their use is rarely required and recent evidence suggests they may increase the chance of recurrence. Accordingly, corticosteroids should be avoided unless absolutely necessary to control severe symptoms that do not respond to other measures.

In about 85–90% of patients, a single course of NSAID therapy will effectively control the illness, and pericarditis will resolve without sequelae. In a small number of patients, a recurrence may develop over a period of weeks or months after the initial episode. Recurrences can be managed with repeated courses of an NSAID or colchicine, or both. In difficult cases of recurrent pericarditis, prolonged colchicine therapy has demonstrated efficacy in prophylaxis and should be strongly considered. While corticosteroids in general should also be avoided in chronic, recurrent pericarditis, occasional patients can best be managed with very brief, intensive courses of prednisone at the first sign of symptoms. Rarely, immunosuppressive drugs such as azathioprine and cyclophosphamide may be helpful in these patients, but there is virtually no organized experience with their use.

In rare cases, frequent and severe recurrences despite aggressive medical therapy have prompted pericardiectomy. However, the efficacy of pericardiectomy in this circumstance is unknown and in one small series was reported to only rarely be effective.

Imazio M et al. Colchicine as first-choice therapy for recurrent pericarditis: results of the CORE (COlchicine for REcurrent pericarditis) trial. Arch Intern Med. 2005 Sep 26;165(17):1987–91. [PMID: 16186468]

Imazio M et al. Colchicine in addition to conventional therapy for acute pericarditis: results of the COlchicine for acute PEricarditis (COPE) trial. Circulation. 2005 Sep 27;112(13):2012–6. [PMID: 16186437]
Imazio M et al. Day-hospital treatment of acute pericarditis: a management program for outpatient therapy. J Am Coll Cardiol. 2004 Mar 17;43(6):1042–6. [PMID: 15028364]
Lange RA et al. Clinical practice. Acute pericarditis. N Engl J Med. 2004 Nov 18;351(21):2195–202. [PMID: 15548780]
Spodick DH. Acute pericarditis: current concepts and practice. JAMA. 2003 Mar 5;289(9):1150–3. [PMID: 12622586]

PERICARDIAL EFFUSION

 ESSENTIALS OF DIAGNOSIS

▶ Echocardiographic demonstration of pericardial fluid.

General Considerations

Pericardial effusion can develop as a result of pericarditis or an injury of any kind to the parietal pericardium. It can be encountered in the absence of pericarditis in many clinical settings, such as, uremia, cardiac trauma or chamber rupture, malignancy, AIDS, and hypothyroidism.

Clinical Findings

A. Symptoms and Signs

Clinical manifestations of pericardial effusion are directly related to the absolute volume of the effusion and the rapidity of accumulation. Small, incidental effusions rarely, if ever, cause symptoms or complications, and patients with slowly developing pericardial effusions can accumulate large volumes of fluid without symptoms. With a very slowly accumulating effusion, the pericardium can accommodate 1–2 L or more of fluid without a clinically significant elevation of intrapericardial pressure. Many of these large effusions are discovered incidentally when a chest radiograph is performed. Some may become clinically manifest by compression of adjacent structures or by causing dysphagia, cough, dyspnea, hiccups, hoarseness, nausea, or a sense of abdominal fullness. It is exceedingly rare for a specific cause of large, incidentally discovered effusions to be identified. In contrast, more rapid accumulation of even modest fluid volumes can be associated with increased intrapericardial pressures and life-threatening hemodynamic compromise.

B. Physical Examination

On examination, signs of pericardial effusion are absent in patients who have small effusions without increased pressure. Large effusions may muffle the heart sounds or cause left lower lobe lung dullness to percussion of the chest (Ewart sign) as a result of compression of lung parenchyma.

C. Diagnostic Studies

1. Electrocardiography—The ECG may be entirely normal. Large effusions can cause both reduced voltage and electrical alternans, alternating QRS voltage as a result of a swinging motion of the heart that characteristically occurs at a frequency of half the heart rate. If pericarditis coexists with effusion, the usual findings may be present.

2. Chest radiography—An increase in the cardiac silhouette combined with clear or oligemic lung fields suggests the presence of a significant pericardial effusion, although the chest radiograph can appear entirely normal in the presence of a small to moderate effusion. Very rapidly accumulating fluid may result in only the subtlest of changes in the cardiac silhouette. With slowly accumulating fluid, the cardiac silhouette may assume a globular shape that has been likened to a water bottle. Radiographic differentiation of pericardial effusion and cardiac enlargement may not be possible. Occasionally, the presence of an effusion may cause increased separation of the pericardial fat-pad layers.

3. Echocardiography—Transthoracic echocardiography is the fastest and most accurate means of diagnosing and estimating the size of a pericardial effusion, but it is not accurate in assessing pericardial thickness. The effusion appears as an echo-free space between the moving epicardium and the stationary pericardium. Although M-mode echocardiography can identify effusions as small as 20 mL, two-dimensional echocardiography has the advantage of demonstrating the full distribution of the effusion and identifying a loculated effusion. Quantification of the volume of effusion by echocardiography is not always precise. Small effusions tend to be imaged only posteriorly; a posterior echo-free space, however, may reflect subepicardial fat rather than pericardial effusion. Larger effusions are usually distributed both anteriorly and posteriorly. On occasion, large effusions are associated with an excessive swinging motion of the heart within the fluid-filled pericardium. Transesophageal echocardiography is particularly useful in quantifying the anatomic distribution of effusions, especially when loculated, and is superior to transthoracic echocardiography in imaging the thickness of the pericardium.

4. Cardiac magnetic resonance imaging and computed tomography—Both of these modalities provide highly accurate imaging of pericardial effusions but, in most cases, are not necessary if echocardiographic images are technically satisfactory. However, they are the most accurate methods for delineating the size of effusions, their anatomic distribution, and the thickness of the pericardium. Thus, they are often valuable adjuncts to echocardiography.

▶ Treatment

The management of a pericardial effusion is largely dictated by its size, the presence or absence of hemodynamic compromise from increased intrapericardial pressure (see next section),

and the nature of the underlying disorder (discussed earlier). In most cases, a small or incidentally discovered effusion warrants no specific intervention. At the same time it should be recalled that once an effusion reaches a certain magnitude, even small additional amounts of fluid can cause a marked increase in intrapericardial pressure and rapid clinical deterioration; these patients must be monitored closely. Very large, chronic effusions discovered accidentally usually do not progress. However, some of these will eventually result in cardiac tamponade. Therefore, elective, closed pericardiocentesis may be recommended in these cases. Interestingly, these effusions typically do not recur following removal of the fluid.

Goland S et al. Idiopathic chronic pericardial effusion. N Engl J Med. 2000 May 11;342(19):1449. [PMID: 10809614]

Hoit BD. Management of effusive and constrictive pericardial heart disease. Circulation. 2002 Jun 25;105(25):2939–42. [PMID: 12081983]

Little WC et al. Pericardial disease. Circulation. 2006 Mar 28;113(12):1622–32. [PMID: 16567581]

Oyama N et al. Computed tomography and magnetic resonance imaging of the pericardium: anatomy and pathology. Magn Reson Med Sci. 2004 Dec 15;3(3):145–52. [PMID: 16093632]

CARDIAC TAMPONADE

ESSENTIALS OF DIAGNOSIS

▶ Increased jugular venous pressure with an obliterated *y* descent.

▶ Pulsus paradoxus.

▶ Echocardiographic evidence of right atrial and ventricular collapse.

▶ Equal diastolic pressures in all four cardiac chambers.

▶ General Considerations

Cardiac tamponade exists when increased intrapericardial pressure from accumulation of fluid compromises the filling of the heart, thereby impairing cardiac output. Whether the intrapericardial pressure rises to a level that impedes filling depends on both the rapidity of accumulation and the volume of the effusion. Severe tamponade may thus ensue in the setting of a traumatic effusion where a modest volume of blood fills the pericardial space in a brief time. Conversely, in settings such as myxedema or chronic idiopathic effusions, a slowly accumulating effusion may reach a remarkably large volume without raising the intrapericardial pressure.

▶ Clinical Findings

A. Symptoms and Signs

Patients with cardiac tamponade may complain of dyspnea and chest discomfort. In more severe cases, consciousness may be impaired, and there may be signs of reduced cardiac output and shock. The systemic arterial pressure is typically low, although it may be surprisingly well-preserved on occasion; pulse pressure is usually diminished. The patient with tamponade is typically tachycardiac and tachypneic although bradycardia may ensue in terminal stages. Patients with tamponade are almost always more comfortable sitting upright. If pericarditis coexists, typical pain and a friction rub may be present.

1. Pulsus paradoxus—Pulsus paradoxus, defined as an abnormally large decline in systolic arterial pressure during inspiration, is present in most cases. The term is actually something of a misnomer because the paradoxical pulse represents an exaggeration of the normal small decline in systolic arterial pressure that occurs during inspiration. Pulsus paradoxus is evaluated through careful auscultation of the Korotkoff sounds as the cuff pressure is slowly released. It is measured as the difference in cuff pressure from the point at which sounds are initially heard intermittently during expiration and the point at which the sounds are audible throughout the respiratory cycle and with each ventricular systole. A pulsus paradoxus greater than 10 mm Hg is considered abnormal. In severe tamponade, the peripheral pulse reveals an obvious decrease in the stroke volume and may even disappear on inspiration. The presence of an abnormal pulsus paradoxus is not essential to the diagnosis of cardiac tamponade, and it may be absent in clinical situations where tamponade coexists with cardiac volume overload lesions, such as atrial septal defect or aortic insufficiency. The absence of a pulsus paradoxus in these settings should not dissuade the physician from the correct diagnosis. In addition, pulsus paradoxus can be present when the inspiratory decrease in intrapleural pressure is exaggerated, as in obstructive airway disease. Reversed pulsus paradoxus—a fall in pressure with expiration—can be seen in patients on positive pressure respirators.

2. Jugular venous pressure—The venous pressure is usually markedly elevated, and examination of the jugular venous pulse wave reveals obliteration of the normal y descent. In patients with low-pressure tamponade (see section on Cardiac catheterization), the venous pressure may actually be normal or only mildly elevated.

3. Other findings—Diminished heart sounds can be heard in one-third of cases; a pericardial friction rub may be heard but is absent in most patients. The concept of an inverse relation between the intensity of a pericardial rub (when present) and the size of the effusion cannot be used in assessing individual patients; the relationship is too variable to be reliable.

B. Diagnostic Studies

1. Electrocardiography—Electrocardiography may offer no specific diagnostic clues, although the ECG abnormalities described in pericarditis and pericardial effusion may be seen. The development of electrical alternans almost always indicates a hemodynamically significant effusion.

2. Chest radiography—Chest radiography offers no specific diagnostic signs of tamponade. As mentioned earlier, the cardiac silhouette may be remarkably normal in size in cases where a modestly sized effusion accumulates rapidly. A pericardial fat pad sign is diagnostic of pericardial effusion but does not necessarily indicate tamponade. The lung fields are frequently oligemic. Occasionally, the chest radiograph offers clues to important coexisting conditions, such as aortic dissection or malignancy.

3. Echocardiography—Echocardiography is an invaluable adjunctive tool. It confirms the presence of pericardial fluid and can provide evidence of increased intrapericardial pressure. The most useful echocardiographic sign is diastolic collapse of the right atrium and right ventricle. Though these changes are neither completely sensitive nor specific, they first occur when the pericardial pressure transiently exceeds the intracardiac chamber pressure. They can therefore be useful in identifying patients whose pericardial pressure level should be of concern. Echocardiography is also extremely useful as a guide in pericardiocentesis. The cardiac chambers are small in tamponade and, as discussed above, in extreme cases the heart swings anteroposteriorly within the effusion. Distention of the caval vessels that does not diminish with inspiration is another useful sign.

Doppler velocity recordings demonstrate exaggerated respiratory variation in right- and left-sided venous and valvular flow, with marked inspiratory increases on the right and decreases on the left. Loss of the y descent in the jugular venous pressure is caused by reduced systemic venous inflow during early diastole. Correspondingly, Doppler evaluation reveals that most caval and pulmonary venous inflow occurs during ventricular systole. These flow patterns were found to have a sensitivity of 75% and a specificity of 91% for diagnosing tamponade. The *absence* of chamber collapse is especially useful in excluding tamponade in patients with effusions but its presence is less well-correlated with tamponade than abnormal venous flow patterns. Newer techniques such as tissue Doppler do not yet have a well-defined, additive role in cardiac tamponade.

4. Cardiac catheterization—In the patient with tamponade, cardiac catheterization reveals a depressed cardiac output as well as elevated and equal or near-equal filling pressures in all four chambers. Examination of the atrial pressure waveforms reveals the loss of the normal y descent. The initial presentation and hemodynamic profile of tamponade may, however, be altered by a concomitant state of intravascular volume depletion, a scenario that has been called **low-pressure cardiac tamponade.** This term underscores an important feature of the pathophysiology of pericardial effusions; the hemodynamic effect is a function of both the intrapericardial pressure and the intravascular volume.

Although this syndrome typically occurs in patients undergoing dialysis for chronic renal failure, it can be encountered in any setting of increased intrapericardial fluid and intravascular volume depletion. In these patients, the effusions are ordinarily insufficient to cause major hemodynamic embarrassment; they become significant when intravascular volume is depleted. The diagnosis should be considered in patients who become unusually hypotensive during dialysis. In some cases, volume expansion will result in more typical hemodynamic findings.

▶ Treatment

Drainage of pericardial fluid is the cornerstone of therapy; reflecting the small pericardial reserve volume, draining even modest amounts (100–200 mL) of fluid may result in striking improvement. Drainage is most commonly achieved by subxiphoid percutaneous pericardiocentesis. Although the procedure is effective and safe, there may be complications; the most common serious complication is laceration or puncture of the heart, typically the right ventricle, because of its anterior location. Echocardiography, by confirming the presence of a sufficiently large volume of fluid in an anterior location, can decrease the risk of cardiac puncture. The presence of at least 1 cm of echo-free space anterior to the heart has been recommended as a guideline for the minimum volume of fluid that should be present before percutaneous pericardiocentesis is undertaken. In addition, the patient should be positioned in a semiupright position to allow inferior pooling of the effusion.

Several aspects of the performance of pericardiocentesis also contribute to a safe and successful outcome. The procedure is ideally carried out in the cardiac catheterization laboratory with fluoroscopic guidance and concomitant right-heart catheterization. The latter allows for hemodynamic confirmation of the diagnosis and assessment of the response to therapy. Occasionally, performance of emergency pericardiocentesis may be required at the bedside; however, it is rare for circumstances to be so critical as to preclude confirming the diagnosis with echocardiography.

Intravenous fluids and pressors can be administered as temporizing measures until the procedure can be performed. These modalities usually will not significantly improve the clinical status, however, and should never be used in place of or allowed to interfere with prompt evacuation of the fluid.

Pericardial fluid can also be evacuated through a subxiphoid surgical pericardiotomy performed under local anesthesia; this procedure also permits pericardial biopsy in cases of suspected malignant effusion. The pericardial fluid should be sent for cultures and cytologic examination except when the tamponade is clearly traumatic. The gross appearance of the fluid is not helpful in establishing the cause, and cell counts and chemistries are also of limited value. The risks of pericardiocentesis must therefore be weighed against the likely benefits before performing the procedure solely for diagnostic purposes. Usually a pericardial biopsy is most useful when the diagnosis is unclear.

In some cases, a single pericardiocentesis alleviates the effusion fully, but in most cases, a pericardial catheter should be left in place for continued drainage, typically for 24–48 hours. The catheter can be removed when the rate of drainage decreases and plans for definitive management of the pericardial disease are in place. Subsequent management is largely dictated by the specific cause of the effusion (discussed earlier).

Definitive management of pericardial fluid accumulation in some conditions may require surgical removal of the pericardium or the surgical creation of an opening between the pericardium and left pleura (a pericardial window). A percutaneous balloon technique for creating a pleuropericardial opening has also been described. If tissue is not required for diagnostic purposes, this may be the preferred technique for draining a chronically recurring effusion and preventing tamponade. However, at present, few centers have sufficient experience with this method. Pericardial windows can close in patients with intense inflammation, and pericardial stripping may be required.

Kuvin JT et al. Postoperative cardiac tamponade in the modern surgical era. Ann Thorac Surg. 2002 Oct;74(4):1148–53. [PMID: 12400760]

Spodick DM. Acute cardiac tamponade. N Engl J Med. 2003 Aug 14;349(7):684–90. [PMID: 12917306]

Tsang TS et al. Outcomes of clinically significant idiopathic pericardial effusion requiring intervention. Am J Cardiol. 2003 Mar 15;91(6):704–7. [PMID: 12633802]

Tsang TS et al. Consecutive 1127 therapeutic echocardiographically guided pericardiocenteses: clinical profile, practice patterns, and outcomes spanning 21 years. Mayo Clin Proc. 2002 May;77(5):429–36. [PMID: 12004992]

CONSTRICTIVE PERICARDITIS

ESSENTIALS OF DIAGNOSIS

▶ Markedly elevated jugular venous pressure with accentuated x and y descents and Kussmaul sign.

▶ Pericardial knock on auscultation.

▶ Magnetic resonance, computed tomography, or echocardiographic imaging showing a thickened pericardium.

▶ General Considerations

Constrictive pericarditis can develop as the aftermath of virtually any pericardial injury or inflammation. Cardiac surgery, radiation therapy, and idiopathic causes are currently the most common. Tuberculous constriction, a leading cause in previous decades, is now rare in most of the industrialized world, but it remains significant in underdeveloped countries and may reappear in developed countries if tuberculosis continues to increase. A highly variable length of time—sometimes many years—can elapse between the initial insult and the development of constriction and its clinical manifestations.

The major physiologic perturbation of constrictive pericarditis is thickening, fibrosis, and (especially with tuberculosis) calcification of the pericardium, causing it to encase the heart in a solid, noncompliant envelope that impairs diastolic filling. In early diastole, the ventricles fill normally until the volume limit of the noncompliant pericardium is attained. At that point, diastolic filling halts abruptly. At the same time, the rigid pericardium markedly increases the intracardiac filling pressures. Because contractile function is usually normal, constrictive pericarditis can be considered an extreme example of heart failure that is caused by diastolic dysfunction.

▶ Clinical Findings

A. Symptoms and Signs

Many symptoms of constrictive pericarditis are nonspecific and are related to chronically elevated cardiac filling pressures and chronically depressed cardiac output; symptoms secondary to venous congestion are most common. Ascites, peripheral edema, and symptoms referable to congestion of the gastrointestinal tract and liver (eg, dyspepsia, anorexia, and postprandial fullness) usually develop. Cardiac cirrhosis may be present in extreme cases. Symptoms of left-sided congestion, such as exertional dyspnea, orthopnea, and cough, may occur but are much less frequent. The chronically low cardiac output results in fatigue and, in conjunction with the effects of visceral congestion, wasting.

B. Physical Examination

The patient may have a striking body habitus with a marked contrast between a massively swollen abdomen and edematous lower extremities and a cachectic, wasted upper torso. Ascites, hepatomegaly with prominent hepatic pulsations, and other signs of hepatic failure are common.

Patients with constrictive pericarditis have marked elevation of the jugular venous pressure. In contrast with cardiac tamponade, the x and y descents are prominent, typically resulting in an M or W shape of the venous waves. Kussmaul sign—the loss of normal inspiratory decrease in the jugular venous pressure or even a frank increase with inspiration—may be present. (Kussmaul sign may be seen in other disorders, however, including restrictive cardiomyopathy.) The arterial pulse pressure may be diminished or normal. A pulsus paradoxus is present in perhaps one-third of cases.

Auscultation of the heart can reveal a characteristic early diastolic sound, the pericardial knock. The knock occurs slightly earlier in diastole than a third heart sound and has a higher acoustic frequency.

C. Diagnostic Studies

1. Electrocardiography—Characteristic ECG abnormalities in constrictive pericarditis are nonspecific and include low voltage, T-wave inversions, and P mitrale or atrial fibrillation. Atrioventricular and intraventricular conduction delays or the development of Q waves are related to the extension of calcification into the myocardium and surrounding the coronary arteries.

2. Chest radiography—The cardiac silhouette on chest radiograph can be small, normal, or enlarged. The presence of pericardial calcification is helpful in confirming the diagnosis and suggests tuberculosis as the cause. However, only a small number of patients with constriction have pericardial calcification. Conversely, a calcified pericardium does not always indicate constriction.

3. Echocardiography—Echocardiography demonstrates pericardial thickening in most cases of constriction. As with chest radiography, however, the presence or absence of echocardiographic pericardial thickening neither establishes nor excludes the diagnosis with certainty, and imaging of the pericardium by echocardiography can sometimes be misleading. (Transesophageal echocardiography is more reliable than transthoracic echocardiography for imaging the pericardium.) Echocardiography may be useful in first raising the suspicion of constrictive pericarditis in a patient with heart failure, preserved left ventricular ejection fraction, and normal or small cardiac chamber sizes. In cases with extreme limitation of cardiac filling or when pericardial calcification extends into the myocardium, left ventricular ejection may be impaired. Thus, preserved systolic function is not a prerequisite for diagnosis. A characteristic echocardiographic feature of constrictive pericarditis is the septal "bounce," a stuttering motion of the septum during diastole. A variety of indices using Doppler echocardiography to assess ventricular filling in various stages of diastole have been proposed to distinguish between constrictive pericarditis and restrictive cardiomyopathy. Those that appear most useful are exaggerated respiratory variations of transmitral and hepatic vein flow and isovolumetric relaxation time. Both of these are present in constriction but absent in restrictive cardiomyopathy. Tissue Doppler examination reveals increased E' velocity of the mitral annulus as well as septal abnormalities analogous to the "bounce." Tissue Doppler appears to be at least as sensitive as conventional echocardiography-Doppler for diagnosing constriction.

4. Magnetic resonance imaging and computed tomography—Both of these methods are especially useful for imaging the pericardium. They are more accurate than echocardiography in this regard and provide a much more complete assessment of the appearance of the entire pericardium. Figure 17–3 is an example of a computed tomographic scan from the same patient whose chest radiograph is shown in Figure 17–4. Patients being considered for pericardiectomy should always be evaluated with one of these techniques. Magnetic resonance imaging in particular can be used to discern features of constrictive pericarditis such as the septal bounce and abnormal respiratory variations in

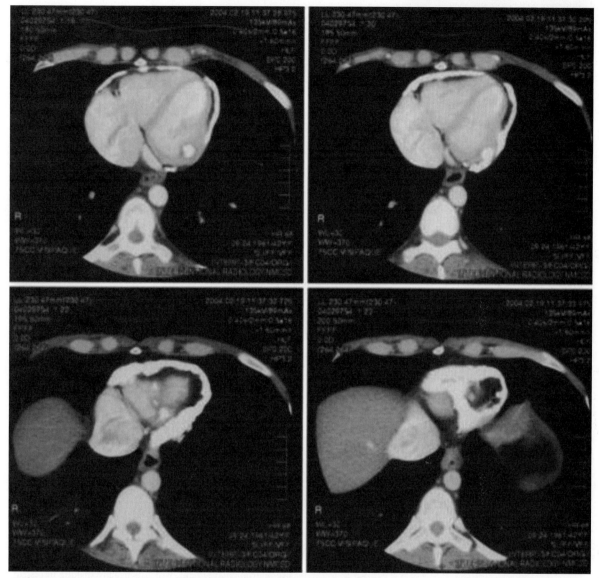

▲ **Figure 17-3.** Computed tomographic scan from same patient as in Figure 17-4 showing a heavily calcified pericardium. (From Cavendish JJ et al. Circulation. 2005;112:e137. Reprinted by permission of the American Heart Association.)

mitral and tricuspid flow. Although the presence of pericardial thickening ordinarily is a key point in distinguishing constrictive pericarditis, occasional cases of constriction in the absence of thickening have been reported.

5. Cardiac catheterization—Cardiac catheterization can help establish the correct diagnosis. It confirms elevated—and usually virtually equal—diastolic pressures in both ventricles. The diastolic pressure waveform has been described as a square root sign, or dip and plateau: an exaggerated early

diastolic downward deflection (the dip) followed by a rapid early pressure rise and plateau. This waveform, however, is not pathognomonic for constriction; it can also be found in restrictive cardiomyopathy. Examination of the right and left atrial waveforms reveals prominent *x* and *y* descents. As with the jugular venous waveform, the appearance of the atrial pressure recording has been likened to a W or an M shape. Several hemodynamic criteria are useful in distinguishing constrictive pericarditis from restrictive cardiomyopathy (Table 17–2). Although the accuracy of any one of these

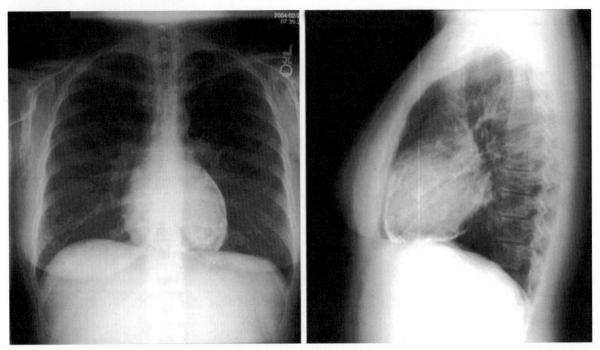

▲ **Figure 17–4.** Chest radiograph showing a heavily calcified pericardium in constrictive pericarditis. (Reprinted with permission from Cavendish JJ et al. Circulation. 2005;112:e137. Reprinted by permission of the American Heart Association.)

criteria is far from perfect, the concordance of all three criteria favoring constriction renders the diagnosis 91% certain. Similarly, if none or only one hemodynamic criterion in favor of constriction is met, the patient has *restriction* with 94% certainty. One-fourth of patients with the appropriate physiology will meet two criteria, making their chances of either diagnosis approximately equal.

6. Endomyocardial biopsy—At the time of cardiac catheterization, endomyocardial biopsy can be performed to search for evidence of infiltrative cardiomyopathy. The finding of amyloidosis, sarcoidosis, or hemochromatosis eliminates the need for further investigation. The finding of myocarditis, however, is not specific, and further studies may be needed.

▶ Differential Diagnosis

With the combined use of Doppler echocardiography, magnetic resonance imaging or computed tomography to image the pericardium, careful hemodynamic studies, and endomyocardial biopsy, it should be possible in the great majority of cases to distinguish constrictive pericarditis from restrictive cardiomyopathy. This distinction is not always possible, however, and such differentiation can sometimes be a major diagnostic challenge. Restrictive cardiomyopathy is a condition that is most commonly caused by infiltrative

diseases of the myocardium such as amyloidosis, sarcoidosis, and hemochromatosis—or, in Africa, by endocardial fibroelastosis. Both constrictive pericarditis and restrictive cardiomyopathy are characterized by impaired diastolic filling of the ventricles. The two differ, however, in the degree of impairment of various phases of diastole. Unlike the rapid early diastolic filling and abrupt halt of constrictive pericarditis, ventricular filling in restrictive cardiomyopathy is impaired uniformly throughout diastole. This physiologic difference underlies many of the features that help distinguish the two diagnoses. Other useful distinguishing features are biatrial enlargement, which is usually striking in restric-

Table 17–2. Hemodynamic Criteria Differentiating Constrictive Pericarditis from Restrictive Cardiomyopathy.

Criteria Favoring Constriction	Predictive Accuracy (%)
Difference between LVEDP and RVEDP < 5 mm Hg	85
RV systolic pressure > 50 mm Hg	70
RVEDP:RV systolic pressure ratio > 0.33	76

LVEDP, left-ventricular end-diastolic pressure; RVEDP, right ventricular end-diastolic pressure; RV, right ventricle.

tive cardiomyopathy and absent in constriction, and markedly increased ventricular wall thickness, which is the rule in most cases of restrictive cardiomyopathy. Last, brain natriuretic peptide levels are helpful; they are elevated in restrictive cardiomyopathy and normal in constriction. The correct differentiation of these two conditions is of paramount importance: Constrictive pericarditis is an eminently treatable disease; cardiac restriction of almost any cause carries a limited prognosis—despite therapy. When the distinction between constriction and restriction remains ambiguous, it may be necessary to proceed to thoracoscopy to permit direct inspection of the pericardium. Pulmonary hypertension causing right heart failure has several similarities with both constrictive pericarditis and restrictive cardiomyopathy. Measurement of the pulmonary artery pressure and vascular resistance establish the diagnosis of pulmonary hypertension.

At the bedside, constrictive pericarditis is sometimes difficult to distinguish from more common causes of congestive heart failure. Disproportionate right-sided failure or ascites out of proportion to peripheral edema may be clues to the presence of constriction. Because of the relative rarity of constriction, it is often not suspected, and congestive heart failure or even noncardiac cirrhosis is diagnosed instead. Because the primary form of therapy for constriction is surgical, it is essential to be sure that the diagnosis of constriction is correct.

▶ Treatment

Although intensive medical management may effectively control symptoms, the long-term prognosis with medical therapy alone is limited: The natural history in most cases is one of advancing severity.

Pericardiectomy is the definitive treatment for constrictive pericarditis. The only exception is early postsurgical constriction which, as discussed earlier, responds well to a course of corticosteroids. In most cases, the procedure is straightforward, and the surgical mortality rate in recent series has ranged from 4% to 11%. Occasionally, however, the dense fibrosis and calcification extend into the epicardium, making identification of a cleavage plane impossible. The operation in this case is associated with excessive hemorrhage and an inability to relieve the compression completely. In other patients, hepatic or cardiac failure may be irreversible. The myocardium may undergo atrophy as a result of long-standing compression, and a low-cardiac-output state may persist after pericardiectomy.

In most cases, patients will exhibit dramatic and sustained improvement, although full improvement may occur only after several months. When symptoms are persistent or recurrent, three possibilities should be considered: myocardial dysfunction resulting from severe, prolonged compression; incomplete or inadequate pericardiectomy; and recurrence of the constriction. In some cases, the inflammatory and fibrotic process involves the epicardial layers and progresses after the pericardium has been removed, leading to a recurrence of constrictive physiology and symptoms.

The combination of constrictive pericarditis and occlusive coronary artery disease is especially difficult to manage. In some cases, the coronary lesions are due to the visceral pericardial process, and stripping the pericardium may damage the coronary arteries. Bypass surgery can be extremely difficult in the presence of the dense calcium. If the coronary obstructions are not corrected, however, the increased myocardial oxygen demands of increased cardiac filling following pericardiectomy may cause postoperative ischemia—which may severely complicate recovery from the surgery.

Ha JW et al. Differentiation of constrictive pericarditis from restrictive cardiomyopathy using mitral annular velocity by tissue Doppler echocardiography. Am J Cardiol. 2004 Aug 1;94(3):316–9. [PMID: 15276095]

Bertog SC et al. Constrictive pericarditis: etiology and cause-specific survival after pericardiectomy. J Am Coll Cardiol. 2004 Apr 21;43(8):1445–52. [PMID: 15093882]

Leya FS et al. The efficacy of brain natriuretic peptide levels in differentiating constrictive pericarditis from restrictive cardiomyopathy. J Am Coll Cardiol. 2005 Jun 7;45(11):1900–2. [PMID: 15936624]

Talreja DR et al. Constrictive pericarditis in 26 patients with histologically normal pericardial thickness. Circulation. 2003 Oct 14;108(15):1852–7. [PMID: 15276095]

Taylor AM et al. Detection of pericardial inflammation with late-enhancement cardiac magnetic resonance imaging: initial results. Eur Radiol. 2006 Mar;16(3):569–74. [PMID: 16249864]

EFFUSIVE-CONSTRICTIVE PERICARDITIS

 ESSENTIALS OF DIAGNOSIS

▶ Echocardiographic demonstration of pericardial fluid.
▶ Persistance of elevated intracardiac filling pressures following pericardiocentesis.

Effusive-constrictive pericarditis combines features of pericardial effusion and constrictive pericarditis. The syndrome is dynamic and may represent an intermediate stage in the development of constrictive pericarditis. The most common causes of effusive-constrictive pericarditis are uremia and metastatic pericardial disease, but any cause of pericarditis can produce this condition. Echocardiography usually shows a small-to-moderate-sized effusion with strands of solid material between the visceral and parietal pericardium. Although effusive-constrictive pericarditis may be suspected on clinical grounds, the diagnosis is established through cardiac catheterization and characterization of the hemodynamics. Effusive-constrictive pericarditis can present as frank tamponade. As the effusion is drained during pericardiocentesis, elevation of intracardiac filling pressures persists and the recorded waveforms may exhibit the classic appearance of constriction.

Although pericardiocentesis may be associated with an improved cardiac output and diminished symptoms, subsequent management is essentially that for pericardial constriction. Thoracotomy with pericardiectomy is indicated to relieve the constriction in symptomatic patients who do not have diagnoses with a very poor short-term prognosis, such as advanced metastatic cancer.

Sagrista-Sauleda J et al. Effusive-constrictive pericarditis. N Engl J Med. 2004 Jan 29;350(5):469–75. [PMID: 14749455]

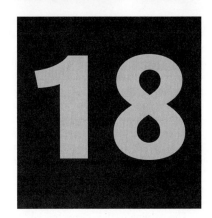

Congestive Heart Failure

18

Prakash C. Deedwania, MD & Enrique V. Carbajal, MD

ESSENTIALS OF DIAGNOSIS

▶ Orthopnea, paroxysmal nocturnal dyspnea, dyspnea at rest and during exertion, fatigue.

▶ Jugular vein distention, peripheral pitting edema, sinus tachycardia, basilar rales or coarse bubbling rales throughout both lung fields, cardiomegaly, S_3 gallop sound, liver enlargement.

▶ Left ventricular systolic or diastolic dysfunction.

▶ General Considerations

Congestive heart failure (CHF) is a complex clinical syndrome characterized by dysfunction of the left, right, or both ventricles and the resultant changes in neurohormonal regulation. This syndrome is accompanied by effort intolerance, fluid retention, and shortened survival. It is often a terminal stage of heart disease, occurring after all reserve capacity and compensatory mechanisms of the myocardium and peripheral circulation have been exhausted. Initially, the syndrome was described as a state of fluid overload with congestion of the lungs caused by a failing heart. It is, however, now well recognized that in many patients the predominant symptom may be a reduction of functional capacity because of poor exercise tolerance associated with limited cardiac reserve.

Heart failure results from myocardial dysfunction that impairs the heart's ability to circulate blood at a rate sufficient to maintain the metabolic needs of peripheral tissues and various organs. It follows myocardial damage when the compensatory hemodynamic and neurohormonal mechanisms are overwhelmed or exhausted and results from the loss of a critical amount of functioning myocardium due to acute myocardial infarction (MI), prolonged cardiovascular stress (hypertension, valvular disease), toxins (eg, alcohol abuse), or infection; in some cases, there is no apparent cause (idiopathic cardiomyopathy).

Heart failure is a relatively common clinical disorder, estimated to affect more than 5 million patients in the United States. Each year, new cases of CHF develop in about 550,000 patients. Morbidity and mortality rates are high; annually, approximately 1 million patients require hospitalization for CHF, approximately 6.5 million hospital-days. Each year 50,000 to 60,000 patients die of this condition.

Approximately one-third to one-half of the deaths in patients with CHF are secondary to the progression of cardiac insufficiency and its associated conditions. The remainder of the patients with CHF die of sudden cardiac death, presumably related to electrical instability and ventricular arrhythmias and other cardiovascular conditions as well as from noncardiovascular causes.

Data describing the natural history of CHF are limited because this condition has not been extensively studied in a prospective manner. The Framingham heart study showed that men in whom clinical symptoms of CHF developed had a 62% probability of dying within 5 years of the onset of symptoms. Subsequent studies in patients with dilated or congestive cardiomyopathy indicate that heart failure is a progressively deteriorating condition, with 20–40% of patients dying within 5 years after the onset of illness; other studies show that patients with advanced CHF (New York Heart Association [NYHA] class IV) have a 40–50% annual mortality rate.

▶ Pathophysiology & Etiology

When an excessive workload is imposed on the heart by increased systolic blood pressure (pressure overload), increased diastolic volume (volume overload), or loss of myocardium, normal myocardial cells hypertrophy in an effort to enhance contractile force of the normal areas. The subsequent alterations in biochemistry, electrophysiology, and contractile function lead to mechanical alterations of myocardial function: The rate of contraction slows, the time to develop peak tension increases, and myocardial relaxation is delayed. Peak force development may be well preserved with enough viable myocardium and adequate time for the development of force. Thickening of the ventricular wall limits the rate of ventricular filling (diastolic dysfunction), which is worsened by increased heart rate because it shortens the duration of ventricular filling. The force of myocardial contraction is eventually reduced as cell loss and hypertrophy continue, leading to significant geometric ventricular alterations and increased volumes. This process of chamber dilatation or hypertrophy is known as cardiac remodeling.

After the initial compensatory phase, the increase in intracavitary volume is usually associated with further reductions in ventricular ejection fraction (progressive systolic dysfunction) and eventually with abnormalities in the peripheral circulation from activation of various neurohormonal compensatory mechanisms.

The ensuing CHF is characterized by a reduced contraction response to increase in volume (flattened Frank-Starling curve) and a reduced left ventricular ejection fraction (LVEF). The abnormal neurohormonal responses lead to increased systemic sympathetic tone and activation of the renin-angiotensin system. Production of angiotensin increases, causing peripheral vasoconstriction. The increase in peripheral arterial resistance limits cardiac output during exercise. The increased levels of angiotensin II also stimulate release of aldosterone by the adrenal glands, enhancing sodium retention and thus leading to fluid retention and peripheral edema.

Myocardial (pump) failure and CHF are not necessarily closely related in time. Patients are often initially asymptomatic, with the signs and symptoms of CHF developing only after several months of myocardial failure and decreased ejection fraction. Cardiac output does not increase adequately during exercise, but it can be normal at rest during this period. Although patients may be asymptomatic or slightly symptomatic at rest, with the ejection fraction unchanged, alterations in peripheral vasculature occur with slowly rising peripheral resistance during exercise. Exercise performance slowly becomes limited because the peripheral vasculature cannot meet the increased metabolic needs of exercising skeletal muscles.

Although the precise mechanism by which hemodynamic responses and neurohormonal factors interact to cause progressive clinical deterioration in CHF is unknown, the hemodynamic and neurohormonal abnormalities that increase cardiac wall stress can lead to cell slippage, morphologic myocardial cell changes, and structural remodeling of the heart. The dilatation of the ventricular cavity and change in its shape can eventually lead to mitral regurgitation. The increase in cardiac pressures and volume may also trigger myocardial ischemia, especially in patients with underlying coronary artery disease (CAD).

The myocardial hypertrophy can enhance cardiac metabolic demands and may increase the risk of ischemia in patients with CAD. In addition, prolonged activation of neurohormonal axes may be deleterious to the heart in an independent manner: High concentrations of norepinephrine and angiotensin II can exert direct toxic effects on myocardial cells. The heightened activity of the sympathetic nervous and renin-angiotensin systems can have adverse electrophysiologic effects and may induce lethal cardiac arrhythmias—particularly in patients with electrolyte imbalances (Table 18–1).

Hunt SA et al; American College of Cardiology/American Heart Association Task Force on Practice Guidelines (Writing Committee to Update the 2001 Guidelines for the Evaluation and Management of Heart Failure). ACC/AHA 2005 guideline update for the diagnosis and management of chronic heart failure in the adult: a report of the American College of Cardiology/American Heart Association Task Force on Practice Guidelines (Writing Committee to Update the 2001 Guidelines for the Evaluation and Management of Heart Failure). Circulation. 2005 Sep 20;112(12):e154–235. [PMID: 16160202]

A. Types of Heart Failure

1. Chronic and acute heart failure—The manifestations of heart failure depend on the rate at which the syndrome develops and whether sufficient time has elapsed for fluid to accumulate in the interstitial spaces. Generally, if the underlying cardiac abnormality develops slowly, compensatory mechanisms have time to become activated, and the patient will be able to adjust to the altered cardiac output. If the underlying condition develops rapidly or an acute precipitating factor is present, the result may be inadequate organ perfusion or acute congestion of the venous bed draining into the affected ventricle, causing sudden cardiac decompensation, with a concomitant reduction in cardiac output and an acute onset of symptoms.

In chronic heart failure, adaptive mechanisms are gradually activated and cardiac hypertrophy develops. These changes allow the patient to adjust to and tolerate a reduction in cardiac output with less difficulty. When the onset of left-heart failure is gradual, the right heart develops higher pressures in response to higher pulmonary resistance; the acute onset of similar increases in pulmonary resistance may produce acute right-heart failure. A patient with chronic heart failure may achieve compensation but then experience acute decompensation as a result of a precipitating condition (Table 18–2).

Table 18–1. Sequence of Events during Hemodynamic Adaptations in Heart Failure.

Increase in
Ventricular end-diastolic volume and pressure
Atrial volume and pressure
Atrial and ventricular contractility (Starling law)
Volume and pressure in adjacent venous system
Capillary pressure and secondary transudation of fluid
Interstitial and extracellular fluid volume
Lymphatic flow from interstitial spaces

Table 18–2. Common Precipitating Factors in Heart Failure.

Lack of compliance (diet, drugs)
Uncontrolled hypertension
Myocardial infarction and ischemia
Cardiac arrhythmias
Multifocal atrial tachycardia
Atrial fibrillation, flutter
Ventricular tachycardia
Fluid overload
Pulmonary embolism
Pulmonary infection
Systemic infection
Endocrine abnormalities
Environmental factors
Inadequate therapy
Emotional stress
Blood loss, anemia

2. Left- and right-sided heart failure—Heart failure is more often limited to one side when the onset is abrupt (eg, in acute MI). The venous reservoir capacity is smaller on the left than is the systemic venous system on the right, and increased venous pressures and associated symptoms occur after a relatively smaller accumulation of fluid on the left.

Although the disease process may involve only one ventricle initially, biventricular failure usually follows, especially when the left ventricle is the site of initial damage. Both ventricles have a common interventricular septum, and biochemical changes are not confined to the stressed ventricle but involve the opposite ventricle as well. In addition, because all four cardiac chambers are enclosed in the pericardial sac, when the size of any chamber suddenly increases the opposite chambers are compressed, and the filling pressure of the normal ventricle rises (this is usually defined as ventricular interdependence). Right-sided failure often follows left-heart failure, but left-heart failure rarely follows isolated right-heart failure (eg, atrial septal defect, cor pulmonale) without a concomitant separate abnormality of the left heart (eg, CAD with ischemia or infarction). In patients with left ventricular (LV) failure, subsequent right-heart failure may relieve the respiratory symptoms (exertional dyspnea, orthopnea, nocturnal dyspnea) generally associated with left-heart failure.

3. High-output and low-output heart failure—Most cases of heart failure are associated with a low-output state. High-output heart failure, which is less common, is usually associated with a hyperkinetic circulatory state usually due to increased demand on the heart from another condition, such as anemia or thyrotoxicosis. These states usually trigger heart failure when superimposed on underlying heart disease. Unlike the vasoconstriction seen in the low-output state, high-output failure is associated with vasodilatation. Although the cardiac index is usually higher than normal (> 4 L/min/m^2), it is

generally lower than before the onset of heart failure and is obviously insufficient to meet the increased oxygen demands.

4. Backward and forward heart failure—Increased pressure in the system draining into one or both ventricles (backward failure), inadequate cardiac output in a forward direction (forward failure), or both conditions account for the clinical manifestations of heart failure. An important tenet of the backward failure theory is the development of right-heart failure as a consequence of LV failure. The elevation of LV diastolic, left atrial, and pulmonary venous pressures causes backward transmission of pressure and leads to pulmonary hypertension that ultimately causes right ventricular failure and increasing systemic venous pressure. Forward failure may account for many of the clinical manifestations of heart failure, such as mental confusion from decreased cerebral perfusion, fatigue and weakness from decreased skeletal muscle perfusion, and sodium and water retention with secondary venous congestion from decreased renal perfusion. The retention of sodium and water, in turn, augments extracellular fluid volume and ultimately leads to congestive symptoms of heart failure that are secondary to accumulation of fluid in various organs and peripheral tissues.

The mechanisms that lead to both forward and backward failure operate in most patients with chronic heart failure. Based on the underlying pathophysiologic process, hemodynamic abnormalities, and abruptness of disease process (eg, acute MI, acute pulmonary embolism), however, one or the other may initially be predominant. Early in the process of heart failure, cardiac output may be normal at rest. During stress, such as physical exercise and other periods of increased metabolic demand, however, the cardiac output fails to rise normally, the glomerular filtration rate declines, and the renal mechanism for salt and water retention becomes activated. Ventricular filling pressure as well as pressures in the atrium and venous system behind the affected ventricle may rise abnormally during periods of stress. This may cause transudation of fluid and symptoms of tissue congestion during exercise. In such early stages, physical rest may induce diuresis and relieve symptoms in many patients with mild heart failure; excessive and repeated strenuous physical activities will worsen the compromised hemodynamic state and cause progression of heart failure.

5. Diastolic and systolic heart failure—The symptoms and signs of heart failure can be caused by either an abnormality in systolic function that leads to reduced ejection of blood from the heart (systolic heart failure) or an abnormality in myocardial diastolic function that leads to decreased ventricular filling (diastolic heart failure), or both. Reduced LV filling caused by diastolic dysfunction leads to decreased stroke volume and associated symptoms of low cardiac output, whereas increased filling pressures lead to symptoms of pulmonary congestion. Thus, some characteristics of heart failure (eg, the inability of the left ventricle to provide adequate forward output to meet the demands of the skeletal muscles during exercise while maintaining normal filling pressures) may result primarily from diastolic dysfunction, which, in some patients, can occur with normal LV systolic function. There are no exact data on the prevalence of diastolic dysfunction leading to heart failure in the presence of normal systolic function. Several studies have shown, however, that as many as 40% of all patients with a clinical diagnosis of heart failure may have preserved LV systolic function, and many of these patients have evidence of diastolic dysfunction. Several factors can predispose to an increased risk of diastolic dysfunction in the presence of normal LV systolic function (Table 18–3).

B. Causes

The most common causes of CHF in the United States are CAD, systemic hypertension, nonischemic dilated cardiomyopathy, and valvular heart disease. Other frequent causes are myocarditis and diabetes mellitus, but there are a great many less common causes. Although diabetes can predispose to CHF, the risk of CHF most commonly appears to result from some form of diabetic cardiomyopathy, particularly in insulin-dependent diabetics. Recent data suggest that the increased (twofold to tenfold) risk for CHF in diabetes patients is independent of associated CAD or hypertension and appears to be highest among women.

Many patients with heart failure have identifiable precipitating factors (see Table 18–2). The most common cause of cardiac decompensation in heart failure patients appears to be insufficient attention to the prescribed treatment regimen, eg, inadequate restriction of sodium, excessive physical activity, and noncompliance with prescribed drug therapy. Cardiac arrhythmias, including atrial or ventricular tachyarrhythmias with or without associated CAD, are common in patients with heart failure and can also precipitate or intensify the signs and symptoms of CHF. Profound and inappropriate bradycardia in the presence of decreased cardiac output and atrioventricular (AV) dissociation in patients with complete AV block can

Table 18–3. Factors Associated with Left Ventricular Diastolic Dysfunction.

Hypertension
Coronary artery disease
Myocardial ischemia
Scarring and hypertrophy secondary to myocardial infection
Left ventricular hypertrophy
Dilated cardiomyopathy
Volume overload
Elevated afterload
Myocardial fibrosis
Restriction to filling
Constrictive pericarditis
Obliterative cardiomyopathy
Myocardial infiltrative diseases (eg, amyloidosis)

also precipitate CHF because the ventricular rate is insufficient to maintain cardiac output in an already compromised heart. Acute infections, especially pneumonia, bronchitis, or other pulmonary infections, can also precipitate heart failure. Patients with heart failure are also at increased risk for pulmonary emboli, especially when confined to bed. Other precipitating factors include physical and emotional stress, cardiac inflammation, unrelated illnesses (especially hepatorenal disorders), cardiac depressants (alcohol and other toxins), sodium-retaining drugs (nonsteroidal antiinflammatory drugs), recurrent myocardial ischemia, and progressive worsening of the underlying cardiac disorder itself.

Jessup M et al. Heart failure. N Engl J Med. 2003 May 15;348(20): 2007–18. [PMID: 12748317]

Redfield MM et al. Burden of systolic and diastolic ventricular dysfunction in the community: appreciating the scope of the heart failure epidemic. JAMA. 2003 Jan 8;289(2):194–202. [PMID: 12517230]

▶ Clinical Findings

A. Symptoms and Signs

1. Shortness of breath—Dyspnea, or breathlessness (a subjective feeling of air hunger), is the earliest and most frequent symptom in CHF. Initially, dyspnea on exertion will be noted by a change in the extent of physical activity that causes shortness of breath. As heart failure worsens, the intensity of exertion required will decrease. Paroxysmal nocturnal dyspnea, orthopnea, and eventually dyspnea at rest will progressively develop in a patient with heart failure.

The severity of dyspnea becomes less prominent in LV failure after right ventricular failure develops. In general, dyspnea is less prominent in right ventricular failure because pulmonary congestion is not present. However, when the failure advances, severe dyspnea can develop even in patients with predominantly right ventricular failure. This is presumably a consequence of the reduced cardiac output and poor perfusion of respiratory muscles and associated hypoxia, leading to metabolic acidosis.

Paroxysmal nocturnal dyspnea (PND) occurs after the patient has been asleep and in the supine position for some time. Suddenly, the patient wakes up with a sensation of choking and air hunger; assuming an upright posture usually relieves the symptoms. Frequently, the patient will feel better after opening a window or going outside to catch a breath of fresh air. PND usually precedes orthopnea; it may be associated with bronchospasm and wheezing (cardiac asthma) and can be confused with an attack of bronchial asthma, especially in patients with prior known chronic obstructive pulmonary disease (COPD). Most severe episodes of PND can cause a feeling of intense suffocation and may leave the patient gasping for breath. The uncomfortable sensation may persist for 30 minutes or more after the patient has assumed an upright posture. PND is primarily caused by mobilization of interstitial fluid (especially in patients with edema) from infrathoracic locations during recumbency. The result is increased circulating blood volume and increased pulmonary venous pressure.

Orthopnea is defined as dyspnea that occurs—often within a few minutes—when the patient assumes a supine position; sitting up or standing usually improves the symptoms. The most severely affected patients usually sleep sitting upright in a chair. Orthopnea has the same cause as PND, but it represents more severe cardiac impairment.

A **dry or nonproductive cough** may occasionally occur. This is due to pulmonary congestion and in patients with heart failure is usually relieved by successful treatment of the heart failure. Certain drugs used to treat heart failure, such as angiotensin-converting enzyme (ACE) inhibitors, can also cause cough.

2. Fatigue and weakness—Other common symptoms of heart failure include fatigue and generalized weakness, particularly in the limbs. These symptoms are secondary to low cardiac output with decreased perfusion of skeletal muscles and can occur with exertion or at rest; they may be worsened after eating because of the increased splanchnic demand for blood flow, which may stress the limited reserve. Low-output syndromes can be present, without evidence of pulmonary congestion, and limit performance during exercise testing. Extreme thirst, an often-overlooked symptom, is associated with activation of the arginine-vasopressin system and hyponatremia in patients with heart failure.

3. Nocturia and oliguria—Nocturia is a common and early symptom in heart failure. Renal filtration of sodium and water is decreased in patients with compromised LV function, in part, because of the redistribution of blood flow away from the kidneys in the upright position and during physical activity. Urine formation is enhanced in the recumbent position when renal stimulus for vasoconstriction decreases and venous return to the heart increases. Oliguria is associated with a markedly reduced cardiac output and is usually a sign of terminal heart failure; it indicates a poor prognosis.

4. Cerebral symptoms—Elderly patients with advanced heart failure may have confusion, memory impairment, anxiety, headaches, insomnia, nightmares and, occasionally, disorientation, delirium, and hallucinations. These cerebral symptoms are predominantly related to a reduced cardiac output and poor perfusion of brain and other neurologic tissues.

5. Abdominal symptoms—Gastrointestinal complaints may develop in patients with heart failure as a result of hepatic congestion and edema of the abdominal wall and intra-abdominal organs. Congestion of abdominal organs may be present with ascites, abdominal fullness and enlargement, early satiety, bloating, anorexia, nausea, vomiting, constipation, and upper abdominal discomfort. The abdominal discomfort is usually described as a dull ache or heaviness that can be enhanced or reproduced by upper abdominal or hepatic palpation. This is consistent with the likely cause, the

stretching of the hepatic capsule. Patients can frequently detect early reaccumulation of fluid by the recurrence of abdominal fullness before the signs become obvious. This symptom can be easily overlooked, however. Asking the patient about a recent change in waist size or a tightening of the clothing at the waist is often helpful.

B. Physical Examination

In general, patients with heart failure of recent onset appear acutely ill but well nourished. Patients with chronic heart failure, on the other hand, frequently appear malnourished, and occasionally cachectic. This appearance arises from anorexia that is secondary to hepatic and intestinal congestion or sometimes to drug therapy (digitalis) and may be, in part, caused by reasons that are unclear. Rarely, patients may experience impaired absorption of fat and, in some cases, a protein-losing enteropathy. Patients may have increased body metabolism from increased myocardial oxygen consumption, excessive work of breathing, or elevated levels of circulating catecholamines and other neurohormones. The combination of reduced caloric intake and increased energy expenditure can lead to a reduction of tissue mass and thus, in severe cases, to cachexia. In the terminal stage, a patient with advanced heart failure may resemble a patient with widespread malignancy.

Evidence of increased sympathetic activity is frequent in patients with heart failure. There may be pallor and coldness of the limbs and cyanosis of the digits because of vasoconstriction. The patient may also have diaphoresis and abnormal distention of the superficial veins. Sinus tachycardia is often observed and usually develops in an effort to maintain the cardiac output when heart failure is decompensated or the stroke volume is significantly decreased.

Sustained periodic or cyclic respirations with regularly alternating phases of hyperpnea and apnea in a smooth crescendo-decrescendo manner (Cheyne-Stokes) can be seen in patients with heart failure. This represents an altered neurogenic control of respiration, usually from intracranial causes, but it is facilitated by a combination of pulmonary congestion, the prolonged circulation time from lung to the brain, and decreased sensitivity of the respiratory center to hypercapnia and hypoxia. Moist rales heard initially at the lung bases result from the transudation of fluid into the alveoli that subsequently moves into the airways. In pulmonary edema, coarse bubbling rales and wheezes are heard over both lung fields and may be accompanied by frothy sputum, with or without bloodstaining. Hydrothorax (pleural effusion) is usually bilateral and can intensify the severity of dyspnea by further reducing vital capacity. Stony dullness on percussion is characteristic of pleural effusion on one or both sides. Shifting dullness can often be found with pleural effusion when the patient moves from the sitting to the lateral decubitus position. Breath sounds over the area of effusion are diminished or absent, but occasionally high-pitched bronchial sounds are present. An accompanying pleural rub usually indicates associated pulmonary infarction, infection, or inflammatory response. Hydrothorax usually is reabsorbed slowly as heart failure improves; in some cases, the pleural effusion persists for many days after the symptoms disappear.

Approximately 5 L of extracellular fluid must accumulate before peripheral edema occurs in heart failure. Pitting edema is common, with the fluid accumulating in a symmetric manner; in general, it initially involves the dependent portions of the body with higher venous pressure. This is typically noted in the feet and ankles of ambulatory patients and in the sacral area of bedridden ones. Late in the course of heart failure, edema may become massive and generalized (anasarca); it can involve the upper extremities, the thoracic and abdominal walls, and the genital area. Occasionally, with acute accumulation of edema or associated trauma, skin rupture and extravasation of fluid can occur. Chronic edema results in increased pigmentation, reddening, and induration of the skin of the lower extremities.

Cardiomegaly, with a laterally displaced, enlarged, and sustained ventricular impulse may be found on physical examination, but this is a nonspecific finding and can be absent, particularly in patients with acute heart failure. The decrease in ventricular compliance may initially become apparent by the presence of a late diastolic atrial sound (S_4 gallop). A protodiastolic sound (S_3 gallop) occurs in patients with more advanced heart failure and is caused by acute deceleration of ventricular inflow after the early filling phase. An S_3 gallop, however, can also be detected in other conditions such as mitral and tricuspid regurgitation and a left-to-right shunt. Gallop sounds are more readily audible in the presence of a rapid heart rate. The presence of a third heart sounds appears to be associated with an increased risk of death, death from pump failure, and hospitalization for heart failure. Systolic murmurs are common in heart failure and are largely secondary to mitral or tricuspid regurgitation that can result from ventricular dilatation. These murmurs frequently diminish or disappear after adequate treatment and reduction of ventricular size.

Systemic venous hypertension can be detected by abnormal distention of the internal jugular veins. Although the jugular venous pressure normally declines on inspiration, it can rise in patients with right-heart failure (Kussmaul sign). Persistent elevation of the jugular venous pressure is one of the earliest and most reliable signs of right-heart failure. The inability of the right ventricle to accept transient increases in venous return (hepatojugular reflux) is observed during transient compression (30 seconds) of the upper abdomen. Systolic pulsations of the liver may be felt in patients with tricuspid regurgitation. Liver enlargement and tenderness on palpation are marked by epigastric fullness and dullness to percussion in the right upper quadrant. These findings may persist after other signs of heart failure have disappeared because it takes longer for hepatic congestion to disappear. In some cases, the liver enlargement does not disappear

because of structural changes in patients with long-standing heart failure. The presence of an elevated jugular venous pressure appears to be associated with an increased risk of death, death from pump failure, and hospitalization for heart failure.

Pulsus alternans is common in patients with CHF; when severe, it can be detected by sphygmomanometry or by palpation of peripheral pulses, particularly the femoral pulse. This sign is characterized by a regular rhythm of alternating strong and weak pulsations. Sometimes the weak beat may be so small that the aortic valve does not open and no aortic or arterial pulse is produced, resulting in total alternans and a pulse that is only half as fast as the apical beats. With total alternans, a first heart sound will occur, but no second heart sound if both the aortic and pulmonic valves fail to open. Pulsus alternans appears to be due to an alternation in the stroke volume of the left ventricle, possibly because of an incomplete recovery of myocardial cells and thus a decrease in the responsiveness of contracting cells on alternate beats. It can be persistent or paroxysmal, or it may occur only after a premature beat or with the Valsalva maneuver.

The hemodynamic response to the Valsalva maneuver has been found useful in the clinical evaluation of patients with heart failure. In this maneuver, the blood pressure cuff is inflated to just about 15 mm Hg above the systolic blood pressure before the maneuver. In a normal response, the Korotkoff sounds disappear during sustained maneuver and reappear after completion of the maneuver. An abnormal response, in which blood pressure sounds either do not disappear or are maintained throughout the maneuver, has been found in patients with CHF. In normal patients, the decrease in blood pressure during the maneuver is associated with tachycardia and the increase in blood pressure after release with bradycardia. Variation in heart rate is lost in patients with CHF.

Drazner MH et al. Prognostic importance of elevated jugular venous pressure and a third heart sound in patients with heart failure. N Engl J Med. 2001 Aug 23;345(8):574–81. [PMID: 11529211]

C. Laboratory Findings

In severe heart failure, neurohormonal compensatory mechanisms frequently lead to hyponatremia and other significant electrolyte abnormalities, even without the use of diuretics, which (especially the thiazide type) may contribute to hyponatremia.

Congestion of the liver is often associated with abnormalities of liver function tests with elevated levels of liver enzyme values, particularly serum aspartate aminotransferase. A concomitant increase in serum alanine aminotransferase or other hepatocellular enzymes documents that the liver is the source of the enzyme elevation. Serum alkaline phosphatase, a hepatobiliary enzyme, may be elevated and is commonly associated with hyperbilirubinemia or even prolongation of prothrombin time as a result of decreased hepatic synthesis of clotting factors. Hyperbilirubinemia of 15–20 mg/dL and aspartate aminotransferase elevation more than 10 times normal can be seen with acute hepatic congestion in patients with decompensated heart failure.

D. Diagnostic Studies

1. Electrocardiography—Changes in the 12-lead electrocardiogram (ECG) are generally nonspecific. Sinus tachycardia is usually present in uncompensated heart failure or in end-stage disease with a low stroke volume that requires tachycardia to maintain the cardiac output. Isolated premature ventricular beats are common, and complex ventricular arrhythmias can be detected in most patients during prolonged (24- to 48-hour) Holter monitoring. ECG findings suggestive of atrial and ventricular chamber enlargement may be evident. Intraventricular conduction delays are also common and include left bundle branch block as well as other, nonspecific repolarization changes.

2. Chest radiography—Cardiomegaly (cardiothoracic ratio > 50%) can be found on chest film in 87% of patients when primary dilated cardiomyopathy is first diagnosed. The lower lobes of the lung are normally better perfused than are the upper lobes; with heart failure, there is progressive vasoconstriction of vessels in the lower lobes and redistribution of the pulmonary flow to the upper lobes. Interstitial and perivascular edema develop with acute increases in pulmonary capillary wedge pressure above 20–25 mm Hg; bronchovascular markings at the bases are prominent. Interstitial edema can present as perivascular or peribronchial edema (initially in perihilar and then in peripheral zones). Kerley lines, spindle-shaped linear opacities at the periphery of the lung bases, occur in the later stages of heart failure; pleural fluid can produce discrete interlobular-type linear opacities and subpleural fluid accumulation between the lung and adjoining pleura. The accumulation of fluid in major and minor lung fissures can be of considerable size and may be incorrectly diagnosed as a tumor mass in the lung. These "phantom tumor" shadows, however, have smooth margins and disappear with resolution of CHF. With acute increases in pulmonary capillary wedge pressures above 25 mm Hg, alveolar edema or pleural effusions, or both may occur. Chronic heart failure patients may show elevated pulmonary capillary pressures in the range of 25–35 mm Hg or more without interstitial or alveolar edema, reflecting associated increased lymphatic flow. After therapy that lowers pulmonary capillary pressure, there may be a delay of 24–48 hours before improvement and clearing of pulmonary infiltrates can be seen on chest radiograph.

3. Echocardiography—The Doppler echocardiographic examination is regarded as the most useful test in evaluating patients with heart failure, in establishing the type of cardiomyopathy (dilated, restrictive, hypertrophic) and in evaluating the possible primary or secondary causes (valvular disease, LV aneurysm, intracardiac shunts) of heart failure. It can not only provide the information about the size of all cardiac chambers and LV systolic function but also gives information about valvular function, stenotic or regurgitant lesions as well as reasonable estimates of both right- and left-sided pressures.

4. Exercise stress testing—Exercise stress testing, using a bicycle ergometer or treadmill with a progressively increasing load, can be helpful in evaluating CHF. However, the degree of LV functional impairment at rest cannot be inferred from and does not always correlate with exercise capacity measured by exercise tolerance testing. Such testing allows for close observation of the patient during graded exercise and can detect obvious difficulty in breathing at a low level of exercise or a higher workload. A more prolonged exercise assessment of heart failure patients should include monitoring the maximum oxygen consumption and anaerobic threshold (the point during exercise testing at which the respiratory quotient rises as a result of the production of excess lactate) during exercise. These measurements can be used to classify the severity of heart failure, follow the progress of the patient, and assess the efficacy of therapeutic maneuvers.

5. Radionuclide ventriculography—This method is helpful in documenting the severity of LV systolic dysfunction and indicating whether the wall motion abnormalities are global or regional. This test is especially helpful in patients in whom technical difficulties for echocardiography are present; it can, for example, be obtained easily even in obese patients and in those with advanced COPD. Comparison of right and LV stroke volumes is also helpful in establishing the severity of regurgitant lesions.

6. Cardiac catheterization—Left-heart catheterization and angiography are necessary when the presence and extent of CAD need to be determined. Right-heart catheterization may be useful in evaluating and selecting patients with refractory heart failure who require customized treatment. In addition, right-heart catheterization can also help evaluate the presence of any intracardiac shunts related to congenital or acquired atrial/ventricular septal defects.

▶ Differential Diagnosis

Many patients with heart failure also have lung disease; the symptoms are often similar, making differentiation between cardiac and pulmonary dyspnea difficult. In the advanced stages of chronic lung disease, patients may experience orthopnea while recumbent; this position may interfere with the descent of the diaphragm or the maximal use of accessory respiratory muscles. Orthopnea can also be precipitated in patients with bronchiectasis or severe bronchitis when excessive secretions pool in the recumbent position. Although PND can occur in chronic lung disease, it is usually relieved by clearing the secretions—without necessarily assuming an upright position. Tachypnea associated with heart failure is characterized by rapid shallow breathing caused by the reduction in vital capacity that results when air in the lungs is replaced by blood, interstitial fluid, or both (stiff lungs syndrome). The prolonged expiratory phase seen in COPD is usually absent, however. Bronchoconstriction and wheezing from heart failure without significant pulmonary disease (cardiac asthma) is frequently associated with wet secretions (bubbly sounds, frothy sputum from bronchial congestion) and cool, dusky, and diaphoretic skin that is caused by generalized vasoconstriction.

It is important to look for both pulmonary conditions (eg, pulmonary embolism, and precipitating causes of heart failure (eg, excessive salt and fluid intake) when dyspnea suddenly worsens. Occasionally, dyspneic symptoms observed in a patient without cardiac or pulmonary illness may be related to anxiety disorders. The breathing pattern of a neurotic or anxious patient, however, is not regular, rapid, or shallow but irregular during rest or with exertion; it is usually deep and sighing. The patient may complain of lightheadedness, paresthesias, blurred vision, lump in the throat, and chest constriction—usually from hyperventilation.

▶ Treatment

A new approach to the management of patients with heart failure incorporates a new classification of heart failure that identifies four stages (A to D) involved in the development of the heart failure syndrome (Figure 18–1). Stage A includes patients without symptoms but who are identified as being at risk for heart failure. Stage B encompasses patients without symptoms but with LV hypertrophy or evidence of impaired LV function. Stage C includes patients with evidence of structural heart disease in whom symptoms of heart failure have developed. Stage D comprises patients suffering from severe, refractory heart failure. This classification emphasizes the development and progression of the disease and complements the functional NYHA classification (class I to IV) used in appraising the severity of symptoms in patients with heart failure stages C or D.

Management of heart failure requires a treatment approach reaching into multiple areas, which includes evaluation and application of general measures, use of pharmacologic agents, and consideration of nonpharmacologic interventions, including device therapies and cardiac transplantation.

A. General Measures

1. Preventive strategies—Therapeutic strategies to prevent (stages A and B) heart failure should be aimed at improving impaired ventricular function before symptoms develop. Detecting and controlling hypertension, managing the metabolic abnormalities associated with diabetes, and adequately treating myocardial ischemia should be initiated before damage to the myocardium occurs.

2. Correction of precipitating factors—Some of the most important reversible causes of heart failure include endocrine abnormalities, valvular dysfunction, intracardiac shunts, and other high-output states; bradyarrhythmias or tachyarrhythmias, systemic hypertension, myocardial toxins (eg, ethanol consumption), and various cardiotoxic drugs. Heart failure can also be secondary to pericardial disease, infectious or ischemic events, poor compliance with medical treatment plan, and suboptimal medical treatment. In all these situations, the obvious therapeutic approach is correction of the precipitating factors and treatment of any reversible underlying cause.

3. Changes in activity and diet—A few consistent modifications in lifestyle can help reduce both the symptoms of heart failure and the need for additional medication. In moderate-to-severe CHF, restriction of physical activities and bed rest often help improve the clinical condition temporarily. Appropriate restriction of physical activity reduces cardiac workload, improves symptoms, and allows the patient to engage in day-to-day activities without promoting physical deconditioning. No data are available to indicate that prolonged bed rest has any significant effect on the natural history of CHF. On the other hand, long-term moderate exercise training in patients with stable chronic heart failure may result in beneficial effects in functional capacity and improved survival.

4. Exercise training—Exercise is often associated with a feeling of well-being. In patients with heart failure, exercise training can lead to an increased exercise ability and improved symptom scores. However, there are little, if any, data to determine the effect of exercise on long-term outcomes in patients with heart failure.

5. Dietary measures—Dietary caloric restriction is particularly necessary in overweight patients because weight reduction lowers demands on the heart and can provide significant relief of symptoms.

Restricting sodium helps reduce water retention, with a concomitant reduction in cardiac work. A moderate sodium restriction (1.5–2 g/day) is usually necessary to achieve therapeutically meaningful results.

Reducing emotional stress and providing psychological support will also benefit patients with heart failure who must deal not only with the fear of increased mortality but also with an altered quality of life: restricted physical activities, changes in dietary habits, and long-term use of medications.

Cook NR et al. Long term effects of dietary sodium reduction on cardiovascular disease outcomes: observational follow-up of the trials of hypertension prevention (TOHP). BMJ. 2007 Apr 28;334(7599):885. [PMID: 17449506]

Piepoli MF et al; ExTraMATCH Collaborative. Exercise training meta-analysis of trials in patients with chronic heart failure (ExTraMATCH). BMJ. 2004 Jan 24;328(7433):189. [PMID: 14729656]

B. Pharmacologic Treatment

Several pharmacologic agents have been used in cases of CHF due to ventricular systolic dysfunction. These include

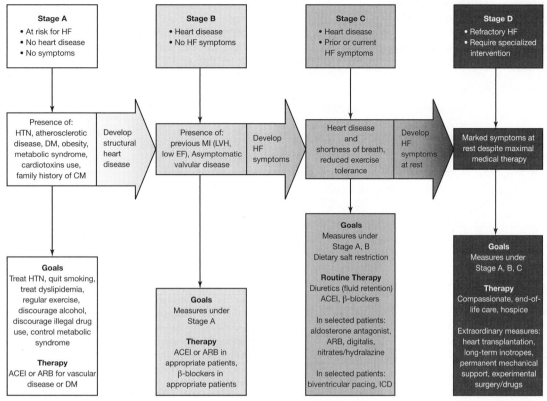

▲ **Figure 18–1.** Stages in the development of heart failure and recommended therapy. ACEI, angiotensin-converting enzyme inhibitors; ARB, angiotensin receptor blocker; CM, cardiomyopathy; DM, diabetes mellitus; EF, ejection fraction; HF, heart failure; HTN, hypertension; ICD, implantable cardioverter-defibrillator; LVH, left ventricular hypertrophy; MI, myocardial infarction. (Modified from Hunt SA et al. Circulation. 2005;112:e154.)

diuretics, inotropic drugs (direct and indirect), vasoactive drugs, and β-blockers (Table 18–4).

1. Diuretics—Diuretics provide rapid symptomatic relief of moderate-to-severe congestive symptoms. The drugs promote excretion of sodium and water and help lower plasma volume, reducing congestion in the pulmonary and systemic vascular beds and thereby improving symptoms and functional capacity. The usual goal is a ventricular filling pressure that will maintain cardiac output and relieve pulmonary congestion without causing orthostatic hypotension; the optimal pressure depends on how quickly the heart failure developed. It should be noted that overdiuresis can significantly reduce intravascular volume and cardiac output (forward cardiac failure); fluids should be given to restore optimal intravascular volume and hemodynamic parameters monitored in such cases.

Of the many diuretic agents available, oral agents are preferred in cases of mild fluid retention, whereas intravenous diuretics are generally recommended for severe, progressive, or refractory heart failure. Current diuretic agents include thiazides, loop diuretics, and potassium-sparing agents.

Thiazides inhibit the active transport of chloride as well as the passive movement of sodium. Some thiazides (eg, metolazone) also appear to block sodium reabsorption, producing an excretion of sodium with associated kaliuresis. Metolazone can be used with a loop diuretic in cases that appear resistant to therapy with a single agent.

Thiazides are generally not effective when the creatinine clearance falls below 30–40 mL/min, as is frequently seen in severe heart failure. Metolazone appears to keep its efficacy with a glomerular filtration rate as low as 10 mL/min.

Loop diuretics—furosemide, bumetanide, and ethacrynic acid—increase sodium excretion by 20–25% and enhance free water clearance. The loop diuretics are effective unless there is severe renal dysfunction and are generally preferred in severe CHF (NYHA classes III–IV) when the patient is unresponsive to other diuretics. For patients who do not seem to respond until a certain drug dosage has been reached, higher and less frequent doses of loop diuretics may be more effective than lower but more frequent doses.

Table 18–4. Pharmacologic Agents Used in Patients with Congestive Heart Failure.

Class	Group	Commonly Used Agent(s)
Diuretics	Thiazide diuretics	HCTZ
	Loop diuretics	Furosemide
	Potassium sparing diuretics	Spironolactone
Cardiac glycosides	Digitalis preparations	Digoxin
Inotropic drugs		Dobutamine
Vasoactive drugs	Vasodilators	Hydralazine
		Isosorbide
	ACE inhibitors	Enalapril
		Captopril
		Lisinopril
		Fosinopril
		Ramipril
		Benazepril
	Angiotensin II receptor blockers	
		Losartan
		Candesartan
		Irbesartan
		Valsartan
β-Blockers		Metoprolol CR/XL
		Carvedilol
Antiarrhythmic drugs		Amiodarone
		Dofetilide
Aldosterone receptor antagonists		Spironolactone
		Eplerenone
Natriuretic peptides		Nesiritide
Vasopressin receptor antagonists		Tolvaptan

ACE, angiotensin-converting enzyme; CR/XL, controlled release/extended release; HCTZ, hydrochlorothiazide.

A major advantage of loop diuretics is their safety and availability in intravenous form.

Potassium-sparing diuretics such as spironolactone (an aldosterone receptor blocker), triamterene, and amiloride decrease active sodium reabsorption and potassium excretion and could potentiate hyperkalemia; this is rare when the potassium-sparing diuretic is combined with a loop diuretic.

Brater DC. Pharmacology of diuretics. Am J Med Sci. 2000 Jan;319(1):38–50. [PMID: 10653443]

A. ELECTROLYTE ABNORMALITIES—Acute diuresis with both intravenous and short-term oral agents has been associated with increases in plasma renin and aldosterone activity as well as increased plasma norepinephrine levels. Patients with heart failure are thus at risk for developing electrolyte abnormalities from neurohormonal stimulation secondary to the use of diuretic agents. Hyponatremia in advanced CHF can be caused by a combination of diuretic therapy, neurohormonal activation, and enhanced vasopressin activity.

Although it is thought that potassium-sparing diuretics used in combination with loop or thiazide diuretics may partially limit excess potassium excretion, supporting data are limited. Another concern is that use of potassium-sparing diuretics in combination with ACE inhibitors may produce hyperkalemia, especially in patients with renal insufficiency.

The excretion of magnesium appears to parallel closely that of potassium. Ongoing treatment with thiazide diuretics can lead to hypomagnesemia, which can potentially lead to life-threatening cardiac arrhythmias in patients with CHF. This problem is further magnified in patients who have concomitant hypokalemia because a combined deficiency of potassium and magnesium not only potentiates the risk of ventricular arrhythmia, but hypokalemia cannot be corrected in some cases until the magnesium levels are restored.

Diuretics used with an ACE inhibitor are usually associated with fewer adverse neurohormonal and metabolic abnormalities.

B. ELECTROLYTE SUPPLEMENTATION—In diuretic-induced hypokalemia associated with a metabolic alkalosis and some chloride deficiency, the preferred salt for supplementation is potassium chloride. Although the usual daily dose for heart failure patients receiving diuretic therapy is 8–24 mEq of potassium, recent data indicate that these patients may have significantly lower potassium reserves, initially requiring 20–80 mEq daily to restore the potassium balance. The dose should be adjusted regularly, particularly during concomitant therapy with an ACE inhibitor or a potassium-sparing diuretic.

Long-term therapy with a thiazide or loop diuretic in patients with heart failure can lead to hypomagnesemia. Some studies have suggested that magnesium supplementation is highly effective in controlling the complex ventricular arrhythmias that can ensue in these patients. Although the antiarrhythmic action of magnesium needs to be confirmed in large-scale clinical trials, it appears reasonable to use magnesium supplementation in patients who exhibit life-threatening ventricular arrhythmias during vigorous diuretic therapy.

C. LIMITATIONS OF DIURETIC THERAPY—Although diuretics can relieve symptoms of pulmonary and systemic venous congestion, they cannot maintain most patients with heart failure in a compensated state for long periods. During the initial period of hospitalization, some patients may need larger doses of diuretics to start diuresis; doses can generally be decreased once diuresis has begun or during periods of bed rest. Somewhat larger doses may be required when the patient once again assumes routine daily activities. Patients with heart failure should be cautioned to watch for increases in weight (approximately 1–2 kg in 3 days), which can indicate retention of sodium and water. Such a weight increase should prompt the patient to seek medical help for adjustments in the diuretic dosage. This vigilance will help avoid frequent hospitalization or the need for emergency treatment, particularly in the advanced stages of heart failure. Patients with severe heart failure should also use nonsteroidal antiinflammatory agents with caution because their use may interfere with diuretic action and decrease natriuresis.

There is no evidence that treatment with most diuretics reduces mortality or alters the natural history of the disease. However, recent evidence suggests a beneficial role for spironolactone in treating moderate to severe heart failure.

Gheorghiade M et al; Efficacy of Vasopressin Antagonism in Heart Failure Outcome Study With Tolvaptan (EVEREST) Investigators. Short-term clinical effects of tolvaptan, an oral vasopressin antagonist, in patients hospitalized for heart failure: the EVEREST Clinical Status Trials. JAMA. 2007 Mar 28;297(12):1332–43. [PMID: 17384438]

Konstam MA et al; Efficacy of Vasopressin Antagonism in Heart Failure Outcome Study With Tolvaptan (EVEREST) Investigators. Effects of oral tolvaptan in patients hospitalized for worsening heart failure: the EVEREST Outcome Trial. JAMA. 2007 Mar 28;297(12):1319–31. [PMID: 17384437]

2. Vasopressin receptor antagonists—Tolvaptan (a nonpeptide vasopressin V_2 receptor antagonist) has been shown to improve congestive symptoms by increasing urinary output and decreasing body weight without adverse effects such as hyponatremia, hypokalemia, or worsening renal function.

Tolvaptan has been approved for treatment of clinically significant hyponatremia, hypokalemia, or worsening renal function. However, further studies are needed to clarify the clinical role of nonpeptide vasopressin V_2 receptor antagonists in the management of patients with LV systolic dysfunction and heart failure.

3. Inotropic agents

A. Digitalis glycosides—Glycosides of digitalis, which have been used in the treatment of heart failure for more than 200 years, are the most frequently used inotropic agents and the only oral positive inotropic preparation approved for treatment of heart failure. Digitalis glycosides, of which digoxin is the agent most commonly used, relieve symptoms by improving cardiac performance through increased myocardial contractility, improved LV function, and increased cardiac output and renal perfusion. Neurohormonal modulating actions have also been reported.

The beneficial effect of digitalis glycosides in patients with heart failure complicated by the occurrence of atrial fibrillation has been well documented and is generally well accepted

by most clinicians. The results of several studies indicate that in patients with heart failure, digitalis does exert sustained beneficial hemodynamic effects accompanied by improvement in both clinical status and exercise tolerance.

(1) Dosage and administration—Although digoxin can be given intravenously or orally, the intravenous route is preferred for patients with supraventricular tachyarrhythmia and fast ventricular rate. The initial intravenous dose is 0.5 mg given slowly over 10–20 minutes. If necessary, additional doses (0.25 or 0.125 mg) can be given after 4 hours. Younger patients generally require a total dose of about 1 mg for a full effect; smaller doses are recommended for the elderly and for patients with smaller total body mass. Although the therapeutic effect of oral digitalis occurs over a relatively prolonged period, it is less likely to result in overdose and toxicity. To achieve a more rapid effect orally, 1.0–1.25 mg of digoxin is given over 24 hours. Preferably, a slower effect should be achieved by giving daily maintenance doses (0.125–0.25 mg). The daily requirements of digoxin may be smaller for patients with renal insufficiency because the drug is excreted primarily by the kidneys and has a half-life of 36–48 hours. The levels of digoxin may be reduced by some antibiotics and cholestyramine; however, quinidine, verapamil, and amiodarone may increase serum digoxin levels and the digoxin dosage will need to be adjusted accordingly.

(2) Digitalis toxicity—Digitalis intoxication may occur in as many as 30% of patients hospitalized for the treatment of heart failure. Common findings are nausea, vomiting, anorexia, malaise, drowsiness, headache, insomnia, altered color vision, or arrhythmia. Almost all known cardiac arrhythmias can be caused by digitalis; they are facilitated by hypokalemia, which is often associated with the concomitant use of diuretics. The most common are premature ventricular beats, junctional tachycardia, second- or third-degree heart block, and paroxysmal atrial tachycardia with block. Digoxin toxicity is usually confirmed by the reversal of symptoms or cessation of arrhythmias after withdrawal of digoxin therapy for 48 hours. Severe toxicity can be reversed quickly with digoxin immune Fab.

(3) Clinical outcomes—Randomized controlled trials have shown that digoxin does not decrease mortality from heart failure but does reduce the rate of hospitalization for worsened heart failure.

B. Inotropes (sympathetic receptor agonist, dopamine agonist, β_1-partial agonist)—Myocardial catecholamine levels are depleted in patients with advanced heart failure, probably as a result of the chronic state of increased sympathetic stimulation. Several sympathomimetic amines have been used in an effort to improve the cardiac function associated with such depletion. The clinical use of sympathetic receptor agonists, however, has been limited by both their adverse effects and progressive loss of efficacy as patients become tolerant to them.

Dopamine and dobutamine are quite useful for short-term treatment of hospitalized patients with acute decompensated heart failure. Although intermittent intravenous dobutamine can improve hemodynamic parameters and decrease the rate of hospitalization, such treatment may reduce survival, especially in patients with preexisting episodes of ventricular tachycardia.

Thus, intermittent low-dose dobutamine therapy with careful supervision should be restricted to patients with refractory heart failure who have not responded to all other therapeutic choices. The aim of such treatment should be the temporary relief of severe symptoms.

> Mebazaa A et al; SURVIVE Investigators. Levosimendan vs dobutamine for patients with acute decompensated heart failure: the SURVIVE Randomized Trial. JAMA. 2007 May 2;297(17):1883–91. [PMID: 17473298]

4. Vasoactive drugs

A. VASODILATORS—These drugs are used to treat patients with CHF who remain symptomatic after administration of diuretics and digitalis; vasodilators are especially useful in patients with a dilated left ventricle, normal or increased systemic blood pressure, increased systemic vascular resistance, or valvular regurgitation. In general, these drugs are classified as venous, arterial, or mixed-vascular dilators; they have also been broadly classified as direct-acting drugs (eg, nitrates, hydralazine, minoxidil, nitroprusside) or neurohormonal antagonist drugs (eg, ACE inhibitor, α- and β-adrenoreceptor blockers, serotonin antagonists, angiotensin receptor blockers [ARB]), which block the vasoconstrictive actions of neurohormonal agents and have no direct vasodilator action. Although in the past vasodilators were primarily used in managing severe CHF, they are now widely accepted for use in mild-to-moderate heart failure. Although most vasodilators produce acute beneficial hemodynamic effects, some (eg, α-blocker prazosin) have been found to be no better than treatment with placebo during large clinical trials.

(1) Venous vasodilators—Nitrates have a greater effect on venous capacitance (venodilation) than on the arterial system. Intravenous administration, however, may produce significant arteriolar vasodilatation. Prolonged or sustained use of nitrates can lead to pharmacologic tolerance and offset its beneficial hemodynamic effects. Tolerance can develop during therapy with any nitrate preparation, whether oral, transcutaneous, or intravenous. The long-term beneficial effects of nitrates have been documented only with intermittent administration of oral preparations. Nitrate tolerance may be minimized by providing a daily nitrate-free interval of 8–12 hours and by using the smallest effective dose.

Isosorbide dinitrate. Long-term administration of isosorbide has been associated with significant improvement in hemodynamic parameters, exercise capacity, and relief of symptoms in moderate-to-severe heart failure. Although isosorbide dinitrate is the only direct-acting vasodilator that produces a sustained decrease in LV filling pressure, it is also the least likely to produce activation of endogenous neurohormones. Abrupt withdrawal after long-term oral therapy may be associated with a rebound phenomenon and should be avoided.

Close monitoring of blood pressure during the initial stages of nitrate therapy is advised in patients with preexisting low systemic blood pressure, suspected normal or low central venous or LV filling pressure (eg, that secondary to overdiuresis), the presence of significant pulmonary hypertension, or a previous history of orthostatic hypotension. Patients in whom significant exertional or nocturnal dyspnea develop may be given sublingual nitroglycerin for acute relief of the dyspnea; this therapy causes rapid and significant pulmonary vasodilatation with pooling of blood in both the pulmonary and systemic vascular beds. Oral nitrate preparations are easy to use, provide sustained systemic venous and pulmonary vascular effects, and are well tolerated. When used alone, these agents produce only modest clinical improvement in severe heart failure, however, and are usually considered as an adjunct to therapy with other vasodilators or ACE inhibitor.

Isosorbide dinitrate (80–160 mg/day), used in combination with hydralazine in patients with moderate CHF due to systolic functioning, is associated with a modest reduction in the risk of mortality and an improvement in LVEF.

(2) Arterial vasodilators—Hydralazine and minoxidil are direct-acting smooth muscle relaxants that seem to dilate arterioles predominantly. During treatment with these drugs, the systemic vascular resistance decreases and the cardiac output increases both at rest and during exercise. These beneficial hemodynamic effects unfortunately do not always translate into sustained clinical benefits. When used in combination with nitrates, hydralazine and minoxidil have shown a short-term increase in cardiac output and decrease in LV filling pressure. Clinical trials, however, have not shown a significant difference in exercise tolerance between placebo and hydralazine or minoxidil in patients with heart failure.

In patients with severe heart failure, hydralazine treatment is associated with a decrease in systemic vascular resistance and with increased stroke volume and cardiac output; it has little effect on the pulmonary capillary wedge pressure or right atrial pressure. Patients who have dilated left ventricles appear to have a better hemodynamic and clinical response than do patients with lesser degrees of enlargement. Studies have shown marked improvement in cardiac index and stroke work with a mild but significant reduction in LV filling pressure and an improvement of prerenal azotemia in patients with ventricular enlargement; rarely did significant reflex tachycardia or hypotension develop. In contrast, clinical deterioration characterized by findings suggestive of decreased tissue perfusion (eg, confusion, weakness, lethargy, worsening azotemia, ventricular arrhythmia, hypotension, or tachycardia) can develop in patients with smaller ventricles who are treated with hydralazine. Hydralazine can produce headaches, flushing, palpitations, nausea, vomiting, myocardial ischemia, and lupus-like syndrome at the required dosage of 200–800 mg/day.

(3) Clinical outcomes—In patients with moderate CHF, the combination of hydralazine (150–300 mg/day) and isosorbide (80–160 mg/day) results in an increase in LVEF and a lower risk of death.

The combination hydralazine-isosorbide should be considered a second-line therapy to be given to patients who do not seem to tolerate other therapies, including ACE inhibitors and β-blockers.

> Taylor AL et al; African-American Heart Failure Trial Investigators. Combination of isosorbide dinitrate and hydralazine in blacks with heart failure. N Engl J Med. 2004 Nov 11;351(20):2049–57. [PMID: 15533851]

5. Angiotensin-converting enzyme inhibitors

A. CLINICAL EFFECTS—In patients with heart failure, inhibition of angiotensin-converting enzyme produces a moderate increase in cardiac output with a concomitant significant decrease in right and left ventricular filling pressures, pulmonary and systemic vascular resistances, and mean arterial pressure, without increasing the heart rate (Table 18–5). Other beneficial effects include a reduction in the incidence of ventricular arrhythmias; decreased end-systolic and end-diastolic dimensions; and sustained improvements in symptoms, exercise duration, and quality of life.

Differences among various ACE inhibitors are primarily related to pharmacokinetic and hemodynamic properties. Both enalapril and lisinopril have delayed onset of action and

Table 18–5. Beneficial Hemodynamic and Neurohumoral Effects of Angiotensin-Converting Enzyme Inhibitor in Congestive Heart Failure.

Hemodynamic changes	
Central venous pressure	↓
Pulmonary capillary venous pressure	↓
Systemic vascular resistance	↓
End-diastolic LV dimension	↓
End-systolic LV dimension	↓
Stroke volume	↑
Cardiac output	↑
Cardiac index	↑
Neurohormonal activity	
Norepinephrine	↓
Vasopressin	↓
Angiotensin II	↓
Aldosterone	↓ or no change
Serum potassium	↑ or no change

LV, left ventricular.

prolonged duration of hemodynamic effects (compared with captopril). Hypotension is delayed and prolonged and can reduce systemic perfusion, compromising both renal and cerebral functions. Because the hypotension caused by captopril is shorter in duration, it rarely compromises organ perfusion.

B. SAFETY OF ANGIOTENSIN-CONVERTING ENZYME INHIBITORS—The major differences in safety appear to be the potential adverse effects of the long-acting agents on renal and cerebral function. Renal function, however, usually returns to baseline or stabilizes at a new steady state despite continued treatment with the ACE inhibitor, except in rare instances when membranous glomerulonephritis occurs. Based on the available data, it seems that renal complications secondary to ACE inhibitor therapy occur predominantly in patients with previous renal disease and those receiving large doses. In most cases, discontinuing treatment or decreasing the dosage of the ACE inhibitor rapidly resolves the proteinuria and renal dysfunction, and this decline in renal function appears to be of little clinical significance. In major clinical trials, the incidence of discontinuation of ACE inhibitor therapy because of impairment in renal function has been low (1–3%); in some studies it was equivalent to that seen with placebo. The longer-acting ACE inhibitors, however, may be associated with a higher risk of renal dysfunction.

Some patients may be very sensitive to the hypotensive effects of ACE inhibitors, particularly patients who are initiating therapy and who are dependent on the renin-angiotensin-aldosterone system for blood pressure maintenance. This includes patients with hyponatremia or hypovolemia, those receiving high-dose diuretic therapy, and those with bilateral renal artery stenosis. The hypotension usually subsides with continued therapy and can be partly avoided by reducing the diuretic dosage for several days before initiating treatment with an ACE inhibitor. This therapy should be started under close medical supervision, and patients considered at risk for severe hypotension should be monitored closely for the first 2 weeks of treatment. Some investigators recommend a period of brief hospitalization and close observation during the initiation of enalapril therapy until a maintenance dose is achieved.

Clinical outcomes—Numerous clinical trials have shown that ACE inhibitors reduce all cause mortality, cardiovascular death, sudden death, heart failure deaths, worsened heart failure, and subsequent hospitalizations. Based on these findings, ACE inhibitors are well established as first-line therapy for all patients with LV dysfunction and heart failure (NYHA I–IV), including heart failure associated with acute MI. In addition, there is evidence that ACE inhibitors are beneficial for asymptomatic patients with reduced LV function and patients with normal LV function with known vascular disease or at high risk for vascular disease.

6. Angiotensin II receptor blockers—The ARBs provide
direct blockade of angiotensin II type-1 (AT$_1$) receptor activation. This action results in the effective blockade of the

potentially harmful effects of angiotensin II on tissues. This action takes place regardless of angiotensin II generation by ACE-dependent pathways or ACE-independent (alternative) pathways (Figure 18–2). In addition, this effect is achieved without accumulation of bradykinin, which is considered to be responsible for some adverse reactions associated with the use of ACE inhibitors, such as persistent cough, angioedema, and significant hypotension.

Theoretically, the use of these drugs should be associated with beneficial effects on clinical outcomes similar to those seen during ACE inhibitor therapy and with fewer side effects. The ARBs have produced favorable hemodynamic effects during short- and long-term administration. Also, randomized clinical trials comparing ARBs with ACE inhibitors have generally shown equivalent or enhanced benefits.

Cohn JN et al; Valsartan Heart Failure Trial Investigators. A randomized trial of the angiotensin-receptor blocker valsartan in chronic heart failure. N Engl J Med. 2001 Dec 6;345(23):1667–75. [PMID: 11759645]

Pfeffer MA et al; CHARM Investigators and Committees. Effects of candesarten on mortality and morbidity in patients with chronic heart failure: the CHARM-Overall programme. Lancet. 2003 Sep 6;362(9386):759–66. [PMID: 13678868]

Pitt B et al. Effect of losartan compared with captopril on mortality in patients with symptomatic heart failure: randomised trial—the Losartan Heart Failure Survival Study ELITE II. Lancet. 2000 May 6;355(9215):1582–7. [PMID: 10821361]

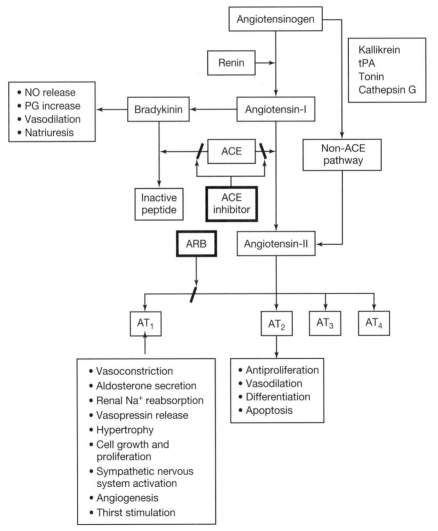

▲ **Figure 18–2.** Renin-angiotensin system cascade and angiotensin II receptors. ACE, angiotensin-converting enzyme; ARB, angiotensin receptor blocker; AT_1–AT_4, angiotensin II types 1–4; NO, nitric oxide; PG, prostaglandins; tPA, tissue plasminogen.

Yusuf S et al. Effects of an angiotensin-converting enzyme inhibitor ramipril, on cardiovascular events in high-risk patients. Heart Outcomes Prevention Evaluation Study Investigators. N Engl J Med. 2000 Jan 20;342(3):145–53. [PMID: 10639539]

7. β-Blockers—Although first-generation β-blocking agents (with a nonselective affinity for β_1- or β_2-receptors) are not well tolerated in heart failure, nonselective third-generation β-blockers with vasodilator activity (bucindolol and carvedilol) as well as the β_1-selective agent metoprolol are generally well tolerated by patients with CHF. Clinical studies demonstrate that prolonged β-blockade improves hemodynamic and clinical function in patients with chronic heart failure. The beneficial effects are seen in patients with idiopathic dilated cardiomyopathy as well as in those with ischemic cardiomyopathy. The findings from recent trials evaluating β-blockers in patients with varying degrees of heart failure indicate that these drugs exert a beneficial effect on LV function and improve survival as well as clinical symptoms. These findings have led to the recommendations in all guidelines for use of β-blockers in the management of heart failure (NYHA II–IV).

Dargie HJ. Effect of carvedilol on outcome after myocardial infarction in patients with left ventricular dysfunction: the CAPRICORN randomised trial. Lancet. 2001 May 5;357(9266):1385–90. [PMID: 11356434]

Flather MD et al; SENIORS Investigators. Randomized trial to determine the effect of nebivolol on mortality and cardiovascular hospital admission in elderly patients with heart failure (SENIORS). Eur Heart J. 2005 Feb;26(3):215–25. [PMID: 15642700]

Hjalmarson A et al. Effects of controlled-release metoprolol on total mortality, hospitalizations, and well-being in patients with heart failure; the Metoprolol CR/XL Randomized Intervention Trial in congestive heart failure (MERIT-HF). MERIT-HF Study Group. JAMA. 2000 Mar 8;283(10):1295–302. [PMID: 10714728]

Packer M et al. Effect of carvedilol on survival in severe chronic heart failure. N Engl J Med. 2001 May 31;344(22):1651–8. [PMID: 11386263]

8. Aldosterone receptor blockers—Spironolactone is a renal competitive aldosterone antagonist. It inhibits the effect of aldosterone by competing for the aldosterone-dependent sodium-potassium exchange site in the distal tubule cells. This increases the secretion of water and sodium, while decreasing the excretion of potassium. Eplerenone is a relatively selective mineralocorticoid receptor blocker that prevents the binding of aldosterone.

Based on the findings from clinical trials, patients with evidence of advanced heart failure (NYHA III or IV) or with post-MI CHF should receive treatment with an aldosterone receptor blocker.

Pitt B et al; Eplerenone Post-Acute Myocardial Infarction Heart Failure Efficacy and Survival Study Investigators. Eplerenone, a selective aldosterone blocker, in patients with left ventricular dysfunction after myocardial infarction. N Engl J Med. 2003 Apr 3;348(14):1309–21. [PMID: 12668699]

9. Natriuretic peptide—The recombinant human B-type (brain) natriuretic peptide, nesiritide, is an agent with vasodilator, natriuretic, and diuretic effects that has been shown to improve symptoms in patients with acutely decompensated heart failure. However, nesiritide may be associated with an increased risk of death within 30 days. Thus, treatment with nesiritide is not recommended for routine use in patients with decompensated heart failure.

Sackner-Bernstein JD et al. Short-term risk of death after treatment with nesiritide for decompensated heart failure: a pooled analysis of randomized controlled trials. JAMA. 2005 Apr 20;293(15):1900–5. [PMID: 15840865]

Yancy CW et al; FUSION II Investigators. The Second Follow-up Serial Infusions of Nesiritide (FUSION II) trial for advanced heart failure: study rationale and design. Am Heart J. 2007 Apr;153(4):478–84. [PMID: 17383282]

10. Antiarrhythmic drugs—Patients with heart failure are at risk for sudden death presumably associated with complex ventricular arrhythmia. There has been interest in evaluating therapies targeted at reduction of this arrhythmic risk in heart failure.

The class III antiarrhythmic agents amiodarone and dofetilide have each been evaluated in patients with heart failure and found not to improve mortality. They can be useful for managing hemodynamically significant atrial and ventricular tachyarrhythmias.

11. Antiischemic therapy—Coronary artery disease is the most common cause of heart failure in the United States. While most cases of heart failure associated with CAD are secondary to mechanical complications from MI (eg, pump failure, mitral regurgitation, cardiac rupture), some cases are a result of transient ventricular dysfunction related to episodes of reversible myocardial ischemia. Although not all episodes of myocardial ischemia in a given patient are associated with the development of heart failure, it seems that relatively prolonged ischemic episodes are associated with significant abnormalities of ventricular function or mitral regurgitation from transient papillary muscle dysfunction. Conventional agents for the treatment of heart failure (eg, digitalis, ACE inhibitors, vasodilators) may prove ineffective in such cases; however, antiischemic drugs, which relieve and help prevent myocardial ischemia, will effectively improve and prevent the development of symptoms of heart failure. This may help explain, in part, why β-blockers appear to be excellent drugs in patients with ischemic heart disease who suffer from recurrent episodes of angina-equivalent symptoms consistent with heart failure. These episodes may be triggered by and parallel the development of transient episodes of silent myocardial ischemia. Signs and symptoms of heart failure may be frequently present in elderly patients during episodes of silent myocardial ischemia. Such episodes are a common occurrence in patients with documented CAD. Simultaneous evaluation of ECG and ventricular function show that ischemic ECG changes are associated with transient depression of LVEF in some patients. Some periods of ischemia may have such a long duration that contractile function is markedly and chronically depressed (hibernating myocardium). Although irreversible myocardial damage usually does not occur in these settings, restoration of contractility may be delayed for days or weeks after the ischemia is relieved. The phenomenon of myocardial stunning is frequently observed after successful reperfusion therapy with thrombolytic agents in patients with acute MI and may also lead to transient symptoms of heart failure.

C. Nonpharmacologic Treatment

1. Myocardial revascularization—Heart failure associated with myocardial ischemia may be improved by myocardial revascularization through relief of myocardial ischemia. Thus, evidence of ischemia should always be sought in patients with CAD and heart failure.

2. Ventricular aneurysmectomy—Although patients with CAD usually experience chest pain in association with a LV aneurysm, heart failure may be present instead. These latter patients should be considered for surgical aneurysmectomy and myocardial revascularization. Left ventricular aneurysmectomy is usually beneficial in attenuating the symptoms of heart failure and can possibly improve survival.

3. Cardiac pacing—Patients with heart failure frequently have associated intraventricular conduction delay or left bundle branch block. These cardiac conduction abnormalities can trigger mechanical dyssynchrony of the ventricular contraction and adversely affect cardiac performance.

Pacing in patients with heart failure is a new concept that could lead to improved clinical outcomes. The benefits would be attained through improving the pattern of ventricular activation, reducing ventricular dyssynchrony, and optimizing synchronization between atrial and ventricular contractility. This treatment modality has been called cardiac resynchronization or biventricular pacing. Uncontrolled, primarily unblinded as well as recently blinded, studies in patients with heart failure who underwent cardiac resynchronization have revealed an improvement in acute hemodynamic performance, exercise capacity, and quality of life during active pacing.

4. Implantable cardiac defibrillator devices—In patients considered at risk for complex ventricular arrhythmia and sudden death, which includes patients with both ischemic and idiopathic dilated cardiomyopathy as well as a LVEF < 35%, implantable cardioverter defibrillators (ICD) have been shown to prolong survival (Table 18–6). These devices are combined with biventricular pacing in the same device.

Bardy GH et al; Sudden Cardiac Death in Heart Failure Trial (SCD-HeFT) Investigators. Amiodarone or an implantable cardioverter-defibrillator for congestive heart failure. N Engl J Med. 2005 Jan 20;352(3):225–37. [PMID: 15659722]

Bristow MR et al; Comparison of Medical Therapy, Pacing, and Defibrillation in Heart Failure (COMPANION) Investigators. Cardiac-resynchronization therapy with or without an implantable defibrillator in advanced chronic heart failure. N Engl J Med. 2004 May 20;350(21):2140–50. [PMID: 15152059]

Cleland JG et al; Cardiac Resynchronization-Heart Failure (CARE-HF) Study Investigators. The effect of cardiac resynchronization on morbidity and mortality in heart failure. N Engl J Med. 2005 Apr 14;352(15):1539–49. [PMID: 15753115]

Table 18–6. Studies That Have Evaluated the Impact of ICD Therapy in Patients with Heart Failure.

Name	Death Benefit	Sudden Death Benefit	Receiving β-Blocker (control arm; %)	Receiving β-Blocker (ICD arm, %)
MADIT-1	Yes	No	5	27
CABG-PATCH	No	Yes	19.8	16
MUSTT	No	Yes	51	29
MADIT-2	Yes	Yes	70	70
CAT	No	No	3.7	4
AMIOVIRT	No	No	50	53
DEFINITE	No	Yes	84.3	85.6
DINAMIT	No	Yes	86.5	87
SCD-HeFT	Yes	NA	79	82

AMIOVIRT, Amiodarone Versus Implantable Cardioverter-Defibrillator: Randomized Trial in Patients With Nonischemic Dilated Cardiomyopathy and Asymptomatic Nonsustained Ventricular Tachycardia; CABG Patch, Coronary Artery Bypass Graft Patch trial; CAT, Cardiomyopathy trial; DEFINITE, Defibrillators in Non-ischemic Cardiomyopathy Treatment Evaluation trial; DINAMIT, Defibrillator in Acute Myocardial Infarction Trial; ICD, implantable cardiac defibrillator; MADIT-I, Multi-center Automatic Defibrillator Trial; MADIT-II, Multi-center Automatic Defibrillator Trial; MUSTT, Multicenter Unsustained Tachycardia Trial; SCD-HeFT, Sudden Cardiac Death in Heart Failure trial.

Ezekowitz JA et al. Implantable cardioverter defibrillators in primary and secondary prevention: a systematic review of randomized, controlled trials. Ann Intern Med. 2003 Mar 18;138(6):445–52. [PMID: 12639076]

Higgins SL et al. Cardiac resynchronization therapy for the treatment of heart failure in patients with intraventricular conduction delay and malignant ventricular tachyarrhythmias. J Am Coll Cardiol. 2003 Oct 15;42(8):1454–9. [PMID: 14563591]

Varma C et al. Pacing for heart failure. Lancet. 2001 Apr 21;357(9264):1277–83. [PMID: 11418172]

5. Cardiac transplantation—Patients with severe heart failure with a limited life expectancy might be considered candidates for heart transplantation (Table 18–7). The conventional criteria for consideration of heart transplantation for patients suffering from heart failure include advanced heart failure (NYHA III–IV) with objective evidence indicating severe limitation of functional ability and an estimated poor 1-month prognosis in the face of optimized or maximized medical therapy, low-output state or refractory cardiac failure requiring frequent or constant use of inotropes, cardiogenic shock or low-output hemodynamic state with reversible end-organ dysfunction requiring mechanical circulatory support, recurrence of or rapidly progressing heart failure unresponsive to optimized or maximized vasodilator and diuretic therapies.

The shortage of donor hearts, however, makes transplantation unavailable to most patients with end-stage heart failure, and many patients die while waiting for a donor organ. Furthermore, the stringent criteria used to select potential candidates make many patients ineligible. The qualification criteria are intended to identify the patients who are at highest risk and who may derive the greatest benefit from heart transplantation. Some patients, however, spontaneously improve while waiting for a suitable donor; this improvement has been accompanied by prolonged survival during the relatively short follow-up period. Furthermore, advances in medical and surgical therapies have been associated with improvement in clinical outcomes for patients with advanced heart failure. Compared with 10–20 years ago, these newer drug therapies have cast some uncertainty over the benefits of cardiac transplantation compared with other treatment options in advanced heart failure.

Deng MC et al. Effect of receiving a heart transplant: analysis of a national cohort entered on to a waiting list, stratified by heart failure severity. Comparative Outcome and Clinical Profiles in Transplantation (COCPIT) Study Group. BMJ. 2000 Sep 2;321(7260):540–5. [PMID: 10968814]

Freudenberger R et al. Characteristics of patients referred for cardiac transplantation: implications for the donor organ shortage. Am Heart J. 2000 Dec;140(6):857–61. [PMID: 11099988]

Koerner MM et al. Cardiac transplantation: the final therapeutic option for the treatment of heart failure. Curr Opin Cardiol. 2000 May;15(3):178–82. [PMID: 10952425]

6. Circulatory-assist devices—These devices can offer additional options for the treatment of patients with severe

Table 18–7. Criteria for Cardiac Transplantation.

End-stage heart disease with poor (6–12 month) prognosis and refractory to aggressive tailored medical or any other surgical treatment
NYHA functional class III or IV
Age 60–65 years (various programs)
Pulmonary vascular resistance < 3 RU or < 2.5 RU after intravenous nitroprusside
Strong self-motivation and psychosocial support
Absence of
Malignancy
Active infection
Active peptic ulcerative disease
Pulmonary infarction within 6 weeks
Advanced insulin-dependent diabetes mellitus with end-organ damage (relative)
Kidney or liver dysfunction beyond that expected from severe CHF
Advanced peripheral vascular disease
Collagen vascular diseases
Active alcoholism or substance abuse

CHF, congestive heart failure; NYHA, New York Heart Association; RU, resistance units.

heart failure who deteriorate despite aggressive pharmacologic therapy and who may be considered candidates for heart transplantation. In general, the reasons for assisting circulation with these devices are to provide ventricular assistance and allow the heart to rest and recover its function in cases of expected recovery and to provide circulatory assistance as a bridge to cardiac transplantation in patients with extensive acute MI, acute myocarditis, or advanced end-stage heart disease or failure on whom recovery of adequate cardiac function is not expected. Several devices, which include extracorporeal membrane oxygenation, univentricular and biventricular extracorporeal nonpulsatile devices; extracorporeal and implantable pulsatile devices; the total artificial heart; and many others, are in various stages of development, and some are currently available for cardiac mechanical support. They are generally classified according to the extent of cardiac support achieved from the degree of stroke volume generated by the device and the length of support provided.

The use of assisted circulation is associated with risk of complications as bleeding, right-sided heart failure, renal insufficiency, infection, air- and thromboembolic events, and progressive multisystem organ failure. Some of these complications, particularly infection and renal failure, carry an increased risk of death. Patients may become ineligible for heart transplantation if they develop severe complications during the period of mechanically assisted circulation.

The concept of "bridge to recovery" might become a goal for ventricular assist devices; however, several issues, particularly reliability for long-term use, need to be determined prior to widespread and extended use of these devices in advanced heart failure.

It is also important to keep in mind that mechanical circulatory support is expensive and can greatly tax the available resources and personnel; it should therefore be considered only in exceptional situations where reversal of the underlying condition or early transplantation is expected.

Rose EA et al; Randomized Evaluation of Mechanical Assistance for the Treatment of Congestive Heart Failure (REMATCH) Study Group. Long-term mechanical left ventricular assistance for end-stage heart failure. N Engl J Med. 2001 Nov 15;345(2):1435–43. [PMID: 11794191]

▶ Prognosis

Heart failure is a complex clinical syndrome associated with adverse clinical outcome and increased likelihood of death. It can develop at various points in the natural history of a number of cardiac disorders and systemic illnesses. In general, the prognosis of patients with heart failure is closely related to the degree of ventricular dysfunction, the amount of oxygen consumption during exercise, and the extent of activation of neurohormonal axes, including the sympathetic nervous system and the renin-angiotensin-aldosterone system. Newer strategies in the treatment of heart failure are based on these and other factors that influence both the pathogenesis and prognosis of heart failure. Despite better diagnostic techniques and treatment options, however, heart failure remains a progressively deteriorating condition associated with increased morbidity and mortality.

Some clinical parameters may be useful in identifying CHF patients at an increased risk for mortality, including severity of LV dysfunction (measured as ejection fraction), circulating levels of neurohormones (particularly norepinephrine), abnormalities of heart rate (fixed rapid rate), NYHA functional class, and complex atrial and ventricular tachyarrhythmias. The prognosis also appears to vary according to the cause of the underlying heart failure. For example, patients with ischemic heart failure have a worse prognosis than those with peripartum cardiomyopathy.

Because the prognosis of patients with heart failure is quite guarded, the ideal therapeutic strategy should be directed at its prevention. This includes prompt intervention in individuals considered at risk for heart failure when evidence of impaired LV function is first detected.

Hunt SA et al; American College of Cardiology/American Heart Association Task Force on Practice Guidelines (Writing Committee to Update the 2001 Guidelines for the Evaluation and Management of Heart Failure). ACC/AHA 2005 guideline update for the diagnosis and management of chronic heart failure in the adult: a report of the American College of Cardiology/American Heart Association Task Force on Practice Guidelines (Writing Committee to Update the 2001 Guidelines for the Evaluation and Management of Heart Failure). Circulation. 2005;112:1825–52.

Heart Failure with Preserved Ejection Fraction

Sanjiv J. Shah, MD

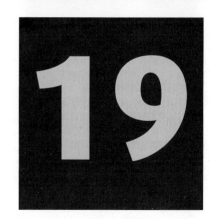

19

ESSENTIALS OF DIAGNOSIS

▸ Symptoms and signs of heart failure with preserved left ventricular ejection fraction (LVEF > 50%).

▸ Presence of an underlying cause of heart failure with preserved ejection fraction (eg, comorbidities such as hypertension, coronary artery disease, diabetes, chronic kidney disease; or underlying valvular heart disease, restrictive cardiomyopathy, or specific myocardial diseases such as amyloidosis).

▸ The diagnosis of diastolic heart failure, which is the most common cause of heart failure with preserved ejection fraction, requires definite clinical evidence of heart failure, LVEF > 50%, and objective evidence of LV diastolic dysfunction by echocardiography or cardiac catheterization.

▶ General Considerations

Heart failure with preserved ejection fraction (HFpEF) is an increasingly common, debilitating syndrome of the elderly, and it carries a high rate of morbidity and mortality. HFpEF accounts for nearly 50% of all hospitalizations for heart failure, and two large epidemiologic studies have confirmed that patients with HFpEF have a mortality rate that is nearly identical to heart failure with low ejection fraction.

HFpEF is the preferred term for patients with a normal ejection fraction who have the syndrome of heart failure, because HFpEF highlights the fact that heart failure is a syndrome and not a distinct clinical or pathophysiologic entity. Many investigators and experts have used the term "diastolic heart failure" for HFpEF in the past. However, this term is not ideal for two main reasons. First, there is ample evidence that patients with HFpEF have abnormalities in systolic function (as defined by tissue Doppler imaging), and many patients with heart failure and low ejection fraction

have abnormal diastolic function. Second, in the clinical setting, patients with heart failure are currently classified into two categories: low ejection fraction (< 50%) and preserved ejection fraction (> 50%). By calling HFpEF "diastolic heart failure," clinicians may not consider the entire differential diagnosis of HFpEF (of which pure diastolic dysfunction is only one cause). HFpEF has also previously been called "heart failure with preserved systolic function" or "heart failure with normal systolic function." As stated above, it is now clear that many patients with HFpEF have abnormalities in systolic function; therefore, HFpEF is a better term.

The most recent American Heart Association/American College of Cardiology (AHA/ACC) guidelines have used the term "heart failure with normal ejection fraction." This term is also not ideal because there is considerable controversy regarding the exact cutoff for a "normal" ejection fraction. Therefore, HFpEF is a slightly better term and was used in the most recent Heart Failure Society of America guidelines on the management of patients with heart failure. Finally, HFpEF has the advantage of being an easy mnemonic for patients to remember. HFpEF sounds like "HUFF-PUFF," which helps patients understand this disease, in which dyspnea and fatigue are two of the most common symptoms.

Chinnaiyan KM et al. Curriculum in cardiology: integrated diagnosis and management of diastolic heart failure. Am Heart J. 2007 Feb;153(2):189–200. [PMID: 17239676]

Heart Failure Society of America. Evaluation and management of patients with heart failure and preserved left ventricular ejection fraction. J Card Fail. 2006 Feb;12(1):e80–5. [PMID: 16500575]

Hunt SA et al; American College of Cardiology; American Heart Association Task Force on Practice Guidelines; American College of Chest Physicians; International Society for Heart and Lung Transplantation; Heart Rhythm Society. ACC/AHA 2005 Guideline Update for the Diagnosis and Management of Chronic Heart Failure in the Adult: a report of the American College of Cardiology/American Heart Association Task Force on Practice Guidelines (Writing Committee to Update the 2001 Guidelines for the Evaluation and Management of Heart Failure): developed in collaboration with the American College of Chest Physicians and the International Society for Heart and Lung Transplantation: endorsed by the Heart Rhythm Society. Circulation. 2005 Sep 20;112(12):e154–235. [PMID: 16160202]

▶ Pathophysiology

Since HFpEF is heterogeneous, there is no single mechanism that can explain the pathophysiology of the HFpEF syndrome. In some patients with HFpEF, such as those who have the signs and symptoms of heart failure due to severe valvular disease or pericardial disease (ie, constrictive pericarditis), pathophysiology is relatively straightforward and well-defined. However, in most patients with HFpEF, pathophysiologic abnormalities cannot be ascribed to a single well-defined mechanism. Instead, these patients typically have one or more of the following underlying pathophysiologic processes: (1) Diastolic dysfunction due to impaired LV relaxation, increased LV diastolic stiffness, or both; (2) LV enlargement with increased intravascular volume, which may be due to extracardiac factors such as renal insufficiency; (3) abnormal ventricular-arterial coupling with increased ventricular systolic stiffness and increased arterial stiffness. In addition, left ventricular hypertrophy and coronary artery disease are especially important in the pathophysiology of patients with HFpEF.

A. Diastolic Dysfunction

Diastolic dysfunction occurs when the ventricle loses its normal ability to suction blood from the left atrium. When the ventricle relaxes abnormally, filling is delayed and left atrial emptying is incomplete. An abnormally stiff ventricle worsens the problem by also impeding left atrial emptying. The end result is abnormally high left atrial and LV diastolic pressures. The LV loses its suction and instead of "pulling"

blood from the left atrium and pulmonary veins, it now relies heavily on left atrial contraction so that the LV can fill and distend appropriately, and recoil in systole. This is one reason why atrial fibrillation is tolerated so poorly in patients with advanced LV diastolic dysfunction with resultant elevation of left atrial pressure, pulmonary vascular congestion, and poor cardiac output.

In patients with HFpEF who have substantial diastolic dysfunction as a cause of their symptoms, the pressure–volume curve is shifted up and to the left (Figure 19–1). In these patients, even small increases in central blood volume or vascular (arterial or venous) tone can result in significant increases in left atrial volume and pulmonary venous pressures. Patients with an upward and leftward shift in the LV diastolic pressure–volume relationship tend to have a high relative wall thickness (high LV mass/volume ratio), increased fibrosis and scar of the LV myocardium due to ischemia, infarction, infiltrative disease, or radiation, and impaired active relaxation of the myocardium (due to abnormal myocyte calcium homeostasis).

B. Left Ventricular Enlargement and Increased Intravascular Volume

Left ventricular enlargement is a key predictor of heart failure, regardless of ejection fraction. However, patients with isolated diastolic heart failure are often thought to have small LV volumes. This apparent discrepancy can be explained by the underlying cause of HFpEF and diastolic heart failure. It is likely that patients with significant coronary disease or myocardial ischemia (even in the absence of epicardial coronary disease) suffer from increased LV enlargement. In addition, many patients with LV enlargement have increased intravascular volume due to comorbidities such as chronic kidney disease, anemia, and obesity.

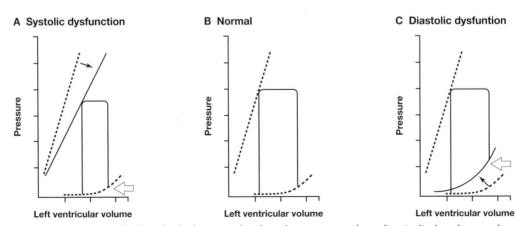

▲ **Figure 19–1.** In patients with diastolic dysfunction, the diastolic pressure–volume line is displaced upward and to the left (Panel C, black arrow); there is diminished capacity to fill at low left-atrial pressures. The ejection fraction is normal and the end-diastolic pressure is elevated (Panel C, open arrow). (Reproduced, with permission, from Aurigemma G et al. Clinical practice: Diastolic heart failure. N Engl J Med 351:1097–1105. © Massachusetts Medical Society 2004. All Rights reserved.)

Thus, LV enlargement and increased intravascular volume cause symptoms of HFpEF by a pathophysiologic mechanism that is distinct from pure LV diastolic dysfunction.

C. Abnormal Ventricular-Arterial Coupling

Ventricular-arterial coupling describes the interaction between ventricular stiffness and central arterial stiffness. In healthy patients, young and old, arterial and ventricular elastance (stiffness) are matched in order to maintain optimal cardiac efficiency. However, with increasing age, ventricular stiffness is elevated and results in decreased contractile reserve, thereby rendering elderly patients susceptible to heart failure, blood pressure lability, and decreased exercise tolerance. Some patients with HFpEF appear to be particularly susceptible to abnormal ventricular-arterial coupling. These patients have the age-related increases in ventricular stiffness described above, but instead of matched ventricular and arterial stiffness, ventricular stiffness rises out of proportion of arterial stiffness, which results in poor cardiac efficiency. These patients tend to have high pulse pressure, and they tend to be most sensitive to diuretics whereby small changes in blood volume result in large changes in blood pressure (either significantly hypertensive or hypotensive).

D. Left Ventricular Hypertrophy

Left ventricular hypertrophy contributes substantially to the pathophysiology of HFpEF and is an important risk factor. Left ventricular hypertrophy limits coronary flow reserve, increases LV diastolic stiffness, and impairs LV relaxation. Patients with LV hypertrophy suffer from an inability to adequately utilize the Frank-Starling mechanism. Therefore, inadequate preload and chronotropic incompetence can lead to decreased cardiac output, with resultant lightheadedness, dizziness, and exercise intolerance. Finally, because of increased LV wall thickness, the subendocardium is especially vulnerable to ischemia in patients with and without epicardial coronary disease due to decreased coronary blood flow during exercise. Subendocardial ischemia can cause both systolic and diastolic dysfunction in these patients and further exacerbate HFpEF.

E. Coronary Artery Disease

Approximately 40% of patients with HFpEF have concomitant coronary artery disease. In these patients, coronary disease is often severe, involving multiple epicardial coronary arteries. Patients with prior myocardial infarction, ongoing ischemia, or stable chronic coronary disease can all present with HFpEF. Myocardial ischemia causes calcium sequestration in diastole, which results in impaired LV relaxation and increased LV filling pressures. In areas of prior infarction or ongoing ischemia, regional systolic dysfunction and dysynchrony can further exacerbate abnormal loading conditions and create a mixture of systolic and diastolic dysfunction. Furthermore, patients with chronic coronary artery disease often have LV remodeling with resultant ventricular enlargement, a known risk factor for increased mortality and heart failure, despite ejection fraction. Preservation of ejection fraction occurs even in patients with prior infarction due to hypertrophy and hyperdynamic function of non-infarcted areas.

Patients with coronary disease suffer from a vicious cycle of abnormalities that contribute to HFpEF. As noted above, ischemia can cause impaired LV relaxation and increased LV filling pressures. Impaired LV relaxation in turn can also adversely affect coronary blood flow and coronary flow reserve, which exacerbates ischemia. Increased LV filling pressures results in extravascular compression of the small intramyocardial coronary vessels, which can cause subendocardial ischemia. Increased LV end-diastolic pressure can also result in poor epicardial coronary blood flow. Thus, ischemia begets worsening LV diastolic function, which begets more ischemia.

Borlaug BA et al. Impaired chronotropic and vasodilator reserves limit exercise capacity in patients with heart failure and a preserved ejection fraction. Circulation. 2006 Nov 14;114(20):2138–47. [PMID: 17088459]

Kliger C et al. A clinical algorithm to differentiate heart failure with a normal ejection fraction by pathophysiologic mechanism. Am J Geriatr Cardiol. 2006 Jan–Feb;15(1):50–7. [PMID: 16415647]

Maurer MS et al. Left heart failure with a normal ejection fraction: identification of different pathophysiologic mechanisms. J Card Fail. 2005 Apr;11(3):177–87. [PMID: 15812744]

Sohn DW et al. Hemodynamic effects of tachycardia in patients with relaxation abnormality: abnormal stroke volume response as an overlooked mechanism of dyspnea associated with tachycardia in diastolic heart failure. J Am Soc Echocardiogr. 2007 Feb;20(2):171–6. [PMID: 17275703]

Zile MR et al. Diastolic heart failure—abnormalities in active relaxation and passive stiffness of the left ventricle. N Engl J Med. 2004 May 6;350(19):1953–9. [PMID: 15128895]

▶ Clinical Findings

The first step in caring for a patient with HFpEF is to ensure the correct diagnosis (see section on Differential Diagnosis below). Several criteria for the diagnosis of HFpEF exist. All require signs and symptoms of heart failure and objective evidence of preserved ejection fraction ($\geq 50\%$).

A. Risk Factors

1. Age—Patients with HFpEF are almost universally elderly, and aging has several effects on cardiovascular structure and function that are pertinent to HFpEF patients. Aging reduces the diastolic filling rate as a result of prolonged relaxation, which results in left atrial overload and pulmonary venous hypertension. Arterial stiffness increases with age, resulting in increased afterload and load-dependent diastolic dysfunction. In addition, stiffening of the central arteries (which is especially common in women) leaves them less capable to handle changes in blood volume, thereby increasing susceptibility to hypotension, lightheadedness, and dizziness.

Finally, aging reduces exercise capacity by increasing ventricular end-systolic chamber elastance (stiffness), which results in decreased ability to augment contractility with exercise.

2. Hypertension—Hypertension is the most important risk factor for HFpEF and is present in most patients with HFpEF. Hypertensive emergency with flash pulmonary edema is a common presentation of HFpEF. Hypertension leads to LV hypertrophy, which causes impaired relaxation, poor coronary flow reserve, and increased diastolic stiffness, all of which exacerbate HFpEF. Hypertension is also a potent risk factor for epicardial coronary disease, which often complicates HFpEF. Ischemia causes both increased LV stiffness and impaired LV relaxation. Many patients with HFpEF have symptoms of chronic angina. Alternatively, recurrent heart failure may be an anginal equivalent in many patients with concomitant HFpEF and coronary disease.

3. Obstructive sleep apnea—Obstructive sleep apnea is a common comorbidity in patients with HFpEF, and it can result in worsening LV hypertrophy and pulmonary hypertension. In addition, patients with HFpEF may also have sleep-disordered breathing (such as Cheyne-Stokes respirations) due to their heart failure. Finally, increased upper airway edema due to generalized heart failure may actually cause obstructive sleep apnea, a finding that has been shown to improve with diuretic therapy. All of the above contribute to nocturnal microarousals and hypoxia, which result in poor sleep quality, which in turn worsens daytime fatigue and exercise intolerance. Therefore, there should be a low threshold to perform a sleep study on the patient with HFpEF.

4. Other clinically important risk factors—Other clinically important risk factors for HFpEF include coronary artery disease, diabetes, chronic kidney disease, obesity, atrial fibrillation, anemia, and chronic obstructive pulmonary disease. All of these comorbidities have their own signs and symptoms that can complicate presentations of HFpEF, and add to diagnostic, prognostic, and therapeutic complexities.

B. Symptoms and Signs

Symptoms and signs of HFpEF are identical to those in patients with heart failure with reduced ejection fraction (systolic heart failure) and include dyspnea, fatigue, peripheral pitting edema, and jugular vein distention (see Chapter 18). Exercise intolerance and acute decompensated heart failure are two common presentations of HFpEF.

1. Exercise intolerance—Exercise intolerance is one of the main symptoms of HFpEF and one of the most debilitating. In patients with HFpEF, there are many reasons for exercise intolerance, including the following:

- Almost all patients with HFpEF have increased LV diastolic or left atrial pressures, or both. These pressure increases are transmitted to the pulmonary veins, which can cause decreased lung compliance, which is exacerbated by exercise.

- Increased LV diastolic pressure during exercise can limit subendocardial blood flow at a time when there are increased myocardial demands, thereby worsening diastolic function. Poor myocardial perfusion is even worse in patients with LV hypertrophy, which is very common in patients with HFpEF.

- Patients with HFpEF have an abnormal stroke volume response to tachycardia with blunted increase in cardiac output with exercise. Inadequate cardiac output can increase lactate production and worsen muscle fatigue.

2. Acutely decompensated HFpEF—The most common factor in acute decompensation is uncontrolled, severe hypertension. Other common clinical findings associated with acute decompensated HFpEF include arrhythmias; noncompliance with medications or salt restriction, or both; acute coronary syndrome; renal insufficiency; valvular regurgitation or stenosis; and infection (eg, pneumonia, urinary tract infection). It is important to recognize the clinical factors associated with acute decompensation because preventing hospitalization is one of the most important goals in patients with HFpEF.

C. Diagnostic Studies

The diagnosis of primary diastolic heart failure requires invasive or echo-Doppler evidence of diastolic dysfunction (abnormal relaxation, filling, diastolic distensibility, or stiffness). With a comprehensive approach to the assessment of diastolic function by echocardiography, the diagnosis of diastolic dysfunction can be made reliably, as discussed below. Table 19–1 lists a standardized battery of diagnostic and prognostic tests for patients being evaluated for HFpEF.

1. Echocardiography—Echocardiography is the most important tool in diagnosing diastolic dysfunction and evaluating for other etiologies of HFpEF, such as valvular, pericardial, and coronary disease. All patients with possible or confirmed HFpEF should undergo comprehensive Doppler echocardiography with tissue Doppler imaging. Besides assessment of diastolic function (see below), all patients should be evaluated for increased LV mass and increased relative wall thickness (= [septal thickness + posterior wall thickness] / end-diastolic dimension > 0.45). Assessment of pulmonary artery systolic pressure; right atrial pressure (from size and collapsibility of the inferior vena cava); and right ventricular size, function, and thickness is important in evaluation of pulmonary hypertension.

It is critically important to understand that no one abnormality on echocardiography can diagnose diastolic dysfunction, and age must be factored into the diagnosis, since almost all parameters of diastolic function are age-dependent. Only the proper combination of echocardiographic abnormalities can make the diagnosis of diastolic dysfunction (Figure 19–2). Figure 19–3 displays an algorithm for the diagnosis of diastolic dysfunction, which requires comprehensive assessment of diastolic function, including mitral inflow, tissue Doppler

Table 19–1. Diagnostic Evaluation of Heart Failure with Preserved Ejection Fraction.

Cardiac imaging
Two-dimensional/M-mode echocardiography
Doppler echocardiography
Tissue Doppler imaging
Contrast-enhanced cardiovascular MRI
Laboratory testing
Complete blood count with evaluation of anemia (if present)
Comprehensive chemistry panel (including liver function tests, albumin, total protein)
Fasting glucose, hemoglobin A_{1c}
Fasting lipid panel
B-type natriuretic peptide (or NT-proBNP)
Urine microalbuminuria
Serum and urine protein electrophoresis
Exercise testing
Cardiopulmonary exercise testing
Noninvasive evaluation of coronary artery disease (eg, stress echocardiography)
Diastolic stress echocardiography
Cardiac catheterization
Coronary angiography (if pretest probability is high or if stress test is abnormal)
Invasive hemodynamic testing to confirm elevated LV diastolic pressure, evaluate for constriction versus restriction, evaluate for pulmonary hypertension, and dynamic testing (systemic or pulmonary vasodilator challenge, fluid challenge)
Endomyocardial biopsy (in selected cases)
Other
Pulmonary function testing
Sleep study

imaging of the mitral annulus, left atrial volume, and pulmonary venous flow. The first step in evaluating diastolic function by echocardiography is to examine mitral inflow. In most patients, the ratio of early (E) to late (A) mitral inflow velocities (E/A ratio) < 0.75 signifies impaired relaxation (grade I diastolic dysfunction), especially if the patient is younger than 70 years and tissue Doppler E' is < 10 cm/s at the lateral annulus. In these patients, exercise stress echocardiography (see below) can help evaluate the functional significance of impaired LV relaxation. If the E/A ratio is > 1.5 and early mitral deceleration time is < 150 ms in an elderly patient, the diagnosis is grade III diastolic dysfunction. These patients universally should have an E' velocity < 10 cm/s at the lateral mitral annulus.

If the E/A ratio is 0.75–1.5 or if the E/A ratio is > 1.5 and early mitral deceleration time is > 150 ms, the question of normal versus pseudonormal mitral inflow arises. In these cases, an E/E' ratio > 15 or E' velocity < 10 cm/s usually signifies pseudonormal mitral inflow (grade II diastolic dysfunction). In these patients, left atrial volume index should be increased (> 28 mL/m^2). Absence of left atrial enlargement should cause reconsideration of the diagnosis of diastolic dysfunction. In patients who do not meet these criteria,

further evaluation with Valsalva maneuver, pulmonary venous flow, or flow propagation velocity can all be used to help differentiate normal versus pseudonormal mitral inflow. Increased left atrial volume index and LV mass index can both provide clues to the presence of diastolic dysfunction in these patients. Even with all of these criteria for LV diastolic dysfunction, there is a subset of patients in whom diastolic function is indeterminate. In addition, there are patients in whom diastolic function is difficult or impossible to assess noninvasively. These patients include those with atrial fibrillation, tachycardia or tachyarrhythmia, moderate or greater mitral regurgitation, mitral stenosis, mitral annuloplasty ring, mitral valve prosthesis, and mitral annular calcification.

It is important to note that although Doppler echocardiography is a powerful noninvasive tool for the assessment of diastolic function, diastolic dysfunction is not synonymous with diastolic heart failure. Many asymptomatic patients have abnormal diastolic function, but since they do not have signs and symptoms of heart failure, they should not be diagnosed incorrectly with diastolic heart failure. In addition, all Doppler echocardiographic variables for the assessment of diastolic function, except perhaps tissue Doppler E' velocity, are extremely load sensitive, and therefore convey more information about preload and afterload than true intrinsic diastolic stiffness. Therefore, it is always important to consider all clinical data, including clinical history and physical examination when making the diagnosis of diastolic heart failure or HFpEF.

2. B-type natriuretic peptide (BNP)—BNP may also have a role in the diagnosis of HFpEF. The Breathing Not Properly Study showed that a BNP > 100 pg/mL had a high sensitivity and negative predictive value for the diagnosis of HFpEF. Therefore, the diagnosis of HFpEF is unlikely in patients presenting to the emergency department with dyspnea and a BNP < 100 pg/mL. However, there is considerable overlap of BNP values in patients with and without HFpEF, especially in elderly women, since BNP increases with age, worsening renal function, and in women. To complicate matters, morbid obesity has been associated with low BNP values, which may be due to BNP clearance receptors on adipocytes. A gray-zone BNP of 100–500 pg/mL is common and is of little help diagnostically. Furthermore, in HFpEF outpatients who are stable, BNP is less useful since it may not be elevated. Therefore, BNP, like Doppler echocardiography findings, must be considered within the context of the patient, and cannot be used as a stand-alone diagnostic test for HFpEF.

3. Exercise testing—Since exercise intolerance is a key symptom in HFpEF, exercise testing is extremely valuable in these patients. Although many patients who are being evaluated for HFpEF may not be able to withstand a Bruce protocol exercise test given their advanced age and multiple comorbidities, low-intensity and bicycle stress protocols are very feasible. There are two simple exercise tests that are very helpful in evaluating patients with HFpEF: cardiopulmonary

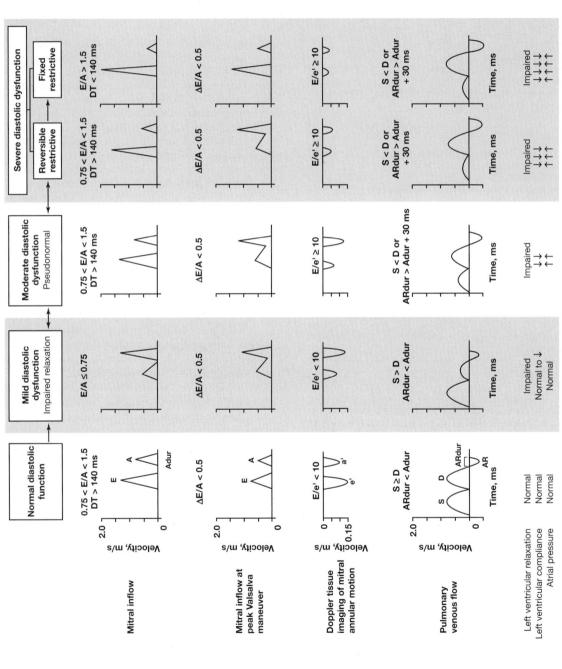

▲ **Figure 19–2.** Echo-Doppler criteria for grading diastolic function. (Reproduced, with permission, from Redfield MM et al. Burden of systolic and diastolic ventricular dysfunction in the community: appreciating the scope of the heart failure epidemic. JAMA 2003;289:194–202. © American Medical Association 2003. All Rights reserved.)

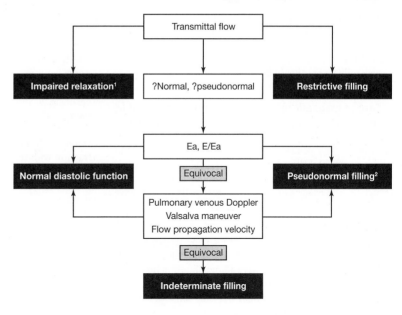

▲ **Figure 19–3.** Echo-Doppler categorization of diastolic function in patients with normal left ventricular ejection fraction. (Reproduced, with permission, from Mottram PM et al. Assessment of diastolic function: what the general cardiologist needs to know. Heart. 2005;91:681–95. © BMJ Publishing Group Ltd & British Cardiovascular Society 2005. All Rights reserved.)

[1]Consider exercise testing to assess functional significance.
[2]Reconsider if normal left atrial size.

exercise testing (CPET) and diastolic stress echocardiography. Studies have shown that on CPET, patients with HFpEF have reduced exercise tolerance, low peak workload, and low peak oxygen consumption (VO_2). Exertional dyspnea is prominent in HFpEF and a VO_2 provides objective evidence of reduced exercise tolerance. Therefore, CPET can provide objective evidence of exercise limitation and can confirm the diagnosis of HFpEF. In addition, CPET is useful in differentiating cardiac from pulmonary components of dyspnea and decreased exercise tolerance. Often, CPET is coupled with pulmonary function testing which also helps evaluate for pulmonary dysfunction, which is very common in elderly patients with HFpEF.

Stress echocardiography for the evolution of diastolic function is a relatively new approach that aims to look for increases in LV filling pressures with exercise. The diastolic evaluation stress can be combined with traditional exercise stress echocardiography. Therefore, one test can diagnose coronary disease and exercise-induced LV diastolic dysfunction. Patients are either tested with a treadmill or bicycle stress protocol. Baseline images are obtained in the parasternal long axis, parasternal short axis, and apical two-chamber, four-chamber, and three-chamber (long-axis) views for assessment of wall motion. Baseline images should also include Doppler assessment of early mitral inflow (E) and tissue Doppler imaging of the septal mitral annulus (E'). At peak stress, wall motion analysis should come first, after which the patient should undergo repeat assessment of mitral inflow and mitral annular velocities. In patients with exercise-induced diastolic dysfunction, LV filling pressures

remain elevated for several minutes, which is advantageous since the heart rate must come down to below 100 bpm in order to prevent E and A (and E' and A') merging on mitral inflow and tissue Doppler imaging, respectively. At peak exercise, an E/E' ratio > 13 (using E' at the septal annulus) suggests exercise-induced increase in LV filling pressures and is diagnostic of exercise-induced diastolic dysfunction.

4. Stress testing for the evaluation of coronary artery disease—All patients with HFpEF should undergo evaluation for coronary artery disease. Exercise stress echocardiography is ideal since patients can be evaluated for the presence of coronary artery disease and exercise-induced diastolic dysfunction with one test. However, adenosine or dipyridamole pharmacologic stress imaging is the test of choice in patients who cannot exercise and in institutions where nuclear myocardial perfusion imaging is superior. Dobutamine stress echocardiography can be performed, but in patients with significant LV hypertrophy, this test may have reduced sensitivity for the detection of wall motion abnormalities.

5. Cardiac catheterization—In patients with a high pretest probability for coronary artery disease and in patients with abnormal results of stress testing, coronary angiography should be performed. LV diastolic pressures should be measured in all patients to confirm the diagnosis of elevated LV pressures. Simultaneous right- and left-heart catheterization can be extremely valuable in the assessment of patients with HFpEF and is often underutilized. Invasive assessment in the cardiac catheterization laboratory is currently the gold standard for hemodynamic assessment, allows accurate assessment of cardiac output, and can be very helpful in evaluating for restrictive cardiomyopathy, constrictive pericarditis, or pulmonary hypertension. In addition, dynamic maneuvers such as fluid challenge, nitroprusside challenge, and pulmonary vasodilator testing (with inhaled nitric oxide or intravenous adenosine) can be valuable in specific circumstances.

6. Cardiac magnetic resonance imaging (MRI)—Cardiac MRI will likely play a key role in the assessment of HFpEF in the future. Currently, cardiac MRI is the gold standard for assessment of LV volumes, left atrial volume, and LV mass. In addition, cardiac MRI can evaluate for focal areas of fibrosis (hyperenhancement), aortic enlargement and dissection (which is important since most patients with HFpEF have significant hypertension), and pericardial thickness.

7. Endomyocardial biopsy—In cases where cardiac MRI or echocardiography shows significant LV hypertrophy but the patient has low voltage QRS complexes on electrocardiogram or the patient does not have a long-standing history of hypertension, it is important to perform endomyocardial biopsy to evaluate for a potentially treatable cause of HFpEF.

Burgess MI et al. Diastolic stress echocardiography: hemodynamic validation and clinical significance of estimation of ventricular filling pressure with exercise. J Am Coll Cardiol. 2006 May 2;47(9):1891–900. [PMID: 16682317]

Guazzi M et al. Cardiopulmonary exercise testing in the clinical and prognostic assessment of diastolic heart failure. J Am Coll Cardiol. 2005 Nov 15;46(10):1883–90. [PMID: 16286176]

Ha JW et al. Diastolic stress echocardiography: a novel noninvasive diagnostic test for diastolic dysfunction using supine bicycle exercise Doppler echocardiography. J Am Soc Echocardiogr. 2005 Jan;18(1):63–8. [PMID: 15637491]

Kasner M et al. Utility of Doppler echocardiography and tissue Doppler imaging in the estimation of diastolic function in heart failure with normal ejection fraction: a comparative Doppler-conductance catheterization study. Circulation. 2007 Aug 7;116(6):637–47. [PMID: 17646587]

Kirkpatrick JN et al. Echocardiography in heart failure: applications, utility, and new horizons. J Am Coll Cardiol. 2007 Jul 31;50(5):381–96. [PMID: 17662389]

Lund LH et al. Peak VO$_2$ in elderly patients with heart failure. Int J Cardiol. 2008 Apr 10;125(2):166–71. [PMID: 18067981]

Oh JK et al. Diastolic heart failure can be diagnosed by comprehensive two-dimensional and Doppler echocardiography. J Am Coll Cardiol. 2006 Feb 7;47(3):500–6. [PMID: 16458127]

▶ Differential Diagnosis

When considering the differential diagnosis in a patient with HFpEF, it is important to first make sure that the diagnosis of heart failure is correct. Mimickers of heart failure include pulmonary disease, obesity, and anemia, all of which can cause shortness of breath and exercise intolerance. Edema, whether confined to the lower extremity or more generalized, has a large differential diagnosis beyond heart failure, and includes venous insufficiency or obstruction (eg, venous thrombosis), liver disease, renal disease (eg, nephrotic syndrome), thyroid disease, and protein-losing enteropathies.

Once the diagnosis of heart failure is confirmed, it is important to make sure that the LVEF has been accurately measured, and that ejection fraction is truly preserved. A multiplanar imaging modality (most commonly two-dimensional echocardiography) with quantitative measurement of ejection fraction (ie, biplane method of discs) is essential for ensuring accurate quantitation of LV systolic function. An increasingly common group of patients with HFpEF are those with a prior history of severe systolic dysfunction (often with LVEF < 25%) who have recovered ejection fraction with medical or device therapies, but who continue to have mild-to-moderate symptoms of heart failure. These patients may have episodic or reversible LV systolic dysfunction, such as patients with tachycardia-induced, alcoholic, viral, or tako-tsubo cardiomyopathy.

Once patients are categorized as true HFpEF, the differential diagnosis is broad. Table 19–2 lists the various causes of HFpEF. It is also important to recognize common comor-

Table 19–2. Etiologies of Heart Failure with Preserved Ejection Fraction.

HFpEF with abnormal diastolic function
Hypertensive heart disease
Coronary artery disease
Prior myocardial infarction,
Inducible myocardial ischemia, or
Severe chronic, stable multivessel coronary disease
Restrictive cardiomyopathy
Radiation-induced cardiac injury
Infiltrative diseases (amyloidosis, sarcoidosis, hemochromatosis)
Metabolic storage diseases (eg, Fabry disease)
Endocardial fibrosis
Primary diabetic cardiomyopathy (in the absence of hypertension and coronary disease)
Idiopathic
Hypertrophic cardiomyopathy
Obstructive
Nonobstructive
Other causes of HFpEF
Primary valvular heart disease
Aortic stenosis
Aortic regurgitation
Mitral stenosis
Mitral regurgitation
Mimickers of obstructive valvular disease (eg, left atrial myxoma, cor triatriatum)
Pericardial disease
Constrictive pericarditis
Cardiac tamponade
Primary right ventricular dysfunction
Pulmonary arterial hypertension
Right ventricular myocardial infarction
Arrhythmogenic right ventricular dysplasia
Congenital heart disease
High-output cardiac failure
Severe anemia
Thyrotoxicosis
Arteriovenous fistulae

bidities in patients with HFpEF, which may act in concert to cause signs and symptoms of heart failure. The most important comorbidities include hypertension, diabetes, coronary artery disease, chronic kidney disease, obesity, anemia, and atrial fibrillation, and it is common for multiple comorbidities to coexist in a single patient with HFpEF. Furthermore, many patients have more than one of the aforementioned etiologies of HFpEF. For example, it is not uncommon for an elderly patient to have HFpEF with hypertension, diabetes, chronic kidney disease, severe coronary artery disease, and moderate mitral regurgitation.

▶ Prevention

HFpEF often represents the culmination of several underlying comorbidities such as hypertension, diabetes, coronary artery disease, chronic kidney disease, and obesity. Therefore, it is imperative to aggressively treat these risk factors in patients who may be at risk for HFpEF. Aggressive control of hypertension is probably the most important factor in preventing HFpEF, and is a class I ACC/AHA recommendation for treatment and prevention of HFpEF.

The VALsartan In Diastolic Dysfunction (VALIDD) trial showed that improvement in diastolic function is related to decreases in blood pressure irrespective of type of antihypertensive therapy, and these findings underscore the importance of aggressive blood pressure control in patients with hypertension in order to improve diastolic function. Many studies have shown that lowering blood pressure reduces heart failure events, and VALIDD adds to these studies by showing improvement in diastolic function with aggressive control of hypertension.

Poor control of diabetes has been associated with increased incidence of heart failure (regardless of type of heart failure). Although there is a tight association between poor glycemic control and incidence of heart failure, it is unclear whether tight control of diabetes will reduce HFpEF. In the absence of randomized controlled data, patients with diabetes should be treated aggressively with tight glycemic control, although vigilance is needed to prevent hypoglycemic episodes. Tight glycemic control results in prevention of microvascular complications, particularly diabetic nephropathy, which can result in fluid overload and heart failure.

Treatment of ischemia is an attractive target for prevention of HFpEF. However, there is little data on whether or not there is a benefit of revascularization. In the Coronary Artery Surgery Study (CASS) database, patients with HFpEF had a higher mortality compared with those with preserved ejection fraction but no heart failure. However, there were no differences in survival between patients with HFpEF who underwent surgical revascularization and those who underwent medical therapy for multivessel coronary disease. Therefore, patients with symptomatic angina and significant coronary disease should be treated with medications or revascularization, or both, but whether doing so will prevent HFpEF remains to be seen.

Iribarren C et al. Glycemic control and heart failure among adult patients with diabetes. Circulation. 2001 Jun 5;103(22):2668–73. [PMID: 11390335]

Solomon SD et al. Effect of angiotensin receptor blockade and antihypertensive drugs on diastolic function in patients with hypertension and diastolic dysfunction: a randomised trial. Lancet. 2007 Jun 23;369(9579):2079–87. [PMID: 17586303]

▶ Treatment

A. Nonpharmacologic Therapy

All patients should keep a diary of daily weight and blood pressure. These two parameters are of extreme importance in evaluating for underdiuresis and overdiuresis. When patients are educated about looking for increased weight gain and increasing blood pressure, they can alert their health care provider in a timely fashion in order to allow for intervention prior to progression of heart failure, which invariably leads to hospitalization.

After undergoing cardiopulmonary exercise testing, all symptomatic patients should be referred for cardiac rehabilitation for exercise training. Although there are no adequate clinical trials evaluating exercise therapy, the downside of endurance training is minimal.

B. Pharmacologic Therapy

Treatment of HFpEF remains ill-defined. Unlike heart failure with reduced ejection fraction, there is a paucity of randomized controlled trial data to guide treatment. To date, there are only very few randomized trials in patients with HFpEF. These include the DIG trial, the CHARM-Preserved trial, and the Hong Kong Diastolic Heart Failure Study.

In the DIG trial, digoxin did not decrease mortality, and although there was a trend toward decreased hospitalization, there was also a trend toward increased unstable angina. Digoxin increases systolic energy demand and adds to calcium overload in diastole and may be deleterious to patients with HFpEF; therefore, it is generally not recommended. If digoxin is necessary for rate control in patients with HFpEF who have atrial fibrillation, digoxin concentration should be kept at 0.5–0.9 ng/mL since higher concentrations were associated with increased mortality in the DIG trial.

In the CHARM-Preserved trial of mostly younger male patients with ejection fraction > 40%, candesartan, an angiotensin receptor blocker, was associated with a slight decrease in hospitalization but no difference in mortality when compared with placebo.

In the Hong Kong Diastolic Heart Failure Study, 150 patients with HFpEF were randomized to diuretics, diuretics plus irbesartan, or diuretics plus ramipril, and were monitored for 1 year.

Quality of life, symptoms, rate of recurrent hospitalization, and systolic and diastolic blood pressure were similar in all three groups. However, the irbesartan and ramipril groups were better than diuretics alone in reducing BNP and improving LV systolic and diastolic longitudinal LV function. Whether these changes translate into improved long-term outcomes is unknown.

Since extensive randomized controlled trial data for HFpEF are not available, treatment of HFpEF relies on extrapolation of therapies for heart failure with reduced ejection fraction, nonspecific relief of congestion, and ameliorating the underlying disease processes and comorbidities. Table 19–3 lists the most important treatment priorities for patients with HFpEF, as outlined below.

For symptomatic relief, the most important first step is to reduce the congestive state. Salt restriction and vasodilator therapy (angiotensin-converting enzyme [ACE] inhibitors, angiotensin receptor blockers, or hydralazine/nitrates) make up the cornerstone of treatment. Diuretics and other forms of fluid removal (eg, dialysis, ultrafiltration) are often needed, but as the acute congestive episode resolves, it is important to minimize diuretic therapy, since overdiuresis activates a heightened neurohormonal response and aggravates the cardiorenal syndrome.

From an electrophysiologic standpoint, it is important, whenever possible, to maintain atrial contraction and atrioventricular synchrony. Therefore, patients with atrial fibrillation or atrial flutter should undergo cardioversion or ablation. When necessary, patients should undergo pacemaker therapy to ensure atrioventricular synchrony, although caution must be used to avoid prolonged right ventricular pacing since this can ultimately lead to LV systolic dysfunction.

In most patients, it is ideal to promote bradycardia and avoid tachycardia. Tachycardia increases myocardial oxygen demand and decreases coronary perfusion time, which promotes diastolic dysfunction due to ischemia even in the absence of epicardial coronary disease. In addition, the time allotted for LV relaxation is decreased and diastolic filling time is decreased when tachycardia is present. By inducing relative bradycardia (eg, heart rate 50–60 bpm), coronary perfusion is optimized, and LV relaxation and diastolic filling time are both increased. Patients who benefit most from this type of treatment are most likely those who have impaired LV relaxation and prolonged early mitral inflow deceleration times. In patients with more severe, end-stage HFpEF, such as severe restrictive cardiomyopathy, increased heart rate may be the most important factor maintaining cardiac output, since stroke volume is often severely decreased. These patients invariably have a very high early mitral inflow velocity and short deceleration time. Although tachycardia should be avoided, heart rates of 80–90 bpm are often required in order to maintain adequate cardiac output. In these patients, overzealous β-blockade or calcium channel blocker therapy can result in a precipitous decline in cardiac output.

Most patients with HFpEF will benefit from rate control therapy with medications such as β-blockers and non-dihydropyridine calcium channel blockers (verapamil, diltiazem). In the absence of adequate randomized controlled trials, β-blockers with proven benefit in heart failure (meto-

Table 19–3. Treatment of Heart Failure with Preserved Ejection Fraction.

Treat underlying causes and precipitating factors
Treat congestion and edema
  Diuretics
  Ultrafiltration or dialysis (when diuretics are insufficient)
  Salt restriction
  Vasodilator therapy
Aggressively treat hypertension
  Use long-acting β-blockers (eg, carvedilol, metoprolol succinate), ACE inhibitors or angiotensin receptor blockers, and thiazide diuretics whenever possible
  Avoid clonidine
Control heart rate and rhythm
  Goal heart rate ~60 bpm (use caution in patients with advanced diastolic dysfunction who require increased heart rates to maintain cardiac output)
  Maintain sinus rhythm (cardioversion, ablation)
  Pacemaker therapy (when necessary) to maintain atrioventricular synchrony
Treat comorbidities
  Myocardial ischemia (medications, revascularization)
  Dyslipidemia (preferably with statins for pleiotropic benefit)
  Anemia
  Chronic kidney disease
Nonpharmacologic therapy
  Instruct patients to keep diary of daily weight and blood pressure
  Prescribe exercise training (cardiac rehabilitation) in mild-to-moderate heart failure to improve functional status and decrease symptoms
  Treat obstructive sleep apnea, sleep-disordered breathing, and nocturnal hypoxia

prolol succinate, carvedilol, bisoprolol) should be used as first-line agents in patients with HFpEF. A good rule of thumb to follow when choosing β-blockers is that metoprolol succinate is a good agent in patients who have problems with rate control (eg, atrial fibrillation) and those with low or normal blood pressure. In patients who have severe hypertension, carvedilol is the agent of choice since it has potent antihypertensive effects due to its α-adrenergic blockade properties.

As stated above, all patients should be evaluated for myocardial ischemia, and when present, ischemia should be treated aggressively with revascularization, β-blockers, nitrates, and dihydropyridine calcium channel blockers. Hypertension should be treated aggressively with goal blood pressure < 130/80 mm Hg. Control of hypertension is the only proven therapy for prevention of HFpEF, and therefore is essential in all patients. HFpEF patients commonly have severe hypertension, and when they are referred, they may be taking four or five or more antihypertensive medications. The number of medications should be kept to a minimum in order to avoid the dangers of polypharmacy and adverse drug-drug interactions. In addition, minimizing medications will often promote increased patient compliance.

Patients with HFpEF and severe hypertension are often taking medications such as clonidine and minoxidil, while other medications with proven cardiovascular benefits, such as β-blockers and ACE inhibitors, are not titrated to maximum doses. Therefore, patients with significant hypertension should ideally be treated with carvedilol, metoprolol succinate, or bisoprolol, and maximum dose of an ACE inhibitor or angiotensin receptor blocker, unless contraindicated. Most patients will also benefit from a thiazide diuretic such as hydrochlorothiazide or chlorthalidone. Routine use of more potent thiazides, such as metolazone, should be avoided since these medications often exacerbate the cardiorenal syndrome. In select patients with resistant hypertension, spironolactone may have substantial antihypertensive effects, and in these cases hyperaldosteronism should be excluded.

In patients with severe, resistant hypertension who cannot be treated adequately with a combination of β-blockers, ACE inhibitors, and thiazide diuretics, the following steps should be taken: (1) ensure medication compliance, (2) ensure euvolemia since fluid overload will exacerbate hypertension, and (3) look for causes of secondary hypertension. Using these steps, most patients will have adequately controlled blood pressure with two or three medications. In patients who need an additional agent, the combination of hydralazine and nitrates is a good option given their beneficial effects in heart failure. If tolerated and not associated with increased lower extremity edema, dihydropyridine calcium channel blockers may also be used to treat severe hypertension. These agents are often useful in patients who have significant chronic kidney disease since they may not be able to take ACE inhibitors, angiotensin receptor blockers, or aldosterone antagonists.

Besides beneficial antihypertensive effects, β-blockers, ACE inhibitors, and angiotensin receptor blockers attenuate neurohormonal activation, which may be beneficial in HFpEF. In addition, ACE inhibitors, angiotensin receptor blockers, and spironolactone may prevent fibrosis and may promote regression of LV hypertrophy. Statins may have pleiotropic benefit in heart failure, and all HFpEF patients with dyslipidemia or coronary risk factors should be treated with a statin. Interestingly, in a large study of Medicare beneficiaries discharged with a primary diagnosis of heart failure and documentation of preserved ejection fraction, statins were associated with increased survival irrespective of total cholesterol, coronary disease, diabetes, hypertension, or age.

1. Caveats—Patients with HFpEF often live in a delicate balance between symptomatic congestion (due to inadequate diuresis) and poor cardiac output (due to overdiuresis). The latter causes lightheadedness, dizziness, fatigue, and worsening renal dysfunction due to decreased renal perfusion. Since patients with HFpEF rely on increased LV filling pressures to maintain cardiac output, they tend to be very sensitive to overdiuresis with small decreases in LV diastolic pressure resulting in large decreases in stroke volume. Therefore, it is important to start low and go slow with diuretic therapy. Many patients typically require frequent visits in order to find a diuretic regimen that results in optimal symptom control without exacerbating the cardiorenal syndrome.

In patients with hypertrophic cardiomyopathy, verapamil may be beneficial, and therefore may be used as first-line therapy before β-blockade. Alternatively, verapamil is contraindicated in amyloidosis. Thiazide diuretics can exacerbate hyperglycemia and hyperuricemia, which are often present in elderly patients with HFpEF. Positive inotropes should be avoided in general because they promote calcium influx into cardiac myocytes, which worsens diastolic function. In addition, many of these patients have hypercontractile ventricles with small LV volumes. Therefore, positive inotropes frequently cause cavity obliteration with resultant obstruction of forward flow and decreased cardiac output. In patients with HFpEF who have non-ST elevation acute coronary syndromes, mortality is increased and patients are often undertreated. Therefore, all efforts should be made to treat this high-risk group (including an early invasive approach) using evidence-based guidelines.

Aside from treatment of hypertension, coronary disease, and atrial fibrillation (as listed above), it is important to treat other underlying comorbidities such as diabetes, metabolic syndrome, obesity, chronic kidney disease, and anemia. In addition, many patients with HFpEF have concomitant chronic obstructive pulmonary disease, which should also be treated aggressively in order to improve symptoms of breathlessness.

2. Drugs to avoid—In all patients with HFpEF, it is important to avoid polypharmacy at all costs since adverse events increase and compliance decreases with increased numbers of medications. In addition, medications should always be carefully scrutinized as causes of signs and symptoms of heart failure. For example, calcium channel blockers and thiazolidinediones (eg, rosiglitazone, pioglitazone) can cause significant edema, nonsteroidal antiinflammatory drugs can cause renal failure, and hydroxychloroquine (which is frequently used in rheumatologic diseases such as systemic lupus erythematosus and rheumatoid arthritis) can cause a restrictive cardiomyopathy. In the elderly cohort of patients with HFpEF, medications for Parkinson disease are common, and these agents have been shown to cause valvular disease. Certain foods and herbal supplements can also be deleterious in patients with HFpEF. Licorice can cause mineralocorticoid excess, ginseng interferes with warfarin, and ginseng also falsely elevated digoxin levels. Treatment of gout is difficult since NSAIDs are contraindicated in patients with HFpEF and colchicine is dangerous since many of these patients are elderly and have abnormal kidney function. In these patients, corticosteroid injection directly into the involved joint, a short pulse of oral corticosteroids, or gentle opioid therapy may be the best treatment options.

Ahmed A et al. Effects of digoxin on morbidity and mortality in diastolic heart failure: the ancillary digitalis investigation group trial. Circulation. 2006 Aug 1;114(5):397–403. [PMID: 16864724]

Bennett KM et al. Heart failure with preserved left ventricular systolic function among patients with non-ST-segment elevation acute coronary syndromes. Am J Cardiol. 2007 May 15;99(10):1351–6. [PMID: 17493458]

Martinez-Selles M. Treatment of heart failure with normal ejection fraction in patients with advanced chronic heart failure. Eur J Heart Fail. 2007 Dec;9(12):1223. [PMID: 18006377]

Shah R et al. Effect of statins, angiotensin-converting enzyme inhibitors, and beta blockers on survival in patients >or=65 years of age with heart failure and preserved left ventricular systolic function. Am J Cardiol. 2008 Jan 15;101(2):217–22. [PMID: 18178410]

Yip GW et al. The Hong Kong diastolic heart failure study: a randomized control trial of diuretics, irbesartan and ramipril on quality of life, exercise capacity, left ventricular global and regional function in heart failure with a normal ejection fraction. Heart. 2008 May;94(5):573–80. [PMID: 18208835]

Yusuf S et al. Effects of candesartan in patients with chronic heart failure and preserved left-ventricular ejection fraction: the CHARM-Preserved Trial. Lancet. 2003 Sep 6;362(9386):777–81. [PMID: 13678871]

▶ Prognosis

Once hospitalized for heart failure, patients with HFpEF have a high mortality. Five-year mortality is high, and is similar to heart failure with reduced ejection fraction. Two large epidemiology studies of patients hospitalized with HFpEF have shown that survival is only 30–40% after 5 years. Studies of outpatients with HFpEF display a lower mortality, but one that is again similar to that of patients with heart failure and reduced ejection fraction. Rates of hospitalization and readmission are similarly high in patients with HFpEF and heart failure with reduced ejection fraction.

Despite the abundance of studies now showing a high rate of mortality in HFpEF, the cause of death remains unclear. Predictors of death in patients hospitalized with HFpEF include increased age, male gender, increased serum creatinine, decreased hemoglobin, decreased blood pressure, increased respiratory rate, and hyponatremia. In addition, diabetes, peripheral arterial disease, cancer, dementia, and end-stage renal disease requiring hemodialysis are all independent predictors of death in HFpEF. In the CHARM trial echocardiographic substudy, evidence of moderate or greater diastolic dysfunction was strongly associated with adverse outcomes. In the DIG trial, worsening heart failure and arrhythmias were the leading causes of death in all heart failure patients, regardless of ejection fraction. However, noncardiovascular causes of death were more frequent in patients with HFpEF, due to their advanced age. A retrospective analysis of the Duke Databank for Cardiovascular Disease found that 8% of deaths in patients with HFpEF were due to sudden cardiac death. This finding was mirrored in another study of 357 patients with HFpEF in whom 8% died due to sudden cardiac death.

Cause of death in HFpEF is most likely multifactorial. Although some patients may die of heart failure and pulmonary edema, most patients are not dying of LV pump failure, and many may be dying of arrhythmias or sudden cardiac death. Even more may be dying of important age-related comorbidities such as cancer and dementia. Until we learn more about cause of death in patients with HFpEF, it is important for health care providers to understand the importance of comorbidities in the prognosis of these patients. Therefore, although evaluation of treatment of HFpEF is extremely important, attention to comorbidities and a multidisciplinary approach to patients with HFpEF will likely lead to the best possible outcome in these patients.

Al-Khatib SM et al. Incidence and predictors of sudden cardiac death in patients with diastolic heart failure. J Cardiovasc Electrophysiol. 2007 Dec;18(12):1231–5. [PMID: 17883404]

Bhatia RS et al. Outcome of heart failure with preserved ejection fraction in a population-based study. N Engl J Med. 2006 Jul 20;355(3):260–9. [PMID: 16855266]

Bursi F et al. Systolic and diastolic heart failure in the community. JAMA. 2006 Nov 8;296(18):2209–16. [PMID: 17090767]

Fonarow GC et al; OPTIMIZE-HF Investigators and Hospitals. Characteristics, treatments, and outcomes of patients with preserved systolic function hospitalized for heart failure: a report from the OPTIMIZE-HF Registry. J Am Coll Cardiol. 2007 Aug 21;50(8):768–77. [PMID: 17707182]

Owan TE et al. Trends in prevalence and outcome of heart failure with preserved ejection fraction. N Engl J Med. 2006 Jul 20;355(3):251–9. [PMID: 16855265]

Persson H et al. Diastolic dysfunction in heart failure with preserved systolic function: need for objective evidence:results from the CHARM Echocardiographic Substudy-CHARMES. J Am Coll Cardiol. 2007 Feb 13;49(6):687–94. [PMID: 17291934]

Shah SJ et al. Heart failure with preserved ejection fraction: treat now by treating comorbidities. JAMA. 2008;300:431–3. [PMID: 18647986]

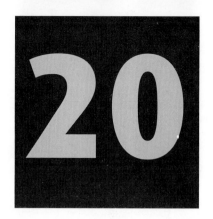

Supraventricular Tachycardias

Byron K. Lee, MD & Peter R. Kowey, MD

ESSENTIALS OF DIAGNOSIS

▶ Heart rate greater than 100 bpm.
▶ Rhythm is supraventricular in origin.

General Considerations

Supraventricular tachycardias (SVTs) are rapid rhythm disturbances originating from the atria or the atrioventricular (AV) node. In the absence of a bundle branch block, there is intact conduction to the ventricles via the right and left bundles leading to a narrow and normal appearing QRS. Therefore, these arrhythmias are also often called narrow complex tachycardias. Since many of the SVTs are episodic, many clinicians also refer to this group of arrhythmias as paroxysmal SVTs. Radiofrequency ablation has become an important therapeutic option in the management of SVTs because of its ability to eliminate these arrhythmias safely. Table 20–1 outlines the pharmacologic therapy for SVTs.

Pathophysiology & Etiology

Arrhythmias occur as a result of three main mechanisms: reentry, which is most common; enhanced or abnormal automaticity; and triggered activity.

Reentrant arrhythmias sustain themselves by repetitively following a revolving pathway comprising two limbs, one that takes the impulse away from, and one that carries it back to the site of origin. For reentry to exist, an area of slow conduction must occur, and each limb must have a different refractory period (see the discussion on AV nodal reentrant tachycardia). In this situation, pacing (by inducing refractoriness in one limb of the circuit) can typically initiate a reentrant tachycardia. Once established, pacing can also terminate the tachycardia by interfering with impulse propagation in one of the limbs.

The second mechanism, **automaticity,** refers to spontaneous and, often, repetitive firing from a single focus, which may either be ectopic or may originate in the sinus node. It should be noted that automaticity is an intrinsic property of all myocardial cells. This mechanism comprises two subcategories. **Enhanced automaticity** is defined as a focus that fires spontaneously and may originate in the sinus node, subsidiary pacemakers in the atrium including the Eustachian ridge, Bachmann bundle, coronary sinus and AV valves, the AV node, His-Purkinje system, and the ventricles. **Abnormal automaticity** is usually secondary to a disease process causing alterations in ionic flow that produces a lower (ie, more positive) resting diastolic membrane potential. Threshold potential is therefore more easily attained, thereby increasing the probability of a sustained arrhythmia.

The third mechanism, **triggered arrhythmias,** depends on oscillations in the membrane potential that closely follow an action potential. In the absence of a new external electrical stimulus, these oscillations, or **after-depolarizations,** cause new action potentials to develop. Thus, each new action potential results from the previous action potential. These arrhythmias can be produced by early or late after-depolarization, depending on the timing of the first after-depolarization relative to the preceding action potential (the one that spawned the triggered activity). In **early after-depolarizations,** membrane repolarization is incomplete, which allows an action potential to be initiated by a subthreshold stimulus. This type is often associated with electrolyte disturbance and may be the mechanism responsible for arrhythmogenesis related to the prolonged-QT syndrome and torsades de pointes caused by quinidine. With **delayed after-depolarization,** membrane repolarization is complete, but an abnormal intracellular calcium load causes spontaneous depolarization. The reason for the high calcium levels is unclear, but it can be related to inhibition of the sodium pump by drugs such as digoxin. In either type of arrhythmia, the process may be repetitive and lead to a sustained tachycardia.

Table 20-1. Antiarrhythmic Drugs for Supraventricular Tachycardias.

Agent	Indication	Intravenous Dose	Oral Dose	Adverse Effects	Drug Interactions
Class Ia					
Quinidine	AF, AFL, AVNRT, AVRT	6–10 mg/kg over 20–30 min	200–400 mg q4-6h; q8h with long-acting preparations	Hypotension (especially IV), ventricular proarrhythmia, GI disturbance, thrombocytopenia	↑ digitalis level; ↑ warfarin effect; ↑ metoprolol, propranolol, propafenone levels
Procainamide	AF, AFL, AVNRT, AVRT	*Bolus:* 15 mg/kg given as 20 mg/min; *Infusion:* 2–4 mg/min	50 mg/kg/day q3-4h; twice daily dosage with long-acting preparation	GI disturbance, hypotension, SLE, agranulocytosis, FUO hemolytic anemia, myasthenia gravis aggravation, ventricular proarrhythmia	↑ Procainamide level with cimetidine, quinidine, and amiodarone
Class 1c					
Flecainide	AF, AFL, AT, AVNRT, AVRT	N/A	50–200 mg q12h	Ventricular proarrhythmia, CHF, GI disturbance CNS (dizziness, tremor, light-headedness)	↑ digitalis level; ↑ flecainide level with amiodarone, cimetidine, norpace, propranolol; ↓ flecainide level with smoking
Propafenone	AF, AFL, AVNRT, AVRT	N/A	150–300 mg q8h	GI disturbance, CNS (dizziness), metallic taste, CHF, first-degree AVB, IVCD, positive ANA	Synergism with β-blockers
Class II (IV)					
Esmolol	Ventricular rate control for AF, AFL, ST, AT	*Bolus:* 500 mcg/kg over 1–2 min; *Infusion:* 50–200 mcg/kg/min	N/A	CHF, AVB, bradycardia, bronchospasm	
Propranolol	Ventricular rate control for AF, AFL, ST, AT	1–5 mg at 1 mg/min	20–320 mg/day q6h, q8h, q12h or once daily, depending on preparation	CHF, AVB, bradycardia, bronchospasm	
Class III					
Sotalol	AF, AFL, AVNRT, AVRT, AT	N/A	80–160 mg q12h	Dyspnea, fatigue, dizziness, CHF, bradycardia, ventricular proarrhythmia, bronchospasm	Synergism with Ca^{2+} antagonists or β-blockers
Amiodarone	AF, AFL, AVNRT, AVRT, AT	*Bolus:* 150 mg over 10 min; *Infusion:* 1 mg/min × 6h, then 0.5 mg/min	100–400 mg once daily	Pulmonary toxicity, CHF, tremor, bradycardia, ↑ LFTs, corneal deposits, skin discoloration, GI intolerance, hyper-/hypothyroidism	↑ digoxin levels; ↑ warfarin effect; ↑ quinidine, prox/NAPA, flecainide; ↑ phenytoin level
Ibutilide	AF, AFL	1 mg bolus over 10 min second bolus, if needed, after 10-min wait	N/A	Ventricular proarrhythmia, hypotension, GI disturbance	
Dofetilide	AF, AFL	N/A	125–500 mcg twice daily modified by algorithm	Ventricular proarrhythmia, headache, chest pain, nausea, dizziness	Contraindicated with verapamil, cimetidine, ketoconazole, trimethoprim

Class IV					
Diltiazem	AF, AFL, AVNRT, AVRT, AT, MAT	*Bolus:* 0.25 mg/min over 2 min then 0.35 mg/kg in 15 min if needed *Infusion:* 5–15 mg/h	90–360 mg/day in 1–4 divided doses, depending on preparation	Hypotension, bradycardia, CHF, AVB	Synergism with β-blockers
Verapamil	AF, AFL, AVNRT, AVRT, AT, MAT	2.5–20 mg over 20 min in divided doses	40–120 mg q8h; 240–360 mg once daily of long-acting preparation	Hypotension, bradycardia, CHF, AVB	Synergism with β-blockers
Class V					
Adenosine	SVT diagnosis AVNRT, AVRT, AT termination	6 mg IV rapid bolus followed by 12 mg × 2 if needed. Half dosage if administered in central line	N/A	Chest tightness, facial flushing, dyspnea, AVB	↑ activity by dipyridamole ↓ activity by theophylline
Digoxin	Ventricular rate control for AF, AFL, AT (generally not very effective in active patients)	Up to 1.0 mg bolus in divided doses followed by 0.125–0.375 mg/day	0.125–0.375 mg/day in single dose	GI disturbance, conduction defects, atrial/ventricular arrhythmias, headache, visual disturbances	↑ *Digoxin level:* amiodarone, quinidine, verapamil, indomethacin, spironolactone, alprazolam, erythromycin, tetracycline ↓ *Digoxin level:* antacids, cholestyramine, rifampin, neomycin ↑ Risk of digitalis toxicity with potassium depleting diuretics

AF, atrial fibrillation; AFL, atrial flutter; ANA, antinuclear antigen; AT, atrial tachycardia; AVB, atrioventricular block; AVNRT, atrioventricular nodal reentrant tachycardia; AVRT, atrioventricular reciprocating tachycardia; CHF, congestive heart failure; CNS, central nervous system; FUO, fever of unknown origin; GI, gastrointestinal; IV, intravenous; IVCD, intraventricular conduction delay; LFT, liver function tests; MAT, multifocal atrial tachycardia; N/A, not applicable; NAPA, N-acetyl procainamide; SLE, systemic lupus erythematosus; ST, sinus tachycardia.

▶ General Diagnostic Approach

A systematic approach to interpreting the 12-lead electrocardiogram (ECG) will allow accurate determination of the type of SVT in most cases (Figure 20–1). The first step is to determine whether the rhythm is regular or irregular. If it is irregular, the rhythm is likely either atrial fibrillation, atrial flutter with variable conduction, or multifocal atrial tachycardia (MAT). The appearance of the P waves will usually distinguish between these three entities. In atrial fibrillation, there is chaotic atrial activity. In atrial flutter, P waves are seen at rate of 240–320 bpm. In MAT, there are P waves preceding each QRS complex, and there are at least three different P wave morphologies.

If the SVT is regular, there are several different types of SVT to consider. The SVT could be sinus tachycardia, sinus node reentry, atrial flutter, atrial tachycardia, AV nodal reentrant tachycardia (AVNRT), junctional tachycardia, or atrioventricular reciprocating tachycardia (AVRT). The type of regular SVT can be usually identified by examining four aspects of the 12-lead ECG: (1) onset and termination, (2) heart rate, (3) P wave morphology, and (4) R-P relationship. The onset and termination can be sudden or gradual. Sinus tachycardia and junctional tachycardia typically have very gradual onset whereas the other SVTs usually start and stop more suddenly.

Rate can also be helpful since sinus tachycardia cannot typically go over 220-age bpm and the heart rate in atrial flutter is often a multiple of 300. P wave morphology can be helpful since retrograde P waves (negative in the inferior leads: II, III, and AVF) favor AVNRT and junctional tachycardia. Finally, R-P relationship refers to the distance from the R wave to the next P wave during tachycardia. If this distance is longer than the P-R interval, the SVT is termed "long R-P," whereas if this distance is short, it is termed "short R-P" (Figure 20-2).

SINUS TACHYCARDIA & SINUS NODE REENTRY

1. Sinus Tachycardia

 ESSENTIALS OF DIAGNOSIS

- ▶ Onset and termination: Gradual.
- ▶ Heart rate: 100 to (220 – age) bpm.
- ▶ P wave: Identical to normal sinus rhythm P wave.
- ▶ R-P relationship: Long.

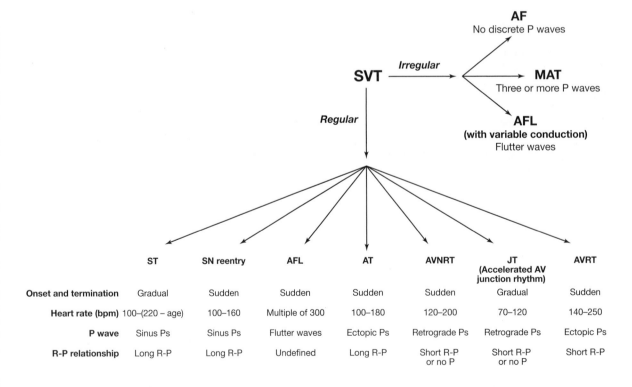

	ST	SN reentry	AFL	AT	AVNRT	JT (Accelerated AV junction rhythm)	AVRT
Onset and termination	Gradual	Sudden	Sudden	Sudden	Sudden	Gradual	Sudden
Heart rate (bpm)	100–(220 – age)	100–160	Multiple of 300	100–180	120–200	70–120	140–250
P wave	Sinus Ps	Sinus Ps	Flutter waves	Ectopic Ps	Retrograde Ps	Retrograde Ps	Ectopic Ps
R-P relationship	Long R-P	Long R-P	Undefined	Long R-P	Short R-P or no P	Short R-P or no P	Short R-P

▲ **Figure 20–1.** Algorithm for distinguishing supraventricular tachycardias. AF, atrial fibrillation; AFL, atrial flutter; AT, atrial tachycardia; AVNRT, atrioventricular nodal reentrant tachycardia; AVRT, atrioventricular reciprocating tachycardia; JT, junctional tachycardia; MAT, multifocal atrial tachycardia; SN, sinus node; ST, sinus tachycardia; SVT, supraventricular tachycardia.

► General Considerations

When the sinus node fires at a rate of more than 100 bpm, the rhythm is, with one exception, considered sinus tachycardia (see section on Sinus Node Reentry). The onset and termination of sinus tachycardia is invariably gradual. The range for heart rate in sinus tachycardia is 100 to (220 – age) bpm; faster rates usually imply a different cause. Confirming that the tachycardic P waves are identical in morphology and axis to the normal sinus rhythm P waves is essential to the diagnosis. Like normal sinus rhythm, the R-P relationship in sinus tachycardia is typically long R-P, unless the patient has a very long P-R interval seen on the baseline ECG.

Sinus tachycardia is usually a physiologic response, activated when the body requires a higher heart rate to meet metabolic demands or maintain blood pressure. Common causes are exercise, hypotension, hypoxemia, heart failure, sepsis, fever, hyperthyroidism, fluid depletion, and blood loss.

The heart rate achieved is proportional to the intensity of the stimulus, but the rapidity with which the heart rate increases and decreases is a function of how quickly the stimulus is applied and withdrawn.

► Treatment

Vagal maneuvers slow the tachycardia gradually but only while being performed; when the vagal stimulus is removed, the heart rate gradually returns to where it started.

Attempting to slow the heart rate pharmacologically can be detrimental because it counteracts the compensatory mechanism provided by the tachycardia. Therefore, management is usually focused on treating the underlying cause of the sinus tachycardia.

2. Sinus Node Reentry

ESSENTIALS OF DIAGNOSIS

- ► Onset and termination: Sudden.
- ► Heart rate: 100–160 bpm.
- ► P wave: Identical to normal sinus rhythm P wave.
- ► R-P relationship: Long.

► General Considerations

This uncommon rhythm accounts for less than 5% of SVTs. It uses the sinus node or perinodal tissue as a critical part of the reentrant circuit, producing P waves identical to those seen during normal sinus rhythm. The heart rate usually falls between 100 and 160 bpm. Like sinus tachycardia, R-P relationship is typically long R-P. Unlike sinus tachycardia, sinus node reentry is initiated by an ectopic beat rather than a physiologic stimulus and possesses the characteristics typical of a reentrant circuit. It therefore begins and ends

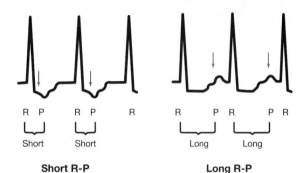

R	P		R	P		R		R		P	R		P	R
Short		Short				Long			Long					

Short R-P   **Long R-P**

▲ **Figure 20–2.** *Short R-P* refers to a regular supraventricular tachycardia (SVT) where the R-P interval is shorter than the P-R interval. *Long R-P* refers to a regular SVT where the R-P interval is longer than the P-R interval.

abruptly and responds to vagal maneuvers and pharmacologic interventions by terminating rather than slowing.

► Treatment

The arrhythmia can be terminated quickly with intravenous adenosine, verapamil, or diltiazem, or via carotid massage. Long-term treatment uses β-blockers and calcium channel blockers. The largest reported series of patients treated with catheter ablation described success in all 10 patients. No complications were reported. Other smaller series described similar efficacy.

ATRIAL FLUTTER

ESSENTIALS OF DIAGNOSIS

- ► Onset and termination: Sudden.
- ► Heart rate: Usually a multiple of 300.
- ► P waves: Flutter waves at 250–340 bpm.
- ► R-P relationship: Undefined due to flutter waves.
- ► Prominent neck vein pulsations of about 300/min.

► General Considerations

Atrial flutter is usually associated with organic heart disease and is second in frequency only to atrial fibrillation in postcoronary bypass surgery patients, with an incidence of up to 33%. With a typical atrial rate of 300 bpm (range: 250–340), atrial flutter produces a "sawtooth" appearance (F waves). As is the case with atrial fibrillation (see Chapter 21), the ventricular rate depends on conduction through the AV node. Unlike atrial fibrillation, the ventricular impulses are transmitted at some integer fraction of the atrial rate. In rare circumstances,

1:1 conduction may occur. Fixed 2:1 or 4:1 block is the usual scenario. However, variable block can also occur, leading to one of the three types of irregular SVTs. If flutter is suspected but F waves are not clearly visible, vagal maneuvers or pharmacologic agents, such as adenosine, can help unmask the flutter waves by enhancing the degree of AV block.

▶ Pathophysiology

Atrial flutter occurs in a variety of forms; the most common is isthmus-dependent counterclockwise atrial flutter; followed by the isthmus-dependent clockwise atrial flutter; and then the atypical, nonisthmus-dependent variety. The counterclockwise flutter is recognized electrocardiographically by negative F waves in leads II, III, and aVF; and positive F waves in V_1. The single reentrant wavefront proceeds up the interatrial septum in a caudocranial direction, across the roof of the right atrium, down the lateral wall and across the inferior wall (Figure 20–3). Clockwise flutter, on the other hand, has positive F waves in leads II, III, and aVF; and negative F waves in lead V_1. The reentrant circuit in this case moves in the reverse direction. In both these types of atrial flutter, the atrial rates range between 250 and 340 bpm.

▶ Clinical Findings

Symptoms attributable to atrial flutter are secondary to the ventricular response in addition to any underlying cardiac diseases. Dizziness, palpitations, angina-type chest pain, dyspnea, weakness, fatigue and, occasionally, syncope may be the presenting symptoms. In those patients with poor left ventricular function, overt congestive heart failure may ensue.

Clinical evaluation is similar to that described for atrial fibrillation (see Chapter 21), but underlying heart disease is detected more often with atrial flutter than with fibrillation.

▶ Prevention

Several antiarrhythmic agents can prevent recurrences of atrial flutter. It appears that both class Ia and Ic agents are effective. Class III agents, such as sotalol and amiodarone, can also work very well. Dofetilide, a newer class III agent, which blocks the rapid form of the delayed rectifier current, Ik_r, has also been found effective in converting to and maintenance of sinus rhythm. Its administration requires initiation in the hospital and a monitored setting. Drugs that are contraindicated with its use include verapamil, ketoconazole, cimetidine, trimethoprim, prochlorperazine, megestrol, and hydrochlorothiazide. With regard to safety, dofetilide has a proarrhythmic event rate of approximately 0.9%, which is less than the 3.3% seen in patients with congestive heart failure or the 2.5% in patients with previous ventricular tachycardia.

It should be emphasized that an AV nodal blocking agent should be started before initiating a class I drug. If the AV node is unblocked, a type I agent could facilitate conduction of atrial flutter by improving nodal conduction or by slowing the flutter rate and paradoxically increasing the ventricular response.

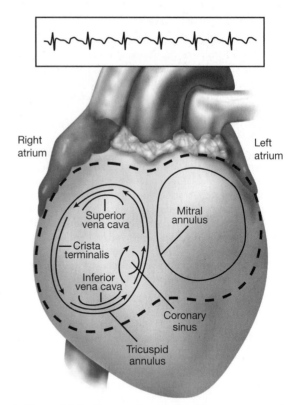

▲ **Figure 20–3.** The reentry circuit of the common variety of atrial flutter (type II). The right and left atria are shown in the left anterior oblique projection. The reentry circuit is confined to the right atrium and circulates in a counterclockwise direction within it (*arrows*). The area between the tricuspid annulus and the inferior vena cava is the critical isthmus that is targeted for ablation of this type of atrial flutter. Also shown is a recording of counterclockwise atrial flutter in lead II, demonstrating the "sawtooth" pattern of flutter waves (rate, 250/min) characteristic of this type of atrial flutter. (Reprinted, with permission, from Morady F. N Engl J Med. 1999;340:534. Copyright © 1999 Massachusetts Medical Society. All rights reserved.)

▶ Treatment
A. Conversion

Once the diagnosis of atrial flutter is made, assessment of the patient's status will dictate whether to perform cardioversion immediately. Immediate cardioversion can be accomplished with synchronized DC cardioversion, rapid atrial pacing to interrupt the macroreentrant circuit, or intravenous infusion of an antiarrhythmic agent. For DC cardioversion, as little as 25 J may be all that is required; however, at least 50 J is recommended to avoid extra shocks, and 100 J will terminate almost all episodes of atrial flutter. The major drawback with DC cardioversion is the need to administer sedation.

Rapid atrial pacing is another method that may terminate the arrhythmia. Pacing is best performed in the right atrium at a rate faster than the flutter rate, which allows the circuit to be entered by the pacing impulse. If the extrinsic pacing rate exceeds the rate that can be sustained through the zone of slow conduction, the flutter wavefront can be interrupted and will no longer be present when the pacing is stopped. If the patient has a pacemaker or implantable cardiac defibrillator with an atrial lead, pace termination can be done painlessly via the device. An alternative method uses a swallowed transesophageal electrode. Because of the interposed tissue, a high current is often necessary to capture and pace the atrium reliably, which may cause significant discomfort to the patient. Of note, overdrive pacing may precipitate atrial fibrillation, which usually terminates spontaneously after several minutes. Should the atrial fibrillation persist, however, it usually is easier to control the ventricular response when compared with atrial flutter.

Finally, rapid pharmacologic cardioversion can be considered with intravenous agents such as ibutilide. Ibutilide is a unique class III antiarrhythmic agent with a rate of conversion of approximately 60% in patients with atrial flutter of less than 45 days duration. Cardioversion can be expected within 30 minutes of administration. The major complication with this agent is the development of torsades de pointes, which can occur in up to 12.5% of patients, with 1.7% requiring cardioversion for sustained polymorphic ventricular tachycardia. These occur primarily within the first hour after administration. Procainamide is another intravenous agent that can be given to pharmacologically convert atrial flutter.

B. Rate Control

In general, controlling the ventricular rate in atrial flutter is more difficult than in atrial fibrillation. β-Blockers and calcium channel blockers are moderately effective in controlling the rate. Digoxin is less helpful since it only weakly blocks the AV node conduction. Intravenous amiodarone has been shown to be at least as efficacious as digoxin.

C. Catheter Ablation and Other Modalities

The reentrant circuit in typical atrial flutter has been successfully mapped and includes an area of slow conduction called the isthmus, which is bound by the tricuspid annulus, the inferior vena cava, and the os of the coronary sinus (Figure 20–3). Ablation in the isthmus region interrupts the reentrant circuit and has been shown to be highly efficacious (90–100%) in permanently eliminating atrial flutter. In cost-effective analysis, ablation appears to be the preferred approach over cardioversion and pharmacologic prevention. Non–isthmus-dependent atypical atrial flutters can be more difficult to ablate. However, with current three-dimensional mapping systems (electroanatomic and noncontact high

resolution) even these types of atrial flutter are being ablated with high success rates.

If attempts to cure flutter fail, the ventricular rate can be controlled by transcatheter ablation of the AV node or His bundle. With a long-standing flutter, there may be a subsequent improvement in left ventricular function.

D. Stroke Prophylaxis

Whether atrial flutter is the source of peripheral embolization and stroke is an unsettled issue because most of the published studies pool their data from patients with atrial flutter and fibrillation, and most studies are retrospective in design. However, mounting evidence indicates that the risk of embolic stroke is more significant than previously thought. In addition, many patients have bouts of both atrial fibrillation and flutter, thereby necessitating aspirin or anticoagulant therapy. The current recommendation is to treat patients with atrial flutter just as atrial fibrillation in terms of stroke prophylaxis.

Calkins H et al. Results of catheter ablation of typical atrial flutter. Am J Cardiol. 2004 Aug 15;94(4):437–42. [PMID: 15325925]

Ellenbogen KA et al. Efficacy of intravenous ibutilide for rapid termination of atrial fibrillation and atrial flutter: a dose dependent study. J Am Coll Cardiol. 1996 Jul;28(1):130–6. [PMID: 8752805]

Falk RH et al. Dofetilide: a new pure class III antiarrhythmic agent. Am Heart J. 2000 Nov;140(5):697–706. [PMID: 11054613]

Feld G et al. Radiofrequency catheter ablation of type 1 atrial flutter using large-tip 8- or 10-mm electrode catheters and a high-output radiofrequency energy generator: results of a multicenter safety and efficacy study. J Am Coll Cardiol. 2004 Apr 21;43(8):1466–72. [PMID: 15093885]

Nakagawa H et al. Characterization of reentrant circuit in macroreentrant right atrial tachycardia after surgical repair of congenital heart disease: isolated channels between scars allow "focal" ablation. Circulation. 2001 Feb 6;103(5):699–709. [PMID: 11156882]

MULTIFOCAL ATRIAL TACHYCARDIA

 ESSENTIALS OF DIAGNOSIS

▶ Heart rate: Up to 150 bpm.

▶ P waves: Three or more distinct P waves in a single lead.

▶ Variable P-P, P-R, and R-R intervals.

▶ General Considerations

Multifocal atrial tachycardia is an irregular SVT that constitutes less than 1% of all arrhythmias. It is related to pulmonary disease in 60–85% of cases, with chronic obstructive pulmonary disease (COPD) exacerbation being the most common. In addition, MAT is precipitated by respiratory failure, acute decompensated cardiac function, and infection. It has also been reported to be associated with hypokalemia, hypomagnesemia, hyponatremia, pulmonary embolism, cancer, and valvular heart disease, as well occurring in the postoperative setting. It occurs in children and adults. Distention of the right atrium from elevated pulmonary pressures causes multiple ectopic foci to fire, with ventricular rates not usually exceeding 150 bpm. Whether this rhythm is due to abnormal automaticity or triggered activity is uncertain, but the ability of verapamil to suppress the ectopic atrial activity by virtue of its calcium-channel-blocking properties supports the latter assumption.

Three ECG criteria must be met to diagnose MAT (Figure 20–4): (1) The presence of at least three distinct P wave morphologies recorded in the same lead. (2) The absence of one dominant atrial pacemaker. (3) Varying P-P, P-R, and R-R intervals.

Multifocal atrial tachycardia is often misdiagnosed as atrial fibrillation. Although both are irregular, the former has distinct P waves with an intervening isoelectric baseline. In fact, MAT may progress to atrial fibrillation.

▶ Treatment

The primary treatment for MAT should be directed at the underlying disease state. Oral and intravenous verapamil and several formulations of intravenous β-blockers have been effective to varying degrees in either slowing the heart rate (without terminating the rhythm) or in converting the arrhythmia to sinus rhythm. Intravenous magnesium and potassium, even in patients with serum levels of these electrolytes within the normal range, convert a significant percentage of these patients to sinus rhythm. Digoxin is not effective in treating this condition. Moreover, treatment with digoxin may precipitate digitalis intoxication. In addition, if the arrhythmia is secondary to delayed after-depolarizations, further aggravation may occur with digitalis because this drug increases delayed after-depolarizations. Medications that cause atrial irritability, such as theophylline and β-agonists, should be withdrawn whenever possible.

Application of radiofrequency energy for both AV node modification and AV node ablation with subsequent implantation of a pacemaker have been reported. The numbers of patients in the studies were very small, and there are no long-term results. Nevertheless, ablation of the AV junction has been shown to reduce symptomatic MAT, resulting in improved quality of life, reduced hospital admissions for recurrent symptomatic MAT, and improved left ventricular function.

▶ Prognosis

Because of the severity of the precipitating underlying diseases, MAT portends a poor outcome. Mortality during the hospitalization when the arrhythmia is first diagnosed is between 30% and 60%, with death being attributed to the disease state rather than the tachycardia itself. In one study of patients with pulmonary disease who were admitted for acute respiratory failure, the in-hospital mortality rate for those with MAT was 87%, compared with 24% for those in a different rhythm.

Bradley DJ et al. The clinical course of multifocal atrial tachycardia in infants and children. J Am Coll Cardiol. 2001 Aug;38(2):401–8. [PMID: 11499730]

Ueng KC et al. Radiofrequency catheter modification of atrioventricular junction in patients with COPD and medically refractory multifocal atrial tachycardia. Chest. 2000 Jan;117(1):52–9. [PMID: 10631199]

ATRIAL TACHYCARDIA

 ESSENTIALS OF DIAGNOSIS

- ▶ Onset and termination: Sudden.
- ▶ Heart rate: 100–180 bpm.
- ▶ P wave: Distinct P waves that differ from sinus P waves.
- ▶ R-P relationship: Long.

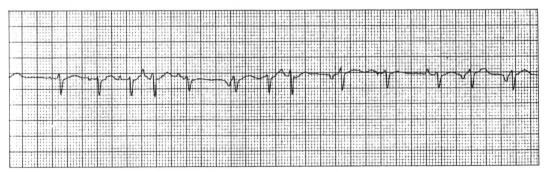

▲ **Figure 20–4.** Multifocal atrial tachycardia. The presence of at least three distinct P-wave morphologies, the absence of one dominant pacemaker focus, and varying P-P, R-R, and PR intervals establish the diagnosis. (Reprinted, with permission, from Goldberger A, Boldberger E. *Clinical Electrocardiography. A Simplified Approach.* St. Louis: Mosby Year Book, 1990.)

▶ General Considerations

Atrial tachycardia originates from an ectopic site in the atrium and, therefore, the P waves are usually quite different than the sinus P waves. It has been demonstrated that these arrhythmias arise from well-defined anatomic regions, including the crista terminalis, the tricuspid and mitral annuli, the right and left atrial appendage, and the region within or surrounding the pulmonary veins. In situations where the P wave is identical to the sinus P wave, the SVT is usually designated to be sinus node reentry or sinus tachycardia. The onset of atrial tachycardia is typically sudden; however, there can be some acceleration at the beginning, which is called the "warm-up" phase. Rates can range from 100 bpm to 180 bpm. The R-P relationship is usually long, unless there is a very long P-R interval, which can sometimes be appreciated on the baseline ECG. The episodes may either be brief and self-terminating or chronic and persistent, eventually leading to a tachycardia-induced cardiomyopathy if left untreated. Short nonsustained bursts of atrial tachycardia can be seen in 2–6% of young adults on Holter evaluations.

In those patients with paroxysmal sustained atrial tachycardia, there is a higher likelihood of associated organic heart disease, including coronary artery disease, valvular heart disease, congenital heart disease, and other cardiomyopathies. Frequently, a transient automatic tachycardia will be present, the cause of which can usually be determined from the associated clinical setting. Some of the most frequent causes include acute myocardial infarction, in which case it is seen in 4–19% of patients, electrolyte disturbances (especially hypokalemia), chronic lung disease or pulmonary infection, acute alcohol ingestion, hypoxia, and use of cardiac stimulants (theophylline, cocaine). Short, unsustained bursts of paroxysmal atrial tachycardia that last only a few seconds can be seen in adults without concomitant heart disease.

The form that occurs almost exclusively, and not uncommonly, in children, is a continuous tachycardia with heart rates of about 175 bpm. Symptoms are severe, and congestive heart failure frequently develops as a result of a tachycardia-induced cardiomyopathy. The arrhythmia may be transient in younger children, but when it persists in older children, it should be considered permanent. Fortunately, if the tachycardia can be terminated, cardiac function returns to normal. When it appears in adults, the continuous variety manifests milder symptoms.

Atrial tachycardias may have an automatic, triggered, or microreentrant mechanism. Although precisely defining the basic mechanism of a particular atrial tachycardia may be difficult, understanding their basic principles may help with choosing therapy.

▶ Treatment

A. Pharmacologic Therapy

Although there are no large-scale trials in the medical treatment of atrial tachycardias, reported data show that β-blockers and calcium channel blockers are at least partially effective, particularly if the underlying mechanism of the tachycardia is abnormal automaticity or triggered activity. Because of their safety profile, these drugs are usually first-line medical therapy.

Other antiarrhythmic drugs may be effective in treating some patients with atrial tachycardias. However, there are no large-scale trials comparing the drugs or even trials comparing drugs to placebo. Therefore, drug therapy is largely empiric and drug choice is determined more by side-effect profile and risk of proarrhythmia than by suspected efficacy. The use of class IC antiarrhythmic drugs may be somewhat successful. Flecainide and propafenone are often well tolerated in patients without structural heart disease and thus can be considered a reasonable first-line antiarrhythmic therapy. Quinidine and procainamide are less well tolerated. Class Ib agents are generally not effective for atrial tachycardias; however, there may be a small subset of lidocaine-sensitive atrial tachycardias in which mexilitine may be effective. Sotalol may also be effective, in part because of its inherent β-blocker (class II) properties. It is generally better tolerated than quinidine and may provide rate control during recurrences. Nevertheless, because sotalol also has class III properties, it will prolong the QT interval and may predispose patients to torsades de pointes, similar to quinidine and procainamide. Amiodarone may be effective, especially in resistant tachycardias. In addition, it is the least proarrhythmic and is generally used as first-line drug therapy in patients with depressed left ventricular function. Newer class III drugs, such as dofetilide, may be effective for atrial tachycardias, but there is little data about their use in atrial arrhythmias, except atrial fibrillation and atrial flutter.

B. Ablation

Ablation for atrial tachycardias has been proven safe and effective, with reported success rates between 77% and 100%. It also has been shown to improve patient quality of life scores. Therefore, ablation should be indicated for all symptomatic patients who have persistent symptoms despite medical therapy or intolerable side effects from medicines. Furthermore, patients who are not willing to undergo medical therapy should also be considered. Recently, the use of electromagnetic and noncontact mapping systems has significantly improved ablative therapy by decreasing fluoroscopic time, mapping time, and number of radiofrequency applications, thereby increasing efficacy.

Kalman JM et al. Localization of focal atrial tachycardias–back to the future...when (old) electrophysiologic first principles complement sophisticated technology. J Cardiovasc Electrophysiol. 2007 Jan;18(1):7–8. [PMID: 17240545]

Natale A et al. Ablation of right and left atrial tachycardias using a three-dimensional nonfluoroscopic mapping system. Am J Cardiol. 1998 Oct 15;82(8):989–92. [PMID: 9794361]

Sanders P et al. Characterization of focal atrial tachycardia using high-density mapping. J Am Coll Cardiol. 2005 Dec 6;46(11):2088–99. [PMID: 16325047]

Scheinman MM et al. The 1998 NASPE prospective catheter ablation registry. Pacing Clin Electrophysiol. 2000 Jun;23(6):1020–8. [PMID: 10879389]

Schmitt H et al. Diagnosis and ablation of focal right atrial tachycardia using a new high-resolution, non-contact mapping system. Am J Cardiol. 2001 Apr 15;87(8):1017–21. [PMID: 11306000]

ATRIOVENTRICULAR NODAL REENTRANT TACHYCARDIA

ESSENTIALS OF DIAGNOSIS

▶ Onset and termination: Sudden.

▶ Heart rate: Usually 120–200 bpm but can be faster; neck pulsations correspond to heart rate.

▶ P waves: Retrograde P waves; P waves not visible in 90% of cases.

▶ R-P relationship: Short, if P waves visible.

▶ General Considerations

Atrioventricular nodal reentrant tachycardia is more common in women than in men. Heart rates usually fall in the range of 120–200 bpm, although rates up to 250 bpm have been recorded. Palpitations are almost universally reported. A feeling of diuresis, noted with other supraventricular arrhythmias, is significantly more common in AVNRT and has been correlated with elevated right atrial pressures and elevated atrial natriuretic peptide. Neck pulsations are common (Brugada phenomenon) and are secondary to simultaneous contraction of the atria and ventricles against closed mitral and tricuspid valves. Dizziness and lightheadedness can occur but frank syncope is very rare. Sudden death has been reported but is extremely rare. Although symptoms may occur at any age, the distribution of when the tachycardia and symptoms commonly appear appears to be bimodal. The initial episode may begin during the second decade of life, only to disappear and then reappear during the fourth and fifth decades of life.

▶ Pathophysiology

Conduction from the right atrium to the ventricles is normally over a singular AV nodal pathway, with no route of reentry back into the atrium. In persons with dual AV nodal pathways, an atrial impulse may travel antegrade from the atrium over one limb of the AV node and then back to the atrium over another limb in a retrograde fashion. When only one cycle occurs, a single echo beat, in the form of a retrograde P wave, may be seen on the ECG. If this echo beat can again penetrate the AV node antegrade, the cycle can perpetuate itself, leading to AVNRT. It is estimated that dual AV nodal pathways exist in up to one-fourth of the population, but only a fraction of these people ever manifest a tachycardia.

If each limb of the circuit conducted impulses equally, echo beats and sustained AVNRT would not occur. An atrial impulse traveling down both limbs at the same speed would cause each limb to be refractory when that impulse reached the bottom of the node, preventing the impulse in each limb from going back up the other. Instead, the limbs have varying conduction speeds (Figure 20–5A) and refractory periods. The faster conducting limb, called the β or fast pathway, has a longer refractory period, whereas the reverse is true for the second limb, called the α or slow pathway.

A premature atrial depolarization may initiate the tachycardia if it finds the fast pathway refractory; the premature impulse can then reach the ventricles through the slow pathway. The ECG manifestation of this is a P-R interval that exceeds the baseline P-R by as much as 50–300% of its value in sinus rhythm. At the same time that it enters the His–Purkinje system and the ventricles, the slow pathway impulse heads retrograde up the fast pathway, where it may block (Figure 20–5B) or continue to produce an atrial echo beat with a retrograde P wave and a short R-P interval. If the slow pathway cannot propagate another impulse antegrade because of refractoriness, only a single atrial echo beat will occur (Figure 20–5C). If the slow pathway has recovered excitability, the circuit can again be entered. Perpetuation of this cycle will lead to a sustained episode of AVNRT (Figure 20–5D). Ventricular ectopic beats can also initiate AVNRT by a similar mechanism.

Conduction up the fast pathway is usually so rapid that retrograde atrial depolarization is simultaneous or almost simultaneous with antegrade ventricular activation. This causes the low-amplitude P wave to become obscured in the much higher amplitude QRS complex. Therefore, the P wave is not visible 50–60% of the time. In 20–30% of cases, the P wave distorts the terminal portion of the QRS causing a pseudo-S wave in the inferior leads and a pseudo-R' in lead V_1, and in approximately 10% of cases the P wave distorts the initial portion of the QRS complex (Figure 20–6). Since the P wave usually occurs simultaneous to or just after the QRS, the common variety of AVNRT is a short R-P tachycardia.

The common type of AVNRT that is described above is also called **slow–fast** AVNRT. "Slow-fast" refers to the antegrade and retrograde limbs of conduction during the tachycardia, respectively. Distinctly more unusual, or **fast–slow** AVNRT, is seen in approximately 5–10% of cases. Here the slow pathway has the longer refractory period, which causes it to become blocked antegrade and then to be used as the return path to the atrium. In contrast, to slow-fast AVNRT, which is short R-P, fast-slow AVNRT is usually long R-P. A third and even rarer variety of AVNRT is the **slow–slow** form in which the retrograde limb is slower than most typical slow pathways, leading to P waves midway between the QRS complexes. Therefore, this type of AVNRT can be long or short R-P.

AVNRT, once initiated, can perpetuate itself without the participation of either the atria or ventricles. Therefore, on rare occasions, the tachycardia can occur with a 2:1 block in

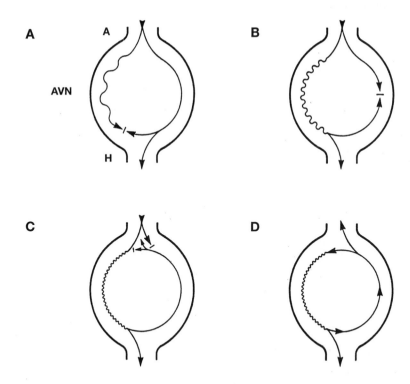

▲ Figure 20–5. Schematic presentation of impulse propagation along with the fast (*straight line*) and slow (*wavy line*) conducting pathways. A sinus atrial impulse preferentially negotiates the His bundle via the fast pathway (**A**). Because of the longer refractoriness of the fast pathway, an atrial premature beat may block it while engaging the His bundle via the slow pathway and then penetrate the fast pathway retrograde (**B**). Depending on the recovery of tissue ahead, the returning impulse may produce a single echo beat (**C**) or sustained arrhythmia (**D**). A, atrium; AVN, atrioventricular node; H, His bundle. (Reprinted, with permission, from Akhtar M. Supraventricular tachycardias. In: Josephson ME, Wellens HJJ, eds. *Tachycardias: Mechanisms, Diagnosis, Treatment.* Philadelphia: Lea & Febiger, 1984.)

either direction leading to two atrial depolarizations for every ventricular depolarization or two ventricular depolarizations for every atrial depolarization.

▶ Prevention

Prevention of AVNRT is directed at slowing or blocking conduction in either the fast or slow pathway. Typical AV nodal blocking agents such as β-blockers, calcium channel blockers, and digoxin are most effective on the antegrade slow pathway. The more potent class Ia antiarrhythmic drugs may be necessary to inhibit conduction in the retrograde fast pathway. Class Ic drugs, and amiodarone and sotalol (class III) affect both pathways.

▶ Treatment

A. Vagal Maneuvers

Vagal maneuvers should be considered, barring any contraindications, before embarking on medical therapy. The Valsalva maneuver and carotid sinus massage can immediately terminate the tachycardia by increasing refractory time in the AV node. In patients over 50 years old, bruits should be ruled out before carotid sinus massage to avoid embolic stroke. Medications may render the arrhythmia more susceptible to termination with vagal maneuvers. Therefore,

these can be attempted immediately after each round of drug therapy if the tachycardia persists.

B. Pharmacologic Therapy

Terminating an acute episode of AVNRT in the hospital setting has been made simpler with the availability of intravenous adenosine, which reaches and acts on its target within seconds of administration. With a clinical half-life of 10 seconds, commonly reported sensations such as breathlessness, chest heaviness, and flushing disappear quickly. The routine dosage is 6 mg followed by up to two more boluses of 12 mg. If adenosine is ineffective, intravenous verapamil can be used, but it takes longer to act. Diltiazem, given as intravenous bolus, can also be effective in aborting the tachycardia. Hypotension occurs with about a 10% incidence and is usually rapidly reversed with fluid administration. Although intravenous β-blockers, procainamide, and digoxin are other second-line choices, they can be advantageous in recurrent cases because of their slower clearance from the body.

C. Radiofrequency Modification in Slow–Fast AVNRT

Radiofrequency lesions delivered via a catheter can be directed at either the fast or slow pathway; the latter is preferred since it is associated with a lower risk of complete heart block.

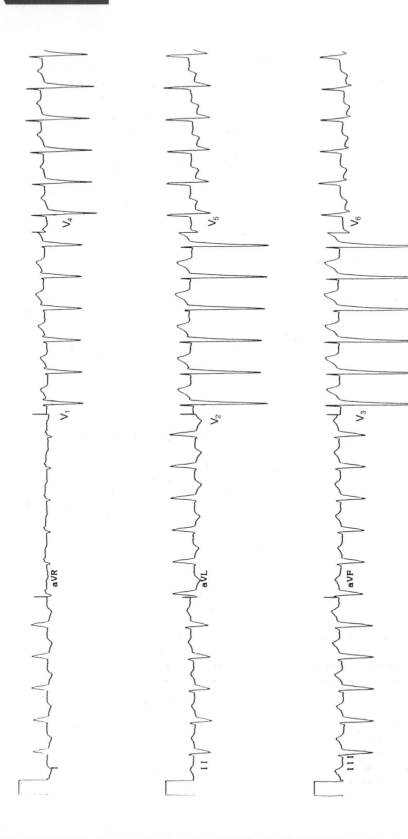

▲ **Figure 20–6 A:** Supraventricular tachycardia without easily identifiable P waves but with pseudo R' in lead V₁ compatible with atrioventricular nodal reentrant tachycardia. (*continued*)

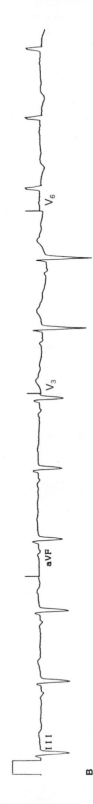

▲ **Figure 20–6** (*continued*) **B:** Postconversion tracing. Note normal QRS in lead V$_1$ when patient displays normal sinus rhythm.

The inferior origin of the slow pathway is variable within the triangle of Koch, but it is usually anterior and superior to (and sometimes within) the os of the coronary sinus. These anatomic landmarks and gross intracardiac electrogram patterns can be used to position the ablation catheter for successful modification of the AV node. The fast pathway is left unaltered and can still be used for transmission of sinus impulses to the ventricles. Long-term freedom from recurrent AVNRT is about 95%, and the risk of complete heart block as a result of inadvertent fast pathway or nodal damage is 0–5%.

A relatively new form of ablation is cryoablation, using a supercooling catheter, which can reversibly or permanently damage endocardial tissue. This novel approach allows for testing the acceptability of a particular ablation site. Should heart block occur prior to irreversible tissue damage, then rewarming can be performed with no untoward effects.

Gupta·D et al. Cryoablation compared with radiofrequency ablation for atrioventricular nodal re-entrant tachycardia: analysis of factors contributing to acute and follow-up outcome. Europace. 2006 Dec;8(12):1022–6. [PMID: 17101629]

Skanes AC et al. Cryothermal ablation of the slow pathway for the elimination of atrioventricular nodal reentrant tachycardia. Circulation. 2000 Dec 5;102(23):2856–60. [PMID: 11104744]

Wu J et al. Mechanisms underlying atrioventricular nodal conduction and the reentrant circuit of atrioventricular nodal reentrant tachycardia using optical mapping. J Cardiovasc Electrophysiol. 2002 Aug;13(8):831–4. [PMID: 12212708]

JUNCTIONAL TACHYCARDIA (ACCELERATED AV JUNCTIONAL RHYTHM)

 ESSENTIALS OF DIAGNOSIS

▶ Onset and termination: Gradual.

▶ Heart rate: 70–120 bpm.

▶ P waves: Retrograde.

▶ R-P relationship: Short, if P waves visible.

▶ General Considerations

Unlike AVNRT, which presents with recurrent tachycardia episodes of sudden onset, junctional tachycardia, which is sometimes also called nonparoxysmal junctional tachycardia (NPJT), is not episodic and starts almost imperceptibly. It is easily differentiated from AVNRT by a heart rate between 70 bpm and 120 bpm, gradual onset and termination, and lack of termination with vagal maneuvers. Although heart rates of less than 100 bpm can be seen, it is, nevertheless, a tachycardia because the rates are faster than the 40–60 bpm seen with a junctional escape rhythm.

▶ Clinical Findings

The heart rate at onset is just slightly faster than that of the rhythm preceding it, with gradual acceleration until the final rate is achieved. AV dissociation is common, occurring in 85% of cases caused by digoxin (see following discussion). When the conduction to the atria is intact, retrograde P waves may appear immediately before or after the QRS complex, or they may be obscured within the QRS. Discharge from the AV node is regular, but if antegrade second-degree AV block (almost always the result of digoxin excess), exit block, or atrial capture beats coexist with junctional tachycardia, the rhythm will appear irregular. Enhanced vagal tone or vagolytic agents will either slow down or speed up the arrhythmia, respectively.

Usually seen in the setting of organic heart disease, the cause of this rhythm is almost always identifiable. At one time, digoxin excess accounted for up to 85% of cases of junctional tachycardia. Awareness of the drug's side effects and the availability of other AV nodal blocking agents have diminished the incidence. Nevertheless, in those patients being treated with digoxin for atrial fibrillation, clinicians should suspect this arrhythmia when the ECG demonstrates a regularized ventricular response. Acute inferior infarction accounts for 20% of junctional tachycardia, and this rhythm may be present in up to 10% of all infarcts in this location, with onset usually within the first 24 hours and disappearance in several days. Junctional tachycardia may follow open heart surgery (valve replacement more often than bypass surgery), or it can be caused by myocarditis (especially rheumatic) and, rarely, congenital heart disease. In all cases, the tachycardia resolves along with the acute underlying event or with digoxin withdrawal.

▶ Treatment

Treatment is usually directed at the underlying causative factor. Because the rhythm rarely causes deleterious hemodynamic effects, treatment of the rhythm itself is usually not indicated. If digoxin toxicity is the cause, it should be withdrawn. If digoxin is not the cause, digoxin, β-blockers, or calcium channel blockers can be used to slow down the rate if necessary. Catheter ablation can also be performed but it carries a risk of complete heart block since the origin of the arrhythmia is near the AV node. However, cryoablation has been used in this setting and may be safer.

Hamdan MH et al. Role of invasive electrophysiologic testing in the evaluation and management of adult patients with focal junctional tachycardia. Card Electrophysiol Rev. 2002 Dec;6(4):431–5. [PMID: 12438824]

Law IH et al. Transcatheter cryothermal ablation of junctional ectopic tachycardia in the normal heart. Heart Rhythm. 2006 Aug;3(8):903–7. [PMID: 16876738]

ATRIOVENTRICULAR RECIPROCATING TACHYCARDIA

 ESSENTIALS OF DIAGNOSIS

▶ Onset and termination: Sudden.

▶ Heart rate: 140–250 bpm.

▶ P wave: Ectopic.

▶ R-P relationship: Short.

▶ Delta wave on baseline ECG if bypass tract conducts antegrade.

1. Bypass Tracts & the Wolff-Parkinson-White Syndrome

▶ General Considerations

Congenital bands of tissue that can conduct impulses but lie outside the normal conduction system are called accessory pathways, or bypass tracts. These pathways are responsible for a variety of mechanistically distinct tachycardias by providing preferential conduction between different areas within the heart.

▶ Epidemiology

Accessory pathways are quite prevalent in the general population with a 2:1 male:female predominance. The presence of a bypass tract, however, does not mean that a tachyarrhythmia is a certainty because less than half of those persons with documented bypass tracts ever sustain an arrhythmia. The actual number depends on the population studied and varies from 13% in a healthy outpatient population to 80% in the hospital setting.

Approximately 5–10% of patients with documented bypass tracts have concomitant structural heart disease. Ebstein anomaly is the most common, accounting for 25–50% of the anomalies in this group. Of patients with Ebstein anomaly, 8–10% have coexistent bypass tracts, mostly on the right side. The association of right-sided accessory pathways with structural heart disease is strong: 45% of patients with right-sided (and only 5% of those with left-sided) pathways display some type of heart disease.

A familial tendency toward bypass tracts has been seen in some instances, with a fourfold to tenfold increase in incidence among first-degree family members.

▶ Pathophysiology

A. Anatomy

Anatomically, the atria and ventricles are in apposition, separated by an invagination known as the AV groove. Paroxysmal tachycardias mediated by accessory pathways that cross the groove and electrically link the atria and ventricles, when combined with a short P-R interval (< 0.12 seconds), a wide QRS, and secondary repolarization abnormalities, define the Wolff-Parkinson-White syndrome. When this ECG pattern is seen without the tachycardia, it is called Wolff-Parkinson-White pattern or ventricular preexcitation.

Although the most common site of insertion is between the lateral aspect of the left atrium and left ventricular myocardium, pathways can cross the AV groove anywhere in its course (except the region between the aortic and mitral valves) to connect the left or right atrium to its respective ventricle (Figure 20–7). In noting the distribution of accessory pathways, 46–60% are located in the left free wall, 25% within the posteroseptal space, 13–21% in the right free wall, and 2% in the anteroseptal space. Each location produces a distinct ECG pattern (Figure 20–8), but in the 13% of patients with two or more bypass tracts the ECG tracing can be confounding and show multiple QRS morphologies.

B. Cardiac Electrical Conduction

Unlike the AV node, whose function is to delay atrial impulses en route to the ventricles, most bypass tracts conduct rapidly and without delay, which accounts for the short P-R interval often seen in sinus rhythm in these patients.

Impulses that reach the ventricles over a bypass tract spread through cell-to-cell conduction within the myocardium, activating the ventricles in series rather than in parallel. This relatively slow process is manifested as a wide QRS complex.

Sinus impulses are not restricted to using the AV node or the bypass tract only to reach the lower chambers. Instead, both may contribute to ventricular activation. This produces a QRS that is initially wide, reflecting conduction over the bypass tract, with the latter portion of the QRS appearing normal and narrow, indicating that the remainder of the ventricle has been depolarized via the normal conduction system (the AV node and His-Purkinje system). The initial slurred upstroke of the QRS, a delta wave, indicates ventricular preexcitation, which can be defined as ventricular depolarization that begins earlier than would be expected by conduction over the AV node alone. The degree of preexcitation and P-R shortening depends on the proportion of ventricular activation occurring over the AV node and the bypass tract. This, in turn, is related to two factors. The first is the conduction velocity of the bypass tract relative to the AV node. The faster the bypass tract can conduct impulses to the ventricles in relation to the AV node, the earlier the ventricle will preexcite, and vice versa. The second factor is the location of the tract, and more specifically, its proximity to the sinus node and AV node. A sinus impulse will encounter a right-sided free-wall bypass tract earlier than it will the AV node, and this favors a short P-R interval with a

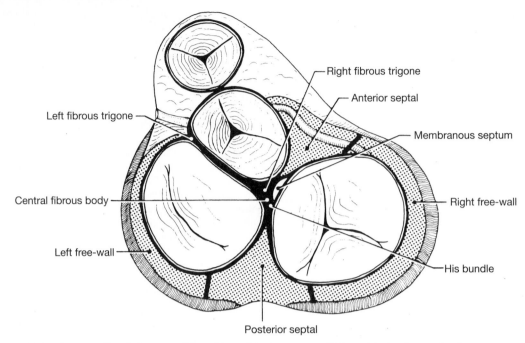

▲ Figure 20–7. Cross-sectional diagram of the atrioventricular groove. Atrioventricular bypass tracts may cross the groove anywhere in its course except in the region bounded by the left and right fibrous trigones. (Reprinted, with permission, from Cox JL et al. J Thorac Cardiovasc Surg. 1985;90:490.)

high degree of ventricular preexcitation (Figure 20–9A). On the other hand, a sinus beat will encounter the AV node early in its course while traveling to a pathway in the lateral left atrium, allowing ventricular activation to occur primarily by the normal conduction system. A narrow, minimally (if at all) preexcited QRS complex with a normal or near-normal P-R interval may be seen (Figure 20–9B). Changes in autonomic tone, by modifying the conduction velocity and refractoriness over both the pathway and the AV node, can produce varying degrees of preexcitation at different times in the same patient (Figure 20–9C).

If the delta wave axis of a maximally preexcited beat is discordant from the accompanying preexcited QRS axis, or if more than one preexcited QRS morphology is noted, there may be multiple bypass tracts.

C. Mechanism

1. Atrioventricular reciprocating tachycardia—An inherent property of accessory pathways is their ability to conduct in a retrograde direction more easily than antegrade. The AV node, on the other hand, conducts more efficiently antegrade. For this reason, reentrant rhythms in this setting most commonly use the AV node to go from atrium to ventricle and the bypass tract to return to the atrium. Orthodromic AVRT, (antegrade conduction over the AV node) accounts for 70–

80% of arrhythmias in patients with AV bypass tracts, with heart rates of 140–250 bpm (Figure 20–10). Antidromic AVRT, in which the atrial impulse is carried to the ventricle over the bypass tract and reenters the atrium via retrograde conduction over the AV node, is rare, occurring in approximately 5–10% of cases. Because conduction to the ventricles during orthodromic AVRT occurs over the normal conduction system, the QRS is narrow, unless bundle branch aberrancy is present. During antidromic AVRT, the QRS is wide and maximally preexcited as a result of the complete lack of AV nodal contribution to ventricular depolarization. When two or more bypass tracts are present, each tract may act as the antegrade or retrograde limb (or both), especially with involvement of the AV node. There is a higher incidence of ventricular fibrillation in patients with multiple accessory pathways. Additionally, multiple pathways are more common in patients with antidromic SVT and in patients with Ebstein anomaly.

Tachycardia is usually initiated by a premature atrial or ventricular beat. In orthodromic tachycardia, a premature atrial beat conducts down the AV node to depolarize the ventricle, and the bypass tract carries the impulse back to the atrium (Figure 20–11). A ventricular premature beat finding the AV node refractory might initiate an identical tachycardia by first conducting up the bypass tract to the atrium. Antidromic tachycardia initiates in an identical fashion but with a reversed direction of conduction.

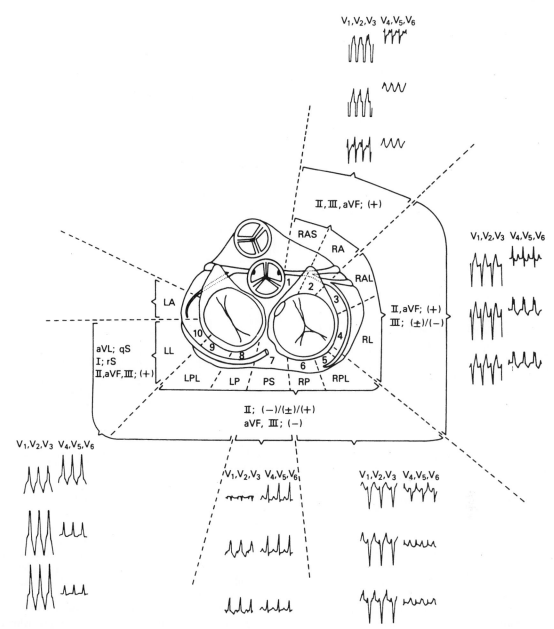

▲ **Figure 20–8.** Single atrioventricular bypass-tract localization based on maximally preexcited electrocardiographic morphology. RAS/RA, right anteroseptal or right anterior accessory pathways; RAL/RL, right anterolateral or right lateral accessory pathways; RP/RPL, right posterior or right posterolateral accessory pathways; PS, posteroseptal accessory pathways; LPL/LP, left posterolateral or left posterior accessory pathways; LL, left lateral accessory pathways; +, positive delta wave; –, negative delta wave; ±, isoelectric delta wave. (Reprinted, with permission, from Fananapazir L et al. Circulation. 1990;81:578.)

Atrial fibrillation accounts for only 19–38% of arrhythmias in the population with accessory pathways, but it is potentially more lethal than the reciprocating tachycardias discussed earlier. It is more common in patients with antegrade conducting accessory pathways and in pathways with a short antegrade refractory period. By virtue of their short refractory periods, bypass tracts (unlike the AV node) have the potential to conduct very rapidly to the ventricles at ventricular rates of 250–

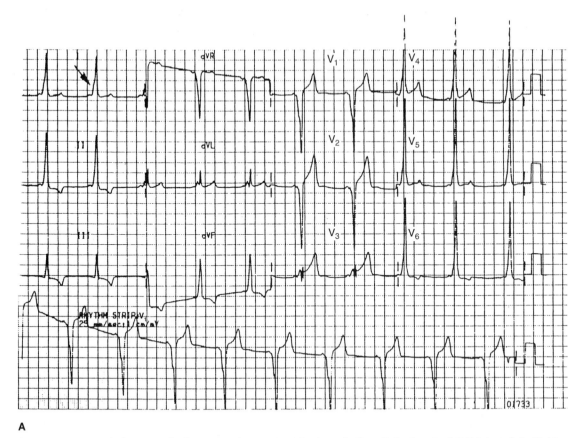

▲ Figure 20–9. Ventricular preexcitation over a bypass tract in sinus rhythm. Note the short P-R interval. **A:** Right anterior bypass tract. The delta wave is positive in most leads (*arrow*), and negative in aVR and V$_1$–V$_3$. (*continued*)

350 bpm (Figure 20–12) with the possibility of causing degeneration to ventricular fibrillation. A reputed marker for sudden death in patients with atrial fibrillation is a shortest preexcited R-R interval of ≤ 250 ms (corresponding to a heart rate of ≥ 240 bpm) between two fully preexcited beats. The finding of a short R-R interval actually has little positive predictive value, however, because sudden death in this syndrome is still rare.

During atrial fibrillation, the ECG reveals an irregular irregular rhythm with QRS complexes of varying morphologies, representing conduction to the ventricles via the AV node (normally conducted narrow complexes), the bypass tract (wide, preexcited complexes), and both (fusion beats, harboring elements of both the normally conducted and preexcited beats). In this setting, the bypass tract may be called a bystander since it is not integral to the tachycardia. Patients with AV bypass tracts have a higher incidence of atrial fibrillation than does the general population, possibly because of the degeneration of reentrant tachycardia or of microreentry within the atrial portion of the bypass tract. It has been shown that ablation of the bypass tract can frequently also eliminate atrial fibrillation.

2. Concealed bypass tracts—Between 15% and 50% of patients with no evidence of preexcitation during sinus rhythm are found to have bypass tracts that conduct only in the retrograde direction. By definition, concealed bypass tracts (their presence cannot be detected by ECG) do not display delta waves on the ECG during sinus rhythm, but they can still support an orthodromic AVRT and account for about 30% of orthodromic tachycardias.

Differentiating orthodromic AVRT from AVNRT on the ECG can be difficult. The incidence of both tachycardias being operative at different times in the same person is reported to be between 1.7% and 7%. Therefore, although the presence of a delta wave on the nontachycardiac tracing makes it statistically unlikely that AVNRT was the documented tachycardia, it does not exclude the possibility completely.

Because of the simultaneous atrial and ventricular activation that occurs during AVNRT, the P waves formed as a result of retrograde conduction to the atrium are usually obscured within the QRS complex. Likewise, because of the short retrograde conduction time via the bypass tract, ortho-

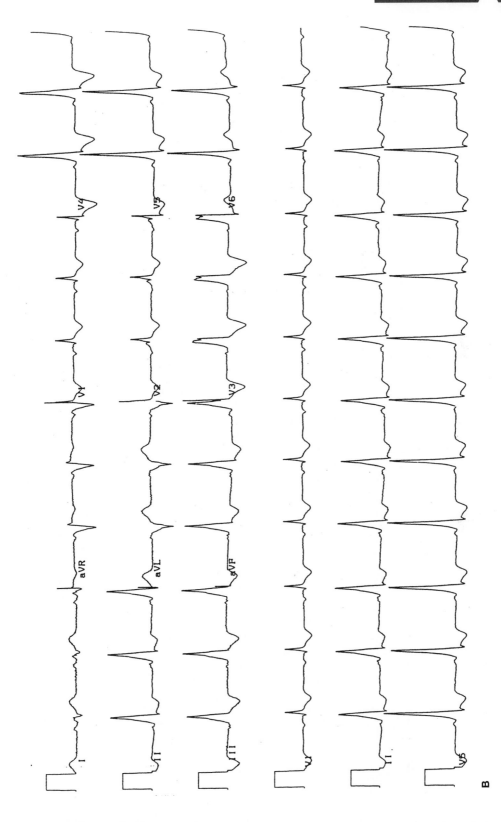

▲ **Figure 20-9.** (*Continued*) **B:** Left lateral bypass tract. The isoelectric delta wave in V₁ gives the appearance of a normal PR interval. Inspection of the simultaneously recorded rhythm strip leads (*lower three panels*) reveals delta wave onset to be at the end of the P wave in leads II and V₅. (*continued*)

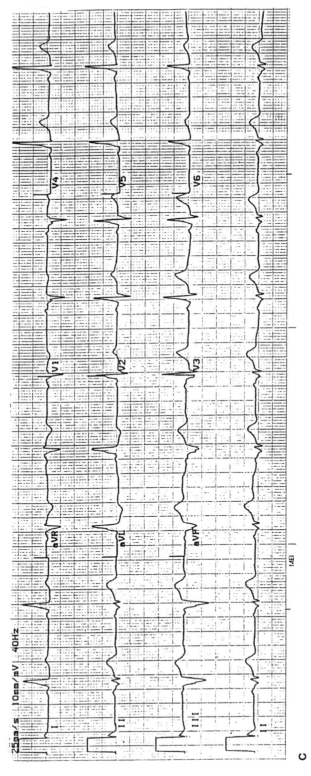

▲ **Figure 20-9.** (*continued*) **C:** A short time after this tracing was obtained the patient exhibited minimal to no preexcitation. This was due to fluctuations in autonomic tone causing enhanced conduction through the AV node.

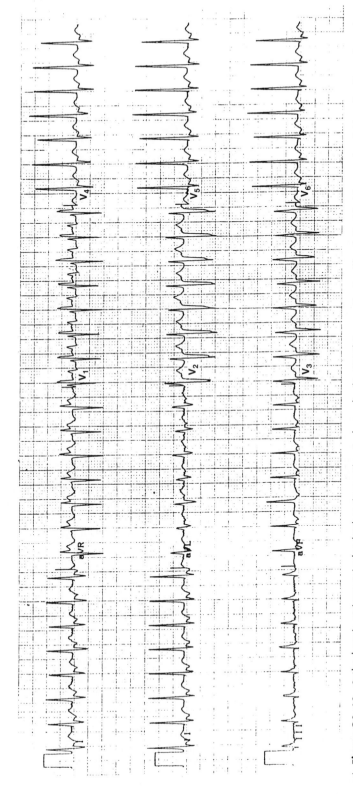

▲ **Figure 20–10.** Orthodromic atrioventricular (AV) reciprocating tachycardia (O-AVRT) in a patient with a left-sided bypass tract. The circuit conducts from atria to ventricles over the AV node and from ventricles to atria retrograde over the bypass tract. This mechanism accounts for the narrow QRS and the retrograde P waves inscribed in the early portion of the T waves. Although the electrocardiogram with common AV nodal reentrant tachycardia may appear similar, a ventriculoatrial conduction time of more than 100 ms, as measured from QRS onset to P wave onset, greatly favors O-AVRT. The time in this tracing is 110 ms.

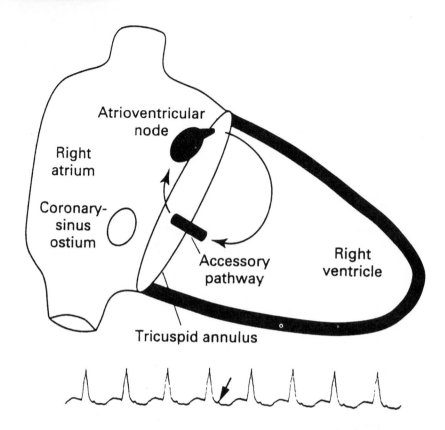

▲ **Figure 20–11.** The reentry circuit of orthodromic reciprocating tachycardia. The atrioventricular (AV) node serves as the antegrade limb of the reentry circuit, and an accessory pathway serves as the retrograde limb. In this case the accessory pathway is located in the free wall of the right ventricle. The wave of depolarization travels from the AV node to the accessory pathway through the ventricle and from the accessory pathway to the AV node through the atrium. Because the ventricles are depolarized by the normal conduction system, the ORS are narrow unless there is a bundle branch block. Also shown is an example of orthodromic reciprocating tachycardia, at a rate of 210 per minute, recoded in lead III. A P wave is present in the left half of the RR cycle (*arrow*) because retrograde conduction through the accessory pathway is more rapid than antegrade conduction through the AV node. (Reprinted, with permission, from Morady F. N Engl J Med. 1999;340:534. Copyright © 1999 Massachusetts Medical Society. All rights reserved.)

dromic AVRT usually is a short R-P tachycardia, albeit somewhat longer than with AVNRT. Usually, the P waves are located within the ST segment, ie, generally, the R-P interval is longer with AVRT than with AVNRT.

▶ **Treatment**

A. Vagal Maneuvers

The management of orthodromic AVRT or antidromic AVRT is similar to that of AVNRT. Since the AV node is an integral part of the reentry circuit in AVRT, blocking the AV node terminates the tachycardia. Therefore, vagal maneuvers such as the Valsalva maneuver or carotid sinus massage can be tried first.

B. Pharmacologic Therapy

Intravenous adenosine almost always terminates these tachycardias. Other AV nodal blocking agents such as β-blockers, calcium channel blockers, and digoxin can also be helpful. Just as in AVNRT, vagal maneuvers can be re-tried after each dose of these longer acting AV nodal blocking agents.

In contrast to orthodromic or antidromic AVRT, patients with atrial fibrillation or atrial flutter and a bystander bypass tract should not be given AV nodal blocking agents. This point is crucial since these types of medicines can precipitate ventricular fibrillation. Blocking the AV node enhances conduction down the bypass tract, making all the complexes wide. Furthermore, the bypass tract can often conduct faster

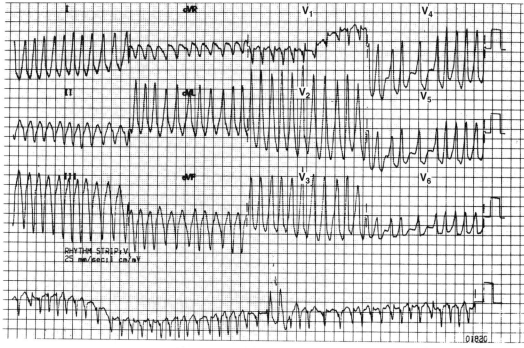

▲ **Figure 20–12.** Atrial fibrillation with antegrade conduction over a left posteroseptal bypass tract. Although most beats are fully preexcited, several of the beats in the rhythm strip are narrower, indicating combined conduction over both the bypass tract and the atrioventricular node. Antidromic atrioventricular reciprocating tachycardia would have a similar appearance on 12-lead electrocardiogram, but the rhythm irregularity and the varying degrees of preexcitation nullify this possibility. (Reprinted, with permission, from Zipes DP. Specific arrhythmias: diagnosis and treatment. In: Braunwald E, ed. *Heart Disease. A Textbook of Cardiovascular Medicine.* Philadelphia: WB Saunders, 1988.)

than the AV node, increasing ventricular rates to sometimes over 200 bpm. The aberrant conduction and rapid rate can lead to disorganized ventricular conduction, resulting in ventricular fibrillation. The drug of choice for patients with atrial fibrillation or atrial flutter and a bystander bypass tract is intravenous procainamide or another drug that preferentially blocks the bypass tract. This shunts more conduction through the AV node, which narrows the QRS complexes and often slows down the overall ventricular rate.

Asymptomatic patients showing delta waves on the ECG generally do not require treatment unless involved in a high-risk profession such as commercial pilots, police officers, and firefighters. Patients with occasional or rare bouts of minimal or mildly symptomatic palpitations from orthodromic or antidromic AVRT can often be safely treated with such agents as β-blockers or calcium channel blockers to prevent recurrent episodes. However, due to the potential of ventricular fibrillation, these AV node blocking agents should be used with great caution or not at all in patients who have also demonstrated atrial fibrillation or atrial flutter.

C. Radiofrequency Catheter Ablation Therapy

Patients who experience significant symptoms such as dizziness, presyncope, or syncope should undergo an electrophysiologic study with concomitant radiofrequency ablation. In addition, patients with frequent symptoms who do not respond to or who wish to avoid drug therapy can also undergo ablative therapy. Recent guidelines indicate that ablation can be considered first-line therapy for patients with symptomatic Wolff-Parkinson-White syndrome.

The right internal jugular or femoral vein ablation approach is used for accessory pathways located on the right side of the heart. Left-sided pathways can be approached from the left ventricle with retrograde technique, or transseptally from within the left atrium using the Brockenbrough technique. A steerable catheter is moved around the mitral or tricuspid annulus until the site of shortest impulse transit between the atrium and ventricle is found. This mapping process localizes the bypass tract. Frequently, an impulse can be recorded directly from the bypass tract, further confirming its localization. Once identified, radiofrequency energy delivered to the tract through the mapping catheter permanently destroys the tract and prevents further transmission of electric impulses over it.

Given its curative potential, a high success rate (95% in experienced hands, even with multiple bypass tracts), and a low complication rate, radiofrequency catheter ablation is now a very common treatment for accessory pathways (Table 20–2). As with other supraventricular arrhythmias, new mapping systems have been developed that decrease fluoroscopy and procedure time as well as allowing the operator to return to specific locations if needed.

D. Surgical Ablation Therapy

In rare instances, patients will have multiple pathways or pathways that are inaccessible to an ablation catheter. These patients may undergo surgical division of their tracts.

2. Other Bypass Tracts

A variety of bypass tracts other than AV tracts (Kent fibers) also exist. Atriohisian fibers connecting the atrium to the His bundle have been demonstrated. This led to the description of the Lown-Ganong-Levine (LGL) syndrome, which refers to those patients with a short P-R interval, normal QRS, and recurrent SVT. However, current data suggest that LGL syndrome does not truly exist since atriohisian pathways have not been shown to support any type of reentry tachycardia.

Atriofascicular fibers, which are also known as Mahaim fibers, typically run from the lateral right atrium to the right bundle branch. The tract is capable of antegrade conduction only, and therefore, only antidromic AVRT is possible. Because the antegrade reentrant circuit engages the right bundle branch, the tachycardia QRS complex typically has a left bundle branch block pattern. Treatment considerations are the same as for Wolff-Parkinson-White syndrome.

Kalarus Z et al. Influence of reciprocating tachycardia on the development of atrial fibrillation in patients with preexcitation syndrome. Pacing Clin Electrophysiol. 2007 Jan;30(1):85–92. [PMID: 17241320]

Kothari S et al. Atriofascicular pathways: where to ablate? Pacing Clin Electrophysiol. 2006 Nov;29(11):1226–33. [PMID: 17100675]

DIFFERENTIATION OF WIDE QRS COMPLEX TACHYCARDIA

With the exception of the AV node, the refractory period of cardiac tissue for a given beat is directly related to the interval between that beat and the preceding beat; the slower the heart rate, the longer the recovery period with each beat. Furthermore, because the stability of refractoriness depends on the stability of the heart rate, a beat-to-beat change in refractoriness accompanies variability in the heart rate.

When an early supraventricular beat occurs in the midst of a regular rhythm, the tissues do not have a chance to

Table 20–2. Complications of Radiofrequency Ablation of Accessory Pathways.[1]

Complication	Incidence (%)
Death	0.08
Nonfatal complications	
Cardiac tamponade	0.5
Atrioventricular block	0.5
Coronary artery spasm	0.2
Mild mitral regurgitation	0.2
Coronary artery thrombosis	0.1
Pericarditis	0.1
Mild aortic regurgitation	0.1
Transient neurologic deficit	0.1
Bacteremia	0.1
Femoral artery complications	
Thrombotic occlusion	0.2
Large hematoma	0.2
Atrioventricular fistula	0.1

[1]The incidence of death is based on unpublished data from the University of Oklahoma, the University of Alabama, the University of Michigan, Duke University, and the University of California, San Francisco. The incidence of nonfatal complications is based on pooled data from seven published studies.

shorten (or reset) their refractory periods; the result may be aberrant conduction (a transient functional refractoriness, or block) in one of the bundle branches. The shorter the interval between the early beat and the preceding one, the greater the probability that the early beat will be aberrant (Ashman phenomenon). Ashman phenomenon is also associated with the irregularity and frequent pauses of atrial fibrillation. Aberrancy may continue for a variable period before normal conduction resumes (Figure 20–13).

Aberrant conduction is often seen at the onset of any SVT that uses the AV node for antegrade conduction. (This excludes tachycardias that conduct antegrade over a bypass tract.) The right bundle branch, with its longer refractory period, is more subject to block than is the left, but occasionally the left bundle becomes refractory earlier. Once the tachycardia has been established and refractory periods stabilized, this normal functional aberrancy may give way to normal conduction, with resumption of a narrow QRS.

Deciding whether a wide-complex tachycardia is supraventricular or ventricular in origin is often difficult. Only when AV dissociation or capture or fusion beats are present can a ventricular rhythm be diagnosed with certainty. The low sensitivities of these findings (20% for AV dissociation) do not provide a firm diagnosis in more than a minority of wide-complex tachycardias, however.

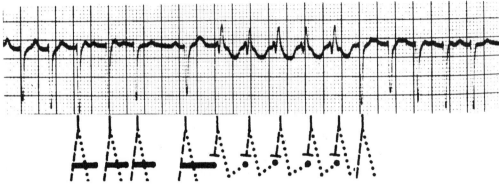

▲ **Figure 20–13.** Atrial tachycardia with Wenckebach (type I) AV block, ventricular aberration from the Ashman phenomenon, and probably concealed transseptal conduction. The long pause of the atrial tachycardia is followed by five QRS complexes with right bundle branch block morphology. The right bundle branch block of the first QRS reflects the Ashman phenomenon. The aberration is perpetuated by concealed transseptal activation from the left bundle into the right bundle, with block of the antegrade conduction of the subsequent sinus impulse in the right bundle. Foreshortening of the R-R cycle, a manifestation of the Wenckebach structure, disturbs the relationship between transseptal and antegrade sinus conduction, and right bundle branch conduction is normalized. In the ladder diagram below the tracing, the solid lines represent the His bundle; the dashes, the right bundle branch; and the dots, the left bundle branch. The solid horizontal bars denote the refractory period. Neither the P waves nor the AV node is identified in the diagram. (Reprinted, with permission, from Fisch C. Electrocardiography and vectorcardiography. In: Braunwald E, ed. *Heart Disease. A Textbook of Cardiovascular Medicine.* Philadelphia: WB Saunders, 1988.)

Classic criteria that examine V_1 when a right bundle branch block pattern is present, the QRS width and axis, the presence of positive or negative concordance across the precordium, and various combinations of QRS patterns in different leads may support a diagnosis, but they have been found lacking in diagnostic power because of their low sensitivity, low specificity, or both. A proposed algorithm separates supraventricular from ventricular tachycardia with 99% sensitivity and 97% specificity. However, this algorithm, which is also known as the "Brugada criteria," has had lower sensitivity and specificity in recent studies.

Lau EW et al. Comparison of two diagnostic algorithms for regular broad complex tachycardia by decision theory analysis. Pacing Clin Electrophysiol. 2001 Jul;24(7):1118–25. [PMID: 11475829]

OTHER SUPRAVENTRICULAR ARRHYTHMIAS

1. Sinus Node Arrhythmia

 ESSENTIALS OF DIAGNOSIS

- ▶ Cyclic heart rate variation with respiration.
- ▶ P-P interval variability ≥ 160 ms or 10%.
- ▶ P-wave morphology identical to normal sinus rhythm P wave.

▶ **General Considerations**

A cyclic increase and decrease in heart rate normally accompanies inspiration and expiration, respectively, and the irregularity in rhythm (mediated by vagal tone) is often imperceptible. More marked degrees of rate excursion can occur, especially at slower heart rates, but these are not considered to be sinus arrhythmia unless the shortest and longest P-P interval varies by 0.16 seconds or more, or by 10% or more. This respiratory form of sinus arrhythmia is common in younger people. It becomes less prevalent with increasing age and in conditions associated with autonomic dysfunction, such as diabetes mellitus. Enhancement of vagal tone with agents such as digoxin and morphine may cause sinus arrhythmia.

▶ **Treatment**

Because of its benign nature, no treatment is required for sinus arrhythmia.

2. Wandering Atrial Pacemaker

 ESSENTIALS OF DIAGNOSIS

- ▶ Progressive cyclic alteration in P wave morphology.
- ▶ Heart rate: 60–100 bpm.

▶ General Considerations

The presence of more than one pacemaker within the atria (which may or may not include the sinus node) causes variation in the P-P interval, P wave morphology, and the P-R interval. The heart rate remains within the normal range.

There is controversy over the cause of this rhythm. Some authorities believe that wandering atrial pacemaker and multifocal atrial tachycardia are the same rhythm artificially separated by heart rate, and that both are attributable to underlying pulmonary disease. Others believe that it is an exaggerated form of a respiratory sinus arrhythmia, with the uncovering of latent atrial and sinus node pacemakers when the primary sinus node pacemaker cycles to a slow rate with expiration.

The significance ascribed to a wandering atrial pacemaker should probably be interpreted in the setting in which it is seen. In those with lung disease, it may simply be a reflection of that process: In the elderly, it may suggest sinus node disease or sick sinus syndrome, and in the young and athletic heart, it may represent heightened vagal tone.

▶ Treatment

The rhythm itself is usually benign and typically requires no intervention. If the rhythm is secondary, treating the underlying etiology may be warranted.

Atrial Fibrillation

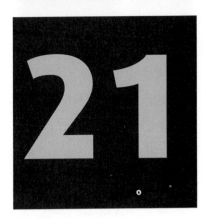

Melvin M. Scheinman, MD

ESSENTIALS OF DIAGNOSIS

▶ Irregularly irregular rhythm.
▶ Absence of P waves on the electrocardiogram.

▶ General Considerations

Atrial fibrillation, the most common sustained clinical arrhythmia, is diagnosed by finding an irregularly irregular ventricular rhythm without discrete P waves (Figure 21–1). The QRS complex is usually narrow, but it may be wide if aberrant conduction or bundle branch block is present. Atrial fibrillation associated with the Wolff-Parkinson-White syndrome may occur with very rapid ventricular rates and may be life-threatening. This arrhythmia is diagnosed by its very rapid irregular rate associated with wide preexcited QRS complexes and requires emergency treatment (see Long-term approach).

▶ Epidemiology

Approximately 4% of the population over age 60 years has sustained an episode of atrial fibrillation, with a particularly steep increase in prevalence after the seventh decade of life. Risk factors for development of atrial fibrillation include heart failure, hypertensive cardiovascular disease, coronary artery disease, and valvular heart disease. Moreover, both sustained and paroxysmal atrial fibrillation have important implications for the development of a cerebrovascular accident (CVA) or other systemic emboli. It is estimated that 15–20% of CVAs in nonrheumatic patients are due to atrial fibrillation.

▶ Clinical Findings

A. Symptoms and Signs

When called on to manage new-onset atrial fibrillation, it is important to establish the precipitating factors because the type of associated condition determines long-term progno-

sis. In some patients, episodes of atrial fibrillation may be initiated by caffeine, alcohol, or marijuana use. Atrial fibrillation may result from acute intercurrent ailments. For example, this arrhythmia may develop in patients with hyperthyroidism or lung disease, or after either cardiac or pulmonary surgery, especially in older patients. Atrial fibrillation is also seen in patients with acute pulmonary embolism, myocarditis, or acute myocardial infarction, particularly when the last condition is complicated by either occlusion of the right coronary artery or heart failure. When atrial fibrillation occurs in these settings, it almost always abates spontaneously if the patient recovers from the underlying problem. Hence, management usually involves administration of drugs to control the heart rate, and long-term antiarrhythmic therapy is generally not needed.

Alternatively, atrial fibrillation may occur in association with structural cardiac disease. Important associated conditions include rheumatic mitral stenosis, hypertension, hypertrophic cardiomyopathy, or chronic heart failure. In contrast to patients with acute intercurrent ailments, those with structural heart disease may expect (even with antiarrhythmic therapy) many recurrences and chronic atrial fibrillation may supervene.

Lone fibrillation is the term used to describe patients with atrial fibrillation not associated with known cardiac conditions or noncardiac precipitants. The natural history of the atrial fibrillation for those with lone atrial fibrillation is similar to that in patients with structural cardiac disease, in that episodes of atrial fibrillation are likely to recur and, eventually, the arrhythmia may become sustained.

B. Physical Examination

The initial evaluation of new-onset atrial fibrillation includes a detailed history focusing on possible precipitating factors as well as the presence of organic cardiac disease. As such, the initial evaluation includes, at a minimum, a careful physical examination, 12-lead electrocardiogram, chest radiograph, echocardiogram, and tests of thyroid function. Further test-

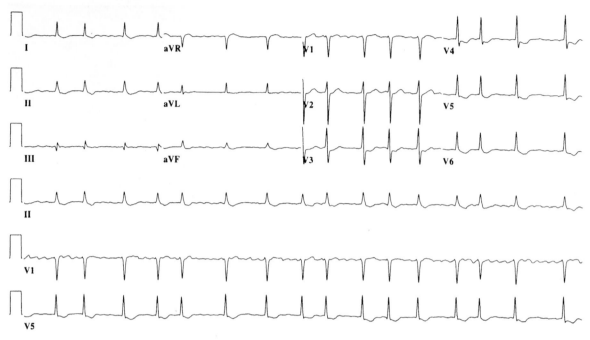

▲ **Figure 21-1.** The 12-lead electrocardiogram shows the typical rapid irregular rhythm seen with atrial fibrillation.

ing will depend on various aspects of the history or physical examination. For example, if atrial fibrillation is usually precipitated by exercise, then an exercise treadmill test is appropriate. In the patient with frequent episodes of paroxysmal atrial fibrillation, a 24-hour to 48-hour Holter recording may discern whether atrial fibrillation was triggered by another arrhythmia such as a premature atrial complex alone or whether the fibrillation was preceded by an episode of supraventricular tachycardia. In addition, patients with vagally mediated fibrillation will typically have episodes either after heavy meals or during sleep. These clues may help identify those patients who may respond to specific approaches (see Treatment).

▶ Treatment

The objectives of therapy include (1) achieving rate control, (2) restoring sinus rhythm (where feasible), and (3) decreasing the risk of CVA. The principles of treatment discussed in this chapter largely follow those promulgated in the recent ACC/AHA/ESC guidelines.

A. Rate Control

If the patient has atrial fibrillation and a rapid rate associated with severe heart failure or cardiogenic shock, emergency direct-current cardioversion is indicated. For patients with atrial fibrillation associated with rapid rate but with stable hemodynamics, attempts to achieve acute rate control are

indicated. Drugs to slow the ventricular rate in patients with atrial fibrillation (Table 21–1) include digitalis preparations, calcium channel blockers (verapamil or diltiazem), and β-blockers. If rapid rate control is desired, then calcium channel blockers and β-blockers are far more effective than digitalis, which may require many hours before rate control is achieved. In addition, a common misconception is that digitalis therapy is associated with acute conversion to sinus rhythm, but carefully controlled studies have shown that conversion to sinus rhythm is no more likely with digoxin than with placebo. As emphasized later, digitalis and intravenous calcium channel blocker therapy are contraindicated in patients with Wolff-Parkinson-White syndrome and atrial fibrillation. Intravenous diltiazem has been shown to be safe and effective for patients with atrial fibrillation and a modest degree of heart failure.

In patients with a known history of congestive heart failure, use of intravenous β-blockers or calcium channel blockers may aggravate the cardiac failure. In this subset, digitalis or intravenous amiodarone would be the preferred agents for rate control.

B. Long-Term Antiarrhythmic Therapy and Elective Cardioversion

For patients who have had a single, initial episode of atrial fibrillation with no significant hemodynamic problems, no specific therapy is required because repeat episodes may not

Table 21–1. Intravenous Pharmacologic Agents for Heart Rate Control in Atrial Fibrillation.

Drug	Loading Dose	Onset	Maintenance Dose	Major Side Effects
Diltiazem	0.25 mg/kg IV over 2 min	2–7 min	5–15 mg/h infusion	Hypotension, heart block, HF
Esmolol	0.5 mg/kg over 1 min	5 min	0.05–0.2 mg kg^{-1} min^{-1}	Hypotension, heart block, bradycardia, asthma, HF
Metoprolol	2.5–5 mg IV bolus over 2 min; up to 3 doses	5 min	NA	Hypotension, heart block, bradycardia, asthma, HF
Propranolol	0.15 mg/kg IV	5 min	NA	Hypotension, heart block, bradycardia, asthma, HF
Verapamil	0.075–0.15 mg/kg IV over 2 min	3–5 min	NA	Hypotension, heart block, HF
Digoxin	0.25 mg IV each 2 h, up to 1.5 mg	2 h	0.125–0.25 mg daily	Digitalis toxicity, heart block, bradycardia

HF, heart failure.
Reprinted, with permission, from Fuster V et al. J Am Coll Cardiol. 2001;38:266i.

occur for many years. In contrast, patients who manifest frequent recurrences may be candidates for long-term antiarrhythmic therapy with class IA (quinidine, procainamide, and disopyramide), class IC (propafenone and flecainide), or class III (sotalol, amiodarone, and dofetilide) agents, all of which are more effective than placebo in maintaining sinus rhythm (Table 21–2).

C. Antiarrhythmic Drug Therapy for Atrial Fibrillation

For patients with lone atrial fibrillation, use of any of the antiarrhythmic drugs listed is appropriate. In general, the class IC agents (flecainide or propafenone) are the first choice in terms of efficacy and lowest incidence of side effects. It would be wise, for example, to withhold amiodarone as a first-line drug in view of the potential for adverse effects. Only two drugs have been proved safe for patients with severe congestive heart failure: dofetilide and amiodarone.

For patients with atrial fibrillation associated with coronary artery disease, consider use of sotalol as initial drug therapy. This agent has class III antiarrhythmic effects and is a potent β-blocker. Class IC drugs should not be used in patients with significant structural cardiac disease or in those with ischemic heart disease. They have, however, been found to be safe and effective for patients with hypertension and atrial fibrillation.

In addition, extra cardiac factors are very important in the choice of antiarrhythmic drugs. For example, dose adjustments are mandatory for patients with renal insufficiency. This is especially true for procainamide, sotalol, and dofetilide. Dofetilide, for example, requires hospital admission, calculation of the creatinine clearance, and drug titration according to the QT corrected for heart rate as well as renal function. An algorithm for antiarrhythmic drug usage is summarized in Figure 21–2.

Even with drug therapy, recurrence rates for atrial fibrillation approach 50% per year (as opposed to recurrences with

Table 21–2. Typical Doses of Drugs Used to Maintain Sinus Rhythm in Atrial Fibrillation, Listed Alphabetically.

Drug	Daily Dosage	Potential Adverse Effects
Amiodarone	100–400 mg	Photosensitivity, pulmonary toxicity, polyneuropathy, GI upset, bradycardia, torsades de pointes (rare), hepatic toxicity, thyroid dysfunction
Disopyramide	400–750 mg	Torsades de pointes, HF, glaucoma, urinary retention, dry mouth
Dofetilide	500–1000 mcg	Torsades de pointes
Flecainide	200–300 mg	Ventricular tachycardia, congestive HF, enhanced AV nodal conduction (conversion to atrial flutter)
Procainamide	1000–4000 mg	Torsades de pointes, lupus-like syndrome, GI symptoms
Propafenone	450–900 mg	Ventricular tachycardia, congestive HF, enhanced AV nodal conduction (conversion to atrial flutter)
Quinidine	600–1500 mg	Torsades de pointes, GI upset, enhanced AV nodal conduction
Sotalol	240–320 mg	Torsades de pointes, congestive HF, bradycardia, exacerbation of chronic obstructive or bronchospastic lung disease

AV, atrioventricular; GI, gastrointestinal; HF, heart failure.
Reprinted, with permission, from Fuster V et al. J Am Coll Cardiol. 2001;38:266i.

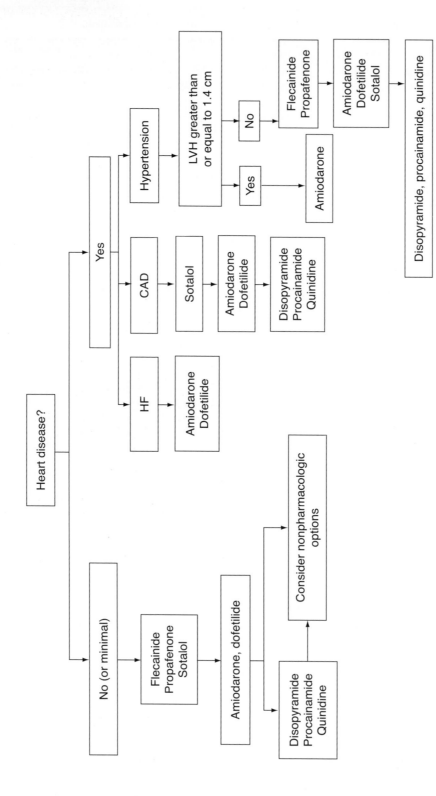

▲ **Figure 21–2.** Antiarrhythmic drug therapy to maintain sinus rhythm in patients with recurrent paroxysmal or persistent atrial fibrillation. Drugs in boxes are listed alphabetically and not in order of suggested use. CAD, coronary artery disease; HF, heart failure; LVH, left ventricular hypertrophy.

placebo therapy of 75% per year). In addition, these agents may be associated with significant side effects. For class IA drugs, these include induction of torsades de pointes, especially for those with congestive heart failure. For example, a meta-analysis compared quinidine with placebo for patients with atrial fibrillation and found that death from all causes was higher in the groups treated with quinidine. In addition, in the Stroke Prevention in Atrial Fibrillation (SPAF) trials, substantial numbers of patients were treated with antiarrhythmic agents; in patients with heart failure, those treated with class I drugs had significantly increased mortality rates compared with those not treated with antiarrhythmic drugs. Great care must be exercised in the use of these agents, balancing the benefits against the potential for adverse effects. General rules include avoidance of all class IA drugs or sotalol for patients with congestive heart failure and avoidance of class IC agents for patients with structural heart disease. In addition, sotalol is contraindicated for patients with severe depression of the left ventricular ejection fraction and severe left ventricular hypertrophy. Patients with significant sinus node or atrioventricular (AV) conduction disease may require pacemaker therapy before use of antiarrhythmic drugs because these drugs may further depress sinus node or AV conduction. The only drugs that appear to be both effective and safe for patients with heart failure and atrial fibrillation are amiodarone and dofetilide. Amiodarone is associated with a host of both cardiac (eg, severe sinus bradycardia or arrest or AV block) and noncardiac (eg, thyroid abnormalities, pulmonary fibrosis) adverse effects, but low-dose amiodarone (ie, 200 mg/day) appears to be effective and very well tolerated. Dofetilide has a narrow therapeutic window and can cause life-threatening arrhythmias; it can be used in patients with atrial fibrillation and congestive heart failure but requires a 2–3 day in-hospital stay for monitoring of the agent.

1. Chemical cardioversion—Recent studies have emphasized the use of drugs for acute conversion of atrial fibrillation. It has been shown that intravenous ibutilide or intravenous dofetilide (not available in the United States) are effective for conversion of approximately 35% of patients with atrial fibrillation. It should be emphasized that this drug should be used only in a monitored environment. The usual dose is 1 mg over 10 minutes, followed by a 10-minute interlude, followed by an additional 1 mg over 10 minutes if necessary. Facilities with intravenous management, and a defibrillator should be readily available because the incidence of sustained torsades de pointes is 1–2%. Ibutilide should be avoided for patients with severe heart failure or bradycardia.

A. Other drugs for chemical cardioversion—Other drug combinations have also been found effective. For example, it has been found that use of large oral doses of either flecainide (300 mg) or propafenone (600 mg) may terminate up to 80% of episodes of atrial fibrillation within 2 hours (pill-in-the-pocket). This approach should be used only in patients who are pretreated with β-blocking drugs and in the absence of significant cardiac disease or heart failure.

B. Anticoagulant therapy—The risk of CVA in patients with nonrheumatic atrial fibrillation is 4–7% per year. Patients at particularly high risk include those over age 70 years or with hypertension, a history of heart failure, increased left atrial size, diabetes, or prior CVA. The risks of CVA are similar in patients with paroxysmal versus chronic atrial fibrillation. Numerous studies have documented the remarkable efficacy of warfarin in decreasing the risk of emboli by 45–85% in patients with nonrheumatic atrial fibrillation with a low risk of significant hemorrhage, provided the international normalized ratio (INR) is in the range of 2.0 to 2.5. Still controversial is the need for anticoagulant therapy in younger patients with lone atrial fibrillation because the risk of emboli is very low in this group.

The role of aspirin therapy for patients with atrial fibrillation remains controversial. In one study, 75 mg of aspirin failed to decrease the stroke risk compared with placebo (5.5%/year). In contrast, the SPAF I trials showed that a higher dose of aspirin, 325 mg, appeared to be of benefit in patients under 75 years of age. In a follow-up study (SPAF II), the incidence of stroke was higher with aspirin (4.8%) compared with warfarin (3.6%). The SPAF III trials demonstrated that aspirin (325 mg/day) and fixed low-dose warfarin (1, 2, or 3 mg) were ineffective for stroke prevention. Therefore, the weight of current data favors use of warfarin with an INR of 2.0–3.0 as the best strategy to prevent systemic embolization. A number of studies involving use of newer antithrombin agents, are in clinical trials. Initial trials with ximelagatran in patients with atrial fibrillation showed non-inferiority compared with warfarin but it failed FDA clearance because of hepatotoxicity. The advantage of these agents will be to obviate the need for blood testing of INR levels. Trials of aspirin and clopidogrel proved inferior to warfarin.

2. Direct-current cardioversion—Direct-current cardioversion is a very effective technique for restoration of sinus rhythm. Because of the benefits of sinus rhythm in terms of improved cardiac output and decreased risk of embolic phenomena, in general, at least one attempt should be made to restore sinus rhythm. Several precautions are in order. If the patient has a history of recurrent episodes of atrial fibrillation then he or she should be pretreated with an antiarrhythmic agent because reversion to atrial fibrillation after shock therapy is very high. Use of antiarrhythmic drugs before direct-current shock, however, is inappropriate for the patient with an initial episode of well-tolerated atrial fibrillation. Unless urgent cardioversion is required because of hemodynamic decompensation, severe ischemia, or congestive heart failure, it is imperative to follow one of several options for reducing the risk of systemic embolization:

   a. For patients with atrial fibrillation of less than 48 hours duration it would appear to be safe to proceed with application of direct-current shock.

   b. If atrial fibrillation persists for more than 48 h, then the risk of embolization increases and anticoagulants are required prior to ablation. One recommended option for patients with atrial fibrillation of more than 48 hours duration is to perform transesophageal echocardiography (TEE), which is excellent for detecting clots in the left atrium or the left atrial appendage. Evidence from several studies indicates that the finding of either a clot or spontaneous echocardiographic contrast in the left atrium is associated with higher risks of systemic embolization. In the absence of such findings on TEE, systemic emboli are rare. Therefore, patients with recent-onset atrial fibrillation with no evidence of atrial clots or spontaneous contrast by TEE may undergo direct-current cardioversion after initiation of heparin therapy. A recent report from the ACUTE trial showed that treatment of patients with atrial fibrillation treated on the basis of TEE-guided therapy versus a group treated with a 3-week course of anticoagulant therapy had similar rates of thromboembolism (< 1%). It must be appreciated that atrial function is depressed (atrial stunning) after cardioversion and that anticoagulant therapy is recommended for at least 1 month after cardioversion. This is true whether the duration of atrial fibrillation was either less than or greater than 48 hours. For those patients with clot or dense spontaneous echocardiographic contrast with TEE, full anticoagulant therapy with an INR of 2.0–3.0 is recommended for at least 2–3 weeks before cardioversion.

c. An alternative approach is that patients with atrial fibrillation of greater than 48 hours be fully anticoagulated for at least 3 consecutive weeks before attempting direct-current cardioversion and for about 4 weeks afterward to decrease the risk of an embolism after successful reversion to sinus rhythm. This approach tends to be less efficient than the TEE-guided approach for recent-onset atrial fibrillation but is an acceptable alternative treatment for atrial fibrillation.

Direct-current external shock is usually performed in a monitored area under supervision of an anesthesiologist. Pads are placed in an anterior-posterior orientation in order to maximize current delivered to the atrium. It is wise to check the arterial oxygen saturation, serum potassium level, digoxin, or antiarrhythmic blood drug levels before cardioversion. Direct-current shocks beginning with at least 200 J are used in an attempt to achieve sinus rhythm. Multiple shocks of lesser energy are to be avoided. If the patient fails to revert after maximal external shocks (360 J monophasic or 200 J biphasic), then successful cardioversion can almost always be achieved either by the use of a biphasic waveform defibrillator or supplemental doses of ibutilide. Ibutilide has been shown to lower the atrial defibrillation threshold. An attempt at internal cardioversion using small energy shocks delivered between the coronary sinus and the right atrium is seldom necessary because the above-described treatments are almost always effective.

3. Long-term approach—Clinicians should be especially careful to identify patients whose atrial fibrillation might be cured. Examples include patients with hyperthyroidism as well as those in whom other cardiac arrhythmias appear to trigger atrial fibrillation. For example, patients with atrial flutter or paroxysmal supraventricular tachycardia may experience atrial premature impulses during tachycardia that trigger atrial fibrillation. In selected patients, it is possible to apply catheter ablation to cure the underlying supraventricular arrhythmia and, hence, prevent the trigger for atrial fibrillation. Therefore, in the evaluation of patients with atrial fibrillation, initial testing should include obtaining a thyroid-stimulating hormone assay, an echocardiogram, and a 48-hour ambulatory electrocardiogram recording for those with paroxysmal atrial fibrillation. In analyses of these recordings, the clinician seeks evidence for triggering arrhythmias. In addition, the clinician looks for vagal triggers of atrial fibrillation, such as sinus bradycardia associated with sleep or heavy meals, that initially may be treated with vagolytic antiarrhythmic agents such as disopyramide. Alternatively, if atrial fibrillation appears only with enhanced sympathetic tone, such as with exercise, a trial of β-blocker therapy is appropriate.

One important special circumstance is that of atrial fibrillation in the patient with Wolff-Parkinson-White syndrome. These patients may have a very rapid irregular rate and wide complex tachycardia owing to conduction over the accessory pathway (Figure 21–3). After recognition of this entity, appropriate immediate therapy includes use of intravenous ibutilide or procainamide or direct-current cardioversion. It is important to remember that intravenous digoxin and calcium channel blockers are contraindicated. In addition, use of lidocaine, β-blockers, or adenosine is not effective and is contraindicated because they delay appropriate therapy. After the rhythm is stabilized, these patients should undergo catheter ablation of the accessory pathway.

The natural history of atrial fibrillation associated with structural cardiac disease or in patients with lone atrial fibrillation is for spontaneous recurrence of the arrhythmia. Unfortunately, no drug is universally effective, and the decision of how many drugs to try before a judgment is made to terminate antiarrhythmic drugs and focus on rate control depends on how symptomatic the patient is during atrial fibrillation. If the episodes are poorly tolerated, then multiple drug trials or even various ablative procedures may be required (see section on Nonpharmacologic Treatment of Atrial Fibrillation). On the other hand, if rate control can be readily achieved with drugs, such as digoxin, β-blockers, or calcium antagonists that block AV nodal conduction and the patient has a good symptomatic outcome, then an acceptable alternative is to use drugs that control rate combined with long-term anticoagulant treatment. A large, randomized trial (AFFIRM) compared the strategy of rate control and anticoagulation versus maintaining sinus rhythm with antiarrhythmic drugs. The AFFIRM trial randomized over 4000 patients

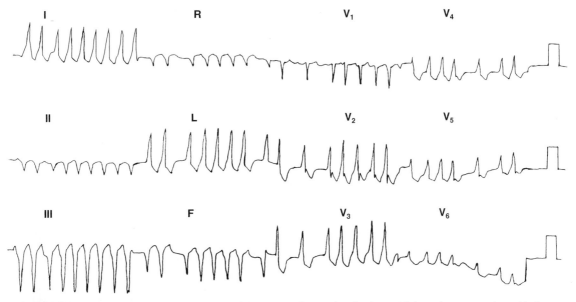

▲ **Figure 21–3.** The 12-lead electrocardiogram shows a rapid irregular rhythm with broad QRS complex. This is pathognomonic of atrial fibrillation in a patient with Wolff-Parkinson-White syndrome. This arrhythmia requires urgent treatment. Acceptable therapy includes use of intravenous ibutilide or procainamide or direct-current shock.

with atrial fibrillation to either rate or rhythm control. The patient cohort consisted in large measure of older (mean age 69 years) patients who were not very symptomatic. They found no difference in mortality or quality of life between groups. The rhythm control group had a higher incidence of hospitalizations and episodes of torsades de pointes. In addition, stroke risk was related to presence of no or inadequate anticoagulant treatment. This study showed that for most patients with atrial fibrillation, rate control was equally effective as rhythm control and that long-term anticoagulation therapy is required for both groups.

D. Nonpharmacologic Treatment of Atrial Fibrillation

Because pharmacologic therapy for atrial fibrillation is not ideal, a number of nonpharmacologic treatment modalities have been introduced. For atrial fibrillation that proves refractory to drug management, one time-tested approach is catheter ablation of the AV junction and permanent pacemaker insertion.

Patients with persistent tachycardia may suffer from a tachycardia-induced cardiomyopathy with left ventricular failure superimposed on their native cardiac disease. Hence, in the management of chronic atrial fibrillation, rate control is an important objective that must be achieved either via AV nodal blocking drugs or, failing these, with catheter ablative procedures. Catheter ablation of the AV junction involves insertion of an electrode catheter in the region of the His

bundle with application of radiofrequency energy in order to destroy AV conduction. The chief benefit of this technique is achievement of perfect rate control without need for drugs. The drawbacks include the need for permanent pacing and a continued need for anticoagulant therapy.

For most of these patients, especially for those with left ventricular ejection fraction greater than 40%, single chamber pacing appears to be sufficient. In some patients, left ventricular function may deteriorate and biventricular pacing may be helpful (PAVE trial).

It has been shown that atrial-based pacing systems will decrease the incidence of atrial fibrillation in patients with the tachycardia-bradycardia syndrome. In addition, pacing may allow for safe use of antiarrhythmic drugs. In patients with vagally mediated atrial fibrillation, atrial pacing may be effective in decreasing episodes of atrial fibrillation. Experimental studies have shown that either dual-site atrial pacing (ie, from coronary sinus and right atrium) or from the atrial septum in conjunction with antiarrhythmic therapy, may suppress atrial fibrillation, but this technique has not been shown to be clinically useful.

An innovative approach to the management of atrial fibrillation involves use of an internal atrial defibrillator. This device has been shown to be safe and effective in conversion of atrial fibrillation in 85% of instances. The chief drawback is that although the energy required for internal defibrillation is quite low, nevertheless, internal shocks are painful and not well tolerated. Currently, atrial defibrillators are combined with ventricular defibrillators and may prove to be very helpful for patients with infrequent episodes of atrial fibrillation. "Stand alone" atrial internal defibrillation has been abandoned.

A number of surgical centers are currently using the maze procedure to try to cure atrial fibrillation. This procedure involves placing transmural lesions over both atria in such a manner that the fibrillatory impulses cannot complete a reentrant circuit. The maze procedure involves all of the risks of major open-heart surgery. This procedure should be considered for patients with atrial fibrillation who require cardiac surgery for correction of valvular diseases, coronary artery disease, or congenital heart disease.

In some patients with paroxysmal atrial fibrillation, a rapidly firing ectopic focus, often near the pulmonary veins, may cause atrial fibrillation. The current experience using catheter ablative procedures to cure atrial fibrillation has been validated by a number of studies. It was found that attempts to ablate a specific focus within the pulmonary vein resulted in a long-term success rate of 50–60% but was associated with an unacceptably high incidence of pulmonary vein stenosis (2–8%). Currently most groups have advocated use of pulmonary vein isolation, which involves placement of a number of lesions around the ostium of the pulmonary vein in order to isolate discharges from pulmonary venous focus. Isolation procedures for at least three of the four pulmonary veins are associated with short-term success rates of 70–90% and are associated with a zero incidence of pulmonary vein stenosis. Pulmonary vein isolation is currently reserved for highly symptomatic patients with atrial fibrillation that is resistant to multiple drug trials.

More recent trials have emphasized the use of wide area ablative lesions around the pulmonary veins as well as use of lesions connecting the left atrial roof and isthmus. In addition, a number of groups have designed lesions to ablate areas of fractionated potentials. These potentials are thought to be derived from the pivot points of random reentrant circuits or from activation of vagal ganglion, or both. The ablative procedures have matured, and in the current ACC/AHA/ESC guidelines, these procedures may be used after failure of a single drug therapy.

European Heart Rhythm Association; Heart Rhythm Society; Fuster V et al. ACC/AHA/ESC 2006 guidelines for the management of patients with atrial fibrillation—executive summary: a report of the American College of Cardiology/American Heart Association Task Force on Practice Guidelines and the European Society of Cardiology Committee for Practice Guidelines. (Writing Committee to Revise the 2001 Guidelines for the Management of Patients With Atrial Fibrillation). J Am Coll Cardiol. 2006 Aug 15;48(4):854–906. [PMID: 16904574]

Haissaguerre M et al. Localized sources maintaining atrial fibrillation organized by prior ablation. Circulation. 2006 Feb 7;113(5):616–25. [PMID: 16461833]

Hart RG et al. Atrial fibrillation and thromboembolism: a decade of progress in stroke prevention. Ann Intern Med. 1999 Nov 2;131(9):688–95. [PMID: 10577332]

Jäis P et al. Long-term evaluation of atrial fibrillation ablation guided by noninducibility. Heart Rhythm. 2006 Feb;3(2):140–5. [PMID: 16443526]

Oral H et al. Noninducibility of atrial fibrillation as an end point of left atrial circumferential ablation for paroxysmal atrial fibrillation: a randomized study. Circulation. 2004 Nov 2;110(18):2797–801. [PMID: 15505091]

Wood MA et al. Clinical outcomes after ablation and pacing therapy for atrial fibrillation: a meta-analysis. Circulation. 2000 Mar 14;101(10):1138–44. [PMID: 10715260]

Wyse DG et al; Atrial Fibrillation Follow-up Investigation of Rhythm Management (AFFIRM) Investigators. A comparison of rate control and rhythm control in patients with atrial fibrillation. N Engl J Med. 2002 Dec 5;347(23):1825–33. [PMID: 12466506]

Conduction Disorders & Cardiac Pacing

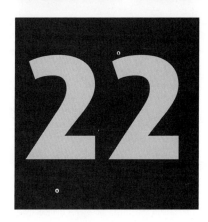

Richard H. Hongo, MD & Nora Goldschlager, MD

ESSENTIALS OF DIAGNOSIS

Sinus node dysfunction ("sick sinus syndrome")

► Sinus bradycardia: Sinus rate of less than 60 bpm.

► Sinoatrial exit block, type I: Progressively shorter P-P intervals, followed by failure of occurrence of a P wave.

► Sinoatrial exit block, type II: Pauses in sinus rhythm that are multiples of basic sinus rate.

► Sinus arrest, sinus pauses: Failure of occurrence of P waves at expected times.

Atrioventricular (AV) block

► First degree: Prolonged PR interval more than 0.2 seconds.

► Second degree
  • Type I: Progressive increase in PR interval, followed by failure of AV conduction and nonoccurrence of a QRS complex
  • Type II: Abrupt failure of AV conduction not preceded by increasing PR intervals.

► High degree: AV conduction ratio 3:1 or greater.

► Complete: Independent atrial and ventricular rhythms, with failure of AV conduction despite temporal opportunity for it to occur.

General Considerations

The clinical presentation of patients with conduction system disease is determined by the existence of three underlying abnormal conditions: bradycardia, inability to increase the heart rate in response to increases in metabolic needs, and atrioventricular (AV) dyssynchrony (inappropriately timed atrial and ventricular depolarization and contraction sequences).

Pathophysiology & Etiology

A. Sinus Node Dysfunction

Sinus node dysfunction ("sick sinus syndrome") is usually due to a degenerative process that involves the sinus node and sinoatrial (SA) area (Table 22–1). Often, the degenerative process and associated fibrosis also involve the AV node and its approaches as well as the intraventricular conduction system; as many as 25–30% of patients with sinus node dysfunction have evidence of AV and bundle branch conduction delay or block.

Respiratory sinus arrhythmia, in which the sinus rate increases with inspiration and decreases with expiration, is not an abnormal rhythm and is most commonly seen in young healthy persons. Nonrespiratory sinus arrhythmia, in which phasic changes in sinus rate are not due to respiration, may be accentuated by the use of vagal agents, such as digitalis and morphine, and is more likely to be observed in patients who are older and who have underlying cardiac disease, although the arrhythmia is not itself a marker for structural heart disease; its mechanism is unknown. Ventriculophasic sinus arrhythmia is an unusual rhythm that occurs during high-grade or complete AV block; it is characterized by shorter P-P intervals when they enclose QRS complexes. The mechanism is not known with certainty but may be related to the effects of the mechanical ventricular systole: the ventricular contraction increases the blood supply to the sinus node, thereby transiently increasing its firing rate; the resulting increase in intra-atrial pressure causes inhibition of the sinus rate. Ventriculophasic sinus arrhythmia is not a pathologic arrhythmia and should not be confused with premature atrial depolarizations or SA block. None of the sinus arrhythmias indicates sinus node dysfunction.

Sinus node dysfunction is present when marked sinus bradycardia, pauses in sinus rhythm (sinus arrest), SA block, or a combination of these exist (Figures 22–1 through 22–5). Some clinically normal individuals without structural heart disease can experience significant sinus bradycardia and

Table 22–1. Causes of Sinus Node Dysfunction.

Idiopathic
  Degenerative process
  Normal aging
Acute myocardial ischemia or infarction
  Right or left circumflex coronary artery occlusion
    Jarisch-Bezold reflex
Medications
  β-Blockers
  Rate-sparing calcium channel blockers
    Diltiazem, verapamil
  Digitalis (with high prevailing vagal tone)
  Class I antiarrhythmic agents
  Class III antiarrhythmic agents (amiodarone, sotalol)
  Clonidine

prolonged sinus pauses under conditions of high vagal tone such as sleep. In some patients a trigger, such as vomiting or coughing, can be identified; in other patients, high levels of acetylcholine may be responsible. Vagal stimulation, often from an identifiable trigger (Table 22–2), is commonly responsible for significant sinus bradyarrhythmias occurring in patients in an intensive care setting.

SA block may take the form of progressive delay in transmission of the sinus-generated impulse through the SA node to the atrium, finally resulting in a nonconducted sinus impulse and an absent P wave on the surface electrocardiogram (ECG) (Wenckebach, or type I second-degree exit block; see Figures 22–1 and 22–4), or abrupt failure of transmission of the sinus impulse to the atrium (type II second-degree exit block; see Figure 22–1). In type I second-degree exit block, there is less incremental delay with each successive impulse transmission through the SA nodal tissue (similar to type I AV nodal block); thus, the P-P intervals become progressively shorter until a P wave fails to occur. In type II second-degree exit block, abrupt failure of sinus impulse conduction to the atria can take the form of 2:1, 3:1 (and so on) SA block. Fixed 2:1 SA exit block cannot be distinguished from sinus bradycardia on the surface ECG.

Bradycardia-tachycardia syndrome is characterized by episodes of both bradycardias and supraventricular tachycardias (Figure 22–6). The bradycardia is due to sinus node dysfunction (sinus arrest or SA exit block) with associated junctional or ventricular escape rhythms. The supraventricular tachycardias may be atrial tachycardia, atrial flutter, atrial fibrillation, AV reciprocating tachycardia, or AV nodal reentry tachycardia (see Chapter 20); more than one type of tachycardia may occur in the same patient. Bradycardia-tachycardia syndrome represents a diffuse disease of the conduction system of the heart but is not necessarily associated with structural heart disease.

Sinus bradycardia not uncommonly results from medications, particularly β-blockers, the rate-sparing calcium chan-

nel-blocking agents verapamil and diltiazem, and some commonly used antiarrhythmic agents such as sotalol and amiodarone (see Figure 22–2). If these medications are necessary to treat the patient, permanent cardiac pacing is indicated.

The natural history of sinus node dysfunction is one of variable progression to an absence of identifiable sinus activity, with the process taking from 10 to 30 years. The condition itself is not associated with a high risk of arrhythmic death, although the morbidity caused by a sudden onset of bradycardia can be considerable. The ultimate prognosis for the patient with sinus node dysfunction depends on the presence and severity of underlying heart disease, rather than on the bradyarrhythmia itself.

B. Atrioventricular Nodal-His Block

Like sinus node dysfunction, AV nodal-His block and bundle branch block (BBB) are often the result of sclerodegenerative processes. These processes can also involve the approaches to the AV node. Acquired AV nodal block is often due to acute ischemia and infarction (especially involving the inferior wall and right ventricle), infection, trauma, and medications (Table 22–3).

The AV node, or junction, is made up of three regions: atrionodal, central compact, and nodal-His. Cells of the atrionodal region have a relatively fast depolarization rate (45–60/min) and are responsive to autonomic nervous system input, whereas cells of the nodal-His region have a slower depolarization rate (about 40/min) and are generally unresponsive to autonomic influences. The site of origin of a junctional rhythm will therefore determine its rate, responsiveness to vagal and adrenergic input, and consequently the presence and severity of clinical symptoms.

The natural history of patients with AV block depends on the underlying cardiac condition; however, the site of the block and the resulting rhythm disturbances themselves contribute to the prognosis. First-degree AV block has little prognostic import. Persistent second-degree (types I and II), high-degree, and complete AV block can all be associated with adverse outcomes, including death, unless the arrhythmias are vagally mediated or are due to other reversible causes.

▶ Clinical Findings
A. Symptoms and Signs

The symptoms resulting from conduction disorders reflect cerebral hypoperfusion, low cardiac output at rest or during exercise, and rarely hemodynamic collapse. Symptoms, which are often subtle, can be episodic or chronic and can change over time. Because a patient often adapts activity levels to compensate for the impairment in heart rate response, significant symptoms may not be evident unless the patient is closely questioned about specific activities and effort tolerance, or the clinician actually observes the patient during performance of activities of daily living such as walking or during formal treadmill exercise tests.

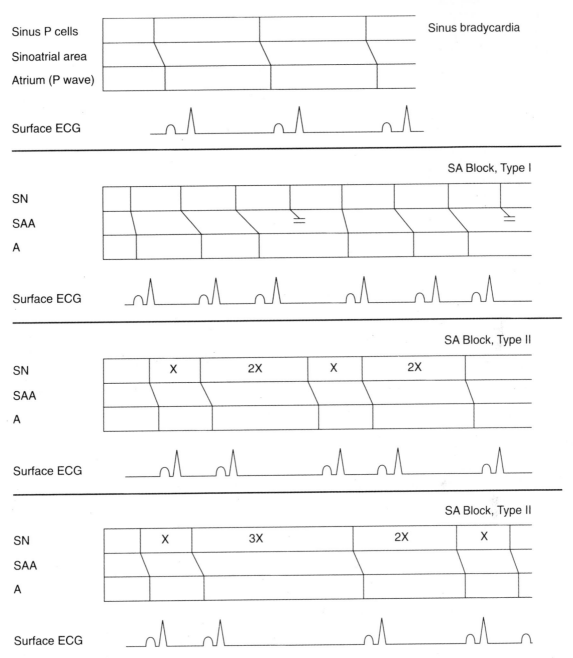

▲ **Figure 22–1.** Ladder diagrams illustrating sinus bradycardia and sinoatrial block, types I and II. ECG, electrocardiogram; SA, sinoatrial; SAA, sinoatrial area; SN, sinoatrial node.

Syncope is the classic symptom of cerebral hypoperfusion due to bradycardia; however, symptoms of presyncope such as dizziness, lightheadedness, and confusion reflect the same pathophysiology and warrant the same aggressive approach to diagnosis and management. It should be emphasized that patients with cerebral hypoperfusion often have impairment of memory surrounding the presyncopal or syncopal episodes and may therefore be unable to provide an adequate history of the events.

Patients with sinus node dysfunction or AV block, in whom the escape pacemaker is unresponsive to autonomic nervous system input, cannot increase their heart rate in

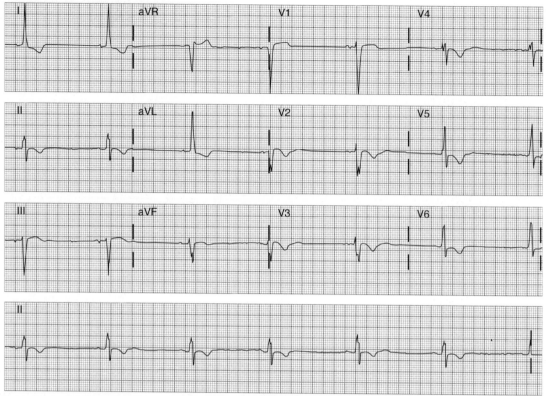

▲ **Figure 22–2.** This 83-year-old woman was being treated for congestive heart failure and was receiving 200 mg/day of amiodarone for episodes of nonsustained ventricular tachycardia. She complained of profound effort fatigue but no symptoms of heart failure. Electrocardiogram reveals an atrial bradycardia at a rate of about 38/min. The P waves vary in morphology, suggesting some wandering of the atrial pacemaker. Left axis deviation and a left intraventricular conduction delay with ST and T wave abnormalities are present. The atrial bradycardia was presumed to be due to the amiodarone, which was discontinued, resulting in appreciable increase in a stable sinus rhythm, with amelioration of the patient's effort fatigue.

response to increases in oxygen demand. They are, therefore, intolerant of effort and will report symptoms of exercise-related breathlessness, weakness, and fatigue. These symptoms, which can be disabling, are often confused with other conditions such as hypothyroidism, medication, underlying heart disease, deconditioning, or simply old age.

During periods of AV block, the atria and ventricles often depolarize and contract asynchronously. There is variable increase in atrial pressures and volumes depending on the degree to which the AV valves are open or closed at the onset of ventricular systole. The resulting atrial stretch and secretion of atrial natriuretic peptide produce reflex systemic hypotension and cerebral hypoperfusion. In addition, the increases in left atrial and pulmonary venous pressures can cause shortness of breath and pulmonary venous congestion, including frank pulmonary edema. The mistaken diagnosis of refractory left ventricular dysfunction is not infrequently made in this situation.

Patients who have the bradycardia-tachycardia syndrome (see Figure 22–6) have symptoms referable to both the

bradycardia and the tachycardia. During tachycardia the patient can experience uncomfortable palpitations and, at times, symptoms of cerebral hypoperfusion from excessively rapid heart rates.

More rarely, bradycardias can lead to a potentially lethal form of polymorphic ventricular tachycardia known as bradycardia- or pause-dependent ventricular tachycardia (Figure 22–7); the tachycardia is triggered in the setting of QT interval prolongation brought on by the longer RR intervals associated with either bradycardia or pause. Symptoms in these patients can include not only palpitations, presyncope, and syncope but also cardiac arrest.

B. Physical Examination

The physical examination of the patient with bradycardia reflects the origin of the QRS rhythm and the AV relationship more so than the heart rate per se. Junctional or ventricular escape rhythms resulting from atrial bradycardia

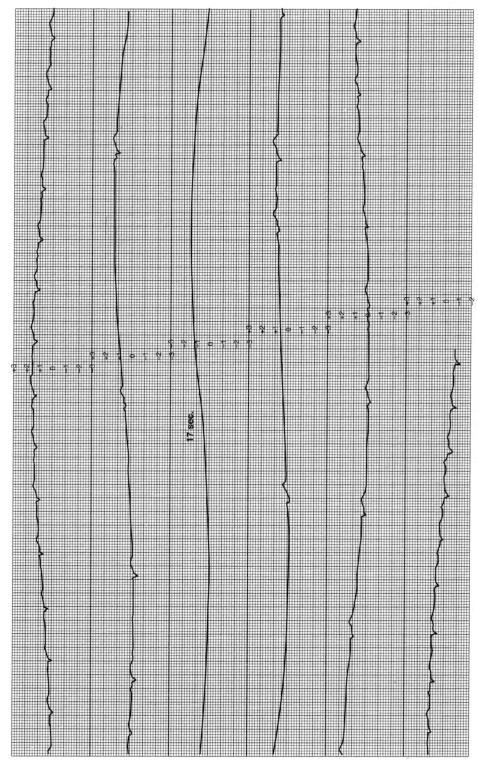

▲ **Figure 22–3.** Continuous modified lead-II ambulatory electrocardiographic recording in a patient with recurrent presyncopal spells. Sinus rhythm is present in the top strip; the second strip shows marked sinus slowing, followed by a 17-second period of sinus arrest without the appearance of a QRS escape rhythm. Sinus rhythm reappears in the fourth strip, gradually increasing its rate until stable rhythm is restored in the bottom strip. The absence of an escape rhythm raises the possibility of diffuse disease of the conduction system and impulse-generating tissue.

MCL

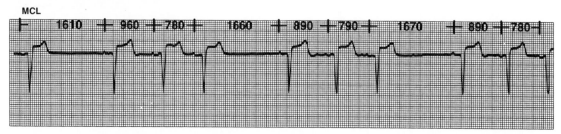

▲ **Figure 22–4.** Progressive decrease in P wave cycle lengths followed by a pause in P wave rate, indicating type I second-degree sinoatrial block. The pauses in sinus rate are less than twice the preceding sinus cycle lengths, satisfying the criteria for Wenckebach periodicity. MCL, modified chest lead.

or AV block produce AV dyssynchrony. This results in varying degrees of atrial contribution to ventricular filling, as well as varying stroke outputs and systolic blood pressures. Because AV dyssynchrony causes changes in the positions of the mitral and tricuspid valves relative to their fully closed or open positions, the intensity of the first heart sound will vary, as will the audibility of atrial gallop (S$_4$) sounds and the intensity of semilunar valve systolic ejection murmurs and AV valve regurgitant murmurs.

Examination of the venous pulse contour in the neck can reveal cannon *a* waves and prominent *cv* waves, and the diagnosis of AV block can occasionally be made by recognizing these findings. Central venous pressure elevation (not to be confused with *a* and *cv* waves) is a fairly common physical finding independent of the venous pulse contour.

The carotid pulse may vary in volume, and even upstroke velocity, in patients with AV dyssynchrony. Examination of

the chest may disclose rales, which reflect increased pulmonary venous pressure and valvular regurgitation rather than systolic or diastolic ventricular dysfunction. The liver may be enlarged and may pulsate because of transmitted *a* and *cv* waves. Peripheral edema may also be present if the AV dyssynchrony is chronic.

These same physical findings can also occur in patients who are being paced by a single-chamber ventricular system during sinus rhythm because AV dyssynchrony will be present under these circumstances. In these patients, the symptoms of weakness, fatigue, and congestive heart failure, together with physical findings indicating AV dyssynchrony, constitute the pacemaker syndrome; this is treated by changing the implanted single-chamber ventricular pacing system to a dual-chamber system in which sensing of the atrial rhythm triggers a paced ventricular response to restore AV synchrony (see section Permanent pacing).

Continuous MCL$_1$ Rhythm Strips

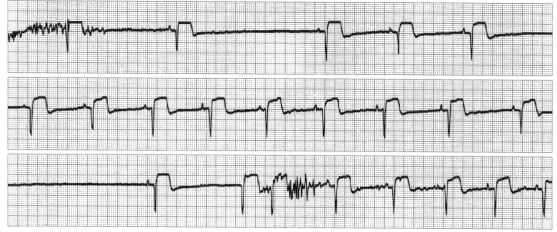

▲ **Figure 22–5.** Irregular pauses in sinus rate, which occur abruptly and are not multiples of a basic sinus-cycle length. Best characterized as sinus pauses rather than sinoatrial block or sinus arrest, this rhythm indicates the existence of sinus node dysfunction. MCL$_1$, modified chest lead.

Table 22–2. Conditions Associated with Vagally Mediated Bradyarrhythmias.

Highly conditioned state
Sleep
Vomiting, retching
Suctioning
Nasal intubation
Gastric intubation
Urination
Defecation
Coughing
Swallowing
Central nervous system trauma with high intracranial pressure
Isotonic exercise conditioning

Table 22–3. Causes of Acquired AV Nodal-His Block.

Idiopathic
Degenerative process
Ischemic heart disease (inferior wall, septal area, right ventricle)
Calcific aortic and mitral valve disease
AV nodal/His ablative procedures
Medications
Digitalis, β-blockers, calcium channel blockers (verapamil, diltiazem), sotalol, amiodarone
Infections (including aortic valve endocarditis)
Inflammatory diseases (myocarditis)
Infiltrative diseases
Amyloidosis, neoplasm, sarcoidosis, hemochromatosis
Collagen-vascular diseases
Trauma
Aortic valve surgery

AV, atrioventricular.

C. Diagnostic Studies

1. Sinus node dysfunction

A. Electrocardiography—The P waves inscribed on the surface ECG represent atrial depolarizations. Sinus node depolarization precedes atrial depolarization and is not seen on the surface ECG. The P waves that result from sinus-generated impulses must be inferred from their morphology and axis.

The sinus P wave has a mean frontal plane axis of +15 to +75° and is upright in leads I/II/aVF, inverted in lead aVR, and variable in leads III and aVL. In the horizontal plane, the sinus P wave can be inverted in lead V_1 but is upright in leads V_3–V_6. Respiratory variation in the sinus P wave contour can be seen in the inferior leads and should not be confused with wandering atrial pacemaker, which is unrelated to breathing and therefore not phasic. Sinus arrhythmia is present when the P wave morphology is normal and consistent and the P-P intervals vary by more than 0.16 seconds. SA block exists when some impulses generated by the sinus pacemaking cells do not exit the SA node to depolarize the atria; in the absence of atrial depolarization, a P wave will not be inscribed on the surface ECG. High-degree SA block, in which most of the sinus impulses fail to exit the SA node to the atrium, is inscribed on the surface ECG as pauses in sinus rhythm. These pauses often cannot be differentiated from sinus arrest caused by failure of impulse generation. If the pauses

between sinus P waves are multiples of a basic rate, however, the diagnosis of type II second-degree SA block can be made.

B. Electrophysiologic studies—Sinus node function can be evaluated in the electrophysiology laboratory by means of simultaneous surface and intracardiac electrographic recordings made during basal conditions, physiologic and pharmacologic interventions, and atrial pacing. This evaluation can be undertaken in patients with either symptomatic sinus bradycardia or bradycardia-tachycardia syndrome. It can also be used in patients with recurrent syncope of unclear etiology, although the diagnostic yield is limited. Measurements include the intrinsic heart rate, the sinus node recovery time (SNRT), the SA conduction time (SACT), and the response to parasympathetic (vagal) stimulation, as assessed by carotid sinus massage.

The intrinsic heart rate (ie, the rate independent of autonomic influences) is the sinus rate during pharmacologic denervation of the sinus node using a β-blocker and atropine. The intrinsic heart rate is sometimes used to distinguish healthy persons from those with sinus node dysfunction.

Sinus node recovery time is the interval between the end of a period of pacing-induced overdrive suppression of sinus

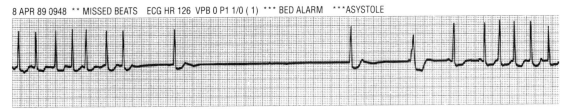

8 APR 89 0948 ** MISSED BEATS ECG HR 126 VPB 0 P1 1/0 (1) *** BED ALARM ***ASYSTOLE

▲ **Figure 22–6.** Lead II rhythm strip characteristic of bradycardia-tachycardia syndrome, recorded from a patient with palpitations and intermittent dizzy spells.

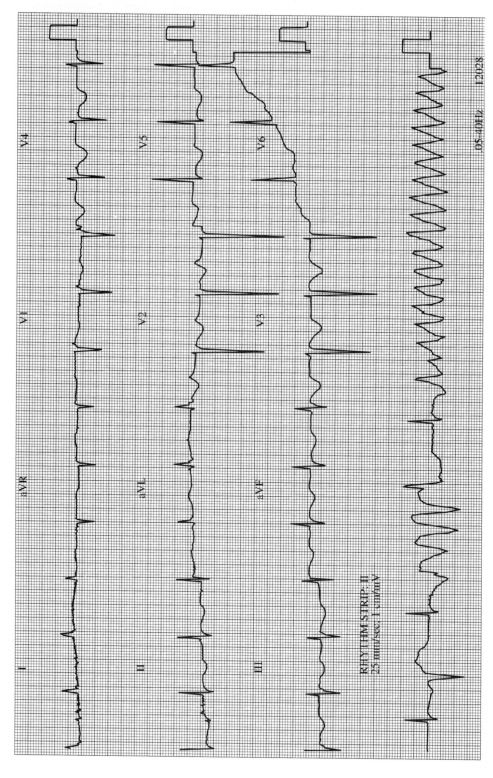

RHYTHM STRIP: II
25 mm/sec; 1 cm/mV

.05–40Hz   12028

▲ **Figure 22–7.** Pause-dependent ventricular tachycardia causing loss of consciousness in a patient with syncopal and presyncopal spells. Note the markedly prolonged QT interval associated with the longer RR cycle lengths.

node activity and the return of sinus node function, manifested on the surface ECG by a postpacing sinus P wave. The measured SNRT depends on several factors, among them the proximity of the pacing catheter to the sinus node, the SACT, the presence or absence of SA entrance block, and local neurohormonal influences. In normal persons, atrial pacing at rates of 120–130 bpm for 30 seconds or more is followed by a return of sinus node activity at a reproducible interval, with the basic sinus rate generally being achieved within three postpacing beats. The usual SNRT is less than 1.5 seconds, although considerable variation may exist depending on the prevailing autonomic tone. The corrected sinus node recovery time can be calculated by subtracting the basic sinus rate from the sinus node recovery time; it is usually between 350 and 550 ms. In patients with sinus node dysfunction, sinus node recovery times are not reproducible and tend to be longer after more prolonged periods of pacing; return to the basic sinus rate within three postpacing beats is also inconstant and may be followed by additional (secondary) pauses in rate.

SA conduction time reflects the time taken by a premature atrial-pacing stimulus delivered near the sinus node area to traverse the atrial tissue to reach the sinus node and prematurely depolarize it, the time to the formation of the next sinus impulse following the premature depolarization, and the return of the sinus-generated impulse through atrial tissue to the recording electrode. The SA conduction time is often prolonged in patients with clinical evidence of sinus node dysfunction other than sinus bradycardia alone.

Because the electrophysiologic tests of sinus node function are neither specific nor sensitive, they can show abnormal results in patients without sinus bradycardia and normal results in those with symptomatic sinus node disease. The test results should not, therefore, be relied on in isolation when making clinical decisions regarding either diagnosis or treatment.

Some of the problems of poor sensitivity and specificity can be overcome by recording the sinus node electrogram from an electrode catheter positioned in the vicinity of the sinus node at the junction of the superior vena cava and the right atrium. The sinus node electrogram cannot be reproducibly recorded in as many as 50% of patients, however, and both T and U waves interfere with it. Sinus node electrography can distinguish between SA exit block and sinus arrest, however, and studies have shown that most pauses in sinus rhythm are due to SA exit block. Notwithstanding these technologic advances, the diagnosis of sinus node dysfunction often remains a clinical one.

C. EXERCISE TESTING—Treadmill exercise testing can be of substantial value in assessing chronotropic response ("competence") to increases in metabolic needs in patients with sinus bradycardia in whom sinus node dysfunction is suspected. The definition of chronotropic incompetence is not agreed on, but it is reasonable to designate it as consisting of either an inability to achieve a heart rate exceeding 75% of age-pre-

dicted maximum (220 – age), or 100–120/min at maximum effort. Irregular (and nonreproducible) increases, and even decreases, in sinus rate during exercise can also occur but are rare. Similarly rare are abrupt changes in rate occurring during the postexercise recovery period. Chronotropic incompetence can result from medications (see Table 22–1) and should be distinguished from intrinsic sinus node dysfunction.

The Bruce treadmill exercise protocol, which is usually used to diagnose the presence and severity of coronary artery disease, is generally inappropriate for patients with sinus node dysfunction, in whom the goal is to assess heart rate at lower workloads expected to be encountered during average daily activities. Specific protocols, such as the chronotropic assessment exercise protocol (CAEP), have therefore been developed for this purpose. In addition to documenting chronotropic incompetence, treadmill exercise testing can be used to aid in optimal programming of rate-adaptive cardiac pacemakers that are usually required in these patients.

2. Atrioventricular block

A. ELECTROGRAPHY AND ELECTROCARDIOGRAPHY—The advent of intracardiac His bundle electrography has provided important information regarding normal and abnormal AV conduction in humans. The technique involves positioning a multipolar electrode catheter across the tricuspid valve in proximity to the AV nodal-His bundle to record electrical activity as it passes through these structures. Because of its location, the catheter records electrical activity at the level of the low right atrium, His bundle, and proximal right bundle branch in addition to ventricular electrical activity. The sinus node pacemaker cells normally initiate the cardiac impulse but is not registered on either the surface ECG or the His bundle electrogram. The onset of the P wave on the surface ECG signifies the beginning of atrial depolarization; because the intracardiac electrode catheter lies at the level of the low right atrium, the early portions of atrial depolarization will not be detected by it; as the atrial depolarization wavefront passes through the region in which the catheter is located (the low right atrium), a deflection is registered (A). As the impulse traverses the His bundle another deflection is registered, representing its depolarization (H). The His bundle deflection is followed by a ventricular deflection (V), which is registered at the time the wavefront of ventricular depolarization reaches the electrodes and often follows the onset of inscription of the QRS complex on the surface ECG.

His bundle electrography is useful in indicating the site of AV conduction delay or block. Normally, the conduction time through the AV node is 90–150 ms, and the conduction time through the His-Purkinje system is 35–55 ms. In a patient with a prolonged PR interval, a prolonged AH interval signifies delayed impulse conduction within the AV node, and a prolonged HV time represents delayed impulse conduction within the His bundle or the bundle branches. Conduction delay within the His bundle itself manifests as more than one His deflection ("split" His deflections).

In **first-degree AV block** (a delay in conduction between the atria and the ventricles), all atrial impulses are conducted to the ventricles; it is characterized by a prolonged PR interval that exceeds 0.2 seconds (Figure 22–8). The components of the PR interval are interatrial conduction (10–50 ms), AV nodal conduction (90–150 ms), and intra-His and His-Purkinje conduction (35–55 ms). The conduction delay in first-degree AV block can thus represent prolonged interatrial, AV nodal, or His-Purkinje conduction, and the bundle recordings help clarify the location of the delay.

In patients with a QRS complex that is narrow and normal-appearing, first-degree AV block is AV nodal in more than 85% and is intra-His in under 15%. In patients with a wide QRS complex, first-degree AV block is AV nodal in less than 25%, infranodal in about 45%, and at more than one site in about 33%.

In **second-degree AV block,** not all atrial impulses are conducted to the ventricles. The ratio of P waves to QRS complexes describes the AV conduction ratio. **Type I (Wenckebach) second-degree AV block** is present when the conduction of atrial impulses to the ventricles is progres-

sively delayed because of AV (generally AV nodal) refractoriness, with eventual failure of conduction of an atrial impulse. The AV conduction ratio in type I second-degree AV block can be 2:1, 4:3, 8:7, and so on; this ratio is also referred to as a **Wenckebach period**. Because type I second-degree AV block usually occurs within the AV node, the PR interval of the first conducted P wave of the Wenckebach period is often prolonged, and because this conduction disturbance does not involve the bundle branches, the QRS complexes are expected to be narrow and normal-appearing unless preexisting bundle branch disease exists.

In a typical, or classic, Wenckebach period, the PR intervals progressively lengthen, the R-R intervals progressively shorten, and the R-R interval encompassing the nonconducted P wave is less than twice the preceding R-R interval. Typical Wenckebach periods are usually seen with low AV conduction ratios (3:2, 4:3, and 5:4), but as the AV conduction ratio increases (exceeding 6:5), more and more Wenckebach sequences are atypical and do not follow the rules. If the sinus rate is not constant, for example in vagal bradycardias, sequences that resemble Wenckebach conduction often occur;

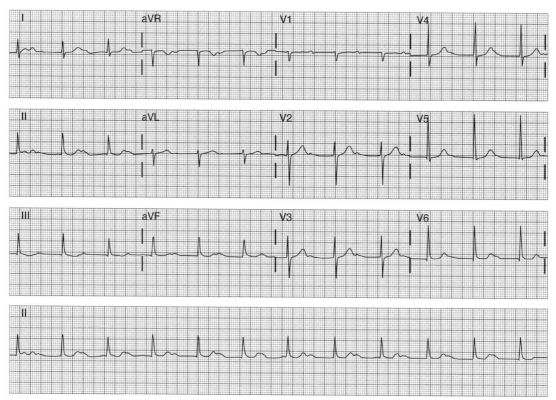

▲ **Figure 22–8.** Sinus rhythm with marked first-degree atrioventricular (AV) block. All P waves are conducted to the ventricles. The PR intervals are about 0.48 seconds. The RP intervals are shorter than the PR intervals, which, in some patients, can cause symptoms due to suboptimal AV contraction sequences. Despite the length of the PR intervals, this conduction disturbance is generally benign; evolution to second-degree AV block can take years.

they should, however, not be considered type I second-degree AV block, in which the sinus rate must be constant for the diagnosis to be made.

In **type II second-degree AV block,** atrial impulses intermittently fail to be transmitted to the ventricles but without progressive conduction delay prior to the conduction failure. Because prior conduction delay from the atria does not occur, the failure of antegrade conduction is often abrupt and unpredictable. In contrast to type I second-degree AV block, in which the conduction delay is usually in the AV node, the conduction delay in type II second-degree AV block can be within the His bundle or, more commonly, distal to the His bundle in the bundle branches. If the block is within the His bundle, the QRS complexes will be narrow and normal-appearing, or only mildly aberrant, unless preexisting BBB is present. If the block is infra-His, the QRS complexes will show a BBB pattern. In contrast to type I second-degree AV block, the PR interval of the conducted P waves is constant and often (but not always) normal (Figure 22–9).

Second-degree AV block with a 2:1 AV conduction ratio may represent either type I or type II AV block (Figures 22–10 and 22–11). Two consecutive PR intervals are not recorded, so the presence or absence of progressive PR prolongation cannot therefore be ascertained, and distinguishing the diagnoses may be difficult. If the PR interval of the conducted P waves is prolonged and the QRS complexes are narrow and normal-appearing, type I second-degree AV block (intra-AV nodal) is probably present. If the PR interval of the conducted P waves is normal and the QRS complexes have a BBB pattern, type II second-degree AV block (infra-His) is probably present. If the PR interval of the conducted P wave is prolonged and the QRS complexes have a BBB pattern, or if the PR interval of the conducted P wave is normal and the QRS complexes appear normal, it may not be possible to distinguish between the two types, and more than one site of AV block may also be present. Altering the AV conduction ratio by means of carotid sinus massage (to produce sinus and AV nodal slowing) or intravenous atropine (to enhance sinus rate and AV nodal conduction) will often allow identification of the nature of the AV block and thus its location (see Figure 22–9).

In **high-degree AV block** the AV conduction ratio is 3:1 or greater, and atrial impulses are only occasionally conducted to the ventricles. In contrast, in **complete AV block,** no atrial impulses are conducted to the ventricles despite temporal opportunity for this to occur, and the atria and ventricles are depolarized by their respective pacemakers, independent of each other (Figure 22–12). The atrial rate in complete AV block is almost always faster than the ventricular rate. The QRS rhythm, or the escape rhythm, originates distal to the site of block and may be in the AV junction, His bundle, bundle branches, or distal Purkinje system. The morphology of the QRS complexes and their rate will depend on their site of origin. A narrow QRS complex escape rhythm originates from the junction. On the other hand, a wide QRS complex rhythm is not a reliable guide to the origin of the rhythm because rhythms originating in the longitudinally separated predivisional region of the His bundle can have a wide QRS complex.

If the atrial rate is not sinus, the existence of advanced or complete AV block is diagnosed by the presence of a slow ventricular rate with varying intervals between the QRS complexes or by a slow and regular rate (Figure 22–13), respectively. Atrial fibrillation and flutter are commonly associated with advanced AV block and slow QRS rates. The rate of the ventricular rhythm, as well as the QRS-complex morphology, will depend on the site of origin of the rhythm. The regularity of the rhythm indicates that it is not being stimulated by the atrial rhythm but by an independent pacemaker originating below the level of conduction block.

In **vagotonic block,** a high degree of vagal tone, such as occurs with sympathetic withdrawal during sleep or in highly conditioned athletes, may be associated with slowing of the sinus rate; pauses in sinus rhythm; variable degrees of delay in AV conduction manifested by prolongation of PR intervals (often irregular); and failure of conduction of P waves, resembling type I or II second-degree AV block (Table 22–4). It is important to recognize vagotonic block because it often occurs in normal individuals as well as in patients with inferior or right ventricular myocardial infarction, or any other clinical condition in which hypervagotonia is present (see Table 22–2). It not uncommonly accompanies the use of certain medications, notably β-blocking agents, some antihypertensive drugs, and, occasionally, digitalis. It can also be seen during swallowing (deglutition bradycardia), coughing (tussive bradycardia), and yawning. In the critical care setting, vagotonic block (and bradycardia) can occur during endotracheal suctioning or esophagogastric intubation, and in patients with elevated intracranial pressure.

B. EXERCISE TESTING—Unlike the value of exercise testing in sinus node dysfunction to both document this diagnosis and evaluate chronotropic competence, exercise testing is generally not useful in patients with AV block. The response of the AV node to vagolysis and increased sympathetic drive that occurs with exercise is enhancement of AV conduction. Thus, patients with first-degree AV block and type I second-degree AV block are expected to have shorter PR intervals during exercise; and, if type I second-degree AV block is present, to develop higher AV conduction ratios (eg, 3:2 at rest becoming 6:5 during exercise). Patients with 2:1 AV conduction in whom the site of conduction block may be uncertain can benefit from exercise testing by observing whether the AV conduction ratio increases in a Wenckebach-like manner (eg, to 3:2 or 4:3) or decreases (eg, to 3:1 or 4:1) (see Figure 22–9). In the latter case, the increase in the sinus rate finds the His-Purkinje system refractory, causing the higher degrees of block. This response is always abnormal because it indicates intra- or infra-His block, which will require permanent cardiac pacing.

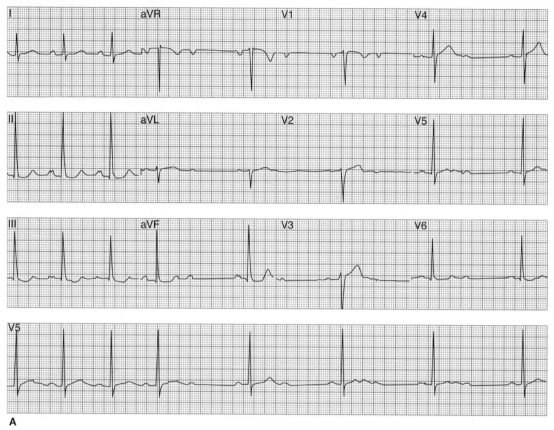

A

▲ **Figure 22–9.** **A:** This electrocardiogram was recorded in a patient with presyncopal spells who was about to undergo exercise treadmill testing. The atrial rhythm is sinus at a rate of about 68/min. The PR intervals of the conducted QRS complexes are all about 0.24 seconds. The QRS complexes are narrow, and nondiagnostic ST and T wave abnormalities are present. 2:1 atrioventricular (AV) conduction develops abruptly during the recording. The prolonged PR intervals of the conducted P waves, as well as the narrow morphology of the QRS complexes (indicating absence of bundle branch system disease), could suggest that the 2:1 AV conduction represents type I second-degree (Wenckebach), which is usually AV nodal; intra-His block, however, is suggested by the absence of prolongation of the PR intervals prior to the nonconducted P waves. Changing of the AV conduction ratio from 2:1 to 3:2, 5:4, etc, would help establish the presence of type I second-degree AV block. This could be achieved by atropine or exercise testing, during which adrenergic drive would be expected to facilitate AV conduction. (*continued*)

▶ **Treatment**

The major reversible causes of conduction system disturbances are high vagal tone and medications. High vagal tone, whether or not it is accompanied by withdrawal of sympathetic tone, can cause or contribute to both atrial and ventricular bradycardia. Vagally mediated bradycardias are usually transient and not accompanied by symptoms of presyncope or frank syncope, and no treatment is needed. If necessary, intravenous atropine can be used to facilitate AV nodal conduction to avoid ventricular bradycardia; however, the atropine-induced increase in atrial rate can lead to a paradoxical slowing of ventricular rate as a result of more

rapid stimulation of, and encroachment on, the refractory period of the AV conduction system ("time-dependent" refractoriness). Moreover, the effects of intravenous atropine are short-lived, and its long-term use is accompanied by significant side effects.

In contrast to the majority of vagally mediated bradycardias, some vasovagal episodes (hypotension with variable degrees of bradycardia or asystole) can be frequent, abrupt, unpredictable, and disabling.

These highly symptomatic episodes, also referred to as neurocardiogenic, neurovascular, or neurally mediated syncopal syndromes, can require heart rate support with oral theophylline or ephedrine. They can also require permanent

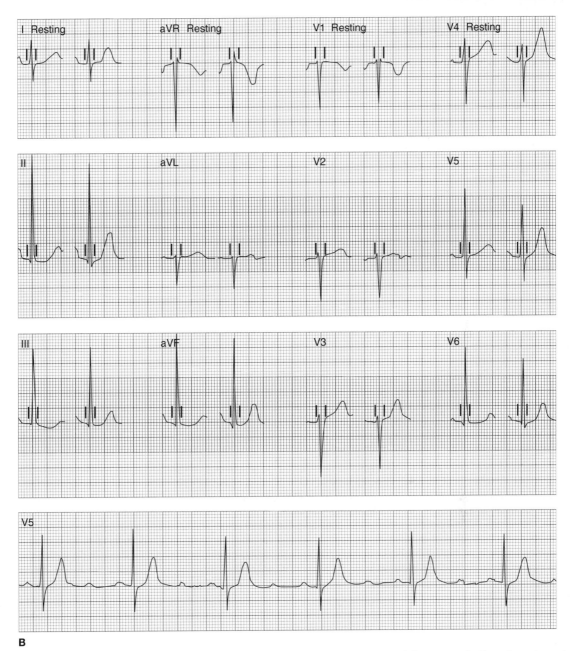

B

▲ **Figure 22–9.** (*Continued*) **B:** The patient achieved stage IV of the Bruce protocol during treadmill testing. The atrial rate was 150/min. At peak effort and for the first 2 minutes of the postexercise recovery period, 3:1 atrioventricular (AV) block developed abruptly, and was associated with the patient's typical presyncopal symptoms. AV block developing during exercise, although decidedly rare, is always abnormal and, if the QRS complexes are narrow or normal-appearing, indicate intra-His block. Permanent cardiac pacing is required.

dual-chamber cardiac pacing, using special algorithms to detect an abrupt fall in heart rate and respond with tachypacing until the spontaneous heart rate increases. Intravascular

volume support with fluids, support hosiery, and even mineralocorticoids can also be helpful. Because left ventricular baroreceptor stimulation (from vigorous systolic ventricular

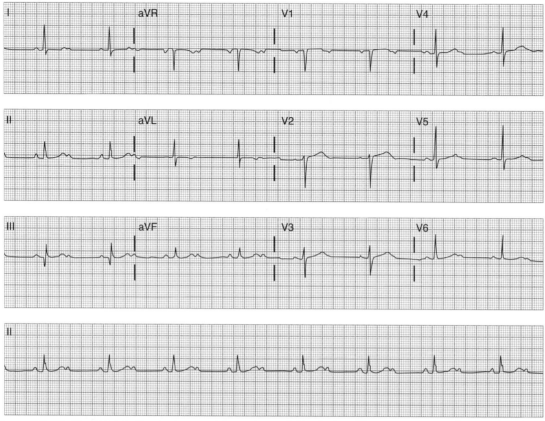

▲ **Figure 22–10.** The atrial rhythm is sinus, and 2:1 atrioventricular (AV) conduction is present. The PR intervals of the conducted beats are normal at about 0.19 seconds. The QRS complexes are narrow and normal-appearing. The 2:1 AV conduction could represent either type I second-degree (Wenckebach) or type II second-degree AV block. When type I second-degree AV block is present, the PR intervals of the conducted complexes are often prolonged and the QRS complexes narrow and normal-appearing, whereas in type II second-degree AV block the PR intervals of the conducted complexes are generally normal and the QRS complexes broad, indicating bundle branch disease. In this tracing, the PR intervals are normal. The site of block cannot be known with certainty from this tracing, and manipulation of the AV conduction ratio by atropine or exercise, which facilitate AV conduction, might be required. Type I second-degree AV block generally does not require cardiac pacing because it is occurring within the AV node; if the block is within the His bundle (which might require electrophysiologic study to document), however, permanent cardiac pacing is indicated.

contraction) and its consequent reflex peripheral vasodilation play a role in this syndrome, drugs having negative inotropic effects (eg, β-blockers, disopyramide) have been used in management, although there is evidence that these agents have limited efficacy. α-Agonists, such as midodrine, have also been used. In addition, because a central effect is recognized, anticholinergic agents and serotonin reuptake inhibitors have been considered.

Commonly used medications that cause or contribute to bradycardia do so by enhancing vagal tone (eg, digitalis), reducing the facilitation of AV conduction that results from sympathetic tone (eg, β-blockers and antiarrhythmia agents with β-blocking properties, such as sotalol and propafenone), or direct action on SA and AV conduction tissue

(eg, verapamil and diltiazem). Simple withdrawal of these medications will reverse the bradycardia, although the process may require several days. If the offending medications are necessary to treat another condition such as angina pectoris and cannot be discontinued, permanent cardiac pacing will be required (Table 22–5).

It is important to exclude AV nodal blocking medications, such as digitalis preparations, β-blockers, and some calcium channel blockers, as a cause of, or contributor to, slow ventricular rates in atrial fibrillation and flutter; withdrawal of these drugs or reduction in dosage is associated with reversal of the AV block, and permanent cardiac pacing may not be required. If the ventricular rhythm is slow in the absence of these agents, intrinsic AV conduction system

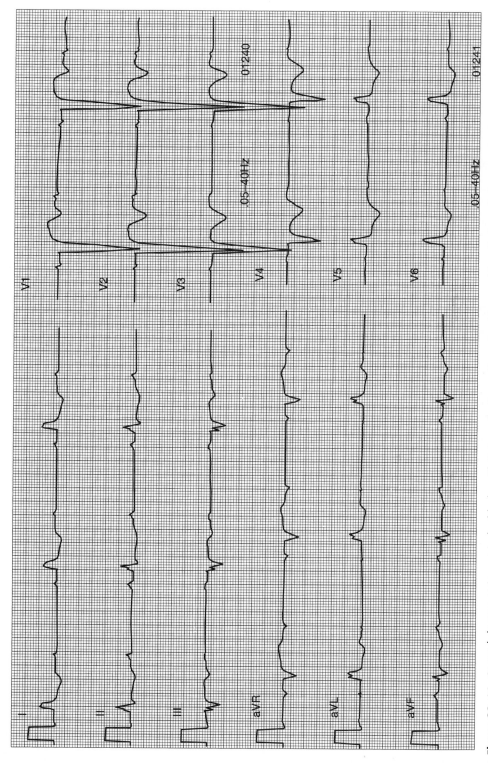

▲ **Figure 22–11.** Second-degree atrioventricular block, with 2:1 conduction ratio and evidence of bundle branch disease. The first-degree block of the conducted P waves and the left bundle branch block pattern of the conducted QRS complexes make localization of the site of block difficult; electrophysiologic study may be necessary to decide whether permanent cardiac pacing is required.

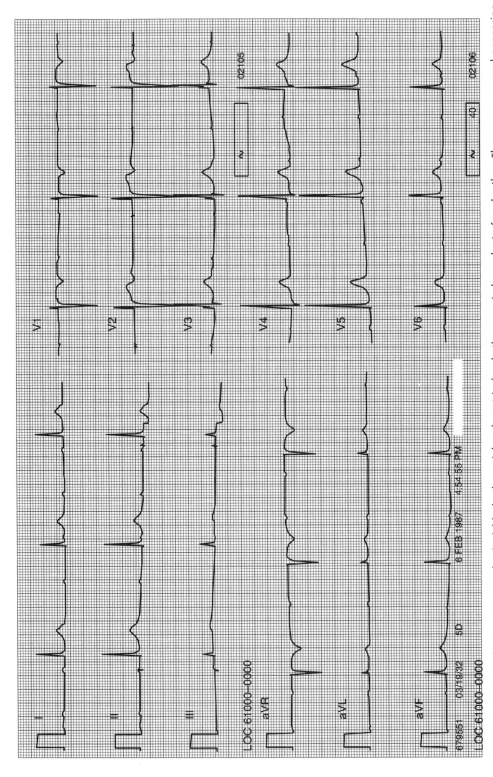

▲ **Figure 22–12.** Complete atrioventricular (AV) block. The atrial and ventricular rhythms are independent of each other. The narrow, normal-appearing QRS complexes suggest that the AV block is within the AV node or the His bundle.

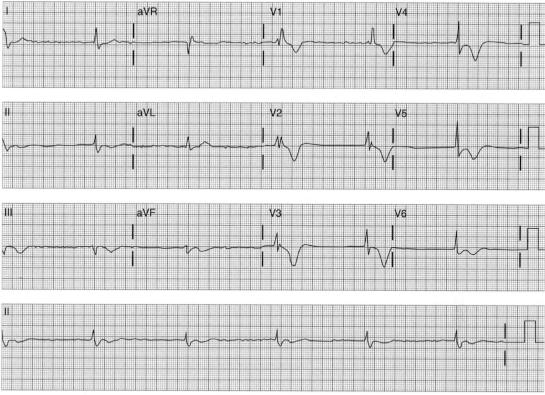

▲ **Figure 22–13.** The atrial rhythm is fibrillation. The QRS rhythm is regular at a rate of about 33/min and displays a right bundle branch block pattern. The regularity of the rhythm indicates complete atrioventricular (AV) block, and the rate and morphology suggest a ventricular focus of origin. This rhythm could be due to digitalis toxicity or to the effects of calcium channel or β-blockers; if offending medications cannot be discontinued, permanent cardiac pacing is indicated. This rhythm and rate are also seen in the absence of medications and after radiofrequency ablation of the AV node to treat uncontrolled ventricular rate in patients with atrial fibrillation; permanent cardiac pacing is required.

disease is likely to be present, and permanent cardiac pacing will usually be indicated. Electrical cardioversion of the atrial arrhythmia should be undertaken with caution, if at all, in patients with slow ventricular rates in the absence of medication; because of the diffuse underlying conduction disease, postcardioversion bradycardia or even asystole can occur.

In bradycardia-tachycardia syndrome, prolonged pauses in rhythm frequently occur following an abrupt termination of the tachycardia. These pauses are often associated with symptoms of cerebral insufficiency, and cardiac pacing is frequently required. Alternatively, elimination of the tachycardia by radiofrequency ablation can potentially avert the need for cardiac pacing; severity of the underlying sinus node dysfunction, however, may still make cardiac pacing necessary.

Although cardiac pacing using AAIR or DDDR devices (see section Permanent pacing) may serve to suppress the tachycardias to some degree, treatment with antiarrhythmic agents is usually required. Control of the ventricular rate is also required, but AV nodal blocking agents are often only

partially effective in achieving this control; moreover, their use can be associated with significant side effects. Radiofrequency AV node ablation, together with dual-chamber cardiac pacing, has thus emerged as a useful and cost-effective technique in the management of this rhythm disturbance. Current pacemakers used to treat the bradycardia-tachycardia syndrome use a special algorithm to switch from a DDD or DDDR mode of operation to a VVI, VVIR, DDI, or DDIR mode on sensing an atrial tachyarrhythmia, and back again to DDD or DDDR mode when a normal atrial rate is sensed.

A. Cardiac Pacing

Temporary or permanent cardiac pacing, in which an electrical stimulus depolarizes cardiac tissue, is indicated when bradycardia causes symptoms of cerebral hypoperfusion or hemodynamic decompensation. Occasionally, patients with bradycardia-dependent ventricular tachycardia require pacing to prevent the pauses in rhythm that lead to the tachyar-

Table 22–4. Diagnostic Clues to Vagally Mediated Atrioventricular Block.

Concomitant slowing of sinus rate
Changing PR intervals, often with irregularity of sinus rates
Atypical Wenckebach periods, often with inconstant PP intervals
Inconstant escape rates
Inconstant escape foci
Transient nature of episodes
Reversed or abolished by intravenous atropine or an increase in sympathetic tone

rhythmia (Tables 22–5 and 22–6, see Figure 22–7). Although emergency pacing can be accomplished temporarily by transcutaneous pacing systems, in all but the most critical situations stable temporary pacing is best ensured by the transvenous insertion of electrodes into the right atrium, right ventricle, or both. Permanent cardiac pacing is also usually performed through the transvenous route; in some circumstances, however, epicardial placement of electrodes via thoracotomy or a subxiphoid approach is still used.

1. Temporary pacing

A. Transmyocardial pacing—Transmyocardial pacing involves the percutaneous placement of cardiac pacing wires into the ventricular cavity or onto the ventricular wall through a transthoracic needle. The reliability of this technique is poor, and it is a highly invasive procedure with significant potential morbidity. Transmyocardial pacing is performed only in an emergency setting, usually during cardiac arrest, when transvenous pacing cannot be accomplished rapidly or when transcutaneous pacing is unavailable or unsuccessful. The reported incidence of successful capture with transthoracic pacing varies from 5% to 90%; typically it is 21–40%.

Often, however, because of the clinical circumstances in which this type of pacing is used, electrical capture is not followed by mechanical systole. The major complications of transthoracic pacing include myocardial or coronary artery laceration, pericardial tamponade, pneumothorax, and hepatic or gastric damage. Transthoracic pacing should therefore be reserved for situations of the utmost gravity where no other pacing system is feasible or available. External (transcutaneous) pacing should always be tried first, because it is probably as efficacious (if not more so) and is associated with significantly less morbidity. Transthoracic pacing should never be used in awake or stable patients.

B. Transcutaneous pacing—This method, in which electrical current is delivered to the heart through the skin via large surface electrodes, is usually reserved for standby prophylaxis in patients recognized to be at high risk for bradycardia, for example during inferior and large anterior wall acute myocardial infarctions (Table 22–7), and in some patients with suspected sinus node dysfunction who are undergoing elective cardioversion. Because of its ease of use and relative efficacy, this pacing modality has virtually eliminated the need for transmyocardial pacing in emergency situations.

The transcutaneous pacing system uses two large, low-impedance surface electrodes placed on the anterior and posterior chest walls. A long pacing stimulus output of 20–40 ms (not programmable by the operator) and current output of more than 100 mA (programmable by the operator) are often necessary to overcome the impedance offered by the chest wall, muscle and bone, and intrathoracic structures. The transcutaneous pacemaker paces the ventricle and inhibits its output when it senses spontaneous ventricular electrical activity, thus functioning in VVI (demand) mode (see section Permanent pacing). Because the pacing pulses are 40 ms in duration and the current output is large, they create a deflection on the surface ECG recording that should not be confused with QRS complexes. If ventricular depolarization (capture) is occurring, the pacer output pulse will be followed by a QRS complex that is best seen on the pacemaker generator's oscilloscope and strip-chart recording. Significant distortion, or total obscuration, of the paced QRS complex can exist on the bedside rhythm monitor or surface ECG recording. Ventricular capture should always be verified by palpating the

Table 22–5. Common Indications for Permanent Cardiac Pacing.

Acquired AV block
High-grade or complete
With symptoms (including symptoms resulting from necessary medications)
With asystole ≥ 3 seconds, or rate of escape pacemaker < 40/min in awake patients
Second-degree
Type II
Type I in patients with symptoms
Acute myocardial infarction
With persistent second- and third-degree AV block
With transient second- and third-degree AV block and bundle branch block
Sinus node dysfunction
With symptoms (including symptoms resulting from necessary medications)
With rates < 40/min
With symptomatic chronotropic incompetence
Carotid sinus hypersensitivity
With syncope during carotid sinus massage
With asystole > 3 seconds during carotid sinus massage
With hypersensitive cardioinhibitory response in patients with unexplained recurrent syncope
Neurocardiogenic syncope
With symptomatic bradycardia documented spontaneously or during tilt-table testing

AV, atrioventricular.
Adapted, with permission, from Gregoratos G et al. J Am Coll Cardiol. 2002;40:1703.

Table 22–6. Common Uses for Temporary Cardiac Pacing.

Therapeutic
To provide adequate heart rate in patients with symptomatic brady-cardia from sinus node dysfunction or high-degree and complete AV block while awaiting definitive therapy
To terminate some supraventricular and ventricular tachycardias by overdrive suppression or entrainment (eg, atrial flutter, monomorphic ventricular tachycardia)
Prophylactic
To prevent high-degree AV block in some patients with acute myocardial infarction, and in some patients after cardiac surgery (eg, aortic valve replacement)
To prevent bradycardia-dependent ventricular tachycardia
Diagnostic
To determine the site of AV block
For evaluation for optimal type of permanent pacing system

AV, atrioventricular.

pulse. Skeletal muscle twitching occurs at a stimulus output of 30 mA, but ventricular capture does not usually occur until 35–80 mA; sedation of the awake patient is usually required to mitigate the painful muscle contractions.

Transcutaneous cardiac pacing can be effective in up to 70% of patients and has its best use in an emergency when pacing of short duration is required or as a bridge to permanent cardiac pacemaker implantation. The majority of pacing failures (specifically, failure to capture) occur in patients during the advanced stages of cardiopulmonary arrest. The likelihood of successful transcutaneous pacing in patients with cardiac arrest of more than 15 minutes duration is approximately 33–45%. Failure to capture can also occur after prolonged (hours to days) pacing and likely represents changes in impedance; repositioning of the electrodes can restore pacing capability.

C. TEMPORARY TRANSVENOUS PACING—Although transcutaneous pacing offers ease of use, rapid initiation of pacing therapy, and very low complication rates, transvenous pacing is far more stable and better tolerated if pacing is needed for longer than 20–30 minutes. Transvenous pacing is usually performed by placing a catheter in the right ventricle. In rare cases where temporary atrial pacing is also required, catheters can be positioned in the right atrium or in the proximal portion of the coronary sinus.

Venous access can be obtained by several approaches. The internal jugular, subclavian, and femoral veins are all potential sites for introduction of the pacing catheter into the right heart. The median cubital and basilic veins can also be used, but these sites are associated with a high incidence of lead dislodgement (because of arm motion) and are rarely, if ever, used today.

Prior to obtaining venous access, the existence of a bleeding diathesis or coagulopathy should be excluded or corrected

if possible. If this is not possible, the femoral vein should be considered as the initial access site because it is easier to apply pressure and achieve hemostasis in this region if a complication occurs. The presence of a prosthetic tricuspid valve is a contraindication to right ventricular pacing; in this circumstance, left ventricular pacing can be performed by positioning the pacing catheter in the left ventricular veins via the coronary sinus. Other factors, such as the patient's pulmonary status, location of dialysis shunts, previous neck surgery, or radiation therapy should be taken into account when considering the appropriate site for venous access.

Ventricular capture thresholds should be < 2 mA and ideally < 1 mA (or < 1 V) in stable lead positions and should not change with coughing or deep breathing. Atrial leads are typically less stable, and capture thresholds around 2 mA (or 1–2 V) are acceptable. The presence of myocardial infarction, ischemia, antiarrhythmic drug therapy, hyperkalemia, and other metabolic derangements can increase capture thresholds.

Sensing thresholds can be affected by myocardial ischemia or infarction, hyperkalemia, and class I antiarrhythmic agents, leading to undersensing ("failure" to sense). Ectopic ventricular depolarizations are often undersensed because of poor signal quality. These considerations need to be borne in mind when setting the sensitivity of the pacemaker.

A daily chest radiograph and paced 12-lead ECG should be obtained and compared with prior studies to check for possible lead migration. Pacing and sensing thresholds should be checked at least daily, with any significant changes being investigated for possible lead migration, lead disconnection from the pulse generator, or change in the patient's clinical status. Battery status should be monitored by the appropriate biomedical personnel, and batteries replaced as needed. Temporary leads and access sites should be changed at least every 3 or 4 days to decrease the risk of infection and venous thrombosis.

Although temporary transvenous pacing is relatively low risk, there are potentially serious complications. Complica-

Table 22–7. Conditions Considered Risks for High-Degree or Complete Atrioventricular Block during Acute Myocardial Infarction.[1]

Inferior-wall MI, especially if it involves the interventricular septum, posterior wall, and right ventricle, with first-degree AV block; second-degree AV block, type I (usually intra-AV nodal); or second-degree AV block, type II (often intra-His)
Extensive anteroseptal MI, with new bifascicular block with a normal PR interval or with first-degree AV block; second-degree AV block, type II; first-degree AV block with bifascicular block (not known to be old); or alternating bundle branch block

[1]The incidence of AV block during acute myocardial infarction has decreased considerably in the current era of fibrinolytic and direct percutaneous revascularization therapies.
AV, atrioventricular; MI, myocardial infarction.

Table 22–8. Some Programmable Functions and Parameters of Cardiac Pacemakers.[1]

Standby rate (base rate, low rate limit): The rate at which the patient is paced unless the spontaneous rhythm is faster

Upper rate limit: The highest rate at which the ventricles are paced 1:1 in response to the atrial rate

AV interval: The interval between the paced or sensed P wave and the delivery of the ventricular pacing stimulus

Atrial refractory period: The time after a sensed P wave or delivery of an atrial output pulse during which the atrial channel is refractory to electrical signals; the refractory period that follows a paced QRS complex, referred to as the PVARP

Ventricular refractory period: The time after a sensed QRS or ventricular output pulse during which the ventricular channel is refractory to electrical signals

Sensitivity (atrial and ventricular channels): The amplitude of the intrinsic atrial and ventricular depolarizations that are to be sensed

Energy output (atrial and ventricular channels): Volts, current and pulse duration

Modes of function: AAI, VVI, AOO, VOO, VDD, DDI, DOO, DDD, OOO

Sensor on

Sensor off

Sensor-based parameters: Time to achieve peak pacing rate; time to decline to standby rate; criteria for sensor activation

Mode switch on: Upon sensing an atrial tachyarrhythmia, a DDD(R) device will automatically switch to DDI(R) or VVI(R) mode of function, and will automatically switch back to DDD(R) mode upon sensing normal atrial rhythm

Mode switch off

---

[1]Pacemaker codes: A, atrium; D, dual; I, inhibited; V, ventricle. PVARP, postventricular atrial refractory period.

tion rates range from 4%–20% and include pneumothorax, hemothorax, arterial puncture, air embolism, serious bleeding, myocardial perforation, cardiac tamponade, nerve injury, thoracic duct injury, arrhythmias, infection, and thromboembolism. The risk of complications is increased if pacing is initiated in emergent situations. To minimize risk, transvenous pacing should be accomplished when the patient is relatively hemodynamically stable.

2. Permanent pacing—Because of the complexity of pacing system design, an identification code has been developed that describes the function of currently available pacemaker generators. The "mode" code consists of three primary letters. The first letter stands for the chamber in which pacing is occurring: A for atrium, V for ventricle, and D for dual, or both. The second letter stands for the chamber in which sensing of the electrical signal occurs: A, V, D, or O for neither. The third letter refers to the mode of response of the generator to the sensed signal: I for inhibited output, D for both inhibited and triggered output delivered in response to a sensed signal (eg, a paced ventricular complex delivered in response to a sensed P wave), and O for not applicable. Most currently available pacing systems incorporate one or two

sensors that allow the pacing rate to increase and decrease with changes in metabolic need; sensor-based pacing systems thus adapt the pacing rate to the activities of daily living. Pacing systems with this feature add an R following the three primary letters (eg, AAIR, DDDR), indicating the existence of rate-adaptive capability. Current pacemakers have numerous functions that can be altered noninvasively by a programmer; such units are described as having multifunction programmability (Table 22–8). Several of the newer temporary pulse generators also have such features.

A. MODES OF PACING

(1) Asynchronous pacing (VOO, AOO, DOO)—In the asynchronous mode of pacemaker function no electrical signals are sensed, and the pulse generator delivers output pulses without regard to any electrical activity occurring spontaneously within the heart (Figure 22–14). Because the native cardiac rhythm is not sensed, competitive rhythms (paced and native depolarizations) can result. Asynchronous pacemaker generators are no longer manufactured; however, the asynchronous pacing mode can be programmed; it also occurs whenever a magnet is placed over an implanted generator to evaluate pacing function. With a magnet in place, asynchronous pacing and concomitant occurrence of the spontaneous rhythm result in iatrogenic parasystole (Figure 22–15). At the energy output of today's generators (1.5–7.5 V), induction of repetitive ventricular or atrial rhythms are usually not observed, although this possibility exists, especially if myocardial ischemia or electrolyte imbalance is present.

(2) Single-chamber demand pacing [VVI(R), AAI(R)]—Both sensing and pacing circuits are present in these units. When a spontaneous intracardiac signal is sensed, VVI and AAI pulse generators will inhibit their output and no pacemaker stimulus artifact will appear. Electrical signals sensed by demand pacemaker generators can originate not only from the heart but also from the environment (electrocautery, cellular telephones), from the patient (muscle potentials), or from the pacing system itself (lead fracture or insulation breaks). Such sensed signals may cause inhibition of output, leading to pauses in paced rhythm; this phenomenon is termed "oversensing" (Tables 22–9 and 22–10), a problem which can generally be corrected by noninvasive programming or, in the case of lead fracture or insulation break, by replacement of the lead. Current generator design and programming capability have not only helped to reduce problems of oversensing but have also simplified their correction.

The pacing function of a demand pulse generator cannot be evaluated if the patient's spontaneous rhythm exceeds the programmed standby (base) rate of the generator. Applying a magnet over the pulse generator converts it to an asynchronous mode of function, and capture (stimulation) of the atria or ventricles by the pacemaker can be confirmed, provided that the pacing stimuli fall outside the refractory period of the cardiac tissue. Conversely, if the patient's rhythm is continu-

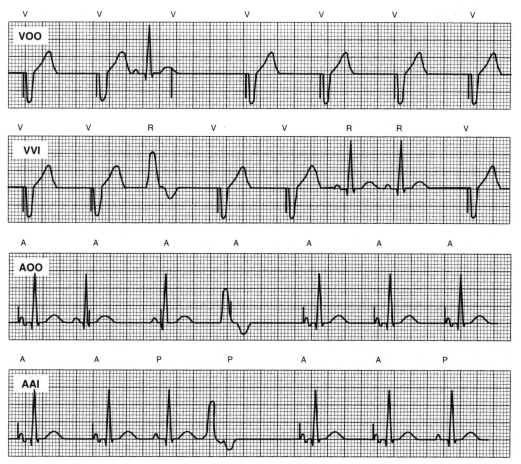

▲ **Figure 22–14.** Schematic illustrations of various pacing modes. (See section Permanent pacing for explanation of symbols.) A, atrial pacing stimulus; P, spontaneous P wave; R, spontaneous QRS; V, ventricular pacing stimulus. (*continued*)

ally paced, the sensing function of the generator cannot be evaluated. Programming the device to a lower rate may allow the emergence of a spontaneous cardiac rhythm, which should then be sensed, resulting in inhibition of pacemaker output.

Continuous single-chamber ventricular pacing will result in AV dyssynchrony (unless during atrial fibrillation). Although the symptoms attributable to bradycardia are alleviated through ventricular rate suppport from the pacemaker, this may be replaced by symptoms due to AV dyssynchrony, or pacemaker syndrome. Either single-chamber atrial pacing (with intact AV conduction) or dual-chamber pacing are solutions to avoid pacemaker syndrome.

(3) Single-lead P-synchronous pacing (VDD)—These are systems in which electrodes for both the atrium and the ventricle are located on a single lead. The lead is positioned in the right ventricular apex where the tip electrodes sense and pace the ventricle; atrial electrodes are located on the lead body, at the level of the atrium and only sense. When the atrial electrodes sense an electrical signal, a ventricular pacing stimulus is delivered after a programmable AV delay that corresponds to the PR interval. If a spontaneous QRS complex occurs, the ventricular output is inhibited. Tracking of the atrial rhythm in a 1:1 relationship allows the ventricular paced rate to change with the sinus rate. The programmed upper rate is the maximum ventricular paced rate that can occur in a 1:1 relationship to atrial activity, and prevents rapid ventricular paced rates should the atrial rate become too fast. If the atrial rate exceeds the upper rate limit, the paced ventricular rate can become irregular because of an electronic Wenckebach protection, can slow to one-half the programmed upper rate limit, or can fall back gradually until 1:1 tracking can resume. This last feature results in disengagement of the tracking function, which causes transient AV dyssynchrony (Figure 22–16).

If no atrial activity is sensed, as occurs in sinus bradycardia, these pulse generators pace the ventricles on demand at

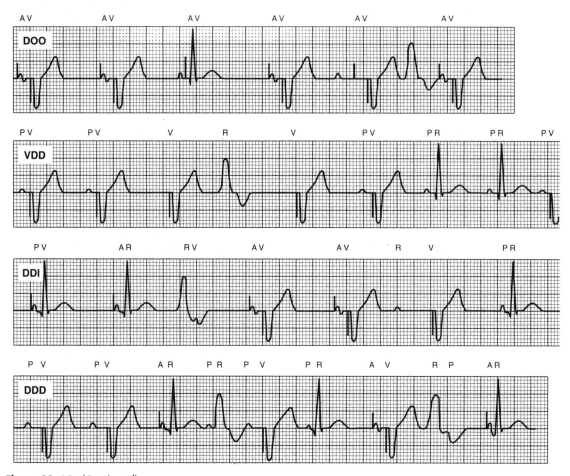

▲ **Figure 22–14.** (*Continued*)

the programmed standby rate; atrial pacing does not occur. Thus, at slow atrial rates the pacing system behaves as though it were a VVI system, and AV synchrony is lost (see Figure 22–14). Although this pacing system seems ideal for patients with normal sinus rhythm and AV block, atrial bradycardia, which occurs commonly over ensuing years, either spontaneously or as a result of medications, makes the VDD device ultimately suboptimal for most patients.

(4) Dual-chamber pacing [DDD(R)]—These pacing systems are capable of sensing and pacing in both the atrium and the ventricle on demand (see Figure 22–14). They therefore approach the physiology of normal AV conduction in many patients who require cardiac pacing. The ability to sense retrograde atrial depolarizations can lead to ventricular stimulus delivery and ventricular pacing in response; if the paced ventricular depolarization travels retrograde to the atrium to depolarize it, the process can become repetitive. This event creates an artificial extra-AV-nodal bypass tract,

causing a pacemaker-mediated tachycardia. Specific algorithms have been designed to terminate these tachycardias and are automatic once they have been programmed.

Dual-chamber devices depend on a stable atrial rhythm for optimum function. Because of their potential for rapid paced ventricular rates, these systems should not be used with atrial arrhythmias such as chronic fibrillation or flutter, multifocal tachycardia, or refractory automatic tachycardia; single-chamber VVI(R) devices should be used instead.

If the atrial tachyarrhythmias are paroxysmal, however, a programmed "mode switch" feature should be turned on that automatically changes the mode from DDD(R) to either DDI(R) or VVI(R) modes when a rapid atrial rate is detected; this takes away the ability to track the atrial rate as long as the atrial tachyarrhythmia persists (Figure 22–17). Studies have established that in patients with bradycardia, compared with ventricular pacing, atrial-based pacing reduces the incidence of atrial fibrillation and may reduce stroke.

A. Without Magnet

B. With Magnet   F   NC   NC   F   NC   NC

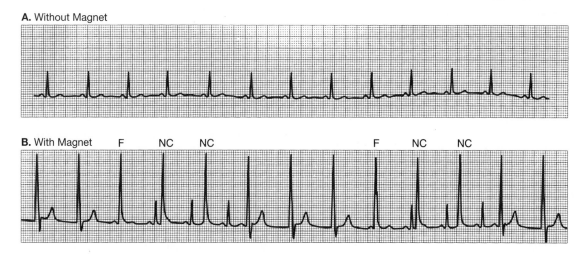

▲ **Figure 22–15.** A VVI pacing system. **A:** Normal sinus rhythm is present. Sensing function is presumed to be normal because no ventricular pacing artifacts are occurring. **B:** With a magnet in place over the pulse generator, ventricular pacing stimuli are emitted asynchronously, resulting in a rhythm that competes with the sinus rhythm. The large magnitude of the pacing artifacts indicates that the lead configuration is unipolar. The large unipolar stimulus obscures the resulting QRS complex; however, because T waves are present following some of these pacing stimuli, capture is confirmed. Both sensing and pacing functions are normal. F, fusion complexes, with ventricular depolarization resulting from both sinus and paced impulses. NC, noncapture because of pacing stimuli falling in the refractory period of ventricular muscle.

Rate-adaptive pacing systems are appropriate for patients with persistent or refractory atrial arrhythmias who are not candidates for DDD devices and for patients whose sinus node dysfunction prevents rate acceleration, but who would benefit from an increase in paced atrial or ventricular rates in response to increases in metabolic demand. Current sensors measure muscle activity, minute ventilation, and QT interval; sensors to measure other parameters (eg, right ventricular dP/dt [rate of rise of pressure within the right ventricle]) are under development. Changes within the sensor's established parameters, designed to reflect physiologic needs, result in changes in paced rates. Sensor-based pacing rates depend on the individual sensor used, however; for example, if an activity sensor is being used, the paced rate can increase in response to body vibrations that are unrelated to actual physical activity. This can cause problems in hospitalized patients, especially those in intensive care units. Several manufacturers, therefore, currently incorporate two sensors into their pacemakers to confirm the need for appropriate changes in pacing rate. For example, the activity sensor input can be confirmed by a more physiologic sensor such as minute ventilation, resulting in a more specific and accurate response to the change in pacing rate for the particular change in metabolic need.

Recently, findings from several studies have raised concern that right ventricular pacing can be detrimental, especially in patients with left ventricular systolic dysfunction. The left ventricular dyssynchrony caused by pacing from the right

ventricle is thought to induce further cardiomyopathy and congestive heart failure. Dyssynchrony-induced cardiomyopathy has also been observed in patients with left BBB, where abnormal electrical activation can initiate electrical remodeling that leads to myocardial remodeling; in some patients with left BBB, cardiomyopathy can be reversed with cardiac resynchronization therapy through biventricular pacing.

In patients who do not need continuous ventricular pacing, various parameters can be programmed to minimize unnecessary ventricular pacing. The AV delay can be programmed to automatically extend to allow native AV conduction as much as possible. Another programmable solution is managed ventricular pacing (MVP) mode (Medtronic, Inc., Minneapolis, MN) that maintains AAI(R) mode until AV block is detected, at which time it automatically switches to DDD(R) mode; AAI(R) mode is restored when the pacemaker detects resumption of native AV conduction. In selected patients with advanced congestive heart failure, biventricular pacing can address the dyssynchrony caused by right ventricular pacing.

The type of pacing system implanted is indicated on an identification card supplied to the patient by the manufacturer; patients should carry these cards with them at all times. It is important to note, however, that such information does not guarantee the operation of a particular mode of function, rate, or any parameter that can be programmed by the patient's pacemaker physician. As pulse-generator design and function increase in complexity, it is best to assume that the

Table 22–9. Pacing System Malfunctions, and Clues to Their Recognition.

Failure to sense (undersensing)
Single-chamber systems
    ECG will show earlier-than-expected appearance of pacing-stimulus artifact.
Dual-chamber systems
    Atrial undersensing: Delivery of atrial pacing stimuli despite occurrence of spontaneous P waves; failure to track intrinsic atrial activity at the programmed AV interval
Ventricular undersensing: Delivery of ventricular pacing stimuli despite occurrence of spontaneous QRS complexes
Oversensing
ECG will show inappropriate inhibition of atrial or ventricular output stimuli; oversensing in the atrial channel causes earlier-than-expected ventricular pacing stimuli.
Failure to capture
Pacing stimuli not followed by atrial or ventricular depolarization (assuming muscle tissue is not refractory)
Failure of output
Absence of pacing stimulus outputs, with oversensing excluded

---

AV, atrioventricular; ECG, electrocardiogram.

pacemaker is performing normally until proved otherwise. (There are, of course, malfunctions and "pseudo" malfunctions; these are addressed in the following sections.) Similarly, ECGs in paced patients should be considered to reflect normal device function unless they are interpreted otherwise by personnel experienced in pacemaker electrocardiography.

B. Unipolar and bipolar pacing—Unipolar pacing systems have the cathode (stimulating electrode) in the heart and the anode at the generator. The distance between the cathode and anode in these systems results in the inscription of large pacing artifacts whose direction (pacing-artifact axis) in the frontal plane points toward the anode.

Bipolar pacing systems have both lead electrodes within the heart, usually less than 1 cm apart, in either or both atrium and ventricle. Either the distal (tip) electrode or the proximal (ring) electrode of the lead can serve as the cathode. Because of the small interelectrode distance, the pacing artifacts are small and their direction in the frontal plane reflects the direction of current flow (Figure 22–18).

Electrocardiograms recorded on digital rather than analog ECG machines can show marked variations in the amplitude and polarity of the pacing artifact. Because the digital equipment samples the pacing stimuli at specific time intervals and then recreates them on paper, the inscribed stimulus artifacts are not seen in real time. In some ECG leads, the pacing stimuli may not be visible at all, raising the question of failure of generator output. It is important to recognize this recording artifact in patients with pacemakers to avoid an erroneous diagnosis of pacemaker malfunction. It is equally important to document the morphology of paced complexes so that when the pacing stimuli cannot be seen, normal pacemaker function can be assumed until an accurate evaluation can be made.

Some permanent bipolar pacing systems offer lead polarity that can be programmed to unipolar; therefore, the presence of a bipolar lead on chest radiograph does not ensure bipolar lead function, and the ECG appearance of the pacing artifacts may differ from what is expected.

C. Electrocardiographic patterns of paced complexes—These patterns depend on how the myocardium is depolarized. Paced atrial complexes reflect the sequence of atrial activation initiated by the pacing impulse and thus, in part, the site of the pacing electrode(s). Because the atrial electrodes can be located in the atrial appendage or screwed into any portion of atrial tissue, paced P waves contours and axes will vary.

Pacing from the right ventricular apex produces paced QRS complexes that have a left BBB configuration (the right ventricular myocardium is depolarized before the left) and a superior mean frontal plane axis (the apex of the heart is depolarized before the base; Figure 22–19). Paced QRS complexes usually have a duration of 0.12–0.18 seconds; if they are substantially longer, intrinsic myocardial disease, hyperkalemia, or antiarrhythmic drug therapy (eg, amiodarone) should be suspected.

Pacing from the right ventricular outflow tract also results in QRS complexes that have a left BBB pattern, but the mean frontal plane axis is inferiorly directed (the base

Table 22–10. Causes of Pacemaker Oversensing.

Electromagnetic interference
Power transformers, power lines; welding equipment; household appliances such as razors and garage-door openers (unusual with today's pulse generators), microwave ovens operating at high power; rotating radar detectors; metal-detector gates (older generation designs); transcutaneous nerve stimulators; cardioverting and defibrillating devices (external or implanted internally); diathermy; lithotriptors; electrocautery; electrocoagulation; MRI; ionizing radiation; tasers; cellular telephones if used on the side ipsilateral to the pulse generator (some models); electronic article surveillance monitors
Physiologic intracardiac signals
R wave sensing (AAI[1] systems), T wave sensing (VVI systems), P wave sensing (VVI systems) (unusual)
Physiologic extracardiac signals
Muscle potentials (eg, diaphragm, pectoral)
Signals generated within the pacing system
Leads
Conductor-wire fracture causing a voltage transient; insulation defect
Pulse generator
Afterpotential sensing of late portions of the pacing stimulus itself (unusual); component malfunction

---

[1]Pacemaker codes: A, atrium; D, dual; MRI, magnetic resonance imaging; I, inhibited; V, ventricle.

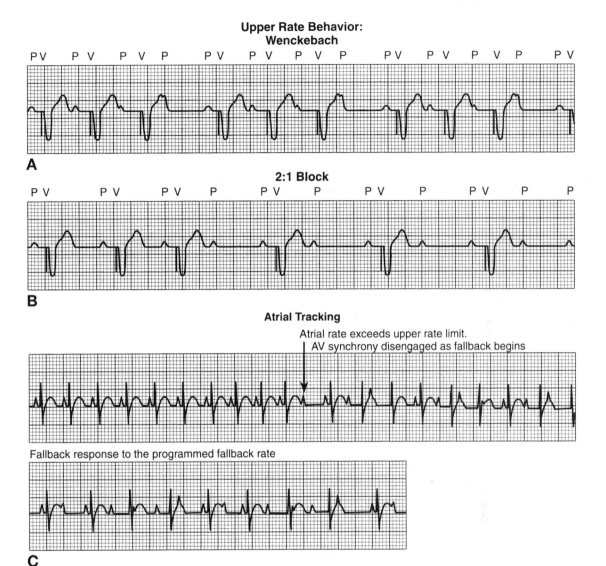

Figure 22–16. Schematic illustration of responses from pulse generators at the atrial-driven upper rate limit. The pacemaker will not allow the ventricular paced rate to exceed this programmed upper rate. Atrial rhythms that can exceed the upper rate limit include sinus tachycardia, atrial tachycardia, atrial flutter, and atrial fibrillation. The pacemaker-mediated tachycardia (see text) will also not exceed the programmed upper rate. **A:** Lengthening of the interval between the sensed P wave and the triggered ventricular-paced complex so as not to violate the upper rate limit (Wenckebach): the P wave that is not followed by a paced QRS complex falls in the refractory period of the atrial channel and is not sensed, resulting in absence (nondelivery) of the ventricular stimulus output. **B:** In 2:1 block, alternate P waves fall in the atrial refractory period and are not sensed: they are not followed by a paced ventricular event. **C:** In fallback, the ventricular paced rate gradually slows once the programmed upper rate has been achieved. During the fallback period, tracking of the atrial rate is disengaged, and AV synchrony is no longer present. The ventricular paced rate will again track the atrial rate once the latter falls below the programmed upper rate. The fallback response avoids abrupt decreases in paced ventricular rate. Pacemakers that function in a rate-adaptive mode can have their sensor-based upper rate limit exceed the above-described upper tracking limit.

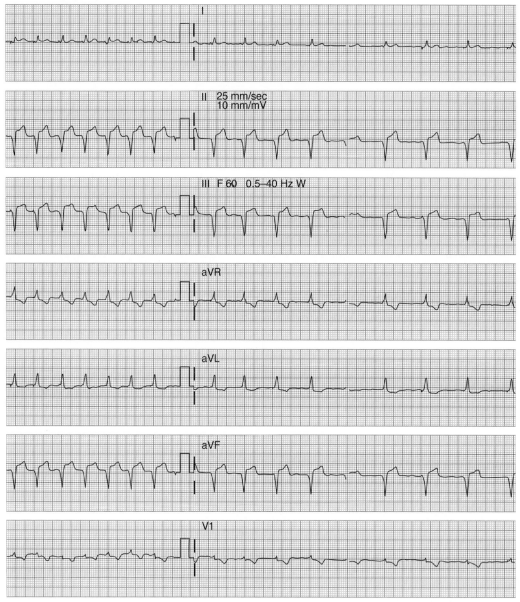

▲ **Figure 22-17.** Depiction of mode-switch operation of a dual-chamber pacemaker. In the initial portion of the rhythm strip, tracking of atrial fibrillation is occurring, resulting in a rapid paced ventricular rate. When the atrial tachyarrhythmia is recognized by the algorithm in the pacemaker, automatic change of mode of function to VVIR takes place, terminating the rapid paced ventricular rate. On sensing restoration of a normal atrial rhythm, the device will automatically restore its dual-chamber mode of operation.

of the heart is depolarized before the apex). Occasionally, pacing from the interventricular septum can result in paced QRS complexes that show an indeterminate conduction delay pattern; they can even be narrow and relatively normal-appearing. This reflects almost simultaneous acti-

vation of both the right and left sides of the interventricular septum.

Pacing from the left ventricular epicardium produces paced QRS complexes having a right BBB pattern, reflecting left ventricular myocardial activation in advance of right

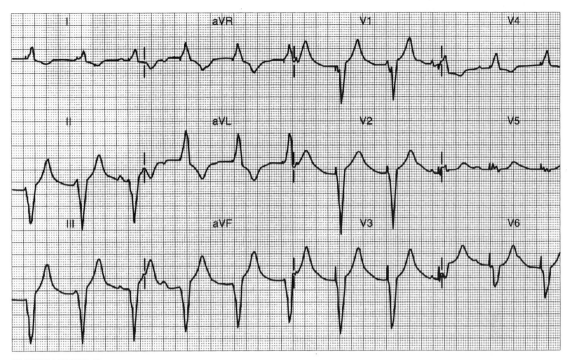

RHYTHM STRIP: II
25 mm/sec; 1 cm/mV

▲ **Figure 22–18.** Bipolar VVI pacing system. All QRS complexes are paced. Note the small magnitude of the pacing artifacts. The simultaneous recordings indicate that in some leads the pacing stimuli are virtually invisible.

ventricular activation. The mean frontal-plane QRS axis will depend on the location of the epicardial electrodes relative to each other (bipolar system) or to the pulse generator serving as anode (unipolar system).

In recent years, left ventricular pacing has been accomplished from the coronary veins approached via the coronary sinus. This technique is used along with simultaneous, or near simultaneous, pacing from the right ventricle in patients with advanced heart failure and wide QRS complexes (> 120 ms) in order to "resynchronize" ventricular depolarization-contraction. The biventricular-paced QRS complexes can be narrower and more normal-appearing than the patient's spontaneous QRS complexes, reflecting electrical resynchronization and suggesting a beneficial result of this therapy; electrical synchrony, however, does not necessarily correlate with mechanical synchrony, and a persistently wide QRS complex does not predict failure of therapy. The mean frontal plane axis of the paced complexes will vary with the location of the electrodes. Because the timing of the two ventricular leads can now be programmed separately, and either lead can be activated first by up to 80 ms, biventricular paced QRS complexes can be preceded by tightly coupled double-pacing artifact (Figure 22–20). Spontaneous QRS complexes occurring in patients with pacemak-

ers often show marked T-wave inversion (Figure 22–21). This phenomenon has been explained as "T-wave memory" or the temporary persistence of abnormal repolarization "learned" by the myocardium during pacing. The ECG abnormality should not be interpreted as acute or chronic myocardial disease (including ischemia and infarction) in the absence of clinical indications.

B. Pacing System Malfunctions

System malfunctions fall into four general categories: (1) undersensing, or failure to sense; (2) oversensing, or sensing unwanted signals; (3) failure to capture and stimulate myocardial tissue; and (4) failure of output. Undersensing of cardiac electrical signals because of poor intrinsic signal quality does not represent sensing failure as such, but rather the inability to detect the suboptimal signal itself; undersensed P waves and QRS complexes are not rare. Premature ventricular complexes (Table 22–9 and Figure 22–22) generate suboptimal signal because they originate from within the myocardium, away from the normal conduction apparatus; they can occur in patients without structural heart disease, during acute myocardial ischemia and infarction, or as a result of drug toxicity and electrolyte imbalance. Undersensed P waves can be caused by

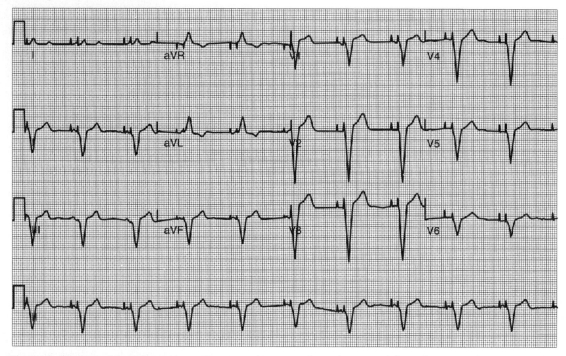

▲ **Figure 22–19.** Atrioventricular pacing with ventricular pacing from the area of the right ventricular apex, yielding superiorly directed paced QRS complexes with a left BBB pattern. The paced P wave morphology and axis are similarly determined by the location of the pacing lead tip.

changes in atrial volume, ectopic atrial rhythms, or retrograde atrial depolarizations. Failure to sense spontaneous complexes and inhibit output results in the delivery of an earlier-than-expected pacing stimulus, which can, on occasion, induce repetitive rhythms.

Ventricular pacing artifacts can sometimes occur after the onset of spontaneous QRS complexes that have a right BBB configuration, raising concern of undersensing. This happens because of delayed conduction in the right bundle branch: the wavefront of ventricular depolarization does not reach the lead electrode in the right ventricular apex in time to inhibit the output of the pacing stimulus. This phenomenon called "pseudofusion" may also be observed in patients with inferior and right ventricular myocardial infarctions and is probably due to the conduction delay resulting from ventricular scarring. The same principles apply to patients who have a left ventricular epicardial electrode and either underlying left BBB or ventricular scarring, and to patients who have a right atrial electrode and an intra-atrial conduction delay. Failure to sense in these cases is due to intrinsic conduction system disease rather than to a malfunctioning unit. The problem is managed by extending the programmed AV delay (in the case of ventricular pseudofusion), programming a higher sensitivity, or, if necessary, by increasing the pacing rate to overdrive the native rhythm.

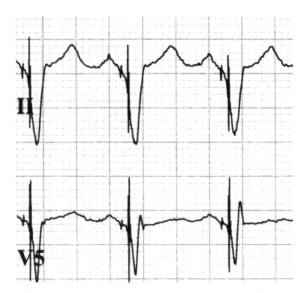

▲ **Figure 22–20.** Lead II and V5 in patient with a biventricular pacing system, programmed with a VV timing set to LV first by 60 ms. Two distinct ventricular stimulus output artifacts are seen tightly coupled at the onset of the paced QRS complex, following a sensed P wave.

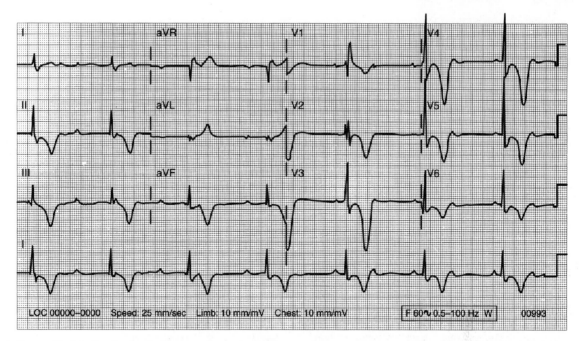

▲ **Figure 22–21.** Twelve-lead electrocardiogram in patient with a DDD pacing system, temporarily programmed to a rate of 30 bpm to permit emergence of the native rhythm. The intrinsic rhythm is sinus with complete atrioventricular block and right bundle branch block. Because no pacing artifacts are occurring, sensing function is normal in both atrium and ventricle. The deeply inverted T waves in the inferior and precordial leads represent a nonspecific abnormality commonly observed in patients with pacemakers; they do not represent myocardial injury.

Oversensing describes sensing of unwanted electrical signals such as T waves, myopotentials, environmental signals (eg, electrocautery; see Table 22–10). Programming the pulse generator (or the temporary pacing unit) to only sense electrical signals of larger magnitude will often solve the problem. When a programmer is not immediately available, placing a magnet over the generator will temporarily eliminate the oversensing by converting the generator to a non-

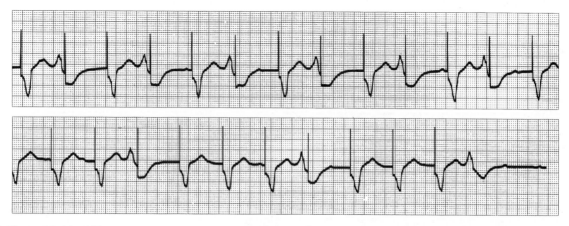

▲ **Figure 22–22.** Failure to sense spontaneous ventricular complexes in a patient with a VVI pacing system. Because the signal quality of depolarization originating in ventricular tissue is often poor, this is not uncommon. Repetitive ventricular beating induced by the stimulus-on-ST complex is, however, rare in stable patients.

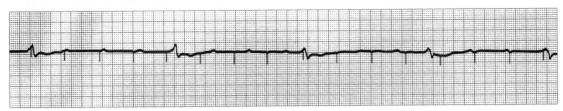

▲ **Figure 22–23.** Failure to capture and sense in a patient following cardiac arrest; a temporary transvenous pacing system had been placed in the right ventricular apex. The QRS complexes are spontaneous and occur at a severely slow rate; they do not follow pacing stimuli.

sensing asynchronous mode. Because competitive rhythms can induce repetitive beating with the magnet in place, these patients should be in a monitored unit.

Failure to pace is when pacing stimuli do not depolarize nonrefractory myocardium (Figure 22–23; Table 22–11). This condition may result from poor electrode position; a subthreshold programmed output; output reduction due to battery depletion; or an increase in myocardial stimulation threshold from acute myocardial infarction, drug toxicity, electrolyte imbalance, cardiopulmonary resuscitation, or fibrosis at the electrode-tissue interface. Pacemaker non-capture can be managed by noninvasive programming of the generator's energy output, surgical repositioning of the lead, or generator exchange, depending on the underlying problem.

The difference between failure to capture when the stimulus artifact is present and a lack of stimulus output should be recognized. If the pacing stimulus has not been delivered (Table 22–12), capture cannot be ascertained. Applying a magnet will aid in determining the cause for the lack of stimulus output.

C. Assessment of Pacing System Function

All patients should have a 12-lead ECG, with and without a magnet applied, to allow identification of spontaneous (where present), purely paced, and fusion P waves and QRS

Table 22–11. Causes and Management of Pacemaker Noncapture.

Tissue refractoriness: Verify capture during temporal opportunity.
Lead dislodgement: Reposition lead, or program lead polarity.
Increase in myocardial stimulation threshold: Program higher energy output; treat underlying cause if possible.
Lead-insulation break: Repair or replace lead; unipolarize lead.
Conductor-wire fracture: Replace lead.
Inappropriately low programmed output: Program higher output.
Generator end of life: Replace generator.

complexes, as well as sensing and pacing functions in both atria and ventricles. The paced rate with a magnet in place may not be the same as the programmed rate, and the mode of function with the magnet in place may differ from the programmed mode (eg, a DDD system may have a magnet mode that is VOO; Figure 22–24).

In addition, all patients should have highly penetrated posteroanterior and lateral chest radiographs in order to assess the leads, and, when possible, to identify the pacemaker's manufacturer and model number.

The number and type (unipolar, bipolar) of leads can be ascertained, as well as the positions of the lead tips and pulse generator. Lead tips lying outside the cardiac silhouette suggest the possibility of myocardial perforation. Occasion-

Table 22–12. Causes of Absence of Pacing Stimulus Output and Response to Magnet Application.

Cause	Response to Magnet
Normal inhibition by P waves and QRS complexes	Pacing stimuli will be delivered asynchronously
Oversensing	Pacing stimuli will be delivered asynchronously
Lead fracture	Pacing stimuli may not be seen if the break in the wire is complete (current does not reach body tissues); may be seen as multiples of a basing pacing rate, or may be seen intermittently (make-break circuit); may have variable amplitude
Lead-generator disconnection or improper connection	Same as for lead fracture
Battery failure (end of life)	Pacing stimuli at slow rate, no visible pacing stimuli, noncapture, failure to sense
Battery component failure	Variable response

A. Without Magnet

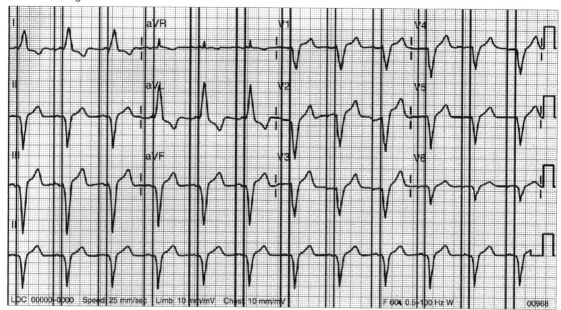

B. With Magnet

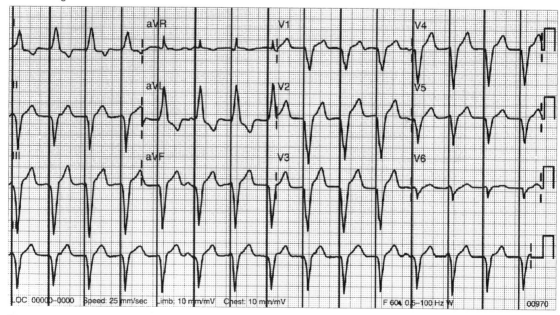

▲ **Figure 22–24. A:** Atrioventricular sequential pacing. The large magnitude of the pacing artifacts indicate unipolar pacing in both chambers. Because atrial pacing stimuli are followed by P waves, and ventricular stimuli are followed by QRS complexes, pacing function is normal in both chambers. Sensing function cannot be evaluated because spontaneous P waves and QRS complexes are not occurring. **B:** Twelve-lead electrocardiogram, recorded with magnet in place. The mode of function is VOO (asynchronous ventricular pacing) at the factory-designated rate of about 88/min. This is normal function for this particular device.

ally, lead insulation degradation, wire fracture, or improper connections between the lead and generator can be seen.

More sophisticated evaluation techniques, such as interrogation of the programmed values of the pulse generator, sensing and pacing threshold determination, and recording of intracardiac electrograms, can be necessary to determine the cause of pacemaker malfunction; these evaluations are best performed by a pacemaker specialist.

Connolly SJ et al; VPS II Investigators. Pacemaker therapy for prevention of syncope in patients with recurrent severe vasovagal syncope: Second Vasovagal Pacemaker Study (VPS II): a randomized trial. JAMA. 2003 May 7;289(17):2224–9. [PMID: 12734133]

Goldschlager N et al; North American Society of Pacing and Electrophysiology (NASPE) Practice Guideline Committee. Environmental and drug effects on patients with pacemakers and implantable cardioverter/defibrillators: a practical guide to patient treatment. Arch Intern Med. 2001 Mar 12;161(5):649–55. [PMID: 11231696]

Gregoratos G et al. ACC/AHA/NASPE 2002 Guideline Update for Implantation of Cardiac Pacemakers and Antiarrhythmia Devices. A report of the American College of Cardiology/American Heart Association Task Force on Practice Guidelines (ACC/AHA/NASPE Committee to Update the 1998 Pacemaker Guidelines). J Am Coll Cardiol. 2002 Nov 6;40(9):1703–19. [PMID: 12427427]

Healey JS et al. Cardiovascular outcomes with atrial-based pacing compared with ventricular pacing: meta-analysis of randomized trials, using individual patient data. Circulation. 2006 Jul 4;114(1):11–7. [PMID: 16801463]

Wilkoff BL et al; Dual Chamber and VVI Implantable Defibrillator Trial Investigators. Dual-chamber pacing or ventricular backup pacing in patients with an implantable defibrillator: the Dual Chamber and VVI Implantable Defibrillator (DAVID) Trial. JAMA. 2002 Dec 25;288(24):3115–23. [PMID: 12495391]

Wood MA et al. Clinical outcomes after ablation and pacing therapy for atrial fibrillation. A meta-analysis. Circulation. 2000 Mar 14;101(10):1138–44. [PMID: 10715260]

Ventricular Tachycardia

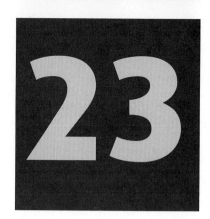

Nitish Badhwar, MD

► Nonsustained: Three or more consecutive QRS complexes of uniform configuration of ventricular origin at a rate of more than 100 bpm.

► Sustained: Lasts more than 30 seconds; requires intervention for termination.

► Monomorphic ventricular tachycardia.

► Polymorphic ventricular tachycardia: Beat-to-beat variation in QRS configuration.

The magnitude of ventricular tachycardia (VT), one of the most common health problems encountered in clinical practice, can best be appreciated in terms of its various clinical manifestations, which include ventricular fibrillation (sudden cardiac death [SCD]), syncope or near syncope, and wide QRS tachycardia.

The most serious is its degeneration into ventricular fibrillation, producing cardiac arrest and SCD that accounts for 200,000 deaths a year. The second most serious clinical presentation is syncope. Although the overall prevalence of VT-related syncope is unclear, it is estimated to be frequent because inducible VT (via electrical stimulation) is the most common arrhythmia detected in patients with unexplained syncope. A high prevalence of SCD (more than 20% incidence within the ensuing 12 months) is noted in patients with syncope from cardiovascular causes, suggesting that undiagnosed VT may be an underlying cause of sudden death in patients with unexplained syncope. The third most significant clinical manifestation of VT is a wide QRS complex tachycardia that is often hemodynamically well tolerated.

DIAGNOSTIC ISSUES

1. Underdiagnosis

Ventricular tachycardia as a cause of morbidity and mortality is grossly underdiagnosed, potentially leading to mis-

management. This may be particularly true when the clinical presentation is unexplained syncope because no concomitant electrocardiographic (ECG) documentation is available. In the case of cardiac arrest or SCD acute myocardial infarction rather than an arrhythmic problem is often assumed to be responsible. Most persons who have suffered sudden death have no evidence of acute myocardial necrosis, even though the episode often occurs in patients with underlying coronary artery disease. Managing the underlying coronary artery disease with no regard to treating the concomitant VT is inadequate.

2. Misdiagnosis

When hemodynamically stable VT is recorded on the surface ECG, it is often misdiagnosed as supraventricular tachycardia (SVT) with aberrant conduction. Any subsequent management is therefore directed toward SVT. Although the exact logic for this line of thinking is unclear, the main reason may be that the hemodynamic stability is associated with the broad QRS rhythm and thus the erroneous belief that the problem cannot be VT.

The clinical presentation of VT depends on many factors, including rate, ventricular function, presence of concomitant coronary artery disease, the presence or absence of cardioactive drugs, and even the patient's posture at the time of onset. Hemodynamic tolerance of VT can, therefore, vary considerably in different situations; at times, it can vary in the same patient, and it is prudent not to exclude the diagnosis of VT on the basis of hemodynamic tolerance alone. It must be understood that approximately 80% of the patients with sustained wide QRS tachycardia have VT. To avoid misdiagnosis, the clinician can either use the established ECG criteria (discussed in the next section) that distinguish VT from SVT with aberrant conduction or simply assume the presence of VT. The assumption of VT is more often correct; it is also safer because misdiagnosing VT as SVT is a riskier judgment error than vice versa.

3. Diagnostic Approach to the Patient with Wide QRS Complex Tachycardia

The diagnosis of wide QRS complex tachycardia by ECG analysis has always been a challenge for clinicians. The differential diagnosis includes VT, SVT with aberrant conduction, and preexcited tachycardia in patients with Wolff-Parkinson-White syndrome (WPW). Figure 23–1 depicts, schematically, the reasons for normal and broad QRS complexes. Preexcited tachycardia results from antegrade activation of the ventricle via an accessory pathway in patients with WPW syndrome, which can present with atrial fibrillation, atrial flutter, atrial tachycardia, atrioventricular nodal reentry tachycardia (AVNRT), or antidromic tachycardia. Preexcited tachycardia is a rare cause of wide QRS complex tachycardia (5–8% of cases); however, the QRS pattern of preexcited QRS complex can be difficult to distinguish from VT because in both instances the QRS starts with muscle-to-muscle conduction. Electrocardiographic artifact can also mimic wide QRS complex tachycardia and be misdiagnosed as VT, leading to expensive testing and even placement of implantable cardioverter-defibrillator (ICD). Clues to the diagnosis include absence of hemodynamic deterioration, an unstable baseline, association with body movement, and ability to march the normal QRS complexes through the artifact ("notches sign") at sinus R-R interval. A number of

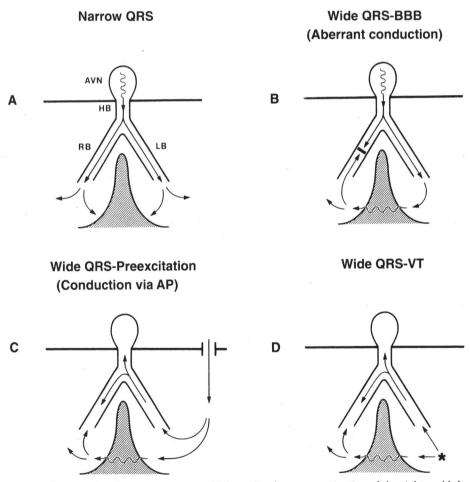

▲ **Figure 23–1.** Mechanism of wide QRS. **A:** Narrow QRS from simultaneous activation of the right and left ventricles. In the three types of wide QRS shown in **B–D,** there is sequential rather than simultaneous activation of the left and right ventricle and a variable amount of muscle-to-muscle conduction. AP, accessory pathway; AVN, atrioventricular node; BBB, bundle branch block; HB, His bundle; LB, left bundle; RB, right bundle. (Reproduced, with permission, from Akhtar M et al. Electrophysiological spectrum of wide QRS complex tachycardia. In: Zipes DP, Jalife J, editors. *Cardiac Electrophysiology. From Cell to Bedside.* Philadelphia: WB Saunders, 1990.)

surface ECG criteria, including the atrioventricular (AV) relationship, the QRS complex duration, specific QRS morphology, and the QRS complex axis, have been established to distinguish VT from SVT with aberrant conduction. These criteria are helpful in arriving at an accurate diagnosis if they are used in a systemic fashion.

▶ Atrioventricular Relationship

In SVT, the arrhythmia arises in the atria or AV junction and reaches the ventricles through the AV node and His-Purkinje system. Because the atrial arrhythmia is the primary event, either a 1:1 AV response or a varying degree of AV block occurs, but in either case the atrial rates equal or exceed ventricular rates. During VT, a retrograde block often leads to either AV dissociation or a varying degree of ventriculoatrial conduction ratios, but the ventricular rates equal or exceed the atrial rate. When AV dissociation can be recognized, it is the most reliable criterion for VT. This criterion lacks sensitivity, however, because the P waves can be identified on the surface ECG in only 25% of patients with VT (Figures 23–2 and 23–3). In patients with slower VT and AV dissociation, intermittent ventricular capture can result in fusion with narrow QRS complexes during wide QRS complex tachycardia. This useful but rarely observed finding is also 100% specific for the diagnosis of VT.

▶ QRS Complex Duration

For the reasons listed earlier, the QRS complex duration is the widest in VT and narrowest in aberrant conduction. To distinguish VT from SVT with aberrant conduction on the basis of QRS duration alone, however, some specific aspects must be considered. In the absence of cardioactive drugs and extensive myocardial fibrosis, aberrancy rarely results in a QRS duration of more than 140 ms with a right bundle branch block (RBBB) pattern (Figure 23–3) or more than 160 ms with a left bundle branch block (LBBB) configuration. In the presence of intramyocardial conduction delay from drugs (such as class I antiarrhythmic agents) and myocardial fibrosis, the QRS width may also exceed these values in SVT with aberrant conduction. Conversely, on a rare occasion, VT can present as a narrow QRS tachycardia (less than 120 ms that is narrower than the conducted QRS complex) when there is near-simultaneous activation of the two ventricles, perhaps from the septum.

▶ Specific QRS Morphology

The prevalence of LBBB versus RBBB morphology among the causes of wide QRS is comparable in both VT and SVT with aberrant conduction; it is therefore of no diagnostic value. The typical RBBB is a triphasic complex best seen in V_1 as rsR' or rSR' pattern and in lead I as qRs, qRS pattern. Similarly, a typical LBBB has no initial q wave in lead I and a small r and a rapid S wave in V_1. Because of the myocardial origin of most forms of VT, however, the QRS appearance is not exactly like a typical LBBB or RBBB. Many ECG criteria, therefore, have exploited this difference to separate VT from aberrant conduction. A study that analyzed the morphology of premature ventricular complexes and aberrantly conducted beats of RBBB morphology in V_1 found that the triphasic RsR' pattern with R' > R was predominant in aberrant conduction (70%) compared with premature ventricular complexes (6%). Monophasic pattern or R > R' was seen in the premature ventricular complex beats. The limitation of that study is that origin of the anomalous beats (SVT

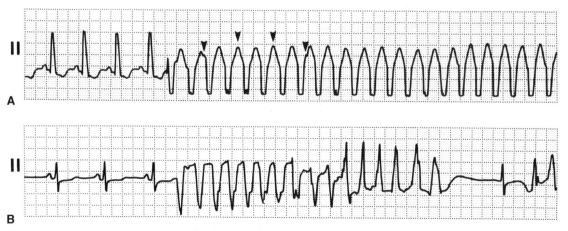

▲ **Figure 23–2. A:** Monomorphic ventricular tachycardia (VT), with a uniform QRS appearance for all complexes. Arrowheads indicate superimposed P waves. **B:** Polymorphic VT, with a beat-to-beat variation in the QRS morphology; QT-interval prolongation follows the termination of the VT episode. (Reproduced, with permission, from Akhtar M. Circulation. 1990;82:1561.)

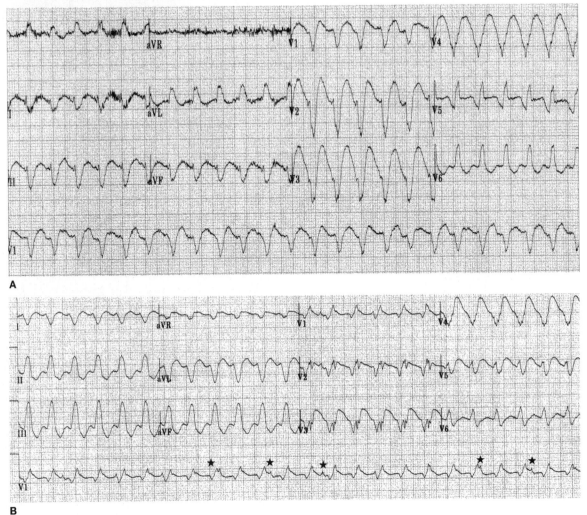

▲ **Figure 23–3. A:** Scar-related ventricular tachycardia (VT), with a left bundle branch block left axis morphology in a patient with ischemic cardiomyopathy and previous myocardial infarction. **B:** Right bundle branch block right axis morphology VT in the same patient at the same rate suggesting that both forms of VT have the same circuit (that revolves around the mitral annulus) with different exits causing the difference in morphology. Atrioventricular dissociation is noted in the rhythm strip on V_1 (*) that is 100% specific for VT.

vs VT) was also based on the ECG (presence or absence of preceding P wave). A retrospective ECG analysis of 70 patients with SVT and 70 patients with VT in whom His bundle recordings were used to determine the site of origin of the wide QRS complex tachycardia found that VT was favored by monophasic or biphasic R waves in V_1 and R:S ratio less than 1 in V_6 in patients with RBBB morphology and any Q wave in V_6 in patients with LBBB morphology. A study of 150 consecutive wide QRS complex tachycardia cases found that 12-lead QRS morphology during wide QRS complex tachycardia was different from that during preexisting bundle branch block in sinus rhythm, favoring a diagno-

sis of VT. The investigators also noted that a positive QRS concordance (positive complexes V_1–V_6) is uncommon in aberrancy, but a negative QRS concordance can occur during aberrant conduction in a small percentage of cases. Another study that evaluated wide QRS complex tachycardia with LBBB morphology in V_1 found that an R wave of > 30 ms, notching in the down stroke of the S wave and an RS (beginning of QRS complex to nadir of S wave) interval > 60 ms in V_1 or V_2, and any Q wave in V_6 favored a diagnosis of VT. In a prospective analysis of wide QRS complex tachycardia (with RBBB and LBBB morphology), the following two criteria for a diagnosis of VT were proposed: (1) absence of

R-S in all precordial leads (2) R-S interval > 100 ms (measured from the beginning of the QRS complex to the nadir of the S wave) in any precordial lead. Finally, the presence of QR complex in any lead during wide QRS complex tachycardia also favors a diagnosis of VT.

▶ QRS Complex Axis

The axis orientation on a 12-lead ECG ranging from normal (−30°–+90°), left (−31°– −90°) or right (+91°– +180°) has significant overlap across the causes of wide QRS complex tachycardia and is of little diagnostic value. The axis range of −91° to 180°, however, is usually not seen in aberrant conduction. The axis location of this extreme during SVT is, therefore, unlikely unless there was a nonarrhythmic reason for it, such as severe right ventricular hypertrophy or lung disease. Similarly, a combination of right axis with LBBB pattern is almost always seen in patients with VT. A previous history of MI and an axis change of more than 40 degrees between sinus rhythm and wide QRS complex tachycardia may independently favor VT over SVT.

▶ History, Physical Examination and 12-Lead ECG

A detailed history and physical examination can provide clues to the diagnosis of wide QRS complex tachycardia. A history of myocardial infarction favors VT as the diagnosis of wide QRS complex tachycardia. The presence of irregular cannon waves and variable intensity of S_1 suggest AV dissociation and are indicative of VT. Carotid massage (performed carefully after ruling out a bruit) that leads to termination of wide QRS complex tachycardia suggests SVT as the mechanism of the arrhythmia (an exception is idiopathic VT arising from the right ventricular outflow tract).

An old ECG in sinus rhythm showing Q waves indicates VT; SVT is the diagnosis if the old ECG shows bundle branch block pattern that matches the 12-lead ECG during wide QRS complex tachycardia; and preexcited tachycardia is inferred from the ECG showing WPW pattern that is similar to wide QRS complex tachycardia ECG pattern. It is essential to obtain a 12-lead ECG during wide QRS complex tachycardia to compare it to the sinus rhythm ECG and look for subtle findings like AV dissociation and narrow beats (fusion and capture) that might not be evident in some leads. Table 23–1 outlines an approach to diagnosing wide QRS complex tachycardia by analyzing the ECG. The first step is to read the ECG with emphasis on rate, regularity (atrial fibrillation with preexcited tachycardia is irregular), axis (extreme northwest axis suggests VT), and morphology in V_1. The next step is looking for AV dissociation (V > A) that is facilitated by marching the sinus P waves at the onset and termination of the wide QRS complex tachycardia if available. Narrow QRS complexes in a wide QRS complex tachycardia (caused by capture and fusion of conducted beats through the AV node-His-Purkinje system) are also 100% specific for VT. The next

Table 23–1. Approach to the ECG with Wide QRS Complex Tachycardia.

1. **Read the ECG:** rate, rhythm, axis, morphology in V_1 (predominantly upright, RBBB; downward, LBBB)
2. **AV dissociation**
3. **Narrow complex beat:** fusion or capture
4. **Brugada criteria:** RS (measured from beginning of QRS to the nadir of S wave) in precordial leads
   a. Absence of RS in all precordial leads favors VT
   b. RS > 100 ms in any precordial lead favors VT
5. **Morphology criteria** (V_1, V_2): classic bundle branch block morphology favors SVT
   a. RBBB (rsR'): R' > r favors SVT
   b. LBBB: Kindwall criteria favors VT
      R > 30 ms, notch in S wave, QRS onset to S > 60 ms Q wave in V_6

AV, atrioventricular; LBBB, left bundle branch block; RBBB, right bundle branch block; SVT, supraventricular tachycardia; VT, ventricular tachycardia.

step is to use the Brugada criteria by evaluating the R-S complexes in precordial leads. Absence of R-S complex in all precordial leads or a R-S greater than 100 ms in one precordial lead favor a diagnosis of VT. The last step is using the morphology criteria for RBBB and LBBB in leads V_1, V_2, and V_6 (as discussed earlier). The morphology criteria have certain limitations as idiopathic VT (fascicular VT, outflow tract VT) and bundle branch reentrant VT can have a typical bundle branch block pattern on the ECG and can be misdiagnosed as SVT with aberrancy while some patients with SVT who take antiarrhythmic medications can have atypical bundle branch block pattern on the ECG, leading to a misdiagnosis of VT.

Miller JM et al. Value of the 12-lead ECG in wide QRS tachycardia. Cardiol Clin. 2006 Aug;24(3):439–51. [PMID: 16939835]

CLASSIFICATIONS OF VENTRICULAR TACHYCARDIA

The spectrum of VT in Table 23–2 lists the two most common varieties encountered in clinical practice and their underlying causes. This classification helps approach the diagnosis in a systematic fashion and directs the physician to specific therapeutic options.

Monomorphic VT is a form of VT in which the QRS complex configuration is uniform from beat to beat in all the surface ECG leads (Figure 23–2A). In **polymorphic VT,** a beat-to-beat variation occurs in the QRS complex configuration in any of the ECG leads (Figure 23–2B). These diagnoses may be difficult, however, when a single-surface ECG lead is recorded. As used in the literature, sustained VT is a tachycardia that lasts for 30 seconds or requires intervention for

Table 23-2. Classification and Causes of Common Ventricular Tachycardias.

Monomorphic ventricular tachycardia
Chronic coronary artery disease
Idiopathic dilated cardiomyopathy
Right ventricular dysplasia
No structural heart disease
    Right bundle branch block configuration
    Left bundle branch block configuration
    Repetitive monomorphic ventricular tachycardia
Other forms
Polymorphic ventricular tachycardia
Prolonged QT interval (torsades de pointes)
    Congenital
    Acquired
Normal QT interval
    Acute ischemia
    Other

termination. The definition does not imply that a prolonged episode of VT lasting less than 30 seconds has any less clinical significance. Nonsustained VT is a term used to describe any three or more consecutive QRS complexes of ventricular origin with a rate of more than 100 bpm. When describing nonsustained VT, it is important to mention the number of complexes and rate in order to convey a clear picture of the event. In this chapter, VT is considered sustained unless specifically stated otherwise.

VT is most commonly associated with structural heart disease; 15–20% of VT episodes reported in various series is seen in patients without structural heart disease and is referred to as idiopathic VT. This distinction is important because the therapeutic approach to VT is different in patients with structural heart disease compared with patients with idiopathic VT in which case catheter ablation can be curative.

VENTRICULAR TACHYCARDIA ASSOCIATED WITH STRUCTURAL HEART DISEASE

1. Monomorphic VT in Association with Chronic Coronary Artery Disease

This is the most common form encountered in clinical practice as well as the most extensively investigated in clinical and electrophysiology laboratories. The underlying substrate is usually an area of fibrosis that provides an anatomic obstacle around which the reentrant impulse can propagate. The extent and architecture of the scar may determine the propensity to VT in a given situation. For example, a homogeneous scar with no surviving conducting tissue is less likely to cause arrhythmias than is fibrosis interspersed with streaks of healthy myocardium. In some situations, acute myocardial ischemia or infarct can produce the conditions of slow conduction and block necessary for reentry. Although nonreentrant mecha-

nisms (eg, abnormal automaticity, triggered activity) may cause VT in these settings, reentry is the most common mechanism.

As myocardial activation spreads from the reentrant circuit, the resultant QRS morphology is determined by the direction of the activation vector. Because of the myocardial origin of this type of VT, some characteristic features are expected: (1) The initial part of the QRS complex will generally be inscribed slowly because of muscle-to-muscle propagation. (2) The resultant QRS width is often markedly increased because of this intramyocardial conduction delay. (3) Because the impulse is not activating the ventricles via the bundle branches, the QRS pattern is not likely to be typical of either the right or LBBB. (4) When there is no septal scar, VT originating in the left ventricle activates the ipsilateral ventricle, followed by the interventricular septum and then the right ventricle. This causes an atypical RBBB pattern. (5) Ventricular tachycardia that originates in the right ventricle shows a LBBB pattern. (6) When the tachycardia originates close to a septal scar, it may show an LBBB pattern even if the reentrant circuit resides in the left ventricle. (7) ECG leads can be used to localize the site of origin of VT from the left ventricle as follows: (a) Positive QRS complex in lead avR and negative in lead V_4 suggests apical site of origin and vice versa for basal sites. (b) Positive QRS complexes in leads II, III, and avF suggest anterior site of origin while negative QRS complex in these leads is seen in VT arising from inferior wall. (c) Positive QRS complex in leads I and avL is seen in VT arising from the septum while a negative QRS in these leads suggests origin from the lateral wall. Figure 23–3 shows scar-related VT in a patient with previous history of myocardial infarction. The VT has one reentrant circuit in the left ventricle with two different morphologies based on different exit sites.

After an initial documentation on the surface ECG, or when VT is suspected by virtue of underlying coronary artery disease and symptoms such as syncope, a further workup is often critical for characterization of VT. Ambulatory monitoring is of limited value because sustained VT is not commonly seen on a daily basis. In most situations, invasive electrophysiologic studies are indicated for these patients for both diagnostic and therapeutic purposes.

2. Monomorphic VT in Association with Idiopathic Dilated Cardiomyopathy

Monomorphic VT associated with idiopathic dilated cardiomyopathy and valvular disease is indistinguishable from VT in chronic coronary artery disease in approximately 60% of patients. The underlying substrate is most probably fibrosis, providing both the anatomic obstacle and the pathway for reexcitation. Invariably, however, these patients have conduction slowing in the His-Purkinje system as a part of the diffuse myocardial disease process, and the baseline ECG shows evidence of nonspecific intraventricular conduction defect. The resultant tachycardia uses the bundle branches and the bundle of His for sustained reentry. Bundle branch reentry could manifest as either an LBBB or RBBB pattern (Figure 23–4). Because ventricular myocardial activation occurs via the bundle branches, a typical LBBB or RBBB configuration is generally noted. Although the prevalence of bundle branch reentry is particularly high in patients with idiopathic dilated cardiomyopathy, it does occur in dilated cardiomyopathy regardless of the underlying pathology.

Bundle branch reentry is also fairly common in patients with aortic and mitral valve disease. Due to the close anatomic relationship between the proximal His-Purkinje system and annuli of these valves, His-Purkinje system conduction delays can occur in association with valvular disease. Frequently, sustained bundle branch reentry is observed soon after valve surgery, probably related to aggregation of local substrata.

3. Monomorphic VT in Arrhythmogenic Right Ventricular Cardiomyopathy

Arrhythmogenic right ventricular cardiomyopathy is a disease that causes fibrofatty infiltration in the right ventricle muscle. Because the left ventricle can be fairly normal

in these patients, arrhythmic problems, primarily VT, are the main manifestations of the underlying cardiac pathology. The amount of fibrosis and fatty infiltration into the right ventricle varies, with eventual dilatation. Genetic abnormalities in plakoglobin, desmoplakin, and the ryanodine receptor have been identified in patients with arrhythmogenic right ventricular cardiomyopathy. The VT is reentrant in nature, similar to other situations with myocardial fibrosis. The QRS morphology is that of an LBBB pattern, but the axis can be right, normal, or leftward. Unless this type of VT is specifically suspected and efforts are made to elucidate right ventricular pathology, the correct diagnosis is likely to be missed. The most common ECG finding is T wave inversion in leads V_1–V_3; presence of delayed depolarization manifested as terminal notch (epsilon wave in V_1–V_3) or timing from nadir of the S wave to the end of the QRS complex > 55 ms are more specific for a diagnosis of arrhythmogenic right ventricular cardiomyopathy (Figure 23–5). This entity should be considered in patients with VT showing an LBBB morphology and left axis when there is no obvious left ventricular pathology.

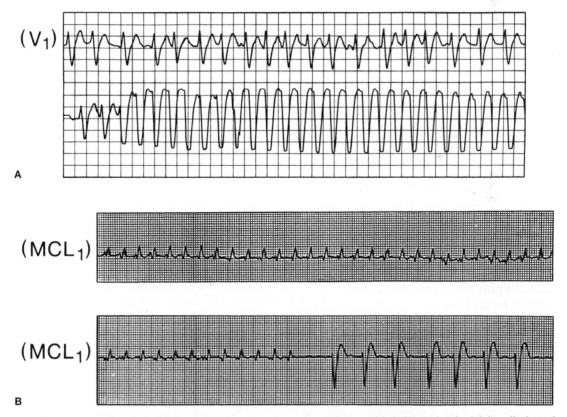

▲ **Figure 23–4.** Bundle branch reentrant ventricular tachycardia with typical left (**A**) and right (**B**) bundle branch morphologies; recorded at different times in a patient with idiopathic dilated cardiomyopathy. Note the underlying intraventricular conduction defect during baseline rhythm, before onset (**A**) and after termination (**B**). (Reproduced, with permission, from Akhtar M. Circulation. 1990;82:1561.)

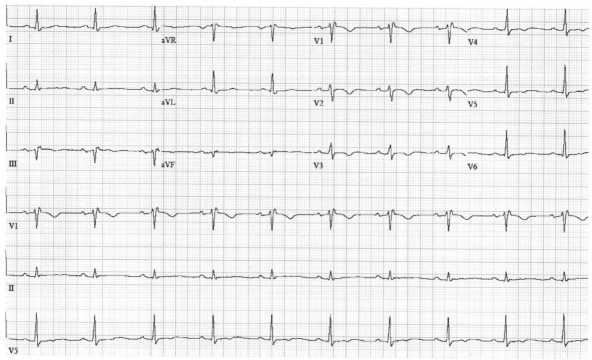

▲ **Figure 23–5.** Twelve-lead electrocardiogram in a patient with arrhythmogenic right ventricular cardiomyopathy showing T-wave inversions in V_1-V_3 and delayed depolarization in V_1.

Many patients with arrhythmogenic right ventricular cardiomyopathy have a VT circuit that arises from the epicardium rather than the endocardium and require a pericardial approach to VT ablation. The diagnosis of arrhythmogenic right ventricular cardiomyopathy is confirmed with MRI or right ventricular angiogram showing fatty infiltration of the right ventricle associated with wall motion abnormalities. Although palpitations and mild hypotension are the usual presentation, syncope and sudden cardiac death do occur in this disease.

4. Monomorphic VT in Patients with Congenital Heart Disease

Ventricular tachycardia can present late in adult life in patients with congenital heart disease (eg, tetralogy of Fallot, aortic stenosis, pulmonary stenosis). The VT is usually due to reentrant circuits between fibrotic scars and healthy myocardium. Tetralogy of Fallot usually leads to enlargement of the right ventricle with VT arising from the right ventricular outflow tract. Severity of pulmonary valvular regurgitation, late surgical repair, and QRS duration greater than 180 ms are risk factors for VT and sudden death in patients with tetralogy of Fallot.

5. Monomorphic VT in Other Forms of Structural Heart Disease

Hypertrophic cardiomyopathy is characterized by hypertrophy and enlargement of the left ventricle especially in the septum. There are fibrotic scars in the ventricle that give rise to VT. Although polymorphic VT is more common in these patients, they can also present with monomorphic VT. This is the most common cause of SCD in persons younger than age 35 years (see Chapter 25). Infiltrative cardiomyopathy associated with sarcoidosis and amyloidosis can manifest with conduction system disease and VT (reentrant VT or automatic VT) that can lead to SCD. Chagas disease is a parasitic disease that is very common in South America. It leads to fibrosis and dilated cardiomyopathy and is the most common cause of VT in South America. Risk factors for mortality in these patients include cardiomegaly on chest radiography, decreased ejection fraction, nonsustained VT on Holtor monitoring, and advanced heart failure. There is a high incidence of epicardial VT in patients with Chagas disease that requires a pericardial approach to VT ablation. Skeletal muscle disorders like myotonic dystrophy and Kearns-Sayre syndrome are associated with degenerative changes in the myocardium and the conduction system that causes AV block and VT. Mitral valve prolapse can ocassionally be associated with fibrotic and degenerative changes in the conduction system and that forms the anatomic basis for VT and sudden death.

VENTRICULAR TACHYCARDIA NOT ASSOCIATED WITH STRUCTURAL HEART DISEASE

Also called idiopathic VT, this condition is being diagnosed more often due to the better understanding of the mechanism and treatment of this form of VT. Table 23–3 enumerates the various causes of idiopathic VT classified as monomorphic and polymorphic VT. The site of origin of idiopathic VT can be diagnosed by a careful analysis of the morphology and axis on the ECG. Depending on the site of origin (eg, left versus right ventricle), the tachycardia may have a different response to therapeutic agents.

1. Idiopathic Left Ventricular Tachycardia or Fascicular VT

This form of VT arises from the fascicles in the left ventricle. Based on the QRS morphology and the site of origin it can be classified as (1) left posterior fascicular VT that has RBBB left axis morphology, (2) left anterior fascicular VT that has RBBB right axis morphology, (3) left upper septal VT (septal VT) that gives rise to a very narrow complex RBBB or LBBB morphology VT. The QRS duration in fascicular VT varies from 140–150 msec and the duration from the beginning of the QRS onset to the nadir of the S-wave (RS interval) in the precordial leads is 60–80 msec unlike VT associated with structural heart disease that is usually associated with longer duration of QRS and RS intervals (Figure 23–6). This makes it difficult to differentiate fascicular VT from SVT with aberrancy using the criteria based on QRS morphology and RS interval.

Most of the affected patients are males (60–70%). The symptoms include palpitations, fatigue, dyspnea, dizziness, and presyncope. Syncope and sudden death are very rare. Most of the episodes occur at rest; however, this form of VT can be triggered by exercise and emotional stress. Because this VT responds to intravenous verapamil, it is often referred to as verapamil-sensitive VT. Radiofrequency catheter ablation is an appropriate management strategy for patients with severe symptoms or those intolerant or resistant to antiarrhythmic therapy with a success rate greater than 92%.

2. Outflow Tract Ventricular Tachycardia

This form of idiopathic VT arises from the outflow tract of the right or the left ventricle. This form of VT is associated with a characteristic ECG morphology of LBBB with inferior axis (Figure 23–7). Lead I has a QS or qR complex in anterior sites and dominant R wave in posterior sites, while avL shows negative complex in septal sites and positive complex in lateral sites. Based on the site of origin, outflow tract VT can

Table 23–3. Idiopathic Ventricular Tachycardia.

Monomorphic Ventricular Tachycardia	Polymorphic Ventricular Tachycardia
Outflow Tract VT	Long QT syndrome
RVOT-VT	Brugada syndrome
LVOT-VT	Short coupled torsades
Aortic cusp VT	Short QT syndrome
Fascicular VT	Catecholaminergic polymorphic VT
LAF-VT	Idiopathic VF
LPF-VT	
Septal VT	
Adrenergic monomorphic VT	
Annular VT	
Mitral annular	
Tricuspid annular	

LAF, left anterior fascicular; LPF, left posterior fascicular; LVOT, left ventricular outflow tract; RVOT, right ventricular outflow tract; VF, ventricular fibrillation; VT, ventricular tachycardia.
Modified, with permission, from Badhwar N et al. Curr Probl Cardiol. 2007;32:7.

be classified as (1) VT that arises from the right ventricular outflow tract, (2) VT that arises from the left ventricular outflow tract, or (3) VT that arises from the aortic cusps (Cusp VT). Cusp VT shows earlier precordial transition (< V₂) and a broader R wave duration in V_1 and V_2. It is important to differentiate right ventricular outflow tract VT from VT associated with arrhythmogenic right ventricular cardiomyopathy that also has an LBBB morphology.

Right ventricular outflow tract VT is more common in women and is usually seen in third to fifth decade of life, while left ventricular outflow tract VT is equally distributed between men and women. Symptoms include palpitations, dizziness, atypical chest pain, and syncope. There are three predominant clinical forms of this syndrome: (1) nonsustained repetitive monomorphic VT alternating with periods of sinus rhythm, (2) paroxysmal exercise-induced sustained VT, and (3) frequent premature ventricular complexes that occasionally present as bigeminal rhythm giving rise to tachycardia-induced cardiomyopathy. In some patients, the tachycardia is provoked by exercise and isoproterenol infusion, suggesting that catecholamines triggered after depolarization may be the underlying mechanism. In most situations, intravenous adenosine will terminate the VT, and triggered activity dependent on cyclic adenosine monophosphate (AMP) may be the mechanism. Immediate termination of right ventricular outflow tract VT can also be achieved with carotid sinus massage, verapamil, and lidocaine. β-Blockers are especially effective for those with exercise-induced outflow tract

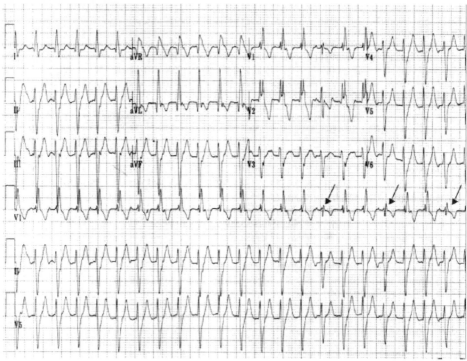

▲ **Figure 23–6.** Twelve-lead electrocardiogram of verapamil-sensitive idiopathic ventricular tachycardia (VT) arising from the left posterior fascicle with a right bundle branch block superior axis morphology. The duration of the QRS complex and the RS interval are narrower than that noted in VT associated with structural heart disease. However, the presence of atrioventricular dissociation and fusion beats (*arrows*) is diagnostic of VT. (Reproduced, with permission, from Badhwar N et al. Curr Probl Cardiol. 2007;32:7.)

VT, and a synergistic action is noted with calcium channel blockers. Antiarrhythmic agents, such as procainamide, flecainide, amiodarone, and sotalol, are also effective in these patients. Catheter ablation using radiofrequency energy to cure patients with outflow tract VT is associated with a high success rate due to the focal origin of this form of VT.

3. Annular Ventricular Tachycardia

Mitral annular VT arises from the mitral annulus in the left ventricle and is associated with RBBB morphology. Palpitations are the presenting manifestation in these patients due to repetitive monomorphic VT or frequent monomorphic premature ventricular complexes. The mechanism is thought to be triggered rhythm that terminates with the administration of intravenous adenosine and verapamil. The ECG in mitral annular VT shows a delta wave–like beginning of the QRS complex similar to that seen in patients with left-sided Wolff-Parkinson-White syndrome. Catheter ablation is associated with a high success rate (> 90%), making it a suitable alternative to drug therapy in these patients.

Recently, VT arising from the tricuspid annulus has been described that is associated with LBBB morphology. Tricus-

pid annulus VT originates more often in the septal region (74%) than in the free wall (26%). The septal VT had an early transition in precordial leads (V_3), narrower QRS complexes, Qs in lead V_1 with absence of "notching" in the inferior leads, while the free wall VT was associated with late precordial transition (> V_3), wider QRS complexes, absence of Q wave in lead V_1, and "notching" in the inferior leads. The success rate for catheter ablation of the free wall VT was 90% compared with 57% in the septal group (since its origin is in close proximity to the normal AV nodal conduction).

Badhwar N et al. Idiopathic ventricular tachycardia: Diagnosis and management. Curr Probl Cardiol. 2007 Jan;32(1):7–43. [PMID: 17197289]

DIAGNOSTIC STUDIES

Patients with sustained VT that is either documented via ECG or suspected from symptoms such as syncope or presyncope should undergo additional studies, which can confirm the diagnosis of wide QRS tachycardia, determine whether VT is the cause of unexplained symptoms, identify the underlying substrate, and determine the direction of therapy.

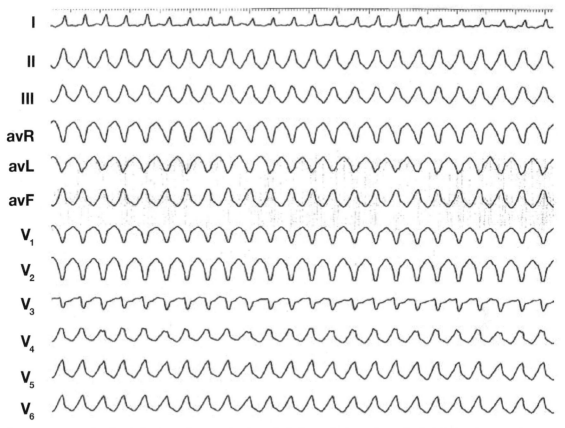

▲ **Figure 23–7.** Twelve-lead electrocardiogram that is typical of ventricular tachycardia (VT) in the absence of structural heart disease, originating in the right ventricular outflow tract. There is left bundle branch block morphology with late transition (V₄) in the precordial leads and an inferior axis in the limb leads. Negative QRS complex in lead avL suggest a septal origin. (Reproduced, with permission, from Badhwar N et al. Curr Probl Cardiol. 2007;32:7.)

In most patients with documented sustained VT, the critical components of the workup include assessment of the nature and extent of any underlying heart disease and an electrophysiologic evaluation. A noninvasive cardiovascular workup includes ambulatory monitoring to detect heart rate variability or a daily fluctuation of arrhythmia; exercise testing to detect coronary artery disease or provoke catecholamine-sensitive VT; and an echocardiographic examination to uncover structural heart disease. Cardiac catheterization is strongly recommended for patients in whom coronary artery disease is suspected. Although a 12-lead ECG is usually adequate to make an accurate diagnosis of VT (versus SVT), the precise nature may not be clear in many patients unless electrophysiologic studies are performed.

When VT is suspected but not documented, its induction in the laboratory is critical to the decision to undertake any therapeutic approach. By inducing or replicating VT in the laboratory, its rate, morphology, origin, hemodynamic tolerance, and response to intravenous drugs can be evaluated.

Catheter ablation using radiofrequency or electrical energy is an effective form of treatment in patients with bundle branch reentry, idiopathic VT, and, in some cases, VT in association with prior myocardial infarction. Thorough electrophysiologic testing is crucial for a successful outcome in these cases.

Many patients with VT have extensive cardiac pathology, including abnormalities of sinus node function and AV conduction. These abnormalities can be further aggravated with the administration of antiarrhythmic drugs. Electrophysiologic studies can frequently identify the nature and determine both the extent of these abnormalities and the need for additional therapeutic interventions (eg, permanent pacing for bradycardia).

Aside from arrhythmia assessment and cardiac substrate identification, the role of further tests in this population is dictated by the initial findings. When reversible abnormalities, such as myocardial ischemia, are detected, every attempt should be made to correct them. Paying separate attention to arrhythmias is critical because monomorphic VT is unlikely to be controlled without addressing specific VT management.

MANAGEMENT OF MONOMORPHIC VENTRICULAR TACHYCARDIA

Because monomorphic VT is most commonly due to underlying myocardial fibrosis, the pharmacologic treatment outlined here primarily relates to this substrate. The same approach can be used in other situations, but it may not be as applicable.

▶ Immediate Termination

The method of VT termination in the acute settings depends on the hemodynamic tolerance of the tachycardia. When the patient loses consciousness or has severe hypotension, a synchronized DC cardioversion should be attempted. Sedation prior to cardioversion is advised in patients who are awake. With hemodynamically well-tolerated VT, there is ample time to gather complete information, including a 12-lead ECG, before initiating therapy. Intravenous amiodarone is the drug of choice for treating VT. VT in association with acute myocardial infarction may respond to lidocaine (2–3 mg/kg). Intravenous procainamide (10–15 mg/kg) at a rate of 50–100 mg/min is also effective, but it can lead to hypotension. Intravenous calcium channel blockers such as verapamil should not be administered unless the supraventricular nature of a sustained wide QRS tachycardia (SVT with aberrant conduction) is certain. The only type of VT that responds to verapamil is uncommon. When VT is triggered or aggravated by exercise, intravenous β-blockers may be tried as the initial therapy unless there are contraindications to their use. If there is any uncertainty regarding the safety of β-blockers in patients with VT, it is somewhat safer to use agents with a short half-life, such as esmolol.

When pharmacologic intervention fails, overdrive termination can be tried. It does require insertion of a pacing catheter but can be quite useful in patients with frequent recurrent VT. Cardioversion is necessary in many situations, particularly if a prolonged VT episode is undesirable, such as in the setting of ischemic heart disease. It should also be emphasized that careful attention should be paid to other factors contributing to ventricular arrhythmogenesis, such as acidosis, hypoxia, electrolyte abnormalities, and the use of drugs. If such factors are involved, pharmacologic treatment alone may fail to control the VT.

▶ Prevention

Although acute termination of VT is relatively straightforward in most situations, the prevention of recurrences is often a challenge. The empiric use of antiarrhythmic drugs is not encouraged because of potential harm to the patient—as well as their unproven efficacy. Because VT represents a potentially life-threatening arrhythmia, establishing an effective form of therapy is desirable before the patient is discharged, especially for patients with VT-related syncope or cardiac arrest. In most situations, the therapy must be individualized, which requires understanding the type of VT, any underlying heart disease, left ventricular function, and the clinical presentation.

A. Pharmacologic Therapy

For monomorphic VT in association with chronic coronary artery disease or any other type of fibrosis, a variety of therapeutic options are now available. These include antiarrhythmic drugs, VT focal ablative therapy, and ICDs. Among the antiarrhythmic drugs, class I agents (Table 23–4) have moderate efficacy; quinidine and procainamide (class Ia) have been used extensively. In recent years, however, their use has progressively declined because of both excessive patient intolerance and lack of efficacy. Class Ib drugs such as mexiletine are weak antiarrhythmic agents when used alone, but they seem more useful in combination with Ia drugs. Class Ic drugs have moderate efficacy but a significant proarrhythmic potential; they are mainly used in patients with idiopathic VT. Exercise-induced VT generally responds well to β-blockers, and serial exercise stress tests can be used to judge drug efficacy. Because other forms of VT in patients with coronary artery disease may respond to β-blockers, they are frequently used alone or in combination with other antiarrhythmic drugs when the patient can tolerate them. At present, class III agents (eg, amiodarone, sotalol, and azimilide) are the most promising antiarrhythmic agents for control of VT and ventricular fibrillation (VF). After a loading dose of 1200–1800 mg/day for 1–2 weeks, amiodarone can be used in a maintenance dose of 200–400 mg/day. It is associated with long-term side effects that can effect the thyroid, lungs, gastrointestinal tract, eyes, skin, genitourinary system, and central nervous system. Baseline thyroid function test, liver function test, pulmonary function test, and ophthalmologic examination should be done in patients when amiodarone therapy is started, with repeat tests every 6 months. The usual daily dose of sotalol is 120–240 mg/day with monitoring of the ECG for QT prolongation during its administration or with any change in dosage. It should be

Table 23–4. Antiarrhythmic Drugs.

Class	Drug
Ia	Quinidine, procainamide, disopyramide
Ib	Mexiletine, lidocaine
Ic	Flecainide, propafenone, others (ethmozine)
II	β-Blockers
III	Amiodarone, sotolol, bepridil
IV	Calcium channel blockers

pointed out that in high-risk patients with coronary artery disease and reduced left ventricular function, none of the antiarrhythmics, including amiodarone, have been shown to decrease mortality compared with placebo. Regardless of the method used, a failure of drug response is usually an indication for nonpharmacologic treatment, which can produce excellent results.

B. Nonpharmacologic Therapy

1. Implantable cardioverter-defibrillators—These devices clearly provide the most effective form of therapy for preventing SCD in patients with VT. The ICD does not prevent VT from occurring, however; it is designed only to terminate the tachycardia or fibrillation. Most episodes of VT can be terminated with overdrive pacing; this form of therapy is usually not perceptible to the patient. There are relatively few contraindications to ICD treatment; these include incessant VT and VF secondary to reversible causes such as antiarrhythmic drugs, electrolyte abnormalities, and acute ischemia. ICDs have demonstrated a remarkable effectiveness in prevention of SCD, with an overall 1-year survival rate of 92% in patients with documented life-threatening ventricular tachyarrhythmias. A meta-analysis of ICD trials showed that the relative risk reduction of sudden death with ICDs in secondary prevention is 50% and that for primary prevention is 37% (see Chapter 25).

2. Surgical ablation—In patients with coronary artery disease and prior myocardial infarction, the VT often originates close to the infarct, thus providing the opportunity for surgical destruction of the VT site of origin. It should be considered in patients undergoing coronary artery bypass surgery who have a ventricular aneurysm or infarction and mappable VT. In patients with a left ventricular ejection fraction of at least 25%, this type of surgery can be carried out with relatively low risk and a cure rate of approximately 75%. There has been a decline in primary surgical therapy for patients with VT with the advent and widespread use of ICDs.

3. Catheter-based ablation—The development of radiofrequency catheter ablation as a therapeutic option for the treatment of arrhythmias has dramatically altered the approach to the tachycardic patient. Since its introduction in 1986, radiofrequency ablation has provided actual cure for thousands of patients with debilitating symptoms from paroxysmal SVTs and certain VTs. ICDs are the standard therapy for sustained VT in patients with structural heart disease. In patients who experience recurrent shocks from the ICD, radiofrequency catheter ablation may be used in an attempt to modify or eliminate the VT circuit and thereby reduce the number of shocks a patient may experience. The success rates for radiofrequency catheter ablation of clinical VT (not all VT foci) range from 64% to 81%.

It is almost always curative, however, for sustained VT from bundle branch reentry from any cause seen in patients with dilated cardiomyopathy. High success rates (85–100%) make radiofrequency catheter ablation a good alternative to drug therapy in patients with idiopathic VT. Radiofrequency catheter ablation is likely to play a greater role in management of VT in the future due to the development of advanced mapping systems, better catheter design, and incorporation of real-time anatomy using CT scan and MRI.

Bardy GH et al; Sudden Cardiac Death in Heart Failure Trial (SCD-HeFT) Investigators. Amiodarone or an implantable cardioverter-defibrillator for congestive heart failure. N Engl J Med. 2005 Jan 20;352(3):225–37. [PMID: 15659722]

European Heart Rhythm Association; Heart Rhythm Society; Zipes DP et al; American College of Cardiology/American Heart Association Task Force; the European Society of Cardiology Committee for Practice Guidelines. ACC/AHA/ESC 2006 guidelines for management of patients with ventricular arrhythmias and the prevention of sudden cardiac death: a report of the American College of Cardiology/American Heart Association Task Force; the European Society of Cardiology Committee for Practice Guidelines (Writing Committee to Develop Guidelines for Management of Patients with Ventricular Arrhythmias and the Prevention of Sudden Cardiac Death). J Am Coll Cardiol. 2006 Sep 5;48(5):e247–346. [PMID: 16949478]

Ezekowitz JA et al. Implantable cardioverter defibrillators in primary and secondary prevention: a systematic review of randomized, controlled trials. Ann Intern Med. 2003 Mar 18; 138(6):445–52. [PMID: 12639076]

Goldschlager N et al. A practical guide for clinicians who treat patients with amiodarone: 2007. Heart Rhythm. 2007 Sep;4(9):1250–9. [PMID: 17765636]

Soejima K et al. Catheter ablation of ventricular tachycardia in patients with ischemic heart disease. Curr Cardiol Rep. 2003 Sep;5(5):364–8. [PMID: 12917050]

POLYMORPHIC VENTRICULAR TACHYCARDIA

Recognition of polymorphic VTs and their distinction from the monomorphic variety represent the crucial first step toward appropriate management. These tachycardias tend to be rapid; they generally produce symptoms of hypotension and can readily degenerate into VF. At least two types can be recognized that must be distinguished by the presence or absence of prolonged myocardial recovery.

1. Polymorphic VT in the Setting of Prolonged QT Interval

This condition is often referred to as torsades de pointes. It can be congenital or acquired. Although the precipitating factor can differ between the two varieties, both show a prolonged QT (QTc) interval and slow, prominent, or unusual-looking T waves.

▶ Clinical Findings

Congenital long QT syndrome (LQTS) can occur with deafness (Jervell and Lange-Nielsen syndrome) or without deafness (Romano-Ward syndrome). It is mainly characterized by episodes of torsades de pointes that are often triggered by adrenergic stimulation, which can be brought about by physical exertion or mental or emotional stress. The QT interval prolongation may be subtle and can be unmasked by long pauses or adrenergic stimuli such as exercise. The electrophysiologic mechanism may be early after-depolarization for initiation and reentry for sustenance. The clinical presentation includes episodes of lightheadedness, near syncope, syncope and, in some cases, cardiac arrest. There are no obvious associated cardiac abnormalities. Characteristic patterns of QT prolongation on the ECG provide a clue to the three most common forms of LQTS (Figure 23–8). It is now clear that congenital LQTS is caused by ion channel defects. LQT_1 and LQT_2 are K^+ channel abnormalities, but LQT_3 is an Na^+ channel mutation. At least eight genetic mutations at different loci have been identified. Congenital LQTS has been proposed as one of the causes of sudden infant death syndrome; however, most of these patients have the first event around 9 to 12 years of age. LQT_1 and LQT_2 account for 80% of the cases. LQT_3 is only seen in 10% of the cases, but it accounts for most of the lethal cases of LQTS. Exercise and sudden auditory stimuli are triggers for LQT_1 and LQT_2, respectively, while LQT_3 patients have most of the events during sleep at slower heart rates. Female sex, congenital deafness, baseline QT interval > 500 msec, a prolonged interval from the peak of the T wave to the end of the T wave, and males with LQT_3 are associated with a high risk of sudden death.

Acquired LQTS can be caused by a variety of pharmacologic agents and metabolic factors (a partial list is given in Table 23–5). These patients have a partial defect in the K^+ channel I_{Kr} that becomes a complete defect in the presence of the offending agents. The main ECG abnormality is that of prolonged QT interval and often an unusual appearance of the T wave, frequently referred to as the slow wave (Figure 23–9). The QT interval prolongation may not always be striking at the normal rates but should show a measurable increase after a pause, for example, following a premature beat. Once it is manifested by any individual, however, extreme caution must be exercised because a recurrence is likely if challenged with the same triggers. This can be triggered in animal models by slow heart rates, hypokalemia, and quinidine. It is likely that each of these makes an independent contribution and that a combination of the three could be particularly arrhythmogenic. The actual list of potentially offending agents may be quite long because many pharmacologic agents have not been tested for such adverse side effects as prolongation of the QT interval, and only the widely known culprits are listed in Table 23–5.

▶ Management

The key to managing torsades de pointes related to acquired prolonged QT interval is recognizing it. Frequently, these patients have underlying monomorphic VT that is being treated with antiarrhythmic agents. The emergence of torsades de pointes in this setting may not be interpreted correctly as a side effect of the medication but as a lack of sufficient control that requires more aggressive but similar therapy. When the proper diagnosis is made, the treatment is withdrawal of the offending agent and replacement of electrolytes. Intravenous magnesium has been shown to decrease early after-depolarizations. The prompt replacement of potassium and calcium is also critical. Because hemodynamic stability is necessary to excrete the offending pharmacologic agent, the immediate suppression of torsades de

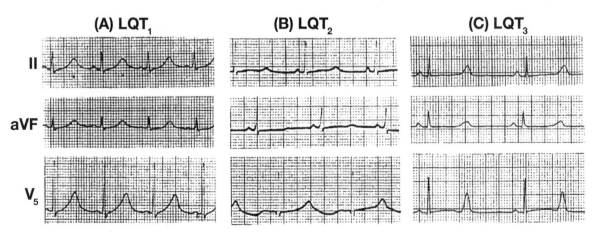

▲ **Figure 23-8.** Genotype specific T-wave morphology on electrocardiogram (ECG) in long QT syndrome (LQTS) patients. **(A)** ECG in LQT_1 showing broad-based T waves. **(B)** ECG in LQT_2 showing low amplitude T waves with notches. **(C)** ECG in LQT_3 showing extended ST segment with relatively narrow peaked T waves. (Reproduced, with permission, from Moss AJ et al. Circulation. 1995;92:2929.)

Table 23–5. Causes of Acquired Long QT Syndrome.

Antiarrhythmic drugs
Class Ia
    Quinidine (I_{Kr}, I_{To}, and I_{Ks}), disopyramide, procainamide
Class III
    Sotalol (I_{Kr}, I_{To}), d-sotalol, amiodarone (I_{Kr}, I_{Ks}), ibutilide, dofetilide (I_{Kr})
Antibiotics
Macrolides (erythromycin [I_{Kr}], clarithromycin, clindamycin), trimetho-
    prim-sulphamethoxazole, pentamidine, imidazoles (ketoconazole)
Histamine receptor antagonists
Terfenadine,[1] astemizole[1] (I_{Kr})
Serotonin receptor antagonists
Ketanserin (I_{Kr}, I_{To})[2]
Serotonin receptor inhibitors
Sertindole (I_{Kr}),[2] zimeldine[2]
Diuretics
Indapamide (I_{Ks})
Psychiatry drugs
Antidepressants (tetra/tricyclic), antipsychotic (phenothiazines,
    haloperidol, sertindole)
Cholinergic antagonists
Cisapride (I_{Kr}), organophosphates (insecticides)
Inotropic drugs
Amrinone, milrinone
Poisons
Arsenic, organophosphates (insecticides, nerve gas)
Metabolic abnormalities
Hypokalemia (I_{Kr}), hypomagnesemia, hypocalcemia
Bradyarrhythmias
Complete atrioventricular block, sick sinus syndrome
Starvation
Anorexia nervosa, "liquid protein" diets, gastroplasty, ileojejunal
    bypass
Nervous system injury
Subarachnoid hemorrhage, thalamic hematoma, right neck dissection
    or hematoma, pheochromocytoma

[1]Withdrawn from the US market.
[2]Not available in the United States.

pointes is desirable and can be accomplished with overdrive pacing or using such drugs as isoproterenol or atropine. When it is related to pauses and bradycardia, pacemaker support may be needed.

The mainstay of long-term treatment in congenital LQTS is β-blockade, and up to 5 mg/kg/day of propranolol (or 1 mg/kg/day of nadolol) may be necessary in some situations. Because cardiac slowing can also be arrhythmogenic, permanent pacing is often performed and is the therapy of choice in LQT$_3$ where β-blockers are contraindicated. Specific drugs that block the culprit ion channels include nicorandil in LQT$_1$, potassium supplements and spironolactone in LQT$_2$, and mexiletine in LQT$_3$. Clearly, drugs that prolong the QT interval must be avoided. Left stellate sympathectomy has been carried out with variable success in difficult cases. In individuals with recurrent syncope or cardiac arrest, ICDs remain a viable option to prevent SCD.

2. Polymorphic VT with a Normal QT Interval

It is not uncommon to see short episodes of polymorphic VT without any QT interval prolongation. Sustained forms of such arrhythmias can lead to VF. The true nature of this problem can be readily appreciated by observation of the QT interval prior to the tachycardia and, more reliably, following the pause that ensues after termination of VT. If no QT prolongation is noted, the following possibilities must be entertained.

Acute ischemia should be suspected with polymorphic VT in the presence of a normal QT interval. Although the exact prevalence of this type of VT is unknown, it is probably more common than realized. The VT tends to be rapid and has a tendency to degenerate into VF (Figure 23–10). Acute ischemia must be excluded in all patients with polymorphic VT in association with normal QT interval. The acute ischemia might be related to underlying coronary stenosis or coronary artery spasm brought about by a variety of factors. Prompt diagnosis and therapy are critical for preventing VT-related SCD in these patients. The workup includes coronary arteriography and an assessment for coronary artery spasm. The traditional diagnostic criteria—history of chest pain or obvious ST abnormalities—may not be present prior to the episode. A high index of suspicion is likely to lead to a correct diagnosis. This type of VT can seldom be induced in the laboratory, and the electrophysiologic mechanism for it remains unclear. The treatment, in essence, is directed toward eliminating myocardial ischemia; it might include myocardial revascularization or antiischemic drugs such as β-blockers or calcium channel blockers.

Polymorphic VT with normal QT interval can also occur in patients without substrates for myocardial ischemia but with chronic fibrosis or hypertrophy; sometimes, it can occur with no obvious pathology. It is prudent to exclude all the previously mentioned correctable causes before a diagnosis of this idiopathic variety is made. In some cases, the polymorphic VT may be inducible, suggesting a reentrant nature. Although such an arrhythmia can occur in patients with healed myocardial infarction, it is also sometimes seen in patients with hypertrophic and congestive cardiomyopathy. This type of polymorphic VT does not provide a reliable end point for drug testing or VT surgery. Antiarrhythmic drugs, particularly amiodarone, may be useful as are ICDs in preventing SCD in this population.

PROGNOSIS

Ventricular tachycardia as a warning sign for SCD differs vastly in various clinical situations. The initial presentation and the left ventricular function are, perhaps, the most important determinants. Recurrent cardiac arrest or SCD is more likely in patients who have had a previous similar

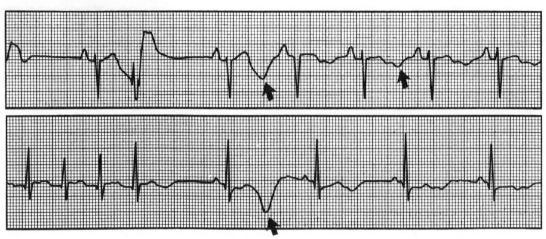

▲ **Figure 23–9.** Prolonged QT interval with slow wave. The T wave has an unusual appearance, and both the QT-interval prolongation and T-wave morphologic abnormality are more pronounced after the pause. The slow wave is indicated by the arrows. (Reproduced, with permission, from Jackman WM et al. Prog Cardiovasc Dis. 1988;31:115.)

presentation, and syncope resulting from VT also carries a poor prognosis. On the other hand, SCD in the event of VT recurrence is less likely in patients with hemodynamically well-tolerated VT. Reduced left ventricular function and VT carry a worse prognosis than does either alone.

Chiang CE et al. The long QT syndromes: genetic basis and clinical implications. J Am Coll Cardiol. 2000 Jul;36(1):1–12. [PMID: 10898405]

Priori SG et al. Risk stratification in the long-QT syndrome. N Engl J Med. 2003 May 8;348(19):1866–74. [PMID: 12736279]

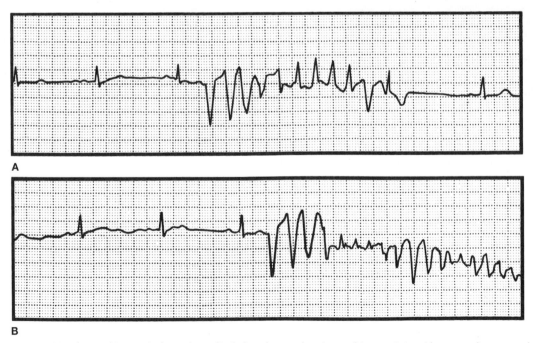

A

B

▲ **Figure 23–10.** Polymorphic ventricular tachycardia (VT) and normal QT interval in a patient with severe three-vessel disease. **A:** Several nonsustained polymorphic VT episodes. **B:** Degeneration to ventricular fibrillation, requiring DC cardioversion.

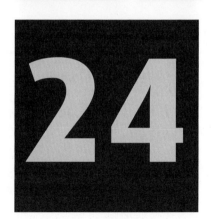

Syncope

Michael H. Crawford, MD

ESSENTIALS OF DIAGNOSIS

▶ Sudden, unexpected, and transient loss of consciousness and postural tone.

▶ Spontaneous and full recovery.

▶ General Considerations

Syncope can be defined as a sudden, transient loss of consciousness and postural tone that fully resolves spontaneously without specific intervention (eg, cardiopulmonary resuscitation [CPR], electrical or chemical cardioversion). The common pathophysiologic mechanism responsible for most syncopal spells is a transient reduction in cerebral blood flow and cerebral hypoperfusion. Reduced cerebral blood flow from cardiovascular and neurocardiogenic causes accounts for most cases in which a diagnosis can be made. Even when cerebral blood flow is normal, a reduced delivery of such essential cerebral nutrients as oxygen and sugar can occasionally cause altered consciousness.

Syncope is a common condition experienced by up to 50% of adults in a lifetime. It is responsible for about 3% of hospital admissions and 4% of emergency department visits. Physicians are frequently consulted to evaluate this symptom and—more commonly—presyncope, dizziness, or lightheadedness, which may have a similar pathogenesis.

Syncope has many causes (Table 24–1), most of which have a benign prognosis. Because cardiac causes are associated with greater morbidity and mortality, early recognition of structural heart disease or other cardiogenic causes is important in order to prevent sudden death or injury.

▶ Pathophysiology & Etiology

A. Cardiac Causes

1. Obstruction to blood flow—Any obstructive structural lesion of the left or right side of the heart can critically reduce the cerebral blood flow. Exertional symptoms are common with obstructive lesions because cardiac output does not rise normally with exercise and cerebral perfusion is not maintained. Obstruction to left ventricular outflow occurs with aortic valve stenosis, mitral stenosis, left atrial myxoma, prosthetic aortic or mitral valve dysfunction, and hypertrophic cardiomyopathy. The ventricular arrhythmias that can occur with valvular heart disease may be responsible for both exertional and nonexertional syncope as well as sudden death.

Lesions that obstruct flow through the right side of the heart include right atrial myxoma, pulmonary stenosis, tricuspid stenosis, pulmonary hypertension, and pulmonary emboli. Limitations to right ventricular outflow diminish the cardiac output and the ability to increase the output with exertion. Exertional syncope is common with severe pulmonary hypertension and severe pulmonic stenosis.

Some congenital heart diseases, such as tetralogy of Fallot, can cause syncope caused by obstruction to flow. These patients frequently have left-to-right shunts that can suddenly reverse with exertion, lessening systemic arterial oxygenation and resulting in hypoxia, which can contribute to syncope.

Nonexertional syncope can be the result of pulmonary emboli (hypoxia and obstruction of right ventricular outflow) and aortic dissection with pericardial tamponade, which impedes right ventricular filling and decreases cardiac output.

2. Electrical disturbances

A. Bradyarrhythmias and atrioventricular block— Both bradyarrhythmias and tachyarrhythmias can cause transient decreased cardiac output with resultant cerebral hypoperfusion. Bradycardias result in symptoms when the rate is so slow that the compensatory increase in stroke volume is inadequate to maintain blood pressure. Periods of ventricular asystole as short as 5 seconds can cause syncope (from the ensuing cerebral hypoperfusion). Mechanisms of symptomatic ventricular bradycardia and asystole include sinus node disease (sinus exit block, sick sinus syndrome, marked sinus bradycardia, or sinus arrest) and second- or third-degree

Table 24–1. Major Causes of Syncope.

Cardiac
Obstruction to blood flow
Valvular stenosis
Hypertrophic cardiomyopathy
Prosthetic valve dysfunction
Atrial myxoma
Congenital heart disease
Pericardial tamponade
Pulmonary hypertension
Pulmonary emboli
Pump failure (myocardial infarction or ischemia)
Arrhythmias (decreased cardiac output)
Bradyarrhythmias
Sinus bradycardia
Sick sinus syndrome
Atrioventricular block (Adams-Stokes attacks)
Pacemaker malfunction
Drug-induced bradyarrhythmia
Tachyarrhythmias
Ventricular tachycardia
Supraventricular tachycardia
Torsades de pointes
Neurocardiogenic
Vasovagal
Vasodepressor
Carotid sinus hypersensitivity
Situational (tussis, micturition, defecation, deglutition)
Other Causes
Seizures
Drugs
Hypoglycemia
Hypoxia
Hypovolemia
Cerebral vascular insufficiency
Extracranial vascular disease
Orthostatic hypotension
Neuralgia
Psychogenesis
Hyperventilation

atrioventricular (AV) block. Syncope from Mobitz II second-degree AV block with paroxysms of several consecutive P waves that fail to conduct to the ventricle is called an **Adams-Stokes** attack. Medications can also cause syncope, and any patient with syncope from bradycardia must be thoroughly questioned regarding medications. Calcium channel blockers, digoxin, β-blockers (including optical formulations), sympatholytics, primary antiarrhythmics, and other medications can all decrease heart rate and increase AV block—enough to cause symptoms in susceptible patients.

Pacemaker malfunction is another possible cause. If a pacemaker was previously implanted for sinus node disease or high-degree AV block and the patient has a recurrence of syncope, there may be a pacemaker system problem, such as battery failure or lead fracture.

B. Tachyarrhythmias—Transient decreased cardiac output during ventricular or supraventricular tachycardias results when the ventricular rate is fast enough to decrease diastole significantly and thus decrease ventricular filling (preload). Concomitant peripheral vasodepression with resultant hypotension may also play a role in the pathophysiology of syncope with supraventricular arrhythmias.

Ventricular tachycardia occurs most frequently in patients with organic heart disease, particularly coronary artery disease with previous myocardial infarction. Ventricular tachycardia is an important and ominous cause of syncope because ventricular tachycardia usually precedes ventricular fibrillation. Symptoms and prognosis are related to the degree of underlying myocardial dysfunction, and the rate and duration of the arrhythmia.

Supraventricular arrhythmias are more likely to cause palpitations and presyncope than true syncope. Although they occur often in young patients with structurally normal hearts, they are also prevalent in structurally abnormal hearts. As with ventricular arrhythmias, the severity of the symptoms is related to the ventricular rate of the arrhythmia and the degree of underlying myocardial dysfunction. Mechanisms associated with syncope include atrial arrhythmias (fibrillation, flutter, tachycardia) with rapid ventricular response, AV nodal reentrant tachycardia, and supraventricular arrhythmias associated with accessory pathways.

Torsades de pointes is a rapid polymorphic ventricular arrhythmia classically known to cause syncope in association with class I antiarrhythmic drugs. Because this arrhythmia can also cause sudden cardiac death, it is very important to understand the reversible conditions that can precipitate it. Most cases of torsades de pointes are associated with acquired long-QT syndromes that can occur with several drugs (class Ia and III antiarrhythmics, erythromycin, certain antihistamines, and tricyclic antidepressants), electrolyte abnormalities (hypomagnesemia, hypokalemia, hypocalcemia), myocardial ischemia, and central nervous system disorders. Rarely, long QT syndrome occurs congenitally, in hereditary forms of prolongation of the QT interval (with or without associated deafness).

B. Neurocardiogenic Causes

1. Vasovagal syncope—This is the most common mechanism of syncope in young, otherwise healthy individuals, constituting approximately 60% of cases. The underlying mechanism is a paradoxical autonomic reflex resulting in profound hypotension (vasodepression) that is often associated with bradycardia (vasovagal). The underlying pathophysiology of vasovagal syncope has been elucidated with the aid of tilt-table testing (see the section on Diagnostic Studies). This technique provides a controlled means of reproducing vasovagal syncope and serves as a means to guide medical therapy. Before the development of tilt-table testing, the diagnosis of vasovagal syncope was largely a matter of exclusion.

Despite extensive study by numerous investigators, several controversies still remain regarding the underlying pathophysiology of vasovagal syncope. When one stands, a significant amount of venous pooling occurs, which can shift from 300 to 800 mL of blood away from the central circulation. To counteract this gravitational effect, baroreceptors in the carotid sinus, aortic arch, and left ventricle sense decreased stretch (low pressure) and send afferent neural messages to the vasomotor center in the brainstem's medulla, which in turn sends efferent stimuli to increase peripheral sympathetic and cardiac tone (vasoconstriction and increased heart rate and contractility) and decrease vagal tone. This is the normal neural reflex arc that maintains cerebral arterial pressure and prevents hypotension or syncope with orthostatic changes.

It is believed that this reflex arc goes awry in susceptible individuals, resulting in a mixed response of vasodepression (hypotension) and cardiac inhibition (bradycardia). This symptomatic reflex arc, commonly known as a vasovagal episode, can occur as pure vasodepression or, rarely, pure cardiac inhibition; the classic mixed response is most common, with hypotension often preceding the bradycardia.

Vasovagal syncope is often, but not always, preceded by predisposing factors such as fear, pain, injury, fatigue, prolonged standing, or such medical procedures as venipuncture. During the initial phase, it is believed that blood pressure and heart rate increase in response to circulating catecholamine increase, sympathetic nerve stimulation, and vagal withdrawal. This is abruptly followed by hypotension, bradycardia, and syncope caused by inhibition of sympathetic vasoconstrictor and cardiac stimulatory activity and increases in vagal tone.

Although the exact pathophysiology is not understood, two conditions are thought to bring on the paradoxical reflex in susceptible individuals: reduced left ventricular filling (an empty ventricle) from decreased venous return; and increased left ventricular pressure from increased contractility caused by cardiac stimulation from circulating catecholamines. A vigorously contracting empty ventricle is thought to paradoxically increase left ventricular pressure (mimicking hypertension), which is sensed by left ventricular stretch receptors (C fibers). This afferent neural arc to the nucleus tractus solitarius in the medulla results in an efferent arc that paradoxically decreases sympathetic and increases vagal tone, causing hypotension and bradycardia, respectively. Because both the sinus node and AV node are richly innervated with autonomic nerves, bradycardia can be caused by both vagal depression of sinus node automaticity and decreased AV nodal conduction with AV block. Assuming a supine posture provides spontaneous resolution because the gravitational effects on cerebral blood flow are immediately neutralized. Figure 24–1 shows a two-lead ambulatory recording of a classic vasovagal episode in a patient with previously undiagnosed syncope.

Vasovagal syncope is usually considered a benign form that can often be treated with patient education and avoidance of the precipitant. Some individuals, however, have frequent severe spells that result in injuries and, rarely, sudden death. Several therapies (discussed later) are available for patients who require intervention.

2. Carotid sinus hypersensitivity—The carotid sinus has baroreceptors located in the internal carotid artery just above the bifurcation of the common carotid artery. These are sensitive to stretch and pressure and give rise to afferent impulses to the vasomotor center in the medulla. In susceptible individuals, particularly the elderly, activation of this reflex results in vagal efferent stimulation, which causes marked bradycardia or AV block (the cardioinhibitory response) with vasodepression (from efferent sympathetic inhibition). In contrast to vasovagal syncope, the cardioinhibitory response is usually dominant. Syncope from carotid sinus hypersensitivity usually is suggested by historical factors: precipitation with turning the head, shaving the neck, or wearing a tight shirt collar. Spontaneous attacks can also occur. Full consciousness is usually regained in less than a minute after attaining a supine position. When syncope from carotid sinus hypersensitivity is suspected, carotid sinus massage (CSM) can be used to diagnose this condition; hypersensitivity is generally defined as cardiac asystole of 3 seconds or more or a decline in systolic blood pressure of at least 50 mm Hg.

3. Situational—The pathophysiologic mechanisms of syncope associated with micturition, defecation, coughing, and swallowing are not precisely elucidated. It is suggested that the vagal-sympathetic autonomic reflex (hypotension and bradycardia) is involved, with afferent neural stimulation coming from the involved viscera. The Valsalva maneuver (used during micturition, defecation, and coughing) is thought to contribute to hypotension by decreasing venous return, which decreases cardiac output.

In micturition syncope, which classically occurs on waking, a combination of physiologic changes that occur during sleep (eg, sudden decompression of the bladder, decreased heart rate and blood pressure) may contribute to syncope. Tussive syncope classically occurs in middle-aged men who drink alcohol, smoke, have chronic lung disease, and experience paroxysms of severe cough; it is thought to be largely due to decreased venous return caused by the Valsalva-like action of coughing. Deglutition syncope is believed to be entirely due to dysfunction of the afferent-efferent reflex arc and is associated with structural abnormalities of the esophagus (eg, diverticula, diffuse esophageal spasm, achalasia, stricture) and heart (acute rheumatic carditis, myocardial infarction).

C. Orthostatic Hypotension

Volume depletion, medications, and autonomic dysfunction (primary and secondary) can all lead to cerebral hypoperfusion and syncope in the standing position. Primary chronic autonomic dysfunction is associated with Shy-Drager syndrome, Parkinson disease, and other rare dysautonomias. Secondary autonomic dysfunction with syncope has been described with diabetes mellitus, anemia, amyloidosis, multiple sclerosis, and HIV infection. Medications that commonly cause orthostatic hypotension include diuretics, antihypertensives (angiotensin-converting enzyme [ACE] inhibitors, β-blockers, calcium channel blockers), and ethanol.

Essential to the diagnosis of orthostatic hypotension is evaluation of postural changes in blood pressure. Normal reflex mechanisms maintain blood pressure on standing (see discussion of neurocardiogenic syncope). The inability to maintain cerebral flow when standing or sitting upright, with resultant hypotension, dizziness, or syncope, is called orthostatic hypotension. Quantitatively, it has been defined as a 20 mm Hg or greater decline in systolic pressure or a 10 mm Hg or greater decline in diastolic pressure on assuming an upright position. Because this finding is frequent and asymptomatic in the elderly, the clinical diagnosis of syncope from orthostatic hypotension requires the presence of symptoms with blood pressure changes.

D. Psychiatric Disorders

Syncope has been well described in patients with several psychiatric disorders, including anxiety disorder with panic attacks, major depression, somatization, and substance abuse. Unfortunately, these patients may also present with pseudo or fictitious syncope. Syncopal episodes with these disorders are often associated with hyperventilation.

E. Neuralgia

Both glossopharyngeal and trigeminal neuralgia can precipitate syncopal spells through paradoxical neural reflexes. Glossopharyngeal neuralgia is characterized by severe unilateral pain in the oropharynx or ear precipitated by swallowing, chewing, or coughing. Syncope is thought to occur through an afferent reflex arc involving the glossopharyngeal nerve, with resultant efferent vagal stimulation that causes a cardioinhibitory response (bradycardia or asystole). Trigeminal neuralgia involves a reflex arc as well, with paroxysmal facial pain episodes precipitating vasodepressor, cardioinhibitory, or mixed responses.

F. Syncope of Unknown Cause

No cause of syncope may be found in about one-third of patients, even after extensive evaluations.

▶ Clinical Findings

A. History and Physical Examination

According to several prospective studies, the initial clinical evaluation establishes the cause of syncope or suggests the necessary diagnostic test in up to 85% of the patients in whom a diagnosis will eventually be made. A detailed history and physical examination are therefore essential parts of the initial clinical evaluation. Relevant historical information includes all details leading up to the event, precipitating factors (micturition, cough, exertion), premonitory symptoms (aura), onset (sudden or slow), associated symptoms (palpitations, chest pain, headache), activity (at rest or with exercise), position (standing, sitting, changing position), and details about the episode (injury, incontinence, rapid recovery versus postictal state) and the frequency and severity of the events. The history should include factors suggestive of cardiac or other systemic illnesses, such as a family history of cardiac illness, arrhythmias, syncope, sudden death, or pacemaker implantation. Because about 10% of syncope is caused by the use of medications and recreational drugs, information regarding their use, prescribed dosages, and the amount actually taken is very important. All witnesses to the event (family, friends, bystanders) should be thoroughly interviewed because they can often supply details that the patient cannot. These witnesses may be able to provide information about the patient's complaints just prior to the event and observations during both the event (eg, pulse rate and rhythm, color, presence of spontaneous breathing, seizures, or seizure-like activity) and recovery. Electrocardiographic (ECG) recordings made by paramedics at the scene or recorded en route to the hospital and in the emergency department may provide important clues.

All patients need a complete cardiac, peripheral vascular, and neurologic examination, including an assessment of positional blood pressure and heart rate. Cardiac murmurs may be suggestive of structural heart disease, such as valvular stenosis. Differential blood pressure and pulse intensity may suggest aortic dissection or subclavian steal syndrome. Focal neurologic findings may point to seizure, stroke, or transient ischemic attack. The development of similar symptoms with upright posture and a corresponding decrease in blood pressure implicates orthostatic hypotension.

Several bedside maneuvers can be used to provoke syncope or presyncopal symptoms in appropriate patients. Arm flexion and extension may be used to provoke symptoms of

▲ **Figure 24–1.** Consecutive two-lead rhythm strips recorded from a patient wearing an ambulatory monitor during a vasovagal near-syncope spell, illustrating the classic response. **A:** In his diary, the patient indicates that he is possibly passing out. Because heart rate and rhythm are normal, the symptom is due to initial hypotension from vasodepression. **B:** As the episode proceeds, sinus bradycardia develops from vagal cardiac inhibition. **C:** Later still sinus rhythm is completely suppressed, resulting in a junctional escape rhythm; *open arrow* shows first junctional beat. **D:** Vagal inhibitory effect on the AV node is also shown because a sinus beat did not conduct to the ventricle (*solid arrow*). **E:** Complete resolution to normal sinus rhythm, correlated with spontaneous full recovery.

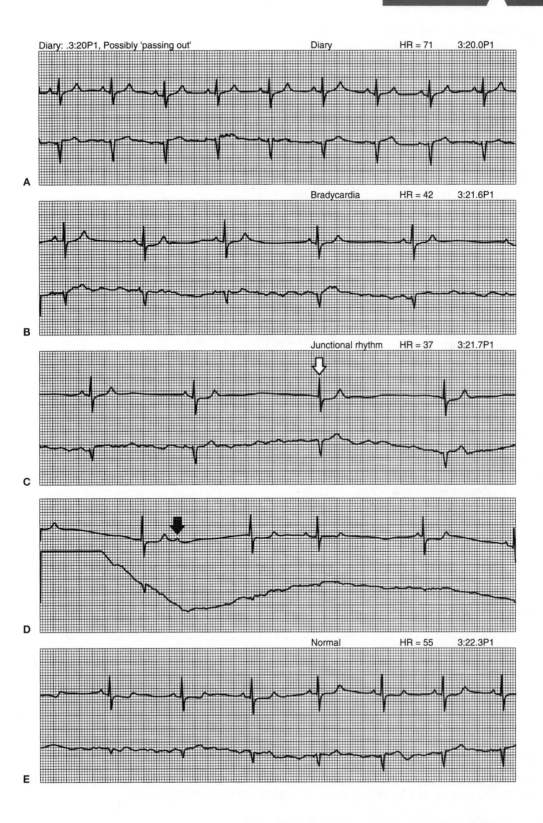

Diary: .3:20P1, Possibly 'passing out'   Diary   HR = 71   3:20.0P1

A

Bradycardia   HR = 42   3:21.6P1

B

Junctional rhythm   HR = 37   3:21.7P1

C

D

Normal   HR = 55   3:22.3P1

E

subclavian steal syndrome; neck flexion and extension may elicit the symptoms of vertebrobasilar insufficiency. Open-mouthed hyperventilation for 1–3 minutes may elicit symptoms described in the history. Carotid sinus massage (when not contraindicated by presence of bruits or known carotid arteriosclerotic disease) can be performed at the bedside with ECG and blood pressure monitoring. Although the technique is not standardized, carotid massage is usually performed with the patient in the supine position, with 5 seconds of firm massage of each carotid body. Note that simultaneous bilateral massage is never done. A positive test is defined as at least 3 seconds of asystole with hypotension or reproduction of symptoms. Because of the high false-positive rate for CSM in the elderly, the diagnosis of carotid sinus hypersensitivity should only be considered if clinical events are associated with activities that press or stretch the carotid sinus.

Toxicology screens and medication levels may provide useful information, and should be ordered if suggested by the patient's or the witness's history. Figure 24–2 outlines a suggested diagnostic approach.

B. Noninvasive Diagnostic Studies

1. Electrocardiography—A 12-lead ECG should be part of the routine clinical evaluation of syncope. A normal 12-lead ECG generally portends a good prognosis, with a very low incidence of either cardiogenic causes or diagnostic findings during invasive electrophysiologic testing. Unfortunately, the initial ECG rarely establishes arrhythmia as the cause unless complete heart block, ventricular tachycardia, or another abnormality is present at the time of the tracing. Given the unpredictably episodic nature of syncopal spells and the fact that most patients recover completely from them prior to the ECG, it is rare that the 12-lead ECG is diagnostic. More often, certain findings will suggest the possibility of a specific diagnosis. For example, Q waves suggestive of previous myocardial

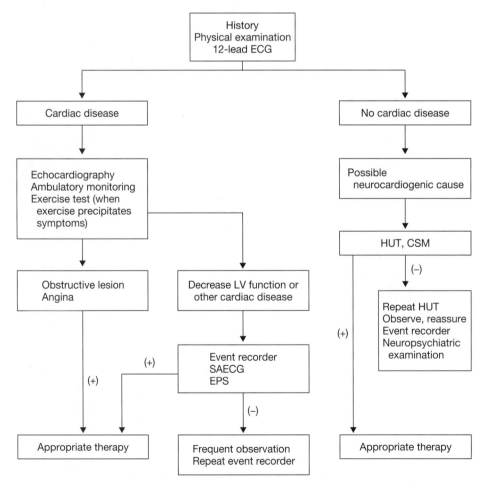

▲ **Figure 24–2.** Diagnostic approach to syncope. CSM, carotid sinus massage; ECG, electrocardiogram; EPS, electrophysiologic study; HUT, head-up tilt-table testing; LV, left ventricular; SAECG, signal-average ECG.

infarction correlate with abnormal electrophysiologic studies and the presence of inducible ventricular arrhythmias. Delta waves suggestive of Wolff-Parkinson-White syndrome make supraventricular tachycardia a very likely diagnosis. A long QT interval suggests torsades de pointes, and bifascicular block correlates with abnormal electrophysiologic findings, including high-degree AV block and inducible ventricular arrhythmias.

The most common abnormalities found in patients with syncope are bifascicular block, prior myocardial infarction, left ventricular hypertrophy, sinus bradycardia, and first-degree or Wenckebach AV block. Although these findings are all nonspecific, they may suggest a cardiac cause. The ECG or rhythm strips recorded by paramedics, the emergency department, or hospital ward lead to a specific diagnosis in about 10% of patients. The most common diagnoses include ventricular tachycardia and bradyarrhythmias caused by sinus node dysfunction or high-degree AV block.

2. Echocardiography—If the history, physical examination, and ECG do not suggest the diagnosis, or if underlying heart disease is suspected, an echocardiogram is a valuable diagnostic tool. Echocardiography may diagnose the likely cause of syncope (aortic stenosis, hypertrophic heart disease); but, more commonly, it is useful in directing further evaluation. Because morbidity and mortality with syncope are directly related to the presence and severity of structural heart disease, the echocardiogram can aid the physician in assessing the patient's prognosis and the necessity for further invasive evaluation. For example, the finding of a low left ventricular ejection fraction suggests ventricular arrhythmias and would be an indication for further electrophysiologic evaluation or an implantable defibrillator. Unsuspected findings on echocardiography are reported in 5–10% of unselected patients with syncope. Although this is similar to the ECG, the cost of the study limits it to persons with no obvious cause or suspected underlying heart disease.

3. Exercise stress testing—Exercise stress testing may be useful in patients with exertional symptoms. Exertional hypotension may occur as a result of underlying structural heart disease, chronotropic incompetence, or severe conduction disease resulting in AV block with increased atrial rates. Supraventricular and ventricular arrhythmias may be provoked with exercise. Hypotension and bradycardia at the termination of exercise can be diagnostic of reflexive vasomotor instability. Also, exercise or other forms of stress testing in those that cannot exercise may detect myocardial ischemia; a potential substrate for ventricular arrhythmias.

4. Ambulatory monitoring—Prolonged ECG monitoring can be useful for documenting transient bradyarrhythmias or tachyarrhythmias. The most common method used is a Holter ambulatory ECG recording. Typically, two surface ECG leads are recorded for a period of 24 to 48 hours. Holter recording can be particularly helpful in diagnosing bradyarrhythmias, such as significant sinus pauses and transient high-degree AV block. When interpreting Holter recordings, clinicians must recognize that several abnormalities can occur in healthy, asymptomatic patients, and correlation with symptoms is often essential. Premature atrial and ventricular contractions, brief and paroxysmal atrial tachycardia, episodic AV Wenckebach block, sinus bradycardia, sinus pauses of up to 3 seconds especially when asleep, and nonsustained ventricular tachycardia can all be seen in normal, asymptomatic patients. Sinus pauses of longer than 3 seconds, Mobitz II AV block, complete heart block, and frequent nonsustained ventricular tachycardia are far less prevalent.

Because the correlation of symptoms with an arrhythmia in patients with syncope provides the most valuable information, it is essential for the patient to keep an accurate diary of symptoms and activity during the recorded interval. Ambulatory monitoring is often useful in excluding arrhythmia mechanisms of syncope when patients experience syncope or presyncope without associated arrhythmias. Conversely, ambulatory monitoring may reveal significant conduction abnormalities or arrhythmias when the patient is asymptomatic. Frequent sinus pause of ≥ 3 seconds with associated atrial fibrillation indicates significant sinoatrial dysfunction. Asymptomatic Mobitz II AV block suggests distal conduction disease, with the possibility of prolonged AV block resulting in Adams-Stokes attacks. Nonsustained ventricular tachycardia in patients with significant left ventricular dysfunction (ejection fraction < 40%) correlates with a risk of sudden death from sustained ventricular arrhythmias and warrants further electrophysiologic evaluation (see section on Invasive Electrophysiology Studies).

A significant limitation of Holter ambulatory ECG recording is how infrequently patients experience either syncope or associated symptoms during the test. The results of studies suggest that Holter monitoring captures the heart rhythm during spontaneous syncope in only 4–10% of patients. For this reason, external ambulatory loop recorders have been used extensively for the evaluation of syncope. These devices record a single ECG lead continuously and can be worn by a patient for weeks. When activated by the patient or an observer, a rhythm strip is saved that includes several minutes surrounding the syncopal or presyncopal episode (Figure 24–3). The rhythm strip is sent to the laboratory using trans-telephonic equipment for added convenience for the patient and physician. Loop recorders are useful for evaluating patients with episodic syncope, presyncope, or dizziness, with or without associated palpitations.

For patients with infrequent symptoms, small loop recorders can be implanted under the skin and have a battery life of 1 year. They can be activated by the patient or a companion remotely, but newer models automatically record abnormal rhythms. This feature is especially valuable for patients who are rapidly incapacitated by their symptoms and cannot reliably activate a device. Although implantable loop recorders were once reserved as a last-resort diagnostic strategy, some physicians recommend earlier implantation because studies have shown diagnostic yields up to 87%.

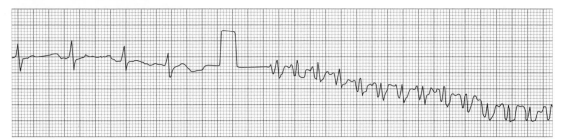

▲ **Figure 24–3.** Event recorder monitor strip received from a patient with a prior history of syncope, recurrent presyncope, and structural heart disease. The patient underwent an electrophysiology study and was found to have inducible monomorphic ventricular tachycardia that was treated with an implantable cardioverter-defibrillator.

5. Head-up tilt-table testing—Gravitational shifts in blood volume have long been recognized as a stimulus to neurocardiogenic syncope (also known as vasomotor, vasovagal, neurally mediated, or neurocardiogenic syncope). The use of the tilt table as a provocative maneuver in the diagnosis of unexplained syncope is decreasing because of concerns about the sensitivity, diagnostic yield, and reproducibility of the test. In patients with a normal cardiac evaluation, the pretest probability of neurocardiogenic syncope is high, so tilt-table testing is unlikely to be of value. The technique starts with monitoring the fasting patient for 10 minutes in the horizontal position, using noninvasive brachial or finger blood pressure, oxygen saturation, continuous ECG, and if somatization disorder is suspected, electroencephalogram (EEG) (true syncope can be differentiated from malingering). The patient is then tilted 60–80 degrees for up to 45 minutes; in children and adolescents, positive tests tend to occur sooner, and a period of 30 minutes is sufficient. The tilt produces a shift in blood volume distribution away from the central circulation and thorax to dependent peripheral vessels. This causes a decrease in central venous pressure, ventricular filling, stroke volume, and mean arterial blood pressure. Normally, activation of the baroreceptor-vasomotor reflex (described above) and renin-angiotensin system and release of catecholamines results in maintenance of blood pressure through increased heart rate and vasoconstriction. Monitoring of a normal passive tilt would show a small decrease in systolic blood pressure, with an increase in diastolic blood pressure, mean arterial pressure, and heart rate. All of these are considered normal adjustments to gravitational stress.

The test is considered positive if syncope or presyncope occurs with hypotension, with or without bradycardia. The patient is then quickly placed in the horizontal position, where normal compensatory mechanisms restore blood pressure and consciousness. The test is considered negative if symptoms and hemodynamic abnormalities fail to occur by 45 minutes of tilt. The tilt can be repeated with a provocative agent, such as the β-agonist isoproterenol, in selected patients (discussed later).

As previously discussed, various degrees of hypotension and bradycardia secondary to a paradoxical reflex that increases vagal tone and decreases sympathetic tone develop in susceptible patients. Both hypotension and bradycardia are present (a mixed response) in most patients. Hypotension usually predominates, however, and tends to occur before bradycardia (as shown in Figure 24–1). Hypotension that occurs alone, without bradycardia, is considered a purely vasodepressor response. Rarely, a patient may have a purely cardioinhibitory response (asystole).

The test has been shown to be 80–90% reproducible and specific, with a low false-positive rate (< 10%) in asymptomatic individuals. However, sensitivity ranges from 25% to 80% depending on the population studied. The 2006 AHA/ACCF scientific statement of the evaluation of syncope no longer recommends routine tilt-table testing for undiagnosed syncope. However, there are some patients in whom the diagnosis is unknown after a cardiac evaluation and the history is not helpful. Some of these patients would benefit from a tilt-table test, whereas in others a presumptive diagnosis of neurocardiogenic syncope is adequate.

6. Other testing—Routine laboratory tests (blood counts and chemistries) rarely reveal useful diagnostic information. Unless specifically suggested by the history and physical examination, it is not recommended in the evaluation of syncope. Likewise, EEG, CT, or MRI studies are of little use in patients whose history is not suggestive of a neurologic cause. These tests should be considered only in those patients whose neurologic history and physical examination are suggestive of seizure or other neurologic condition. Although routinely performed, the usefulness of transcranial Doppler ultrasonography in patients with syncope is unclear. Transient ischemic attacks rarely result in syncope without other associated symptoms. In patients with bruits on physical examination, ultrasonography is reasonable and may be useful in leading to a diagnosis.

C. Invasive Electrophysiology Studies

An invasive electrophysiology study (EPS) uses multielectrode catheters inserted percutaneously and guided under fluoroscopy or by magnetic sensors to specific cardiac locations. Electrode recording and pacing protocols are then performed to assess the patient's conduction system, including sinoatrial and AV nodal function and the distal conduction system (His-Purkinje). In addition, supraventricular and ventricular arrhythmias may be induced and their mechanisms determined in susceptible patients. In selected patients, ablation of the arrhythmic substrate with radiofrequency energy can be performed, often curing the patient of the condition.

Because patients are generally supine and sedated during EPS, one significant limitation is the inability to definitely correlate induction of arrhythmias with syncope; however, a rapid tachycardia associated with a significant decrease in systolic blood pressure generally supports the clinical importance of inducible arrhythmias. Induction of certain arrhythmias, such as atrial fibrillation, atrial flutter, polymorphic ventricular tachycardia, and ventricular fibrillation, can be a nonspecific finding. Asymptomatic patients with normal hearts can have all these induced with aggressive stimulation protocols.

The AHA/ACCF scientific statement on the evaluation of syncope does not recommend routine EPS in patients without underlying heart disease. It does recommend EPS in patients with cardiac disease and syncope that remains unexplained after appropriate evaluation, especially if the ejection fraction is reduced. In addition, EPS is reasonable in patients with recurrent unexplained syncope without structural heart disease and a negative head-up tilt test. In patients with no structural heart disease, normal ECG, normal ambulatory monitoring, and recurrent syncope not associated with injury, EPS is usually not diagnostic. EPS is not indicated in patients with a known cause of syncope for whom treatment will not be guided by electrophysiology testing.

The most significant finding at EPS is the induction of ventricular tachyarrhythmias. In addition, the induction of supraventricular tachycardias with associated hypotension is considered a positive study. Other significant findings include a prolonged corrected sinus node recovery time longer than 1000 ms, prolongation of the His-to-ventricle activation interval greater than 100 ms (normally 35–55 ms), or induction of infra-Hisian conduction block during rapid atrial pacing. These three findings are associated with significant bradyarrhythmias. Unfortunately, the diagnostic sensitivity of EPS for bradyarrhythmias is low, and further ambulatory monitoring is often necessary after a nondiagnostic EPS.

Ermis C et al. Comparison of automatic and patient-activated arrhythmia recordings by implantable loop recorders in the evaluation of syncope. Am J Cardiol. 2003 Oct 1;92(7):815–9. [PMID: 14516882]

Gula LJ et al. External loop recorders: determinants of diagnostic yield in patients with syncope. Am Heart J. 2004 Apr;147(4):644–8. [PMID: 15077079]

Krahn AD et al. Cost implications of testing strategy in patients with syncope: randomized assessment of syncope trial. J Am Coll Cardiol. 2003 Aug 6;42(3):495–501. [PMID: 12906979]

Rockx MA et al. Is ambulatory monitoring for "community-acquired" syncope economically attractive? A cost-effectiveness analysis of a randomized trial of external loop recorders versus Holter monitoring. Am Heart J. 2005 Nov;150(5):1065. [PMID: 16290999]

Shen WK et al. Syncope Evaluation in Emergency Department Study (SEEDS): a multidisciplinary approach to syncope management. Circulation. 2004 Dec 14;110(24):3636–45. [PMID: 15536093]

Strickberger SA et al; American Heart Association Councils on Clinical Cardiology, Cardiovascular Nursing, Cardiovascular Disease in the Young, and Stroke; Quality of Care and Outcomes Research Interdisciplinary Working Group; American College of Cardiology Foundation; Heart Rhythm Society; American Autonomic Society. AHA/ACCF Scientific Statement on the evaluation of syncope: from the American Heart Association Councils on Clinical Cardiology, Cardiovascular Nursing, Cardiovascular Disease in the Young, and Stroke, and the Quality of Care and Outcomes Research Interdisciplinary Working Group; and the American College of Cardiology Foundation: in collaboration with the Heart Rhythm Society: endorsed by the American Autonomic Society. Circulation. 2006 Jan 17;113(2):316–27. [PMID: 16418451]

▶ Differential Diagnosis

A. Seizure

True seizures are rarely established as the cause of a syncopal event, although they are frequently considered. A history of loss of bowel or bladder tone, witnessed convulsions, a preceding aura, and slow recovery with prolonged postictal state strongly suggest seizure. Syncope occurs frequently without a preceding aura or loss of sphincter tone and characteristically has a rapid spontaneous recovery without postictal state.

Some factors blur the distinction between these two entities: convulsions may occur with syncope (from cerebral anoxia or ischemia), the episode may be unwitnessed, the patient may not be able to recall associated symptoms, and the patient may have temporal lobe epilepsy, in which loss of consciousness is not associated with tonic-clonic movements. Temporal lobe epilepsy can also cause arrhythmias. Electroencephalography is indicated when the history cannot provide a clear distinction between syncope and seizure.

B. Metabolic Disorders and Hypoxia

Any condition that starves the cerebrum of essential nutrients (electrolytes, oxygen, glucose) or markedly changes pH can cause somnolence or coma. These conditions are not usually associated with spontaneous recovery (ie, without intervention); they tend to be longer lasting, and treatment is directed at the underlying abnormality. Hypoglycemia in outpatient diabetics, resulting from excessive insulin injection, can cause somnolence with a normal pulse and blood pressure; it is rapidly correctable with glucose.

C. Cerebral Vascular Insufficiency and Extracranial Vascular Disease

Although altered states of consciousness are known to occur with cerebral vascular events, true syncope is an uncommon presentation. Diseases of the intracranial and extracranial vessels can cause strokes and transient ischemic attacks, rarely syncope. Focal neurologic defects found during the physical examination are clues to the presence of cerebral vascular insufficiency, and differential peripheral arterial pressures or bruits suggest extracranial arterial disease. The extracranial arteries most commonly involved are the vertebrobasilar (occlusion), carotids (occlusion, emboli), aortic arch (dissection), and subclavian artery (stenosis), which may produce the subclavian steal syndrome.

D. Psychiatric Disorders with Hyperventilation and Pseudoseizure

Psychiatric illnesses are an important cause of syncope, especially in younger patients with multiple episodes and no organic heart disease. Depression, anxiety attacks, somatization disorder, panic disorder, and substance abuse (eg, alcohol, cocaine, sedatives) have all been associated with syncopal spells. In addition, pseudoseizure that may or may not be associated with true seizure disorder may be present.

Hyperventilation may cause syncope by producing hypocapnia and metabolic alkalosis, both of which stimulate cerebral arterial chemoreceptors to produce cerebral arterial vasoconstriction and decrease blood flow. Hyperventilation is frequently associated with such psychiatric illnesses as anxiety, depression, and panic attacks, but it can also occur sporadically in patients without psychiatric disease. A history of rapid breathing and perioral numbness is suggestive. A monitored hyperventilation maneuver that reproduces the patient's symptoms helps confirm the diagnosis.

▶ Treatment

Medical therapy is primarily targeted toward tachyarrhythmias, and pacemakers are generally used for bradyarrhythmias. In some situations, however, both are needed. For example, in sick sinus syndrome, a pacemaker is needed to prevent sinus bradycardia and pauses, and antiarrhythmic medications are needed to prevent the tachycardia (paroxysmal atrial fibrillation and flutter). Moreover, antiarrhythmic drugs can exacerbate bradycardia in some patients and necessitate implantation of a pacemaker to prevent medication-induced bradycardia and syncope.

A. Pharmacologic and Nonpharmacologic

Supraventricular arrhythmias can be treated with an assortment of antiarrhythmic medications (sodium channel blockers, β-blockers, potassium channel blockers, calcium channel blockers) with a wide range in therapeutic efficacy. Inherent in the medical treatment of arrhythmias, unfortunately, is a consistently high rate of side effects and the occurrence of proarrhythmia, worsening the arrhythmia or creating new arrhythmias such as torsades de pointes. Sustained ventricular arrhythmias can be suppressed with antiarrhythmic drugs; however, recent studies favor their use only in combination with an implantable cardioverter-defibrillator (ICD) in most patients.

Coronary artery, valvular, and other structural heart disease can usually be managed medically. If the disease has reached the point of causing syncope, however, it is usually severe enough to warrant surgical intervention or, percutaneous revascularization.

Neurocardiogenic and situational syncope can be treated in a number of ways (Table 24–2). Education and avoidance of known precipitants are a first step. α-Agonists, such as ephedrine or midodrine, can be used to enhance vasoconstriction and counteract the vasodilation portion of the reflex arc. β-Blockers (eg, metoprolol, pindolol) have been used effectively; they are thought to work by decreasing inotropy and preventing the afferent loop of the paradoxical reflex arc. Propantheline and scopolamine have been used for their anticholinergic effects against the vagal efferent loop of the reflex. The sodium channel blocker disopyramide has been used successfully, although its mechanism of action against neurocardiogenic syncope is poorly understood. Theophylline, an adenosine antagonist, has also been used successfully (adenosine is thought to be a mediator of vasodepression in the reflex arc). Some success has been reported using the antidepressants (serotonin reuptake inhibitors) fluoxetine and sertraline. Although the mechanism of action is not fully understood, serotonin is believed to play a central role in the development of vasovagal syncope. Volume expansion with liberalization of salt and water intake, administration of the mineralocorticoid

Table 24–2. Medical Treatment of Neurocardiogenic Syncope.

Class	Drug	Dosage Range
α-Agonists	Ephedrine	24 mg, two to four times daily
	Etilefrine	15–30 mg/day
	Midodrine	2.5 mg, two or three times daily, up to 40 mg/day
β-Blockers	Metoprolol	25–100 mg, twice daily
	Pindolol	5–30 mg, twice daily
Anticholinergics	Propantheline	7.5–15 mg, three times daily
	Scopolamine patch	1.5 mg over 3 days
Sodium channel blocker	Disopyramide CR	150–300 mg, twice daily[1]
Adenosine antagonist	Theophylline	200–450 mg, twice daily[1]
Serotonin antagonist	Sertraline	50–200 mg/day
Antidepressant	Fluoxetine	20–80 mg/day
Mineralocorticoid	Fludrocortisone	0.1 mg/day

[1]Dose can be guided by serum levels.
CR, controlled release.

fludrocortisone, and the use of thigh-high elastic stockings are effective because they can augment venous return. Also, isometric exercise such as handgrip and leg tensing can raise systemic blood pressure and prevent syncope if applied as soon as premonitory symptoms are appreciated.

None of these therapies has been shown to have any particular therapeutic advantage over the others. The specific therapy chosen should be based on the patient's age, lifestyle, and medication side effects. Each therapy can be given an empiric trial until an effective agent is found, or a repeat tilt-table test response can be used as a guide to long-term therapy.

When drug-induced syncope is suspected, the offending agent should be discontinued and the patient monitored closely for recurrence. In the case of documented or suspected torsades de pointes, the underlying drug; electrolyte abnormality; or thyroid, neurologic, or cardiac cause must be sought and corrected. Intravenous magnesium, lidocaine, or isoproterenol or temporary ventricular pacing can be used to stabilize a patient with torsades de pointes while the underlying problem is corrected.

B. Electrophysiologic Therapies

Implantable devices, such as the ICD and pacemakers, surgical procedures, and catheter ablation have all been used to treat syncope in appropriate patients. Besides causing syncope, ventricular tachycardia has the potential to degenerate to ventricular fibrillation. Many electrophysiologists consider syncope with ventricular tachycardia to be aborted sudden cardiac death. For this reason, patients with structural heart disease, documented ventricular tachycardia, and associated syncope are best treated with an ICD; moreover, patients with structural heart disease, syncope of unknown origin, and inducible ventricular arrhythmias during EPS are also most commonly treated with an ICD. The device continuously monitors the patient's heart rate and can apply a DC shock to convert ventricular fibrillation or tachycardia to sinus rhythm. ICDs have been found to reduce the likelihood of mortality in appropriate patients when compared with antiarrhythmic drugs. Although an ICD does not always prevent syncope, it effectively prevents sudden cardiac death. In addition, an ICD can terminate some ventricular tachycardias with rapid ventricular antitachycardia pacing (ATP). This therapy is painless and often unnoticed by the patient.

Ventricular tachycardia with associated ventricular aneurysm has also been successfully treated with open heart surgical ablation. With the development of nonthoracotomy ICD implantation, surgical ablation has become less common. In addition, nonsurgical catheter ablation techniques have been developed that allow for the treatment of some selected patients in the electrophysiology laboratory. In most patients, surgical or catheter ablation is used to reduce frequent appropriate ICD shocks and does not replace ICD therapy.

Single- and dual-chamber pacemakers are very effective in reducing symptomatic recurrences and preventing sudden death in patients with syncope caused by bradyarrhythmias

from sinus node dysfunction, sick sinus syndrome with bradyarrhythmias and tachyarrhythmias, high-degree AV block, and carotid sinus hypersensitivity. Pacemaker therapy has been shown to have little role in treating neurocardiogenic syncope, largely because vasodepression is often the dominant component of the reflex and is not corrected by pacing. Pacemaker implantation may occasionally be appropriate for these patients if temporary pacing shows that the symptoms can be minimized (converting syncope to dizziness only) or if the episodes are purely cardioinhibitory. It may also be considered if multiple medications have been ineffective in severely diseased patients with mixed (vasodepressive and cardioinhibitory) episodes and the desired goal is to convert syncopal to presyncopal spells by abolishing the cardioinhibitory component.

In the past decade, electrophysiologic percutaneous catheter techniques using radiofrequency energy as an ablative source have been more than 95% effective in curing patients with supraventricular arrhythmias from AV nodal reentry or accessory pathways. Although successful ablation of atrial tachycardias, atrial flutter, some ventricular tachycardias, and even atrial fibrillation can be performed in selected patients, recurrence is not uncommon. In the case of atrial fibrillation with an uncontrollably rapid and symptomatic ventricular response, creation of complete heart block with catheter ablation and implantation of an activity-modulated ventricular pacemaker can effectively ameliorate symptoms.

Connolly SJ et al; VPS II Investigators. Pacemaker therapy for prevention of syncope in patients with recurrent severe vasovagal syncope: Second Vasovagal Pacemaker Study (VPS II): a randomized trial. JAMA. 2003 May 7;289(17):2224–9. [PMID: 12734133]

Lu CC et al. Water ingestion as prophylaxis against syncope. Circulation. 2003 Nov 25;108(21):2660–5. [PMID: 14623807]

Sheldon R et al; POST Investigators. Prevention of Syncope Trial (POST): a randomized, placebo-controlled study of metoprolol in the prevention of vasovagal syncope. Circulation. 2006 Mar 7;113(9):1164–70. [PMID: 16505178]

van Dijk N et al; PC-Trial Investigators. Effectiveness of physical counterpressure maneuvers in preventing vasovagal syncope; the Physical Counterpressure Manoeuvres Trial (PC-Trial). J Am Coll Cardiol. 2006 Oct 17;48(8):1652–7. [PMID: 17045903]

▶ Prognosis

The studies to date suggest that mortality rates in patients with syncope are strongly correlated with the presence or absence of underlying structural heart disease. Dividing syncope patients into three groups is helpful for assessing their prognosis. In patients with cardiac causes of syncope, mortality is high at 1 year, ranging from 18% to 33%. In patients with noncardiac causes of syncope, 1-year mortality is much lower and ranges from 0% to 12%. Patients in whom syncope remains of unknown origin (despite an appropriate directed workup) do fairly well with a 6% 1-year mortality rate. The incidence of sudden death in the cardiac patients is also much higher than in the other two groups. Recurrence rates in all three groups are similar: up to 15% per year. Recurrences do not predict an increase in mortality, although they are associated with increased morbidity (eg, fractures, soft tissue injury).

Recurrent syncope of unknown origin remains a difficult management problem. Patients with multiple atraumatic episodes and structurally normal hearts are more likely to have psychiatric illness or neurocardiogenic syncope and less likely to have electrophysiologic abnormalities at EPS. Memory-loop event recorders (to rule out bradyarrhythmias and tachyarrhythmias), tilt-table testing, and neuropsychiatric evaluation are probably the best means of evaluating these patients further. Patients with syncope of unknown origin and no structural heart disease have an excellent prognosis. They need to be reassured, but close follow-up and episodic reevaluation are also recommended. Intensive follow-up and reevaluation are needed for the patient with underlying heart disease and syncope of unknown origin. Such patients are not rare, and therapy should be directed at likely causes (such as EPS-induced sustained ventricular tachycardia). Empiric therapy (such as antiarrhythmic medication to suppress ventricular ectopy) is not without significant risk, however, and cannot be recommended as a general approach.

Kapoor WN. Syncope. N Engl J Med. 2000 Dec 21;343(25):1856–62. [PMID: 11117979]

Sudden Cardiac Death

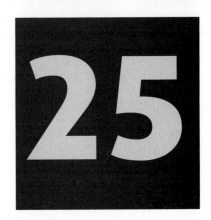

John P. DiMarco, MD, PhD

ESSENTIALS OF DIAGNOSIS

► Unexpected death occurring within an hour of onset of symptoms.

► Primary electrical mechanisms include ventricular fibrillation, ventricular tachycardia, asystole, and pulseless electrical activity.

▶ General Considerations

Each year in the United States, more than 250,000 individuals die suddenly of some form of cardiovascular disease. Because of the many advances made during the past 30 years in clinicians' ability to identify and modify the risk factors associated with sudden death, to resuscitate victims of cardiac arrest, and to prescribe specific antiarrhythmic therapy to prevent recurrences, age-adjusted sudden death mortality rates have declined dramatically. However, the number of elderly individuals in the population has increased, and sudden cardiac arrest remains an important problem.

In a simplistic sense, any death can be considered sudden. For general clinical purposes, however, the term "sudden cardiac death" is usually reserved for those deaths in which the patient had stable cardiac function until the terminal event, with death occurring within a short time (often defined as less than 1 hour) of the onset of symptoms. Some experts prefer the term "instantaneous death," namely, death with immediate collapse without preceding symptoms. Instantaneous death is usually assumed to be due to primary arrhythmia, but other catastrophic events, such as a massive pulmonary embolism, the rupture of an aortic aneurysm, or a stroke, can also cause instantaneous death. It is also important to note that not all arrhythmic deaths are sudden. For example, a patient who is resuscitated from a cardiac arrest may die days or weeks later from complications of the arrest. This death would be due to an arrhythmia but would

not meet the standard definition for instantaneous or sudden death.

Effective evaluation and treatment of patients at risk for cardiac arrest and sudden death require an understanding of the responsible pathophysiologic mechanisms, the strategies proposed for primary prevention, the techniques and results of resuscitation, and the treatment modalities for secondary prevention in survivors of an initial episode.

Rosamond W et al; American Heart Association Statistics Committee and Stroke Statistics Subcommittee. Heart disease and stroke statistics—2008 update: a report from the American Heart Association Statistics Committee and Stroke Statistics Subcommittee. Circulation. 2008 Jan 29;117(4):e25–146. [PMID: 18086926]

▶ Pathophysiology & Etiology

A number of different electrophysiologic mechanisms may be responsible for sudden cardiac death. When ambulatory electrocardiographic (ECG) recordings from the time of an out-of-hospital cardiac arrest are examined, ventricular fibrillation and rapid ventricular tachycardia are the most commonly documented initial arrhythmias. Bradyarrhythmias, including atrioventricular block, asystole, or electromechanical dissociation, are also observed. The prevalence of these latter arrhythmias is higher in the setting of progressive and advanced underlying heart disease; in the elderly; and in patients whose sudden death is precipitated by an acute catastrophe, such as a pulmonary embolism, an acute myocardial infarction, rupture of a major vessel, or a major neurologic insult. The focus of this chapter will be principally those sudden deaths for which an arrhythmia was the primary cause.

A. Coronary Artery Disease

Although sudden death occurs in all forms of heart disease, in the United States and Europe, coronary artery disease is the most common cardiac diagnosis seen in sudden death victims

(Table 25–1). Several mechanisms can produce potentially fatal arrhythmias among patients with coronary artery disease, and it is often difficult to define the precise factors that underlie a given episode. At one extreme is the patient with a previously normal ventricle who has an acute occlusion of a major epicardial coronary artery in whom ventricular fibrillation then develops during the first minutes of an acute infarction. This patient represents an example of pure ischemic injury without associated prior scar. At the other end of the spectrum is the patient with a history of a single-vessel occlusion and an old myocardial infarction, in whom postinfarction scarring has provided the anatomic substrate for a rapid reentrant ventricular tachycardia that results in hemodynamic collapse and sudden death. Acute ischemia need not be involved. In coronary artery disease, the individuals at highest risk for sudden death have both multivessel disease and myocardial scarring from one or more prior infarctions. Even in such individuals, sudden cardiac arrest may be the first clinical manifestation of the disease. As treatment of acute myocardial infarction has become more aggressive during the past 20 years, the nature of the typical scar that results from a myocardial infarction has also changed. Dense scar tissue with aneurysm formation, the classic substrate associated with uniform morphology ventricular tachycardia, is now seen less often. After pharmacologic or mechanical reperfusion, the current standards of therapy, the infarct zone shows mostly patchy fibrosis, and in such areas disorganized arrhythmias predominate. In patients with this complex substrate, sudden death is thought to result from a complex interaction between some triggering event, such as ischemia, autonomic nervous system dysfunction, electrolyte imbalance, or drug toxicity, and the unstable electrophysiologic milieu created by prior infarction.

Autopsy and clinical studies have highlighted this complexity. Coronary artery thrombi or plaque rupture may be detected in up to 50% of sudden death victims, but new Q wave myocardial infarctions will develop in only about 25% of patients resuscitated from an out-of-hospital cardiac arrest. Angiographic studies in cardiac arrest survivors have shown that a high proportion of persons have long, diffusely irregular, and ulcerated coronary lesions similar to those seen in patients with acute coronary syndromes. Therapy directed at ischemia reduces the incidence of sudden death. Aggressive surgical revascularization has been shown to decrease late sudden death mortality. In the Coronary Artery Bypass Graft (CABG-Patch) trial, no survival benefit over control was seen in patients who received an implantable cardioverter defibrillator (ICD) at the time of their revascularization surgery. Based on this confusing overall picture, it is prudent in any individual with coronary disease to consider ischemia as an important, potentially reversible risk factor for sudden death, even in the absence of clinical angina. In previously asymptomatic individuals, coronary artery disease may still be the cause of sudden death. Significant coronary artery disease may be asymptomatic or unrec-

Table 25–1. Cardiac Conditions Associated with Sudden Death.

Diseases of the coronary arteries
Atherosclerotic
Acute ischemia or infarction
Prior myocardial infarction
Congenital coronary anomalies
Others
Spasm
Arteritis
Dissection
Diseases of the aorta
Marfan syndrome
Aortic aneurysm
Diseases of the myocardium
Hypertrophic cardiomyopathies
Dilated cardiomyopathies
Valvular heart disease
Arrhythmogenic right ventricular cardiomyopathy
Congenital heart disease
Infiltrative cardiomyopathy
Primary pulmonary hypertension
Myocarditis
Chagas disease
Neuromuscular disorders with cardiac involvement
Primary electrophysiologic disorders
Long-QT syndrome: acquired and congenital
Brugada syndrome
Catecholaminergic polymorphic ventricular tachycardia
Preexcitation syndromes
Congenital atrioventricular block
Other
Drug ingestion
Commotio cordis
Electrolyte disorders
Diet related

ognized, and the general population contains a large number of such individuals. Up to 50% of all sudden cardiac deaths due to coronary artery disease may occur in individuals not previously known to have the condition.

Other diseases of the coronary arteries are rare causes of sudden death. An anomalous origin of a coronary artery may give rise to either myocardial scarring with late ventricular tachycardia or to arrhythmias mediated by acute intermittent ischemia. Similar mechanisms affecting patients with coronary artery spasm, embolism, trauma, dissections, or arteritis may cause sudden death.

B. Hypertrophic Cardiomyopathy

In hypertrophic cardiomyopathy, sudden death tends to occur in young adults who often have had no prior cardiac symptoms. There appears to be an excess of events during vigorous exercise. Teenagers or young adults in some kindreds with familial hypertrophic cardiomyopathy have a higher incidence of sudden death than do older members. In other families, sudden death in young adults is uncommon but may occur after heart failure has developed.

Several clinical risk factors for sudden death in patients with hypertrophic cardiomyopathy have been determined. These include a family history of sudden death; recurrent, unexplained syncope; nonsustained ventricular tachycardia during ambulatory monitoring; hypotension during exercise; and severe (> 30 mm) left ventricular hypertrophy. Genetic studies of patients with hypertrophic cardiomyopathy have revealed mutations in the genes for more than 10 myocardial proteins. Some mutations (eg, those in troponin T) may be associated with a high risk of sudden death even in the absence of marked left ventricular hypertrophy. Polymorphic ventricular tachycardia or ventricular fibrillation, rather than monomorphic ventricular tachycardia with a scar-related intramyocardial circuit, is thought to be the initial arrhythmia at the time of cardiac arrest in patients with hypertrophic cardiomyopathy. Due to the severe hypertrophy and conduction system disease seen in patients with hypertrophic cardiomyopathy, sustained ventricular tachycardia due to reentry in the His-Purkinje system may occur and result in hemodynamic collapse with sudden death. Patients with hypertrophic cardiomyopathy are also at risk for sudden death due to atrioventricular block and supraventricular arrhythmias because any change in rhythm that produces significant ischemia in the hypertrophied ventricular wall may degenerate to a fatal arrhythmia.

C. Nonischemic Dilated Cardiomyopathy

Nonischemic dilated cardiomyopathy is the primary cardiac diagnosis in about 10% of patients who have been resuscitated after cardiac arrest. Sudden death accounts for about half of all deaths in patients with this diagnosis. In contrast to the situation in some forms of hypertrophic cardiomyopathy, sudden death tends to occur relatively late in the course of dilated cardiomyopathy, after hemodynamic symptoms have been present for some time. A variety of arrhythmias have been implicated in patients with this condition; both monomorphic and polymorphic ventricular tachycardias are seen in patients with nonischemic dilated cardiomyopathies. Intraventricular conduction delays may lead to ventricular tachycardia caused by macroreentry in the His-Purkinje system. In patients with this arrhythmia, catheter ablation of one of the bundle branches may be curative. In patients with cardiomyopathies and very advanced heart failure, bradyarrhythmias, rather than tachyarrhythmias, are the initial recorded rhythm in up to 50% of cardiac arrests.

D. Other Cardiac Diseases

In valvular heart disease, sudden death can occur in several ways. Sudden death is usually related to exertion in young adults with congenital aortic stenoses. In other forms of valvular heart disease, sudden death is usually a late occurrence seen in patients with advanced heart failure and

ventricular hypertrophy. Although symptomatic atrial and ventricular arrhythmias are common in patients with mitral valve prolapse, truly life-threatening arrhythmias are rare, except in the presence of some complicating condition, such as a long QT syndrome, electrolyte imbalance, or drug toxicity. In pulmonary hypertension, sudden death may occur from hemodynamic causes, bradyarrhythmias, or tachyarrhythmias.

Arrhythmogenic right ventricular cardiomyopathy (ARVC) is a regional myopathy with primarily right ventricular involvement. When genetic studies have been performed, mutations in one of the desmosomal proteins are often found. These patients usually have a left bundle branch block morphology ventricular tachycardia. Symptoms and signs of right ventricular dysfunction may or may not be present in patients with ARVC and ventricular tachycardia, and the clinical course is highly variable.

In most forms of **congenital heart disease,** sudden arrhythmic death in the absence of severe heart failure, ventricular hypertrophy, or hypoxemia is uncommon. However, late ventricular tachycardia that arises from the right ventriculotomy scar or the septal repair may develop in some patients who have undergone a successful surgical repair of Fallot tetralogy.

E. Inherited Arrhythmia Syndromes

The **congenital long-QT syndrome** is a family of disorders characterized by prolongation of cardiac repolarization with a prolonged QT interval on the scalar ECG and a tendency to develop polymorphic ventricular tachycardia that may degenerate to ventricular fibrillation. The most common types of the long QT syndrome are caused by mutations in genes that encode ion channel proteins. The resultant ion channel dysfunction causes a prolonged repolarization phase of the ventricular action potential. This promotes polymorphic ventricular tachycardia triggered by oscillations in the action potential called early after-depolarizations. Electrolyte imbalance, bradycardia or pauses, sudden sympathetic stimulation, and drug effects all may further prolong repolarization in individuals with these mutations and trigger acute episodes. It is important to recognize patients with the long-QT syndrome because standard antiarrhythmic drugs may worsen their condition.

A **short QT syndrome** caused by a gain in function mutation in a repolarizing potassium current that is associated with sudden death has also been described.

The **Brugada syndrome** is another familial condition associated with sudden death. These individuals have an incomplete or complete right bundle branch block on their ECG with ST-segment elevation in V_1 and V_2. These patients will manifest spontaneous episodes of polymorphic ventricular tachycardia and ventricular fibrillation, often during sleep. Some patients with Brugada syndrome have a mutation in the sodium channel gene (SCN5A) with a decrease in the inward sodium current during the plateau phase of the action potential. The unusual ECG manifestations are believed to be due to more pronounced ion channel dysfunction in the right ventricular epicardium.

Catecholaminergic polymorphic ventricular tachycardia is a rare syndrome in which bursts of rapid ventricular tachycardia occur during sympathetic stimulation or exercise. This syndrome is genetically heterogenous, with mutations in the genes encoding the cardiac ryanodine receptor type II and calsequestrin.

Shah M et al. Molecular basis of arrhythmias. Circulation. 2005 Oct 18;112(16):2517–29. [PMID: 16230503]

F. Drug-Induced Arrhythmias

Drug toxicity can also result in sudden death. A variety of medications can affect cardiac electrophysiology and lead to fatal arrhythmias. Even when prescribed for atrial fibrillation or supraventricular tachycardia, all antiarrhythmic drugs may be associated with a proarrhythmic response in the ventricle. Other cardiac and noncardiac drugs can also cause arrhythmias. The most common mechanism is I_{Kr} blockade. Multiple factors are often required for drug-induced proarrhythmia. Risk factors include electrolyte disturbances, age, female gender, genetic polymorphisms or mutations, left ventricular hypertrophy, and bradycardia.

Patients with severe electrolyte disturbances and abnormal dietary histories (eg, anorexia nervosa and liquid protein diets) are also susceptible to potentially fatal ventricular arrhythmias even in the absence of significant heart disease.

G. Other Arrhythmias

Several electrophysiologic abnormalities can produce sudden death without associated major structural heart disease. **Supraventricular arrhythmias,** if associated with very rapid ventricular rates, can cause hemodynamic collapse and degenerate to ventricular fibrillation. Atrial fibrillation with rapid conduction over an accessory pathway in a patient with **Wolff-Parkinson-White syndrome** is the supraventricular arrhythmia most frequently associated with sudden death, but other supraventricular arrhythmias have also occasionally been implicated. Although sudden death due to a ventricular preexcitation syndrome is rare, it may be the first clinical manifestation of the condition.

Bradyarrhythmias may also be associated with sudden death. In **congenital complete heart block,** the escape pacemaker may deteriorate over time, with ventricular arrhythmias appearing as the patient's bradycardia becomes more and more inappropriate. Most previously healthy adults in whom a bradycardia develops as a result of sinus node dysfunction or heart block will have some functioning escape pacemaker that can, at least briefly, support vital organs. Therefore, sudden death is uncommon with these arrhythmias in the absence of severe ventricular dysfunction, another complicating disease, electrolyte imbalance, drug toxicity, or a prolonged delay in treatment of the bradycardia.

A recently recognized syndrome of sudden death in young individuals with structurally normal hearts is **commotio cordis.** Ventricular fibrillation develops after the patient receives a sharp blow to the chest, often while engaged in sports. Animal models have shown that a critically timed and placed chest impact during a vulnerable portion of the T wave can initiate ventricular fibrillation. It is assumed that a similar mechanism is responsible for the human syndrome.

Not all ventricular arrhythmias in patients with structurally normal hearts carry a risk for sudden death. Sudden death is very rare in individuals with structurally normal hearts who initially present with a stable **monomorphic ventricular tachycardia.** The two most common forms of sustained monomorphic ventricular tachycardia in patients with structurally normal hearts arise either from the right ventricular outflow tract with a left bundle branch block pattern and an inferior axis or from the inferior septal region with a right bundle branch block and left axis pattern. Both these forms of ventricular tachycardia are usually hemodynamically well tolerated and rarely result in hemodynamic collapse.

▶ Management of Cardiac Arrest: Initial Resuscitation

The introduction of transthoracic defibrillation 40 years ago sparked the development of community-based programs to resuscitate persons who suffered cardiac arrest out of the hospital. A successful system involves both an educated lay public that can provide at least basic cardiopulmonary resuscitation (CPR) and an organized structure to provide advanced life support in the field. Because the time period for delivering effective therapy to the person suffering cardiac arrest is very short, even the best community programs will have survival-to-hospital discharge rates of only 20–30%. Several factors have been identified with a favorable outcome. Probably the most important is the time from cardiac arrest to restoration of an organized cardiac rhythm. If an effective rhythm is not restored within 4–8 minutes, survival with well preserved neurologic function becomes unlikely. Bystander CPR can extend this window for survival by a few minutes.

Because early defibrillation is the key to survival, community programs to speed defibrillation have been widely introduced but with modest results. Initial efforts involved emergency medical technicians trained in both basic and advanced cardiac life support who responded to the emergency call. The success of these programs was limited by the ability of these trained responders to reach the patient within the first critical minutes after the arrest.

Public access to automatic external defibrillators (AEDs) offers the potential to improve survival further for out-of-hospital cardiac arrest patients. When an AED is connected to an unconscious individual by electrode pads placed on the chest, a microprocessor within the device analyzes the patient's rhythm. Ventricular fibrillation and rapid ventricular tachycardia are accurately identifiable as "shockable" rhythms, and the AED instructs the rescuer to push a button to deliver a shock. AEDs designed for home use by minimally trained lay family members are now commercially available, and a wearable vest AED that does not require a rescuer for activation has recently been introduced. Bystander CPR techniques have also evolved, with the current emphasis placed on maintenance of effective chest compression.

A discussion of the techniques for basic and advanced cardiac life support are beyond the scope of this chapter. For patients with ventricular tachycardia or fibrillation, early cardioversion or defibrillation is the key to survival. For patients with asystole or pulseless electrical activity, the prospects for survival are dismal unless some reversible cause can be identified and immediately corrected.

▶ Management of Cardiac Arrest Survivors: In-Hospital Phase

Even in communities that have effective programs for pre-hospital cardiac care, only a fraction of cardiac arrest patients will survive to hospital admission. Optimal management for these survivors of an episode of cardiac arrest requires a systematic approach. First, potential complications of the resuscitation must be identified and treatment instituted. Next, the probable cause, including reversible precipitating events, the nature and severity of any underlying heart disease, and the arrhythmia probably responsible for the episode, should be determined. Finally, therapy can be selected and its potential for success evaluated.

A. Complications of Resuscitation

Only a fraction of cardiac arrest survivors who receive early defibrillation will be alert and oriented with full recovery of function at the time of hospital admission. Most patients will have pulmonary, cardiac, or neurologic complications resulting from the period of arrest or the resuscitation itself. Pulmonary complications are usually due either to aspiration of gastric contents or to mechanical injury to the thoracic cage during closed-chest compressions. The chest wall should be carefully inspected, palpated, and stabilized, if necessary. In extreme cases, bony thoracic fractures may result in a flail chest, or hepatic or splenic lacerations may occur. Chest radiography may be helpful in detecting aspiration, but repeated examinations may be necessary to document the delayed appearance of infiltrates. If a central line has been placed, the chest radiograph is also useful to confirm catheter position and to exclude a pneumothorax. Mechanical ventilation is often required in the early period after admission to allow adequate oxygenation and pulmonary cleansing; this may require the use of muscle relaxants and sedation.

Cardiac arrest produces a period of global cardiac ischemia, frequently resulting in a period of cardiac stunning, defined as a reversible depression in cardiac systolic function. This has two important implications. First, inotropic or even mechanical (eg, intra-aortic counterpulsation) support may be necessary to maintain vital organ perfusion during the early phase after resuscitation. Second, any acute assessment of ventricular function may overestimate the amount of permanent dysfunction. Thus, a low ejection fraction measured in the first several days after arrest may not be an accurate gauge of eventual cardiac function. ECG and enzymatic data obtained after an arrest are often difficult to interpret. It is usually wise to reserve a definite diagnosis of an acute infarction as the primary event for those patients with chest pain preceding collapse and documented ST-segment elevation or new Q waves. Without a documented new infarction, it may be hoped that the patient's cardiac function will eventually recover to its status before the arrest, but this may take several weeks. Arrhythmias are frequently seen during the period immediately after resuscitation. They may be similar to those that originally produced the arrest, or they may be new rhythm disturbances caused by poor hemodynamic function and multiorgan failure. No single therapy will be predictably effective against these arrhythmias, and antiarrhythmic agents, β-adrenergic blockers, positive inotropic agents, and other measures to improve hemodynamic function must be tried. Recent studies using intravenous amiodarone prior to hospital admission have demonstrated improvements in rates of return of spontaneous circulation and survival-to-hospital admission but no clear benefit in survival-to-hospital discharge.

Neurologic damage occurs quickly during a cardiac arrest. Unless defibrillation with restoration of spontaneous circulation was almost immediate, patients will be unconscious when admitted to the hospital, and an accurate evaluation of the potential for functional recovery is often difficult in this early stage. Brainstem reflexes may be preserved, but their presence does not necessarily predict a favorable outcome. Generalized or focal seizure activity, decerebrate or decorticate posturing, and involuntary respiratory efforts may make mechanical ventilation difficult. Neuromuscular blocking agents, anticonvulsants, and sedation are often required, further hampering any ability to make an accurate neurologic assessment. In the absence of some severe concomitant disease, it is usually wise to withhold any decisions concerning the withdrawal of support for at least 24 hours. Recent studies have demonstrated that mild hypothermia (32–34 °C for 12–24 hours) improves neurologic recovery in unconscious resuscitated cardiac arrest patients. The prognosis is good for patients who regain consciousness within 72 hours of arrest, and many of them will recover completely with minimal or no long-term neurologic impairment. If coma persists longer than 72 hours, few patients survive. Those who do will often have persistent severe motor and cognitive deficits. Decisions about prolonged artificial support of these latter patients are often difficult and require that a variety of medical, ethical, and social factors be taken into consideration.

ECC Committee, Subcommittees and Task Forces of the American Heart Association. 2005 American Heart Association Guidelines for Cardiopulmonary Resuscitation and Emergency Cardiovascular Care. Circulation. 2005 Dec 13;112(24 Suppl1):IV1–203. [PMID: 16314375]

Eisenberg MS et al. Cardiac resuscitation. N Engl J Med. 2001 Apr 26;344(17):1304–13. [PMID: 11320390]

Nolan JP et al. European Resuscitation Council guidelines for resuscitation 2005 Section 4. Adult advanced life support. Resuscitation. 2005 Dec;67 Suppl 1:S39–86. [PMID: 16321716]

Sanders AB. Therapeutic hypothermia after cardiac arrest. Curr Opin Crit Care. 2006 Jun;12(3):213–7. [PMID: 16672779]

SOS-Kantos study group. Cardiopulmonary resuscitation by bystanders with chest compression only (SOS-KANTO): an observational study. Lancet. 2007 Mar 17;369(9565):920–26. [PMID: 17368153]

B. Diagnostic Studies

1. Noninvasive evaluation for structural heart disease— Once the patient has recovered to the point that long-term survival seems likely, efforts should be made to define fully the type and extent of underlying cardiac disease.

A. Electrocardiography—Although the ECG usually provides the first information available, the initial ECG after defibrillation may be misleading. Transient ST-segment elevation in leads with prior Q waves is common and does not always signify a new infarction as the primary cause of the arrest. Only if ST elevation has been documented during normal rhythm before the arrest, or if new Q waves appear, should a definite diagnosis of an acute infarction be made. This distinction is critical for two reasons: (1) patients with a new ST elevation myocardial infarction are candidates for acute mechanical or pharmacologic reperfusion, and (2) the prognosis associated with resuscitated ventricular fibrillation precipitated by a new acute infarction is not significantly different than that associated with an infarct of similar size without arrest. If in doubt, acute phase cardiac catheterization may be necessary. More commonly, the ECG after resuscitation will show such evidence of chronic disease, including old Q waves, conduction defects, or hypertrophy. ST segment and T-wave abnormalities appear in virtually all patients following resuscitation and are of limited significance. The ECG may also be useful in the diagnosis of congenital and acquired long-QT syndromes, the Brugada syndrome, preexcitation syndromes, cardiomyopathies, and congenital heart disease.

B. Echocardiography—Echocardiography performed in the coronary care unit can provide a noninvasive assessment of cardiac function and anatomy shortly after resuscitation. An early, two-dimensional echocardiogram can provide valuable information about chamber size, valvular abnormalities, and ventricular function. Serial studies are often helpful in documenting recovery of function after an initial period of stunning.

C. Other noninvasive tests—Other noninvasive tests may also be appropriate in some cases. Magnetic resonance imaging is particularly valuable in patients with arrhythmogenic right ventricular cardiomyopathy and with myocarditis. Positron emission tomography, magnetic resonance imaging, and isotope perfusion scans may be useful for assessing viability in regions of poor ventricular function. Preserved viability may influence decisions concerning the appropriateness of any attempts at revascularization.

2. Invasive evaluation for structural heart disease— Cardiac catheterization provides the most complete assessment of the structure, function, and blood supply of the heart, and it should be performed in virtually all survivors of cardiac arrest. Coronary artery disease is found in about 80% of cardiac arrest patients in the United States and Europe. In coronary disease, unanticipated cardiac arrest occurs primarily in two clinical settings: acute infarction and transient ischemia, with and without healed prior infarction.

The prognosis of a patient who survives a cardiac arrest in the acute phase of a myocardial infarction is determined by the total amount of ventricular damage, the severity of residual ischemia, and the completeness of recovery from any noncardiac complications of the arrest. Treatment of these patients should be similar to that for other acute infarct patients, and special steps to define long-term antiarrhythmic therapy are not required. The role of ischemia in cardiac arrest patients without new Q wave infarction is controversial. As noted earlier, long, ulcerated coronary artery lesions are often seen on coronary angiograms in cardiac arrest survivors and at autopsy in those who suffered sudden death. If these lesions are seen in patients with totally normal ventricular function, ischemia from these lesions alone may be responsible for the arrest. Correcting the ischemia through revascularization is the most appropriate—and sometimes the only required—therapy. More commonly, both a potential for acute ischemia and a fixed scar will be present, and a complex interaction between the two will be responsible for the event.

3. Diagnosis of arrhythmias—A variety of arrhythmias can cause cardiac arrest and sudden death. Supraventricular arrhythmias with rapid ventricular rates and primary bradyarrhythmias are infrequent causes of cardiac arrest. However, it is important to identify patients with these arrhythmias because they will require a different therapeutic approach. Ventricular tachycardia and ventricular fibrillation are the most common causes of out-of-hospital cardiac arrest, and the evaluation and treatment of these arrhythmias will be the focus of the rest of this chapter.

A. Noninvasive evaluation—The role of noninvasive testing in patients who have suffered cardiac arrest is limited because a history of cardiac arrest has already placed them in a high-risk group. Noninvasive tests, however, are often used to assess the risk for future events in patients with known cardiac disease.

Exercise testing may be useful in some cases of exercise-induced ventricular tachycardia or in some patients with cardiac arrest to determine the presence of inducible ischemia. Abnormal prolongation of the QT interval in patients with the long-QT syndrome and the appearance of arrhythmias in patients with congenital heart block may also be useful markers of future risk. In most cases, however, exercise testing is used to provide information about the potential for ischemia, rather than to diagnose the mechanism of arrhythmia or to guide therapy.

Ambulatory ECG monitoring is rarely useful in cardiac arrest survivors, but the presence of frequent and complex ventricular premature beats and abnormal heart rate variability are risk factors for sudden death during follow-up in patients with many forms of heart disease. In population studies, frequent or complex ventricular ectopy is associated with an increased risk of both sudden and nonsudden cardiac death. Unfortunately, the prognostic value of ambulatory ECG monitoring data in any individual patient is limited by poor day-to-day reproducibility of the data. The use of antiarrhythmic drug therapy guided by suppression of ventricular ectopic activity has not been shown to improve survival. Other noninvasive tests have been used to risk stratify patients. Tests that assess microvolt T-wave alternans during exercise, late potentials on a signal averaged ECG, heart rate variability and baroreceptor sensitivity have been proposed, but their value in individual patients is controversial.

B. Invasive evaluation—Invasive evaluation involves a baseline electrophysiologic study that uses programmed electrical stimulation to initiate and characterize the patient's arrhythmia. As ICDs have become more accepted as the most effective therapy to prevent cardiac arrest, electrophysiologic studies have been relegated to a secondary role. They are now used to help define an arrhythmia mechanism if either an unusual mechanism of arrhythmia or an arrhythmia that might be susceptible to ablation is suspected. The ability to identify an effective antiarrhythmic drug by serial testing is limited, and the failure rate of drug therapy selected by the technique is unacceptably high. Electrophysiologic studies are useful for characterizing the effects of drug therapy on tachycardias. Drug therapy may change the rate of many ventricular tachycardias and can affect defibrillation thresholds. Data obtained from electrophysiologic studies during drug therapy can be used to guide programming of ICDs.

▶ Treatment of Cardiac Arrest Survivors

Treating the cardiac arrest survivor requires a comprehensive strategy that must consider both aggressive and appropriate management of the underlying cardiac disease process as well as specific antiarrhythmic therapy.

A. Antiarrhythmic Drug Therapy

The role of antiarrhythmic drugs in the treatment of cardiac arrest survivors has changed substantially in the last 15 years. This change in strategy has been based on the results of randomized clinical trials for the primary and secondary prevention of sudden death. These trials have shown that therapy with class I antiarrhythmic drugs does not improve,

and may worsen, survival when used for primary prevention in patients after myocardial infarction. When used in patients with a history of sustained ventricular tachycardia or ventricular fibrillation, class I drugs are inferior to sotalol and amiodarone. The latter drugs have, in turn, been shown to be less effective for improving survival than is therapy with an ICD.

Antiarrhythmic drugs, however, are still valuable for individual patients. Unstable arrhythmias are common in the immediate period after resuscitation. Intravenous amiodarone and β-blockers are the most effective treatments in this setting. Many patients with an ICD, in the absence of drug therapy, may have frequent episodes of sustained or nonsustained ventricular tachycardia that would trigger ICD therapy. Sotalol, a class III agent with β-adrenergic blocking activity, and amiodarone have been shown in randomized trials to decrease the frequency of ICD therapy. The usual dosage range for sotalol is 120–160 mg twice daily. Sotalol is cleared by the kidneys, and the dose should be adjusted in patients with renal insufficiency. d, l-Sotalol is a potent β-adrenergic blocker, and bradycardia may limit therapy. Sotalol may also lower defibrillation thresholds. Amiodarone is usually administered with a loading dose of 5–10 g in the first 1–2 weeks of therapy, followed by a daily dose of 200-300 mg. Common adverse reactions during amiodarone therapy include thyroid dysfunction, photosensitivity and skin discoloration, neuromuscular complaints, and abnormal liver function tests. Amiodarone-induced pulmonary toxicity can be life-threatening if unrecognized and occurs in approximately 1–2% of patients in the first year of therapy and in 0.5% of patients per year thereafter. Some patients will not be candidates for or will not desire ICD therapy. In those cases, sotalol or amiodarone would be the drugs of choice. Effective pharmacologic treatment to prevent ischemia and heart failure progression is also critical to long-term management.

B. Revascularization

Revascularization may play an important role in the care of both survivors of cardiac arrest and patients at risk for sudden death. In patients with ischemic heart disease and chronic stable angina, coronary revascularization decreases sudden death rates, with the greatest benefits being observed in patients with multivessel disease and depressed left ventricular function. Among cardiac arrest survivors, revascularization is indicated in patients with evidence of active ischemia or extensive areas of hibernating, dysfunctional but viable, myocardium. If no significant prior scarring is evident, revascularization alone may provide effective therapy for selected patients. In the presence of prior scarring, however, revascularization alone may not be effective at preventing future arrhythmias. Cardiac transplantation plays an important role in patients with both arrhythmias and intractable ischemia or severe heart failure and in patients whose arrhythmias cannot be controlled with any less drastic form of therapy.

C. Surgical or Catheter Ablation

Direct surgical or catheter approaches have been developed to eliminate or ablate the myocardial areas where the reentry circuit responsible for ventricular tachycardia arises. Both approaches involve induction of tachycardia using programmed stimulation, mapping to determine critical portions of the tachycardia circuit, and either resection or ablation at the sites identified. Map-guided surgical resection procedures are no longer commonly performed due to the high mortality associated with these operations. Although catheter ablation has been successfully used in patients with sustained ventricular tachycardia, the highest success rates have been in patients with well-tolerated tachycardias or no structural heart disease. At present, the most frequent use of catheter ablation in cardiac arrest patients is as an adjunct treatment to reduce the frequency of arrhythmias in patients who also have ICDs. New ablation approaches designed to isolate large areas of arrhythmogenic myocardium are now being studied and may be effective in some patients with rapid and unstable arrhythmias.

Catheter ablation of an accessory atrioventricular connection will be curative in patients with cardiac arrest in association with atrial arrhythmias. In patients with ventricular tachycardia caused by macroreentry in the His-Purkinje system, ablation of the right bundle will eliminate further episodes.

D. Implantable Cardioverter Defibrillators

The first ICD was implanted for clinical use in 1980. Primitive by today's standards, the early devices clearly demonstrated the validity of the concept that a totally implanted device could be used to terminate life-threatening arrhythmias automatically. Advances in defibrillator technology have extended the applications of these devices, and ICD therapy is now considered the main therapeutic option for cardiac arrest survivors and for primary prevention in many high-risk patients.

An ICD has two basic components: the ICD generator and a lead system for pacing and shock delivery. An ICD generator contains sensing circuits, memory storage, capacitors, voltage enhancers, a telemetry module, and a control microprocessor. Advances in miniaturization and complexity in all of these components have permitted a tremendous reduction in the size of the generator itself despite increased functionality. The original implantable defibrillator was designed to recognize the disorganized electrical activity characteristic of ventricular fibrillation only. The ability to recognize ventricular tachycardia was added shortly thereafter. Subsequent generations of devices have added extensive programming options, antitachycardia pacing, single- and dual-chamber rate-responsive pacing for bradycardia, biphasic defibrillation waveforms, enhanced arrhythmia detection features, innovations in lead systems, and cardiac resynchronization. The original systems required a thoracotomy to place epicardial

patches and, as a result, the implant procedure itself was associated with substantial morbidity and mortality rates. After transvenous leads were developed that allowed successful defibrillation and the generator size was reduced, subcutaneous implants in the pectoral region became standard. Current systems can be implanted by electrophysiologists using local anesthesia in a cardiac laboratory.

From the point of their introduction, there was little doubt that ICDs were very effective for terminating episodes of ventricular tachycardia and ventricular fibrillation. Initially, they were implanted chiefly in patients who did not respond to antiarrhythmic drug therapy as assessed by repeat ECG monitoring or electrophysiologic testing. As the limitations of antiarrhythmic drugs became more apparent, ICDs began to be used as the first treatment option. Three large randomized secondary prevention trials have compared ICD therapy with antiarrhythmic therapy in survivors of cardiac arrest or hemodynamically unstable ventricular tachycardia (Table 25–2). In the Antiarrhythmics versus Implantable Defibrillator (AVID) study, 1016 patients were randomly assigned to either drug therapy (amiodarone or, rarely, sotalol) or an ICD. Survival analysis showed a decrease in total mortality rates of 39%, 27%, and 31% at follow-up points of 1, 2, and 3 years, respectively. The Cardiac Arrest Study Hamburg (CASH) randomly assigned 346 cardiac arrest survivors to either an ICD or drug therapy with one of three agents: amiodarone, metoprolol, or propafenone. The propafenone arm was terminated early due to an excessive mortality rate among those patients. At 2-year follow-up, the mortality rate was 37% lower in the ICD group than in the combined metoprolol and amiodarone group. In the Canadian Implantable Defibrillator Study (CIDS), 659 patients with cardiac arrest, sustained ventricular tachycardia, or inducible ventricular tachycardia with unexplained syncope were treated with either an ICD or amiodarone. The mortality rate at 2-year follow-up was 19.7% lower in the ICD group. These three studies provide convincing evidence that an ICD should be first-line therapy in a cardiac arrest survivor.

ICD therapy has a number of limitations, however. An ICD terminates arrhythmias by using either antitachycardia pacing or direct current shocks. The latter produce significant discomfort, and patients who receive multiple shocks report significant negative effects on their quality of life. Although an ICD may be programmed to use various pacing strategies that may decrease arrhythmia frequency, these steps are not always effective, and antiarrhythmic drugs are often required as adjunctive therapy. Sotalol, amiodarone, and β-adrenergic blockers are the agents most commonly used to decrease shock frequency in patients with an ICD. Disease progression often limits the usefulness of an ICD, and the most effective use of ICDs in patients with far advanced disease is controversial. Hardware deterioration, although rarely life-threatening, continues to be a problem and may lead to the need for multiple invasive procedures. Finally, ICD therapy is very costly. Estimates of added cost

Table 25–2. Implantable Cardioverter Defibrillator Trials.

Trial	#	Age (years)	LVEF	Follow-up (months)	Mortality Control (%)	Mortality ICD (%)	Relative RR (%)	Absolute RR (%)	NNT (36 months)
Secondary Prevention									
AVID	1016	65	0.35	18	24	16	31	8.2	9
CIDS	659	64	0.34	36	30	25	23	4.3	23
CASH	228	58	0.45	57	44	36	23	8.1	20
Primary Prevention									
MADIT	196	63	0.26	27	39	16	54	22.8	3
MADIT II	1232	64	0.23	20	20	14	31	5.4	10
DEFINITE	458	58	0.21	29	14	8	35	5.2	24
SCD-HeFT	1676	60	0.25	46	28	22	23	6.8	23
CABG-Patch	900	64	0.27	32	21	23	7 (increase)	1.7 (increase)	
DINAMIT	674	62	0.31	30	17	19	8 (increase)	1.7 (increase)	

AVID, Antiarrhythmics Versus Implantable Defibrillator; CABG-Patch, Coronary Artery Bypass Graft-Patch Trial; CASH, Cardiac Arrest Study Hamburg; CIDS, Canadian Implantable Defibrillator Study; DEFINITE, Defibrillators in Nonischemic Cardiomyopathy Treatment Evaluation; DINAMIT, The Defibrillator in Acute Myocardial Infarction Trial; ICD, implantable cardioverter defibrillator; LVEF, left ventricular ejection fraction; MADIT I and II, Multicenter Automatic Implantable Defibrillator Trials I and II; NNT, number needed to treat; RR, risk reduction; SCD-HeFT, Sudden Cardiac Death in Heart Failure Trial.

over drug therapy per quality of life year saved in the AVID and CIDS populations exceeded $100,000.

European Heart Rhythm Association; Heart Rhythm Society, Zipes DP et al; American College of Cardiology; American Heart Association Task Force; European Society of Cardiology Committee for Practice Guidelines. ACC/AHA/ESC 2006 guidelines for management of patients with ventricular arrhythmias and the prevention of sudden death: a report of the American College of Cardiology/American Heart Association Task Force and the European Society of Cardiology Committee for Practice Guidelines (Writing Committee to Develop Guidelines for Management of Patients With Ventricular Arrhythmias and the Prevention of Sudden Cardiac Death). J Am Coll Cardiol. 2006 Sep 5;48(5):e247–346. [PMID: 16949478]

DiMarco JP. Implantable cardioverter-defibrillators. N Engl J Med. 2003 Nov 6;349(19):1836–47. [PMID: 14602883]

▶ Identification of Patients at Risk

Even in communities with the most advanced systems for emergency response and out-of-hospital resuscitation, only a fraction of patients are resuscitated and survive to hospital discharge without significant residual deficits. In many areas, it is logistically impossible to rescue more than a small fraction of persons who suffer cardiac arrest. It is, therefore, important to be able to identify patients at high risk for sudden death and to determine the specific interventions that would be effective in this population.

A. Risk-Assessment Studies

The most comprehensive assessments of factors that predict risk for future sudden death have been undertaken in populations of patients with recent myocardial infarction. In general, laboratory or clinical findings of residual ischemia, ventricular dysfunction, and electrical instability have been associated with an adverse prognosis. A number of findings have been identified as markers for chronic electrical instability. The presence of frequent or complex ventricular premature beats (VPBs) is a risk factor for sudden death after myocardial infarction. An increase in risk can be identified in patients with as few as 3–6 VPBs per hour on a 24-hour ambulatory recording. Poor day-to-day reproducibility in both the frequency and patterns of spontaneous ventricular arrhythmias limits the value of this finding in individual patients. Other findings during ambulatory monitoring may be useful. A decrease in the normally observed variability in R-R intervals during ambulatory ECG monitoring is a marker for heightened adrenergic tone and an increased risk of sudden death. The signal-averaged ECG is used to detect abnormal delays of ventricular activation that would be indistinguishable from noise in a routine ECG. These late potentials are frequently seen in patients with sustained monomorphic ventricular tachycardia and are predictors of mortality in patients after myocardial infarction. Microvolt alternation in T-wave amplitude during exercise is another finding thought to be a marker of increased risk. Decreased baroreceptor sensitivity and abnormal heart rate variability have also been used to identify high-risk patient subgroups. All proposed noninvasive tests have been limited by a fairly low positive predictive accuracy, and their use in individual patient decisions is controversial. Current guidelines for ICD implantation are evidence-based, with arrhythmia history, left ventricular ejection fraction, and New York Heart Association (NYHA) functional class the bases for the indications.

B. Primary Prevention of Sudden Death

Primary prevention of sudden death remains an elusive goal. Although many risk factors have been identified, it has been difficult to show in clinical trials that therapy directed at any single risk factor is effective. β-Adrenergic blocking agents, cholesterol-lowering drugs, and angiotensin-converting enzyme (ACE) inhibitors have been shown to decrease both sudden and nonsudden deaths in patients with heart failure or after myocardial infarction, but these agents are not thought to treat arrhythmias in a specific fashion. Clinical trials have shown that class I antiarrhythmic drugs did not decrease sudden death mortality rates. In fact, the most definitive study—the Cardiac Arrhythmia Suppression Trial (CAST)—showed a higher mortality rate among patients who were randomized to drug therapy after it was shown that their spontaneous VPBs could be suppressed. Several studies using empirically prescribed amiodarone have reported improved survival after myocardial infarction, but the largest, placebo-controlled studies—the European and Canadian Amiodarone Myocardial Infarction Trials (EMIAT and CAMIAT) and the Sudden Cardiac Death–Heart Failure Trial (SCD-HeFT)—have not shown any benefit.

Dofetilide and azimilide have been tested in patients after myocardial infarction, and dofetilide in patients with chronic heart failure. Treatment with these two drugs showed no change in mortality rates. Cardiac resynchronization therapy in patients with advanced heart failure and a wide QRS has been shown to improve NYHA functional class, decrease hospitalizations, and reduce sudden and nonsudden cardiac deaths.

Randomized trials have indicated that ICD therapy for primary prevention of sudden death is effective in many populations. Summary data from a number of clinical trials are shown in Table 25–2, and the current indications for ICD insertion accepted by the Center for Medicare Services are shown in Table 25–3. The most recent trials have used entry criteria based primarily on left ventricular ejection fraction (below 30% or 35%) and NYHA functional class. Most primary prevention trials have reported relative risk reductions in a range similar to those seen in the secondary prevention trials (20–30%). The CABG-Patch Trial and the Defibrillators in Acute Myocardial Infarction Trial (DINAMIT) failed to show benefit in patients who received their ICD either at the time of coronary revascularization or within 40 days of an acute myocardial infarction, respectively. These trials resulted in the specific exclusion of these conditions in the current guidelines.

Table 25–3. Indications and Contraindications for Implantable Cardioverter Defibrillator Therapy.

I. Indications for Secondary Prevention
  A. Documented episode of cardiac arrest due to ventricular fibrillation (VF), not due to a transient or reversible cause
  B. Documented sustained ventricular tachyarrhythmia (VT), either spontaneous or induced by an electrophysiology (EP) study, not associated with an acute myocardial infarction (MI) and not due to a transient or reversible cause
II. Indications for Primary Prevention
  A. Documented familial or inherited conditions with a high risk of life-threatening VT, such as long QT syndrome or hypertrophic cardiomyopathy
  B. Coronary artery disease with a documented prior MI, a measured left ventricular ejection fraction (LVEF) < 35%, and inducible, sustained VT or VF at EP study. (The EP test must be performed more than 4 weeks after the qualifying MI.)
  C. Documented prior MI and a measured LVEF < 30%
  D. Patients with ischemic dilated cardiomyopathy, documented prior MI, New York Heart Association (NYHA) class II and III heart failure, and measured LVEF < 35%
  E. Patients with nonischemic dilated cardiomyopathy > 9 months, NYHA class II and III heart failure, and measured LVEF < 35%
  F. Patients who meet all current Centers for Medicare & Medicaid Services coverage requirements for a cardiac resynchronization therapy (CRT) device and have NYHA class IV heart failure
  G. Patients with nonischemic dilated cardiomyopathy > 3 months, NYHA class II and III heart failure, and measured LVEF < 35%
III. Exclusions
  A. NYHA classification IV without CRT
  B. Cardiogenic shock or symptomatic hypotension while in a stable baseline rhythm
  C. Had a coronary artery bypass graft or percutaneous transluminal coronary angioplasty within past 3 months
  D. Had an enzyme positive MI within past 40 days
  E. Clinical symptoms or findings that would make them a candidate for coronary revascularization
  F. Any disease, other than cardiac disease (eg, cancer, uremia, liver failure), associated with a likelihood of survival less than 1 year
  G. Patients must not have irreversible brain damage from preexisting cerebral disease

Modified from Pub 100-03 Medicare National Coverage Determinations. Chapter 1, Part 1, Section 20.4 (Rev. 29, 03-04-05).

Connolly SJ et al. Meta-analysis of the implantable cardioverter defibrillator secondary prevention trials. AVID, CASH, and CIDS studies. Antiarrhythmics vs Implantable Defibrillator study. Cardiac Arrest Study Hamburg. Canadian Implantable Defibrillator Study. Eur Heart J. 2000 Dec;21(24):2071–8. [PMID: 11102258]

Connolly SJ et al; Optimal Pharmacological Therapy in Cardioverter Defibrillator Patients (OPTIC) Investigators. Comparison of beta-blockers, amiodarone plus beta-blockers, or sotalol for prevention of shocks from implantable cardioverter defibrillators: the OPTIC study: a randomized trial. JAMA. 2006 Jan 11;295(2):165–71. [PMID: 16403928]

Nanthakumar K et al. Prophylactic implantable cardioverter-defibrillator therapy in patients with left ventricular dysfunction: a pooled analysis of 10 primary prevention trials. J Am Coll Cardiol. 2004 Dec 7;44(11):2166–72. [PMID: 15582314]

Pulmonary Embolic Disease

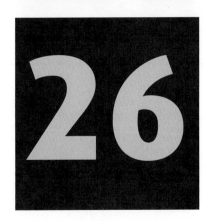

Rajni K. Rao, MD

ESSENTIALS OF DIAGNOSIS

▶ Otherwise unexplained dyspnea, tachypnea, or chest pain.

▶ Clinical, ECG, or echocardiographic evidence of acute cor pulmonale.

▶ Positive chest CT angiography scan with contrast.

▶ High-probability ventilation-perfusion lung scan or high-probability perfusion lung scan with a normal chest radiograph.

▶ Positive venous ultrasound of the legs with a convincing clinical history and suggestive lung scan.

▶ Diagnostic contrast pulmonary angiogram.

General Considerations

The term "venous thromboembolism" (VTE) encompasses both pulmonary embolism (PE) and deep venous thrombosis (DVT) and accounts for more than 250,000 hospitalizations per year in the United States. Venous thromboembolism constitutes one of the most common causes of cardiovascular and cardiopulmonary illnesses in Western civilization. Pulmonary embolism causes or contributes to at least 50,000 deaths per year in the United States, a rate that has probably remained constant for the past three decades. For those who survive PE, further disability includes the potential development of chronic pulmonary hypertension or chronic venous insufficiency. After a VTE event, patients and their physicians are concerned about the presence of an occult carcinoma, the risk of a recurrent PE after anticoagulation therapy has been discontinued, and whether the patients' family members are at risk for VTE.

Etiology

"Primary" PE occurs in the absence of surgery or trauma. Patients with this condition often have an underlying hyper-coagulable state, although a specific thrombophilic condition may not be identified. A common scenario is a clinically silent tendency toward thrombosis, which is precipitated by a stressor such as prolonged immobilization, oral contraceptives, pregnancy, or hormone replacement therapy. Recently, there has been an increased appreciation of the risks of VTE among patients with medical illnesses, including cancer (which itself may be associated with a hypercoagulable state), congestive heart failure, and chronic obstructive pulmonary disease.

The prevalence of "secondary" PE is high among patients undergoing certain types of surgery, especially orthopedic surgery of the hip and knee, gynecologic cancer surgery, major trauma, and craniotomy for brain tumor. Pulmonary embolism in these patients may occur as late as a month after discharge from the hospital.

A. Thrombophilia

Principal thrombophilic risk factors for VTE are listed in Table 26–1. The two most common genetic mutations that predispose to VTE are the factor V Leiden and the pro-thrombin gene. Both are autosomal-dominant. Whether factor V Leiden predisposes to recurrent VTE after anticoagulation is discontinued remains controversial. The pro-thrombin gene mutation is associated with an increased risk of recurrent VTE after discontinuation of anticoagulation, especially in patients who have coinherited the factor V Leiden mutation.

Elevated levels of homocysteine are usually easily treated with folate. The presence of anticardiolipin antibodies suggests the need for prolonged and intensive anticoagulation.

Screening for deficiencies of antithrombin III, protein C, and protein S is a low-yield strategy that produces positive findings in less than 5% of patients. Heparin decreases the antithrombin III level, whereas warfarin, pregnancy, and oral contraceptives decrease the protein C and S levels, thereby resulting in potentially spurious diagnoses of these hypercoagulable states.

Table 26–1. Thrombophilic Risk Factors for Venous Thromboembolism.

Common
Factor V Leiden
Prothrombin gene mutation
Anticardiolipin antibodies (including lupus anticoagulant) as a feature of the antiphospholipid antibody syndrome
Hyperhomocysteinemia (usually due to folate deficiency)
Uncommon
Antithrombin III deficiency
Protein C deficiency
Protein S deficiency
Mutations of cystathionine β-synthase or methylene tetrahydrofolate reductase (MTHFR)
High concentrations of Factors VIII or XI (or both)

B. Women's Health

Pulmonary embolism poses a special threat for women because VTE is associated with the use of oral contraceptives, pregnancy, and hormone replacement therapy.

One-third of pregnancy-related VTE occurs postpartum. The risk of DVT is present throughout pregnancy and increases during the third trimester. Of all antepartum DVT, about one-fifth occur during the first trimester, one-third during the second trimester, and almost half during the third trimester. After delivery, two of the most important risk factors for VTE are increased maternal age and cesarean section. Emergency cesarean section increases the VTE risk by about 50% compared with elective cesarean section.

Thrombophilia increases the risk of VTE during pregnancy and puerperium. Among women with a history of VTE during pregnancy or puerperium in one study, the prevalence of factor V Leiden was 44% and the prevalence of the prothrombin gene mutation was 17%. Compared with controls, the Leiden mutation increased the risk of VTE ninefold, and the prothrombin gene mutation increased the risk by a factor of 15. The combination of the Leiden and prothrombin gene mutations increased the VTE risk to more than 100 times that seen in the controls. Irrespective of factor V Leiden, pregnancy itself causes hypercoagulability because it induces a relative state of activated protein C resistance.

Hormone replacement therapy also predisposes to VTE. In 1996, three separate large data sets implicated hormone replacement therapy as doubling, tripling, or even quadrupling the risk of VTE. As with oral contraceptives, the risk of VTE peaks during the first year of hormone replacement therapy.

Gerhardt A et al. Prothrombin and factor V mutations in women with a history of thrombosis during pregnancy and the puerperium. N Engl J Med. 2000 Feb 10;342(6):374–80. [PMID: 10666427]

Miles JS et al. G20210A mutation in the prothrombin gene and the risk of recurrent venous thromboembolism. J Am Coll Cardiol. 2001 Jan;37(1):215–8. [PMID: 11153741]

Nguyen A. Prothrombin G20210A polymorphism and thrombophilia. Mayo Clin Proc. 2000 Jun;75(6):595–604. [PMID: 10852421]

Wicki J et al. Predicting adverse outcome in patients with acute pulmonary embolism: a risk score. Thromb Haemost. 2000 Oct;84(4):548–52. [PMID: 11057848]

▶ Clinical Findings

Pulmonary embolism is often difficult to diagnose. Despite the availability of lung scanning, chest computed tomographic (CT) scanning, and pulmonary angiography, many emboli are not discovered until postmortem examination. Appreciation of the clinical settings that make patients susceptible to PE and maintenance of a high degree of clinical suspicion are, therefore, of paramount importance.

An integrated diagnostic approach for cases of suspected PE (Figure 26–1) has been shown to be useful. The diagnostic workup should begin by quantifying the clinical suspicion with a precise clinical scoring algorithm. If the patient has no obvious acute comorbid illnesses, such as acute myocardial infarction, metastatic cancer, sepsis, or recent surgery, then a plasma D-dimer level should be obtained. If the D-dimer ELISA is normal (< 500 ng/mL), then the diagnosis of PE is almost always excluded. To pursue the diagnosis of PE with imaging tests, chest CT scanning is the single most useful examination, but a normal lung scan is also very reliable. If a diagnostic dilemma persists because of an equivocal chest CT scan, then venous ultrasonography of the legs can be undertaken. If the ultrasound is negative and the clinical suspicion remains very high, then pulmonary angiography is indicated in centers where pulmonary angiograms can be accurately interpreted.

A. Symptoms and Signs

The most common symptoms or signs of PE are nonspecific: dyspnea, tachypnea, chest pain, or tachycardia. Patients with life-threatening PE are apt to have dyspnea, syncope, or cyanosis rather than chest pain. Less than one-third of patients with PE have symptoms of a DVT. Massive PE should be suspected in hypotensive patients who have evidence of, or predisposing factors for, venous thrombosis and clinical findings of acute cor pulmonale (acute right ventricular failure), such as distended neck veins, an S_3 gallop, a right ventricular heave, tachycardia, or tachypnea.

Patients with severe chest pain or hemoptysis usually have anatomically small PE near the periphery of the lung. This is where innervation is greatest and where pulmonary infarction is most likely to occur from a dearth of collateral bronchial circulation.

Clinical scoring systems—Traditionally, the clinical likelihood of PE has been estimated subjectively by "gestalt" as low, moderate, or high. However, quantitative clinical scoring systems have been devised. This approach provides standardization and objectivity. If widely used, clinical

Brigham and Women's Hospital Integrated Approach

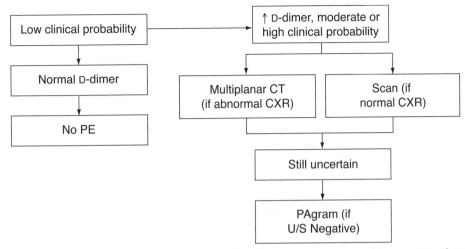

▲ **Figure 26–1.** Strategy for diagnosing pulmonary embolism. CT, computed tomographic scan; CXR, chest x-ray film; PAgram, pulmonary angiogram; PE, pulmonary embolism; U/S, ultrasound.

scoring systems will improve communication among members of the health care team when they are considering the diagnosis of PE.

The Ottawa Scoring System has a maximum of 12.5 points (Table 26–2). The greatest emphasis is placed on the presence of signs or symptoms of DVT (3 points) and whether an alternative diagnosis is unlikely (3 points). If the score exceeds 4 points, the overall likelihood of PE being confirmed with imaging tests is 41%. However, if the score is 4 points or less, the likelihood of PE is only 8%. Although this scoring system has the advantage of simplicity and rapidity, it offers a somewhat subjective approach with regard to the important, heavily weighted category of "alternative diagnosis unlikely." The Geneva Scoring System is more objective but also more complex (Table 26–3).

B. Diagnostic Studies

1. Nonimaging studies

A. ELECTROCARDIOGRAPHY—Electrocardiograms (ECG) may show evidence of acute cor pulmonale, manifested by a new S_1 $Q_3 T_3$ pattern, new incomplete right bundle branch block, right axis deviation, or right ventricular ischemia or strain with ST-segment depressions in the right precordial leads.

B. ARTERIAL BLOOD GASES—Neither measurement of room air arterial blood gases (Figure 26–2) nor calculation of the alveolar-arterial oxygen gradient (Figure 26–3) is useful in excluding the diagnosis of PE. Among patients in whom PE is suspected, neither test helped differentiate patients with a confirmed PE at angiography from those with a normal pulmonary angiogram. Therefore, arterial blood gases should not be obtained as a screening test for suspected PE.

C. PLASMA D-DIMER ENZYME-LINKED IMMUNOSORBENT ASSAY—Endogenous fibrinolysis, although ineffective in preventing PE, almost always causes the release of D-dimers from fibrin clot in the presence of established PE. Therefore, elevated levels of the D-dimer enzyme-linked immunosorbent assay (ELISA) serve as a highly sensitive screening test for patients in whom PE is suspected. However, such results are not specific and are elevated in many other conditions, such as myocardial infarction, pneumonia, cancer, sepsis, or the postoperative state. Normal D-dimer ELISA levels have a high negative predictive value in patients in whom acute PE is suspected. Among patients with a normal D-dimer level, the likelihood of no PE is approximately 95%. The combination of low clinical

Table 26–2. Ottawa Scoring System.

Signs or Symptoms	Points
Clinical signs and symptoms of DVT (minimum of leg swelling and pain with palpation of the deep veins)	3.0
An alternative diagnosis is less likely than PE	3.0
Heart rate greater than 100 bpm	1.5
Immobilization or surgery in the previous 4 weeks	1.5
Previous DVT or PE	1.5
Hemoptysis	1.0
Malignancy (on treatment, treated in the last 6 months or palliative)	1.0

DVT, deep venous thrombosis; PE, pulmonary embolism.
Reprinted, with permission, from: Wells PS et al. Thromb Haemost. 2000;83:416.

Table 26–3. Geneva Diagnostic Scoring System–Multivariate Predictors of Pulmonary Embolism and Development of the Clinical Score.

Variable	Logistic Regression Coefficients	Adjusted Odds Ratio (95% CI)	P	Point Score
Age, years				
60–79	0.6	1.9 (1.3–2.7)	.002	+1
≥ 80	1.0	2.8 (1.8–4.4)	< .001	+2
Previous PE or DVT	1.1	3.0 (2.1–4.4)	< .001	+2
Recent surgery	1.5	4.6 (2.6–8.3)	< .001	+3
Pulse rate > 100/min	0.5	1.6 (1.1–2.2)	.008	+1
Paco$_2$ mm Hg				
< 36 mm Hg	1.1	2.9 (1.9–4.4)	< .001	+2
36–40 mm Hg	0.6	1.9 (1.1–3.2)	.02	+1
Pao$_2$ mm Hg				
< 50	2.0	7.2 (3.2–15.8)	< .001	+4
50–59	1.4	3.9 (2.2–6.8)	< .001	+3
60–72	1.0	2.6 (1.6–4.2)	< .001	+2
73–82	0.6	1.8 (1.1–2.9)	.03	+1
Chest radiograph				
Platelike atelectasis	0.7	1.9 (1.3–2.9)	.001	+1
Elevation of hemidiaphragm	0.5	1.6 (1.1–2.4)	.02	+1

DVT, deep venous thrombosis; PE, pulmonary embolism.
Adapted, with permission, from Wicki J, et al. Arch Intern Med. 2001;161:92.

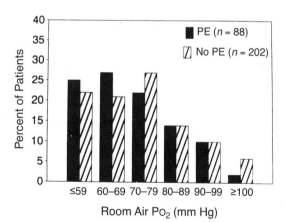

▲ **Figure 26–2.** Distribution of partial pressure of oxygen in arterial blood (Po$_2$) while breathing room air. The group included 88 patients with angiographically proven pulmonary embolism and no preexisting cardiac or pulmonary disease and 202 patients in whom PE was excluded with normal pulmonary angiograms. (Reprinted, with permission, from Stein PD et al. Chest. 1991;100:598.)

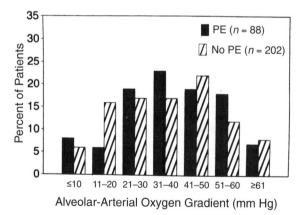

▲ **Figure 26–3.** Distribution of alveolar-arterial oxygen gradient among 88 patients with angiographically proven pulmonary embolism and no preexisting cardiac or pulmonary disease and 202 patients in whom PE was excluded with normal pulmonary angiograms. (Reprinted, with permission, from Stein PD et al. Chest. 1991;100:598.)

suspicion, ideally quantified with a validated scoring system, and a normal D-dimer ELISA, makes PE exceedingly unlikely.

D. Troponin levels—Screening for troponins is now the standard blood test for cardiac injury, and it is obtained routinely when acute myocardial infarction or unstable angina is suspected. Circulating troponin indicates irreversible myocardial cell damage and is much more sensitive than creatine kinase or its myocardial muscle isoenzyme. Cardiac markers of injury should not be used, however, as a primary diagnostic test for acute PE. Nevertheless, elevation of cardiac troponin is an adverse prognostic factor in patients with acute PE and is associated with a markedly increased mortality rate and requirement for inotropic support and mechanical ventilation. Troponin elevation also correlates with ECG evidence of right ventricular strain. This suggests that release of troponin from the myocardium during PE may result from acute right ventricular microinfarction due to pressure overload, impaired coronary artery blood flow, or hypoxemia caused by the PE.

2. Imaging studies

A. Chest radiography—Chest radiography can help exclude diseases such as lobar pneumonia, pneumothorax, or cardiogenic pulmonary edema, which can have clinical presentations that mimic acute PE. However, patients with these disorders can also have concomitant PE.

B. Radionuclide lung scanning—This study has served as the principal diagnostic imaging test for PE but is now with increasing frequency being superseded by chest CT scanning.

Lung scanning is most useful when unequivocally normal or when highly suggestive of PE (Figure 26–4). Neither intermediate nor low-probability scans (in the presence of high clinical suspicion) exclude PE. For example, with the combination of a low-probability scan and high clinical suspicion for PE, the likelihood of PE is 40%. When lung scanning is performed, the ventilation scan is being used less frequently than previously because its contribution to the diagnostic decision is only marginally better than the combination of a perfusion scan and chest radiograph.

C. Chest computed tomographic scanning—The chest CT is diagnostic of PE when an intraluminal pulmonary arterial filling defect is surrounded by contrast material. Computed tomographic scanning has two major advantages over lung scanning: (1) directly visualizing thrombus and (2) establishing alternative diagnoses on CT images of the lung parenchyma that are not evident on chest film.

Conventional chest CT scanning relies on imaging a series of consecutive sections of the chest. With the introduction of spiral chest CT scanning, patients can be scanned continually. As patients are advanced through the spiral CT scanner, the x-ray source and single-row detector array rotate around them. These scans are performed during a single breath-hold, thereby eliminating respiratory motion artifact that previously limited thoracic imaging. Overlap data from adjacent slices are acquired, thus reducing the possibility of missed pathology. Scans are performed in less than 30 seconds, and excellent vascular opacification with the contrast agent can usually be achieved (Figure 26–5).

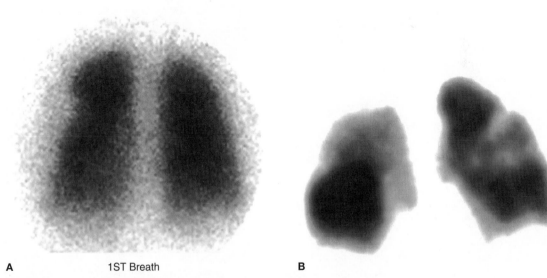

A   1ST Breath   B

▲ **Figure 26–4.** Lung scan for a 63-year-old woman who presented with idiopathic pulmonary embolism. The lung scan showed **A:** normal ventilation and **B:** multiple segmental perfusion defects, indicating a ventilator perfusion mismatch and high probability of pulmonary embolism.

However, the major limitation has been failure to detect PEs beyond third-order pulmonary arterial branches.

Further innovations occurred with the introduction of multidetector CT scanners, which acquire four slices simultaneously during each rotation of the x-ray source. Multidetector CT improves resolution from 5 mm to 1.25 mm and allows for better visualization of subsegmental vessels. Compared with conventional spiral CT, the sensitivity of multirow detector scanners for the diagnosis of acute PE increases from about 70% to 80–90%. In the PIOPED II study, which used multidetector CT angiography, the sensitivity and specificity was 83% and 96%, respectively. The positive predictive value was 96% with a concordant clinical assessment. The addition of CT venography to image DVTs improves the sensitivity from 83% to 90% with no change in specificity. In order to answer concerns that CT angiography could miss clinically important PEs in the branch pulmonary arteries, another randomized trial directly compared CT angiography with $\dot{V}/\dot{Q}$ scanning. In this study, CT was found to be noninferior. Pulmonary embolism was diagnosed in more patients in the CT group than in the $\dot{V}/\dot{Q}$ scanning group. The risk of VTE during 3-month follow-up after having a negative imaging study was 0.4% for CT and 1% for $\dot{V}/\dot{Q}$ scan.

Occasionally, determining whether a pulmonary embolus represents the residua of prior PE or a new event may be challenging. A systematic review of the literature has shown that over half of patients with PE will still have a defect on either CT scan or radionuclide imaging 6 months after diagnosis.

D. Venous ultrasonography—In combination with color Doppler imaging, venous ultrasonography is known as duplex sonography and is the principal diagnostic imaging test for suspected acute DVT. Sonographic evaluation uses compression ultrasound along the full length of the femoral, popliteal, and calf veins. The transducer is held transverse to the vein and, normally, the vein collapses with gentle manual compression. The compressed vein appears as if it is winking. The main criterion for diagnosing DVT

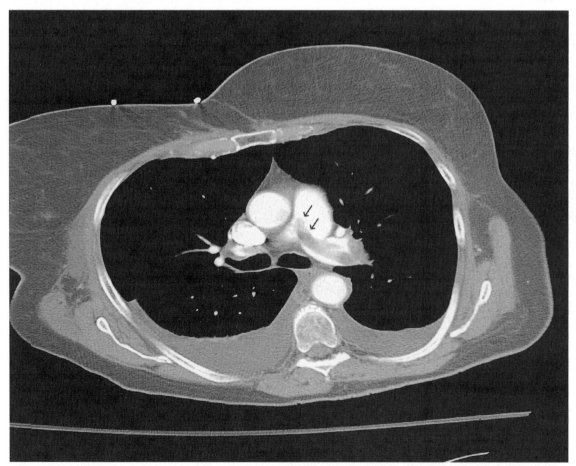

▲ **Figure 26–5.** Spiral computed tomography scan of massive bilateral pulmonary arterial filling defects (*arrows*) in the main pulmonary arteries of a 72-year-old woman who suffered acute pulmonary embolism after general surgery.

is lack of compression of a deep vein. This diagnosis can be confirmed by direct visualization of thrombus on ultrasound or by abnormal venous flow on Doppler examination (eg, loss of physiologic respiratory variation or loss of the expected augmentation of blood flow during calf compression).

Among symptomatic patients, duplex sonography is very accurate, with high sensitivity and specificity. Its sensitivity decreases when assessing asymptomatic patients. Major limitations include an inability to image pelvic vein thrombosis directly, lower sensitivity for diagnosing isolated calf DVT, and difficulty diagnosing an acute DVT superimposed upon a chronic one. Magnetic resonance imaging may be useful under these circumstances.

Importantly, many patients with PE do not have evidence of leg DVT, probably because the thrombus has already embolized to the pulmonary arteries. Therefore, PE is not necessarily ruled out if the clinical suspicion is high and imaging evidence of DVT is lacking.

E. Echocardiography—Echocardiography should not be used routinely to diagnose suspected PE because most patients with PE have normal echocardiograms. However, the echocardiogram, like the troponin level, is an excellent tool for risk stratification and prognostication. Echocardiography is useful diagnostically when the differential diagnosis includes pericardial tamponade, right ventricular infarction, and dissection of the aorta as well as PE.

Imaging a normal left ventricle in the presence of a dilated, hypokinetic right ventricle strongly suggests the diagnosis of PE (Figure 26–6). The presence of right ventricular mid-free wall akinesis with sparing of the apex (the McConnell sign) has been found to be highly specific for acute pulmonary embolism. Echocardiographic findings in PE patients are listed in Table 26–4.

The pulmonary arterial systolic pressure can be estimated by measuring the peak velocity of the tricuspid regurgitant jet obtained with Doppler echocardiography. The gradient across the tricuspid valve can be estimated by using the modified Bernoulli equation, $P = 4V^2$, where V is the peak velocity of the regurgitant jet, and P represents the peak pressure difference between the right atrium and right ventricle. The estimated right atrial pressure is added to the gradient to obtain an estimate of pulmonary arterial systolic pressure. The pulmonary artery systolic pressure may be low, normal, or mildly elevated in the setting of acute pulmonary embolism. Significant pulmonary hypertension suggests a subacute or chronic process. The incidence of chronic thromboembolic pulmonary hypertension following a first episode of PE is low overall (~1%), but in patients with unexplained persistent dyspnea after PE, the incidence may be as high as 4% after 2 years. Echocardiography to measure pulmonary artery pressure and exclude chronic thromboembolic pulmonary hypertension should be obtained for patients with persistent unexplained dyspnea following treatment of PE.

Transesophageal echocardiography for suspected PE is best reserved for critically ill patients. Transesophageal echocardiography diagnoses PE by direct visualization of thrombus, assesses its extent, and provides guidance regarding its

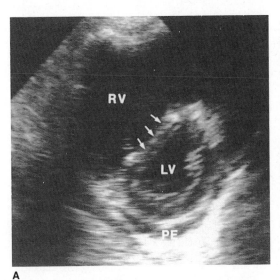 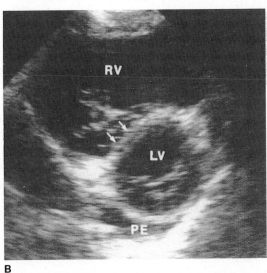

A   B

▲ **Figure 26–6.** Parasternal short-axis views of the right ventricle (RV) and left ventricle (LV) in **A:** diastole and **B:** systole. Diastolic and systolic bowing of the interventricular septum (*arrows*) into the left ventricle is evident, which is compatible with right ventricular volume and pressure overloads, respectively. The right ventricle is appreciably dilated and markedly hypokinetic, with little change in apparent right ventricular area from diastole to systole. PE, small pericardial effusion. (Reprinted, with permission, from Come PC. Chest. 1992;101[Suppl]:151S.)

Table 26–4. Abnormal Echocardiographic Findings in Pulmonary Embolism.

Abnormal Finding	Description
Right ventricular dilatation and hypokinesis	Associated with leftward septal shift; the ratio of the RVEDA to LVEDA exceeds the upper limit of normal (0.6). Associated with right atrial enlargement and tricuspid regurgitation.
Septal flattening and paradoxical septal motion	Right ventricular contraction continues even after the left ventricle starts relaxing at end-systole; therefore, the interventricular septum bulges toward the left ventricle.
Diastolic left ventricular impairment with a small difference between left ventricular area during diastole and systole, indicative of low cardiac output	Due to septal displacement and reduced left ventricular distensibility during diastole; consequently, Doppler mitral flow exhibits a prominent A wave, much higher than the E wave, with an increased contribution of atrial contraction to left ventricular filling.
Direct visualization of PE	Only if PE is large and centrally located; much more easily visualized on transesophageal than on transthoracic echocardiography.
Pulmonary arterial hypertension detected by Doppler flow velocity in the right ventricular outflow tract	Shortened acceleration time, with peak velocity occurring close to the onset of ejection. Biphasic ejection curve, with midsystolic reduction in velocity.
Right ventricular hypertrophy	With mildly increased right ventricular thickness (often about 6 mm, with 4 mm as upper limit of normal); clear visualization of right ventricular muscle trabeculations.
Patent foramen ovale	When right atrial pressure exceeds left atrial presure, the foramen ovale may open and cause worsening hypoxemia or stroke.

LVEDA, left ventricular end-diastolic area; PE, pulmonary embolism; RVEDA, right ventricular end–diastolic area.

surgical accessibility. Transesophageal echocardiography may also have a valuable role in detecting unexplained sudden cardiac arrest and pulseless electrical activity due to acute PE. In a series of 1246 patients who suffered cardiac arrest, 5% of cases were caused by PE; of those with PE, 63% of cardiac arrest cases were caused by pulseless electrical activity. Therefore, when pulseless electrical activity is present, PE should be considered.

F. PULMONARY ANGIOGRAPHY—This imaging method is rapidly becoming a lost art and is being undertaken primarily for therapeutic interventions (such as suction catheter embolectomy) rather than to solve diagnostic dilemmas. Most diagnostic questions can be resolved with the new generation chest CT scanners, which provide resolution to subsegmental branches. A constant intraluminal filling defect seen in more than one projection is the most reliable angiographic diagnostic feature for PE.

Pulmonary angiography can almost always be accomplished safely, although the risk may be increased in patients with severe pulmonary hypertension. Selective angiography should be performed, with the equivocal portion of the perfusion lung scan or chest CT scan serving as a road map. To avoid damaging the intima of the pulmonary artery, soft, flexible catheters with side holes should be used, rather than stiff catheters with end holes. Low-osmolar contrast agents minimize the transient hypotension, heat, and coughing that often occur with conventional radioactive contrast agents.

Anderson DR et al. Computed tomographic pulmonary angiography vs ventilation-perfusion lung scanning in patients with suspected pulmonary embolism: a randomized controlled trial. JAMA. 2007 Dec 19;298(23):2743–53. [PMID: 18165667]

Becattini C et al. Incidence of chronic thromboembolic pulmonary hypertension after a first episode of pulmonary embolism. Chest. 2006 Jul;130(1):172–5. [PMID: 16840398]

Giannitsis E et al. Independent prognostic value of cardiac troponin T in patients with confirmed pulmonary embolism. Circulation. 2000 Jul 11;102(2):211–7. [PMID: 10889133]

Kürkciyan I et al. Pulmonary embolism as cause of cardiac arrest: presentation and outcome. Arch Intern Med. 2000 May 22;160(10):1529–35. [PMID: 10826469]

McConnell MV et al. Regional right ventricular dysfunction detected by echocardiography in acute pulmonary embolism. Am J Cardiol. 1996 Aug 15;78(4):469–73. [PMID: 8752195]

Meyer T et al. Cardiac troponin I elevation in acute pulmonary embolism is associated with right ventricular dysfunction. J Am Coll Cardiol. 2000 Nov 1;36(5):1632–6. [PMID: 11079669]

Nijkeuter M et al. Resolution of thromboemboli in patients with acute pulmonary embolism: a systematic review. Chest. 2006 Jan;129(1):192–7. [PMID: 16424432]

Pattynama PM et al. Second-generation, subsecond multislice computed-tomography: advancing the role of helical CT pulmonary angiography in suspected pulmonary embolism. Semin Vasc Med. 2001 Nov;1(2):195–204. [PMID: 15199503]

Pengo V et al; Thromboembolic Pulmonary Hypertension Study Group. Incidence of chronic thromboembolic pulmonary hypertension after pulmonary embolism. N Engl J Med. 2004 May 27;350(22):2257–64. [PMID: 15163775]

Stein PD et al; PIOPED II Investigators. Multidetector computed tomography for acute pulmonary embolism. N Engl J Med. 2006 Jun 1;354(22):2317–27. [PMID: 16738268]

van Belle A et al; Christopher Study Investigators. Effectiveness of managing suspected pulmonary embolism using an algorithm combining clinical probability, D-dimer testing, and computed tomography. JAMA. 2006 Jan 11;295(2):172–9. [PMID: 16403929]

Wells PS et al. Derivation of a simple clinical model to categorize patients probability of pulmonary embolism: increasing the models utility with the SimpliRED D-dimer. Thromb Haemost. 2000 Mar;83(3):416–20. [PMID: 10744147]

Wicki J et al. Assessing clinical probability of pulmonary embolism in the emergency ward: a simple score. Arch Intern Med. 2001 Jan 8;161(1):92–7. [PMID: 11146703]

▶ Prevention

Pulmonary embolism is easier and less expensive to prevent than to diagnose or treat; therefore, virtually all hospitalized patients should receive prophylaxis against VTE. Unfortunately, such prophylaxis is underutilized, even for high-risk patients. Furthermore, prophylaxis, even when instituted, may not be effective. Nonetheless, prevention programs should be established at all hospitals to ensure that adequate measures are implemented. Nurses and physicians must collaborate to achieve this goal by instituting protocols that are both streamlined and standardized. In addition, quality assurance personnel should adopt a proactive stance to encourage the development of such programs.

The preventive measures should be based on an assessment of the patient's level of risk for PE and whether the optimal strategy will be nonpharmacologic, pharmacologic, or combined modalities. Because the risk of PE continues after discharge from the hospital, prophylaxis should be continued at home among those patients at moderate or high risk for VTE.

1. Nonpharmacologic prevention—The most commonly used nonpharmacologic measures are graduated compression stockings and intermittent pneumatic compression devices ("boots"). Vascular compression with either stockings or boots is effective among surgical patients, because it counters the otherwise-unopposed perioperative venodilation that appears causally related to postoperative venous thrombosis. Even among low-risk general surgery patients, graduated compression stockings can substantially reduce the frequency of venous thrombosis and should therefore be considered first-line prophylaxis against PE in all hospitalized patients, except those with peripheral arterial occlusive disease whose condition may be worsened by vascular compression.

Intermittent pneumatic compression boots, which provide intermittent inflation of air-filled cuffs, prevent venous stasis in the legs; they also appear to stimulate the endogenous fibrinolytic system. Because it appears that graduated compression stockings and intermittent pneumatic compression boots work through somewhat different—although complementary—mechanisms, these modalities can be used in combination in patients at moderate or high risk for venous thrombosis.

2. Pharmacologic prevention—Anticoagulant drugs can be used instead of—or in addition to—nonpharmacologic prophylaxis (Table 26–5).

Table 26–5. FDA–Approved Low–Molecular Weight Regimens for Orthopedic and General Surgery Prophylaxis.

Indication	Drug and Dose	Duration	Timing of Initial Dose
Hip replacement ("USA-style") with enoxaparin	Enoxaparin 30 mg q12h or 40 mg q24h	≤ 14 days	12–24 h postoperatively, providing that hemostasis has been achieved
Hip replacement ("European-style") with enoxaparin	Enoxaparin 40 mg q24h	≤ 14 days	12 h ± 3 h preoperatively
Hip replacement with dalteparin (option #1)	Dalteparin 2500 units preoperatively and first dose postoperatively, followed by 5000 units q24h	≤ 14 days	First dose within 2 h preoperatively; second dose at least 6 h after the first dose, usually on the evening of the day of surgery; omit second dose on the day of surgery if surgery is done in the evening
Hip replacement with dalteparin (option #2)	Dalteparin 5000 units q24h	≤ 14 days	First dose on the preoperative evening; second dose on the evening of the day of surgery (unless surgery is done in the evening)
Extended hip prophylaxis	Enoxaparin 40 mg q24h	An additional 3 weeks after initial hip replacement prophylaxis	After the initial hip replacement prophylaxis regimen has been completed
General surgery with enoxaparin	Enoxaparin 40 mg q24h	≤ 12 days	2 h preoperatively
General surgery with dalteparin (moderate risk for venous thromboembolism)	Dalteparin 2500 units q24h	5–10 days	1–2 h preoperatively
General surgery with dalteparin (high risk for venous thromboembolism: option #1)	Dalteparin 5000 units q24h	5–10 days	Preoperative evening
General surgery with dalteparin (high risk for venous thromboembolism: option #2)	Dalteparin 2500 units preoperatively and first dose postoperatively, followed by 5000 units q24h	5–10 days	First dose 1–2 h preoperatively; second dose 12 h later

3. Future directions—Many hospitals use protocol-driven prophylaxis for all hospitalized patients, especially for medical patients hospitalized in intensive care units. The emphasis on preventive strategies includes the time of hospital discharge or transfer to a skilled nursing facility or rehabilitation hospital. Orders to prescribe these prophylactic measures often are prompted by a computerized order entry system that reminds physicians about the need for prophylaxis.

▶ Risk Stratification

Not all PEs are created equal. The most important concept in PE management is that acute PE spans a wide range of risk, from small asymptomatic emboli to massive thromboembolism with catastrophic cardiovascular collapse and death due to right ventricular failure. Therapy must be geared to patient risk. Low-risk patients will do well with anticoagulation alone, whereas high-risk patients may require thrombolysis or embolectomy in addition to anticoagulation.

Investigators in Geneva have developed a clinical risk score to predict adverse outcomes after PE (Tables 26–6 and 26–7). The maximum number of points, based on clinical parameters, is 8. Those patients scoring 5 or more points had a more than 50% likelihood of a major adverse clinical event, such as recurrent thromboembolism, major bleeding, or death. Other nonimaging markers of poor prognosis include hypoxemia despite oxygen supplementation, physical examination evidence (accentuated pulmonic component of the second heart sound or left parasternal heave, or distended neck veins) of pulmonary hypertension or right ventricular strain, or an elevated troponin level.

The most important imaging test for risk stratification is echocardiographic assessment of right ventricular function. Even if the initial systemic blood pressure is normal, patients with echocardiographic evidence of right ventricular dysfunction may develop cardiogenic shock within 24 hours; these patients may have a high mortality rate. In contrast, the mortality rate is low in normotensive patients with normal right ventricular function on echocardiography.

Table 26–6. Geneva Point Score to Assess Pulmonary Embolism Prognosis.

Variable	Point Score
Cancer	+2
Heart failure	+1
Prior DVT	+1
Hypotension	+2
Hypoxemia	+1
DVT on ultrasound	+1

DVT, deep venous thrombosis.
Modified, with permission, from Wicki J et al. Thromb Haemost. 2000;84:548.

Pulmonary hypertension, as estimated by Doppler echocardiography, that persists for more than 5 weeks after the diagnosis of PE is associated with an adverse long-term prognosis.

Biomarkers that reflect right ventricular strain or ischemia may also be useful tools to assess risk. The combination of either an elevated brain-natriuretic peptide (BNP) or an elevated troponin level in conjunction with echocardiographic evidence of right ventricular dysfunction increases the odds of an in-hospital complication by tenfold. Elevated levels of these biomarkers should prompt an echocardiogram to look for right ventricular dysfunction.

▶ Treatment

A. Heparin

Unfractionated heparin is the standard initial treatment for isolated PE. The FDA has not approved any LMWH for primary symptomatic PE without associated DVT.

Although unfractionated heparin has served as the standard foundation of PE treatment for more than 40 years, this anticoagulant has important limitations. Its variable protein

Table 26–7. Geneva Adverse Outcome Score.

Number of Points	Number of Patients	Cumulative %	Percent of Patients with Adverse Outcome (n)
0	52	19.4	0 (0)
1	79	48.9	2.5 (2)
2	49	67.2	4.1 (2)
3	56	88.1	17.8 (10)
4	22	96.3	27.3 (6)
5	7	98.9	57.1 (4)
6	3	100	100 (3)

Reprinted with permission from: Wicki J et al. Thromb Haemost. 2000;84:548.

binding leads to an often unpredictable dose response and makes it a drug that is difficult to administer properly in everyday clinical practice. Subtherapeutic levels of heparin increase the risk of recurrent PE, while excessive levels of heparin increase the risk of major bleeding. Unfractionated heparin for PE treatment is usually ordered as an intravenous bolus followed by a continuous intravenous infusion. The required dose is unpredictable and must be adjusted according to the activated partial thromboplastin time. In general, the target partial thromboplastin time is 60–80 seconds. Heparin is usually administered as a bolus of 5000–10,000 units followed by a weight-based hourly infusion (Table 26–8).

Patients being treated with heparin who have a subsequent drop in platelet count should be evaluated for heparin-induced thrombocytopenia. The platelet count may decline within hours or, more commonly, 5–10 days after exposure to heparin. Patients with known or suspected heparin-induced thrombocytopenia should be treated with either direct thrombin inhibitors (such as lepirudin, argatroban, or bivalirudin) or heparinoids (such as danaparoid). Heparin, LMWH, and warfarin monotherapy should be avoided in the setting of known or suspected heparin-induced thrombocytopenia.

B. Low-Molecular-Weight Heparin

Low-molecular-weight heparins (LMWHs) have revolutionized the initial management of venous thromboembolism (Table 26–9). The use of LMWHs to treat DVT has dramatically converted the therapy of this illness from a 5- to 6-day hospitalization to primarily outpatient or overnight in-hospital management. In the United States, two LMWHs are approved for treatment of patients with symptomatic DVT, with or without PE: enoxaparin and tinzaparin (Table 26–10). The FDA-approved outpatient therapy for DVT with the LMWH enoxaparin is 1 mg/kg twice daily, or a once daily dose of 1.5 mg/kg. Low-molecular-weight heparins appear to be safer than unfractionated heparin because osteopenia and heparin-induced thrombocytopenia occur far less often. They

have a much more predictable dose response than unfractionated heparin and can usually be administered on the basis of weight alone, without any blood testing to modify the dose. They have a minimal effect on the partial thromboplastin time. Renal insufficiency (particularly a creatinine clearance < 30 mL/min), low body weight, massive obesity, elderly age, and pregnancy increase the risk of incorrect dosing, resulting in either over- or under-anticoagulation. Avoidance of LMWH, dose-adjustment, or monitoring of anti-factor Xa activity may be necessary in these patients (Table 26–11). Even though dose-adjustment is not recommended for patients with mild to moderate renal insufficiency ($Cl_{cr} \geq 30$ mL/min), spontaneous bleeding from standard weight-based dosing of LMWHs may develop in such patients.

In a meta-analysis of randomized DVT treatment trials comparing LMWHs with unfractionated heparin, LMWHs were found to be more effective and safer. Their use resulted in fewer recurrent thromboemboli, less bleeding, less thrombocytopenia, and an improved quality of life and patient satisfaction. The strategy of using LMWHs was also more cost-effective. The 2007 American College of Physicians (ACP) guidelines thus recommend the initial use of LMWH in lieu of unfractionated heparin for the inpatient or outpatient treatment of DVT.

C. Thrombolysis

Pulmonary embolism thrombolysis remains controversial because large clinical trials using survival as an end point have not been conducted. A definitive clinical trial is long overdue. Nevertheless, successful thrombolysis usually reverses right heart failure rapidly and safely, thereby preventing a downhill spiral of cardiogenic shock. Thrombolysis may also prevent chronic pulmonary hypertension over the long term and thus improve exercise tolerance and quality of life. It is certain that thrombolysis should be considered only for those patients at high risk for an adverse clinical outcome with anticoagulation alone. Although no precise indications currently exist in the absence of massive PE with cardiogenic shock, the clinician should be wary of conservative manage-

Table 26–8. Unfractionated Heparin Weight–Based Nomogram for Acute Venous Thromboembolism.

PTT	Repeat Bolus	Stop Infusion (min)	Rate Change	Repeat PTT (h)
< 35	70 units/kg[1]	0	Increase 3 units/kg/h	6
35–59	35 units/kg[2]	0	Increase 2 units/kg/h	6
60–80 target	0	0	No change	6
81–100	0	0	Decrease 2 units/kg/h	6
> 100	0	60	Decrease 3 units/kg/h	6

[1]Maximum bolus 10,000 units.
[2]Maximum bolus 5000 units.
PTT, activated partial thromboplastin time; measured in seconds.

Table 26–9. Comparison of Unfractionated Heparin versus Low–Molecular–Weight Heparin.

Characteristic	UFH	LMWH
Molecular weight (average in daltons)	15,000	5000
Ratio of anti-Xa to anti-IIa (thrombin) activity	1	> 1
Metabolism	Hepatic	Renal
Bioavailability	Fair	Excellent
Frequency of subcutaneous administration	X2–X3/day	X1–X2/day
Frequency of heparin-induced thrombocytopenia	1–2%	0.1–0.2%
Osteoporosis after prolonged exposure	Rare	Very rare
Laboratory assay of anticoagulant effect	Activated partial thromboplastin time	Anti-Xa level
Reversal of anticoagulant effect	Protamine	Protamine
Spinal or epidural anesthesia	OK	Heed the FDA warning

FDA, Food and Drug Administration.

ment in the presence of risk factors for a poor prognosis (Table 26–12).

For patients with massive PE and cardiogenic shock, thrombolysis can be life-saving. While thrombolysis for massive PE with shock is a widely accepted treatment, thrombolysis for submassive PE remains controversial. Echocardiography helps identify a subgroup of PE patients with impending right ventricular failure who appear to be at high risk for adverse clinical outcomes if treated with heparin alone. Right ventricular dysfunction can also be inferred when right ventricular dilatation is seen on CT scan. The combination of elevated cardiac biomarkers (which likely indicate right ventricular infarction or strain) along with echocardiographic evidence of right ventricular dysfunction predicts a poor outcome in acute submassive PE.

Catheter-directed thrombolysis, in which the thrombolytic agent is delivered directly to the pulmonary arterial circulation through a side-hole catheter, can be efficacious, but there is insufficient evidence to recommend this treatment option at this time.

D. Embolectomy

Patients at high risk for an adverse outcome with anticoagulation alone should be considered for embolectomy if they have contraindications to thrombolytic therapy. Embolectomy can be performed as a catheter-based procedure in the interventional laboratory or in the operating room. Clinical success has been reported, but randomized trials are lacking. Catheter embolectomy has a very limited application because it cannot successfully remove large amounts of thrombus, due to limitations in available catheter devices.

Surgical embolectomy for acute PE should be considered for patients who would otherwise receive thrombolytic therapy but who have contraindications to this treatment modality. The operation is best performed on a warm beating heart with continuous TEE monitoring, after performing a median sternotomy and placing the patient on cardiopulmonary bypass. The embolus should be removed under direct visualization, never "blindly." With experience, all lobar and most segmental pulmonary artery branches can be visualized. It is crucial to refer high-risk PE patients as soon as their prognosis with anticoagulation has been established. Taking a "watch and wait" approach and delaying referring until the onset of cardiogenic shock requiring pressors yields poor results.

To manage severe chronic thromboembolic pulmonary hypertension due to prior PE, a separate and more technically challenging operation can be performed, a pulmonary thromboendarterectomy. This operation is only performed in highly specialized centers. If successful, this operation can reduce and possibly cure pulmonary hypertension. This surgery requires careful dissection of the old thrombus, which has turned whitish and hardened, from the walls of the pulmonary arteries. Complications include pulmonary arterial perforation and hemorrhage; pulmonary steal syndrome, in which blood rushes from previously well-perfused lung tissue to newly perfused tissue; and reperfusion pulmonary edema. For patients who are not candidates for pulmonary thromboendarterectomy, balloon pulmonary angioplasty can be considered.

Table 26–10. FDA-Approved Low-Molecular-Weight Heparins for the Initial Treatment of DVT (with or without Asymptomatic PE).

Enoxaparin 1 mg/kg twice daily
Enoxaparin 1.5 mg/kg once daily
Tinzaparin 175 units/kg once daily

DVT, deep venous thrombosis; FDA, Food and Drug Administration; PE, pulmonary embolism.

Table 26–11. Low–Molecular–Weight Heparin Weight–Based Nomogram for Enoxaparin in the Presence of Renal Insufficiency or Marked Obesity.

Renal Insufficiency Creatinine Clearance (mL/min)	Enoxaparin Dose	Anti-Xa Monitoring (Heparin Level)[1]
> 70	1 mg/kg q12h	None
35–69	0.75 mg/kg q12h	3–6 h after the third injection
< 35	1 mg/kg q24h	3–6 h after the third injection
Obese Weight	**Enoxaparin Dose**	**Anti-Xa Monitoring (Heparin Level)[1]**
< 100 kg	1 mg/kg q12h	None
100–130 kg	1 mg/kg q12h	3–6 h after the first injection
> 130 kg	130 mg q12h	3–6 h after the first injection

[1]Therapeutic level is 0.5–1.0 units/mL.

E. Inferior Vena Caval Filters

There are two indications for placing an inferior vena caval filter for patients with acute PE: (1) concomitant major bleeding requiring transfusion or any intracranial hemorrhage that precludes the use of anticoagulant therapy, (2) recurrent PE despite prolonged intensive anticoagulation. Though filters reduce the frequency of PE, they do not halt the thrombotic process and are associated with a doubling of the rate of DVT.

F. Warfarin

Warfarin is the standard oral anticoagulant used in the United States. Warfarin dosing is adjusted according to a standardized prothrombin time by using the international normalized ratio (INR). For PE and DVT, the target INR is ordinarily between 2.0 and 3.0. Unfortunately, warfarin treatment is limited by a narrow therapeutic window. Too little anticoagulant effect leads to thromboembolism, and excessive anticoagulation leads to bleeding. The drug is plagued by a long list of interactions with other drugs that either decrease or increase warfarin's anticoagulant effect. The consumption of vitamin K-containing foods such as green leafy vegetables decreases the anticoagulant effect, whereas the ingestion of alcohol increases the likelihood of hemorrhage.

Optimal warfarin dosing can be facilitated by understanding the following factors. First, use of acetaminophen in high doses may lead to an unintended increase in the INR. Second, warfarin should be initiated in a dose of about 5 mg once daily for an average sized adult, rather than initiating much higher loading doses. Third, since 2–3% of patients have a genetic mutation that results in slow metabolism of warfarin, the INR should be tested after several doses of warfarin, rather than waiting for 5 days after initiation of therapy. Pharmacogenetic testing to help guide initial warfarin dosing is being studied and may become common practice in the future. Finally, for patients who require long-term anticoagulation, point-of-care fingerstick INR testing machines can be prescribed for home use for patients who are able to be trained to self-adjust their warfarin doses based on the results of the INR.

Although warfarin is the most commonly used drug for long-term outpatient anticoagulation, for select patient populations, such as those with cancer, difficult to control INR values, or recurrent embolism despite therapeutic INR, long-term LMWH may be preferable to warfarin.

1. Reversal of warfarin—When the INR exceeds 5.0 in the absence of clinical bleeding, warfarin should be withheld and oral vitamin K administered, usually in a dose of 2.5 mg. Although oral vitamin K is preferable, it may be given subcutaneously when gastrointestinal absorption is uncertain. Occasionally, patients will require immediate reversal of excessive anticoagulation. This can be accomplished by the emergency administration of fresh frozen plasma, usually two units. However, to ensure continued reversal, vitamin K should be administered concomitantly.

Table 26–12. Pulmonary Embolism Patients at High Risk (in the Absence of Systemic Arterial Hypotension and Cardiogenic Shock).

Physical findings of right ventricular dysfunction (eg, distended neck veins, accentuated P_2, tricuspid regurgitation murmur)
Electrocardiographic manifestations of right ventricular strain (eg, new right bundle branch block, new T-wave inversion in leads V_1-V_4)
Right ventricular dilatation and hypokinesis or akinesis on echocardiogram
Patent foramen ovale
Free-floating right-heart thrombi
Doppler echocardiographic pulmonary arterial systolic pressure > 50 mm Hg
Elevated troponin level
Age > 70 years
Cancer
Congestive heart failure
Chronic obstructive pulmonary disease

2. Optimal duration of anticoagulation—The optimal duration of anticoagulation for patients with acute PE remains extremely controversial. The ACP guidelines recommend that anticoagulation be continued for 3–6 months for VTE due to transient risk factors (such as postoperative state) and for > 12 months or indefinitely for recurrent VTE. For first-time idiopathic VTE, ie, PE that occurs without relation to cancer, surgery, or trauma, the optimal duration of anticoagulation is not known. Although several trials have shown that extended duration (beyond 3–12 months) of anticoagulant therapy for idiopathic VTE does reduce the rate of VTE recurrence, the follow-up has only been for 4 years, and therefore the risk-benefit ratio needs to be determined on a case-by-case basis. Further research will be required to identify those patients prospectively who are at highest risk for recurrence after discontinuation of anticoagulation.

G. Adjunctive Measures

Occasionally, PE patients will require ventilatory assistance for respiratory failure or will rarely require pulmonary artery catheterization to determine optimal fluid management. Most patients with acute PE, however, can be cared for in an intermediate care or step-down unit. Most will benefit from supplemental oxygen. Opioids usually do not relieve the chest discomfort. Nonsteroidal antiinflammatory agents are often effective, and combining them with anticoagulation usually does not pose an undue risk of bleeding complications.

Patients with PE and concomitant DVT of the leg should wear below-knee graduated compression stockings (ideally 30–40 mm Hg or, if not tolerated, 20–30 mm Hg), to provide leg support while ambulating, for a minimum of 1 year after DVT diagnosis. The stockings help prevent distention of the vein wall and may mitigate the syndrome of chronic venous insufficiency—most often characterized by leg swelling and discomfort—that most DVT patients experience.

H. Venous Thromboembolism in Pregnancy

The risk of VTE is increased fivefold during pregnancy. There is insufficient evidence to definitively guide the management of VTE during pregnancy. Warfarin should be avoided in early pregnancy because it may lead to embryopathy between 6 and 12 weeks of gestation. Unfractionated heparin and LMWH are not associated with embryopathy because they do not cross the placenta. However, prolonged unfractionated heparin use may lead to osteoporosis and is inconvenient. The correct dosing of LMWH may be difficult to determine by weight during pregnancy; thus, anti-Factor Xa levels may need to be monitored periodically to ensure adequacy of dosing.

I. Counseling

Although PE can be as devastating emotionally and physically as myocardial infarction, the burden on individual patients may be even greater because the general public does not have as good an understanding of PE, particularly in terms of the potential incomplete recovery from it and long-term disability it engenders. Young patients with PE repeatedly voice a common theme. Although they appear healthy, they have actually suffered a life-threatening illness. Because of their youth and healthy appearance, others may not empathize with their fears and feelings about the illness.

Virtually all patients with PE will wonder why they were stricken with the illness and whether they harbor an underlying coagulopathy (or "bad" gene) that predisposed them. When anticoagulation is discontinued after an adequate course of therapy, patients are often fearful of recurrent PE.

Agnelli G et al; Warfarin Optimal Duration Italian Trial Investigators. Three months versus one year of oral anticoagulant therapy for idiopathic deep venous thrombosis. Warfarin Optimal Duration Italian Trial Investigators. N Engl J Med. 2001 Jul 19;345(3):165–9. [PMID: 11463010]

Aklog L et al. Acute pulmonary embolectomy: a contemporary approach. Circulation. 2002 Mar 26;105(12):1416–9. [PMID: 11914247]

Arepally GM et al. Clinical practice. Heparin-induced thrombocytopenia. N Engl J Med. 2006 Aug 24;355(8):809–17. [PMID: 16928996]

Binder L et al. N-terminal pro-brain natriuretic peptide or troponin testing followed by echocardiography for risk stratification of acute pulmonary embolism. Circulation. 2005 Sep 13;112(11):1573–9. [PMID: 16144990]

Campbell IA et al. Anticoagulation for three versus six months in patients with deep vein thrombosis or pulmonary embolism or both: randomised trial. BMJ. 2007 Mar 31;334(7595):674. [PMID: 17289685]

Fedullo PF et al. Chronic thromboembolic pulmonary hypertension. N Engl J Med. 2001 Nov 15;345(20):1465–72. [PMID: 11794196]

Feinstein JA et al. Balloon pulmonary angioplasty for treatment of chronic thromboembolic pulmonary hypertension. Circulation. 2001 Jan 2;103(1):10–3. [PMID: 11136677]

Gibson NS et al. Prognostic value of echocardiography and spiral computed tomography in patients with pulmonary embolism. Curr Opin Pulm Med. 2005 Sep;11(5):380–4. [PMID: 16093809]

Grifoni S et al. Short-term clinical outcome of patients with acute pulmonary embolism, normal blood pressure, and echocardiographic right ventricular dysfunction. Circulation. 2000 Jun 20;101(24):2817–22. [PMID: 10859287]

Hron G et al. Identification of patients at low risk for recurrent venous thromboembolism by measuring thrombin generation. JAMA. 2006 Jul 26;296(4):397–402. [PMID: 16868297]

Lee AY et al; Randomized Comparison of Low-Molecular-Weight Heparin versus Oral Anticoagulant Therapy for the Prevention of Recurrent Venous Thromboembolism in Patients with Cancer (CLOT) Investigators. Low-molecular-weight heparin versus a coumarin for the prevention of recurrent venous thromboembolism in patients with cancer. N Engl J Med. 2003 Jul 10;349(2):146–53. [PMID: 12853587]

Logeart D et al. Biomarker-based strategy for screening right ventricular dysfunction in patients with non-massive pulmonary embolism. Intensive Care Med. 2007 Feb;33(2):286–92. [PMID: 17165016]

Merli G et al; Enoxaparin Clinical Trial Group. Subcutaneous enoxaparin once or twice daily compared with intravenous unfractionated heparin for treatment of venous thromboembolic disease. Ann Intern Med. 2001 Feb 6;134(3):191–202. [PMID: 11177331]

Palareti G et al; PROLONG Investigators. D-dimer testing to determine the duration of anticoagulation therapy. N Engl J Med. 2006 Oct 26;355(17):1780–9. [PMID: 17065639]

Pinede L et al; Investigators of the "Durée Optimale du Traitment AntiVitamines K" (DOTAVK) Study. Comparison of 3 and 6 months of oral anticoagulant therapy after a first episode of proximal deep vein thrombosis or pulmonary embolism and comparison of 6 and 12 weeks of therapy after isolated calf deep vein thrombosis. Circulation. 2001 May 22;103(2):2453–60. [PMID: 11369685]

PREPIC Study Group. Eight-year follow-up of patients with permanent vena cava filters in the prevention of pulmonary embolism: the PREPIC (Prevention du Risque d'Embolie Pulmonaire par Interruption Cave) randomized study. Circulation. 2005 Jul 19;112(3):416–22. [PMID: 16009794]

Schwarz UI et al. Genetic determinants of response to warfarin during initial anticoagulation. N Engl J Med. 2008 Mar 6;358(10):999–1008. [PMID: 18322281]

Segal JB et al. Management of venous thromboembolism: a systematic review for a practice guideline. Ann Intern Med. 2007 Feb 6;146(3):211–22. [PMID: 17261856]

Snow V et al; American College of Physicians; American Academy of Family Physicians Panel on Deep Venous Thrombosis/Pulmonary Embolism. Management of venous thromboembolism: a clinical practice guideline from the American College of Physicians and the American Academy of Family Physicians. Ann Intern Med. 2007 Feb 6;146(3):204–10. [PMID: 17261857]

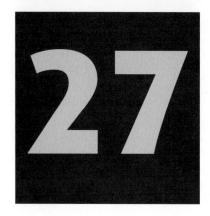

Pulmonary Hypertension

David D. McManus, MD & Teresa De Marco, MD

ESSENTIALS OF DIAGNOSIS

Pulmonary hypertension

▶ A loud pulmonic valve closure (P₂), a right-sided S₄, or a right ventricular heave.

▶ Electrocardiographic evidence of right ventricular hypertrophy.

▶ Presence of sustained elevation in mean pulmonary artery pressure ≥ 25 mm Hg at rest or ≥ 30 mm Hg with exercise.

Pulmonary arterial hypertension

▶ A subset of pulmonary hypertension.

▶ Elevated mean pulmonary artery pressure ≥ 25 mm Hg.

▶ Pulmonary arterial wedge pressure ≤ 15 mm Hg.

▶ Elevated pulmonary vascular resistance > 3 Wood units or > 240 dynes × s × cm⁻⁵

Pulmonary hypertension (PH) is caused by a wide array of conditions that increase pulmonary arterial (PA) pressure either passively or through vasoconstriction with or without vascular remodeling. The natural history of PH is heavily influenced by its underlying cause. In the United States, PH most commonly results from left-sided heart disease or chronic lung disease. Pulmonary arterial hypertension (PAH) is a less common but serious condition associated with a dismal prognosis. Diagnosis of PAH requires a high index of clinical suspicion. If PAH is considered likely, echocardiography and right-heart catheterization are commonly used diagnostic tests. Selection of therapies for patients with PH is complex but largely predicated on an understanding of the underlying disease and on the severity of the patient's symptoms. Prompt referral to specialty centers for patients with PAH is often crucial for confirmation of diagnosis, early initiation of appropriate therapy, and monitoring of response to treatment.

▶ General Considerations

Pulmonary hypertension is a pathologic state defined by a sustained elevation in the mean PA pressure of 25 mm Hg or greater at rest. The PA systolic pressure is normally 20–30 mm Hg and the PA diastolic pressure is normally 8–12 mm Hg. Normal mean PA pressure is 12–16 mm Hg. Normal pulmonary arterial wedge pressure (PAWP) is 8–12 mm Hg. The small arteriovenous pressure gradient generated by blood flow across the pulmonary circulation is a byproduct of such variables as total vascular surface area and pulmonary vascular compliance. This pressure gradient, termed the "pulmonary vascular resistance" (PVR), is quantified using **Ohm's law** [PVR = (mean PA – PAWP) / cardiac output (CO). Pulmonary arterial hypertension is a subset of PH marked by persistent elevation in the mean PA pressure and PVR. Significant advances have been made over the past decade in improving clinicians' understanding of the clinical profile, pathobiology, and treatment of PAH.

▶ Classification & Pathogenesis

The World Health Organization has proposed a system to categorize PH into five groups on the basis of underlying etiology (Table 27–1). Pulmonary hypertension can also be categorized on a hemodynamic basis at right heart catheterization (Figure 27–1). Pulmonary hypertension is characterized based on the mean PA pressure: mild (25–40 mm Hg), moderate (41–55 mm Hg), or severe (> 55 mm Hg).

A. Pulmonary Arterial Hypertension

Pulmonary arterial hypertension is hemodynamically precapillary in origin (Figure 27–1). Pulmonary arterial hypertension is defined by a progressive and sustained elevation of the mean PA pressure ≥ 25 mm Hg at rest (or ≥ 30 mm Hg with exercise), in the presence of a PAWP ≤ 15 mm Hg and PVR > 3.0 Wood units (240 dynes × s × cm⁻⁵).

Pulmonary arterial hypertension is caused by a disparate group of diseases that converge to produce intrinsic pulmo-

Table 27–1. Revised Classification System for Pulmonary Hypertension.

Group 1: Pulmonary arterial hypertension
- Idiopathic
- Familial
- Associated with:
  Connective tissue disease
  Congenital systemic-to-pulmonary shunts
  Portal hypertension
  HIV infection
  Drugs and toxins
  Other (thyroid disorders, glycogen storage disease, Gaucher disease, hereditary hemorrhagic telangiectasia, hemoglobin-opathies, myeloproliferative disorders, splenectomy)
- Associated with significant venous or capillary involvement
  Pulmonary veno-occlusive disease
  Pulmonary capillary hemangiomatosis
- Persistent pulmonary hypertension of the newborn

Group 2: Pulmonary hypertension with left-sided heart disease
- Left-sided atrial or ventricular heart disease
- Left-sided valvular heart disease

Group 3: Pulmonary hypertension associated with lung disease and/or hypoxemia
- Chronic obstructive pulmonary disease
- Interstitial lung disease
- Sleep-disordered breathing
- Alveolar hypoventilation disorders
- Long-term exposure to high altitude
- Developmental abnormalities

Group 4: Pulmonary hypertension due to chronic thrombotic and/or embolic disease
- Thromboembolic obstruction of proximal pulmonary arteries
- Thromboembolic obstruction of distal pulmonary arteries
- Non-thrombotic pulmonary embolism (tumor, parasites, foreign material)

Group 5: Miscellaneous
- Sarcoidosis, histiocytosis X, lymphangiomatosis, compression of pulmonary vessels (adenopathy, tumor, fibrosing mediastinitis)

---

nary arterial disease (Table 27–1). Pulmonary arterial hypertension results in progressive cardiopulmonary deterioration, right heart failure, and death. While the prognosis for patients with PAH is affected by its underlying cause, overall survival is poor. Figure 27–2 shows survival characteristics in patients with different subtypes of PAH.

The prevalence of PAH in the United States is estimated to be between 50,000 and 100,000. Of these, only 15,000 to 25,000 are appropriately diagnosed and treated. Multicenter registry data suggest that most patients with PAH are women (with a 2:1 female to male ratio), with a mean age of 50 years. Seventy-five percent of patients with PAH have symptoms at rest or with minimal exertion. The mean duration of symptoms prior to diagnosis is 27 months.

Three processes contribute to PA luminal narrowing in PAH: vasoconstriction, arterial remodeling, and thrombosis in situ (Figure 27–3). In persons at risk for PAH, pulmonary

vascular injury leads to endothelial cell and vascular smooth muscle cell dysfunction. Endothelial dysfunction results from up-regulation of vasoconstrictive and pro-proliferative mediators (ie, endothelin-1, serotonin, and thromboxane) and down-regulation of vasodilatory and anti-proliferative mediators (ie, nitric oxide, prostacyclin, and smooth muscle cell potassium channels).

The homeostatic balance normally present in the PA tree is disrupted in PAH. Vasoconstriction and vascular injury can lead to vascular remodeling and in situ thrombosis. Pulmonary arterial hypertension promotes thrombus formation as a result of increased platelet activation, increased blood stasis, up-regulation of plasminogen activator inhibitor-1 and reduced fibrinolytic activity. The cellular processes that have been implicated in the pathogenesis of PAH are summarized in Figure 27–4.

Pulmonary arterial hypertension encompasses the disorder previously referred to as primary pulmonary hypertension, or PH of unknown cause. Primary pulmonary hypertension is now subdivided into idiopathic and familial variants. Idiopathic and familial PAH are rare disorders with a prevalence of 15 cases per million per year and an incidence of 1–2 cases per million per year. Idiopathic and familial PAH afflict predominantly young women, with a mean age at diagnosis of 35 years. These are progressive disorders with a high mortality (median life expectancy 2.8 years from diagnosis).

Mutations in the bone morphogenetic protein receptor (*BMPR*)-*2* gene have been identified in approximately 50% of patients with familial PAH. Those who inherit the mutation have a 10% risk of developing PAH. The genetic pattern of inheritance is autosomal dominant with incomplete penetrance and anticipation (subsequent generations manifest the disease at an earlier age).

Diseases associated with PAH include collagen vascular diseases (especially systemic sclerosis), congenital systemic-to-pulmonary shunts, portal hypertension, HIV infection, drug (notably anorexinogens) and toxin exposures, and other disorders as delineated in Table 27–1.

For those patients in whom PAH develops secondary to collagen-vascular disease, the prognosis is extremely poor. In patients with PAH associated with systemic sclerosis, for instance, the 1-year survival is approximately 50%.

Congenital systemic-to-pulmonary shunts result from ventricular or atrial septal defects, anomalous pulmonary venous drainage, patent ductus arteriosus, or an aorto-pulmonary window. Systemic-to-pulmonary shunts expose the pulmonary vasculature to a persistent high-flow state. This can lead to PA endothelial dysfunction, mediator activation, and reactive vasoconstriction. Vascular remodeling ensues and can progress to the point that shunt reversal occurs. Shunt reversal worsens hypoxemia and further exacerbates PAH.

Pulmonary arterial hypertension develops in approximately 5–10% of patients with portal hypertension. Porto-pulmonary hypertension can interfere with eligibility for liver transplantation because it is associated with high perioperative mortality.

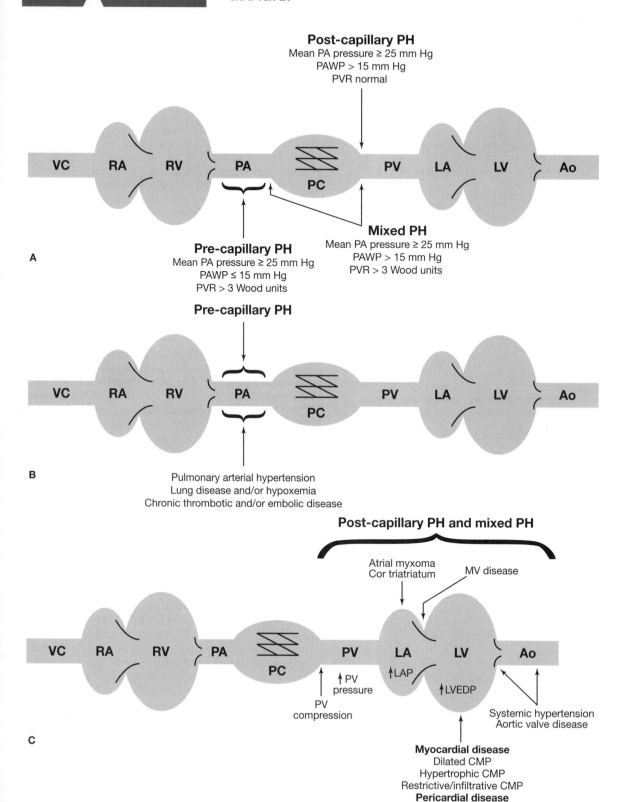

▲ **Figure 27–1.** Hemodynamic classification of pulmonary hypertension. **A:** Pulmonary hypertension may result from pathology in pre-capillary or post-capillary pulmonary circulation. **B:** Common causes of pre-capillary PH. **C:** Common causes of post-capillary and mixed PH. Ao, aorta; CMP, cardiomyopathy; LA, left atrium; LV, left ventricle; LVEDP, left ventricular end-diastolic pressure; PA, pulmonary artery; PAWP, pulmonary arterial wedge pressure; PC, pulmonary capillaries; PH, pulmonary hypertension; PV, pulmonary veins; PVR, pulmonary vascular resistance; RA, right atrium; RV, right ventricle; VC, vena cava.

It is estimated that PAH develops in 1 of every 200 patients with HIV infection. Those patients with HIV in whom PAH develops have a particularly ominous prognosis (see Figure 27–2). Methamphetamine use is also associated with the development of PAH. The diet drug fenfluramine, which has been removed from the US market, has also been associated with increased likelihood of PAH.

The disorders discussed thus far, while distinct, result in pulmonary endothelial and vascular smooth muscle cell dysfunction, maladaptive arterial remodeling, and increased vascular resistance. While prognosis of PAH varies based on the underlying disease, presence of significant PAH significantly increases the morbidity and mortality of all associated conditions.

B. Pulmonary Hypertension with Left-Sided Heart Disease

Elevation of left-sided cardiac filling pressures can lead to PH through passive congestion and retrograde transmission of elevated pressure to the PA tree. This is termed "post-capillary pulmonary hypertension" (see Figure 27–1A,C). Post-capillary PH is characterized hemodynamically by a mean PA pressure ≥ 25 mm Hg, PAWP > 15 mm Hg, and a normal PVR. Elevation of left-sided cardiac filling pressures may result from aortic or mitral valve dysfunction, myocardial disease, pericardial disease, atrial myxoma with obstruction, or pulmonary vein compression. With

chronic elevation of pulmonary venous pressures, up-regulation of inflammatory cytokines, as well as vasoconstrictive and pro-proliferative mediators, results in **reactive** vasoconstriction. Elevation of PA pressure can therefore exist out of proportion to left-sided filling pressures. This entity is referred to as **mixed pulmonary hypertension** and is characterized hemodynamically by a mean PA pressure ≥ 25 mm Hg, PAWP > 15 mm Hg, and a PVR > 3 Wood units (240 dynes × s × cm^{-5}).

Since the PVR is normal in pure post-capillary PH, therapies that reduce the left-sided cardiac filling pressure (ie, diuretics or vasodilator agents, or both) will result in normalization of the PA pressure. This is not the case if mixed pulmonary hypertension has developed. Targeted vasodilator therapy can often improve reactive PA vasoconstriction in this setting. However, pulmonary vascular remodeling can result in "fixed" mixed PH that is refractory to vasodilator therapy. Maladaptive arterial remodeling can pose a significant problem in patients receiving heart transplantation. Acute right heart failure may occur when an unconditioned donor right ventricle is exposed to irreversibly high PVR post-transplantation.

C. Pulmonary Hypertension Associated with Lung Diseases and Hypoxemia

Pulmonary hypertension is also associated with diseases that affect the lung parenchyma such as chronic obstructive pulmo-

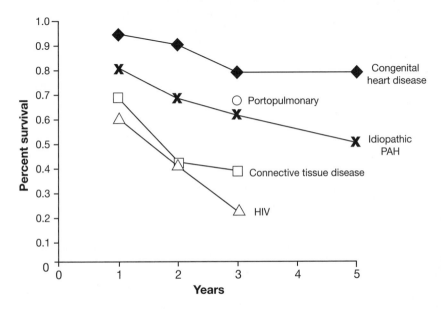

▲ **Figure 27–2.** Survival in pulmonary arterial hypertension (PAH) based on underlying etiology. (Reprinted, with permission, from McLaughlin VV. Chest. 2004;126[1 Suppl]:78S.)

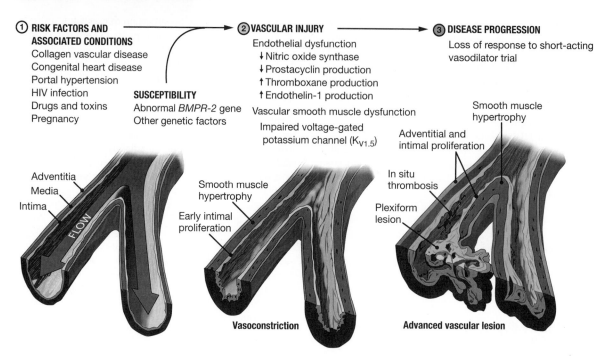

▲ **Figure 27–3.** Pathogenesis of pulmonary arterial hypertension. (Data from Gaine S. JAMA. 2000;284:3160.)

nary disease (COPD) and interstitial lung disease (ILD). Pulmonary hypertension secondary to lung disease is hemodynamically pre-capillary in origin (see Figure 27–1A,B). Several factors contribute to the development of PH in this setting. Disruption of capillary networks results in a decrease in the overall surface area of the pulmonary vascular bed and thereby increases PVR. Hypoxemia directly triggers pulmonary vasoconstriction and indirectly contributes to pulmonary vascular remodeling by resulting in up-regulation of pro-proliferative mediators. Hyperviscosity secondary to hypoxia-induced erythrocytosis can worsen PH. Sleep-disordered breathing, alveolar hypoventilation disorders, and prolonged exposure to high altitude are other causes of PH associated with hypoxemia.

Treatment of these disorders is based on correction of the underlying disorder, provision of supplemental oxygen, and management of cor pulmonale. Some experts suggest potential benefit of targeted pulmonary vasodilator therapy in ILD. Evidence-based data for the use of these agents for PH associated with lung disease are lacking.

D. Pulmonary Hypertension due to Chronic Thrombotic or Embolic Diseases

A massive, sudden pulmonary embolus may significantly increase pulmonary pressures and cause hemodynamic collapse secondary to acute right ventricular failure. This scenario leads to death in approximately 20–40% of patients with acute pulmonary embolism. The presence of severe PH in this setting portends a poor prognosis and predicts an increased likelihood of chronic thromboembolic PH.

Chronic thromboembolic PH occurs in a small percentage (0.1%–3.8%) of patients who survive an episode of pulmonary embolism. In fact, most patients with pulmonary embolism experience complete resolution of thromboemboli within 30 days. In patients with chronic thromboembolic PH, however, these thrombi do not resolve and instead undergo organization and incomplete recanalization. Small vessel arteriopathy and in situ thrombosis may also contribute to disease progression. Chronic thromboembolic PH has a slow, progressive course and often leads to right ventricular hypertrophy before symptoms develop. Diagnosis of chronic thromboembolic PH often requires use of ventilation-perfusion lung scans or high-resolution computed tomography (CT) scans. Pulmonary angiography is often necessary to establish the location and extent of thromboembolic disease.

E. Miscellaneous

This category of PH encompasses disorders that are hemodynamically pre-capillary in origin and includes sarcoidosis, histiocytosis X, lymphangiomatosis, and pulmonary vein compression.

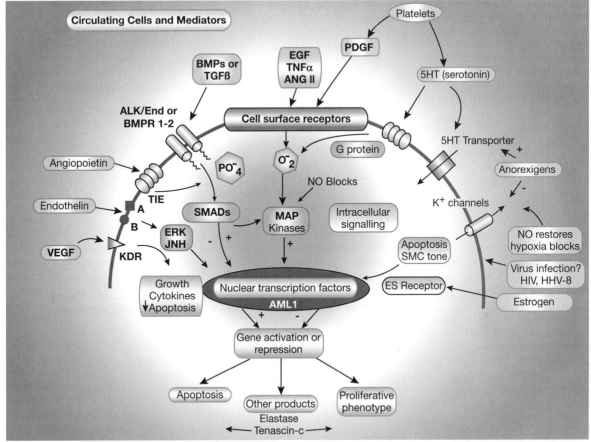

▲ **Figure 27–4.** Some cellular processes implicated in the pathogenesis of pulmonary arterial hypertension. VEGF indicates vascular endothelial growth factor; its receptor is KDR. Endothelin is vasoactive and acts through calcium channels and ERK/Jun kinases. TIE is the angiopoietin receptor, a system found to be upregulated in pulmonary vascular disease. Alk1 and BMPR1-2 are TGF receptors. Alk1 mutations cause hereditary hemorrhagic telangiectasia and some cases of PH. Epidermal growth factor, tumor necrosis factor, angiotensin II, and platelet-derived growth factor are all proliferative stimuli that act through tyrosine kinase receptors. SMADs are regulatory proteins that activate nuclear transcription factors and interact with MAP kinases. AML1 is a nuclear transcription factor. (Reprinted, with permission, from Newman JH. Circulation. 2004;109:2947.)

F. Pathophysiologic Consequences of Pulmonary Hypertension

Chronic PH, regardless of etiology, impacts right ventricular structure and function (Figure 27–5) and presents a pressure-overload state to the right ventricle. In response, the right ventricle undergoes hypertrophic remodeling to maintain cardiac output and compensate for increased afterload. During this initial response to PH, the right ventricle can have supernormal function and normal-to-reduced chamber dimensions. Chronic right ventricular pressure overload results in persistent up-regulation of pro-proliferative neurohormones, endothelin-1, and cytokines. These mediators contribute to the development of maladaptive hypertrophy with fibrosis and diastolic dysfunction.

If exposure to elevated PA pressure continues, the right ventricle dilates. This is an ominous sign because it signifies the presence of increased right ventricular wall stress. Increased wall stress, when coupled with increased heart rate, results in increased myocardial oxygen demand. This develops in concert with a reduction in the epicardial-to-endocardial coronary perfusion gradient secondary to increased right ventricular end-diastolic pressure. In sum, these changes result in a myocardial oxygen supply-demand mismatch and right ventricular ischemia. Right ventricular ischemia worsens systolic function, increases end-diastolic pressure, and promotes

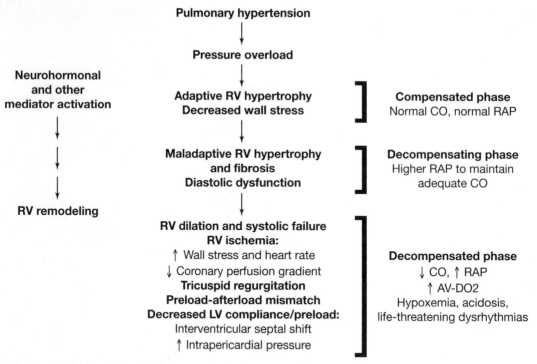

▲ **Figure 27–5.** Pathophysiology of right ventricular dysfunction in pulmonary hypertension. AV-DO$_2$, arteriovenous oxygen differential; CO, cardiac output; LV, left ventricular; RAP, right atrial pressure; RV, right ventricular.

further ventricular enlargement. Tricuspid regurgitation secondary to annular dilatation often occurs and serves to further reduce effective right ventricular forward output.

Right ventricular dilation, in the setting of an intact pericardium, results in a shift of the interventricular septum toward the left ventricle. This, especially when coupled with increased intra-pericardial pressure, impedes left ventricular filling (preload). In turn, when left ventricular filling is impaired, systemic cardiac output is reduced.

Multiple mechanisms contribute to the development of hypoxemia in PH, even when intrinsic pulmonary disease (COPD, chronic thromboembolic PH) is absent. Pulmonary vascular remodeling and in situ thromboses disrupt normal capillary-alveolar gas exchange and raise the alveolar-to-arterial oxygen gradient. Increased pulmonary pressures can increase right atrial pressure and cause shunting through a patent foramen ovale. Because a patent foramen ovale is present in up to 30% of adults, right-to-left shunting should be considered in patients with PH and hypoxemia.

De Marco T et al. Managing right ventricular failure in pulmonary arterial hypertension. Advances in Pulmonary Hypertension. 2005;4(4):16–26.

Gaine S. Pulmonary hypertension. JAMA. 2000 Dec 27;284(24): 3160–8. [PMID: 11135781]

Humbert M et al. Pulmonary arterial hypertension in France: results from a national registry. Am J Respir Crit Care Med. 2006 May 1;173(9):1023–30. [PMID: 16456139]

McLaughlin VV et al. Pulmonary arterial hypertension. Circulation. 2006 Sep 26;114(13):1417–31. [PMID: 17000921]

Moraes DL et al. Secondary pulmonary hypertension in chronic heart failure: the role of the endothelium in pathophysiology and management. Circulation. 2000 Oct 3;102(14):1718–23. [PMID: 11015353]

Newman JH et al; National Heart, Lung and Blood Institute/Office of Rare Diseases. Pulmonary arterial hypertension: future directions: report of a National Heart, Lung and Blood Institute/Office of Rare Diseases workshop. Circulation. 2004 Jun 22;109(24):2947–52. [PMID: 15210611]

Pengo V et al; Thromboembolic Pulmonary Hypertension Study Group. Incidence of chronic thromboembolic pulmonary hypertension after pulmonary embolism. N Engl J Med. 2004 May 27;350(22):2257–64. [PMID: 15163775]

Simonneau G et al. Clinical classification of pulmonary hypertension. J Am Coll Cardiol. 2004 Jun 16;43(12 Suppl S):5S–12S. [PMID: 15194173]

▶ Clinical Findings

A. Symptoms and Signs

One of the major difficulties in PH management is the failure to make an early diagnosis. It takes an average of 2.5 years from symptom onset to PH diagnosis. This results, in part, from the fact that PH often presents with a subtle, nonspecific symptom complex. Pulmonary hypertension most commonly manifests as dyspnea on exertion or fatigue, but it can also manifest as chest pain or syncope (often with exercise). Once right ventricular failure occurs, lower extremity edema and ascites become manifest. The New York Heart Association and World Health Organization have proposed systems for categorizing the severity of symptoms secondary to PH (Table 27–2).

B. Physical Examination

Careful examination of the patient with PH can reveal clues not only about the presence or severity of PH but also about the underlying cause. A loud pulmonic valve closure (P_2) or an early systolic ejection click may be heard as a consequence of marked elevation in PA pressures. With right ventricular hypertrophy and enlargement, a left parasternal lift can be palpated. Another manifestation of right ventricular hypertrophy with diastolic dysfunction is the right ventricular S_4 gallop. A right-sided S_3 is also appreciable in patients with significant elevation in the right ventricular end-diastolic pressure.

Often the holosystolic murmur of tricuspid regurgitation (although frequently without the classically described respiratory variation) and the less common diastolic murmur of pulmonic insufficiency are noted in patients with PH. Jugulovenous distention, peripheral edema, and ascites become manifest in advanced PH with right heart failure. Cool extremities and diminished peripheral pulses are indicative of low cardiac output and peripheral vasoconstriction in severe right ventricular failure.

A murmur of mitral or aortic stenosis, a left-sided S_3, or severe bronchial wheezing and diminished breath sounds

may be clues to the presence of left-sided heart disease or pulmonary parenchymal disease, respectively. Jaundice and spider angiomata may point to the presence of cirrhosis and portal hypertension. Connective tissue diseases may present not only with signs of PH but also with Raynaud phenomenon, arthritis, rashes or other skin changes (ie, sclerodactyly).

C. Diagnostic Studies

1. Electrocardiography—The electrocardiogram (ECG) in patients with significant PH typically suggests right ventricular hypertrophy. There is often a distinct correlation between the amplitude of the R wave in V_1, the R/S ratio in V_1, and the severity of the PH. Classic ECG findings include right axis deviation and right atrial enlargement. Incomplete or complete right bundle branch block is also common. The ECG criteria for right ventricular hypertrophy and a typical ECG in a patient with PH are shown in Table 27–3 and Figure 27–6, respectively. The ECG is not sensitive enough to serve as a screening tool for PH.

2. Chest radiography—Radiographic examination of the chest in a patient with PAH may show enlargement of the main pulmonary artery and its major branches, with distal pruning of peripheral arteries. The retrosternal space is often filled by the hypertrophic right ventricle on lateral projection. Pulmonary venous congestion, left atrial or left ventricular enlargement suggest the presence of a left-sided cause of PH. Hyperinflated lung fields or bullous changes point to a chronic pulmonary disorder with secondary PH. A classic chest radiograph of a patient with PAH is shown in Figure 27–7.

3. Echocardiography—Two-dimensional and Doppler echocardiography are essential to the noninvasive assessment of patients with suspected PH. Echocardiography can demonstrate structural changes such as right atrial or right ventricular enlargement, right ventricular hypertrophy, and PA enlargement. Flattening, or leftward shift of the interventricular septum can also be identified. If the shift occurs during systole, it suggests ventricular pressure overload. If it occurs during diastole, it suggests volume overload. Leftward shift of the septum throughout the cardiac cycle suggests both right ventricular pressure and volume overload (Figure 27–8A,B). The left ventricle is often small and underfilled in PAH, with normal systolic function (Figure 27–8B).

Table 27–2. New York Heart Association and World Health Organization Functional Classes in Pulmonary Hypertension.

Class	Symptoms/Function
NYHA I/ WHO I	No limitation in physical activity.
	Ordinary physical activity does not cause undue dyspnea, fatigue, chest pain, or near-syncope.
NYHA II/ WHO II	Slight limitation in physical activity.
	Ordinary physical activity causes undue dyspnea, fatigue, chest pain, or near-syncope.
NYHA III/ WHO III	Marked limitation in physical activity.
	Less than ordinary physical activity causes undue dyspnea, fatigue, chest pain, or near-syncope.
NYHA IV/ WHO IV	Inability to carry out any physical activity without symptoms.
	Patients manifest signs of right heart failure.
	Dyspnea and/or fatigue may be present at rest.

Table 27–3. Electrocardiographic Criteria for Right Ventricular Hypertrophy.

Right axis deviation (axis > +90 degrees)
R-S amplitude in lead V_1 > 1.0 mm
R-wave amplitude in V_1 ≥ 7 mm
S-wave amplitude in V_1 < 2 mm
qR pattern in precordial lead V_1
R-wave amplitude in lead V_1 + S-wave amplitude in V_5 or V_6 > 10.5 mm
R-S amplitude in V5 or V6 ≤ 1.0 mm

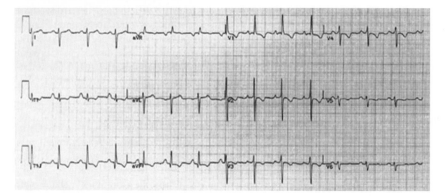

▲ **Figure 27-6.** Electrocardiogram in a patient with pulmonary arterial hypertension and right ventricular hypertrophy.

Tricuspid regurgitation can also be assessed by echocardiography. Using the velocity of the tricuspid regurgitant jet and inferior vena cava dynamics, pulmonary artery systolic pressure (PASP) can be estimated using the modified Bernoulli equation (PASP = $4v^2$ + right atrial [RA] pressure) (Figure 27–8C). Noninvasive PA pressure assessment is not only important in establishing a diagnosis of PH but also in monitoring the patient's response to therapy.

Echocardiography can also be helpful in detecting left-sided heart disease. A dilated, hypocontractile left ventricle, valvular disease, or left atrial myxoma can be identified or excluded on a routine echocardiogram. Color-flow and agitated saline injection can also be used to assess for the existence of congenital intracardiac or intrapulmonary shunts.

4. Lung scintigraphy—Ventilation-perfusion lung scintigraphy is an important screening tool in the evaluation of PH due to chronic thromboembolic disease. In PAH, the lung scan may reveal a normal perfusion pattern or it may show diffuse, patchy ("mottled") perfusion defects. Parenchymal lung disease can also result in perfusion scan abnormalities, but typically, these are matched by ventilatory defects. In chronic thromboembolic PH, however, the lung perfusion scan demonstrates one or more segmental defects mismatched

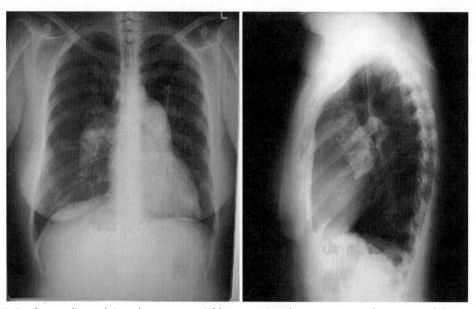

▲ **Figure 27-7.** Chest radiograph in pulmonary arterial hypertension demonstrating enlargement of the central pulmonary arteries with peripheral pruning of the pulmonary vasculature. Also notable is the reduction in the retrosternal air space on the lateral view and the distinct lack of pulmonary pathology.

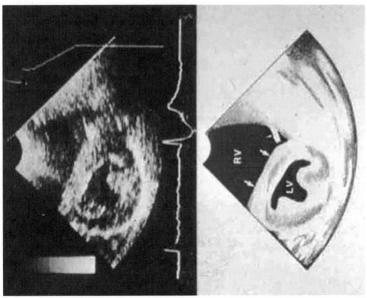

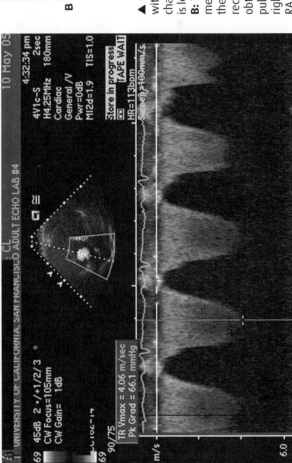

▲ **Figure 27-8.** Transthoracic echocardiogram of a patient with pulmonary arterial hypertension. **A:** This apical four-chamber view demonstrates RA and RV enlargement. There is leftward shifting (flattening) of the interventricular septum. **B:** This parasternal short-axis view demonstrates RV enlargement, a small LV cavity, and leftward shifting (flattening) of the interventricular septum. **C:** This continuous wave Doppler recording shows how the tricuspid regurgitation velocity is obtained by echocardiography and used to estimate the pulmonary artery systolic pressure (PASP = $4V^2$ + RAP). RV, right ventricle; IVS, interventricular septum; LV, left ventricle; RA, right atrium; LA, left atrium; RAP, right atrial pressure.

by the ventilation scan (Figure 27–9). An abnormal ventilation-perfusion scan should prompt further testing with a spiral CT scan or pulmonary angiography.

5. Pulmonary function testing—

Pulmonary function testing is helpful in PH because it can establish the diagnosis of underlying obstructive or restrictive pulmonary disease. Interpretation of pulmonary function test results should be tempered by an awareness that PAH can reduce diffusion capacity. If the total lung capacity is less than 70% of predicted, a high-resolution CT scan should be considered to evaluate for ILD.

6. Computed tomography and magnetic resonance imaging—

CT scans and magnetic resonance imaging (MRI) of the chest can provide useful information in parenchymal lung disorders and several other conditions that can cause PH. Chest CT or MRI scans can demonstrate characteristic findings in patients with fibrosing mediastinitis and cystic fibrosis as well as infiltrative or granulomatous lung diseases.

7. Cardiac catheterization and pulmonary angiography—

Right heart catheterization represents the gold-standard test to establish the diagnosis of PH, ascertain its etiology, establish severity and prognosis, evaluate vasoreactivity, and assist in guiding therapy.

At right heart catheterization, a full cardiopulmonary hemodynamic profile is established by recording the right atrial, right ventricular, PA, and pulmonary arterial wedge pressures as well as measuring the CO. The PVR (mean PA – PAWP/CO) is also determined during right heart catheterization. Arterial and venous oxygen saturations obtained during right heart catheterization are used to detect and determine the severity of shunts. Abnormalities of the left heart, such as aortic or mitral valve disease or left heart failure, will be suggested during right heart catheterization by the presence of an elevated PAWP.

Vasoreactivity testing is an important component of right heart catheterization in PAH. Acute vasoreactivity is tested using inhaled nitric oxide or intravenous prostacyclin or adenosine. A reduction in mean PA pressure > 10 mm Hg with an absolute mean PA pressure ≤ 40 mm Hg suggests that reversible vasoconstriction, rather than fixed vascular remodeling, is the major mechanism for PAH. Less than 15% of patients with idiopathic PAH will respond to acute vasodilator testing, but a positive vasoreactivity trial identifies a subset of patients with superior overall prognosis and greater likelihood of benefit from calcium channel blocker therapy.

Pulmonary angiography is not routinely conducted in patients with PH. When ventilation-perfusion scintigraphy or spiral CT scan suggest chronic thromboembolic disease, pulmonary angiography and angioscopy can determine the extent and location of thromboembolic disease. For this reason, pulmonary angiography is often used as part of the preoperative assessment of patients considered for thromboendarterectomy.

8. Lung biopsy—

A lung biopsy is infrequently required to determine the cause of PH. Lung biopsy can identify injected particulate matter in injection drug users, establish the diagnosis of pulmonary veno-occlusive disease, and may identify causative pathogens in ILD. Due to its substantial morbidity, however, lung biopsy is seldom used. If lung biopsy is obtained in an individual with reversible PH, medial smooth muscle hypertrophy may be noted. In more

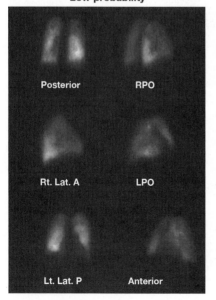

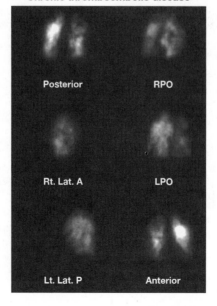

▲ **Figure 27–9.** Perfusion lung scans from a normal patient and a patient with chronic thromboembolic disease. The scan on the left shows uniform perfusion. The scan on the right shows multiple perfusion defects consistent with the diagnosis of chronic thromboembolic disease.

advanced cases, necrotizing arteritis and plexiform lesions can be seen (Figure 27–10).

9. Functional capacity and exercise testing—The use of the World Health Organization's functional classification and symptom-limited exercise testing can be very helpful in the evaluation of patients with PH. Exercise testing, particularly the 6-minute walk test, has been shown to predict mortality and allows for objective assessment of symptom burden. Baseline functional capacity and exercise testing utilizing the 6-minute walk test should be measured prior to initiation of therapy and serially during treatment.

10. Other studies—If sleep apnea is suspected, a full sleep study can be diagnostic. Liver biochemical testing and hepatic ultrasound can help diagnose liver cirrhosis and portal hypertension. If connective tissue diseases (eg, scleroderma, rheumatoid arthritis, systemic lupus erythematosus, mixed connective tissue disease, polymyositis) are suspected, serologic and immunogenetic studies can be helpful. Thyroid function and HIV testing should be performed. Parasitic disease (schistosomiasis or filariasis) should be suspected and tested for in patients from endemic areas with PH. Tissue biopsy, complement fixation, blood smear and skin testing are diagnostic tests of choice in such patients.

Cockrill BA et al. Comparison of the effects of nitric oxide, nitroprusside, and nifedipine on hemodynamics and right ventricular contractility in patients with chronic pulmonary hypertension. Chest. 2001 Jan;119(1):128–36. [PMID: 11157594]

Fleischmann D et al. Three-dimensional visualization of pulmonary thromboemboli in chronic thromboembolic pulmonary hypertension with multiple detector-row spiral computed tomography. Circulation. 2001 Jun 19;103(24):2993. [PMID: 11413092]

McGoon M et al; American College of Chest Physicians. Screening, early detection, and diagnosis of pulmonary arterial hypertension. ACCP evidence-based clinical practice guidelines. Chest. 2004 Jul;126(1 Suppl):14S–34S. [PMID: 15249493]

Miyamoto S et al. Clinical correlates and prognostic significance of six-minute walk test in patients with primary pulmonary hypertension. Comparison with cardiopulmonary exercise testing. Am J Respir Crit Care Med. 2000 Feb;161(2 Pt 1):487–92. [PMID: 10673190]

▶ **Differential Diagnosis**

The differential diagnosis for PAH includes a number of well-defined causes of PH (see Table 27–1). Diagnostic efforts should be pursued vigorously, since PAH can progress rapidly and is associated with substantial morbidity and mortality. An algorithmic approach to diagnosis has been proposed by the American College of Chest Physicians and is shown in Figure 27–11.

Suspicion for PAH should be raised on the basis of clinical history and physical examination, as previously outlined. Initial diagnostic testing should include a baseline ECG and chest radiograph. Two-dimensional and Doppler echocardiography are recommended to noninvasively assess PASP and evaluate biventricular structure and function. Color-flow and agitated saline injection should be utilized to assess for the existence of congenital intracardiac or intrapulmonary shunts.

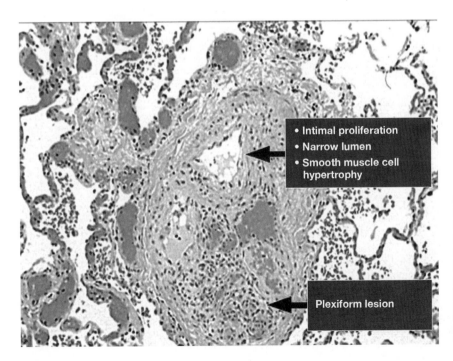

- Intimal proliferation
- Narrow lumen
- Smooth muscle cell hypertrophy

Plexiform lesion

▲ **Figure 27–10.** Pulmonary arterial hypertension results in vascular endothelial cell proliferation and smooth muscle cell (SMC) hypertrophy. Plexiform lesions can develop and predispose to in situ thrombosis. (Reprinted with permission from the American Medical Association. Gaine S, JAMA 2000; 284:3160–3168.)

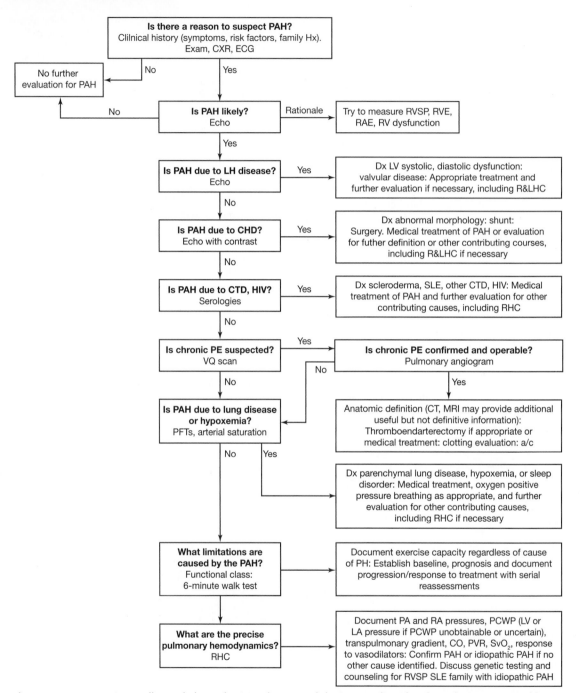

▲ Figure 27–11. American College of Chest Physicians' proposed diagnostic algorithm for pulmonary arterial hypertension. Hx, history; Echo, echocardiography; LH, left heart; CHD, congenital heart disease; CTD, connective tissue disease; PFT, pulmonary function test; TRV, peak velocity of TR jet; RVE, right ventricular enlargement; RAE, right atrial enlargement; RV, right ventricular; Dx, diagnosis; LV, left ventricular; R&LHC, right and left heart catheterization; RHC, right catheterization; PE, pulmonary embolism; a/c, anticoagulation; LA, left atrial; PCWP, pulmonary capillary wedge pressure; CO, cardiac output; PVR, pulmonary vascular resistance; $\bar{S}vo_2$, mixed venous oxygen saturation. (From McGoon M et al. Chest. 2004;126:14S.)

If echocardiography suggests that PH is present and no clear left-sided or congenital lesions have been identified, an evaluation for thromboembolic disease should be conducted. If chronic pulmonary emboli are identified by lung scintigraphy, spiral CT or pulmonary angiography, or both, can be helpful as a confirmatory test and to evaluate for thromboendarterectomy candidacy.

Pulmonary disease can be assessed with chest radiograph, arterial oxygen saturation measurement, pulmonary function testing, and chest CT scan. If sleep apnea or sleep-disordered breathing is suspected, a thorough sleep study should be conducted. A serologic workup for common connective tissue diseases, thyroid disease, liver disease, and HIV is also required.

Assessment of functional capacity and symptom burden should be conducted using the World Health Organization's functional classification and 6-minute walk test. Exercise capacity correlates well with overall prognosis and baseline 6-minute walk test values can help later evaluation of treatment response. Right-heart catheterization is also recommended at this stage in order to document right atrial, pulmonary arterial, and pulmonary arterial wedge pressures. Cardiac output, PVR, and vasoreactivity testing should also be assessed during right heart catheterization. If a patient has an elevated mean PA pressure on right heart catheterization and no cause of PH has been identified, the diagnosis of idiopathic PAH has been made. Genetic testing should be discussed with the patient and family members.

▶ Treatment

A. Pulmonary Arterial Hypertension

Improvement in cardiopulmonary hemodynamics, exercise capacity, functional class, survival, and prevention of clinical worsening are the goals of PAH treatment. General measures in the management of PAH include symptom-limited, regular exercise to maintain skeletal muscle conditioning and overall cardiovascular fitness. Intense exercise should be avoided, especially if the patient with PAH has a history of exercise-induced syncope or presyncope. Patients should avoid high altitude, and supplemental oxygen should be provided for air travel. Since patients with PAH have reduced cardiopulmonary reserve, immunization against influenza and pneumococcus is recommended.

Pregnancy in PAH deserves special attention. Patients with PAH should be counseled to avoid pregnancy because it is associated with significant (30%) mortality. Birth control should be discussed, and contraceptive methods prescribed in women of childbearing age. Hemoglobin levels should be monitored regularly. In patients with Eisenmenger syndrome, erythrocytosis should be treated with phlebotomy only if symptoms of hyperviscosity develop. Patients with PAH should refrain from smoking and adhere to a sodium-restricted diet in setting of right heart failure.

Patients with PAH require supplemental oxygen if they exhibit arterial oxygen desaturation at rest or with minimal exertion. Patients with PAH, particularly idiopathic PAH, should receive oral anticoagulant therapy with a goal international normalized ratio (INR) of 1.5 to 2.5. This recommendation is based on several nonrandomized clinical trials showing improved survival in patients with idiopathic PAH treated with warfarin.

Diuretic therapy is the mainstay of treatment for symptomatic PAH with volume overload. Digoxin may also help improve right-sided hemodynamics and can be an effective rate-controlling agent in the setting of atrial tachyarrhythmia. Digoxin has also been shown to reduce circulating catecholamine levels in patients with chronic PAH. However, no other data exist regarding the efficacy of cardiac glycosides (ie, digoxin) in PAH with right ventricular failure. Digoxin toxicity, especially in patients with severe hypoxia, renal insufficiency or hypokalemia, is well recognized and warrants vigilance.

In patients with PAH and decompensated right heart failure, strategies to improve clinical status include (1) afterload reduction with pulmonary vasodilators, such as oxygen, inhaled nitric oxide, prostanoids, endothelin-receptor antagonists and phosphodiesterase inhibitors, (2) preload reduction with diuretics or ultrafiltration, and (3) augmentation of right ventricular function with inotropic therapy. Intravenous inotropes such as low-dose dobutamine or dopamine (1–2 mcg/kg/min) are of particular benefit in patients with right ventricular failure and hypotension in whom diuretic therapy is ineffective or in whom renal failure has developed (Figure 27–12).

Until 1996, high-dose calcium channel blockers were the only vasodilators available to treat PAH. Calcium channel blocker therapy may reduce PA pressure and right ventricular afterload, thereby improving right ventricular hemodynamics and increasing CO. Vasoreactivity testing identifies a subset of idiopathic PAH patients (less clear for the general PAH cohort) who may benefit from calcium channel blocker therapy. If a patient with PAH has a favorable response to acute vasodilator testing, a hemodynamically monitored trial of an oral calcium channel blocker, such as nifedipine, amlodipine, or diltiazem, may be undertaken. If a reduction in PA pressures occurs with preservation of CO, then the patient can be considered for long-term therapy. Verapamil is contraindicated due to its significant negative inotropic properties. Response to calcium channel blocker therapy should be assessed during a repeat right heart catheterization.

There are several limitations to calcium channel blocker therapy. Use of a calcium channel blocker is not advisable in patients with severe right ventricular failure or hypotension. Empiric calcium channel blocker therapy is contraindicated in the absence of a positive vasoreactivity trial or a favorable hemodynamic response. Lastly, only a small percentage (< 7%) of patients with PAH who have acute vasoreactivity will have a sustained response to long-term calcium channel blocker therapy.

Fortunately, the following drugs have been approved as alternatives for the treatment of PAH: oral bosentan and

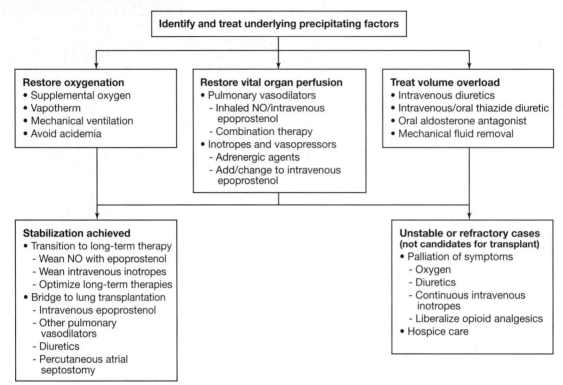

▲ **Figure 27–12.** Management of acute decompensated right ventricular failure in pulmonary arterial hypertension. NO, nitric oxide.

ambrisentan, oral sildenafil, inhalational iloprost, subcutaneous/intravenous treprostinil, and intravenous epoprostenol. These agents target the endothelin, nitric oxide, and prostacyclin pathways (Figure 27–13). These pathways are thought to mediate vascular tone and arterial remodeling. When used appropriately, these newer pulmonary vasodilators can improve symptoms and exercise capacity. Most of these agents delay time to clinical worsening and some (ie, epoprostenol) have been shown to improve survival (Table 27–4).

Endothelin-1 is secreted by vascular endothelial cells and is a potent vasoconstrictor and mediator of smooth-muscle cell proliferation. In addition, endothelin-1 enhances vascular fibrosis, increases platelet aggregation, promotes cardiac myocyte hypertrophy, and increases aldosterone production. Endothelin-1 is secreted in response to a variety of stimuli, including hypoxemia, endothelial sheer and pulsatile stress, and neurohormonal activation as well as PH-related growth factors and cytokines.

Bosentan is an endothelin-A and -B receptor antagonist approved for the treatment of functional class III and IV PAH. Bosentan has been shown to increase 6-minute walk distance, decrease symptom burden and delay clinical worsening in patients with idiopathic PAH and patients with associated PAH secondary to scleroderma (Table 27–4).

Bosentan also appears to have benefit in symptomatic patients with PAH secondary to congenital heart disease and Eisenmenger syndrome.

Transaminitis develops in approximately 11% of patients treated with bosentan. While this is usually reversible, monthly liver function testing in patients treated with bosentan is required. Bosentan has teratogenic properties, and treated patients must avoid pregnancy. Side effects associated with bosentan include nasal congestion, flushing, anemia, and lower extremity edema.

Ambrisentan is a selective endothelin-A receptor antagonist that has recently been approved in the United States for PAH for functional class II and III patients. Ambrisentan significantly improves exercise capacity, delays time to clinical worsening, and improves cardiopulmonary hemodynamics. The incidence of transaminitis is approximately 3% at 1 year. However, monthly liver function testing is necessary. Importantly, ambrisentan has no significant interactions with warfarin or sildenafil. The drug is teratogenic and so, as with bosentan, pregnancy must be avoided. Ambrisentan can cause peripheral edema, nasal congestion, and flushing.

In patients with PAH, nitric oxide bioavailability is significantly reduced. Nitric oxide is secreted by the endothelial cell and diffuses to the smooth muscle cell where it mediates

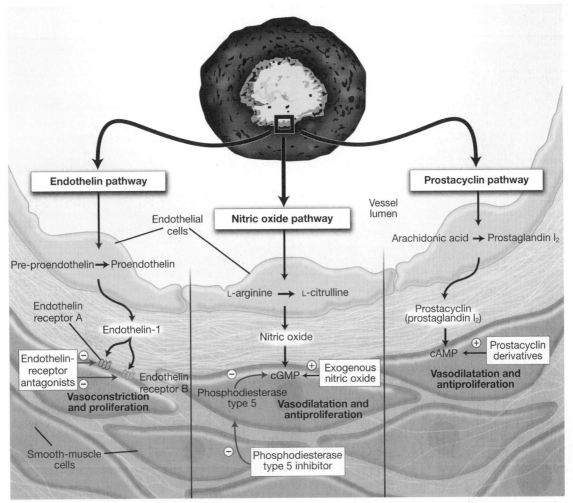

▲ **Figure 27–13.** Therapeutic targets for pulmonary arterial hypertension treatment. cAMP, cyclic adenyl monophosphate; cGMP, cyclic guanyl monophosphate. (Reprinted, with permission, from Humbert M et al. N Engl J Med. 2004;351:1425.)

vasodilation and exerts an anti-proliferative effect via activation of the cyclic guanyl monophosphate (cGMP) pathway.

The nitric oxide pathway can be enhanced by administering exogenous inhaled nitric oxide. It can also be enhanced by inhibiting phosphodiesterase isoform–5, the enzyme responsible for the degradation of cGMP. Sildenafil is an oral phosphodiesterase–5 inhibitor (PDEI-5) known to dilate the PA bed without increasing left-sided filling pressures. It is approved for treatment of PAH patients with functional class II–IV symptoms. When administered long-term, sildenafil improves exercise capacity, reduces symptom burden, and improves cardiopulmonary hemodynamics (Table 27–4). However, sildenafil has not been shown to delay clinical worsening. Sildenafil can cause headache, flushing, dyspepsia, epistaxis, and visual changes.

Prostacyclin (PGI$_2$) is a direct pulmonary and systemic vasodilator as well as inhibitor of vascular remodeling and platelet aggregation. Prostacyclin is secreted by the endothelial cell and exerts its vascular effect by stimulating smooth muscle cell cyclic adenyl monophosphate (cAMP). The PGI$_2$ pathway is down-regulated in PAH. To enhance this pathway, exogenously synthesized epoprostenol (prostacyclin) and other prostanoids can be administered. Current, FDA-approved prostanoids for PAH are administered through intravenous, subcutaneous, or inhalational routes. A summary of the pivotal trials that have led to approval of these agents for PAH is provided in Table 27–4.

Epoprostenol has a short half-life and is unstable if exposed to room temperature or light. It is degraded by gastric pH and must therefore be administered via continuous intravenous

Table 27–4. Summary of Randomized Controlled Trials of Approved Drugs for the Treatment of PH and PAH.

Drug	Study Characteristics	Positive Results	Disadvantages
Endothelin Receptor Antagonists			
Oral bosentan (dual ERA)	*Name:* BREATHE-1 *Design:* Double-blind *Number:* 213 *Indication:* Class III, IV PAH	Improved 6-minute walk distance (44 m) Improved dyspnea Delayed clinical worsening	Hepatic toxicity (4% in study, 11% in PI) Monthly transaminase monitoring Teratogenic anemia Side effects
Oral ambrisentan (selective ERA)	*Name:* ARIES-1 *Name:* ARIES-2 *Design:* Double-blind *Number:* 202 and 192, respectively *Indication:* Class I–IV PAH	Improved 6-minute walk distance (30–51 m) Delayed clinical worsening Improved cardiopulmonary hemodynamics	Hepatic toxicity (0.8 at 12 wks, 2.8% at 1 year) Monthly transaminase monitoring Teratogenic Side effects
Phosphodiesterase-5 Inhibitors			
Oral sildenafil	*Name:* SUPER-1 *Design:* Double-blind *Number:* 278 *Indication:* Class II–IV PAH	Improved 6-minute walk distance (45 m) Improved dyspnea Improved cardiopulmonary hemodynamics	No delay in clinical worsening end point Headache, flushing, dyspepsia, epistaxis, visual disturbance
Prostanoids			
Epoprostenol (prostacyclin)	*Design:* Open-label *Number:* 81 *Indication:* Class III, IV PAH	Improved 6-minute walk distance Improved dyspnea Improved cardiopulmonary hemodynamics Improved survival	Indwelling central line Pump (infection/malfunction) Side effects
Treprostinil (prostacyclin analogue)	*Design:* Double-blind *Number:* 470 *Indication:* Class II–IV PAH	Improved 6-minute walk distance Improved dyspnea Improved cardiopulmonary hemodynamics	Pain, erythema at infusion site Side effects
Inhalational iloprost (prostacyclin analogue)	*Design:* Double-blind *Number:* 203 *Indication:* Class III–IV PH	Improved composite end point of 6-minute walk distance and dyspnea	Administration 6–9 times daily Side effects

ERA, endothelin receptor antagonist; PAH, pulmonary arterial hypertension; PH, pulmonary hypertension; PI, package insert.

infusion. When added to conventional therapy, epoprostenol has been shown to improve exercise capacity, reduce symptom burden, improve cardiopulmonary hemodynamics and reduce mortality in patients with PAH who have NYHA class III–IV symptoms. Major adverse effects of this agent relate to its complex delivery system and include infection, thrombosis, and pump malfunction. Due to its short half-life, brief interruption of epoprostenol infusion can result in rebound PH and cardiopulmonary collapse. Prostanoids, as a class, are known to cause headache, flushing, nausea, vomiting, diarrhea, arthralgias, myalgias, and jaw pain.

Treprostinil is a prostanoid that is pre-mixed, stable at room temperature, and has a longer half-life than epoprostenol. Treprostinil can be administered subcutaneously as well as intravenously. In patients with NYHA class II–IV PAH, treprostinil improves exercise capacity, reduces symptoms,

and improves cardiopulmonary hemodynamics (Table 27–4). Inhalational iloprost has also been shown to improve clinical outcomes in patients with symptomatic PAH. Iloprost must be administered six to nine times daily to maintain efficacy. While iloprost and treprostinil have advantages over epoprostenol, epoprostenol is the only prostanoid shown to reduce mortality in advanced PAH.

Choosing the correct treatment regimen for the patient with PAH relies on an understanding of the underlying disease and of patient-specific factors. Disease severity, as assessed by integration of hemodynamic, clinical, and laboratory parameters, is crucial in selecting the appropriate treatment (Table 27–5, Figure 27–11). Individual patient factors, such as comorbidities (ie, liver disease), concomitant drug therapy, or a history of medication nonadherence, may all influence treatment choice (Figure 27–14).

Table 27–5. Prognostic Factors for Risk of Pulmonary Arterial Hypertension Disease Progression.

Determinant	Higher Risk	Lower Risk
Evidence of RV failure	Yes	No
Progression	Rapid	Gradual
WHO Class	IV	II, II
6-minute walk distance	< 325 m	> 380 m
Brain natriuretic peptide	> 180 pg/mL	< 180 pg/mL
Echocardiographic findings	Pericardial effusion; significant RV dysfunction	Minimal RV dysfunction
Hemodynamics	High RAP, Low CI	Normal/near normal RAP and CI

CI, cardiac index; RAP, right atrial pressure; RV, right ventricular; WHO, World Health Organization.

Invasive treatment options for PAH include atrial septostomy, lung transplantation and combined heart-lung transplantation. Atrial septostomy has been performed as a palliative measure for patients with PAH and right heart failure or recurrent syncope. It is postulated that a right-left shunt in this setting improves left ventricular filling and cardiac output. Atrial septostomy can, however, worsen hypoxia and increases the likelihood of paradoxical embolization. As such, it is recommended that atrial septostomy be performed only at experienced centers. Outcomes with lung and combined heart-lung transplantation are improving. One-year survival posttransplantation is 70% and 5-year survival is 50%. Transplantation is reserved for PAH patients with heart failure and poor quality of life who continue to deteriorate despite maximal medical therapy.

B. Pulmonary Hypertension with Left-Sided Heart Disease

Pulmonary hypertension occurs in 25–30% of patients with left-sided heart disease and is associated with worse outcomes in this population. Treatment is dictated by the underlying

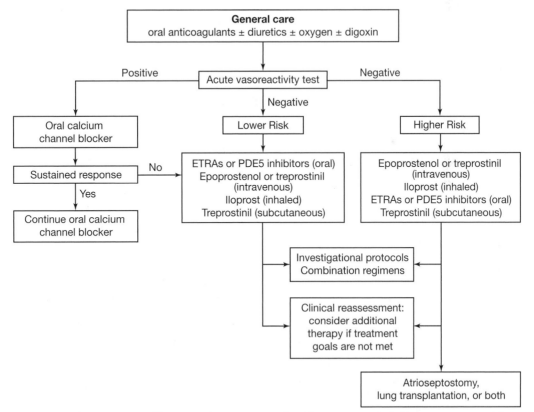

▲ **Figure 27–14.** Pulmonary arterial hypertension treatment algorithm. ETRA, endothelin receptor antagonist; PDE-5, phosphodiesterase-5. (Adapted, with permission, from McLaughlin VV et al. Circulation. 2006;114:1417.)

disease process. Surgical or percutaneous treatment of aortic or mitral valve disease and treatment of coronary artery disease should be aggressively pursued as these interventions can improve left-sided filling pressures, reduce PA pressure, and improve symptoms. Standard therapy for systolic and diastolic heart failure is recommended. Supplemental oxygen is required for those who exhibit systemic oxygen desaturation.

Although limited data are available, oral or intravenous vasodilators (eg, nitrates or sildenafil, nitroprusside, nesiritide, milrinone) are sometimes used for the management of refractory cases of PH with left-sided heart disease. Calcium channel blocker therapy, with the possible exception of amlodipine, is largely avoided in systolic heart failure with PH. Endothelin-receptor antagonists are also avoided in left-sided heart failure because they have been shown to worsen heart failure and increase mortality. Intravenous epoprostenol is also contraindicated in the treatment of advanced systolic heart failure because it has been shown to increase mortality. Mechanical circulatory-assist devices and heart-lung transplantation are other therapies available for PH due to left-sided heart disease.

C. Pulmonary Hypertension Associated with Lung Disease or Hypoxemia

Pulmonary hypertension in persons with lung disease or hypoxemia, or both, is best relieved by treating the underlying disease. In this cohort, correction of hypoxemia is especially important. Bronchodilator therapy should be optimized for patients with obstructive pulmonary disease. Continuous positive airway pressure and weight loss often aid in the treatment of PAH patients with sleep-disordered breathing. Inflammatory conditions that lead to ILD should be sought and aggressively treated with antiinflammatory agents. Specific pulmonary vasodilator therapy is controversial for PH associated with lung disease on the basis of insufficient evidence.

Cor pulmonale, or right heart failure secondary to lung disease, often develops in patients with PH. As previously outlined for PAH, sodium-restriction and diuretics are the mainstays of right heart failure therapy. Digoxin and vasodilator therapy may be considered, although outcome data are lacking. For select, severely symptomatic patients with PH and lung disease, lung transplantation can improve quality of life and survival.

D. Pulmonary Hypertension due to Chronic Thrombotic or Embolic Disease

Patients with chronic thromboembolic PH who have organized, proximal PA thrombi can undergo pulmonary thromboendarterectomy and many achieve normalization of PA pressure. Most patients experience improvement in PA pressure, right heart function, NYHA class, and exercise capacity following pulmonary thromboendarterectomy.

The operative mortality of pulmonary thromboendarterectomy is fairly high, however, with a 30-day mortality rate of 9–12%. Residual PH occurs in approximately 10% of patients after pulmonary thromboendarterectomy and appears to be linked to the degree of small vessel arteriopathy. Pathophysiologic similarities between PAH and chronic thromboembolic PH have prompted investigation into the usefulness of pulmonary vasodilator therapy for PH that persists post–pulmonary thromboendarterectomy and as bridging therapy. Encouraging data are emerging from small nonrandomized trials showing hemodynamic improvement in chronic thromboembolic PH patients with vasodilator therapy. The role for medical treatment in chronic thromboembolic PH is as yet incompletely defined and is an area of ongoing research.

Badesch DB et al. Medical therapy for pulmonary arterial hypertension: updated ACCP evidence-based clinical practice guidelines. Chest. 2007 Jun;131(6):1917–28. [PMID: 17565025]

Galie N et al; Sildenafil Use in Pulmonary Arterial Hypertension (SUPER) Study Group. Sildenafil citrate therapy for pulmonary arterial hypertension. N Engl J Med. 2005 Nov 17;353(20):2148–57. [PMID: 16291984]

Humbert M et al. Treatment of pulmonary arterial hypertension. N Engl J Med. 2004 Sep 30;351(14):1425–36. [PMID: 15459304]

Mclaughlin VV et al. Survival in primary pulmonary hypertension: the impact of epoprostenol therapy. Circulation. 2002 Sep 17;106(12):1477–82. [PMID: 12234951]

Rubin LJ et al. Bosentan therapy for pulmonary arterial hypertension. N Engl J Med. 2002 Mar 21;346(12):896–903. [PMID: 11907289]

Sitbon O et al. Long-term response to calcium channel blockers in idiopathic pulmonary arterial hypertension. Circulation. 2005 Jun 14;111(23):3105–11. [PMID: 15939821]

Thistlethwaite PA et al. Pulmonary thromboendarterectomy surgery. Cardiol Clin. 2004 Aug;22(3):467–78. [PMID: 15302365]

▶ Prognosis

Pulmonary hypertension is a progressive disorder associated with a high mortality rate. The underlying cause of the PH is a key factor in determining the prognosis and natural history of the disease (see Figure 27–2). Patients with PAH associated with connective tissue disease and those with PAH and HIV have the worst prognoses. Patients with congenital heart disease, by contrast, have the best prognosis (6-month survival is 89%). Even for patients with PH due to lung disease or hypoxemia, survival rates vary widely. Patients with PH and emphysema have a 6-month survival of 81% whereas patients with PH and interstitial lung disease have a 6-month survival of 38%.

Clinical features and hemodynamic parameters also strongly influence survival. Markers of poor prognosis in PH include advanced functional class (NYHA III-IV) (Table 27–2), poor exercise capacity (reduced 6-minute walk distance), resting hemodynamics consistent with right ventricular failure (high right atrial pressure, low cardiac output), elevated B-type natriuretic peptide, and presence of a pericardial effusion or significant right ventricular dysfunction on echocardiogram (Table 27–5).

McLaughlin VV et al; American College of Chest Physicians. Prognosis of pulmonary arterial hypertension: ACCP evidence-based clinical practice guidelines. Chest 2004 Jul;126(1 Suppl):78S–92S. [PMID: 15249497]

Congenital Heart Disease in Adults

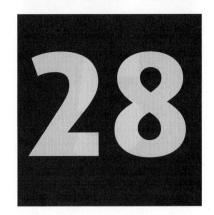

Ian S. Harris, MD & Elyse Foster, MD

▶ **General Considerations**

Congenital cardiac anomalies are the most common birth defects in humans, affecting approximately 0.7 in 100 live births. While the incidence of congenital heart disease is expected to decline as a consequence of improved prenatal diagnosis, the number of patients surviving with congenital heart disease, both in the United States and worldwide, has increased significantly over the past three decades. Over 85% of infants born with cardiovascular anomalies now can expect to reach adulthood. Reduced mortality rates can be attributed to improved diagnostic abilities, enhanced surgical and nonsurgical therapies, and improvements in intensive care. For the first time, the number of adults with congenital heart disease exceeds the number of children with the disorder.

The increase in the number of adults with congenital heart disease requires that the physician managing the care of these patients have improved knowledge of simple and complex anatomy and physiology. Although actual numbers are difficult to ascertain, it has been estimated that approximately 1 million adults in the United States alone currently have congenital heart disease and that the number of patients reaching adulthood with treated congenital heart disease will increase by approximately 9000 per year.

These patients fall into several broad categories: those surviving into adulthood without intervention, those surviving with curative surgical or nonsurgical intervention, and those surviving with palliative surgical or nonsurgical intervention. Nonsurgical interventions may include catheter-based valvuloplasty, stenting, coiling, or device occlusion. The patients who are today making the transition into the adult congenital heart disease population have hemodynamic and cardiac problems differing from those in previous eras. Surgical techniques have evolved, intervention occurs earlier and is often definitive rather than palliative, and a greater number of patients with complex single-ventricle physiology and various modifications of cavopulmonary anastomoses (Glenn shunt, Fontan procedure) will reach adulthood.

Although many patients are referred by pediatric cardiologists, others may seek medical attention for the first time in adulthood. Examples of cardiac pathology that may not be readily apparent in childhood include secundum atrial septal defects (ASD), coarctation of the aorta, Ebstein anomaly of the tricuspid valve, congenitally corrected transposition (ventricular inversion), and coronary artery anomalies.

The risk of infective endocarditis remains an issue of ongoing concern in many patients with congenital cardiac defects. The absolute magnitude of risk varies considerably from one lesion to another and is also dependent on whether the patient has been surgically treated. In 2007, the American Heart Association revised its guidelines regarding infective endocarditis prophylaxis. The revised guidelines suggest a much more conservative approach to the use of prophylactic antibiotics. Broadly speaking, infective endocarditis prophylaxis is now recommended in only three groups of patients with congenital heart disease: (1) those with unrepaired cyanotic congenital heart disease, including patients with palliative shunts and conduits, (2) those with a defect completely repaired (either surgically or by catheter-based intervention) using prosthetic material or device, during the first 6 months after the procedure, and (3) those with repaired congenital heart disease who have residual defects at the site of adjacent to the site of a prosthetic patch or device. The risk of endocarditis in individual lesions is summarized in Table 28–1.

Hoffman JI et al. Prevalence of congenital heart disease. Am Heart J. 2004 Mar;147(3):425–39. [PMID: 14999190]

Perloff JK et al. Challenges posed by adults with repaired congenital heart disease. Circulation. 2001 May 29;103(21):2637–43. [PMID: 11382736]

Thirty-second Bethesda Conference: Care of the adult with congenital heart disease. J Am Coll Cardiol. 2001 Apr;37(5):1166.

Wilson W et al; American Heart Association Rheumatic Fever, Endocarditis, and Kawasaki Disease Committee; American Heart Association Council on Cardiovascular Disease in the Young; American Heart Association Council on Clinical Cardiology;

Table 28–1. Congenital Heart Disease in Adults.

Defect	M:F	Associated Defects	Risk of Endocarditis
Acyanotic			
Bicuspid AV	4:1	Coarctation	High
Valvar PS	1:1	VSD (see TOF), Noonan syndrome	Low (mild PS), intermediate (severe PS)
ASD secundum	1:2	Mitral valve prolapse	Low
ASD primum AV septal defect	1:1	Bridging AV valve leaflets, trisomy 21	Intermediate (with MR)
VSD	1:1	PS (see TOF), AR	Intermediate-high (unoperated or with AR) Low (operated without AR)
PDA	1:2-3	Coexists with many complex syndromes	Low (ligated), intermediate (patent)
Coarctation	2:1	Bicuspid AV	Low (operated[1]), intermediate (without treatment)
C-TGA	M > F	VSD, infundibular PS	Low (isolated C-TGA)
Ebstein anomaly	1:1	ASD PFO	Low-intermediate
Coronary AV fistulae	1:1		Intermediate
Cyanotic			
TOF	1.5:1	RAA, ASD	Intermediate
Eisenmenger syndrome	M < F	VSD, ASD, PDA	Low
Tricuspid atresia	1:1[2]	Pulmonary atresia, ASD, VSD	?
Pulmonary atresia with intact septum	1:1		?
D-TGA	2-4:1	ASD, PFO, PDA, VSD, PS, RAA	Intermediate
Postoperative			
Fontan			Variable
Glenn			Variable
Blalock-Taussig			High
RV-PA conduit			High

[1]Unless there is associated bicuspid AV.
[2]In tricuspid atresia with transposition, M > F.
AR, aortic regurgitation; ASD, atrial septal defect; AV, aortic valve; C-TGV, congenitally corrected transposition of the great vessels; MR, mitral regurgitation; PA, pulmonary artery; PDA, patent ductus arteriosus; PFO, patent foramen ovale; PS, pulmonic stenosis; RAA, right-sided aortic arch; RV, right ventricle; TOF, tetralogy of Fallot; VSD, ventricular septal defect.

American Heart Association Council on Cardiovascular Surgery and Anesthesia; Quality of Care and Outcomes Research Interdisciplinary Working Group. Prevention of infective endocarditis: guidelines from the American Heart Association: a guideline from the American Heart Association Rheumatic Fever, Endocarditis, and Kawasaki Disease Committee, Council on Cardiovascular Disease in the Young, and the Council on Clinical Cardiology, Council on Cardiovascular Surgery and Anesthesia, and the Quality of Care and Outcomes Research Interdisciplinary Working Group. Circulation. 2007 Oct 9;116(15):1736–54. [PMID: 17446442]

Wren C et al. Survival with congenital heart disease and need for follow up in adult life. Heart. 2001 Apr;85(4):438–43. [PMID: 11250973]

ACYANOTIC CONGENITAL HEART DISEASE

The most common acyanotic congenital heart defects include abnormalities of the heart valves and great vessels, ventricular or atrial communications with left-to-right shunting, and such lesions as partial anomalous pulmonary veins and anomalous coronary arteries.

CONGENITAL AORTIC VALVULAR DISEASE

 ESSENTIALS OF DIAGNOSIS

▶ History of murmur since infancy, coarctation repair, or endocarditis.

▶ Early systolic ejection click, harsh crescendo-decrescendo systolic, or early decrescendo diastolic murmur.

▶ Left ventricular hypertrophy.

▶ Abnormal bicuspid or dysplastic aortic valve with stenosis or regurgitation on Doppler echocardiography.

▶ General Considerations

Congenital aortic stenosis is the most common anomaly encountered in the adult population and constitutes approximately 7% of all forms of congenital heart disease. The male:female ratio is approximately 2–3:1. The term "bicuspid aortic valve" is actually a misnomer; a raphe caused by commissural fusion of two leaflets usually exists. The valve is often dysplastic, with thickened, rolled, and calcified leaflets. The predominant pathophysiology results from mildly obstructed nonlaminar (disturbed) flow across the abnormal valve. A left ventricle-to-aorta pressure gradient of variable severity occurs, setting the stage for the inevitable deterioration of the valve with long-term calcium deposition and progressive stenosis or regurgitation. In a study of young adults with aortic stenosis who underwent surgery between the ages of 21 and 38, diastolic murmurs were audible in 75%, and calcification was found at surgery in 75%. The valve is also at risk for endocarditis, which can lead to early destruction and regurgitation. There is a well-recognized association between bicuspid aortic valve and aortic coarctation.

▶ Clinical Findings

A. Symptoms and Signs

The individual with congenital aortic stenosis is usually asymptomatic unless hemodynamically significant stenosis or regurgitation is present. Routine physical examination reveals a normal carotid pulse contour and left ventricular (LV) impulse, a normal S_2, an early systolic click or sound, and an early-peaking systolic murmur. Identifying these patients in the asymptomatic stage is important. Current guidelines do not recommend endocarditis prophylaxis for the native valve. Refraining from high-level isometric exercise is generally believed to preserve valve function and limit valve regurgitation. The presence of a diastolic murmur of aortic regurgitation in a patient with a febrile illness should

alert the clinician to the possibility of endocarditis and prompt the performance of appropriate diagnostic tests (eg, blood cultures, echocardiogram).

Congenital aortic stenosis is progressive; once hemodynamically significant valvular disease develops in a patient, generally in the fifth or sixth decade of life, the symptoms and signs are identical to those of a patient with acquired aortic valvular disease. Dyspnea, chest pain, and exertional syncope are the classic presenting symptoms. When stenosis predominates, the carotid upstroke is delayed and diminished in volume, the systolic click is no longer present, S_2 is single, and the systolic murmur is crescendo-decrescendo, peaking in late systole. The murmur of aortic regurgitation is often present. The finding of upper extremity hypertension should alert the examiner to the possibility of concomitant aortic coarctation.

B. Diagnostic Studies

1. Electrocardiography and chest radiography—The major electrocardiographic (ECG) findings occur in the presence of hemodynamically significant disease and include left ventricular hypertrophy (LVH) with high QRS voltage, left-axis deviation, and repolarization changes; left atrial enlargement may also be present. The chest radiographic findings are nonspecific. With predominant valvular aortic stenosis, the cardiothoracic ratio may be normal, but LV enlargement and calcification may be evident in the region of the aortic valve on the lateral film. A dilated ascending aorta or a prominent aortic knob may be seen. The cardiac silhouette is enlarged in patients with predominant aortic regurgitation. Pulmonary vasculature may be prominent in the presence of congestive heart failure (CHF).

2. Echocardiography—In the child and younger adult, the abnormally thickened leaflets of the congenitally abnormal valve are readily seen, and the bicuspid valve with its ovoid appearance in systole is apparent (Figure 28–1). On M-mode echocardiography, the point of closure may be eccentric. Heavy calcification often obscures the original valve morphology in the older individual with stenosis. The peak systolic gradient in severe aortic stenosis is usually greater than 64 mm Hg (peak velocity > 4 m/s by continuous wave Doppler). Aortic valve area can be accurately calculated by the continuity equation. Severe aortic stenosis is defined as a valve area of less than 1.0 cm² or 0.5 cm²/m². The LV shows concentric hypertrophy with thick walls and normal cavity dimensions, and the LV ejection fraction is usually normal. In cases with reduced ejection fraction, however, the peak gradient across the aortic valve is generally lower.

In hemodynamically significant aortic regurgitation, the high-velocity diastolic color-flow jet is broad at its site of origin below the aortic valve. Spectral Doppler imaging demonstrates a dense diastolic velocity signal with a short pressure half-time (< 400 ms), and diastolic flow reversal can be recorded in the descending aorta. The LV shows eccentric hypertrophy with normal LV wall thickness and a dilated cavity.

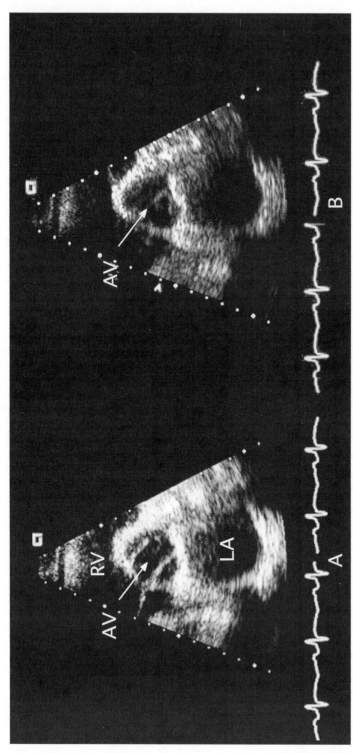

▲ **Figure 28-1.** Transesophageal echocardiographic views of a patient with bicuspid aortic valve. **A:** Systolic frame showing two leaflets of the aortic valve (AV) with an ovoid opening (*arrow*). **B:** Diastolic frame showing the single line of coaptation (*arrow*). LA, left atrium; RV, right ventricle.

In occasional patients with poor precordial windows, transesophageal echocardiography (TEE) may be required to define valve anatomy by demonstrating commissural fusion and asymmetric sinuses of Valsalva. Systolic doming of the leaflets can be easily seen in the long axis view of the LV outflow tract, which also allows measurements to be taken of the aortic valve annulus, sinuses of Valsalva, sinotubular ridge, and ascending aorta.

Cardiac magnetic resonance angiography (MRA) is a possible alternative imaging technique.

3. Cardiac catheterization—Indications for cardiac catheterization in congenital aortic valve disease have changed significantly because most of the diagnostic data are now available noninvasively. According to current guidelines (Circulation. 2006 Aug 1;114(5):e84–231), it is, however, indicated in the following situations:

- "Cardiac catheterization for hemodynamic measurement is recommended for assessment of severity of aortic stenosis in symptomatic patients when noninvasive tests are inconclusive or when there is a discrepancy between noninvasive tests and clinical findings regarding severity of aortic stenosis."

- "Coronary angiography should be performed before valve surgery in men aged 35 years or older, premenopausal women aged 35 years or older who have coronary risk factors, and postmenopausal women."

- "Coronary angiography is recommended before aortic valve replacement in patients with aortic stenosis for whom a pulmonary autograft (Ross procedure) is contemplated and if the origin of the coronary arteries was not identified by noninvasive techniques."

4. Magnetic resonance imaging—Serial imaging with magnetic resonance imaging (MRI) permits accurate and reproducible follow-up of aortic dilatation and is accepted as the standard of care for follow-up of repaired coarctation, a frequent association with a bicuspid aortic valve.

▶ Differential Diagnosis

Subaortic stenosis may be due to an obstructing fibrous membrane in discrete subaortic stenosis, which is more frequently encountered in adults, or by a tubular fibromuscular channel that usually presents in childhood. Aortic regurgitation, commonly associated with discrete membranous subaortic stenosis (in approximately 60% of cases), increases in frequency with age. Regurgitation may occur due to leaflet thickening induced by direct trauma to the aortic leaflets from the high velocity jet or by interference with leaflet closure from the membrane. The aortic valve appearance and the severity and mechanism of aortic regurgitation must be carefully assessed.

Recurrent stenosis caused by regrowth following surgical resection of the fibromuscular ridge is sometimes encountered

in the adolescent or adult. Discrete subaortic stenosis and congenital valvular aortic stenosis must also be distinguished from dynamic LV outflow-tract obstruction caused by hypertrophic obstructive cardiomyopathy (see Chapter 14).

When aortic regurgitation is the predominant lesion and ascending aorta dilatation is present, the condition must be distinguished from Marfan syndrome. This latter condition is characterized by dilatation of the aortic root at the level of the sinuses of Valsalva (Figure 28–2). The aortic valve leaflets are not thickened, and regurgitation is caused by failure of leaflet coaptation caused by the root dilatation. With valvular stenosis, the aorta narrows toward normal at the sinotubular junction, and the descending thoracic aorta is spared. In some patients with a bicuspid aortic valve an underlying abnormality of the medial layer of the aorta above the valve predisposes to the dilatation of the aortic root, which may progress to aneurysm formation or rupture and places the patient at risk for aortic dissection. All components of the vessel wall, smooth muscle, elastic fibers, collagen, and ground substance can be affected and should be recognized as a potential risk in the surgical patient.

▶ Prognosis & Treatment

The natural history of aortic stenosis presenting in childhood depends largely on the severity of the stenosis at the time of diagnosis. During a 25-year follow-up period, approximately one-third of the children with a peak systolic gradient of less than 50 mm Hg who were treated medically required surgery, in contrast to 80% of those with an intermediate gradient (50–79 mm Hg). Of those treated surgically for a gradient of more than 79 mm Hg, approximately one-fourth required reoperation; reoperation was more common in those treated with initial valvotomy (30%) than aortic valve replacement (5%). The overall 25-year survival rate is approximately 85%; sudden death accounts for approximately half of the cardiac-related deaths.

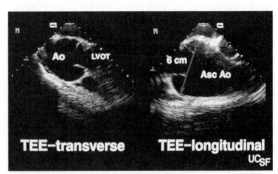

▲ **Figure 28–2.** Transesophageal echocardiographic (TEE) views of the ascending aorta (Asc Ao) measuring 8 cm in a patient with Marfan syndrome. LVOT, left ventricular outflow tract.

Once symptoms of aortic stenosis develop, the prognosis without valve replacement is poor; the 5-year mortality rate is approximately 90%. Although percutaneous valvuloplasty has been successful in children and adolescents, the results in adults (even those with congenitally abnormal valves), have been disappointing. Therefore, surgery with aortic valve replacement, rather than percutaneous valvuloplasty, is generally mandated. Surgery is indicated in the symptomatic patient with a valve area of less than 1.0 cm^2 (or < 0.5 cm^2/m^2). It should be considered in the asymptomatic patient with critical stenosis when the patient requires cardiac surgery (eg, coronary artery bypass surgery) for another lesion. A particularly difficult management decision ensues in the asymptomatic woman with severe aortic stenosis who is contemplating pregnancy. Valve replacement prior to pregnancy should be considered when there is evidence of LV dysfunction or reduced exercise tolerance on objective stress testing.

Patients with a bicuspid aortic valve and concomitant annuloaortic ectasia may show a more rapid progression of aortic regurgitation and require surgical intervention earlier than those patients with pure aortic stenosis.

An ideal substitute for replacing the aortic valve does not exist. Homografts and bioprosthetic valves can develop rapid calcific degeneration, causing valve dysfunction, particularly in the younger cohort of patients. Mechanical valves, although extremely durable, require anticoagulation to reduce the complication of thromboembolism. The risks associated with long-term anticoagulation have made surgical options to avoid the use of mechanical valves desirable alternatives. This is particularly germane to the choice of prosthetic valve in young women of childbearing age, in whom management of anticoagulation can be problematic. The Ross procedure (in which the autologous pulmonary valve replaces the aortic valve, and an aortic or pulmonary homograft replaces the pulmonary valve) has been increasingly performed for a variety of LV outflow tract diseases, including aortic insufficiency and valvar aortic stenosis with or without other forms of obstruction (eg, subaortic stenosis, supravalvar stenosis, and arch hypoplasia). Although the Ross procedure is more complex than simple aortic valve replacement, it can be performed with a low mortality rate in selected patients. Advantages of the pulmonary valve autograft include freedom from anticoagulation and the absence of compromise from host reactions and autograft growth, making it an attractive option for aortic valve replacement in infants and children. It is recognized, however, that the pulmonary homograft will require replacement for degenerative disease and size restriction in children. In adults who are confronting surgery for a stenotic aortic valve in the fifth or sixth decade of life, the Ross procedure has shown to be an acceptable alternative to the usual mechanical or bioprosthetic valve. However, recently recognized problems associated with the Ross procedure include progressive dilatation of the neo-aortic root, pulmonary conduit stenosis, and neo-aortic valve regurgitation. Contraindications to the Ross procedure include advanced three-vessel coronary artery disease, poor LV function, a severely calcified or dilated aortic root, or pulmonary valve pathology.

American College of Cardiology/American Heart Association Task Force on Practice Guidelines; Society of Cardiovascular Anesthesiologists; Society for Cardiovascular Angiography and Interventions; Society of Thoracic Surgeons; Bonow RO et al. ACC/AHA 2006 guidelines for the management of patients with valvular heart disease: a report of the American College of Cardiology/American Heart Association Task Force on Practice Guidelines (writing committee to revise the 1998 Guidelines for the Management of Patients With Valvular Heart Disease): developed in collaboration with the Society of Cardiovascular Anesthesiologists: endorsed by the Society for Cardiovascular Angiography and Interventions and the Society of Thoracic Surgeons. Circulation. 2006 Aug 1;114(5):e84–231. [PMID: 16880336]

Garg V et al. Mutations in NOTCH1 cause aortic valve disease. Nature. 2005 Sep 8;437(7056):270–4. [PMID: 16025100]

Knott-Craig CJ et al. Aortic valve replacement: comparison of late survival between autografts and homografts. Ann Thorac Surg. 2000 May;69(5):1327–32. [PMID: 10881799]

Lambert V et al. Long-term results after valvotomy for congenital aortic valvar stenosis in children. Cardiol Young. 2000 Nov;10(6):590–6. [PMID: 11117391]

Masani N. Transesophageal echocardiography in adult congenital heart disease. Heart. 2001 Dec;86(Suppl 2):II30–II40. [PMID: 11709532]

Niwa K et al. Structural abnormalities of great arterial walls in congenital heart disease: light and electron microscopic analyses. Circulation. 2001 Jan 23;103(3):393–400. [PMID: 11157691]

Raja SG et al. Current outcomes of Ross operation for pediatric and adolescent patients. J Heart Valve Dis. 2007 Jan;16(1):27–36. [PMID: 17315380]

PULMONARY VALVE STENOSIS

 ESSENTIALS OF DIAGNOSIS

▶ History of systolic murmur since infancy.

▶ Systolic ejection click and an early systolic murmur in the second left intercostal space with transmission to the back. S$_2$ may split widely.

▶ ECG evidence of right ventricular hypertrophy.

▶ Dilatation of main and left pulmonary arteries on chest radiograph.

▶ Right ventricular hypertrophy, systolic doming of the pulmonary valve, and a transpulmonic gradient by Doppler echocardiography.

▶ General Considerations

Pulmonary valve, or pulmonic stenosis (PS), is the second most common form of congenital heart disease in the adult. Although many cases are so mild that they require no treatment, it often coexists with other congenital cardiac abnormalities (ASD, ventricular septal defect [VSD], patent ductus arteriosus, or tetralogy of Fallot [TOF]). Pulmonary valve stenosis is characterized by a conical or dome-shaped pliant valve with a narrow outlet at its apex. Right ventricular (RV) outflow is obstructed depending on the size of the orifice, and RV stroke volume may not rise appropriately during exercise. In response to the pressure overload, the RV hypertrophies, with an increase in wall thickness. This compensatory hypertrophy can involve the infundibulum and potentially lead to reversible dynamic subpulmonic stenosis once the valvular stenosis is relieved. If severe stenosis remains untreated, RV failure may ensue. It is important to differentiate pulmonary valve stenosis from stenoses of the peripheral pulmonary arteries and primary infundibular stenosis, often associated with ventricular septal defect (see Tetralogy of Fallot). Pulmonary stenosis from a thickened, dysplastic valve is seen in patients with Noonan syndrome (a heterogeneous malformation syndrome with autosomal-dominant inheritance).

▶ Clinical Findings

A. Symptoms and Signs

The patient with PS usually has exercise intolerance in the form of exertional fatigue, dyspnea, chest pain, or syncope. Right ventricular failure with systemic venous congestion occurs late in the course of the disease. If the foramen ovale is patent or a concomitant ASD exists, shunting of blood from the right atrium to the left may occur, causing cyanosis and clubbing. The volume overload of pregnancy may precipitate right heart failure in patients with severe PS, although mild and even moderate stenosis are usually well tolerated.

In significant PS, the physical examination demonstrates a parasternal RV heave, a delayed and diminished or absent P_2, and a late-peaking crescendo-decrescendo murmur. If the valve is pliable, an ejection click precedes the murmur. This pulmonic ejection sound, best heard in the second left intercostal space, is the only right-sided event that decreases in intensity during inspiration and increases during expiration. As the stenosis becomes more severe, the systolic murmur will peak later in systole and the ejection click moves closer to the first heart sound, eventually becoming superimposed on it. The jugular venous pulse shows a prominent *a* wave, as a result of the diminished RV compliance, but jugular venous pressure is increased only in the late stages when RV failure occurs. Similarly, there may be an RV S_4 gallop early in the course of the disease and a right-sided S_3 in the later stages.

B. Diagnostic Studies

1. Electrocardiography and chest radiography—The ECG demonstrates evidence of right ventricular hypertrophy (RVH) with right-axis deviation, prominent R waves in the right precordial leads, and deep S waves in the left precordial leads (Figure 28–3). There may also be evidence of P-pulmonale with peaked inferior (II, III, aVF) P waves.

The cardiac silhouette on the chest radiograph is normal in mild-to-moderate PS but may become enlarged in severe stenosis when right heart failure occurs. The main and left pulmonary arteries are often dilated. In addition to this "post-stenotic dilatation," dilatation may be seen even in cases of mild PS and may be related to intrinsic abnormalities of the pulmonary artery (idiopathic pulmonary artery dilatation).

2. Echocardiography—The poor near-field resolution of transthoracic echocardiography (TTE) often limits definition of pulmonary valve morphology in the adult patient. When examined from the parasternal short-axis view, the valve may appear thickened (rarely calcified) and usually manifests systolic doming. In the absence of right heart failure, the RV dimension is normal or only mildly increased, but the RV wall thickness is increased (more than 5 mm). In severe cases, the septum may be deviated toward the LV from the pressure overload of the RV. The right atrium and ventricle dilate late in the course of the disease. Saline contrast echocardiography should be performed in all patients with pulmonary valve stenosis to exclude an ASD or a patent foramen ovale.

Color-flow Doppler imaging demonstrates high-velocity flow within the pulmonary artery and is helpful in excluding a VSD or a patent ductus arteriosus. Continuous wave Doppler demonstrates a high-velocity jet across the RV outflow tract (Figure 28–4B). This signal is best obtained from the parasternal short-axis or subcostal short-axis views where flow is axial to the Doppler beam. Pulmonic stenosis is classified as mild when the peak gradient is < 50 mm Hg, moderate when the gradient is 50–79 mm Hg, and severe when the gradient is > 80 mm Hg. Unfortunately, because of the lack of range resolution, continuous wave Doppler cannot localize the level of the obstruction. The morphology of the valve by echocardiography and pulsed wave Doppler mapping may provide localizing information, but additional diagnostic procedures are often necessary.

Transesophageal echocardiography provides excellent definition of the RV outflow tract and pulmonary valve in the basal longitudinal views and excellent images of the atrial septum. As a result, noninvasive methods may now be adequate for establishing the diagnosis, even in adults.

3. Cardiac catheterization—In most patients, cardiac catheterization is therapeutic as well as diagnostic because percutaneous balloon valvuloplasty has virtually replaced surgery for treatment of pulmonary valve stenosis (see below). During right-heart catheterization, the level of the stenosis can be confirmed by pressure monitoring during pullback from the pulmonary artery and supplemented by RV angiography. In valvular stenosis, there is a rise in peak systolic pressure as the catheter tip passes from the pulmonary artery into the infundibulum. In contrast, when the stenosis is in the infundibulum, the systolic pressure increases when the catheter is pulled into the body of the RV. As mentioned earlier, in PS, secondary hypertrophy may result in some degree of infundibular stenosis, and a pressure differential may be

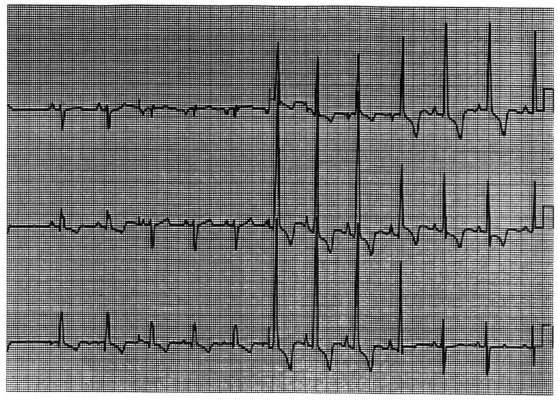

▲ **Figure 28–3.** Electrocardiograph in congenital pulmonic stenosis with severe right ventricular hypertrophy and marked right-axis deviation.

demonstrated at both levels on pullback (Figure 28–5). If the level of obstruction is still uncertain, cine-angiography may show the hypertrophied infundibulum or, alternatively, the domed and thickened pulmonary valve. Of course, both levels of obstruction may coexist.

Unlike aortic valve stenosis, the valve area is not calculated from the Doppler or invasive hemodynamic data, and the gradient alone is used to determine the severity of the obstruction and guide therapy.

▶ Prognosis & Treatment

In severe untreated pulmonary valve stenosis, the average life expectancy is approximately 30 years. The natural history of medically treated mild (gradient < 50 mm Hg) or moderate (gradient 50–79 mm Hg) PS and surgically treated severe (gradient > 80 mm Hg) PS is excellent with a 25-year survival rate of 95%. Surgical valvotomy via a pulmonary artery incision has been extremely effective in long-term relief of pulmonary valve obstruction. Although approximately 50% of patients have mild-to-moderate regurgitation following surgery, it is seldom of hemodynamic significance, and reoperation is rarely necessary.

In children treated conservatively for PS, the likelihood of eventually requiring surgery is dependent on the initial gradient: less than 25 mm Hg, 5%; 25–49 mm Hg, 20%; and 50–79 mm Hg, 76%. In the adult, the indication for treatment of pulmonary valve stenosis is a peak systolic gradient in excess of 50 mm Hg. When the gradient is between 40 and 50 mm Hg, the decision to treat is based on the presence of symptoms, the age of the patient, and the degree of RVH (by echocardiography or electrocardiography). Echocardiography, before and after exercise, may be an important technique to assess RV function in the presence of an increased gradient.

As mentioned above, most patients (including adults) with pulmonary valve stenosis are currently treated with percutaneous balloon valvuloplasty. The Registry of the Valvuloplasty and Angioplasty of Congenital Anomalies has listed 35 patients over the age of 20, among them a 76-year-old man. No significant complications occurred in adult patients, and the gradient was reduced from approximately 70 mm Hg to 30 mm Hg, with about 50% of the residual gradient caused by infundibular hypertrophy. Ongoing assessment of these patients indicate sustained long-term relief of the pulmonary valve gradient with progressive infundibular remodeling causing further reduction in the

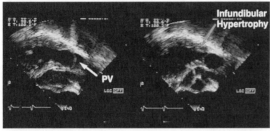

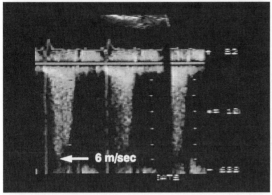

▲ **Figure 28–4. A:** Transesophageal echocardiographic views of a pregnant woman with severe pulmonary valve (PV) stenosis. The left image demonstrates the doming pulmonary valve in systole. The right frame illustrates the severe infundibular hypertrophy. **B:** Continuous wave Doppler recording from the same patient demonstrated a peak velocity of 6 m/s corresponding to a peak transvalvular gradient of 144 mm Hg.

outflow tract gradient over time. Recent technical improvements leading to the development of low profile balloon have decreased the risk of pulmonary regurgitation after dilatation. Based on these results, percutaneous balloon valvuloplasty appears to be the treatment of choice in adults with pulmonary valve stenosis. Severe pulmonary valve insufficiency after either balloon or surgical valvotomy is uncommon, but patients should be evaluated every 5–10 years for this complication. Even when pulmonic stenosis is associated with severe infundibular stenosis and tricuspid regurgitation, the long-term results from balloon valvuloplasty are excellent.

Bashore TM. Adult congenital heart disease: right ventricular outflow tract lesions. Circulation. 2007 Apr 10;115(14):1933–47. [PMID: 17420363]

Brickner ME et al. Congenital heart disease in adults. First of two parts. N Engl J Med. 2000 Jan 27;342(4):256–63. [PMID: 10648769]

Fawzy ME et al. Long-term results (up to 17 years) of pulmonary balloon valvuloplasty in adults and its effects on concomitant severe infundibular stenosis and tricuspid regurgitation. Am Heart J. 2007 Mar;153(3):433–8. [PMID: 17307424]

ATRIAL SEPTAL DEFECT

ESSENTIALS OF DIAGNOSIS

▶ A widely split S_2 without respiratory variation ("fixed split") and a midsystolic murmur are characteristic.

▶ Right ventricular conduction delay ("incomplete right bundle branch block") with vertical QRS axis (ostium secundum ASD) and superior axis (ostium primum ASD) on ECG.

▶ Prominent pulmonary arteries and right ventricular enlargement (decreased retrosternal air space) on chest radiograph. Increased pulmonary vascular markings.

▶ Right ventricular dilatation, increased pulmonary artery flow velocity, and left-to-right atrial shunt by contrast and Doppler echocardiography.

▶ Oxygen step-up within the right atrium; right-sided catheter can pass into the left atrium across the defect.

▶ General Considerations

Atrial septal defects make up 10% of congenital heart disease cases in newborns and are regularly encountered as new diagnoses in adults. The defects vary in size from the smallest fenestrated ASD (a few millimeters) to the largest defect—the complete absence of the atrial septum, or common atrium. The most common interatrial communication is a patent foramen ovale that is anatomically and physiologically not classified as an ASD.

Classification of ASDs is according to location (Figure 28–6): ostium secundum in the region of the fossa ovalis, ostium primum in the lower portion of the atrial septum (actually part of an atrioventricular [AV] canal defect, discussed below), sinus venosus in the upper part of the septum near the entrance of the superior vena cava or at the entrance of the inferior vena cava, and unroofed coronary sinus (communication between the coronary sinus and left atrium). Important associated abnormalities include anomalous drainage of the right upper pulmonary vein into the superior vena cava associated with a superior sinus venosus ASD, a persistent left superior vena cava draining to the coronary sinus with secundum or primum ASDs, and a cleft anterior mitral leaflet and mitral regurgitation associated with an ostium primum ASD. Ostium primum ASD is a common cardiac anomaly in trisomy 21 (Down syndrome) and is part of the spectrum of AV septal "canal" defects (discussed later). There is an approximately 2:1 female predominance for ostium secundum ASDs, while the sex ratio for ostium primum and sinus venosus ASDs is approximately 1:1. An autosomal-dominant inheritance pattern has been demonstrated in some patients with ostium secundum ASD with associated first-degree AV block and cases of ASD

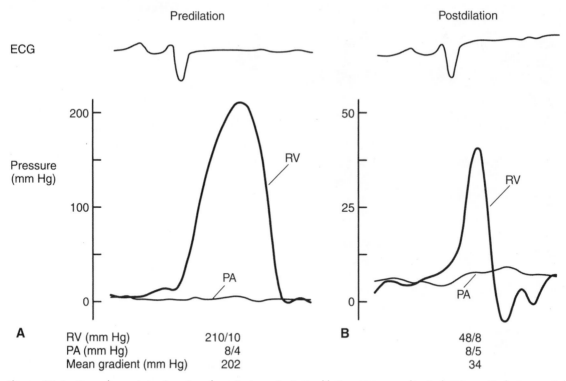

Predilation

Postdilation

ECG

Pressure (mm Hg)

	RV (mm Hg)	PA (mm Hg)	Mean gradient (mm Hg)
A	210/10	8/4	202
B	48/8	8/5	34

▲ **Figure 28–5.** Hemodynamic tracings in pulmonic stenosis. **A:** Predilation: Mean gradient of 202 mm Hg between right ventricle (RV) and pulmonary artery (PA). **B:** Postdilation: Residual gradient of 34 mm Hg between RV infundibulum and pulmonary artery. (Reprinted, with permission, from McGregor J, Ports TA. Catheter balloon valvuloplasty. In: Parmley WW, Chatterjee KD, eds. Philadelphia: Lippincott; 1993.)

in monozygotic twins have been reported. Recent studies have implicated mutations in the genes *gata4*, and *nkx2-5* in non-syndromic ASDs, while point mutations in the gene *tbx5* are known to cause the Holt-Oram syndrome (ASD and limb defects).

The pathophysiologic consequences of an ASD depend on the quantity of blood shunted from the systemic to pulmonary circulation. The size of the shunt is in turn dependent on the size of the defect and the relative compliance of the RV and LV. Little or no shunting occurs immediately after birth because of the high pulmonary vascular resistance (PVR), but as resistance falls, the more compliant RV receives the shunted blood mainly in diastole, when all four chambers are in communication. In the compensated patient with ASD, pulmonary resistance is usually low. The older adult with the LV diastolic abnormalities of hypertension, coronary artery disease, and aging may experience increased left-to-right shunting and, consequently, right heart failure. While pulmonary resistance may increase, the development of Eisenmenger physiology is unusual after the age of 25. Atrial arrhythmias, especially atrial fibrillation, are common over the age of 50.

▶ Clinical Findings

A. Symptoms and Signs

The young adult with an uncorrected ASD and normal pulmonary artery pressures is usually asymptomatic, with normal or minimally diminished exercise tolerance. After the age of 30, however, exertional dyspnea and atypical chest pain increase in frequency. As mentioned earlier, the frequency of atrial arrhythmias increases with age and occurs in a high percentage of patients over the age of 50 who have not been treated surgically. Signs and symptoms of RV failure may occur because of pulmonary hypertension or as a result of long-standing volume overload.

Important findings of the physical examination in an uncomplicated ASD include a prominent RV impulse along the lower-left sternal border; a palpable pulmonary artery; a systolic ejection murmur, caused by increased flow across the pulmonic valve, which does not vary in intensity with respiration; and the almost pathognomonic fixed split second heart sound. When the $Q_p:Q_s$ exceeds 1.5, there may be an associated right-sided diastolic flow rumble and S_3 gallop

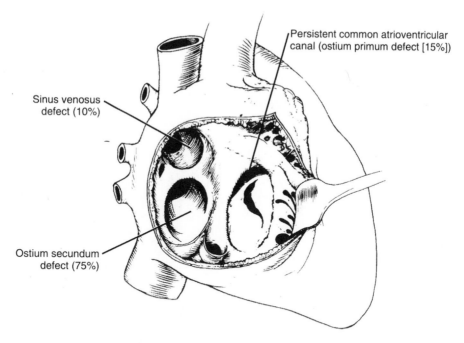

Anatomic features of atrial septal defects.

▲ **Figure 28–6.** Anatomic location of atrial septal defects. (Adapted from Cheitlin M, Sokolow M, McIlroy M. Congenital heart disease. In: *Clinical Cardiology*. Norwalk, CT: Appleton & Lange; 1993.)

from increased flow across the tricuspid valve. The patient with ostium primum ASD usually has a holosystolic murmur of mitral regurgitation. If pulmonary hypertension is present, P_2 is increased and a high-pitched murmur of pulmonary regurgitation (Graham Steell murmur) may be audible. Signs of RV failure with elevated jugular venous pressure and venous congestion may be apparent in the later stages of this disease.

B. Diagnostic Studies

1. Electrocardiography and chest radiography—The ECG shows an RV conduction delay ("incomplete right bundle branch block," IRBBB) in 90% of cases (Figure 28–7). In ostium secundum and sinus venosus ASDs, the QRS axis is vertical or rightward. In the patient with ostium primum ASD, the axis is superior and leftward. Abnormal sinus node function in patients with sinus venosus ASD often results in an ectopic atrial rhythm with a superior P-wave axis.

The chest radiograph shows prominent main and branch pulmonary arteries with a small aortic knob and RV enlargement. The right atrium may appear enlarged. In the absence of pulmonary hypertension, the lung markings are increased as a result of increased pulmonary blood flow.

2. Echocardiography—The findings on TTE include right-heart enlargement and increased pulmonary artery flow. Color-flow Doppler often can identify the interatrial flow, especially in the subcostal four-chamber view. An intravenous saline contrast injection should be used in all patients with these findings to exclude an unsuspected ASD. In the presence of an ASD, a negative contrast effect can be seen in the right atrium as the unopacified left atrial blood is shunted from left to right. A small degree of bidirectional shunting nearly always is present and microbubbles can be seen in the left atrium as a result of right-to-left shunting. The shunting across a patent foramen ovale is purely right to left and occurs only during transient (eg, Valsalva maneuver, coughing) or persistent elevations in right atrial pressure.

Pulmonary artery pressure can be estimated from the peak velocity of the tricuspid regurgitant jet. Echocardiographic measurements may be used to determine shunt flow, eliminating the need for an invasive assessment. In adults, however, the TTE is somewhat limited in quantifying the magnitude of shunts and the size of the defect and in locating sinus venosus defects or anomalous pulmonary veins. As noted earlier, TEE has been found to be more accurate in determining the size and location of atrial communications

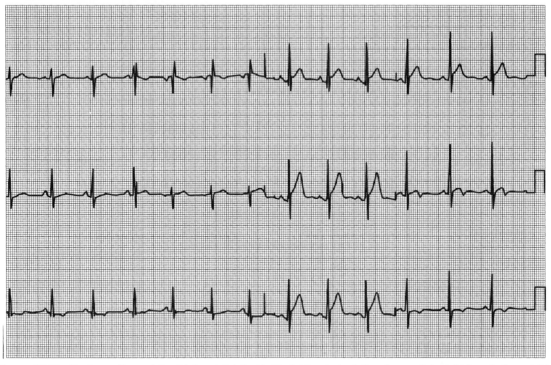

▲ **Figure 28–7.** Electrocardiograph in atrial septal defect with right-axis deviation, incomplete right bundle branch block and right ventricular hypertrophy.

(Figure 28–8). Biplanar and multiplanar transesophageal views are particularly useful in identifying sinus venosus type ASD (Figure 28–9).

3. Cardiac catheterization—In some younger individuals with unequivocally large defects on noninvasive imaging, cardiac catheterization may be avoidable. In others, however, invasive studies may be necessary to accurately quantitate the shunt, measure PVR, and exclude coronary artery disease. Right-heart catheterization with repeated blood sampling for oxygen saturation demonstrates an oxygen step-up (ie, an increase in saturation) from the vena cava to the right atrium. In general, the higher the pulmonary arterial oxygen saturation, the greater the shunt, with a value greater than 90% suggesting a large shunt. The ratio of pulmonary to systemic flow can be calculated by the following formula:

$$\frac{Q_P}{Q_S} = \frac{(SaO_2 - MvO_2)}{(PvO_2 - PaO_2)}$$

Where SaO_2, MvO_2, PvO_2, and PaO_2 are systemic arterial, mixed venous, pulmonary venous, and pulmonary arterial blood oxygen saturations, respectively. Mixed venous O_2 is calculated using the Flamm equation, $[(3 \times SVC) + IVC]/4$, where SVC is the oxygen saturation of blood from the superior vena cava and IVC is the oxygen saturation of blood from the inferior vena cava.

A PVR that is more than 70% of the systemic vascular resistance suggests significant pulmonary vascular disease, and closure is best avoided. Pulmonary vasodilator therapy

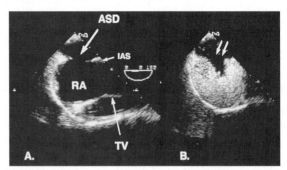

▲ **Figure 28–8.** Transesophageal echocardiogram in a patient with an ostium secundum atrial septal defect (ASD). **A:** The image clearly demonstrates the position of the ASD in the midportion of the interatrial septum (IAS). **B:** The image is obtained after intravenous injection of agitated saline, which opacifies the right atrium (RA). The negative contrast effect produced by the unopacified left atrial blood entering the RA is clearly demonstrated (*double arrow*). TV, tricuspid valve.

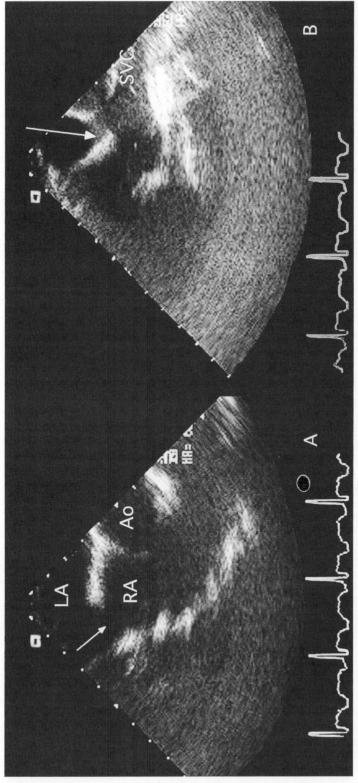

▲ **Figure 28–9.** Transesophageal echocardiography in a 50-year-old man with a sinus venosus atrial septal defect. **A:** Horizontal view showing the defect (*arrow*) in the superior portion of the interatrial septum. **B:** The defect (*arrow*) is clearly demonstrated in this longitudinal plane view. Ao, aorta; LA, left atrium; RA, right atrium; SVC, superior vena cava.

may be used and occasionally pulmonary resistance decreases enough to consider closure.

Prognosis & Treatment

Although patients with an uncorrected ostium secundum ASD generally survive into adulthood, their life expectancy is not normal; older natural history studies showed a 50% survival beyond age 40. The mortality rate after the age of 40 is about 6% per year. Small ASDs (a $Q_p:Q_s$ < 1.5–2:1) may cause problems only in the advanced years, when hypertension and coronary artery disease cause reduced LV compliance, resulting in increased left-to-right shunting, atrial arrhythmias, and potential biventricular failure. In addition, intrinsic abnormalities in LV diastolic function may develop in patients with ASDs unrelated to acquired heart disease. Severe pulmonary hypertension develops during young adulthood in only 5–10% of patients with large shunts ($Q_p:Q_s$ > 2:1). Although most adults with ASDs have mild-to-moderate pulmonary hypertension, the late development of severe pulmonary hypertension in older adults appears to be quite rare. Pregnancy, in the absence of pulmonary hypertension, is usually uncomplicated. Another potential complication of ASD (including even the smallest patent foramen ovale) in the adult patient is paradoxical embolization. Endocarditis is rare in patients with ASD, and prophylaxis is not routinely recommended unless associated lesions with higher risk exist.

The natural history of sinus venosus ASDs is similar to that of ostium secundum defects, although many of these patients have associated partial anomalous pulmonary venous drainage. Adults with an ostium primum ASD are less commonly encountered and may have additional complications resulting from mitral regurgitation caused by the cleft leaflet (see the discussion on AV canal defects, later in this chapter).

Ostium secundum ASDs have been surgically repaired for more than 40 years. No late cardiac deaths occurred in those who had early surgical repair of ASDs (before the age of 18) among patients in a large registry. Patients with elevated pulmonary systolic pressure (> 40 mm Hg) at the time of surgery have the poorest survival rate, especially if they are older than 40 at the time of operation.

Despite the poorer surgical results in adults older than 40 years, closure is superior to medical therapy and is recommended in patients with predominant left-to-right shunts ($Q_p:Q_s$ > 1.5 to 2:1) and PVR less than 10 units/m². Although mortality rates increase when the resistance exceeds this level, surgery can be performed safely in many patients with PVR between 10 and 15 units/m²; pulmonary vasodilator therapy should be considered in these patients before closure. Surgery will improve functional class and eliminate the risk of paradoxical embolization, but closure does not reduce the incidence of atrial arrhythmias.

Percutaneous device closure is widely available, and retrospective studies have suggested comparable results with device closure and surgical closure. Therefore, device closure has become the standard of care for appropriately selected adolescents and adults with ostium secundum defects.

Adult patients with initially small shunts ($Q_p:Q_s$ < 1.5) should undergo continued echocardiographic surveillance because the shunt may increase over time owing to a progressive decline in LV compliance.

In patients with patent foramen ovale who have suffered embolic phenomena, device closure has become a standard intervention although evidence from a randomized controlled trial is lacking. In addition, a correlation has been noted between patent foramen ovale and migraine. However, further study is required before migraine can be considered an indication for patent foramen ovale closure.

Attie F et al. Surgical treatment for secundum atrial septal defects in patients > 40 years old. A randomized clinical trial. J Am Coll Cardiol. 2001 Dec;38(7):2035–42. [PMID: 11738312]

Garg V et al. GATA4 mutations cause human congenital heart defects and reveal an interaction with TBX5. Nature. 2003 Jul 24;424(6947):443–7. [PMID: 12845333]

Hung J et al. Closure of patent foramen ovale for paradoxical emboli: Intermediate term risk of recurrent neurological events following transcatheter device placement. J Am Coll Cardiol. 2000 Apr;35(5):1311–6. [PMID: 10758974]

Patel A et al. Transcatheter closure of atrial septal defects in adults > or =40 years of age: immediate and follow-up results. J Interv Cardiol. 2007 Feb;20(1):82–8. [PMID: 17300410]

Webb G et al. Atrial septal defects in the adult: recent progress and overview. Circulation. 2006 Oct 10;114(15):1645–53. [PMID: 17030704]

VENTRICULAR SEPTAL DEFECTS

 ESSENTIALS OF DIAGNOSIS

▶ History of murmur appearing shortly after birth.

▶ Holosystolic murmur at left sternal border radiating rightward.

▶ Left atrial and LV or biventricular enlargement.

▶ High-velocity color-flow Doppler jet across VSD.

▶ Increased pulmonary flow velocities.

General Considerations

Because of the tendency for many VSDs to close spontaneously (see later discussion) and the tendency of larger defects to appear in early childhood as CHF, it is relatively uncommon to encounter adults with previously undiagnosed VSDs of hemodynamic consequence. Ventricular septal defects in adults are usually either small and hemodynamically insignificant or large and associated with Eisenmenger syndrome. The importance of identifying the former is that they pose an ongoing risk of endocarditis and the potential complication of progressive aortic regurgitation. Eisenmenger syndrome is discussed later in this chapter.

Classifications of VSDs can be based on anatomic location or physiology. The anatomic classification includes defects of both the membranous and muscular portions of the ventricular septum (Figure 28–10). Membranous VSDs can be subdivided into supracristal (also known as doubly committed subarterial), perimembranous (the inlet portion of the membranous septum), and malalignment (found in TOF with an overriding aorta) defects. The muscular VSDs, often multiple, may be located in the inlet or outlet regions or within the trabecular portion of the septum. Classifying VSDs physiologically is based on the size of the defect as well as the relative vascular resistances within the systemic and pulmonary circulation. A high-pressure gradient exists across a small restrictive VSD, with normal or mildly elevated pulmonary artery pressure and predominant left-to-right shunting. A large nonrestrictive VSD permits equalization of RV and LV pressures with obligatory pulmonary hypertension (in the absence of RV outflow-tract obstruction) and bidirectional shunting. The smallest VSD (maladie de Roger) is characterized by a hemodynamically insignificant shunt, a loud murmur, and an intermediate-to-high risk of endocarditis.

In the infant, left-to-right shunting occurs only when PVR falls below systemic vascular resistance, and the murmur usually becomes audible in the first month of life. With a large nonrestrictive defect, PVR may not fall; if the defect is not surgically closed by age 2, irreversible pulmonary hypertension may ensue. The volume overload caused by a large restrictive VSD may cause CHF in the first 6 months of life. Approximately 40% of VSDs close spontaneously by age 3, and a smaller percentage close before age 10. Generally, the smaller defects are more likely to close, but even in infants with heart failure, 7% will experience spontaneous closure.

Three late complications of VSD are worth mentioning. Tricuspid regurgitation may rarely result when the septal leaflet of the tricuspid valve is deformed by the ventricular septal aneurysm that causes spontaneous closure of a perimembranous VSD. Aortic regurgitation is common in patients with doubly committed subarterial VSDs (supracristal, or outlet, VSDs), as a result of herniation of the right aortic sinus into the defect; it also occurs in those with perimembranous VSDs. Infundibular PS from hypertrophy of the RV outflow tract can develop, functionally dividing the RV into inflow and outflow segments, a condition termed "double-chambered right ventricle." If a sufficient pressure gradient develops, RV systolic pressure can exceed LV systolic pressure and right-to-left shunting can occur across the VSD. The resultant hypoxia may only occur during exercise.

▶ Clinical Findings

A. Symptoms and Signs

The young adult with an uncorrected VSD and normal pulmonary artery pressures is usually asymptomatic, with normal or minimally diminished exercise tolerance. Like those with ASDs, exertional dyspnea often develops in

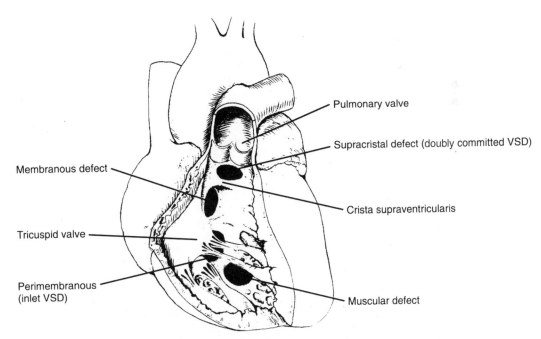

▲ **Figure 28–10.** Anatomic location of ventricular septal defects (VSDs). (Adapted, with permission, from Way LW, Doherty GM. Current Surgical Diagnosis & Treatment. McGraw-Hill, 2003.)

patients with VSDs after the age of 30 when the Q_p:Q_s exceeds 2–3:1. Individuals with smaller shunts rarely report symptoms. The most disabled group with pulmonary hypertension and cyanosis (Eisenmenger physiology, or syndrome) will be discussed later.

Physical findings depend on the size of the VSD. The patient with uncomplicated VSD is acyanotic, and the LV apical impulse is displaced laterally and may be hyperdynamic. A holosystolic murmur occurs, often associated with a systolic thrill, heard best in the fourth or fifth intercostal space along the left sternal border, with radiation to the right parasternal region. Because of the increased flow across the mitral valve, an S_3 gallop and a diastolic rumble may be present. Additional signs of tricuspid insufficiency (prominent jugular venous v wave and systolic murmur) or aortic valve regurgitation (diastolic blowing murmur, increased arterial pulses) will be present in patients with these complications.

B. Diagnostic Studies

1. Electrocardiography and chest radiography—In the presence of a large shunt, the ECG is suggestive of LVH or biventricular hypertrophy, with biphasic QRS complexes in the transitional precordial leads. Evidence of left or right atrial enlargement is present in only about 25% of patients.

Cardiac enlargement with an increased cardiac silhouette is evident on chest radiograph only in the presence of a large left-to-right shunt. In the absence of pulmonary hypertension, there is evidence of pulmonary vascular engorgement with a plethora of the peripheral vasculature as well as enlargement of the proximal vessels. Left atrial enlargement may be evident on the lateral chest radiograph.

It is important to remember that in most adults with a small VSD (< 1.5–2:1 shunt), both the ECG and radiograph are normal, even in the presence of a loud murmur. On the other hand, the presence of pulmonary hypertension alters the ECG and radiograph findings.

2. Echocardiography—Two-dimensional and Doppler echocardiography can usually define the location and often the size of a VSD, although accurate Doppler shunt quantitation may not be possible in the adult. There is evidence of left atrial and LV dilatation. The right-heart chamber dimensions are usually normal, although the main pulmonary artery may appear dilated. The presence of RVH usually signifies pulmonary hypertension or associated PS (with right-to-left shunting and cyanosis). Usually only the largest defects, often located in the membranous septum, can actually be visualized echocardiographically (Figure 28–11). The aneurysmal pouch of a ventricular septal aneurysm may be seen in the parasternal short-axis view just below the aortic valve in the inlet portion of the septum near the septal leaflet of the tricuspid valve. Saline contrast administration shows a negative contrast effect within the RV, and a small degree of bidirectional shunting is sometimes present, with microbubbles appearing in the LV.

Color-flow Doppler imaging demonstrates a high-velocity (aliased) systolic jet across the ventricular septum into the RV. The location of the jet provides the best guide to the location of the defect. In the parasternal short-axis view, the jet from a membranous VSD may be seen in the region of the tricuspid valve (perimembranous) or toward the pulmonary artery (doubly committed subarterial, or supracristal). Muscular VSD jets are best seen in the apical or subcostal four-chamber views (Figure 28–12).

In continuous wave Doppler, the peak velocity of the jet across the ventricular septum provides the peak systolic LV-RV gradient (using the modified Bernoulli equation). Subtracting this gradient from the systolic blood pressure gives the peak RV systolic pressure. In the absence of a pressure gradient across the RV outflow tract—including the pulmonary valve (which should be carefully sought)—the RV systolic pressure is equivalent to the pulmonary artery systolic pressure. Additional Doppler evidence of the left-to-right shunt is found in the increased pulmonary artery flow velocity.

In the postrepair patient, the VSD patch may or may not be apparent, depending on the size of the original defect. Once endothelialized, the patch may not cause acoustic shadowing (or distal echo blockout). Color-flow Doppler may demonstrate patch leaks at the peripheral suture lines of the patch in a small percentage of patients. Spontaneous closure of a VSD involving juxtaposed tricuspid valve tissue may cause significant tricuspid regurgitation. Varying degrees of aortic regurgitation may be present and are most often associated with membranous or supracristal VSDs.

3. Cardiac catheterization—Although the diagnosis is often made noninvasively, the decision to close a VSD rests on accurate measurements of the shunt ratio and the level of PVR. Catheterization is therefore often necessary for therapeutic decision making.

Right-heart catheterization with sequential measurements of oxygen saturation reveals a step-up within the body of the RV. As with an ASD, the higher the RV oxygen saturation, the greater the degree of shunting. For the calculation of Q_p:Q_s, the same formula is used as for ASD, except that the mixed venous blood sample is drawn from the right atrium. Pulmonary artery pressures and vascular resistance should be measured and a gradient across the RV outflow tract, including the infundibulum and the pulmonary valve, must be excluded. Left ventriculography in the cranial left anterior oblique projection will reveal the location of the defect as contrast enters the RV.

▶ Prognosis & Treatment

As previously mentioned, adults with large, uncorrected VSDs are uncommonly encountered. With an uncorrected VSD, the overall 10-year survival rate after initial presentation is 75%. Survival is adversely affected by functional class greater than New York Heart Association I, cardiomegaly,

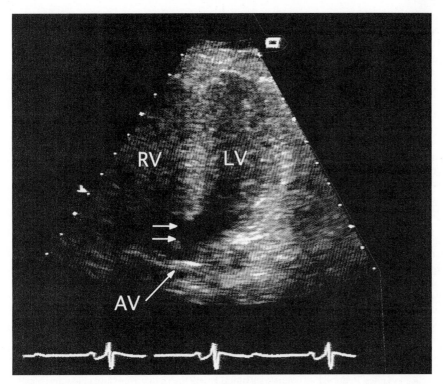

▲ **Figure 28–11.** Transthoracic echocardiogram in a 40-year-old woman with a large membranous ventricular septal defect (*double arrow*). The right ventricle (RV) was enlarged because of pulmonary hypertension. AV, aortic valve; LV, left ventricle.

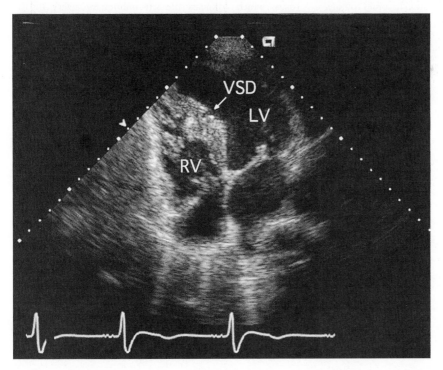

▲ **Figure 28–12.** Transthoracic echocardiogram in a 45-year-old woman with a small muscular ventricular septal defect (VSD). LV, left ventricle; RV, right ventricle.

and elevated pulmonary artery pressure (> 50 mm Hg). As in patients with ASD, surgery is generally recommended when the magnitude of the systemic-to-pulmonary-shunt ratio exceeds 2:1. Other indications for surgery may include recurrent endocarditis and progressive aortic regurgitation.

In patients with small VSDs treated either conservatively or with surgery, outcomes are identical for patients with a Q_p:Q_s < 2.0, normal PVR, no LV volume overload or VSD-related aortic regurgitation, and no symptoms of exercise intolerance.

Surgery for closure of VSDs has been available for more than 40 years, and long-term follow-up data are available. Surgery prior to age 2—even in infants with a large VSD, high pulmonary blood flow, and preoperative pulmonary hypertension—almost always prevents the development of pulmonary vascular obstructive disease. In patients who underwent surgery during the 1960s and 1970s, there is an approximately 20% incidence of residual left-to-right shunt and a persistent risk of endocarditis. Ventricular arrhythmias and RBBB are more common with a repair performed via right ventriculotomy (eg, muscular or subarterial VSD); when possible, the right atrium is the preferred approach. The risk of sudden death and complete heart block is low. Most patients who have VSDs repaired in childhood survive to lead normal adult lives.

Devices have been developed for percutaneous closure of both muscular and perimembranous VSDs but are not yet commercially available in the United States. Initial case series suggest high success rates and low complication rates. Reported complications (in nine patients) include conduction anomalies and aortic or tricuspid regurgitation. More extensive follow-up data are needed before device implantation becomes routine.

Gabriel HM et al. Long-term outcome of patients with ventricular septal defect considered not to require surgical closure during childhood. J Am Coll Cardiol. 2002 Mar 20;39(6):1066–71. [PMID: 11897452]

Minette MS et al. Ventricular septal defects. Circulation. 2006 Nov 14;114(20):2190–7. [PMID: 17101870]

PATENT DUCTUS ARTERIOSUS

ESSENTIALS OF DIAGNOSIS

► Continuous machinery-like murmur, loudest below the left clavicle.

► Left ventricular hypertrophy.

► Pulmonary plethora, left atrial and ventricular enlargement; in older adults, calcification of the ductus on chest radiograph.

► Left atrial and ventricular dilatation with normal right-heart chambers on echocardiography.

► Continuous high-velocity color Doppler jet with retrograde flow along lateral wall of main pulmonary artery near left branch.

► General Considerations

The patent ductus arteriosus (PDA) is a remnant of the normal fetal circulation. In the fetal circulation, superior vena cava blood enters the right atrium and characteristically is directed across the tricuspid valve into the RV. It is then delivered into the systemic circulation via the ductus arteriosus, which connects the left pulmonary artery to the descending aorta just distal to the insertion of the left subclavian artery (Figure 28–13). In the normal full-term newborn, the ductus closes within the first 10–15 hours following birth. If the ductus fails to close after birth when PVR falls, the direction of blood flow within the ductus

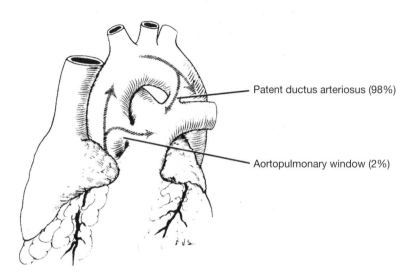

Patent ductus arteriosus (98%)

Aortopulmonary window (2%)

▲ **Figure 28–13.** Anatomic locations of patent ductus arteriosus and aortopulmonary window. (Adapted, with permission, from Cheitlin M, Sokolow M, McIlroy M. Congenital heart disease. In: *Clinical Cardiology.* Norwalk, CT: Appleton & Lange; 1993.)

reverses, producing a left-to-right shunt. Congestive heart failure usually develops within the first year of life in patients with nonrestrictive PDA (large left-to-right shunts). As with VSD, it is relatively unusual—but by no means rare—to encounter an adult with uncorrected PDA.

An anatomic variant of the PDA is the aortopulmonary window (see Figure 28–13), which is usually a relatively large communication between the ascending aorta and the main pulmonary artery. The pathophysiology is similar to that of the PDA and is dependent on the size of the shunt and the level of PVR. The degree of pulmonary hypertension depends on the directly transmitted aortic pressure, which in turn depends on the size of the channel and the amount of pulmonary blood flow. If LV failure occurs, pulmonary venous hypertension may contribute further to the pulmonary hypertension. In a small number of patients, PVR rises above systemic vascular resistance and the shunt reverses. Because the site of the PDA is distal to the left subclavian, the head and neck vessels continue to receive oxygenated blood—but the descending aorta receives the desaturated blood, with the development of differential cyanosis.

When present in isolation, the PDA may lead to heart failure from pulmonary overcirculation. In conjunction with other defects, however, it may represent the sole pulmonary (eg, pulmonary atresia with intact ventricular septum) or systemic (eg, aortic atresia) blood supply, and survival may depend on persistent patency.

▶ Clinical Findings

A. Symptoms and Signs

The mothers of patients with PDA may have a history of maternal rubella, and the patient may have had a murmur since infancy. If CHF has not developed by age 10, most patients will be asymptomatic as adults. Congestive heart failure develops in a few patients in their 20s and 30s, however, and presents as exertional dyspnea, chest pain, and palpitations.

The patient is almost always acyanotic; but when cyanosis and clubbing are present the upper extremities are usually spared. Thus, the lower extremities and sometimes the left hand may show clubbing and cyanosis, but the right hand and head are always pink. The pulse pressure may be widened, and the pulses are collapsing. The LV impulse is hyperdynamic and often laterally displaced. The classic murmur of the uncomplicated PDA is best heard below the left clavicle and gradually builds to its peak in late systole; it is continuous through the second heart sound and wanes in diastole. There may be a pause in late diastole or early systole. With a significant LV volume overload caused by a large shunt, an S_3 gallop and a diastolic murmur of relative mitral stenosis (similar to that of the large VSD) may be present. The murmur varies as PVR increases and shunting reverses, first with a decrease

in the diastolic component and then a decrease in the systolic component. Finally, the murmur is silent and the physical findings are consistent with pulmonary hypertension (see Eisenmenger Syndrome).

B. Diagnostic Studies

1. Electrocardiography and chest radiography—The ECG is normal when the shunt is small; it shows left atrial and ventricular hypertrophy in the presence of a large shunt. When pulmonary hypertension is present and the shunt is predominantly right to left, the ECG may show P-pulmonale, right-axis deviation, and evidence of RVH.

The chest radiograph is also normal in the presence of a small shunt. With a significant shunt, LV prominence is evident with an enlarged cardiac silhouette and pulmonary vascular plethora. In the presence of pulmonary hypertension, pruning of the peripheral pulmonary vessels is present, with prominence of the central pulmonary arteries. The ductus may be calcified in the older adult.

2. Echocardiography—The two-dimensional echocardiogram shows left atrial and ventricular enlargement, but imaging of the ductus itself is usually difficult in the adult. Color-flow Doppler imaging is diagnostic and reveals continuous high-velocity flow within the main pulmonary artery near the left branch. Flow is predominantly retrograde within the pulmonary artery and can be detected by continuous wave Doppler. In an aortopulmonary window, continuous color-flow is detected, but it is most often antegrade, which distinguishes it from the flow through a PDA. Pulmonary artery pressure can be estimated from the almost ubiquitous tricuspid regurgitant jet.

3. Cardiac catheterization—Right-heart catheterization is performed to measure the pulmonary artery pressure, PVR, and the flow ratio (Q_p:Q_s). The oxygen step-up is at the level of the pulmonary artery, and when the ductus is large enough, the descending aorta can be entered from the pulmonary artery. The ductus can also be seen during aortography in the left lateral projection. Because echocardiography is noninvasive and diagnostic, cardiac catheterization may become exclusively therapeutic in the future. Techniques for coil and, more recently, device occlusion are well established and currently represent the treatment of choice for simple PDAs in many institutions. Thus, catheterization should be combined with a therapeutic intervention.

▶ Prognosis & Treatment

Patients who survive into adulthood with a large uncorrected PDA generally have CHF or pulmonary hypertension (with right-to-left shunting and differential cyanosis) by about age 30. Most adults with PDA and normal or only mildly elevated PVR (< 4 units) are either asymptomatic or mildly impaired and can undergo surgical ligation or percutaneous closure with good results. In the group with severely elevated PVR (> 10 units/m^2), survival is poor. Approximately 15% of patients older than 40 years of age may have calcification or aneurysmal dilatation of the ductus, which can complicate surgery. Surgical ligation or percutaneous coil or device occlusion of a PDA can be performed with low morbidity and mortality and is recommended—independent of the size of the shunt—because of the high risk of endocarditis in uncorrected cases. Division of an isolated restrictive PDA in childhood can be curative of congenital heart disease. If repaired after childhood, the morbidity and mortality rates depend on the degree of pulmonary hypertension, LV volume overload, and calcification of the ductus. Unless persistent shunting is present following a surgical ligation, endocarditis prophylaxis is not recommended after the sixth postoperative month.

Masura J et al. Long-term outcome of transcatheter patent ductus arteriosus closure using Amplatzer duct occluders. Am Heart J. 2006 Mar;151(3):755.e7–755.e10. [PMID: 16504649]

Schneider DJ et al. Patent ductus arteriosus. Circulation. 2006 Oct 24;114(17):1873–82. [PMID: 17060397]

COARCTATION OF THE AORTA

ESSENTIALS OF DIAGNOSIS

▶ Elevated systolic blood pressure in the upper extremities (always in right arm); normal or diminished systolic blood pressure in lower extremities (and often left arm); radial-femoral pulse delay.

▶ Left ventricular hypertrophy, LV prominence, "3" sign, rib-notching on chest radiograph.

▶ Visualization of the coarctation by imaging.

▶ Distal aortic pressure drop by Doppler echocardiography or catheterization.

▶ General Considerations

Coarctation of the thoracic aorta predominates in males and is often associated with a congenitally abnormal aortic valve. The most common location is distal to the origin of the left subclavian artery (postductal; Figure 28–14), but

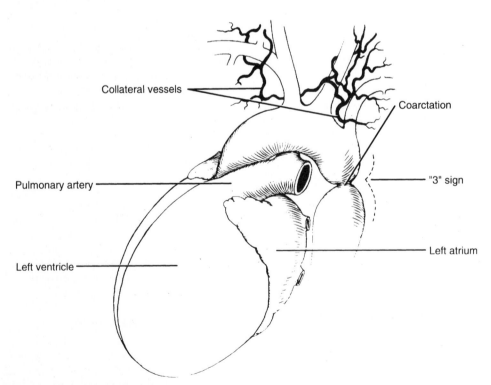

▲ **Figure 28-14.** Anatomic features of aortic coarctation. (Reproduced, with permission, from Cheitlin M, Sokolow M, McIlroy M. Congenital heart disease. In: *Clinical Cardiology*. Norwalk, CT: Appleton & Lange; 1993.)

the narrowing may also be proximal (preductal). Infrequently, a preductal coarctation is present in combination with an anomalous origin of the right subclavian artery, causing reduced pressures in the right upper extremity. There is considerable variability in the degree and extent of narrowing, ranging from a localized shelf to a long tubular narrowing. Multiple discrete sites are rarely encountered. Coarctation of the abdominal aorta is less common than that of the thoracic aorta; it is found equally in males and females and presents with symptoms of claudication. Additional coexisting problems may include congenital mitral valve disease and aneurysms of the circle of Willis (the latter are present in approximately 25% of patients with coarctation). Collateral circulation to the distal aorta develops mainly via the subclavian and intercostal arteries, in addition to the vertebral and anterior spinal arteries.

Aortic coarctation is usually diagnosed during childhood in the asymptomatic phase by routine examination of blood pressure and femoral pulse palpation. Aortic coarctation is approximately two to five times more common in boys than in girls. In cases of severe obstruction, infants may have CHF. Symptoms may arise in the adult during the 20s and 30s, and evidence of coarctation should always be sought in patients of this age group presenting with hypertension. Early detection and repair are highly desirable because repair forestalls the associated accelerated development of coronary artery disease.

▶ Clinical Findings

A. Symptoms and Signs

The adult with uncorrected coarctation is usually asymptomatic. When symptoms occur, they are nonspecific: exertional dyspnea, headache, epistaxis, and leg fatigue. Congestive heart failure can occur in the adult with long-standing hypertension secondary to coarctation. Additional significant complications, usually occurring between the ages of 15 and 40, include aortic rupture or dissection of the proximal thoracic aorta or an aneurysm distal to the coarctation, infective endocarditis on an associated bicuspid aortic valve or endarteritis at the site of coarctation, and cerebrovascular accidents, which are most often due to rupture of an aneurysm of the circle of Willis.

The systolic blood pressure is elevated in the right arm and often the left arm, with reduced systolic blood pressures in the lower extremities. Diastolic blood pressures are not usually affected. Simultaneous palpation of the brachial and femoral pulses reveals delayed arrival of the femoral pulse. Adult patients with highly developed collateral circulation may no longer exhibit these signs, however. The jugular venous pulse is normal, the carotid upstroke is usually brisk, and the aorta may be palpable in the suprasternal notch. Cardiac examination reveals a nondisplaced, but forceful, LV impulse. The first heart sound is normal, and

the aortic component of the second heart sound may be accentuated. A late systolic murmur is present (as a result of the coarctation) that is best heard between the scapulae to the left of the spine. The murmur caused by collateral flow through the intercostal and internal mammary arteries is longer, but it is not necessarily continuous. An ejection click and systolic murmur as well as a blowing diastolic murmur of aortic regurgitation may be associated with a bicuspid aortic valve.

B. Diagnostic Studies

1. Electrocardiography and chest radiography—The ECG is nonspecific, with LVH and, in the later stages, left atrial enlargement. As in other patients with long-standing hypertension, atrial fibrillation may occur.

On the other hand, the radiograph finding of rib notching is highly specific, although it is not 100% sensitive even in adults. Notching is present on the bottom of the rib where the intercostal arteries are located. In preductal coarctation (ie, proximal to the left subclavian artery), the rib notching is present only on the right side, and, in abdominal coarctation, it is limited to the lower ribs. Another classic radiograph finding is the "3" sign, with the dilatated left subclavian artery forming the upper curvature and the dilatated distal aorta forming the lower. There may be radiologic evidence of LV and atrial enlargement.

2. Echocardiography—It is extremely difficult to identify the actual site of the coarctation in the adult patient with precordial two-dimensional echocardiography. Doppler evidence of flow acceleration in the descending aorta from the suprasternal notch, however, can often identify obstruction even when images are suboptimal. The peak systolic velocity can be used to estimate the gradient, but the presence of persistent antegrade flow in diastole (Figure 28–15A) and decreased acceleration time beyond the coarctation provide additional confirmation of hemodynamic significance. Further localization of the coarctation is now possible with imaging of the descending aorta in the longitudinal plane during multiplanar TEE. The anatomy of the aortic valve should be carefully defined, and careful Doppler interrogation for evidence of stenosis or insufficiency is essential.

3. Magnetic resonance angiography and CT angiography—Magnetic resonance angiography can localize and define the extent of narrowing with a high degree of accuracy (Figure 28–15B) and provides estimates of the presence of collateral flow to the distal aorta. Aneurysmal dilatation is visible, and postoperative evaluation is possible. CT angiography provides excellent anatomic definition but cannot provide any physiologic information.

4. Cardiac catheterization—Aortography is necessary only when the diagnosis is not adequately confirmed clinically or the anatomy cannot be fully defined noninvasively. Prema-

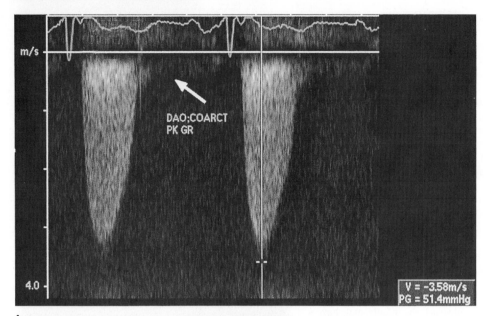

A

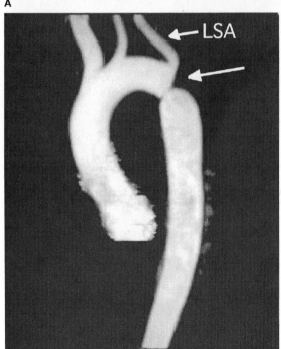

B

▲ **Figure 28–15. A:** Continuous wave Doppler from transthoracic echocardiogram in a patient with coarctation of the descending aorta (DAO). There was a peak gradient (PK GR) of 51.4 mm Hg with runoff in diastole (*arrow*). **B:** Three-dimensional reconstruction of a magnetic resonance angiogram of the thoracic aorta demonstrates a discrete coarctation (*lower arrow*) in the typical location after the take-off of the left subclavian artery (LSA).

ture coronary disease is common, and if it is clinically suspected, coronary arteriography should be performed. Balloon dilatation with or without stent placement across native and recurrent coarctation has been attempted in cases of discrete narrowing (see later discussion).

▶ Prognosis & Treatment

The importance of identifying coarctation in adults lies in the tendency toward LVH and CHF, premature coronary artery disease, and cerebral hemorrhage. In an autopsy series of uncorrected coarctation, 50% of patients had died by about age 30 and 90% by age 60. Proximal aortic rupture and cerebral hemorrhage often occur before the age of 30, and the incidence of CHF continues to increase after the age of 40.

Surgery for correcting coarctation presents a considerable challenge in patients over the age of 15 years because of often-huge intercostal aneurysms and atheromatous changes in the aorta near the shelf. It should be noted that surgical repair even in childhood is often only palliative, and these patients require continued surveillance, particularly in the presence of associated cardiac lesions or preoperative systemic hypertension. Hypertension persists in approximately one-third of patients operated on after the age of 14. The major determinants of long-term survival following repair of aortic coarctation are the presence of associated lesions and the age at operation. The postsurgery cardiac mortality rate after age 20 is approximately 5% in patients with isolated coarctation. Causes of late cardiovascular deaths (in order of frequency) include coronary artery disease, sudden death, aortic regurgitation and heart failure, hypertension and heart failure, and cerebrovascular accidents. Approximately 10% of patients require subsequent cardiovascular surgery, the majority for aortic valve replacement. The incidence of recurrent coarctation requiring surgery or percutaneous intervention varies significantly depending on surgical technique and can be 16–60%, with the highest recoarctation rates generally associated with earlier operation.

The surgical methods of repair have undergone considerable evolution since their initial introduction in the late 1950s. In part this is due to the considerable morphologic variability which has precluded using a single method for correction. The removal of the abnormal coarctation tissue as occurs in an end-to-end anastomosis is most desirable, but depending on other factors a subclavian flap repair or an interposition graft may be necessary. Less reliance is placed on the patch angioplasty because long-term studies have shown late aneurysm formation due to thinning of the posterior wall.

Over the last 10 years, endovascular repair of coarctation has become a popular treatment option. Furthermore, the advent of balloon-expandable stents has reduced the complication rate associated with balloon angioplasty alone. Complications of stent implantation can be classified into three categories: technical (stent migration or fracture, balloon rupture, and overlap of the braciocephalic vessels), aortic (intimal tear, dissection, and aneurysm formation), and peripheral vascular (cerebral vascular accident, peripheral embolization, and injury to access vessels). Compared with surgical therapy, endovascular stenting of native coarctation has a similar morbidity and mortality but is associated with a significantly higher incidence of recoarctation, need for reintervention, and persistent hypertension. In light of these differences, there is ongoing controversy about the best treatment approach for adults and adult-sized adolescents with native coarctation of the aorta. There is general agreement, however, that recoarctation in adults can be managed by percutaneous transluminal balloon angioplasty, with or without stent implantation.

Because of the risk of recoarctation and of complications such as aortic aneurysm, periodic surveillance with MRI or with CT aortography is recommended in the adult after repair, irrespective of technique. It is essential to screen women of childbearing age for post-repair aortic dilatation because the risk of rupture during pregnancy is high. The need to screen for intracranial aneurysms is controversial.

Carr JA. The results of catheter-based therapy compared with surgical repair of adult aortic coarctation. J Am Coll Cardiol. 2006 Mar 21;47(6):1101–7. [PMID: 16545637]

Connolly HM et al. Intracranial aneurysms in patients with coarctation of the aorta: a prospective magnetic resonance angiographic study of 100 patients. Mayo Clin Proc. 2003 Dec;78(12):1491–9. [PMID: 14661678]

Golden AB et al. Coarctation of the aorta: stenting in children and adults. Catheter Cardiovasc Interv. 2007 Feb 1;69(2):289–99. [PMID: 17191237]

EBSTEIN ANOMALY

 ESSENTIALS OF DIAGNOSIS

▶ History of dyspnea, atypical chest pain, or intermittent cyanosis.

▶ Palpitations associated with supraventricular arrhythmias and preexcitation syndrome.

▶ Right parasternal lift, widely split S_1, systolic clicks, and systolic murmur of tricuspid regurgitation (without inspiratory accentuation).

▶ Right atrial enlargement, RV conduction defect of RBBB type, posteriorly directed delta waves with accessory pathway by ECG. Frequent first-degree AV block.

▶ Normal or reduced pulmonary vascularity without pulmonary artery enlargement, right atrial enlargement, normal left-sided cardiac silhouette on chest radiograph.

▶ Apical displacement of septal tricuspid valve leaflet; variable degrees of tricuspid regurgitation originating from apical portion of RV; and enlarged right atrium on echocardiography.

▶ General Considerations

Ebstein anomaly is characterized by deformity of the tricuspid valve with apical displacement of the septal and posterior leaflets (Figure 28–16) and their adhesion to the RV wall. The anterior leaflet is elongated and has been described as sail-like. Tricuspid regurgitation arises from the apically displaced site of leaflet coaptation with considerable variability in the extent of tricuspid leaflet displacement and the degree of tricuspid regurgitation. The portion of the RV proximal to the leaflets is atrialized (thinned), and if the

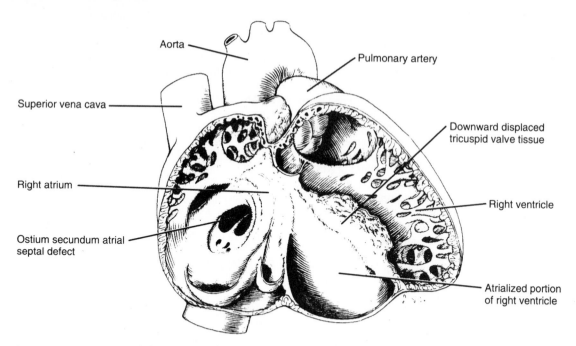

▲ **Figure 28–16.** Anatomy of Ebstein anomaly. (Redrawn with permission from Icon Learning Systems division of Medi-Media USA, Inc.)

remaining RV is diminutive in size, pump function may be inadequate. Cyanosis may be present as a result of right-to-left shunting across an ASD or patent foramen ovale in the presence of significant tricuspid regurgitation or elevated right atrial pressures. Interatrial septal defects, including patent foramen ovales, are the most common associated anomaly, occurring in 80–90% of patients with Ebstein anomaly.

Tremendous variability exists in the morphologic abnormalities and clinical presentation of patients with Ebstein anomaly. In severe cases, CHF or cyanosis may be present during infancy. At the opposite end of the spectrum, a mildly affected adult may be asymptomatic or symptomatic only because of supraventricular tachyarrhythmias. The latter are an important feature of Ebstein anomaly, which is associated with preexcitation in 25–30% of patients. The accessory pathway is usually posteroseptal or posterolateral in location.

▶ **Clinical Findings**

A. Symptoms and Signs

Cyanosis may be the most important clinical feature in early life, but in older patients long-standing RV volume overload and right atrial distention result in CHF. Dysrhythmias, including the Wolff-Parkinson-White syndrome, are frequent. Adult patients may have dyspnea, arrhythmias, decreased exercise tolerance, and intermittent or exercise-

induced cyanosis (with associated right-to-left shunting across an ASD or patent foramen ovale).

Physical examination reveals right parasternal lift, widely split S_1, systolic clicks (from delayed tricuspid valve closure, the "sail" sounds), and the systolic murmur of tricuspid regurgitation. The latter does not usually increase in intensity during inspiration, because the noncompliant RV cannot accept an increase in venous return. On the other hand, the RA is compliant, and systemic venous congestion is uncommon; the jugular venous pulse is therefore usually normal. S_3 and S_4 gallops may be present as may an early diastolic snap from the opening of the elongated anterior leaflet.

B. Diagnostic Studies

1. Electrocardiography and chest radiography—The ECG shows evidence of right atrial enlargement and an RV conduction defect of the RBBB type. The PR interval may be prolonged, except in the presence of an accessory pathway. In 25–30% of patients, ECG findings are consistent with Wolff-Parkinson-White syndrome; the PR interval is short, and delta waves from a posterolateral or posteroseptal bundle of Kent are evident (Figure 28–17). Atrial fibrillation may be present in older patients.

The chest radiograph shows normal or reduced pulmonary vascularity without pulmonary artery enlargement; it also shows cardiac enlargement to the right of the sternum

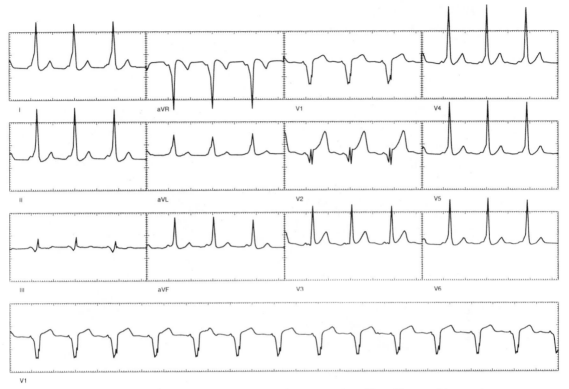

▲ **Figure 28–17.** Electrocardiogram in Ebstein anomaly with associated Wolff-Parkinson-White syndrome.

caused by right atrial enlargement. The LV and left atrium are normal in size.

2. Echocardiography—The classic M-mode description of this anomaly included increased excursion of the anterior tricuspid valve leaflet and delayed tricuspid valve closure (> 40 ms) following mitral valve closure. Two-dimensional and Doppler echocardiography are diagnostic in most adults. The four-chamber apical and subcostal views provide most of the necessary information. The right atrium is enlarged and the RV is usually small, consisting of the atrialized portion and the remaining pumping chamber. The septal, and possibly the posterior, leaflet of the tricuspid valve is apically displaced, and color-flow Doppler imaging shows the regurgitant jet arising from the apical point of coaptation (Figure 28–18). The degree of tricuspid regurgitation can be estimated from the extent of right atrial filling by color-flow and from the density of the continuous wave Doppler signal. The pulmonary artery systolic pressure estimated from the continuous wave tricuspid regurgitation jet is nearly always normal.

Although color-flow imaging may reveal a patent foramen ovale or an ASD, it is mandatory to perform a saline contrast examination to reliably exclude these sources of right-to-left shunting. When precordial echocardiography is

inadequate, TEE can be used to exclude associated lesions of the atrial septum.

3. Cardiac catheterization—During right-heart catheterization, simultaneous recordings of an RV electrogram and a right atrial pressure tracing are obtained with a catheter in the atrialized portion of the RV. This finding is considered pathognomonic of Ebstein anomaly, but catheterization is rarely necessary for diagnosis.

▶ Prognosis & Treatment

The chance of surviving to age 50 is about 50%, with survival dependent on the degree of the anatomic and physiologic abnormalities. As mentioned, 25–30% of patients have supraventricular arrhythmias, many associated with accessory pathways that are now amenable to catheter ablation. Although tricuspid annuloplasty and tricuspid valve reconstruction, with creation of a monocuspid valve, are often possible, tricuspid valve replacement may be required in some patients. Improvement in exercise tolerance following tricuspid valve replacement or repair has been observed, especially in patients with associated ASD. In patients with severe morphologic variants, a Fontan-like procedure (see Palliative Surgical Procedures) may be the only suitable choice. In patients who are symptomatic predominantly on

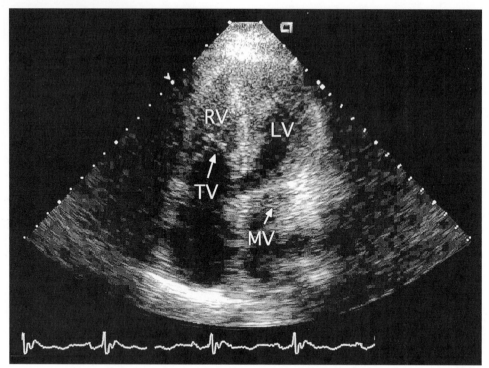

▲ **Figure 28–18.** Transesophageal echocardiogram in a 50-year-old woman with Ebstein anomaly. This four-chamber view shows the apically displaced tricuspid valve (TV) in relation to the normal mitral valve (MV). LV, left ventricle; RV, right ventricle.

the basis of exercise-induced cyanosis, device closure of the interarterial septal defect may be adequate treatment.

Attenhofer Jost CH et al. Ebstein's anomaly. Circulation. 2007 Jan 16;115(2):277–85. [PMID: 17228014]

CONGENITALLY CORRECTED TRANSPOSITION OF THE GREAT ARTERIES

ESSENTIALS OF DIAGNOSIS

▶ Prominent left parasternal impulse, soft S_1, accentuated A_2, soft or inaudible P_2.

▶ PR prolongation, variable degrees of AV block, Q waves in right precordial leads with absence in left precordial leads on ECG.

▶ Absence of left-sided aortic knob on chest radiograph.

▶ Rightward and posterior pulmonary artery with leftward and anterior aorta, apical displacement of right-sided AV valve, coarsely trabeculated left-sided systemic ventricle with moderator band (the morphologic RV) on cardiac imaging.

▶ **General Considerations**

In congenitally corrected transposition of the great arteries (C-TGA, also abbreviated as l-TGA), the visceroatrial relationship is normal with the right atrium to the right of the left atrium (Figure 28–19). The systemic venous blood drains into the right atrium and through a bileaflet (mitral) valve into a morphologic LV pumping into a posterior and rightward pulmonary artery. The pulmonary venous blood drains into the left atrium and through a trileaflet tricuspid valve into a morphologic RV pumping into an anterior and leftward aorta. This occurs because of atrial-ventricular discordance (ventricular inversion), which causes the RV to be located to the left of the LV. The great arteries are transposed, with the aorta arising from the RV and the pulmonary artery rising from the LV. The result is physiologic correction of the circulation, in that oxygenated blood comes into the left atrium, goes to the anatomic right ventricle, and then flows out of the aorta. The patient is acyanotic and is usually asymptomatic in the absence of associated lesions.

The most common complications are complete heart block (occurring with an incidence of approximately 2% per year) and other associated anomalies, most commonly VSD, subvalvular PS, and abnormalities of the systemic AV valve. Coronary anomalies are uncommon, and the coronary cir-

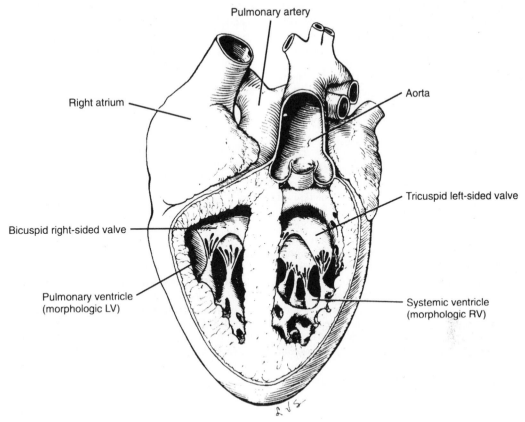

▲ **Figure 28–19.** Anatomy of congenitally corrected transposition of the great arteries. LV, left ventricle; RV, right ventricle. (Redrawn with permission from Icon Learning Systems division of MediMedia USA, Inc.)

culation is usually concordant; that is, a right coronary artery supplies the RV. Eventually, the systemic ventricle (a massively hypertrophied RV) is subject to pump failure, even in cases of isolated C-TGA. The relative degree of PS and the size of the VSD determine whether cyanosis is present. In the absence of PS, the patient with a large VSD may have CHF due to the volume overload of the systemic ventricle and is at risk for pulmonary vascular disease.

The male:female ratio is approximately 1.5:1. While familial recurrence has been reported, no genetic linkage has been identified.

▶ Clinical Findings

A. Symptoms and Signs

Most patients with isolated C-TGA are asymptomatic in childhood and young adulthood. The highly prevalent complication of complete heart block may present with syncope, sudden death or, less dramatically, with exercise intolerance. More often, the clinical picture is dominated by associated lesions.

Exertional dyspnea and easy fatigability may develop with systemic AV valve regurgitation. Pulmonary venous congestion from pump failure of the anatomic RV may occur in middle age.

The physical examination depends largely on the associated anomalies. The left parasternal impulse is prominent as a result of the hypertrophied systemic ventricle. In the presence of a prolonged PR interval, S_1 is diminished in intensity. The proximity of the aorta to the chest wall causes an accentuated A_2; conversely, the posterior displacement of the pulmonary valve causes a soft or inaudible P_2. Systolic thrills occur in the presence of PS, with and without VSD. If PS is present, the murmur is best heard in the third left intercostal space, radiating to the right. The murmur of a VSD is usually typical, but the murmur of left-sided AV valve regurgitation radiates to the left sternal border in C-TGA.

B. Diagnostic Studies

1. Electrocardiography and chest radiography—The ECG and radiologic findings of C-TGA are dominated by its associated lesions. The ECG shows variable degrees of AV block, from simple PR prolongation to complete heart block. The absence of Q waves in leads I, V_5 and V_6 or the presence of Q waves in leads V_4R or V_1 is characteristic of the condition. This pattern results because the ventricular septal depolarization proceeds from the morphologic LV to RV (Figure 28–20). The typical chest radiograph finding in isolated C-TGA is a straight, left upper cardiac border, formed by the ascending aorta and loss of the pulmonary trunk contour.

2. Echocardiography—The anatomic features of isolated C-TGA are usually apparent by TTE, even in adults. Transesophageal echocardiography may be useful in defining the anatomy of associated lesions such as infundibular obstruction and the severity of left-sided AV valve regurgitation. In the basal parasternal short-axis view, the aortic valve is anterior and usually to the left of the pulmonic valve. Because the two great arteries arise in parallel, there is a "figure-eight" appearance, rather than the usual arrangement of the pulmonary artery in long axis surrounding the aortic valve. On careful inspection, the coronary arteries can be identified as they emerge from the aortic root. In the long-axis view (obtained from a more vertical and leftward scan), the aorta arises from the posterior ventricle, and its valve is not in fibrous continuity with the AV valve. The heavily trabeculated and hypertrophied RV with its moderator band is posterior and to the left and the smoothly trabeculated LV is anterior and to the right (Figure 28–21). The systemic AV (anatomi-

cally a tricuspid) valve has three leaflets and septal attachments, is apically displaced, and may show variable degrees of regurgitation. In contrast, the subpulmonary AV (anatomically a mitral) valve has two leaflets and no septal attachments.

It is essential to identify associated lesions because these are the primary determinants of survival, specifically a VSD and infundibular pulmonary valve stenosis. Doppler echocardiography should be used to determine the pulmonary valve gradient and to estimate the degree of pulmonary hypertension. Left-sided Ebstein anomaly may coexist, with the systemic AV valve leaflets displaced apically. Furthermore, morphologic abnormalities of the tricuspid valve are frequently found in patients with C-TGA. Autopsy studies of patients with this lesion have documented tricuspid valve abnormalities in greater than 90% of cases, most commonly an Ebstein-like anomaly with short, thickened chordae tendineae. Clinically significant tricuspid systemic AV valve regurgitation has been reported in 20–50% of patients with C-TGA.

3. Cardiac catheterization—When noninvasive data are diagnostically conclusive, the role of cardiac catheterization is for preoperative evaluation in patients with surgically remediable lesions. The pulmonary artery may be difficult to enter; fluoroscopically, the venous catheter is noted to enter a posterior and rightward vessel. The PVR must be measured to rule out irreversible pulmonary vascular disease in patients with VSD. Although angiography can indicate the

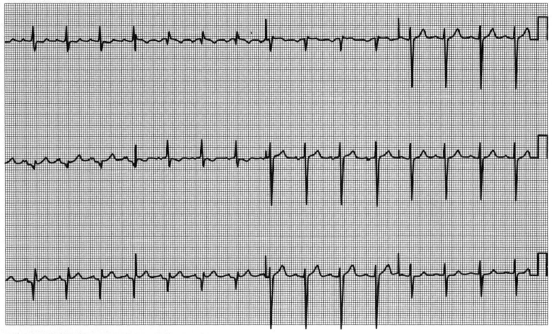

▲ **Figure 28-20.** Electrocardiograph in congenitally corrected transposition of the great arteries with associated pulmonic stenosis and ventricular septal defect.

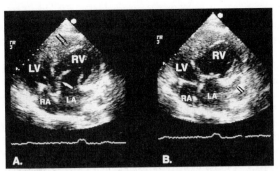

▲ **Figure 28–21.** Apical transthoracic echocardiographic views in a patient with congenitally corrected transposition of the great arteries. **A:** The moderator band is clearly visualized (*double arrow*) in the left-sided morphologic right ventricle (RV). **B:** The narrow based atrial appendage (*double arrow*) clearly identifies this as a left atrium. The right ventricle (RV) is spherically dilated, reflecting the pressure overload of this chamber. The left ventricle (LV) is small and compressed. RA, right atrium. The left-sided atrioventricular (AV) valve is a morphologic tricuspid valve and the right-sided AV valve is a morphologic mitral valve.

abnormally positioned great arteries, it is important only for identification of anomalous coronary arteries, which are infrequently encountered.

▶ Prognosis & Treatment

Survival in congenitally corrected transposition of the great arteries is usually determined by other, associated lesions, but even in its isolated form, survival may not be normal. The natural history and postoperative outcome of patients with C-TGA and the commonly associated lesions of VSD and PS are known to be less satisfactory than those of patients with normal AV connections and similar intracardiac lesions. The propensity for AV conduction abnormalities, for tricuspid valve dysfunction, and the much-debated capability of the RV to function adequately in the systemic circulation may all affect survival.

A frequent feature of C-TGA is the development of complete heart block, estimated to occur at a rate of about 2% per year. Atrioventricular conduction abnormalities of varying degrees are seen in nearly 75% of patients with this anomaly; many will require permanent pacemaker insertion. Periodic surveillance for the development of high-degree AV block is important: sudden death may be the first manifestation of this complication. However, it is the morphologic abnormalities of the tricuspid valve resulting in severe valvular dysfunction/regurgitation which have been shown to be the most critical determinant for survival. The systemic RV in C-TGA appears to be less tolerant than an anatomic LV of similar degrees of valvular incompetence, and there is an

acceleration of the usual vicious cycle of ventricular remodeling, hypertrophy, and dysfunction in response to volume overload. The RVs inability to cope with significant tricuspid regurgitation leads to decreased contractility and annular dilation that in turn exacerbates the degree of regurgitation. Theoretically, the anatomic RV is subject to progressive pump failure from the obligatory pressure overload of the systemic circulation, potentially hastened by systemic hypertension, coronary artery disease, and volume overload from a regurgitant AV valve. Because the circulation is functionally corrected, the indications for surgery are those of the associated lesion requiring surgery (eg, VSD with a $Q_p:Q_s$ of 2:1, VSD with PS causing cyanosis). Repair or replacement of the tricuspid valve may be indicated; however, 10-year survival after surgical intervention is low. A "double switch" operation has been proposed for patients whose tricuspid valves are severely insufficient. An atrial switch combined with an arterial switch (see the section on Transposition of the Great Arteries) in the absence of LV outflow obstruction or with a **Rastelli** procedure (RV to pulmonary artery conduit) has been successfully performed. After surgery, the LV and mitral valve are restored to systemic circulation. Improvement in tricuspid valve function in a low-pressure RV has been documented after these operations. This procedure carries significant risk, and late complications relating to the atrial switch component (baffle obstruction, sick sinus syndrome) are of additional concern. Heart transplantation remains the final option for patients with C-TGA, intractable tricuspid regurgitation, and RV failure.

Graham TP Jr et al. Long-term outcome in congenitally corrected transposition of the great arteries: a multi-institutional study. J Am Coll Cardiol. 2000 Jul;36(1):255–61. [PMID: 10898443]
Warnes CA. Transposition of the great arteries. Circulation. 2006 Dec 12;114(24):2699–709. [PMID: 17159076]

▼ OTHER ACYANOTIC CONGENITAL DEFECTS

Partial anomalous pulmonary venous return usually involves abnormal drainage of the right upper pulmonary vein into the superior vena cava and is often associated with sinus venosus ASD. Other sites of drainage include the coronary sinus and the inferior vena cava (scimitar syndrome). The need for surgical correction depends on the presence or degree of pulmonary venous obstruction and on the size of the shunt, which in turn is related to the number of pulmonary veins draining into the pulmonary circulation.

Atrioventricular septal defects (also known as **endocardial cushion defects** or **AV canal defects,** both terms referring to abnormalities of derivatives of the endocardial cushions of the embryonic AV canal) are particularly common in children born with trisomy 21. These defects include an ostium primum ASD, a membranous VSD, and a mitral valve malformation, consisting of a cleft in the anterior leaflet or anterior and posterior bridging leaflets (Figure 28–22). Irreversible pulmonary vascular disease with shunt reversal may lead to cyanosis (see section on Eisenmenger Syndrome) and is extremely common in the adult who has had no attempt at repair. Residual mitral regurgitation is often encountered following repair. Even when the valve is competent in the early postoperative period, late regurgitation occurs in a small percentage of patients.

Coronary artery anomalies are seen not uncommonly as an isolated defect in the adult patient. They are found in approximately 1% of patients undergoing coronary arteriography and in approximately 0.3% of autopsies. An anomaly of particular importance is the left main coronary artery arising from the pulmonary trunk. This may present in infancy as cardiomyopathy and CHF from myocardial ischemia and systolic dysfunction. Sufficient myocardial collaterals from the right coronary artery may develop in a small number of patients, which allows survival into adulthood. Physical examination may reveal a continuous murmur, and clinical assessment may be remarkable for angina pectoris, myocardial infarction, dyspnea, syncope, and sudden death. Treatments include surgical closure of the left main artery with possible bypass to the left anterior descending artery or primary reanastomosis of the anomalous artery from the pulmonary artery to the aorta or the subclavian artery. There are many anatomic variations of the less severe coronary anomalies. When the left coronary artery arises from the right or noncoronary cusp and passes between the aorta and pulmonary artery, however, the patient is at increased risk for ischemia and sudden death. This diagnosis should be considered in young patients with exertional chest pain. Transesophageal echocardiography may identify anomalous coronary ostia. Although MRA or CT angiography may be diagnostic in skilled hands, coronary angiography is currently the diagnostic gold standard.

Coronary arteriovenous fistulas are more likely than serious coronary anomalies to permit survival to adulthood.

Large fistulas draining into the right side of the circulation may be associated with a sizable shunt and can rarely present with CHF in infancy. Coronary steal may occur, leading to myocardial ischemia. In the adult, there may be a history of exertional dyspnea or chest pain and a continuous murmur on physical examination. Transthoracic echocardiogram detects the dilated fistulous coronary artery in approximately 50% of patients. Abnormal continuous jets within the cardiac chambers (RV is most common) or in the pulmonary artery seen in color-flow Doppler should suggest this diagnosis. Cardiac catheterization showing the dilated coronary artery and fistulous communication confirm the diagnosis.

Congenital **sinus of Valsalva aneurysms** have the potential for catastrophic rupture with development of acute severe aortic regurgitation or pericardial tamponade. Although the perforation may be subacute with mild regurgitation, it nonetheless poses an ongoing risk for endocarditis. Echocardiography, with a transesophageal approach if necessary, is diagnostic. Surgical repair with a pericardial patch is indicated when rupture is present.

Angelini P. Coronary artery anomalies: an entity in search of an identity. Circulation. 2007 Mar 13;115(10):1296–305. [PMID: 17353457]

Taylor AM et al. Coronary artery imaging in grown up congenital heart disease: complementary role of magnetic resonance and x-ray coronary angiography. Circulation. 2000 Apr 11;101(14): 1670–8. [PMID: 10758049]

◤ CYANOTIC CONGENITAL HEART DISEASE

Patients with cyanotic congenital heart disease have arterial oxygen desaturation resulting from the shunting of systemic venous blood to the arterial circulation, or from cardiac anatomy that mandates mixing of systemic and pulmonary

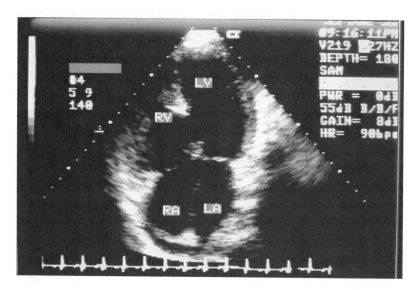

▲ **Figure 28–22.** Apical four-chamber view from a transthoracic echocardiogram in a patient with atrioventricular septal defect and Down syndrome. The crux of the heart is missing, and a large ostium primum atrial septal defect and large ventricular septal defect are evident. LA, left atrium; LV, left ventricle; RA, right atrium; RV, right ventricle.

venous blood. The shunting can occur at the level of the atrium (ASD), the ventricle (VSD), or the great vessels (PDA or aortopulmonary window). If a right-to-left shunt is present, it implies a right-sided obstruction distal to that level, or the presence of pulmonary vascular obstructive disease causing reversal of flow through a previous left-to-right shunting lesion. Thus, right-to-left shunting through an ASD (or patent foramen ovale) may be due to tricuspid atresia, tricuspid stenosis, severe PS, or atresia with an intact ventricular septum or pulmonary vascular disease. Also, in Ebstein anomaly (sometimes classified with acyanotic heart disease) with severe tricuspid regurgitation and an associated ASD or patent foramen ovale, right-to-left shunting is due to the increased right atrial pressure. Right-to-left shunting at the ventricular level (through a VSD) may be due to RV outflow obstruction created by pulmonary valvular or infundibular stenosis (TOF) or increased pulmonary vascular resistance (Eisenmenger syndrome). Right-to-left shunting across a patent ductus is almost always due to pulmonary vascular disease.

In d-transposition of the great arteries (D-TGA), the aorta arises from the RV carrying desaturated blood to the body and the pulmonary artery arises from the LV carrying oxygenated blood to the lungs. The result of D-TGA is complete separation of the pulmonary and systemic circulations. Infants with this condition have severe cyanosis. Survival depends on saturated blood entering the systemic circulation via an intracardiac (ASD or VSD) or interarterial (PDA) communication.

In patients with a single ventricle (double-inlet ventricle), both AV valves are connected to a main, single ventricular chamber. One great artery arises from the main chamber, the other arises from a rudimentary chamber. Because almost complete mixing of the systemic and pulmonary venous return takes place in the single ventricle, the systemic arterial saturation is primarily determined by the amount of pulmonary blood flow. Cyanosis of varying degrees is present from birth.

Untreated cyanotic heart disease carries an extremely high mortality rate in the infant and child; therefore, most patients reaching adulthood have had reparative or palliative surgery. Those who reach adulthood without surgery are usually those with TOF or irreversible pulmonary vascular disease (eg, Eisenmenger syndrome) from underlying congenital cardiac lesions.

The importance of recognizing cyanotic heart disease in the adult lies not only in the potential for possible surgical or nonsurgical intervention but also for appropriate management of the extracardiac manifestations of long-standing cyanosis. The systemic complications of cyanotic heart disease include the development of hematologic and metabolic disorders. Neurologic abnormalities include infectious, hemorrhagic, and hypoxic disorders.

Hematologic disorders in adults with cyanotic congenital heart disease can significantly influence morbidity and mortality rates. Secondary erythrocytosis has been classified as either **compensated** or **decompensated.** Patients with compensated erythrocytosis are in equilibrium with stable hematocrits, no evidence of iron depletion, and few (if any) symptoms of hyperviscosity. Even with hematocrits above 70%, they do not appear to be at increased risk for cerebrovascular accidents and do not require phlebotomy. Patients with decompensated erythrocytosis have increased hematocrits (> 65%) with symptoms. Because iron deficiency and dehydration may also produce hyperviscosity, these conditions should be excluded and, if present, treated before phlebotomy is undertaken. Generally, phlebotomy is not recommended for patients with hematocrits of less than 65%. A bleeding diathesis is also associated with cyanotic heart disease; it is usually mild and requires no specific therapy except for the avoidance of heparin and aspirin. Because severe life-threatening bleeding can occur during surgical procedures, preoperative phlebotomy to attain a hematocrit just below 65% is recommended. Associated abnormalities include thrombocytopenia and hyperuricemia secondary to increased red cell turnover. Urolithiasis and urate nephropathy rarely occur, but gout is common. The last problem can be managed with conventional therapy, taking care to avoid the antiplatelet properties of antiinflammatory agents.

Counseling of the young adult with reference to contraception, pregnancy, and exercise is especially important in this group of patients.

Palliative surgical procedures for complex cyanotic congenital heart disease performed during infancy or childhood in the early years of pediatric cardiothoracic surgery were associated with unique physical findings and specific complications. These procedures, such as aortopulmonary anastomoses (Waterston, Potts, Blalock-Taussig) and atrial switches (Senning and Mustard), are still commonly encountered in adult patients. These procedures may produce unique physical findings and specific complications, which are discussed later (see Palliative Surgical Procedures). Most of these procedures are no longer performed in children, since surgical techniques that optimize physiology and reduce complications have evolved over the years.

Brickner ME et al. Congenital heart disease in adults. Second of two parts. N Engl J Med. 2000 Feb 3;342(5):334–42. [PMID: 10655533]

Foster E et al. Task force 2: special health care needs of adults with congenital heart disease. J Am Coll Cardiol. 2001 Apr;37(5):1176–83. [PMID: 11300419]

TETRALOGY OF FALLOT & PULMONARY ATRESIA WITH VSD

 ESSENTIALS OF DIAGNOSIS

▶ History of exercise intolerance and squatting during childhood.

▶ Central cyanosis, mildly prominent RV impulse, murmur of pulmonic stenosis (with sufficient pulmonary blood flow) and absent P$_2$.

- Mild RVH; occasionally, LVH.
- Chest radiograph shows classic boot-shaped heart (coeur en sabot) in severe cases without left-to-right shunt; LV enlargement and post-stenotic pulmonary artery dilatation in milder cases; right-sided aortic arch in approximately 25% of patients.
- Echocardiogram shows RVH, overriding aorta, large perimembranous VSD, and obstruction of the RV outflow tract (subvalvular, valvular, supravalvular, or in the pulmonary arterial branches).
- Gradient across pulmonary outflow tract, normal pulmonary artery pressures, equalization of RV and LV pressures.
- Possibly anomalous branches of right coronary artery crossing RV outflow tract on coronary angiography.

General Considerations

Tetralogy of Fallot is the most common form of cyanotic congenital heart disease. Without surgical intervention, most patients die in childhood; however, occasionally an acyanotic patient with only mild-to-moderate PS and minimal right-to-left shunting is encountered (pink TOF). Although it is called a tetralogy, only the membranous nonrestrictive VSD and PS contribute to the pathophysiology of this disorder

(Figure 28–23). The severity of PS determines the RV systolic pressure and thus the degree of right-to-left shunting. The PS can be valvular or, more commonly, infundibular with an obstructing muscular band in the RV outflow tract. The other two components of the tetralogy include the aortic override and the secondary RVH. Both cyanotic and acyanotic patients are at high risk for endocarditis, much like patients with complicated VSD.

Common associated anomalies include ASD (15%; the pentalogy of Fallot), right-sided aortic arch (25%, most commonly seen in pulmonary atresia with VSD), and anomalous coronary distribution (about 10%). It is important to identify the origin of the left anterior descending artery from the right coronary cusp preoperatively because the artery courses over the RV infundibulum, a potential incision site for the repair. Tetralogy of Fallot is a form of conotruncal malformation that may occur in conjunction with DiGeorge syndrome. The chromosome 22q11.2 microdeletion is present in as many as 8–35% of patients with TOF and routine screening for the deletion is now recommended for affected patients to guide appropriate management and identify those patients whose offspring will be at increased risk for congenital heart disease. In addition, mutations in the genes encoding the cardiac transcription factor NKX2-5 and the Notch-1 ligand Jagged have been reported in patients with TOF.

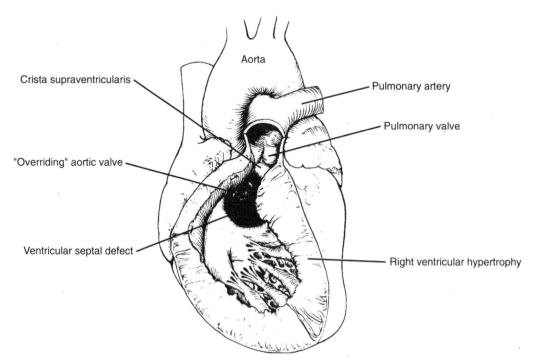

▲ **Figure 28–23.** Anatomy of tetralogy of Fallot. (Adapted, with permission, from Way LW, Doherty GM. Current Surgical Diagnosis & Treatment. McGraw-Hill, 2003.)

▶ Clinical Findings

A. Symptoms and Signs

The patient with TOF was typically a blue baby, cyanotic at birth. There is usually a history of exercise intolerance and squatting during childhood. Characteristic "tet spells," which are typified by episodic faintness and worsening cyanosis, are believed to be due to infundibular spasm and are generally diminished or absent by adulthood. Worsening cyanosis also occurs during exercise because of the associated systemic vasodilation and increased right-to-left shunt.

In severe cases of PS or atresia, the patient may have had life-saving surgical palliation with an aortopulmonary shunt. In the past, total repairs were not attempted until school age, but they are now being performed in infancy in many centers.

Physical examination reveals cyanosis and, less frequently, clubbing. The precordium is generally quiet, although a mild RV heave may be present. The intensity and duration of the pulmonic flow murmur vary with the degree of PS; P_2 is usually absent. In cases of pulmonary atresia with VSD (an extreme form of TOF), a continuous murmur over the back may be audible due to aortopulmonary collaterals. Patients who have had a "classic" Blalock-Taussig shunt, anastomosis of the subclavian to the side of the pulmonary artery, will have an absent pulse in the ipsilateral arm and a continuous murmur as long as the shunt is patent and functioning properly. A "modified" Blalock-Taussig shunt, interposing a small Gore-Tex tube between the subclavian artery and the pulmonary artery, preserves the brachial pulse and is easily occluded at the time of intracardiac repair. In patients who have had intracardiac repair, a low-pitched pulmonary regurgitation murmur is commonly audible. When the murmur occurs only in early diastole, it suggests clinically important residual regurgitation.

B. Diagnostic Studies

1. Electrocardiography and chest radiography—The ECG findings depend on the severity of the PS and the relative degree of shunting. If PS is severe, RVH is usually evident. If the PS is mild and the shunt is predominantly left to right, LVH may be evident. P waves are usually normal. Following intracardiac repair with infundibular resection, RBBB and varying forms of heart block are common. Postoperative atrial and ventricular arrhythmias are well-recognized complications. A QRS duration of > 180 ms has been shown to correlate with significant RV dilatation due to pulmonic regurgitation after surgical repair and to predict sudden cardiac death in patients with repaired TOF.

The radiographic findings also depend on the underlying individual pathophysiology. The typical boot-shaped coeur en sabot is seen when PS is severe and the LV is small. In these cases, pulmonary blood flow is reduced. Post-stenotic pulmonary artery dilatation and a right-sided aortic arch may be visible on chest radiograph.

2. Echocardiography—Transthoracic two-dimensional and Doppler echocardiography demonstrates the features of this defect in its native and repaired state. The typical findings in patients with unrepaired TOF include severe RVH and a thickened, malformed pulmonary valve with post-stenotic dilation. Alternatively, the level of stenosis may be primarily infundibular, with marked hypertrophic narrowing of the RV outflow tract (Figure 28–24). Systolic color-flow aliasing and a continuous wave Doppler gradient are detectable across the RV outflow tract or pulmonic valve. Two-dimensional imaging reveals a perimembranous VSD with evidence of right-to-left shunting by color-flow imaging; the peak velocity of the VSD jet seen by spectral Doppler is usually low reflecting the low interventricular gradient. The aortic root is variably enlarged and overrides the VSD. Aortic insufficiency, usually mild, may be present. Multiplanar TEE is particularly suited to define the anatomy of the RV outflow tract and the pulmonary valve when precordial imaging is difficult. In pulmonary atresia with VSD, aortopulmonary collaterals arising from the descending aorta can also be imaged by TEE.

Complications of TOF repair that can be detected noninvasively by echocardiography include residual outflow obstruction, pulmonary valve regurgitation, RV outflow-tract aneurysms, and VSD patch leak. In rare cases, an anomalous left anterior descending artery that was severed during surgery results in an LV apical aneurysm. Late LV systolic dysfunction has been increasingly recognized after TOF repair and is a risk factor for sudden cardiac death.

3. Magnetic resonance imaging—MRI has become an important noninvasive imaging modality in the assessment of patients with conotruncal anomalies, including TOF. Advantages include the ability to obtain accurate measurements of RV size and ejection fraction, and pulmonic regurgitant fraction.

4. Cardiac catheterization—Cardiac catheterization reveals a gradient across the pulmonary outflow tract, usually normal pulmonary artery pressure, and equalization of RV and LV pressures. Angiography may better define the anatomy of the RV outflow tract and the size of the VSD (this information is usually available noninvasively). Coronary arteriography may demonstrate anomalous origins of the left coronary artery.

5. Other laboratory findings—Arterial saturation is variably reduced, and secondary erythrocytosis is present in the adult who has had no reparative surgery. In those with adequate surgical repair, arterial saturation should be normal.

▶ Prognosis & Treatment

Only 11% of individuals born with this lesion survive without palliative surgery beyond the age of 20, and only 3% survive beyond the age of 40. Because the PS protects TOF patients from the development of pulmonary hypertension, however,

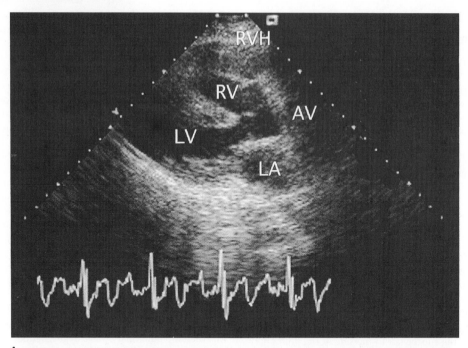

A

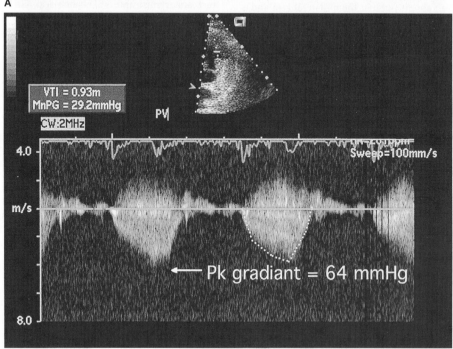

B

▲ **Figure 28–24.** Transthoracic echocardiogram in patient with tetralogy of Fallot. **A:** The parasternal long-axis view shows the ventricular septal defect, overriding aorta. **B:** Continuous wave Doppler signal across the right ventricular outflow tract shows a high-velocity, late-peaking jet. This demonstrates severe outflow tract obstruction. The late peak suggests a component of dynamic obstruction due to the hypertrophied infundibulum. AV, aortic valve; LA, left atrium; LV, left ventricle; Pk, peak; RVH, right ventricular hypertrophy; RV, right ventricle.

they are almost always surgical candidates as adults. Medically, it is important to avoid systemic vasodilator therapy in the patient whose TOF is uncorrected because a reduction in arterial blood pressure can increase right-to-left shunting. Endocarditis is relatively common in unrepaired TOF.

Total intracardiac repair with closure of the VSD and correction of the pulmonary or infundibular stenosis is indicated in the cyanotic patient to reduce symptoms and forestall complications attributable to cyanosis. The infundibulum is incised and resected to alleviate obstruction, with patching of the RV outflow tract or pulmonary annulus when necessary. The indications for surgery in the occasional acyanotic patient with TOF are similar to those of a patient with VSD. Important considerations prior to surgery include the presence of anomalies in the pulmonary and coronary arteries (approximately 15% and 35%, respectively). In pulmonary atresia with VSD, survival depends on the presence of well-developed bronchopulmonary or systemic-to-pulmonary collaterals. **In the rare adult with uncorrected pulmonary atresia with VSD,** surgical repair is either more complicated, requiring multiple procedures, or it is not feasible.

In patients who undergo intracardiac repair for TOF, potentially significant postoperative anatomic sequelae are possible, including residual outflow obstruction, pulmonary valve regurgitation, RV aneurysms, and VSD patch leak. Pulmonary regurgitation may develop as a consequence of surgical repair of the RV outflow tract as well as with placement of a patch to enlarge the pulmonary artery annulus (transannular). Although even substantial regurgitation can be tolerated for long periods, enlargement of the RV eventually occurs, with resultant RV dysfunction, and repair or replacement of the pulmonary valve may be required.

A recent large retrospective study of risk stratification for arrhythmia and sudden death in these patients underscores the importance of vigilant assessment of ECG parameters (QRS duration), and hemodynamic characteristics (pulmonary regurgitation/obstruction) with timely intervention as a means of modifying the risk for sudden cardiac death in these patients. Appropriately timed surgical replacement of the regurgitant pulmonic valve has been shown to stabilize QRS prolongation and to reduce the incidence of ventricular arrhythmias when combined with cryoablation. It is hoped that two current trends in surgery will further reduce the incidence of arrhythmias. The first is avoidance of RV outflow tract incisions by either a transatrial or transpulmonary approach. Secondly, earlier surgical intervention may allow less time for the development of ventricular fibrosis. Given the frequency of ventricular tachycardia and sudden cardiac death in these patients, clinicians should remain vigilant for symptoms of palpitations. Some experts advocate routine annual screening with a Holter monitor and referral for electrophysiologic study upon finding nonsustained ventricular tachycardia or complex ectopy, although no consensus exists at this point.

Bashore TM. Adult congenital heart disease: right ventricular outflow tract lesions. Circulation. 2007 Apr 10;115(14):1933–47. [PMID: 17420363]

Ghai A et al. Left ventricular dysfunction is a risk factor for sudden cardiac death in adults late after repair of tetralogy of Fallot. J Am Coll Cardiol. 2002 Nov 6;40(9):1675–80. [PMID: 12427422]

Knauth AL et al. Ventricular size and function assessed by cardiac MRI predict major adverse clinical outcomes late after tetralogy of Fallot repair. Heart. 2008 Feb;94(2):211–6. [PMID: 17135219]

Pierpont ME et al; American Heart Association Congenital Cardiac Defects Committee, Council on Cardiovascular Disease in the Young. Genetic basis for congenital heart defects: current knowledge: a scientific statement from the American Heart Association Congenital Cardiac Defects Committee, Council on Cardiovascular Disease in the Young: endorsed by the American Academy of Pediatrics. Circulation. 2007 Jun 12;115(23):3015–38. [PMID: 17519398]

Therrien J et al. Impact of pulmonary valve replacement on arrhythmia propensity late after repair of tetralogy of Fallot. Circulation. 2001 May 22;103(2):2489–94. [PMID: 11369690]

EISENMENGER SYNDROME

 ESSENTIALS OF DIAGNOSIS

▶ History of murmur or cyanosis in infancy, symptoms of dyspnea and exercise intolerance since childhood.

▶ Hemoptysis, chest pain, and syncope in the adult.

▶ Clubbing, cyanosis, and prominent P_2.

▶ Compensatory erythrocytosis, iron deficiency, and hyperuricemia.

▶ Right ventricular hypertrophy; large central pulmonary arteries with peripheral pruning on chest radiograph.

▶ Severe right ventricular hypertrophy and right atrial enlargement, elevated pulmonary artery pressures, pulmonary regurgitation.

▶ Detection of bidirectional shunt.

▶ General Considerations

Three related, but not identical, clinical terms bear the name of Eisenmenger. The development of pulmonary hypertension in the presence of increased pulmonary blood flow is called the **Eisenmenger reaction. Eisenmenger syndrome** is a general term applied to pulmonary hypertension and shunt reversal in the presence of a congenital defect, including VSD, ostium primum ASD, AV canal defect, aortopulmonary window, or PDA. **Eisenmenger complex,** as originally described, is the association of a VSD with pulmonary hypertension and shunt reversal. The pulmonary hypertension usually develops before puberty; however, pulmonary vascular disease and the Eisenmenger reaction can occasionally develop after puberty in patients with ostium secundum ASDs.

In approximately 10% of patients with nonrestrictive VSDs, the pulmonary artery pressure does not fall normally in the neonatal period. Therefore, a large left-to-right shunt and CHF are not present. If the VSD goes undetected and the problem is not repaired before the infant reaches the age of 1 year, irreversible pulmonary vascular disease may result. The same is true for the other lesions associated with Eisenmenger syndrome. In patients with ostium secundum ASD, PVR almost always falls to normal levels in the neonatal period, and the development of irreversible pulmonary hypertension is far less common.

Hemoptysis in Eisenmenger syndrome may occasionally be due to bronchitis or pneumonia. Pulmonary infarction, a potentially fatal complication, and pulmonary arteriolar rupture must be excluded. Pregnancy is accompanied by an unacceptably high rate of maternal and fetal mortality and is virtually contraindicated in patients with Eisenmenger syndrome.

▶ Clinical Findings

A. Symptoms and Signs

Patients usually have a history of murmur or cyanosis during infancy. Exertional dyspnea is the most commonly encountered symptom. Chest pain, hemoptysis, and presyncope are less common. Transient bacteremias can result in brain abscess as a result of right-to-left shunting and entry of bacteria into the cerebral circulation without the normal filtering through the pulmonary circulation.

Physical examination reveals cyanosis (differential when the cause is PDA); cardiovascular examination is most remarkable for findings associated with pulmonary hypertension. The LV impulse is not displaced and an RV parasternal heave is present. The jugular venous pressure may be elevated in the presence of RV failure and the *a* wave may be prominent. The first heart sound is normal, and P_2 is markedly accentuated. A systolic murmur of tricuspid regurgitation may be present, and a high-pitched diastolic murmur of pulmonary regurgitation (Graham Steell murmur) is common. In the presence of RV failure, hepatomegaly, ascites, and peripheral edema may be present.

B. Diagnostic Studies

1. Electrocardiography and chest radiography—The ECG shows evidence of right atrial enlargement and RVH with a rightward axis (Figure 28–25A). The presence of a leftward or superior axis suggests an ostium primum ASD or AV canal defect as the underlying cause (Figure 28–25B). Chest radiograph findings include RV enlargement with filling-in of the retrosternal air space, prominent proximal pulmonary arteries with pulmonary oligemia, and pruning of the peripheral pulmonary vessels.

2. Echocardiography—Severe RVH and right atrial enlargement is evident (Figure 28–26A). Right ventricular function may be normal until the late stages of the disease, at which time the right atrium enlarges. The LV appears small and underfilled; the septum deviates toward the LV. The level of shunt can be determined by two-dimensional imaging, aided by color-flow Doppler and saline contrast injection (Figure 28–26B). When a VSD is present, the flow velocity across the defect is low because of pressure equalization between the two ventricles. On the other hand, the tricuspid regurgitant velocity is increased and can be used to estimate the peak RV systolic pressure (Figure 28–26C). Pulmonary insufficiency with a high-velocity regurgitant jet is a frequent finding. Other valvular lesions are uncommon except in ostium primum ASD or AV canal defects, when mitral regurgitation is commonly present.

Eisenmenger syndrome can usually be differentiated from primary pulmonary hypertension noninvasively by TTE, although shunting across a patent foramen ovale may mimic an ASD with Eisenmenger syndrome and a PDA may be missed on color-flow Doppler in the presence of severe pulmonary hypertension. In these cases, further investigation with TEE or cardiac catheterization and sometimes cardiac MRI/MRA may be indicated.

3. Cardiac catheterization—The pathognomonic hemodynamic findings are elevated pulmonary artery pressure, increased PVR, and right-to-left shunting. The degree of residual left-to-right shunt should be measured. Oxygen should be administered during catheterization to determine whether pulmonary vascular reactivity persists. If PVR falls during oxygen or nitric oxide administration, increased left-to-right shunting can be measured. In this case, the patient may be a candidate for pulmonary vasodilator therapy and surgical repair.

4. Other laboratory findings—The arterial oxygen saturation by pulse oximetry or arterial blood gas measurements is markedly decreased. The hematocrit is elevated, with an overall increase in red cell mass. Iron deficiency is common, particularly after injudicious phlebotomies. Hyperuricemia caused by increased red cell turnover may be present.

▶ Prognosis & Treatment

Life expectancy is markedly shortened in patients with Eisenmenger syndrome; however, meticulous medical management can result in improved longevity in adults with this and other forms of cyanotic heart disease. The causes of death include pulmonary infarction with uncontrollable hemoptysis, arrhythmias with sudden death, progressive RV failure, and brain abscess.

Surgical repair is contraindicated when the pulmonary vascular disease is fixed; that is, pulmonary resistance does not fall in response to oxygen or nitric oxide inhalation. In these patients, closure of the VSD (or other defects) increases the work of the RV, with a resultant excessively high mortality rate. Heart-lung transplantation offers hope for the adolescent and young adult with Eisenmenger syndrome, but the results support only guarded optimism. In addition,

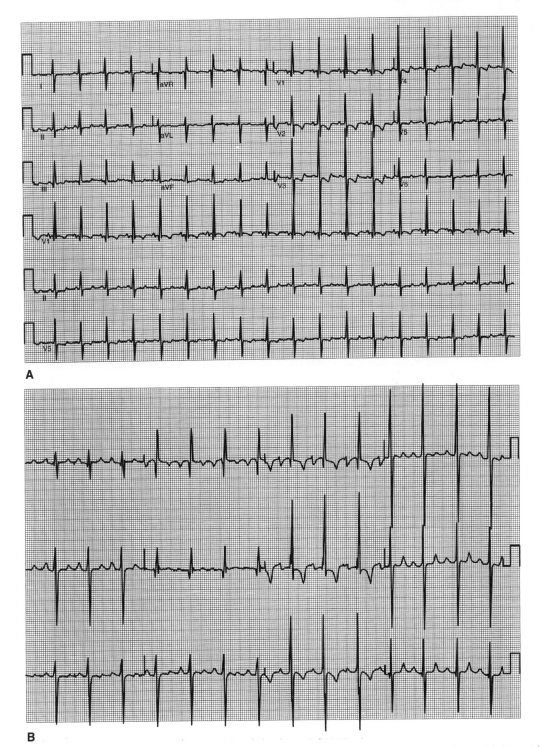

▲ **Figure 28–25. A:** Electrocardiograph in Eisenmenger syndrome from ostium secundum atrial septal defect with right ventricular hypertrophy and right-axis deviation. **B:** Electrocardiograph in Eisenmenger syndrome and atrioventricular canal defect with right ventricular hypertrophy and left anterior hemiblock.

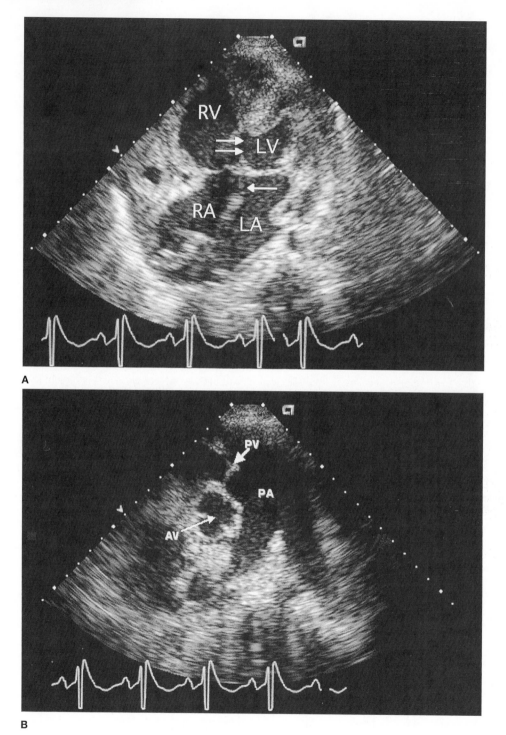

▲ **Figure 28–26. A:** Transthoracic echocardiogram in a 32-year-old woman with Down syndrome. She has Eisenmenger syndrome due to an atrioventricular septal defect. Four-chamber view shows hypertrophied right ventricular (RV) wall, ventricular septal defect (*double white arrow*), and ostium primum atrial septal defect (*single white arrow*). **B:** Parasternal short-axis view showing markedly dilated pulmonary artery (PA). (*continued*)

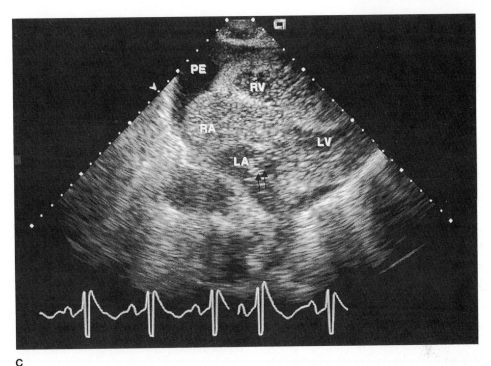

▲ Figure 28–26. (*Continued*) **C:** Subcostal view after intravenous injection of agitated saline. The right atrium (RA) and right ventricle (RV) are opacified and there is rapid appearance of contrast in the left atrium (LA) and ventricle (LV) (*double black arrow*). A moderate pericardial effusion is also noted. AV, aortic valve; PV, pulmonary valve.

some centers are considering the feasibility of intracardiac repair in children after treatment with pulmonary vasodilator therapy to decrease the PVR.

Careful medical management of the complications of cyanotic congenital heart disease is crucial in these patients (see Cyanotic Congenital Heart Disease above). Counseling regarding contraception is crucial in these patients, and pregnancy should be avoided if at all possible (see later discussion).

Diller GP et al. Pulmonary vascular disease in adults with congenital heart disease. Circulation. 2007 Feb 27;115(8):1039–50. [PMID: 17325254]

Galie N et al; Bosentan Randomized Trial of Endothelin Antagonist Therapy-5 (BREATHE-5) Investigators. Bosentan therapy in patients with Eisenmenger syndrome: a multicenter, double-blind, randomized, placebo-controlled study. Circulation. 2006 Jul 4;114(1):48–54. [PMID: 16801459]

TRANSPOSITION OF THE GREAT ARTERIES

 ESSENTIALS OF DIAGNOSIS

▶ History of cyanosis that worsens shortly after birth at the time of ductal closure.

▶ Prominent RV impulse, palpable and delayed A_2; murmurs from associated defects (eg, VSD, PS).

▶ Chest radiograph shows narrowing at base of heart in region of great vessels; prominent pulmonary vascularity unless PVR is increased.

▶ Right atrial enlargement, RVH; occasionally biventricular hypertrophy (with an associated VSD).

▶ Great arteries discordant with anterior and rightward aorta arising from the RV and leftward and posterior pulmonary artery arising from the LV. Atria and ventricles usually in normal position with severe RVH.

▶ General Considerations

The key to the pathophysiology of transposition of the great arteries (D-TGA) is that the pulmonary and systemic circulations exist in parallel rather than in the normal series relationship (Figure 28–27). Survival after birth therefore depends on mixing saturated and desaturated blood via a PDA or an ASD or VSD. If an ASD or VSD does not coexist with D-TGA, an atrial communication must be created (usually percutaneously via an atrial balloon septostomy [the Rashkind procedure]) to permit survival in the newborn once the ductus

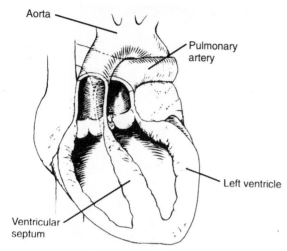

▲ Figure 28–27. Anatomy of transposition of the great arteries. (Reproduced, with permission, from Way LW, Doherty GM. Current Surgical Diagnosis & Treatment. McGraw-Hill, 2003.)

closes. Prostaglandin E_1 may be given to restore or maintain patency of the ductus arteriosus; however, this does not always provide adequate mixing. When a VSD is present, the physiologic consequences depend largely on whether associated PS is present. In the absence of PS, there is a risk of pulmonary vascular disease because of the increased pulmonary blood flow; in the presence of PS, an aortopulmonary shunt may be necessary to increase pulmonary blood flow.

▶ Clinical Findings

A. Symptoms and Signs

More males (3:1) are affected by this condition. There is a history of cyanosis at birth that worsens shortly thereafter when the ductus closes. In the infant with a large VSD, heart failure can occur with lesser degrees of cyanosis. In addition to profound central cyanosis, physical examination reveals a prominent RV impulse, a palpable and delayed A_2, and murmurs caused by associated defects (eg, VSD, PS). The findings usually associated with a large PDA (see previous discussion of PDA) may be absent. The physical examination is often nondiagnostic and may actually provide more information about associated anomalies than about the presence of transposition.

B. Diagnostic Studies

1. Electrocardiography and chest radiography—The ECG usually demonstrates right atrial enlargement, a rightward QRS axis, and RVH. In the presence of a VSD, biventricular hypertrophy may be evident. The chest radiograph shows

narrowing at the base of the heart in the region of the great vessels. In the newborn, prior to surgery, pulmonary vascularity is prominent unless the PVR is increased by the associated pulmonary vascular disease. The RV and right atrium are prominent.

2. Echocardiography—The atria and ventricles are usually in the normal position with severe RVH. The great vessels are discordant with the anterior and rightward aorta arising from the RV, and leftward and posterior pulmonary artery arising from the LV. In the newborn, complete examination, using combined two-dimensional and color-flow Doppler imaging should confirm or exclude the presence of an associated ASD, VSD, or PS. Virtually all surviving adults have had palliative surgical procedures, most often an atrial-switch (Mustard or Senning) operation. In these patients, baffle obstruction and leaks can be detected by color-flow Doppler and contrast echocardiography. Late obstruction of the superior vena cava can be detected by contrast echocardiography with agitated saline injected into an arm vein, opacifying the inferior vena cava. After arterial switch procedures, echocardiography may show regurgitation of the neoaortic valve or stenosis of the neopulmonary valve or branches. Magnetic resonance imaging may also be helpful in determining the anatomy of the vena cava and pulmonary veins.

3. Cardiac catheterization—Invasive studies confirm the noninvasive diagnosis and the presence of associated defects. In the newborn, catheterization with a percutaneous atrial balloon septostomy is therapeutic and usually life-saving as well as diagnostic. The administration of intravenous prostaglandin E_1 to maintain ductal patency may preclude the need for an atrial septostomy if the oxygen saturations are adequate. In the adult with associated VSD, cardiac catheterization may be indicated to determine PVR or the severity of PS.

▶ Prognosis & Treatment

Without treatment, isolated D-TGA carries a mortality rate of greater than 90% in the first year of life. Infants with an ASD, a VSD, or a large PDA have higher oxygen saturations and better survival rates, but early surgery is indicated to prevent the development of irreversible pulmonary vascular disease.

Definitive repair of this defect was first undertaken in the early 1960s. The atrial switch operation (Mustard or Senning) redirects the pulmonary and systemic venous return at the atrial level. The atrial septum is excised, and using either a pericardial or prosthetic baffle, the systemic venous return is directed across the mitral valve into the left ventricle and the pulmonary venous return flows across the tricuspid valve into the RV. The postoperative physiology after an atrial switch procedure is similar to that of patients with C-TGA, in that the RV continues to supply the systemic circulation. Many of these patients have survived to lead productive lives; however, they are potentially faced with significant late postoperative complications, including sick sinus syndrome, atrial and ventricular tachyarrhythmias, baffle obstruction and leaks (approximately 15%), and systemic ventricular dysfunction (10–15%). The late (30-year) mortality rate is approximately 20%. Sudden (presumed arrhythmic) death and systemic ventricular failure are the most common causes of late death. Atrial arrhythmias are particularly common. In a large cohort study, sinus rhythm was present in 77% of patients at 5 years and only 40% of patients at 20 years. Atrial flutter, which is thought to be a marker for sudden death, was present in 14% of patients. Pacemaker implantation, which can pose technical challenges after atrial switch, was required in 11% of patients.

Repair since the early 1980s has favored the arterial switch procedure pioneered by Jatene. This repair reestablishes the LV as the systemic ventricle, and has ameliorated many of such long-term complications of the atrial switch as arrhythmias, RV dysfunction, baffle stenosis, and tricuspid regurgitation.

Follow-up of patients after arterial switch procedures has recently become available. The late mortality rate is low, and good LV function and sinus rhythm have been maintained. Postoperative aortic regurgitation and the potential for development of coronary artery ostial stenosis and late supravalvular narrowing at the anastomotic sites are of concern but will require ongoing assessment.

Kammeraad JA et al. Predictors of sudden cardiac death after Mustard or Senning repair for transposition of the great arteries. J Am Coll Cardiol. 2004 Sep 1;44(5):1095–102. [PMID: 15337224]

Legendre A et al. Coronary events after arterial switch operation for transposition of the great arteries. Circulation. 2003 Sep 9;108 Suppl 1:II186–90. [PMID: 12970230]

Losay J et al. Late outcome after arterial switch operation for transposition of the great arteries. Circulation. 2001 Sep 18;104(12 Suppl 1):I121–6. [PMID: 11568042]

von Bernuth G. 25 years after the first arterial switch procedure: mid-term results. Thorac Cardiovasc Surg. 2000 Aug;48(4):228–32. [PMID: 11005598]

Warnes CA. Transposition of the great arteries. Circulation. 2006 Dec 12;114(24):2699–709. [PMID: 17159076]

TRICUSPID ATRESIA

 ESSENTIALS OF DIAGNOSIS

- ▶ History of either cyanosis (70%) or CHF (30%).
- ▶ Cyanotic patient with absent RV impulse and prominent LV impulse.
- ▶ Oligemic lung fields, right atrial and LV without RV enlargement in retrosternal airspace on chest radiograph.
- ▶ Evidence of LVH, absent or atretic tricuspid valve, ASD, small RV.

▶ General Considerations

Atresia of the tricuspid valve cannot be viewed as a single congenital anomaly. In these patients the tricuspid valve is absent or inperforate, the RV is hypoplastic, and the inflow portion of the RV is absent. Although an atrial communication is invariably present, the additional associated anomalies determine the ultimate pathophysiology and clinical presentation (Figure 28–28). Tricuspid atresia is usually classified according to the presence or absence of pulmonary stenosis and of transposition of the aorta and pulmonary artery. The great arteries are normally related in about 70% of the cases and are transposed in 30%. Pulmonary blood flow is supplied by either a PDA or aortopulmonary collaterals. Palliative surgery in this group is aimed at increasing pulmonary blood flow by a systemic venous or an arterial-to-pulmonary-artery shunt (see Palliative Surgical Procedures). In the 30% of patients born with tricuspid atresia and associated transposition of the great vessels, a VSD is usually present and no pulmonary obstruction is evident. These infants have CHF; pulmonary banding in the first year of life may prevent the development of irreversible pulmonary vascular disease and allow a later intracardiac repair to be performed.

Adult survival without surgical intervention is rare. The clinical condition at presentation depends on the patient's underlying anatomy as well as the adequacy of the palliative procedure.

▶ Clinical Findings

A. Symptoms and Signs

A history of cyanosis predominates in patients with normally related great arteries, restrictive VSD, or PS or atresia. Patients with associated transposition of the great vessels and nonrestrictive VSD usually have a history of CHF from LV volume overload.

Physical examination is highly variable, but the absence of an RV impulse with a prominent LV impulse in a cyanotic patient suggests tricuspid atresia. The second heart sound is often single. A continuous murmur may be present as a result of aortopulmonary collaterals or a Blalock-Taussig shunt.

B. Diagnostic Studies

1. Electrocardiography and chest radiography—The ECG reveals right atrial enlargement and LVH, the only cyanotic lesion associated with LVH at birth. In the adult, the chest radiograph usually shows oligemic lung fields and right atrial and LV prominence without RV enlargement in the retrosternal airspace.

2. Echocardiography and magnetic resonance imaging—Constant echocardiographic features include an absent or atretic imperforate tricuspid valve, ASD, and a small RV. More variable features include the size of the RV, the

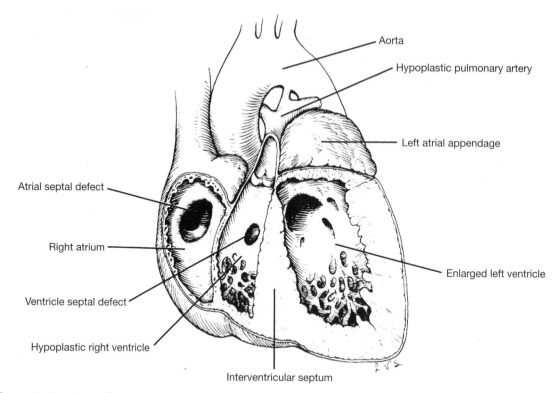

Aorta

Hypoplastic pulmonary artery

Left atrial appendage

Atrial septal defect

Right atrium

Enlarged left ventricle

Ventricle septal defect

Hypoplastic right ventricle

Interventricular septum

▲ **Figure 28–28.** Tricuspid atresia. (Reproduced, with permission, from Cheitlin M, Sokolow M, McIlroy M. Congenital heart disease. In: *Clinical Cardiology*. Norwalk, CT: Appleton & Lange; 1993.)

presence and size of a VSD, the presence of pulmonary atresia or stenosis, and relationship of the great vessels (normal or transposed). Doppler examination can estimate the degree of PS and the gradient across the VSD. When PS is not present, the estimated RV systolic pressure reflects the pulmonary artery systolic pressure. Color-flow Doppler imaging is helpful in confirming the pattern of flow and the site of the VSD (Figure 28–29). Magnetic resonance imaging can also be helpful in defining the anatomy.

3. Cardiac catheterization—Cardiac catheterization is used to determine operability by measuring PVR and the size of the pulmonary arteries. The RV cannot be entered through the right atrium, and the pulmonary artery (in the absence of atresia) must be entered from the LV through the VSD. Catheterization can also be used to assess the patency of palliative shunts.

▶ Prognosis & Treatment

Adults with tricuspid atresia will almost uniformly have undergone one or more operations to separate the pulmonary and systemic circulations. Patients with reduced pul-

monary blood flow generally undergo a bidirectional Glenn procedure (superior vena cava to right pulmonary artery anastomosis) followed by a complete cavopulmonary anastomosis (Fontan procedure). Patients with increased pulmonary blood flow (typically those with associated d-malposition) may undergo pulmonary arterial banding as an initial procedure. The 1-year survival rate among patients who have not undergone palliative surgery is approximately 10%. Patients who have had successful modified Fontan procedures have widely variable outcomes, but routinely survive well into adulthood (see Palliative Surgical Procedures).

Lan YT et al. Outcome of patients with double-inlet left ventricle or tricuspid atresia with transposed great arteries. J Am Coll Cardiol. 2004 Jan 7;43(1):113–9. [PMID: 14715192]

Mair DD et al. The Fontan procedure for tricuspid atresia: early and late results of a 25-year experience with 216 patients. J Am Coll Cardiol. 2001 Mar 1;37(3):933–9. [PMID: 11693773]

Sittiwangkul R et al. Outcomes of tricuspid atresia in the Fontan era. Ann Thorac Surg. 2004 Mar;77(3):889–94. [PMID: 14992893]

Wald RM et al. Outcome after prenatal diagnosis of tricuspid atresia: a multicenter experience. Am Heart J. 2007 May;153(5): 772–8. [PMID: 17452152]

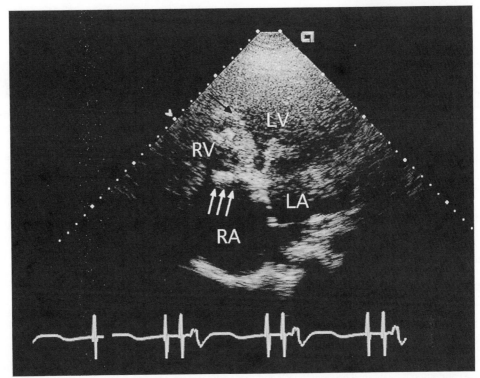

▲ **Figure 28–29.** Transthoracic echocardiogram in a 30-year-old woman with tricuspid atresia. This four-chamber view demonstrates the plate-like imperforate tricuspid annulus (*three white arrows*). The right atrium (RA) is markedly dilated, and the right ventricle (RV) is hypoplastic. A ventricular septal defect (*black arrow*) is noted. LA, left atrium; LV, left ventricle.

PULMONARY ATRESIA WITH INTACT VENTRICULAR SEPTUM

 ESSENTIALS OF DIAGNOSIS

▸ History of cyanosis at birth, worsening at the time of ductal closure.

▸ Single S_2; continuous murmur is rare.

▸ Prominent LV forces.

▸ Oligemic lung fields, enlarged cardiac silhouette on chest radiograph.

▸ Atrial septal defect, small RV, absent pulmonary valve. In adults, a palliative shunt or RV-to-pulmonary-artery conduit.

▶ General Considerations

Pulmonary atresia with intact ventricular septum is rarely encountered in the adult population with congenital heart disease. The pulmonary valve is absent or imperforate, and blood flow is entirely through a PDA in the newborn. As in tricuspid atresia, an atrial communication exists through which the left atrium receives all of the systemic and pulmonary venous return. The volume-overloaded LV pumps the total blood flow into the aorta and, in most cases, all the pulmonary blood flow is received retrograde via the ductus. When the ductus closes, cyanosis may worsen acutely, and pulmonary blood flow must be restored by a palliative shunt. The RV may be diminutive, normal, or increased in size, and the tricuspid valve is, respectively, atretic, normal, or severely regurgitant. The high pressure in the RV is decompressed through dilated coronary circulation (ie, coronary sinusoids) into the left or right coronary artery. The presence of the sinusoids directly relates to RV pressure and inversely to the amount of tricuspid regurgitation. These factors largely determine the clinical and echocardiographic findings.

▶ Clinical Findings

Patients have a history of cyanosis at birth that worsens shortly afterward, at the time of ductal closure. The physical examination is variable, and the findings depend on the size of the RV and the presence of tricuspid regurgitation. The chest radiograph may reveal oligemic lung fields and an enlarged cardiac silhouette, caused by the enlargement of the LV. The main pulmonary artery segment is concave. The echocardiogram most commonly shows an ASD; a hypertro-phied RV wall with a small cavity; a patent but small tricuspid valve; and a thickened, immobile, atretic pulmo-nary valve with no Doppler evidence of blood flow through it. The ductus arteriosus is seen running vertically from the aortic arch to the pulmonary artery (ie, vertical ductus). In adults, a palliative shunt (see section on Tricuspid Atresia) or an RV-to-pulmonary-artery conduit (the Rastelli procedure) is almost always present. Cardiac catheterization reveals systemic or suprasystemic RV pressures, and the catheter cannot be passed from the RV to the pulmonic artery. Angiography of the RV fails to opacify the pulmonary arteries, and contrast may fill the sinusoidal vessels that often communicate with the coronary arteries.

▶ Prognosis & Treatment

Three categories of surgical intervention exist for infants with pulmonary atresia with intact ventricular septum. The inter-vention selected depends on the size of the RV and the presence or absence of coronary sinusoids or coronary artery anomalies. When the RV is of adequate size for anticipated future growth, a connection is established between the RV and main pulmonary artery to prepare for a two-ventricle repair. A systemic-to-pulmonary-artery shunt is performed at the same time. Generally, an RV-to-pulmonary-artery conduit (with or without a valve) can be placed in the older child. Problems from valvular obstruction or degeneration and conduit obstruction caused by pseudo-intimal thickening can be detected by Doppler echocardiography. A two-ventricle repair is not possible in the subset of these patients with severely hypoplastic RVs. Therefore, a systemic-to-pulmonary-artery shunt without the connection to the RV is performed, with anticipation of a Fontan procedure at a later date. Patients who have a rudimentary RV and sinusoidal channels serving as the major source of coronary circulation, with perfusion by desat-urated blood, represent a special problem. Decompression of the RV by connection with the pulmonary artery may result in a reversal of coronary flow into the RV, thereby producing myocardial ischemia. If coronary anomalies are identified by an aortogram, the sinusoids are left alone, and a systemic-to-pulmonary-artery shunt is performed in anticipation of a future Fontan-type operation. Overall, the prognosis in pul-monary atresia is limited, and although palliative surgery improves longevity, these patients require careful surveillance for complications of the surgery in addition to the underlying cyanotic heart disease. An exciting therapeutic innovation of recent years is the development of radiofrequency-assisted valve perforation followed by balloon valvotomy. This has permitted completely percutaneous repair of the defect, pro-vided that there is a patent infundibulum and a non–RV-

dependent coronary circulation. The first patients to have undergone this procedure will be entering adulthood shortly.

▼ OTHER CYANOTIC CONGENITAL HEART DEFECTS

It is increasingly common to encounter adults with complex forms of cyanotic congenital heart disease that have had some sort of palliative surgery. In addition to the conditions already discussed, there are many variants of the single-ventricular and double-outlet-ventricular anomalies. Most common among these are the **double-inlet LV, double-outlet RV,** and **hypoplastic left heart.** The anatomic features of the dominant ventricle that identify it as a right or left ventricle on echocar-diography include the trabeculae (coarse in an RV, smooth in an LV), the presence of the moderator band (RV), the pres-ence of septal attachments of the AV valve (RV), and the presence of conus tissue between the annuli of the AV and subarterial valves (RV). Sometimes a rudimentary second ventricle is present. In the absence of pulmonary or infundib-ular stenosis, pulmonary vascular disease is prevalent; subaor-tic stenosis and AV valve regurgitation are also common. Survival into adulthood is more likely in patients with PS.

The defect in **truncus arteriosus** arises from a failure of the single truncus in the embryo to divide into pulmonary and aortic vessels; and the pulmonary artery, aorta, and coronary arteries arise from a single main trunk. Although the anatomy of this lesion varies, a VSD is always present. The single semilu-nar valve, often with more than three cusps, is usually incompe-tent. The LV is faced with not only the volume overload of both pulmonary and systemic circulations but also that caused by truncal valve regurgitation. The mortality rate in the first year of life from CHF is high. Pulmonary branch stenosis and increased PVR may improve prognosis by decreasing the likelihood of CHF. Treatment consists of closure of the VSD, surgical separa-tion of the pulmonary arteries from the truncus, and placement of a valved conduit to connect them to the RV. Late sequelae include progressive truncal valve regurgitation, progressive pul-monary vascular disease, and the need for conduit revision because of patient growth and valve degeneration.

In **total anomalous pulmonary veins,** the pulmonary venous flow enters the right atrium either directly or by one of many possible connections including the coronary sinus, superior vena cava, inferior vena cava, portal vein, hepatic vein, and ductus venosus. There is an atrial communication, and the degree of cyanosis depends on the size of the ASD and the PVR. If left untreated, most (80%) die within the first year of life. The subdiaphragmatic anomalous veins are more likely to be associated with pulmonary venous obstruc-tion. Surgical correction consists of connecting the common pulmonary venous channel to the left atrium. Obstruction may recur following surgery in those patients in whom obstruction was originally present; in others, the postopera-tive course is usually uncomplicated.

PALLIATIVE SURGICAL PROCEDURES

In cyanotic congenital heart disease associated with diminished pulmonary blood flow, palliative procedures have been aimed at increasing pulmonary blood flow by directly or indirectly shunting blood from the systemic veins or systemic circulation. These procedures have continued to evolve.

The **Fontan procedure** (with its many modifications), the final common pathway for single ventricle repair, precludes the need for an RV by rerouting the venous return from the superior and inferior vena cava directly to the pulmonary circulation, thus separating the systemic and pulmonary venous return. This operation was originally used in patients with tricuspid atresia but currently is the palliative procedure of choice for a variety of congenital heart defects, including hypoplastic left heart syndrome and morphologic single ventricle. The Fontan procedure has also been shown to be an effective palliation for selected adults with single-ventricle physiology when the pulmonary bed has been protected by congenital or palliative (ie, pulmonary band) stenosis. The Fontan procedure performed in adulthood carries a relatively low perioperative risk and leads to relief of cyanosis and improved functional class. However, arrhythmias, protein-losing enteropathy, and progressive systemic ventricular dysfunction remain ongoing concerns. The extracardiac Fontan procedure (direct cavopulmonary anastomosis) may decrease the incidence of arrhythmias. Thromboembolic disease is also a major cause of morbidity and mortality among patients after the Fontan procedure, and this recognition has led some cardiologists to advocate prophylactic anticoagulation in these patients. However, insufficient data exist to support a blanket recommendation on this issue. The modified, or bidirectional, **Glenn procedure** (superior vena cava to confluent pulmonary artery) can be used as a staging procedure for a future Fontan procedure or as a palliative shunt that can increase pulmonary blood flow when a Fontan is contraindicated because of poor ventricular function. Because right atrial distention does not occur, atrial arrhythmias may be less common.

In cyanotic patients with inadequate pulmonary blood flow (eg, TOF, pulmonary and tricuspid atresia), early surgical **systemic-to-pulmonary shunts** are life-saving procedures. The **Waterston** (ascending-aorta-to-pulmonary-artery) and **Potts** (descending-aorta-to-pulmonary-artery) shunts have been abandoned because of the high frequency of pulmonary hypertension, stenosis distal to the shunt sites, and considerable difficulty with surgical take down, but adult patients with these types of shunts are still infrequently encountered. Pulmonary artery pressure can be estimated noninvasively using the brachial artery systolic cuff pressure and continuous wave Doppler echocardiography to measure the gradient between aorta and pulmonary artery across the shunt. The classic **Blalock-Taussig shunt** (subclavian artery anastomosed to the pulmonary artery) has a much lower risk of pulmonary vascular disease, with preferential blood flow into one lung (usually the left). Even when pulmonary vascular disease develops in the ipsilateral lung, the other lung is usually protected and late intracardiac repair may be possible. Because the subclavian artery is diverted, the ipsilateral arm is pulseless. The modified Blalock-Taussig shunt (now more commonly performed) uses a synthetic conduit and maintains perfusion to the arm. These shunts can become obstructed with recurrence of cyanosis, loss of the continuous murmur on physical examination, and decreased flow on Doppler echocardiography.

In the **Rastelli procedure,** extracardiac conduits from the right ventricle to the pulmonary artery may be used in pulmonary atresia and C-TGA with PS, truncus arteriosus, and double-outlet RV with PS. They can be synthetic (heterograft) or cadaveric (homograft) and may or may not contain valves. Problems are caused by valvular obstruction or degeneration and obstruction of shunts, baffles, and conduits. Continued clinical and noninvasive follow-up is essential in this group of patients.

Some further considerations are necessary when dealing with patients with congenital heart disease. Congestive heart failure and arrhythmias may occur as part of the natural history of the congenital defect or as a result of acquired heart disease. In managing CHF in these patients, diuretics must be used judiciously to avoid dehydration, especially in cyanotic patients, who may also be more susceptible to digoxin toxicity. In addition, the benefit of digoxin is unproven in right-heart failure associated with pulmonary vascular disease. Rhythm disturbances are a common source of morbidity among adult patients with congenital heart disease. Intra-atrial reentrant tachycardia (resembling atrial flutter) is particularly common in patients with prior atriotomies and atrial suture lines and is often poorly tolerated. Furthermore, the development of atrial flutter/intra-atrial reentrant tachycardia or atrial fibrillation is a risk factor for sudden death. Modern interventional electrophysiologic techniques, using three-dimensional mapping and radiofrequency ablation, have expanded treatment options, and early electrophysiologic consultation should be considered for patients with complex congenital heart disease and recurrent atrial arrhythmias. Ventricular tachycardia is relatively common in patients with prior ventriculotomies (particularly for TOF repair) and with myopathic ventricles. Clinicians should have a low threshold to perform Holter monitoring in these patients, and some advocate routine annual testing in patients with TOF. Sinus node dysfunction occurs frequently in patients with atrial isomerism or with prior Fontan or atrial switch operations. The resultant bradycardia is associated with a higher rate of intra-atrial reentrant tachycardia or atrial fibrillation in these patients. Atrioventricular node dysfunction is commonly seen in patients as a consequence of surgery and also in patients with AV septal defect and with C-TGA. The indications for pacing are similar to those in the general population, although an awareness of the patient's anatomy is important because patients with atrial switch procedures or single ventricles often require placement of epicardial pacing leads.

GENETIC COUNSELING & PREGNANCY

As many young adults with congenital heart disease have entered or are about to enter their reproductive years, genetic counseling and prepregnancy consultation are an important component of their care. The risk of congenital heart defects increases to 5–10% (higher in specific disorders) in the off-spring of patients with congenital heart disease. Preconception genetic counseling and genetic testing are indicated for patients with syndromic congenital heart disease as well as for patients with nonsyndromic congenital heart disease and a family history of congenital heart disease. In addition, testing for the 22q11 deletion is indicated in patients with TOF, truncus arteriosus, aortic arch anomalies, or VSD who display at least one other feature of the 22q11 deletion syndrome (including dysmorphic facies, cleft palate, hypernasal speech, learning disabilities, behavioral or psychiatric disorders, thymic abnormalities, or hypocalcemia).

Most patients with acyanotic congenital heart disease can successfully carry a pregnancy to term. A small number of conditions place the patient and fetus at high risk during pregnancy. These include unrepaired cyanotic heart disease, Eisenmenger syndrome with severe pulmonary vascular disease/pulmonary hypertension, Marfan syndrome with a dilated aortic root, severe LV outflow obstruction, and moderate to severe systolic dysfunction of the systemic ventricle. Patients with these conditions should be advised against pregnancy. Other patients should be risk-stratified with respect to their tolerance of the anticipated hemodynamic changes of pregnancy and labor, namely expansion of intravascular volume, reduction of vascular resistance, and augmentation of cardiac output. It is therefore helpful to assess exercise tolerance prior to conception. Maternal and fetal mortality rates vary with functional class: in NYHA class I, they are 0% and 0.4%, respectively; in NYHA class IV, the rates are 30% and 6.8%, respectively. Although pulmonary edema occurs less commonly than in patients with acquired heart disease, it may be useful to assess ventricular function noninvasively prepartum and in the early months of pregnancy. Patients with significant congenital heart disease should receive close follow-up during pregnancy by a cardiologist and should receive care in a high-risk obstetric clinic. Fetal echocardiography should be offered when the parent or a previous child is affected. Prophylaxis during vaginal delivery is generally recommended for those at high risk for endocarditis (see Table 28–1). For a complete discussion of pregnancy in patients with heart disease, please see Chapter 31.

RECOMMENDATIONS FOR EXERCISE & SPORTS PARTICIPATION

General recommendations regarding exercise should be individualized to the patient following a complete clinical and noninvasive evaluation. Exercise testing and Holter monitoring should be included in this evaluation to define exercise capacity and detect significant asymptomatic arrhythmias. No exercise restrictions are recommended for patients with small or repaired ASDs, VSDs, or PDAs, repaired AV septal defects, repaired total or partial anomalous pulmonary venous connection, mild PS, repaired coarctation, repaired congenital coronary artery anomalies, or patients with D-TGA who have had an arterial switch procedure. Patients with moderate PS, mild aortic stenosis, completely repaired TOF, or AV septal defect with moderate mitral regurgitation should be restricted to moderate dynamic and isometric exercise. Patients with Ebstein anomaly, D-TGA after atrial switch procedure, C-TGA, or univentricular hearts/Fontan circulation should be restricted to moderate dynamic exercise and mild isometric exercise. Patients with moderate aortic stenosis or TOF with residual disease should be restricted to mild dynamic and static exercise. Patients with Eisenmenger syndrome should be restricted to mild dynamic exercise.

ACQUIRED HEART DISEASE IN ADULTS WITH CONGENITAL HEART DISEASE

It is important not to ignore the presence of acquired heart disease in adults with congenital heart disease. Acquired and congenital heart lesions may interact in unexpected ways, for example, the association of rheumatic mitral stenosis causing increased shunting across an ASD in Lutembacher syndrome. Impaired diastolic function from hypertension or coronary artery disease in a patient with an ASD may also increase the magnitude of the left-to-right shunt. Similarly, increased systemic vascular resistance from hypertension in a patient with a VSD may worsen the shunt. The clinician must exclude coronary artery disease as a cause of chest pain in adults with congenital aortic stenosis and pulmonary hypertension. In addition, the progression of atherosclerotic coronary disease may be accelerated in association with aortic coarctation.

Gatzoulis MA et al. Definitive palliation with cavopulmonary or aortopulmonary shunts for adults with single ventricle physiology. Heart. 2000 Jan;83:51–7. [PMID: 10618336]

Hirth A et al. Recommendations for participation in competitive and leisure sports in patients with congenital heart disease: a consensus document. Eur J Cardiovasc Prev Rehabil. 2006 Jun;13(3):293–9. [PMID: 16926656]

Pierpont ME et al; American Heart Association Congenital Cardiac Defects Committee, Council on Cardiovascular Disease in the Young. Genetic basis for congenital heart defects: current knowledge: a scientific statement from the American Heart Association Congenital Cardiac Defects Committee, Council on Cardiovascular Disease in the Young: endorsed by the American Academy of Pediatrics. Circulation. 2007 Jun 12;115(23):3015–38. [PMID: 17519398]

Walsh EP et al. Arrhythmias in adult patients with congenital heart disease. Circulation. 2007 Jan 30;115(4):534–45. [PMID: 17261672]

Long-Term Anticoagulation for Cardiac Conditions

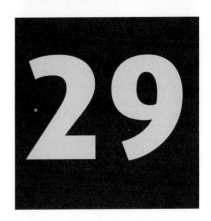

Richard D. Taylor, MD & Richard W. Asinger, MD

▶ **General Considerations**

Long-term anticoagulation is important in the treatment of many cardiac conditions. Intracardiac thrombi can form and lead to devastating consequences as a result of obstruction of blood flow and peripheral embolization. Treatment for intracardiac thrombi involves the use of anticoagulants for both primary and secondary prevention of thrombosis and embolization. There are, however, risks associated with the use of these agents, and an understanding of the risks and benefits of anticoagulant therapy for various cardiac conditions is important.

A. Anticoagulants

These agents affect the coagulation protein cascade to reduce thrombosis. Their greatest use is in primary and secondary prevention of intravascular and intracardiac thrombosis and embolization.

1. Unfractionated heparin—Unfractionated heparin (UFH) binds to antithrombin III, markedly increasing the effect of antithrombin III in neutralizing thrombin. It also inhibits the activation of factors IX and X. The effectiveness of UFH varies greatly from person to person due to its interactions with a number of plasma proteins and the endothelium. Monitoring the effects of full dose UFH on hemostasis is mandatory. Routinely, the activated partial thromboplastin time (aPTT) is used to monitor the effects of UFH, which should be titrated to 1.5–2.0 times greater than control. In certain situations, a higher level of anticoagulation is needed, ie, during coronary interventions. In those instances, the activated clotting time (ACT) is used to monitor its effect, and the dose of UFH is adjusted to keep the ACT 250–300 seconds or greater. When given intravenously, the effects of UFH are immediate. It is usually given as a bolus, followed by a continuous infusion. It may also be given subcutaneously. The effects of UFH will dissipate within 6 hours. Protamine can be given to reverse its effects more quickly. UFH can be given subcutaneously in smaller doses, which

will not affect the aPTT, for primary prevention of deep venous thrombosis in certain high-risk situations.

2. Low-molecular-weight heparin—Low-molecular-weight heparins (LMWHs) are breakdown products of UFH. They have a greater affect on factor X than on thrombin. Low-molecular-weight heparins bind less to plasma proteins than UFH and therefore, the dosing is more predictable. They are more resistant to neutralization by platelet factor 4 than UFH and have less inhibitory affect on platelet function than UFH. Low-molecular-weight heparins have a more predictable affect on coagulation than UFH and laboratory monitoring is usually not necessary. Monitoring the effects of LMWHs is difficult, since the commonly used tests for anticoagulation are not helpful and activated factor Xa levels need to be measured. Low-molecular-weight heparins are usually administered subcutaneously twice daily. They are not easily reversed by protamine. Low-molecular-weight heparin can also be given in smaller doses for the primary prevention of deep venous thrombosis in certain high-risk situations.

3. Oral vitamin K antagonists—Coumarins, or vitamin K antagonists, are the mainstay of oral anticoagulants and have been used for more than 50 years. Warfarin is the most commonly used oral anticoagulant. It blocks the conversion of vitamin K to the active moiety, vitamin K epoxide, which is necessary for the synthesis of factors II, VII, IX, X and proteins C and S. The half-life of warfarin is about 40 hours. It is nearly completely absorbed when given orally and binds to albumin. Its effect on hemostasis is quite variable from person to person and sometimes, for the same person at different times. Warfarin's effect can be influenced by dietary factors, liver disease, congestive heart failure, hypermetabolic states, and numerous drug interactions. Monitoring the anticoagulant effect of warfarin is mandatory. The prothrombin time (PT) is now standardized to an international thromboplastin reagent and is reported as the international normalized ratio (INR), which is used to monitor the effects of warfarin and adjust its dose. Warfarin therapy may be started without a loading dose. It usually takes several days for the optimal or target INR to be achieved. During initiation of therapy, there may be a brief paradoxical hypercoagulable state due to the inhibition of proteins C and S (anticoagulant factors) before the inhibition of the coagulant factors. For this reason, UFH or LMWH may be used as a bridge until a therapeutic INR is achieved. During initiation of warfarin therapy, the INR should be checked frequently until a stable dose of warfarin that achieves the target INR is found. Subsequently, the INR should be monitored at least once a month and more frequently if the dose needs to be adjusted. Monitoring can be done by an individual care provider or through a warfarin clinic. The latter tends to be more organized and efficient. Point of care monitoring of INR is now available and can be done at home. If warfarin needs to be stopped, the INR will normalize in about 3–4 days. If its anticoagulant effect needs to be reversed more quickly, vitamin K can be administered subcutaneously or, preferably, by the oral route. The INR will usually correct in 1–2 days if vitamin K is given. If it is necessary to reverse the effects of warfarin more quickly, fresh frozen plasma or prothrombin concentrate can be given.

B. Risks of Anticoagulant Therapy

Bleeding is the most common serious adverse effect seen with the use of anticoagulant agents. Bleeding complications are more likely to occur in patients who are older; who have a history of previous stroke or gastrointestinal tract bleeding; who have had a recent myocardial infarction; who have anemia, renal insufficiency, serious concurrent illness, or diabetes; or who drink alcohol excessively or take aspirin (Table 29–1). Intracranial hemorrhage is perhaps the most feared complication of anticoagulant therapy. Intracranial hemorrhage that occurs without anticoagulation usually pre-sents suddenly, with rapid progression to the maximal neurologic deficit. Intracranial hemorrhage that occurs while a patient is receiving anticoagulant therapy is more devastating, with continued bleeding and progressive neurologic deterioration. In such situations, reversal of the anticoagulant effect is necessary, as soon as possible.

Thrombocytopenia can complicate the use of UFH and LMWH in two ways. A dose-dependent lowering of the platelet count is usually not serious and does not necessarily require stopping these agents. The second type of thrombocytopenia is termed "heparin-induced thrombocytopenia" (HIT). It is immune-mediated and can be life-threatening due to arterial and venous thrombus formation. An antibody to heparin interacts with a heparin-platelet factor 4 complex on the platelet surface, resulting in platelet destruction. Heparin-induced thrombocytopenia usually starts at least 4 days after heparin initiation unless there has been previous heparin exposure. It is not dose dependent. There is usually at least a 50% reduction in the platelet count. The diagnosis of HIT can be confirmed with the immunoassay for the antibody-heparin-platelet factor 4 complex. Heparin-induced thrombocytopenia is much less common with LMWH than with UFH, occurring about 1/10th as frequently. The treatment for HIT is immediate discontinuation of all heparin, even low doses used to maintain intravenous access. A direct thrombin inhibitor, such as lepuridin or argatroban should be substituted.

Additional rare complications seen with the use of UFH and LMWH include hyperkalemia (due to hyperaldosteronism), osteoporosis, skin necrosis, and alopecia.

Adverse effects seen with warfarin include skin necrosis and teratogenic effects. Skin necrosis due to warfarin is a rare complication seen within the first few days of treatment. It is most likely to occur in patients with protein C and S deficiencies. Because of its teratogenic effects, warfarin should be used cautiously during pregnancy (if at all), especially the first trimester.

Table 29–1. Risk Factors for Bleeding Complications with Anticoagulants.

Age > 65 years
History of hemorrhagic stroke
History of stroke
History of gastrointestinal bleeding
INR > 4.0
Prosthetic heart valve
Recent myocardial infarction
Anemia
Renal insufficiency
Diabetes
High risk for trauma
Concurrent illness
Multiple medications
Unreliable taking of medications
Unreliable medical follow-up
Aspirin use
Excessive alcohol intake

INR, international normalized ratio.

Hirsh J et al. American Heart Association/American College of Cardiology Foundation guide to warfarin therapy. J Am Coll Cardiol. 2003 May 7;41(9):1633–52. [PMID: 12742309]

Hirsh J et al. Oral anticoagulants: mechanism of action, clinical effectiveness, and optimal therapeutic range. Chest. 2001 Jan;119 (1 Suppl):8S–21S. [PMID: 11157640]

Levine MN et al. Hemorrhagic complications of anticoagulant treatment. Chest. 2001 Jan;119(1 Suppl):108S–121S. [PMID: 11157645]

Monagle P et al. Antithrombotic therapy in children: the Seventh ACCP Conference on Antithrombotic and Thrombolytic Therapy. Chest. 2004 Sep;126:(3 Suppl):645S–687S. [PMID: 15383489]

▶ Pathophysiology & Etiology

A. Pathogenesis of Intravascular Thrombi

In the nineteenth century, Virchow theorized that stasis of intracavitary blood, endocardial injury, and a hypercoagulable state were necessary for the formation of intracardiac thrombi. In the normally functioning heart, stasis and thrombosis do not occur, but a high incidence of thrombosis is noted in cardiac chambers that are enlarged or have low flow. Left atrial thrombi complicate mitral stenosis, particularly in persons with atrial fibrillation; left ventricular thrombi complicate acute myocardial infarction, left ventricular aneurysm, and dilated cardiomyopathy. In these clinical settings, there is generalized or localized low flow in either the left atrium or left ventricle.

Acute ST-segment elevation myocardial infarction (STEMI) causes stasis of intracavitary blood (secondary to dysfunction of part of the left ventricle) in the setting of a hypercoagulable state and left ventricular thrombi are common, particularly if reperfusion therapy is not given or is ineffective. These thrombi usually develop at the apex of the left ventricle 2–7 days after infarction; they rarely develop with inferior STEMI or non–ST-segment elevation myocardial infarction (NSTEMI). Because the left anterior descending coronary artery usually supplies the apex, apical stasis occurs with anterior infarction. The apex is the portion of the left ventricle furthest from the inflow and outflow areas, which are the areas with the highest blood flow velocities. Severe apical wall motion abnormalities, such as akinesia and dyskinesia, precede thrombus formation in acute infarction. Endocardial injury that occurs in acute infarction may also contribute to thrombosis.

Myocardial necrosis, including the endocardium, may occur with infarction and contribute to thrombus development. Endocardial abnormalities may also be present in other clinical settings such as atrial fibrillation, in which elevated von Willebrand factor is noted in the left atrium. The introduction of a foreign material, such as a prosthetic valve, can also provide a nidus for thrombus formation. An inflammatory process that involves the myocardium, secondary to myocarditis or noninfectious endocarditis, may be responsible for thrombus formation, particularly when there is a coexistent hypercoagulable state. Reduced ventricular function can also contribute to thrombosis with myocarditis. Eosinophils presumably cause the endothelial injury with Löffler endocarditis that leads to thrombus formation.

The final prerequisite for intracardiac thrombosis is a hypercoagulable state. Activation of the coagulation system can be found in conditions associated with intracardiac thrombi, including acute myocardial infarction and atrial fibrillation. Rare cases have been reported in which, even with normal wall motion and presumably normal blood flow, intracardiac thrombi develop because of a hypercoagulable state. Platelets may also play an active role in the formation of intracardiac thrombi and are activated in such clinical situations as acute infarction and atrial fibrillation.

Although all three of Virchow prerequisites are operative in specific settings, most clinical data indicate a complex interaction exists with stasis the most frequent (or perhaps the most easily demonstrated) factor leading to intracardiac thrombosis.

B. Embolization of Thrombi

The major risk associated with intracardiac thrombi is end organ ischemia due to peripheral embolization. The factors that result in embolization of intracardiac thrombi are poorly understood. The restoration of mechanical function to an area of the heart that was previously non-contractile and the site of thrombus formation may result in embolization. Left ventricular thrombi usually form within the first week of an anterior myocardial infarction. However, embolization due to these thrombi usually occurs 5–21 days following infarction, when the left ventricular function has improved, eliminating stasis of blood flow and expelling the thrombus. Improved myocardial function at the margins of a thrombus could theoretically change the shape of a thrombus from mural to protruding, leading to embolization.

Recovery of the mechanical function of the left atrium following conversion from atrial fibrillation has also been implicated in the embolization of left atrial thrombi. Following conversion of atrial fibrillation to sinus rhythm, the mechanical function of the left atrium may not return for several weeks. During this time, the atrium is stunned, creating a low flow state that may lead to thrombus formation. Embolization of such thrombi may occur several days after successful cardioversion when mechanical function returns. Endogenous or pharmacologic thrombolysis can result in the breakup of thrombi, resulting in embolization. Embolization may be more likely for certain intracardiac thrombi, especially protruding or mobile thrombi. Embolization may also be more likely when larger thrombi are present. Although all the factors that lead to embolization are not known, it is known that embolization is likely to recur in patients who have had embolization in the past.

Peripheral embolization of intracardiac thrombi can be to the brain, extremities, bowel, spleen, and kidneys. The most frequent site recognized clinically is to the brain, resulting in stroke.

An estimated 15% of all ischemic strokes are cardioembolic. The differentiation of thrombotic from embolic stroke is not always possible, and the diagnosis may depend on the clinical setting. Patients with atrial fibrillation, prosthetic heart valves, or left ventricular mural thrombi are more likely to have cardioembolic events, whereas, patients with known carotid artery disease are more likely to have a thrombotic stroke or an artery to artery embolus.

Patients who suffer a cardiogenic cerebral emboli are at risk for recurrent stroke, both in the short- and long-term. Antithrombotic therapy could lower the risk of recurrent stroke, in both the short- and long-term. A serious and potentially life-threatening complication of cerebral emboli is intracerebral bleeding. CT scanning should be performed in patients with a cerebral embolus to identify cerebral hemorrhage or if there are features indicating a high risk of hemorrhagic transformation. The Cerebral Embolism Study Group recommends that patients with cardiogenic cerebral emboli receive anticoagulation if they are not hypertensive and there is no evidence of intracerebral hemorrhage on CT scan at 24–48 hours. A delay of 7 days might be prudent in those with large cerebral infarction to lower the risk of hemorrhagic transformation.

▶ Diagnostic Studies

An intracardiac source of embolization is often suspected clinically, and a number of diagnostic tests can be used to specifically identify intracardiac thrombi.

Echocardiography is an accurate, noninvasive technique for detecting intracardiac thrombi. Transthoracic echocardiography (TTE) is sensitive and specific for detecting left ventricular thrombi (Figures 29–1 and 29–2). Transesophageal echocardiography (TEE) is required to reliably detect left atrial thrombi (Figure 29–3) and atherothrombotic material in the ascending or transverse aorta. Intravenous contrast may help in the correct identification of cardiac masses.

The use of serial echocardiography has greatly enhanced clinicians' knowledge of the natural history of intracardiac thrombosis associated with acute myocardial infarction. The precise onset of the pathophysiologic thrombotic process can be accurately defined for acute myocardial infarction. Doppler studies of blood flow within the left ventricle of patients in whom thrombosis develops have shown that apical patterns of low flow precede thrombosis. Because high-risk factors (anterior infarction and severe apical wall motion abnormality) are present and can be detected prior to thrombus development, it is possible to initiate prophylactic treatment with anticoagulants and decrease the development of thrombus and subsequent systemic emboli.

Spontaneous echo contrast ("smoke") detected in a cardiac chamber represents low flow and early rouleaux formation and is frequently associated with thrombus or subsequent development of thrombus. Patients with spontaneous echo contrast or low flow velocities in the left atrium or its appendage accompanying rheumatic mitral stenosis, prosthetic mitral valves, and nonvalvular atrial fibrillation have a high incidence of left atrial thrombi and thromboembolism.

High-speed contrast CT and MRI can also be used to reliably detect intracardiac thrombus, especially in the left ventricle. However, these techniques require specialized equipment not always available and are expensive. Until now, they are used infrequently for this purpose.

Although intracardiac thrombi are the most common cardiac cause of peripheral embolization, there are other causes, including valvular vegetations due to infectious or noninfectious endocarditis, calcific emboli due to degenerative aortic and mitral valve disease, tumor emboli from left-sided myxoma, and atheroemboli from friable or mobile plaque in the aorta or great vessels. In addition, embolic events can occur due to paradoxical emboli which originate in the venous system and transverse an intracardiac communication (most commonly a patent foramen ovale) (Figure 29–4). All of these conditions are readily identified by TTE or TEE, or both.

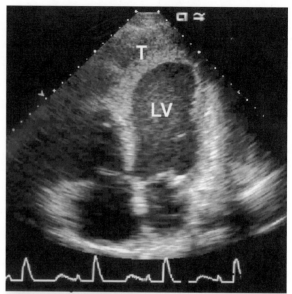
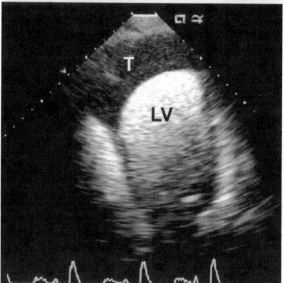

▲ **Figure 29–1.** Mural thrombus (T) in the left ventricle (LV) of a patient with a left ventricular aneurysm following anterior myocardial infarction. Top panel is an apical four-chamber echocardiogram with second harmonic imaging. The thrombus is well imaged but delineation of the underlying wall motion abnormality is difficult to appreciate. Bottom panel is the same view with a lipid based echo contrast agent; note the clearer definition of the thrombus and aneurysm.

Kirkpatrick JN et al. Differential diagnosis of cardiac masses using contrast echocardiographic perfusion imaging. J Am Coll Cardiol. 2004 Apr 21;43(8):1412–9. [PMID: 15093876]

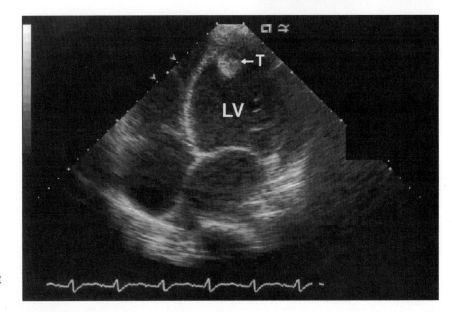

▲ **Figure 29-2.** Apical four-chamber two-dimensional echocardiogram of a patient with dilated cardiomyopathy showing a protruding thrombus (T) at the apex of the left ventricle (LV).

Mollet NR et al. Visualization of ventricular thrombi with contrast-enhanced magnetic resonance imaging in patients with ischemic heart disease. Circulation. 2002 Dec 3;106(23):2873–6. [PMID: 12460863]

Srichai MB et al. Clinical, imaging, and pathological characteristics of left ventricular thrombus: a comparison of contrast-enhanced magnetic resonance imaging, transthoracic echocardiography, and transesophageal echocardiography with surgical or pathological validation. Am Heart J. 2006 Jul;152(1):75–84. [PMID: 16824834]

Thambidorai SK et al; ACUTE investigators. Utility of transesophageal echocardiography in identification of thrombogenic milieu in patients with atrial fibrillation (an ACUTE ancillary study). Am J Cardiol. 2005 Oct 1;96(7):935–41. [PMID: 16188520]

▶ Treatment of Cardiac Conditions Requiring Anticoagulation

Short- and long-term anticoagulation are integral parts of the treatment of many cardiovascular conditions, including

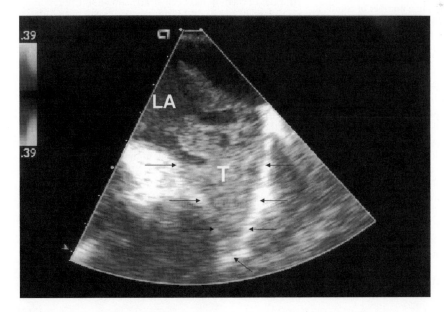

▲ **Figure 29-3.** Transesophageal echocardiogram demonstrating the left atrium (LA) with a large thrombus (T) filling the left atrial appendage. Arrows outline the left atrial appendage.

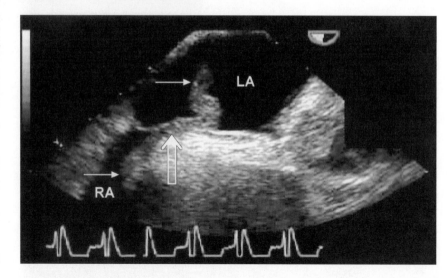

▲ **Figure 29–4.** Transesophageal echocardiogram demonstrating a systemic venous thrombus (T), which has embolized to the heart and lodged in a patent foramen ovale. RA, right atrium; LA, left atrium. Arrows indicate the thrombus; the open arrow indicates the patent foramen ovale.

acute coronary syndromes, stroke, peripheral arterial disease, and venous thromboembolic disease. These conditions are discussed in other chapters. Long-term anticoagulation will be discussed in this chapter for the following conditions: atrial fibrillation, native valvular heart disease, prosthetic heart valves, left ventricular thrombus with acute myocardial infarction, remote myocardial infarction, left ventricular aneurysm, dilated cardiomyopathy, atherosclerotic sources of emboli, paradoxical emboli associated with a patent foramen ovale, and intracardiac devices.

Guidelines have been written by a number of organizations, including the American Heart Association (AHA), American College of Cardiology (ACC), the American College of Chest Physicians (ACCP), and European Society of Cardiology (ESC) for the management of anticoagulation in a number of conditions. These guidelines vary in their content and format; however, their recommendations rarely conflict significantly.

A. Atrial Fibrillation

Atrial fibrillation can result in atrial thrombus formation (most often seen in the left atrial appendage [see Figure 29–3]), which can subsequently result in embolization (most often resulting in ischemic stroke). The incidence of stroke in patients with atrial fibrillation is about 4–5% per year and is about 4–5 times greater than in similar patients who do not have atrial fibrillation. The incidence of stroke with atrial fibrillation is age related. For those aged 50–59 years, the incidence of stroke is about 1.5% per year. For those aged 80–89 years, the incidence increases to more than 20% per year.

Atrial fibrillation is classified as acute and chronic. Acute atrial fibrillation is that which occurs for the first time. Chronic atrial fibrillation can be paroxysmal, persistent, or permanent. In paroxysmal atrial fibrillation, episodes spontaneously revert to normal sinus rhythm. In persistent atrial fibrillation, conversion to normal sinus rhythm requires

cardioversion, either chemical or electrical. In permanent atrial fibrillation, normal sinus rhythm can no longer be restored and the patient remains in atrial fibrillation permanently. The risk of stroke is considered the same for all three categories of chronic atrial fibrillation.

Atrial flutter is much less common than atrial fibrillation. However, the two arrhythmias are often seen in the same individual. Patients with atrial flutter are also at risk for thromboembolism, and therefore, the two arrhythmias are treated the same in terms of anticoagulation.

1. Chronic atrial fibrillation (nonvalvular)—The efficacy of long-term therapy with oral anticoagulants (warfarin) in the primary prevention of stroke in patients with nonvalvular atrial fibrillation has been clearly shown in five randomized controlled trials (Table 29–2). Equal efficacy for anticoagulant therapy has been shown for secondary prevention of strokes in patients with atrial fibrillation. In these studies, strokes occurred primarily in patients who had discontinued anticoagulant therapy or who had an INR below the target goal of treatment.

The risks of anticoagulant therapy in this patient population are considerable. In the randomized trials of anticoagulation, there were more bleeding complications in the anticoagulant arms. However, there were no significant differences in the incidence of major bleeding in those treated with anticoagulants compared with controls. Major bleeding complications were those that resulted in transfusion, hospitalization, death, permanent disability, or an intracranial hemorrhage. The risk of intracranial hemorrhage increases significantly with age greater than 75 years and INRs greater than 4.0.

Randomized studies have also evaluated the effects of aspirin in reducing the incidence of stroke in patients with nonvalvular atrial fibrillation. Some studies compared the effects of aspirin with placebo and others compared aspirin with warfarin. The results of these studies were somewhat

Table 29–2. Ischemic Stroke and Systemic Embolus Rates for Placebo-Controlled Studies of Anticoagulant Therapy for Nonvalvular Atrial Fibrillation.[1]

	AFASAK[2] (n = 1007) (%)	SPAF-1[3] (n = 1330) (%)	BAATAF[4] (n = 420) (%)	CAFA[5] (n = 378) (%)	Spinaf[6] (n = 538) (%)
Placebo	5.5	6.3	3.07	4.6	3.9
Warfarin	2.2	2.3	0.4	3.0	1.0
Aspirin	4.7	3.6	NA	NA	NA
Hemorrhagic rate	0.5	1.5	0.8	2.5	1.3

[1]Intention-to-treat analysis.
[2]Data from Peterson P et al. Lancet 1989;1:175.
[3]Data from Stroke Prevention in Atrial Fibrillation Investigators. Circulation. 1991;84:527.
[4]Data from Boston Area Anticoagulation Trial for Atrial Fibrillation Investigators. N Engl J Med. 1990;323:1505.
[5]Data from Connolly SJ et al. J Am Coll Cardiol. 1991;18:349.
[6]Data from Ezekowitz MD et al. N Engl J Med. 1992;327:1406.
AFASAK, Atrial Fibrillation, Aspirin, Anticoagulation Study; BAATAF, Boston Area Anticoagulation Trial for Atrial Fibrillation; CAFA, Canadian Atrial Fibrillation Anticoagulation Study; NA, no information available; SPAF-1, Stroke Prevention and Atrial Fibrillation Study-1; SPINAF, Stroke Prevention in Nonrheumatic Atrial Fibrillation.

disparate, some showing no benefit of aspirin and one showing a small positive effect that was significantly less than oral anticoagulants. The combination of aspirin and low-dose warfarin has been compared with dose-adjusted warfarin and was not as effective in lowering the incidence of stroke.

The optimal intensity or target INR for anticoagulant therapy in atrial fibrillation should provide efficacy in reducing the incidence of stroke and minimize the risk of complications. The randomized studies varied in the target INRs. Review of the combined studies indicates that the efficacy of treatment is diminished if the INR is less than 2.0. International normalized ratios greater than 4.0 are associated with a higher risk of minor and major bleeding. The usually accepted target INR for the prevention of stroke in atrial fibrillation is 2.0–3.0. In view of the higher risk of anticoagulation in the very elderly, the target INR is at times lowered to 2.0–2.5 in these individuals.

In patients with atrial fibrillation and atherosclerosis, low-dose aspirin (81 mg) is often added to warfarin for added protection from coronary artery disease. This strategy is intuitively sound, although there is little supporting evidence. Patients with chronic atrial fibrillation who undergo percutaneous coronary interventions, particularly the placement of coronary stents, require treatment with clopidogrel in addition to aspirin. Some interventional cardiologists treat with all three agents, while others recommend stopping the aspirin and giving warfarin and clopidogrel during the necessary period following stent placement.

2. Risk of stroke in atrial fibrillation—In choosing to treat a patient who has atrial fibrillation with oral anticoagulants, the balance of risks and benefits needs to be considered. The SPAF investigators, the Atrial Fibrillation Investigators, the AHA/ACC/ECS, and the ACCP have determined risk

factors for stroke in patients with atrial fibrillation. Assessment of patients for these risk factors can be used to decide who should be treated with warfarin. CHADS2 is a modified stroke risk classification that integrates the above schemes (Table 29–3). Congestive heart failure (C), hypertension (H), age greater than 75 years (A) and diabetes (D) are each assigned one point. Patients with previous stroke (S) are assigned two points. The CHADS2 risk assessment assists in determining the approach to antithrombotic treatment (Table 29–4). Lowest risk patients have a score of 0 and do not require warfarin. Intermediate risk patients have a score of 1 or 2 and may or may not be treated with anticoagulants. High-risk patients have a score of 3 or greater and derive the most benefit from anticoagulants. Patients with atrial fibrillation who have had a previous stroke should receive anticoagulation therapy unless there is a contraindication.

Table 29–3. CHADS2 Risk Assessment for Anticoagulation in Nonvalvular Atrial Fibrillation.

Risk	Points
Congestive heart failure	1
Hypertension	1
Age > 75 years	1
Diabetes	1
Stroke	2
	Total number of points:
	0 points, low risk.
	1–2 points, intermediate risk.
	3–6 points, high risk.

Table 29–4. Anticoagulation for Chronic Nonvalvular Atrial Fibrillation by CHADS2 Risk.

Risk	Anticoagulation
Low (CHADS2 = 0)	None or aspirin, 325 mg/day
Intermediate (CHADS2 = 1-2)	Aspirin, 325 mg/day or warfarin, INR 2.0-3.0
High (CHADS2 = 3 or more)	Warfarin, INR 2.0-3.0

INR, international normalized ratio.

The risk of stroke is not different in patients with chronic paroxysmal, persistent, and permanent atrial fibrillation. The decision to treat with oral anticoagulants should be made on the basis of risk factors and not on the classification of atrial fibrillation.

Several studies have compared the outcomes in patients with atrial fibrillation who were treated with a rate control versus a rhythm control strategy. The incidence of stroke was similar for both strategies. Most strokes occurred in patients who were not taking anticoagulants or who were inadequately treated, with subtherapeutic INRs. In some of these studies, patients in the rhythm control strategy could be taken off anticoagulants if they remained in normal sinus rhythm for at least 1 month. Recommendations about stopping anticoagulants when a patient is no longer in atrial fibrillation are somewhat vague. (See below discussion of anticoagulation in regard to cardioversion in atrial fibrillation.) It is known that patients are not always accurate when self-reporting the occurrence of atrial fibrillation based on symptoms. The decision to stop warfarin in patients who are no longer in atrial fibrillation should consider risk factors for stroke and the risk of anticoagulation.

3. Cardioversion of atrial fibrillation—Restoration of sinus rhythm can occur spontaneously or as the result of chemical or electrical cardioversion. Conversion to sinus rhythm can result in systemic emboli through two potential mechanisms. The first is embolization of existing left atrial appendage thrombus, as the mechanical function of the atrium returns. The second is due to the development of left atrial appendage thrombus during the postconversion period, when the atrium is mechanically stunned. Embolization of the newly formed thrombus may occur several days to weeks postconversion, as the mechanical function of the atrium returns. Retrospective studies have shown up to a 5% incidence of embolic events in patients with atrial fibrillation of unknown duration who were not given anticoagulants at the time of cardioversion, compared with less than 1% in those who were given anticoagulants.

There are two approaches to elective cardioversion: the conventional and the TEE-guided approach (Figure 29–5). A randomized study showed that these two approaches were equal in terms of stroke risk. In the conventional approach, patients with atrial fibrillation of unknown or greater than 48 hours duration are treated with warfarin to achieve an INR of 2.0–3.0 for at least 3 weeks before and at least 4 weeks after successful cardioversion. This recommendation applies regardless of risk factors. Continuation of warfarin beyond 4 weeks depends on risk factors for stroke and whether there have been previous episodes of atrial fibrillation. In the TEE-guided approach, patients with atrial fibrillation of unknown or greater than 48 hours duration are treated with UFH to maintain an aPTT of 50–70 seconds or warfarin to maintain an INR of 2.0–3.0 and then undergo a TEE. If no left atrial or left atrial appendage thrombus is seen, cardioversion is performed. If sinus rhythm is restored, warfarin should be continued for at least 4 weeks or longer, depending on risk factors. If a left atrial thrombus is seen on TEE, cardioversion should not be performed. These patients should be treated with warfarin indefinitely. After 3–4 weeks of therapeutic anticoagulation (INR 2.0–3.0), TEE can be repeated. If no thrombus is seen, then cardioversion can be performed.

For patients with atrial fibrillation of known duration of less than 48 hours, cardioversion may be performed without anticoagulation. Whether to administer anticoagulants following cardioversion treatment should be decided on the basis of risk factors and whether there had been previous episodes of atrial fibrillation. For emergency cardioversion (patients with unstable hemodynamics, uncontrolled angina, and congestive heart failure), UFH should be given and the patient should be treated with warfarin for at least 4 weeks or longer after cardioversion, depending on risk factors.

4. Problems in prescribing anticoagulation for atrial fibrillation—A number of studies have shown that warfarin is underprescribed, particularly in elderly patients with atrial fibrillation. Elderly patients are at greatest risk for stroke but also are at greatest risk for bleeding complications from warfarin. Often cited reasons for not prescribing warfarin in those who meet criteria for its use include risk of falls, poor compliance, concurrent illnesses, and history of substance abuse. Applying the results of randomized studies to clinical practice is difficult. Patients who were studied in these clinical trials were quite select, in fact, less than 10% of those screened were included. In addition, most studies included very few patients 80 years of age or older. Patients at high risk for bleeding, such as those with recent gastrointestinal tract bleeding, previous intracranial hemorrhage, recent stroke, renal insufficiency, were not included in these studies. It is also important to note that the protocols of these studies required closer monitoring of patients than is usually done in clinical practice. Patients included in these studies were probably more motivated and compliant than those usually seen in clinical practice. Applying the recommendations derived from these randomized studies requires judgment, and clinicians must consider issues of compliance, risk of trauma and bleeding, and adequacy of follow-up.

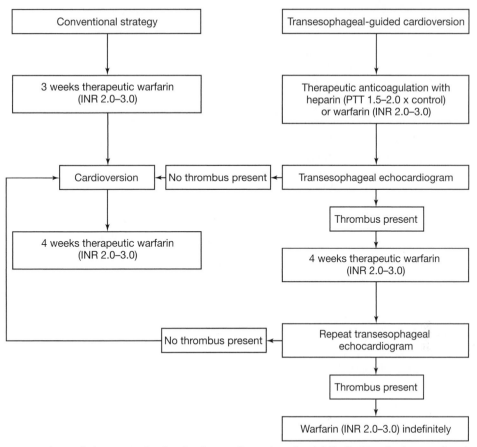

▲ **Figure 29–5.** Anticoagulation strategies for elective cardioversion of atrial fibrillation of unknown duration or lasting longer than 48 hours.

B. Native Valvular Heart Disease

Thromboembolic complications may occur with a number of valvular conditions. Rheumatic mitral valve disease, particularly when accompanied by atrial fibrillation, has a high incidence of embolic events. In contrast, patients with mitral valve prolapse and calcific aortic and mitral valve disease (except when atrial fibrillation is also present) are at low risk for embolic events.

1. Rheumatic mitral valve disease—The risk of thromboembolism due to left atrial thrombi with mitral stenosis and atrial fibrillation is 18 times greater than matched controls. Patients with rheumatic mitral valve stenosis have at least one chance in five of having a clinically detectable embolic event during their lifetime. The risk of systemic emboli is greater in older patients and those with lower cardiac outputs. Atrial fibrillation is common in patients with rheumatic mitral stenosis but thromboembolic complications can also occur in patients with rheumatic mitral stenosis who are in sinus rhythm. The ACCP recommends that all patients with rheu-

matic mitral valve disease and atrial fibrillation or a previous embolic event receive warfarin with a target INR of 2.0–3.0. If an embolic event occurs while a patient is receiving therapeutic anticoagulant therapy, then aspirin 75–100 mg, dipyridamole 400 mg, or clopidogrel 75 mg should be added. In patients with rheumatic mitral stenosis in sinus rhythm, with a left atrial diameter of greater than 5.5 cm by echocardiography, treatment with warfarin with a target INR of 2.0–3.0 has been recommended. For patients with rheumatic mitral stenosis undergoing balloon valvuloplasty, warfarin should be given for 3 weeks before and 4 weeks after the procedure.

Patients with rheumatic mitral regurgitation may be at less risk for thromboembolism than those with mitral stenosis. The increased left atrial flow associated with mitral regurgitation may lessen the likelihood of thrombus formation. There are no specific recommendations for anticoagulation of patients with rheumatic mitral regurgitation. However, most patients with rheumatic mitral regurgitation also have some degree of mitral stenosis. Recommendations for anticoagulation for mitral stenosis apply to these patients.

2. Mitral valve prolapse—A very small number of patients with mitral valve prolapse experience stroke or transient ischemic attacks despite no other identifiable cause. The ACCP recommends that patients with mitral valve prolapse who have had documented but unexplained transient ischemic attacks or strokes receive long-term treatment with aspirin (50–162 mg daily). For patients with mitral valve prolapse who have had systemic emboli or recurrent transient ischemic attacks despite aspirin therapy, long-term treatment with warfarin, with a target INR of 2.0-3.0 is recommended.

3. Calcific mitral and aortic valve conditions—Calcification of the mitral valve annulus and aortic valve occur commonly in elderly individuals. The incidence of stroke in patients with mitral annular calcification is increased. Embolic events associated with fibrocalcific mitral annular disease occur particularly in those with chronic kidney disease. In addition to thromboembolism, calcified spicules can be dislodged from ulcerated calcific plaques. It may not be possible to differentiate thromboembolism from calcific emboli. Occasionally, calcific emboli may be seen on fundoscopic examination. The ACCP recommends that patients with mitral annular calcification complicated by systemic emboli, not documented to be due to calcific emboli, be treated with warfarin with a target INR of 2.0–3.0. Individuals with calcified aortic valves do not have an increased incidence of strokes compared to controls, although they may also be at risk for calcific emboli. Patients with calcification of the aortic valve should not receive warfarin unless they have other indications.

4. Endocarditis—The incidence of embolic events in infective endocarditis is quite high. In the pre-antibiotic era, clinically detected emboli occurred in 70–90% of patients. Currently, the incidence of emboli is 12–40%. In the sulfonamide era, anticoagulant therapy was used to improve penetration of antibiotics into the vegetations. This resulted in a high incidence of cerebral hemorrhage, and the use of anticoagulants was abandoned in this situation.

Infective endocarditis may occur in patients who have been receiving long-term anticoagulant therapy. High-risk patients, such as those with mitral stenosis and atrial fibrillation, mechanical prosthetic valves, or previous embolic strokes, in whom infective endocarditis develops should continue to receive anticoagulation therapy unless there is a hemorrhagic complication.

Nonbacterial thrombotic endocarditis is a condition in which fibrin thrombi are deposited on normal or superficially degenerated cardiac valves. This usually occurs in malignancies, chronic debilitating conditions and acute fulminant diseases such as septicemia and disseminated intravascular coagulation. The reported incidence of systemic emboli in this condition varies from 14% to 91%. Treatment of nonbacterial thrombotic endocarditis should be directed at the underlying condition. The ACCP recommends UFH for patients with nonbacterial endocarditis with systemic or pulmonary emboli.

C. Prosthetic Heart Valves

Prosthetic heart valves may be either mechanical or bioprosthetic. A mechanical valve requires lifelong anticoagulation, whereas, a bioprosthetic valve may not. A mechanical valve prosthesis is more durable than a bioprosthesis and therefore, it is less likely to require repeat valve surgery. Therefore, it is important to evaluate patients for hemorrhagic risk and likelihood of the need for repeat surgery when choosing the type of prosthetic valve. For older patients, the risk of anticoagulation may be greater than the risk of another operation to replace a bioprosthetic valve. For women of childbearing age, the risks of anticoagulation during pregnancy should be considered in selecting the type of prosthetic heart valve.

1. Mechanical prosthetic heart valves—Mechanical prosthetic heart valves include caged-ball, unileaflet tilting-disk, and bileaflet tilting-disk prosthesis. Caged-ball-prosthetic valves are no longer implanted, and patients with these valves are rarely seen. Although flow characteristics vary, all prosthetic valves are foreign material (the sewing ring and the mechanical portions of the prosthesis) placed in the central circulation, providing a potential nidus for thrombus formation. The underlying pathologic process, as well as atrial fibrillation and decreased systolic performance of the left ventricle are important risk factors for post-implant thromboembolism. The risk of thromboembolism varies for the different types of mechanical prosthetic valves. The lowest risk is for the bileaflet tilting-disk and the highest risk is for the caged-ball valves.

The thromboembolic rate of patients with mechanical valves treated with moderate or high intensity anticoagulation is similar. However, the hemorrhagic risk is much higher for those receiving high intensity anticoagulation. Antiplatelet agents may be used in combination with warfarin. The addition of aspirin to warfarin has been shown to lower the incidence of thromboembolism, with some increase in the occurrence of hemorrhagic complications.

Current ACCP recommendations for anticoagulant therapy in patients with a mechanical heart valve are as follows: (1) For patients who have had an aortic valve replacement with a St. Jude or CarboMedics bileaflet valves or a Medtronic Hall unileaflet valve, warfarin with a target INR of 2.0–3.0 should be given. (2) For patients who have had a mitral valve replacement with either a unileaflet or bileaflet valve, warfarin should be given with a target INR of 2.5–3.5. Aspirin in doses of 75–100 mg should be added for patients with high-risk factors for thromboembolism, such as atrial fibrillation, myocardial infarction, or low left ventricular ejection fraction or in patients who have had a systemic embolism despite warfarin with therapeutic INRs.

The AHA/ACC guidelines differ slightly. They recommend that aspirin be used in addition to warfarin in all patients with mechanical valve prosthesis. In patients with bileaflet tilting-disk valves, warfarin should be given with a target INR of

2.5–3.5 for the first 3 months after aortic valve replacement. Subsequently, the target INR should be 2.0–3.0. There is less certain evidence for high-risk patients who cannot take aspirin, that clopidogrel, 75 mg daily, may be substituted or that warfarin be increased to a target INR of 3.0–4.0.

The European College of Cardiology recommends warfarin therapy for mechanical valves based on the thrombogenicity of the different types of valves. For low-risk valves (bileaflet tilting-disk), they recommend a target INR of 2.0–3.0. For intermediate-risk valves (unileaflet tilting-disk), they recommend a target INR of 2.5–3.5. For high-risk valves (caged-ball), they also recommend a target INR of 3.0–4.0, without other risk factors and 3.5–4.5 if there are other risk factors. They recommend the addition of antiplatelet therapy for concurrent arterial disease, coronary artery stenting, recurrent thromboembolism despite treatment of other risk factors and optimization of anticoagulation for caged-ball valves. Table 29–5 summarizes anticoagulation recommendations for mechanical prosthetic heart valves.

An embolic event is the most common adverse consequence seen as a result of thrombosis of a mechanical prosthetic heart valve. Although less frequent, the consequences of hemodynamic compromise resulting from prosthetic valve thrombosis can be insidious or acutely life-threatening. Thrombi affecting mechanical prosthetic valves can either obstruct or prevent closure of the valve. Pannus formation on the sewing ring of the prosthetic valve can cause similar hemodynamic compromise and may be a nidus for thrombus. TTE and TEE are the most sensitive and specific diagnostic tests. Fluoroscopic imaging of prosthetic valve motion can also be useful. According to ACCP guidelines, emergency surgery is reasonable for patients with a thrombosed left-sided prosthetic valve with functional class III–IV symptoms or a large clot burden. Thrombolytic therapy may be considered as first-line therapy for patients with a thrombosed left-sided prosthetic valve and functional class I–II symptoms. Thrombolytic therapy may be considered as first-line therapy in any patient with a left-sided prosthetic valve if emergency surgery is considered to be too high of a risk or is not available. Thrombolytic therapy is reasonable for a thrombosed right-sided prosthetic heart valve in a patient with functional class III–IV symptoms. Unfractionated heparin may be considered an alternative to thrombolytic therapy in a patient with a thrombosed prosthetic valve with a low clot burden and functional class I–II symptoms.

2. Bioprosthetic heart valves—Despite the advantages of bioprosthetic valves in terms of central flow and less-thrombogenic valve material, thromboembolic complications do occur, particularly in the early postoperative period. The presumed mechanism in this setting is thrombus formation on the sewing ring. A randomized trial of two intensities of anticoagulation following bioprosthetic valve replacement showed similar rates of thromboembolism but fewer hemorrhagic complications for low-intensity anticoagulation. In the first 3 months following bioprosthetic valve replacement, warfarin is recommended with a target INR of 2.0–3.0. Unfractionated heparin or LMWH should be given postoperatively until the INR is therapeutic for 2 days. Long-term treatment with warfarin is not necessary following bioprosthetic valve replacement in patients who are in sinus rhythm. Long-term therapy with aspirin is recommended for these patients. If atrial fibrillation is present, these patients should receive warfarin, as the rate of thromboembolism is high without its use. The AHA/ACC Guidelines recommend that patients with a mitral bioprosthesis and risk factors (atrial fibrillation, prior thromboembolic event, left ventricular dysfunction and a hypercoagulable state) should receive warfarin with a target INR goal of 2.0–3.0. It is also recommended that patients with a bioprosthetic valve receive aspirin in addition to warfarin, if high-risk factors are present. Table 29–6 summarizes general recommendations for anticoagulants with bioprosthetic valves.

D. Left Ventricular Thrombus

Left ventricular thrombi can complicate myocardial infarction and nonischemic dilated cardiomyopathy. In acute and remote myocardial infarction, the risk factors for the embolization of ventricular thrombus include anterior myocardial infarction, apical wall motion abnormality, and left ventricular ejection fraction < 40%. No reperfusion in acute myocar-

Table 29–5. Anticoagulation for Mechanical Prosthetic Valves.

Type of Mechanical Prosthetic Valve	Goal of Anticoagulation[1]
Aortic bileaflet tilting disk	INR 2.0–3.0
Aortic unileaflet tilting disk	INR 2.5–3.5
Aortic caged-ball	INR 3.0–4.0
Mitral bileaflet tilting disk	INR 2.5–3.5
Mitral unileaflet tilting disk	INR 2.5–3.5
Mitral caged-ball	INR 3.0–4.0

[1]Add antiplatelet agent if additional risk factors.
INR, international normalized ratio.

Table 29–6. Anticoagulation for Bioprosthetic Valves.

Postoperative Criteria	Anticoagulation
For first 3 months after surgery	Warfarin INR 2–3
After 3 months	
No atrial fibrillation	Aspirin, 325 mg/day
Aortic + atrial fibrillation	Warfarin, INR 2.0–3.0[1]
Mitral + atrial fibrillation	Warfarin, INR 2.0–3.0[1]

[1]Add antiplatelet agent for additional risk factors.

dial infarction is an additional risk factor. In dilated cardiomyopathy, left ventricular ejection fraction < 40% is a risk factor for embolization of left ventricular thrombus. Risk factors for embolization of left ventricular thrombus include protruding or mobile thrombus, a low left ventricular ejection fraction (< 40%), and less than 3 months after acute infarction.

1. Acute myocardial infarction—Postmortem findings of patients with acute myocardial infarction before the reperfusion era indicated a high incidence of left ventricular thrombi, pulmonary and systemic emboli, and coronary artery thrombi. Although embolic events were uncommon, they were frequently devastating, since most (> 80%) were to the central nervous system (87% occur between days 5 and 21 following infarction). The risk of systemic emboli can be decreased with long-term oral anticoagulation, with relatively low risk of hemorrhagic complications. Risk stratification, to identify high- and low-risk groups for the development of thrombus and embolism, can improve the efficacy of anticoagulation following infarction.

Echocardiographic studies have shown thrombus formation to be more common in patients with anterior than inferior myocardial infarction. An even higher risk group can be identified by analysis of the left ventricular apex. Patients with anterior infarction and akinesia or dyskinesia of the apex are at highest risk. On the basis of clinical and echocardiographic data, there appears to be good rationale for long-term (3 months) treatment with oral anticoagulants following anterior infarction in patients who did not receive or achieve reperfusion therapy. Significantly fewer left ventricular thrombi and fewer embolic events develop in patients receiving therapeutic doses of UFH following acute anterior infarction than in those treated with low-dose or no UFH. Studies of long-term oral anticoagulation following infarction have documented that anticoagulant therapy reduces the incidence of stroke and systemic emboli, although most did not report results based on infarct location.

For patients with anterior infarction, with apical akinesis or dyskinesia and reduced left ventricular function, who have not received reperfusion therapy in the form of thrombolytic therapy or percutaneous intervention, initial anticoagulation with UFH followed by warfarin to maintain an INR of 2.0–3.0 for 3 months, in addition to low-dose aspirin (81–162 mg/day), may be given because most systemic emboli occur during this interval. After that time, aspirin (325 mg/day) should be given, particularly if no intracardiac thrombus can be seen by echocardiography.

Because the incidence of ischemic stroke is so low in patients receiving reperfusion therapy, either with thrombolytic or direct percutaneous intervention, it is unclear whether the risk-benefit ratio favors short- or long-term anticoagulation therapy for 3 months following infarction. A reasonable approach is clinical evaluation and echocardiography before the patient is discharged from the hospital. Those with inferior infarction or anterior infarction without akinesia or dyskinesia of the apex and with good left ventricular function should be treated with aspirin alone. Patients with left ventricular thrombus on echocardiography are at high risk for thromboembolism, and oral anticoagulation should be given for a period of 3 months to maintain an INR of 2.0–3.0. If repeat echocardiography shows resolution of the thrombus at 3 months, oral anticoagulation can be stopped. Aspirin and clopidogrel are usually prescribed for patients who have undergone percutaneous coronary intervention with placement of a stent. If warfarin is also prescribed for other indications, there is concern that the risk of bleeding is high. Although there is little evidence to guide therapy, many interventional cardiologists recommend all three agents for a given period, while others use warfarin and clopidogrel and withhold aspirin until clopidogrel is discontinued.

2. Remote infarction with thrombus—Antithrombotic management of remote myocardial infarction (more than 3 months after the acute event) is controversial. Although traditional studies have not indicated a high risk of embolization, some reports indicate that thrombus detected at least 3 months following infarction still carries a risk for embolism. For patients with remote infarction and left ventricular thrombus seen on echocardiography, treatment with warfarin to maintain an INR of 2.0–3.0 is recommended. A repeat echocardiogram at 3 months can be used to determine whether treatment with warfarin should be continued.

3. Left ventricular aneurysm—Although an uncommon complication of myocardial infarction in the reperfusion era, left ventricular aneurysm provides the necessary substrate for thrombus formation (see Figure 29–1). These aneurysms frequently contain thrombus, but systemic embolization is unusual. It is hypothesized that the low incidence of systemic emboli noted when left ventricular thrombus is contained within a discrete aneurysm relates to a smaller surface area of the clot being exposed to circulating blood. It is unclear whether patients with left ventricular aneurysm warrant long-term anticoagulant therapy, particularly if the aneurysm contains flat thrombi. However, documented systemic embolization in patients with left ventricular aneurysm and thrombus should certainly prompt therapeutic anticoagulation to maintain an INR of 2.0–3.0. Recurrent embolization despite therapeutic anticoagulation in this setting is an indication for left ventricular aneurysmectomy.

4. Dilated cardiomyopathy—Dilated cardiomyopathy may be the end result of many types of heart disease. Characteristically, generalized four-chamber cardiac enlargement is present with right and left ventricular dysfunction that can cause stasis in any cardiac chamber. These patients have a high incidence of intracardiac thrombi, particularly in the left ventricle and a high incidence of systemic emboli. In one clinical study, atrial fibrillation was shown to be the only independent predictor for thromboembolism in dilated cardiomyopathy. Another study stressed the importance of severe depression of left ventricular function as a predictor.

The characteristics and the embolic potential of left ventricular thrombi in dilated cardiomyopathy and those in left ventricular aneurysm seem to differ. In dilated cardiomyopathy, left ventricular thrombi have a tendency to protrude and thus expose a greater surface area to circulating blood (see Figure 29–2). Several studies have indicated that thrombi that protrude into the left ventricular cavity or demonstrate free intracavitary motion are associated with a high risk of embolic events. Thrombi in left ventricular aneurysms are frequently mural and contained within the aneurysm; exposure to circulating blood is minimal because of both their containment and flat shape; patients with these features are at low risk for embolization.

Unlike acute infarction, the natural history of left ventricular thrombus complicating dilated cardiomyopathy is unclear because no clinically apparent event marks the initiation of thrombus development. The studies of intracardiac thrombi complicating dilated cardiomyopathy have, in general, consisted of small numbers of patients, varying definitions of dilated cardiomyopathy, varying proportions of patients with coronary artery disease and incomplete reporting of anticoagulation status. Aggregate analyses of these clinical and echocardiographic studies indicate that anticoagulation can reduce the thromboembolic rate. Anticoagulation following a thromboembolic event also appears effective as a secondary prevention measure.

Patients with dilated cardiomyopathy are at highest risk for thromboembolic complications if they have atrial fibrillation, severe left ventricular dysfunction with fractional shortening of less than 10%, previous thromboembolism, or left ventricular thrombus documented by imaging techniques. For patients with these high-risk characteristics, therapeutic warfarin is recommended to maintain an INR of 2.0–3.0.

E. Aortic Atheroma

The aortic arch and descending aorta can be visualized by TEE. Aortic atheroma detected by this technique have been identified as a cause of embolic stroke. In the Stroke Prevention in Atrial Fibrillation Trial, patients who underwent TEE had a 35% incidence of complex aortic plaque greater than 4 mm thick. The risk of stroke at 1 year in these patients was 12–20%. The risk of stroke in patients with atrial fibrillation without complex aortic plaque was 1.2%. Studies have shown that plaque size greater than 4 mm thick and the absence of calcification increase the risk of ischemic events.

Treatment of complex aortic plaque for the primary and secondary prevention of embolic strokes is controversial. One study prospectively compared antiplatelet agents to oral anticoagulants and found a sixfold-higher risk of combined events in patients treated with antiplatelet agents. In another study, patients with complex aortic plaques were evaluated for embolic events. Those treated with hydroxymethylglutaryl coenzyme A (HMG-CoA) reductase inhibitors to lower cholesterol had a significantly lower risk of embolic events than those taking warfarin or aspirin. The ACCP recommends that patients with mobile aortic atheroma and plaques > 4 mm as measured by TEE receive warfarin.

F. Paradoxical Emboli Associated with Patent Foramen Ovale (see Figure 29–4)

Intracardiac shunts have the potential to allow for venoarterial or paradoxical emboli. These shunts may be predominately left to right but there may also be right to left shunting under certain circumstances, such as cough or Valsalva maneuver, which temporarily raises and then lowers intrathoracic pressure increasing right atrial flow. Patent foramen ovale is quite common, occurring in up to 15–20% of the population. Asymptomatic patent foramen ovale can be detected on TTE and TEE. The ACCP recommends that asymptomatic patients should not be treated with anticoagulants. Patients who have an unexplained systematic embolism or transient ischemic attack and demonstrate venous thrombosis or pulmonary embolism and are found to have a patent foramen ovale on echocardiography should be treated with long-term warfarin to maintain an INR of 2.0–3.0 unless patent foramen ovale closure (either surgically or percutaneously) is performed.

G. Pacemakers, Implantable Cardioverter Defibrillators, and Other Intracardiac Devices

Anticoagulant therapy is not usually considered for patients with pacemakers and implantable cardioverter-defibrillators (ICDs). However, a number of thromboembolic complications can occur. The intravascular and intracardiac leads used in these devices are foreign bodies that can act as a nidus for thrombus formation. On rare occasions, swelling of the arm on the side of implantation may develop. Ultrasound or venography may indicate obstruction of the subclavian vein. The treatment for subclavian vein thrombosis is UFH followed by oral anticoagulation. The duration of treatment with anticoagulants varies but is usually for at least 3 months.

Transesophageal echocardiography has demonstrated a high incidence of thrombi on long-term pacing and ICD leads. Often these thrombi are highly mobile. Differentiation from infective endocarditis is mandatory, since the clinical approach and treatment will be affected. The risk for embolization (presumably to the pulmonary artery or systemically if there is a patent foramen ovale) is unknown. There are no guidelines for treating these thrombi with anticoagulation or for removal of the device. If embolic events have occurred or there are other high-risk factors for thromboembolism, it seems reasonable to treat with oral anticoagulants. Followup TEE seems reasonable after at least 3 months of therapeutic anticoagulation to determine whether the thrombus has resolved. There is little evidence or experience to guide the duration of treatment.

Technological advances are leading to the implantation of other new intracardiac devices. Since these devices are foreign bodies, they can act as a nidus for thrombus formation. Percutaneous devise closure of atrial septal defects is available. Current anticoagulation recommendations are for aspirin and clopidogrel for 3 months following the procedure. Warfarin is not recommended. Devices for percutaneous occlusion of the left atrial appendage are currently being investigated in those with nonvalvular atrial fibrillation; the strategy behind these devices is to avoid long-term anticoagulation. These devices are not yet available.

American College of Cardiology; American Heart Association Task Force on Practice Guidelines (Writing Committee to revise the 1998 guidelines for the management of patients with valvular heart disease); Society of Cardiovascular Anesthesiologists, Bonow RO et al. ACC/AHA 2006 guidelines for the management of patients with valvular heart disease: a report of the American College of Cardiology/American Heart Association Task Force on Practice Guidelines (writing Committee to Revise the 1998 guidelines for the management of patients with valvular heart disease) developed in collaboration with the Society of Cardiovascular Anesthesiologists endorsed by the Society for Cardiovascular Angiography and Interventions and the Society of Thoracic Surgeons. J Am Coll Cardiol. 2006 Aug 1;48(3):e1–148. [PMID: 16875962]

Bates SM et al. Use of antithrombotic agents during pregnancy: the Seventh ACCP Conference on Antithrombotic and Thrombolytic Therapy. Chest. 2004 Sep;126(3 Suppl)627S–644S. [PMID: 15383488]

Fuster V et al; American College of Cardiology/American Heart Association Task Force on Practice Guidelines; European Society of Cardiology Committee for Practice Guidelines; European Heart Rhythm Association; Heart Rhythm Society. ACC/AHA/ESC 2006 Guidelines for the Management of Patients with Atrial Fibrillation: a report of the American College of Cardiology/American Heart Association Task Force on Practice Guidelines and the European Society of Cardiology Committee for Practice Guidelines (Writing Committee to Revise the 2001 Guidelines for the Management of Patients With Atrial Fibrillation): developed in collaboration with the European Heart Rhythm Association and the Heart Rhythm Society. Circulation. 2006 Aug 15;114(7):e257–354. [PMID: 16908781]

Gage BF et al. Validation of clinical classification schemes for predicting stroke: results from the National Registry of Atrial Fibrillation. JAMA. 2001 Jun 13;285(22):2864–70. [PMID: 11401607]

Klein AL et al; Assessment of Cardioversion Using Transesophageal Echocardiography Investigators. Use of transesophageal echocardiography to guide cardioversion in patients with atrial fibrillation. N Engl J Med. 2001 May 10;344(19):1411–20. [PMID: 11346805]

Korkeila PJ et al. Transesophageal echocardiography in the diagnosis of thrombosis associated with permanent transvenous pacemaker electrodes. Pacing Clin Electrophysiol. 2006 Nov;29(11):1245–50. [PMID: 17100678]

Singer DE et al. Antithrombotic therapy in atrial fibrillation: the Seventh ACCP Conference on Antithrombotic and Thrombolytic Therapy. Chest. 2004 Sep;126(3 Suppl):429S–456S. [PMID: 15383480]

Van Gelder IC et al; Rate Control versus Electrical Cardioversion for Persistent Atrial Fibrillation Study Group. A comparison of rate control and rhythm control in patients with recurrent persistent atrial fibrillation. N Engl J Med. 2002 Dec 5;347(23):1834–40. [PMID: 12466507]

Wyse DG et al; Atrial Fibrillation Follow-up Investigation of Rhythm Management (AFFIRM) Investigators. A comparison of rate control and rhythm control in patients with atrial fibrillation. N Engl J Med. 2002 Dec 5;347(23):1825–33. [PMID: 12466506]

H. Special Considerations

1. Pregnancy—Warfarin use during pregnancy represents a significant risk of both maternal and fetal complications. Warfarin crosses the placenta and can cause an embryopathy, especially when used between the sixth and twelfth weeks of gestation. Fetal central nervous system abnormalities may occur with maternal warfarin use in any trimester. Unfractionated heparin and LMWH do not cross the placenta, and therefore, their use in pregnancy may be safer for the fetus. However, both are expensive, difficult to administer and are associated with risks of bleeding, osteoporosis and HIT (much less likely with LMWH). Low-dose aspirin (< 150 mg/daily) is considered safe in the second and third trimesters. Warfarin, UFH, and LMWH can safely be administered to the nursing mother, as they do not have an anticoagulant effect in breastfed infants.

When a patient who is receiving long-term warfarin therapy is planning a pregnancy, risks for the fetus should be considered. One approach would be to perform frequent pregnancy tests and substitute UFH or LMWH for warfarin when the patient becomes pregnant. The second approach is to replace warfarin with UFH or LMWH before conception is attempted.

The most common cardiac condition requiring anticoagulation during pregnancy is mechanical prosthetic heart valves. Three different approaches for anticoagulation during pregnancy were evaluated in a review of a number of prospective and retrospective studies (none were randomized): (1) Warfarin throughout the pregnancy. (2) Warfarin throughout pregnancy except replaced by UFH from the sixth through twelfth weeks. Warfarin was then restarted and used throughout the remainder of pregnancy. (3) Unfractionated heparin throughout the pregnancy.

The lowest risk for prosthetic valve thrombosis or systemic embolization was with warfarin use throughout pregnancy, but this strategy was associated with embryopathy in 6.4% of newborns. It appears that warfarin may place the fetus at more risk and the mother at less risk. It is difficult to know if the higher incidence of thrombotic complications with UFH were due to inadequate dosing. There is very little data on the efficacy of LMWH in preventing thrombotic complications during pregnancy. There are medicolegal concerns with the use of warfarin during pregnancy, although it is commonly used in Europe.

The ACCP recommends that women with prosthetic heart valves who are pregnant and routinely require long-term anticoagulants receive adjusted dose LMWH twice a day throughout pregnancy with doses adjusted to keep 4-hour post-injection anti-Xa level at approximately 1.0 to 1.2 units/mL or according to weight. An alternative regimen is for UFH throughout pregnancy in doses adjusted to keep the aPTT at least twice control or to attain an anti-Xa level of 0.35 to 0.70 units/mL. An alternative regimen is to use UFH or LMWH for the first 12 weeks of pregnancy, warfarin until the middle of the third trimester, and then UFH or LMWH for the remainder of the pregnancy. Low-dose aspirin can be added if there are additional high-risk factors. Anticoagulation may be interrupted briefly for delivery and resumed postpartum.

Women of childbearing age who need to have a prosthetic heart valve should consider their desire to become pregnant when making a decision of the type of valve to be implanted. A bioprosthetic valve or native valve repair, which does not require lifelong anticoagulation, would be safer in terms of anticoagulation and pregnancy risks.

2. Interruption of anticoagulation for surgery and invasive procedures—At times anticoagulant therapy needs to be interrupted because of surgery or other invasive procedures. The anticoagulant effects of warfarin persist for several days. During this period, there may be a period of time in which there is inadequate protection from thromboembolism.

Elective and planned surgery and procedures allow for a systematic approach to dealing with anticoagulation issues. Anticoagulants may need to be stopped for the procedure or surgery, and this may place the patient at risk for thromboembolic complications.

The risk of thromboembolism when warfarin is discontinued varies in different cardiac conditions. In each year after the discontinuation of warfarin, the risk of thrombotic complications are as follows: 1% for lone atrial fibrillation and 5% for nonvalvular atrial fibrillation (low risk); 12% for high-risk atrial fibrillation and 10–12% for St. Jude prosthetic aortic valve (intermediate risk); and 22% for a mitral mechanical prosthetic valve and up to 91% for multiple mechanical prosthetic valves (high risk). The recommended approach for periprocedure anticoagulation for low-risk patients is to stop warfarin 4 days before and to restart UFH or LMWH after the procedure (Table 29–7). (Low dose UFH or LMWH can be used before the procedure.) For intermediate-risk patients, the recommended approach is to stop warfarin 4 days before the procedure and start full dose UFH or LMWH 2 days before the procedure. Unfractionated heparin can be stopped 4 hours prior to the procedure. After the procedure, UFH or LMWH and warfarin are started. For high-risk patients, warfarin should be stopped 4 days prior to the procedure with either UFH (target a PTT of two times control) or LMWH started when the INR is 2.0. Unfractionated heparin can be stopped 4 hours prior to the procedure. Anticoagulation with UFH or LMWH and warfarin should be resumed as soon as possible after surgery. The risk for bleeding varies for different procedures. For procedures with a low risk for bleeding,

Table 29–7. Interruption of Anticoagulation for Surgery or Invasive Procedures.

Procedure	Recommendation
Atrial fibrillation and aortic bileaflet prosthesis	Stop warfarin 4 days before procedure
	Restart after the procedure as soon as it is safe
All other mechanical valve prosthesis[1]	Stop warfarin 3-4 days before the procedure
	Start unfractionated heparin when INR = 2.0
	Stop unfractionated heparin 4-6 hours before procedure
	Restart unfractionated heparin and warfarin after the procedure as soon as it is safe

[1]Mitral bileaflet prosthesis, aortic and mitral unileaflet prosthesis, aortic and mitral ball-cage prosthesis.

an INR of 1.5 may be acceptable. Dental procedures generally do not require stopping warfarin.

The ACC/AHA have established guidelines for bridging anticoagulant therapy in patients with mechanical prosthetic valves. For patients who are at low risk for thrombosis (bileaflet tilting-disk prosthetic aortic valves and no additional risk factors for thromboembolism), warfarin should be stopped 48–72 hours before the procedure to allow the INR to fall below 1.5. Warfarin should be restarted 24 hours after the procedure. Bridging with UFH or LMWH is not necessary. For patients who are at high risk for thrombosis (mechanical aortic valve with risk factors for thromboembolism or any mechanical mitral valve prosthesis), warfarin should be stopped more than 72 hours before the procedure; therapeutic doses of intravenous UFH should be started when the INR falls below 2.0 (usually 48 hours before the procedure); UFH is stopped 4–6 hours before the procedure. Unfractionated heparin and warfarin are restarted as soon after the procedure as possible and UFH is stopped when the INR is therapeutic.

Emergency surgery and procedures require a different approach, which usually demands immediate reversal of warfarin effects with fresh frozen plasma or prothrombin concentrate (does not require a large volume load) and restarting anticoagulants when the bleeding risk is acceptably low. The use of vitamin K is discouraged because it may cause a hypercoagulable state.

Kovacs MJ et al. Single-arm study of bridging therapy with low-molecular-weight heparin for patients at risk of arterial embolism who require temporary interruption of warfarin. Circulation. 2004 Sep 21;110(12):1658–63. [PMID: 15364803]

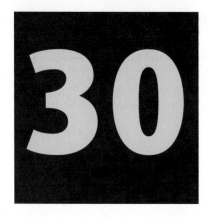

Cardiac Tumors

Bill P.C. Hsieh, MD &

Rita F. Redberg, MD, MSc, FACC, FAHA

▶ An uncommon but important differential diagnosis of cardiac masses.

▶ Diagnosis is suspected by history, physical examination, and imaging characteristics and confirmed by biopsy of mass.

▶ General Considerations

Cardiac tumors arise either as a primary tumor of the heart or more commonly from metastasis of a distant noncardiac primary tumor. Because of the low incidence and nonspecific clinical manifestations, cardiac tumors have often been diagnosed incidentally during evaluation of a seemingly unrelated problem or misdiagnosed as other cardiac conditions. A high index of suspicion in combination with characteristic cardiovascular imaging study are essential for rapid identification of cardiac tumors.

A. Metastatic Cardiac Tumors

Metastatic cardiac tumors are about 40 times more common than primary tumors. Cardiac metastases occur in approximately 5% of patients who die of malignant tumors and are often present as pericardial effusions; myocardial, coronary, and intracavitary involvement occurs with less frequency. The tumor that most often metastasizes to the heart is disseminated malignant melanoma, which occurs in 50–65% of afflicted patients. Other tumors with high predilection for cardiac metastasis are bronchogenic carcinoma, breast cancer, renal cell carcinoma, mesothelioma (by direct extension or hematogenous spread), and lymphoma and leukemia (by lymphatic spread). Rarely, adenocarcinoma of the colon can metastasize to the heart by lymphatic or hematogenous spread, usually affecting first the pericardium and then the myocardium. Cardiac metastases that occur in patients with

colon cancer are usually preceded by involvement of other organs. Metastases to the endocardium have been reported in renal cell carcinoma, adenocarcinoma of the stomach, laryngeal carcinoma, pancreatic cancer, and mucinous adenocarcinoma of the cecum and of the ovary. Renal cell carcinomas can extend into the inferior vena cava, and the tumor thrombus occasionally involves the right atrium (Figure 30–1).

B. Primary Tumors

Primary tumors of the heart are rare, with an incidence from 0.001% to 0.28% reported in unselected autopsy studies. Although myxoma is the most frequent tumor type in adults, rhabdomyomas represent the most common type in the pediatric population.

1. Benign—The majority (75–80%) of primary cardiac tumors are benign and therefore potentially curable (Table 30–1).

McAllister HA, Hall RJ, et al. Tumors of the heart and pericardium. Cur Probl Cardiol 1999;24:57–116. [PMID: 10028128]

A. MYXOMAS—These tumors account for approximately half of benign cardiac tumors and are usually found in patients between 30 and 60 years old, with a mean age of onset of 51 years. They occur predominantly in women; although most are isolated or sporadic, they can also be familial or complex. Less than 10% of myxomas are familial and are apparently transmitted in an autosomal-dominant pattern. Familial myxoma presents earlier in life, with a mean age of onset of 25 years. Complex cardiac myxomas or the familial Carney complex may include such features as multiple pigmented skin lesions (lentigines), myxoid fibroadenomas of the breast, tumors of the pituitary and testes, and primary pigmented nodular adrenocortical disease. Carney complex appears to be genetically heterogenous with gene localization on chromosome 2p16 and chromosome 17q24. The majority of Carney complex appears to be caused by a mutation in the *PRKAR1α* gene that encodes the R1α regulatory subunit of the cyclic adenosine monophosphate-dependent protein kinase A (PKA). Patients with familial

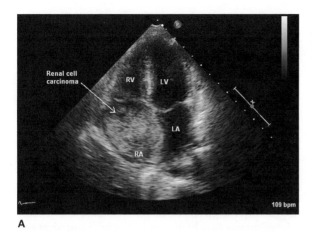

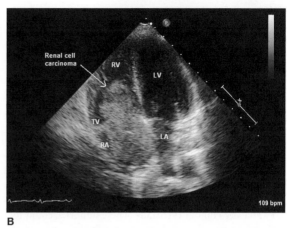

A

B

▲ **Figure 30-1.** Transthoracic echocardiogram in a 65-year-old man with a history of renal cell carcinoma in whom dyspnea and lower extremity edema developed. **A:** The apical four-chamber view shows a large mass most likely representing metastatic renal cell carcinoma in the right atrium. **B:** During diastole, the tumor prolapses through the tricuspid valve. LA, left atrium; LV, left ventricle; RA, right atrium; RV, right ventricle; TV, tricuspid valve.

or complex myxomas are more likely than those with sporadic myxomas to have multiple (30–50%) and recurrent (12–22%) tumors. This occasional recurrence of myxomas and a few reported cases of invasion of surrounding tissue by the tumor suggest that myxomas have some low-grade malignant features.

Macroscopically, myxomas are pedunculated and gelatinous in consistency; the surface may be smooth, irregular, or friable. Friable or villous, myxomas are associated with a higher risk of embolization, whereas larger tumors with a smooth surface tend to present with obstructive cardiovascular symptoms. Microscopically, myxoma is characterized by islands of tumor cells with variable shapes, round, elongated, or polyhedral scattered throughout pale staining extracellular matrix. The tumor cells are thought to be derived from mesenchymal cardiomyogenic precursor cells.

Most myxomas (74%) occur in the left atrium, although they can occur in any chamber (right atrium, 18%; right ventricle, 4%; left ventricle, 4%) or on any valve. They often arise from the endocardial surface of the left atrium with a stalk attached to the interatrial septum close to the fossa ovalis (Figure 30–2). When a myxoma occurs in the ventricles, it almost always originates from the free wall. Although asymp-

Table 30-1. Primary Cardiac Neoplasms.

Benign
Myxoma
Papillary fibroelastoma
Lipoma
Fibroma
Rhabdomyoma
Hamartoma
Hemangiomas
Malignant
Sarcoma
Lymphoma
Malignant fibrous histiocytoma
Benign or Malignant
Mesothelioma
Paraganglioma

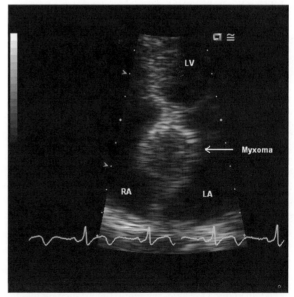

▲ **Figure 30-2.** Transthoracic echocardiogram in an apical four-chamber view showing a mass in the interatrial septum. The mass was resected and found to be an atrial myxoma.

tomatic myxomas have been recognized, most patients experience one or more effects from the classic triad of constitutional, embolic, and obstructive manifestations. (For details, refer to the section on Clinical Findings.)

Kirschner LS et al. Mutations of the gene encoding the protein kinase A type I-alpha regulatory subunit in patients with the Carney complex. Nat Genet. 2000 Sep;26(1):89–92. [PMID: 10973256]

Kodama H et al. Cardiomyogenic differentiation in cardiac myxoma expressing lineage-specific transcription factors. Am J Pathol. 2002 Aug;161(2):381–89. [PMID: 12163362]

Vaughan CJ et al. Tumors and the heart: molecular genetic advances. Curr Opin Cardiol. 2001 May;16(3):195–200. [PMID: 11357016]

B. PAPILLARY FIBROELASTOMAS—These tumors account for 7–8% of cardiac tumors. They are usually discovered postmortem, with an autopsy incidence of 0.002–0.33% although their premorbid detection rate is rising with the increasing use of echocardiography (Figure 30–3). They are usually found in patients older than 60 years of age, although they have been reported in patients from 3 to 86 years old. A profusion of names—cardiac papilloma, papillary fibroma, giant Lambl excrescence, and papillary endocardial tumor—have been used to describe what is properly a papillary fibroelastoma. These tumors (first described as small filiform projections on the cusps of aortic valves) have multiple papillary fronds and look like a sea anemone, attached to the endocardial surface of the valves by a small pedicle.

Papillary fibroelastomas can form a nidus for platelet and fibrin aggregation and lead to systemic or cerebrovascular emboli. They are most commonly identified on the valves, arising on the left-sided valvular structures much more frequently than the right-sided ones. A literature review of 725 reported cases of papillary fibroelastoma found 44% of the tumors arising from the aortic valve, followed by mitral valve in 35%, tricuspid valve in 15% and pulmonary valve in 8%. Other less common locations, such as the chordae, papillary apparatuses, left ventricular septum, left ventricular outflow tract, left ventricular free wall, and the left atrium, have also been reported. Clinical manifestations include such conditions as cerebral embolism, myocardial infarction, sudden death, pulmonary embolism, and syncope. Surgical excision is generally recommended in the symptomatic individual. Mobile tumors have been suggested to be independent predictors of the occurrence of death or nonfatal embolization.

Gowda RM et al. Cardiac papillary fibroelastoma: a comprehensive analysis of 725 cases. Am Heart J. 2003 Sep;146(3):404–10. [PMID: 12947356]

Shahian DM. Papillary fibroelastomas. Semin Thorac Cardiovasc Surg. 2000 Apr;12(2):101–10. [PMID: 10807432]

Sun JP et al. Clinical and echocardiographic characteristics of papillary fibroelastomas: a retrospective and prospective study in 162 patients. Circulation. 2001 Jun 5;103(22):2687–93. [PMID: 11390338]

C. LIPOMAS—These tumors are a common benign cardiac tumor in adults, with a similar incidence to papillary elastoma. They occur as solitary, circumscribed, encapsulated

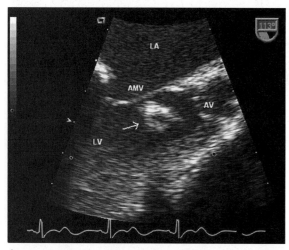

A

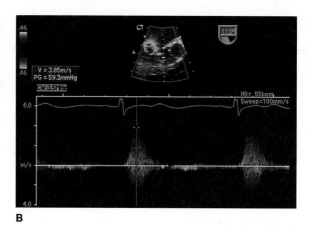

B

▲ **Figure 30–3.** Transesophageal echocardiogram to evaluate a mass found on a transthoracic echocardiogram in a 75-year-old man who suffered from dizziness. **A:** An irregular mass attached to the ventricular side of the anterior mitral leaflet is shown in this 113° long-axis view. The location on the downstream side of the valve and the frond-like surface are highly suggestive of a papillary fibroelastoma (*arrow*). **B:** Doppler signal demonstrating left ventricular outflow tract obstruction caused by the mass during systole. LA, left atrium; LV, left ventricle; AV, aortic valve; AMV, anterior mitral valve leaflet.

tumors with a wide range of size and weight. Being clinically silent, they are mostly found at autopsy. The typical locations are left ventricle (intramuscular, subendocardial, or subepicardial), right atrium, and interatrial septum.

D. Fibromas—Approximately three-quarters of all fibromas occur in the pediatric population. The second most common benign tumor of childhood, they have been reported in patients from age 2 to 57 years. Almost always solitary, fibromas can occur in any chamber but are most commonly found in the ventricular myocardium—usually in the anterior wall of the left ventricle and interventricular septum—and in the right ventricle (Figure 30–4). These tumors are often large, between 4 cm and 7 cm in diameter, and exert a mass effect. They are also associated with ventricular arrhythmias and heart failure; when arising from the ventricular septum, they can be associated with sudden death. Their size can make complete excision difficult.

E. Rhabdomyomas—Rhabdomyomas are the most common benign cardiac tumor in children, usually occurring before the age of 1 year. There are frequently multiple tumors, occurring equally in the right and left ventricles or the atria; the valves are spared (Figure 30–5). They range in size from a few millimeters to a few centimeters and are white to yellow. Rhabdomyomas are often associated with tuberous sclerosis, more frequently seen in those with mutations in *TSC2* gene compared to *TSC1*

gene. Spontaneous regression is well established in the pediatric population, although tumor enlargement and de novo appearance have been observed during puberty. Unless the patient is symptomatic, surgical intervention is often unnecessary. In fact, an intracavitary mass discovered incidentally in a pediatric patient is suggestive of rhabdomyoma until proven otherwise.

Jozwiak S et al. Clinical and genotype studies of cardiac tumors in 154 patients with tuberous sclerosis complex. Pediatrics. 2006 Oct;118(4):e1146–51. [PMID: 16940165]

F. Cardiac hamartomas (oncocytic cardiomyopathy)—Also known as histiocytoid cardiomyopathy or Purkinje cell hamartoma, these tumors are seen in children and infants. Hamartomas occur as flat sheets of cells on the endocardial or epicardial surfaces of the left ventricle and may present as ventricular arrhythmia. As many as 50% of cardiac hamartomas undergo involution with time, and recent data suggest that conservative management is appropriate. Controlling the arrhythmia medically, when possible, obviates the need for surgery.

G. Hemangiomas—Occurring in a wide age distribution from age 2 weeks to 65 years old, hemangiomas can be isolated or be in multiple locations. They are located in any of the cardiac chambers and have been associated with arrhythmias or sudden death.

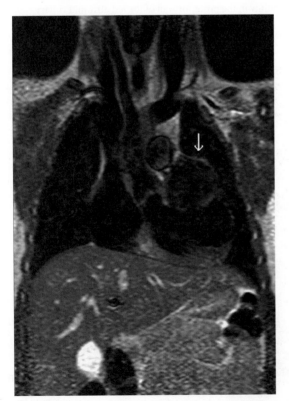

A

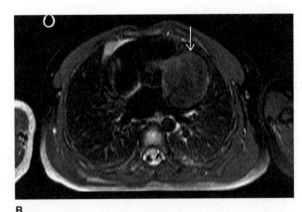

B

▲ **Figure 30–4. A:** Coronal T1-weighted spin-echo magnetic resonance image of the heart through the level of the left ventricular anterior wall and the aortic valve. A mass is visualized emanating from the anterior wall of the left ventricle (*arrow*). The mass is mildly heterogeneous with mild T1 hypointensity relative to the myocardium. **B:** Transaxial T1-weighted image obtained after gadolinium administration. It demonstrates predominantly peripheral enhancement. These findings are suggestive of a cardiac fibroma. (Courtesy of C Higgins.)

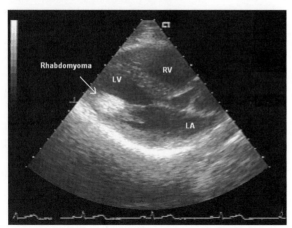

▲ **Figure 30–5.** Transthoracic echocardiogram in parasternal long-axis view showing a rhabdomyoma in the left ventricle of a patient with tuberous sclerosis. LA, left atrium; LV, left ventricle; RV, right ventricle.

Becker AE. Primary heart tumors in the pediatric age group: a review of salient pathologic features relevant for clinicians. Pediatr Cardiol. 2000 Jul–Aug;21(4):317–23. [PMID: 10865004]
Freedom RM et al. Selected aspects of cardiac tumors in infancy and childhood. Pediatr Cardiol. 2000 Jul–Aug;21(4):299–316. [PMID: 10865003]

2. Malignant—Twenty five percent of all primary cardiac tumors have malignant characteristics.

A. Sarcomas—These are the most common malignant cardiac tumors in adults with a predilection for men between the third and fifth decades. Angiosarcomas are the most common, followed by rhabdomyosarcomas, fibrosarcomas, and osteosar-comas. Because angiosarcomas usually occur in the right atrium or pericardium, right-sided failure, pericardial disease, or vena caval obstruction can be the presenting manifestations. The tumor is extensively infiltrative of cardiac structures, and metastatic spread at the time of diagnosis is common (Figure 30–6). The tumor can be diagnosed by lung biopsy if pulmonary metastases are present. Cardiac Kaposi sarcoma is a type of angiosarcoma found in immunocompromised individuals, such as those with AIDS. Angiosarcomas are usually found on the epicardial or pericardial surface. Rhabdomyosarcomas have been reported in all age groups with a male predominance; in children they constitute the most common malignant cardiac tumors. Fibrosarcomas have the characteristic "white fish flesh" appearance, composed of spindle cells. They occur equally in the left and right sides of the heart, are often multiple, extensively infiltrative, and protrude into a cardiac chamber or the pericardium. A valve is affected in half the cases. Osteosarcomas have been found in patients ranging in age from 24 to 67 years. They usually originate in the posterior wall of the left atrium, near the entrance of the pulmonary veins, and can be intramural or intracavitary. Osteosarcomas can metastasize to the thyroid, skin, and lungs. They exhibit the same gross and microscopic appearance as osteosarcoma of the bone. Leiomyosarcomas have rarely been reported in the heart. When they do occur, they are found in an older age group (older than 55 years) and mainly in the posterior wall of the left atrium. Primary cardiac liposarcomas occur in younger patients (28–37 years) and are found in the right atrium or left ventricle and on the mitral valve. Cardiac liposarcomas may also be metastatic in origin.

B. Lymphomas—Although cardiac involvement is seen (at autopsy) in 25% of patients with lymphoma, primary cardiac lymphoma is extremely rare. Largely composed of diffuse large B cell lymphoma, it can involve any area of the heart,

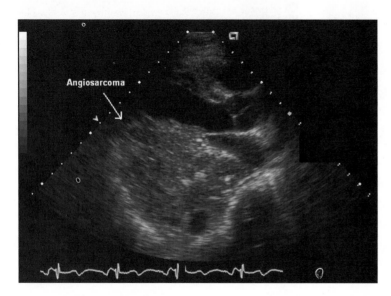

▲ **Figure 30–6.** Transthoracic echocardiogram in a 60-year-old woman who had a 2-month history of dyspnea and palpitations. A parasternal long-axis view shows an infiltrating mass involving the left ventricular posterior wall and left atrium. A biopsy of the mass showed angiosarcoma.

with the highest frequency arising from the right side of the heart, particularly the right atrium. The infiltrative nature of this disorder can lead to conduction abnormalities, large pericardial effusion, and even congestive heart failure symptoms from restriction. A review of 40 reported cases from the literature between 1995 and 2002 showed overall poor prognosis; only 38% of patients achieved complete remission with systemic therapy.

Ikeda H et al. Primary lymphoma of the heart: case report and literature review. Pathol Int. 2004 Mar;54(3):187–95. [PMID: 14989742]

Mejhert M et al. Primary lymphoma of the heart. Scand Cardiovasc J. 2000 Dec;34(6):606–8. [PMID: 11214017]

Tighe DA et al. Primary cardiac lymphoma. Echocardiography. 2000 May;17(4):345–7. [PMID: 10979005]

C. Malignant fibrous histiocytomas—These have been reported to occur in the heart, usually in the left atrium. These are very invasive tumors, with a high likelihood of recurrence after surgical resection.

Schena S et al. Survival following treatment of a cardiac malignant fibrous histiocytoma. Chest. 2000 Jul;118(1):271–3. [PMID: 10893397]

3. Tumors that may be benign or malignant

A. Mesotheliomas—These pericardial tumors present with pericarditis, tamponade, or constriction. Benign mesotheliomas of the atrioventricular node may produce heart block. There is a 2:1 male predominance, and adults are most frequently afflicted. Pericardial mesotheliomas usually cover most of the parietal and visceral surfaces encasing the heart, with only superficial invasion of adjacent myocardium. Unlike pleural mesotheliomas, pericardial mesotheliomas are not linked to asbestos exposure.

Vander Salm TJ. Unusual primary tumors of the heart. Semin Thorac Cardiovasc Surg. 2000 Apr;12(2):89–100. [PMID: 10807431]

B. Paraganglioma—These tumors can produce catecholamines and cause symptoms of heightened sympathetic activity. Most of the tumors originate from the visceral autonomic paraganglia of the left atrial wall. Because they are supplied by multiple cardiac blood vessels, complete excision is difficult. Perioperative α- and β-adrenergic blockade should be performed.

▶ Clinical Findings

A. Symptoms and Signs

Cardiac tumors are challenging to diagnose because there are no specifically identifiable symptoms. The anatomic location and size of the tumor rather than the histopathology determine the clinical findings (Table 30–2). For example, small intracavitary tumors that cause obstruction of flow may pro-

Table 30–2. Clinical Manifestations of Cardiac Neoplasm.

Endocardial
Thromboembolism: cerebral, coronary, pulmonary, systemic
Cavitary obliteration or outflow tract obstruction
Valve obstruction and valve damage
Constitutional manifestations
Myocardial
Arrhythmias, ventricular or atrial
Conduction abnormalities
Electrocardiographic changes
Systolic or diastolic left ventricular dysfunction
Coronary involvement: angina, infarction
Pericardial
Pericarditis and pain
Pericardial effusion
Arrhythmias
Tamponade
Constriction
Valvular
Valvular damage, obstruction, or regurgitation
Congestive heart failure
Sudden death or syncope

duce symptoms earlier than would large, infiltrative intramural tumors. In addition to producing obstruction, arrhythmias, and myocardial dysfunction, cardiac tumors (particularly myxomas, which produce interleukin-6) may also present with constitutional symptoms, such as weight loss, fatigue, fever, arthralgias, or symptoms and signs mimicking vasculitis.

1. Endocardial tumors—Endocardial tumors can lead to embolic events or events related to cardiac obstruction. Emboli may occur to the pulmonary, coronary, carotid, or peripheral circulation. Repeated embolization of right-sided tumors can cause cor pulmonale. Because of their endocardial attachment and mobility as well as the friability of the tumor, myxomas have an embolization rate of 30–40%. Half of these are cerebral emboli, which manifest themselves as transient ischemic attacks, cerebral vascular events, or seizures. Embolic events in a young person without another source should raise the suspicion for a myxoma.

Depending on which cardiac chamber the tumor is located, obstructive symptoms may include congestive heart failure, right-sided venous congestion, syncope, or valvular dysfunction. For example, left atrial myxoma can cause obstruction by intermittently occluding left ventricular inflow and becoming evident as syncope. Myxomas sometimes prolapse into the mitral orifice and cause mitral stenosis or regurgitation, or both.

2. Myocardial tumors—These most commonly cause arrhythmias or disturbances of conduction. For example, new atrioventricular conduction disturbances, such as complete heart block or asystole, can help diagnose a tumor near the atrioventricular node. Atrial fibrillation, atrial flutter, paroxysmal atrial tachycardia with or without block, junctional rhythm, premature ventricular contraction, ventricular tachycardia, and ventricular fibrillation may also be associated with cardiac tumors. Eighty percent of cases of malignant myocardial tumors show ST-segment elevation. There is a close correlation between the electrocardiographic (ECG) lead showing ST elevation and the anatomic location of the infiltration. Inversion of the T wave is a less sensitive and less specific marker of infiltration, occurring in 47% of such cases. When ST-T wave segments remain normal, the infiltration is generally limited to the right side of the heart. Unstable angina with persistent ST-segment elevation from compression of the left main coronary artery can be caused by metastatic lung cancer.

Being nonfunctional myocardium, intramural tumor infiltration can also cause myocardial systolic and diastolic dysfunction. If the tumor grows large enough to protrude into the cavity, mechanical obstruction can ensue.

> Krasuski RA et al. Cardiac rhabdomyoma in an adult patient presenting with ventricular arrhythmia. Chest. 2000 Oct;118(4): 1217–21. [PMID: 11035702]

3. Pericardial tumors—Pericardial tumors can lead to pericardial pain, constriction, pericardial tamponade, and symptoms related to the invasion of contiguous mediastinal structures. Pericardial invasion occurs most often with the contiguous spread of metastatic breast and lung cancers.

> Warren WH. Malignancies involving the pericardium. Semin Thorac Cardiovasc Surg. 2000 Apr;12(2):119–29. [PMID: 10807434]

4. Valvular tumors—These tumors can affect any of the four valves with equal frequency, and the presence of symptoms is common. Mitral valve tumors are more likely than aortic valve tumors to produce serious neurologic symptoms or sudden death. The most common type of valve tumor is the papillary fibroelastoma.

B. Physical Examination

1. Left atrial tumors—Physical findings may include signs of pulmonary congestion; a loud, widely split S_1; an S_4; a holosystolic murmur that is loudest at the apex; a diastolic murmur caused by the obstruction of the mitral valve orifice by the tumor; or a diastolic tumor "plop." The loud S_1 that occurs in patients with left atrial myxoma may be due to delayed mitral valve closure caused by prolapse of the tumor through the valvular orifice. This causes the left ventricular/left atrial pressure curves to intersect at a higher pressure, similar to what is seen in patients with mitral stenosis or a short PR interval. A marked spontaneous variation over short periods with changes in position is characteristic of the diastolic murmur associated with left atrial tumor. The tumor plop is thought to be created by the tumor hitting the endocardial wall or as the excursion of the tumor is halted. Although, in most cases, the plop occurs later than the opening snap of a stenotic mitral valve and earlier than an S_3; so, it can be difficult to distinguish these sounds. Physical findings consistent with mitral stenosis in a patient

without a history of rheumatic fever should raise the possibility of a left atrial tumor.

Overall, myxomas are associated with a mitral diastolic murmur in 75% of cases; mitral regurgitation murmur in 50%; pulmonary hypertension in 70%; right-sided heart failure in 70%; pulmonary emboli in 25%; anemia in 33%; elevated erythrocyte sedimentation rate in 33%; and a third heart sound (the tumor plop) in 33%.

2. Left ventricular tumors—These are often silent and do not become symptomatic until they grow to be quite large. Infiltrative tumors can present as conduction disturbances and arrhythmias.

3. Right atrial tumors—Sometimes associated with elevated jugular venous pressure or right-sided heart failure, right atrial tumors are also often clinically silent and asymptomatic until they become quite large. A diastolic rumble that varies with respiration should raise the possibility of a right atrial tumor. New and rapidly progressive right-sided heart failure, with new murmurs and prominent *a* waves in the jugular venous pulse, also suggests a right atrial tumor.

Elevated right atrial pressure from obstructed blood flow can lead to the opening of a previously closed patent foramen ovale and right-to-left shunting. The arterial oxygen desaturation in these patients can be severe and associated with polycythemia.

4. Right ventricular tumors—Obstruction of the right ventricular outflow tract from tumors is associated with venous congestion, systolic murmur, and right-axis deviation or a right bundle branch conduction abnormality. Acute cor pulmonale can be secondary to metastatic laryngeal carcinoma of the right ventricle, with subsequent tumor emboli to the pulmonary vasculature.

5. Pericardial tumors—Neoplastic pericardial effusions are often painless, although they can be associated with dyspnea and cough, especially if tamponade is present. Other physical findings suggestive of tamponade are tachycardia, tachypnea, narrow pulse pressure and pulsus paradoxus. Pericardial tumors can be associated with a pericardial friction rub or knock.

> Butany J et al. Cardiac tumours: diagnosis and management. Lancet Oncol. 2005 Apr;6(4):219–28. [PMID: 15811617]

C. Diagnostic Studies

Advances in noninvasive imaging techniques have facilitated the early diagnosis of cardiac tumors and increased the accuracy and complexity of information available to both the cardiologist and the cardiac surgeon. Echocardiography, computed tomography (CT), magnetic resonance imaging (MRI), and positron emission tomography (PET) have replaced plain radiographs and angiography.

1. Echocardiography—Echocardiography is the initial diagnostic modality of choice. In general, the sensitivity of both the transthoracic and transesophageal echocardiography is highest for endocardial lesions because the mass is easily distinguished from the echolucent chamber; the sensitivity is slightly lower for intramyocardial lesions and lowest for pericardial tumors. Despite its inconsistency in image quality secondary to varying degree of chest structure interference between different individuals, transthoracic echocardiography offers a superior acoustic window for the left ventricle and, therefore, is more sensitive in detecting a left ventricular tumor. On the other hand, transesophageal echocardiography has the advantage of providing better resolution for valvular and posterior structures that are distant from the anterior chest wall, such as the left and right atria, superior vena cava, and the descending thoracic aorta. Because of its superior image resolution and transesophageal approach, intraoperative transesophageal echocardiography has proven extremely useful to the surgeon for the guidance of tumor resection, particularly in cardiac sarcoma. Increasingly, transesophageal echocardiography is also used to aid cardiac biopsy and guide surgical intervention, helping to ensure that there is no residual tumor and that the repaired structures are free of defects (Figure 30–7). Follow-up echocardiography is recommended after resection of a tumor, particularly a myxoma, where there is a significant recurrence rate of 5%.

Newer echocardiograpic techniques are being increasingly used to determine tissue characterization of the tumor. Perfusion contrast enhancement of the tumor is seen in malignant or vascular tumors, whereas hypoenhancement is indicative of benign tumors or thrombi. Real-time three-dimensional echocardiography provides accurate estimation of the tumor size, compared with two-dimensional transthoracic or transesophageal echocardiography.

Asch FM et al. Real-time 3-dimensional echocardiography evaluation of intracardiac masses. Echocardiography. 2006 Mar;23(3): 218–24. [PMID: 16524392]

Dujardin KS et al. The role of intraoperative transesophageal echocardiography in patients undergoing cardiac mass removal. J Am Soc Echocardiogr. 2000 Dec;13(12):1080–3. [PMID: 11119275]

Jurkovich D et al. Primary cardiac lymphoma diagnosed by percutaneous intracardiac biopsy with combined fluoroscopic and transesophageal echocardiographic imaging. Catheter Cardiovasc Interv. 2000 Jun;50(2):226–33. [PMID: 10842397]

Kirkpatrick JN et al. Differential diagnosis of cardiac masses using contrast echocardiographic perfusion imaging. J Am Coll Cardiol. 2004 Apr 21;43(8):1412–9. [PMID: 15093876]

2. Computed tomography—Conventional, nongated CT scanning is most useful in diagnosing paracardiac masses in the region of the pericardium. It can differentiate tissue types and help identify the type of tumor and its extent within the lungs, mediastinum, pericardium, and cardiac chambers. The evaluation can be improved with contrast enhancement.

Computed tomography is also superior in identifying tumor involvement of the pericardium when there is no pericardial effusion and in identifying nodular pericardial thickening. Computed tomography may be useful when the mediastinum, pleura, and lungs must also be examined to provide therapeutic guidance and management of cardiac tumors. This modality can show a complete cross section of all cardiac, mediastinal, pulmonary, and thoracic structures (in contrast to angiocardiography), without the anatomic restrictions of echocardiography.

Two techniques have been developed to reduce the poor temporal resolution and motion blurring seen in the conventional single slice CT. Multidetector row CT with ECG gating allows a complete chest survey with high-resolution images to be performed in 10–15 minutes. Ultrafast CT and more recently

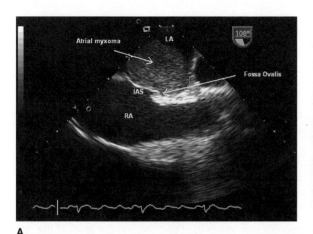

A

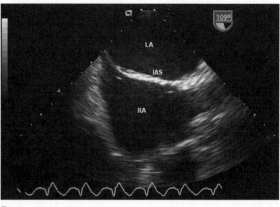

B

▲ **Figure 30–7.** **A:** Intraoperative transesophageal echocardiogram in the bicaval view, showing a left atrial myxoma attaching to the fossa ovalis of the interatrial septum. **B:** Postoperative transesophageal echocardiogram shows complete resection of the atrial myxoma with intact interatrial septum. IAS, interatrial septum; LA, left atrium; RA, right atrium.

electron-beam computed tomography (EB-CT), using continuous high-speed scanning, with 50–100 ms exposures improves the detection of paracardiac and intracardiac masses, and produces images with excellent spatial and density resolution. The technique also allows a movie mode, adding information to the static images; because it avoids superimposition of other tissues, it is useful in evaluating multiple masses.

Albers J et al. In vivo validation of cardiac spiral computed tomography using retrospective gating. Ann Thorac Surg. 2003 Mar;75(3):885–9. [PMID: 12645712]

Grebenc ML et al. Primary cardiac and pericardial neoplasms: radiologic-pathologic correlation. Radiographics. 2000 Jul–Aug;20(4):1073–103. [PMID: 10903697]

Tatli S et al. CT for intracardiac thrombi and tumors. Int J Cardiovasc Imaging. 2005 Feb;21(1):115–31. [PMID: 15915945]

3. Magnetic resonance imaging—Magnetic resonance imaging is a three-dimensional technique that can be used to supplement the information provided by echocardiography about cardiac masses. The high natural contrast between the blood pool and cardiovascular structures allows internal cardiac structures to be visualized by this technique. The direct multiplanar imaging capability of MRI is advantageous in demonstrating vessels and vessel/mass relationships. This capability makes it superior to CT for such areas as the aortopulmonic window and subcarinal region and lesions at the cervicothoracic or thoracoabdominal junction. Magnetic resonance imaging can be useful for surgical planning in questions of chest wall invasion; brachial plexus involvement; and extension to the diaphragm, pericardium, or lung apex. The coronal or sagittal format makes MRI useful in planning radiation therapy. Structures such as the trachea and the superior vena cava can be evaluated in their plane of anatomic orientation. Although MRI may be useful for detecting pericardial tumor involvement, its reconstruction imaging technique often makes small mobile tumors difficult or impossible to visualize.

Magnetic resonance imaging also has the potential for tissue characterization. Fibrous tissue remains at low signal intensity on T_2-weighted image, while tumors have an increased signal intensity. Fat-rich tissues, such as the lipomas, can be accurately characterized by using the fat suppression technique (Figure 30–8). Tumors and thrombi can be distinguished by using the inversion recovery scouting sequence or gadolinium injection, which enhances masses with rich vascular supply. Delayed enhancement with gadolinium injection is indicative of necrosis or nonviable tissues, which are often located in the center of a tumor where the cells have outgrown the blood supply.

Functional assessment should be included as part of a complete MRI study of a cardiac mass. Using long- and short-axis cine imaging, the mobility of the mass and its hemodynamic consequence can be evaluated. Furthermore, myocardial tagging allows examination of intramyocardial strain pattern, which helps differentiate contractile from noncontractile tissue. This is particularly useful in determining whether a segment of intramyocardial thickening represents a tumor, such as rhabdomyoma, or hypertrophied myocardium.

Magnetic resonance imaging correctly identifies the etiology of cardiac masses about 75% of the time, while echocardiography (both transthoracic and transesophageal) only correctly diagnose about one-third of cases. Thus, unless a contraindication exists, a cardiac MRI or chest CT should be performed to supplement the echocardiographic finding of a cardiac tumor. The exception would be when there is sufficient finding to suggest a myxoma on an echocardiogram.

Fieno DS et al. Cardiovascular magnetic resonance of primary tumors of the heart: A review. J Cardiovasc Magn Reson. 2006;8(6):839–53. [PMID: 17060107]

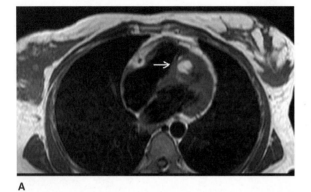 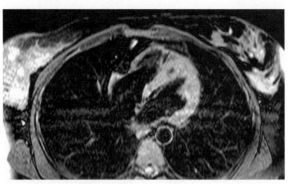

A   B

▲ **Figure 30–8.** T_1-weighted transaxial spin-echo magnetic resonance image of the heart through the level of the interventricular septum. **A:** A high-signal-intensity mass (*arrow*) is seen embedded in the distal anteroseptum. **B:** During fat saturation pulse application, the mass loses its bright signal suggesting the diagnosis of a cardiac lipoma. (Courtesy of C Higgins.)

Gulati G et al. Comparison of echo and MRI in the imaging evaluation of intracardiac masses. Cardiovasc Intervent Radiol. 2004 Sep–Oct;27(5):459–69.[PMID: 15383848]

4. Positron emission tomography—Whole-body 18-fluorodeoxyglucose positron emission tomography (PET) has increasingly been used to diagnose cardiac metastasis in patients with renal cell carcinoma or lung cancer.

Garcia JR et al. Usefulness of 18-fluorodeoxyglucose positron emission tomography in the evaluation of tumor cardiac thrombus from renal cell carcinoma. Clin Transl Oncol. 2006 Feb;8(2):124–8. [PMID: 16632427]

Gates GF et al. Intracardiac extension of lung cancer demonstrated on PET scanning. Clin Nucl Med. 2006 Feb;31(2):68–70. [PMID: 16424687]

▶ Differential Diagnosis

The differential diagnosis of cardiac masses includes tumors, thrombus, nonbacterial thrombotic endocarditis, infective endocarditis, or normal variant intracardiac or extracardiac structures. Imaging features that favor a diagnosis of tumor are a mobile, pedunculated appearance and an associated pericardial effusion. Masses that cross anatomic planes, from myocardium to pericardium or endocardium, are likely to be tumors. Clinical features are crucial in guiding the diagnosis of a cardiac mass. For example, left atrial thrombi are associated with mitral valve stenosis, enlarged left atrium, and atrial fibrillation, while ventricular thrombi are associated with cardiomyopathies or regional wall-motion abnormalities. Right atrial thrombi are seen in the setting of indwelling catheters or pacemaker wires

(Figure 30–9). Nonbacterial thrombotic endocarditis is found in patients with malignancy or systemic lupus erythematosus.

Pericardial cysts can be identified by their unilocular nature and their location in either the right or left costophrenic angle. Diaphragmatic hernia can mimic a left atrial mass on transthoracic echocardiography. Transesophageal echocardiography, on the other hand, can help diagnose the hernia by showing an extracardiac structure indenting the left atrium posteriorly and the swirling nonuniform echo densities within this structure caused by motion of the gastric contents.

Although lipomatous cardiac infiltration can mimic a tumor, it can be distinguished by its characteristic location (atrial septum) and dumbbell-shaped appearance (Figure 30–10). The shape is due to the thin fossa ovalis that separates the lipomatous atrial septum on either side. The incidence of lipomatous septal hypertrophy increases with age and obesity. No intervention is required unless the hypertrophy causes arrhythmias or obstruction.

A number of normal variants of anatomic structures are occasionally confused with tumors. These include the Chiari network, a remnant of the sinus venosus seen in the right atrium; the eustachian valve, the valve of the inferior vena cava (Figure 30–11); the septum spurium, a superior fold of the coronary sinus opening; the thebesian valve, the valve of coronary sinus.

▶ Treatment

A. Pharmacologic Therapy

Surgery remains the mainstay of treatment for all cardiac tumors. Pharmacologic therapy has no role in the management of benign cardiac tumors. In cardiac sarcoma, adjuvant chemotherapy using doxorubicin-containing regimen has been studied to determine whether survival improved after surgical resection. The results from two case series and one

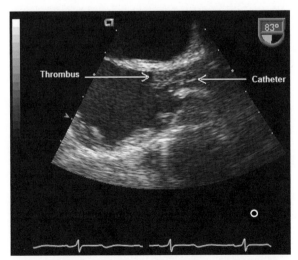

▲ **Figure 30–9.** Transesophageal echocardiogram in a 64-year-old hemodialysis patient for evaluation of fever. The bicaval view shows a thrombus forming around a catheter at the junction of the superior vena cava and the right atrium.

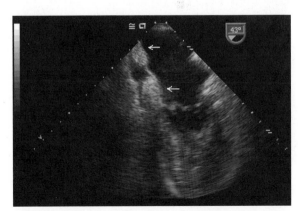

▲ **Figure 30–10.** Transesophageal echocardiogram in 43° long-axis plane showing lipomatous hypertrophy of the interatrial septum (*arrows*). Note the dumbbell-shaped appearance.

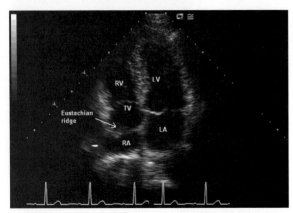

▲ **Figure 30–11.** Transthoracic echocardiogram in an apical four-chamber view showing a prominent eustachian ridge. LA, left atrium; LV, left ventricle; RA, right atrium; RV, right ventricle; TV, tricuspid valve.

large meta-analysis of soft tissue sarcoma all failed to show significant survival benefit from the adjuvant chemotherapy. In fact, in these trials, complete tumor resection was the most predictive factor for longer term survival. The use of chemotherapy in tumor cytoreduction in preparation for surgical resection and palliation of unresectable disease might be of value in selected cases. Unlike sarcoma, primary cardiac lymphoma is thought to be more responsive to chemotherapy. Using CHOP (cyclophosphamide + doxorubicin + vincristine + prednisone)–based regimen, combined with radiation or surgery (or both) in certain cases, one-third of patients may experience complete remission, and a median survival of 1 year has been observed. More recently, promising results have been obtained with monoclonal CD20 antibody (rituximab) and autologous stem cell transplant.

Ikeda H et al. Primary lymphoma of the heart: case report and literature review. Pathol Int. 2004 Mar;54(3):187–95. [PMID: 14989742]
Sato Y et al. Successful treatment of primary cardiac B-cell lymphoma: depiction at multislice computed tomography and magnetic resonance imaging. Int J Cardiol. 2006 Oct 26;113(1):E26–9. [PMID: 17049383]

B. Radiation

Adjuvant radiotherapy can be helpful for prolonging survival if total surgical excision is not successful or curative for malignant tumors. Radiation (compared with repeated pericardiocentesis) may prolong life in patients with pericardial metastases; however, high doses of radiation can lead to cardiac damage.

C. Surgery

Because of embolic complications and the limited capacity of the heart to tolerate space-occupying lesions, most cardiac tumors—benign or malignant—require prompt surgical removal.

1. Benign tumors—Myxomas should be removed expeditiously because of their high embolic potential. Lipomas are often asymptomatic and do not require further treatment. Because large papillary fibroelastomas are a nidus for platelet aggregation, resection is recommended to prevent emboli. Small papillary fibroelastomas, such as Lambl excrescences, on an elderly patient's aortic leaflets need not be resected. Present data suggest a conservative approach to treatment of rhabdomyomas in asymptomatic patients. Although surgery is indicated for symptomatic patients (a large mass can cause inflow and outflow obstruction), it can be difficult because these tumors tend to be multiple, nonencapsulated, and embedded in the myocardium. Patients may need inotropic support in the postoperative period because of the extensive surgical dissection, which often involves the myocardium. Fibromas are often large (4–7 cm in diameter); prompt surgery is recommended. Excision may remove much ventricular myocardium. Complete excision is recommended, because any fibroma that remains may be a focus for ventricular arrhythmias. Reconstructive surgery with a synthetic patch may be necessary.

2. Malignant tumors—Although total surgical resection for sarcoma is often impossible, surgery is done to relieve compressive or obstructive symptoms in some cases. Surgery is rarely performed to remove metastatic tumor masses unless a cure of the primary tumor is highly likely. In addition to high in-hospital mortality rate, surgery for malignant tumors remains palliative without effective adjuvant therapy. Prognosis of malignant cardiac tumor is overall extremely poor.

Almassi GH. Surgery for tumors with cavoatrial extension. Semin Thorac Cardiovasc Surg. 2000 Apr;12(2):111–8. [PMID: 10807433]
Schaff HV et al. Surgery for cardiac myxomas. Semin Thorac Cardiovasc Surg. 2000 Apr;12(2):77–88. [PMID: 10807430]

D. Pericardiocentesis

Symptomatic neoplastic effusions, such those seen in metastatic breast or lung cancer, may require pericardiocentesis, and recurrent effusions may require partial pericardiectomy. Echocardiographic guidance is generally preferred. Instilling isotopes or sclerosing agents such as tetracyclines and chemotherapeutic agents in the pericardial space has been successfully used to prevent such recurrences; recurrence is common after pericardiocentesis for recurrent malignant pericardial disease.

Tsang TS et al. Outcomes of primary and secondary treatment of pericardial effusion in patients with malignancy. Mayo Clin Proc. 2000 Mar;75(3):248–53. [PMID: 10725950]

E. Cardiac Transplantation

Cardiac transplantation can be an alternative therapy for unresectable cardiac tumors, when infiltration by fibroma is too extensive for excision. This approach remains experimental and is limited by the potential for posttransplant recurrence, which may be accelerated by immunosuppressive therapy. In rare cases where radical resection of the tumor and ex vivo repair of the heart is possible, autotransplantation instead of allogenic transplantation should be attempted.

Gowdamarajan A et al. Therapy for primary cardiac tumors: is there a role for heart transplantation? Curr Opin Cardiol. 2000 Mar;15(2):121–5. [PMID: 10963150]
Mery GM et al. A combined modality approach to recurrent cardiac sarcoma resulting in a prolonged remission: a case report. Chest. 2003 May;123(5):1766–8. [PMID: 12740300]

► Prognosis

A. Metastatic Tumors

The prognosis depends on the pathology of the primary tumor, but it is generally poor.

B. Primary Tumors

Surgical resection usually results in cure of benign cardiac tumors. Approximately 1.5% of myxomas (12–22% in patients with familial or syndrome-related myxomas) recur within 10–15 years. Because of this small risk of recurrence, patients should be monitored with periodic echocardiography every 1–2 years for 15 years following the resection.

Long-term results for primary malignant tumors are disappointing, usually because of early metastatic or local spread or recurrence. Mean survival for pericardial mesotheliomas is 6 months to 1 year and for sarcomas, 3 months to 1 year with or without treatment. Localized disease arising from the left atrium with no necrotic tissues is associated with better prognosis in sarcomas. The survival of treated primary cardiac lymphoma can be as long as 5 years, but as short as 1 month if left untreated.

Grebenc ML et al. Primary cardiac and pericardial neoplasms: radiologic-pathologic correlation. Radiographics. 2000 Jul–Aug;20(4):1073–103 [PMID: 10903697].

► Cardiac Toxicities from Oncologic Treatments

Because survival of various oncologic conditions has improved, early, or especially late, adverse cardiac effects related to treatment can develop. Fortunately, because of increasing recognition of some of these potential toxicities, modern treatment protocols have been modified to minimize side effects. Nevertheless, it is important to recognize some of the adverse outcomes related to earlier treatments. At the same time, clinicians need to be cognizant of potential late effects of contemporary therapy (Table 30–3).

A. Chemotherapy

1. Anthracyclines—These drugs are all associated with cardiac toxicities. The most important offending anthracyclines

Table 30–3. Cardiotoxicity Induced by Chemotherapeutic Agents.

Chemotherapeutic Agent	Adverse Effect
Anthracyclines/anthraquinolones	
Doxorubicin/daunorubicin	LV dysfunction Myopericarditis
Epirubicin	LV dysfunction Supraventricular tachycardia
Mitoxantrone	LV dysfunction Arrhythmias
Alkylating agents	
Cisplatin	LV dysfunction Myocardial ischemia Heart blocks
Cyclophosphamide	Hemorrhagic myopericarditis Acute heart failure Arrhythmias
Antimetabolites	
Cytarabine	Pericarditis Angina
5-Fluorouracil	Myocardial spasm Ischemia Ventricular arrhythmias
Antimicrotubules	
Paclitaxel	Sinus bradycardia AV block Ventricular tachycardia
Vinca alkaloids	Myocardial ischemia Myocardial infarction
Biologic response modifiers	
Interferons	Hypotension/LV dysfunction
Interleukin-2	Hypotension/LV dysfunction
Topoisomerase inhibitors	
Etoposide	Hypotension Myocardial ischemia
Differentiation agents	
All-*trans*-retinoic acid	Pericardial effusion Pulmonary edema
Arsenic trioxide	Prolonged QT Torsades de pointes
Monoclonal antibodies	
Trastuzumab	LV dysfunction
Rituximab	Hypotension Arrhythmias

include daunorubicin and doxorubicin. Clinical manifestations include ECG abnormalities, pericarditis, and ventricular dysfunction ocurring rarely during or immediately after the infusion. More commonly, development of nonischemic car-diomyopathy occurs 3 months or even decades after the last dose of anthracycline. The cardiac toxicity is dose-dependent and a threshold cumulative dose of 450 mg/m^2 has been suggested to reduce cardiac toxicities. Other factors predispos-ing to increased risk of cardiotoxicity include age older than 70; preexisting cardiac disease; concurrent or prior chest irradiation; and administration of multiple chemotherapeutic agents, particularly paclitaxel and trastuzumab.

Baseline and serial ventricular function assessment with echocardiography after each dose helps detect subclinical cardiotoxicity. In patients with equivocal results on serial monitoring, endomyocardial biopsy may be necessary. Effec-tive strategies have been developed to reduce the risk of anthracycline cardiotoxicity, including continuous infusion protocol, liposome encapsulation, molecular modification, and dexrazoxane chelation.

2. Trastuzumab—A recombinant humanized IgG mono-clonal antibody that selectively binds to human epidermal growth factor receptor-2 (HER-2) has been reported to cause predominantly asymptomatic ventricular dysfunction in 2–8% of breast cancer patients. The incidence is higher in those receiving concomitant cardiac toxic chemotherapy, and those with older age and history of chest irradiation. Unlike anthracycline toxicity, trastuzumab-related cardiac dysfunc-tion is not dose dependent; prompt resolution of ventricular dysfunction with drug withdrawal or standard heart failure therapy has been reported.

3. Cyclophosphamide—Cyclophosphamide in high-dose protocol, 120–170 mg/kg over 1–7 days can lead to cardiac injury commonly manifesting as decreased QRS amplitude, repolarization abnormalities, tachyarrhythmias, and heart block. Other reported cardiac complications include acute onset heart failure, which occurs in as much as 28% of patients receiving high-dose cyclophosphamide. Hemorrhagic myo-pericarditis leading to pericardial effusion and tamponade, which usually occurs within the first week after the treatment is caused by endothelial capillary damage and red cells extrav-asation. Pericardiocentesis is usually not necessary for hemor-rhagic pericardial effusion. Analgesics and corticosteroids with serial echocardiographic monitoring are effective treatment.

4. Retinoic acid—Retinoic acid produces a syndrome in up to 25% of cases, with manifestations of fever, dyspnea, pleural and pericardial effusion, pulmonary infiltrates, peripheral edema, and transient myocardial dysfunction. This syndrome is usually responsive to corticosteroid therapy.

5. Paclitaxel—Paclitaxel commonly leads to ECG changes and cardiac rhythm disturbances; atrioventricular conduc-tion abnormalities, complete heart block, and even asystole have been reported. Fortunately, these conduction abnor-malities are usually reversible with the termination of treat-ment. Thus, continuous ECG monitoring is advised during treatment.

6. 5-Fluorouracil—This drug is frequently associated with myocardial ischemia. Anginal symptoms with or without objective evidence of myocardial ischemia are common com-plaints. The mechanism of ischemia is unknown, but vaso-spasm has been shown to be a contributive factor. In general, ECG changes resolve following termination of treatment, and anginal symptoms are responsive to conservative medical treatment. Prophylactic treatment with nitrates and calcium channel blockers, stress testing and coronary angiography before commencing 5-fluorouracil (5-FU) therapy may be considered in high-risk patients. Atrial or ventricular arrhyth-mias, ventricular dysfunction unrelated to myocardial is-chemia are other potential complications of 5-FU therapy.

7. Interleukin-2—This immunomodulator produces a cap-illary leak syndrome and causes cardiovascular changes that mimic septic shock syndrome. In severe cases, ventricular arrhthymias and profound cardiac systolic function depres-sion can occur. The syndrome usually subsides after treat-ment cessation and supportive treatment; however, it may take up to 6 days after the last dose for some patients to completely regain normal hemodynamics.

Floyd JD et al. Cardiotoxicity of cancer therapy. J Clin Oncol. 2005 Oct 20;23(30):7685–96. [PMID: 16234530]

Yeh ET et al. Cardiovascular complications of cancer therapy: diagnosis, pathogenesis, and management. Circulation. 2004 Jun 29;109(25):3122–31. [PMID: 15226229]

B. Radiation

Radiation-induced heart disease involves most structures of the heart (Table 30–4). Pericardial involvement is the most common cardiac complication. For patients who had under-gone radiation to the chest, pericardial effusion was reported in 6–30% of the patients. In the past, acute pericarditis was seen in 10–15% of the patients with Hodgkin disease. Today, contemporary delivery of radiation has led to a dramatic decrease of pericardial disease estimated now at about 2–2.5% of patients. However, survivors of past treatment of

Table 30–4. Clinical Manifestations of Radiation-Induced Heart Disease.

Pericardial disease
Acute pericarditis
Delayed pericarditis
Pericardial effusion
Constrictive pericarditis
Myocardial disease
Ventricular dysfunction
Myocarditis
Valvular heart disease
Predominantly mitral and aortic valves
Electrical conduction disturbances
Coronary artery disease

radiation such as the Hodgkin disease survivors are still at risk for late development of pericardial complications such as constrictive pericarditis. A history of past irradiation to the chest (especially with greater than 40 Gy) and unexplained signs or symptoms of right-sided venous congestion should raise the index of suspicion for constrictive pericarditis. Diagnosis may involve a combination of echocardiographic, MRI/CT, and invasive cardiac hemodynamics evaluations. Afflicted patients will often require pericardiectomy.

Furthermore, radiation is associated with an increased incidence of early ischemic heart disease, valvular heart disease, and the development of electrical abnormalities.

Gregor A. How to improve effects of radiation and control its toxicity. Ann Oncol. 2000;11 Suppl 3:231–4. [PMID: 11079146]

Keefe DL. Cardiovascular emergencies in the cancer patient. Semin Oncol. 2000 Jun;27(3):244–55. [PMID: 10864214]

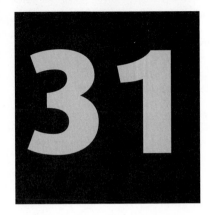

Cardiovascular Disease in Pregnancy

Kirsten Tolstrup, MD, FACC, FASE

ESSENTIALS OF DIAGNOSIS

▶ Pregnancy.

▶ History of heart disease.

▶ Symptoms and signs of heart disease.

▶ Echocardiographic or other objective evidence of heart disease.

▶ General Considerations

Cardiovascular disease occurs in approximately 1% of pregnancies, but the incidence is increasing due to improved prognosis of women with congenital heart disease and a trend toward older maternal age. The unique hemodynamic changes associated with pregnancy make diagnosis and management of heart disease in pregnant patients a challenge to the physicians, who must consider not only the patient but also the risks to the fetus.

In general, the normal hemodynamic changes associated with pregnancy are well tolerated by those who have a normal cardiovascular system, valvular regurgitation, and left-to-right intracardiac shunts. On the other hand, the highest maternal and fetal morbidity and mortality is seen with severe obstructive valvular lesions, severe aortic disease (dilated thoracic aorta or uncorrected coarctation), New York Heart Association (NYHA) class III or IV heart failure, uncontrolled hypertension, and cyanotic congenital heart disease. As a rule, spontaneous vaginal delivery, often with use of vacuum extraction or forceps to facilitate stage 2 of labor to avoid the hemodynamic stress associated with pushing, is preferred. Cesarean section, with few exceptions, should be reserved for obstetric indications.

Stout KK et al. Pregnancy in women with valvular heart disease. Heart. 2007 May;93(5):552–8. [PMID: 16905631]

▶ Cardiovascular Physiology of Normal Pregnancy

Normal pregnancy is accompanied by significant physiologic changes, although underlying mechanisms remain virtually unknown (Table 31–1). The normal signs and symptoms associated with pregnancy, such as shortness of breath, fatigue, and exercise intolerance, may obscure the diagnosis of heart disease. The clinician must, therefore, have a thorough knowledge of these normal changes and the aspects of the history and physical examination that suggest the presence of heart disease.

A. Blood Volume

The increase in maternal blood volume begins as early as the sixth week of pregnancy, peaks at approximately 32 weeks of gestation, and stays at that level (40–50% higher than pregestational levels) until delivery. The plasma volume shows a more rapid and significant rise than the red blood cell mass, accounting for the appearance of *physiologic anemia during pregnancy*. The increased blood volume is maintained until after delivery, when a spontaneous diuresis occurs. At the same time, there is an increased venous return due to the relief of vena caval compression after delivery. These rapid postpartum changes in blood volume are critical for patients with underlying heart disease.

B. Cardiac Output

One of the most significant changes during pregnancy is the increase in cardiac output, which begins to rise during the first trimester and peaks around the twenty-fifth week of gestation and then levels off. Total cardiac output increases up to 50% over pregestational levels. Cardiac output is the product of stroke volume and heart rate. During the early part of pregnancy, the increase in cardiac output is predominantly the result of an increase in stroke volume, augmented by increased intrinsic myocardial contractility. Numerous studies have shown a gradual increase in left ventricular

Table 31–1. Cardiovascular Changes in Normal Pregnancy.

	First Trimester	Second Trimester	Third Trimester	At Term
Blood volume	+	+ +	+ + +	↑ 30–50%
Heart rate	+	+ +	+ + (+)	↑ 15–20 beats/min
Stroke volume	+	+ + (+)	+	
Cardiac output	+	+ + (+)	+	↑ 30–50%
Systolic blood pressure	–	–	No change	↓ 5–10 mm Hg mid pregnancy
Diastolic blood pressure	–	– –	–	
Pulse pressure	+	++	+	
Systemic vascular resistance	–	– – –	– –	
Pulmonary vascular resistance	–	– –	–	
Left ventricular end-diastolic pressure	+	+ +	No change	
Venous compliance and volume	+	+ +	+	
Red blood cell mass	+	+	+	↑ 15–20%

Data from Fujitan S. Crit Care Med. 2005;33:S354.

systolic function attributed to left ventricular afterload reduction due to the low-resistance runoff of the placenta. The rise in left ventricular systolic function begins in early pregnancy, peaks in the twentieth week, and then remains constant until delivery. As pregnancy advances, heart rate increases and stroke volume mildly decreases. The increased cardiac output in late pregnancy is maintained because of the increased heart rate.

A unique aspect of pregnancy is the hemodynamic changes induced by a change in a patient's position. When the patient is in the supine position, the gravid uterus induces profound mechanical compression of the inferior vena cava, decreasing venous return to the heart, and thus, cardiac output. A change from the supine to the left lateral position results in a 25–30% increase in cardiac output because of an increase in stroke volume.

C. Intravascular Pressures and Vascular Resistance

Systolic and diastolic pressures drop during pregnancy. A small decrease in systolic blood pressure begins in the first trimester, peaks at midgestation, and returns to near prepregnancy levels at term. The diastolic blood pressure decreases more than the systolic blood pressure, due to a significant fall in systemic vascular resistance, and results in a wider pulse pressure. The systemic blood pressure increases during pregnancy with the patient's age and parity. It also varies with the patient's position. The highest levels are recorded early in the pregnancy when the patient is upright, and lowest when she is supine. During the latter part of pregnancy, the effect of position on systemic blood pressure depends on the relative degrees of inferior vena cava and

aortic compression. Total vascular resistance, including both the systemic and the pulmonary, decrease during pregnancy. The mechanism for the fall in resistances is poorly understood but is attributed to the low-resistance circulation of the pregnant uterus and to hormonal changes associated with pregnancy.

Fujitani S et al. Hemodynamic assessment in a pregnant and peripartum patient. Crit Care Med. 2005 Oct;33(10 Suppl):S354–61. [PMID: 16215359]

▶ Etiology & Symptomatology

A. Congenital Heart Disease

Because the medical and surgical treatment of uncorrected or surgically corrected congenital heart diseases has improved, more women are surviving into adulthood and may become pregnant. Cardiac complications occur in approximately 11% of these patients, most commonly due to heart failure (in 4.8%) and arrhythmias (in 4.5%). Maternal *mortality* primarily occurs in women with Eisenmenger syndrome. Obstetric complications are not increased, except in cases of hypertension and thromboembolic disease (2%). Premature delivery occurs in about 16%, and children small for gestational age are also common. Overall, offspring mortality is around 4%. The risk of recurrence of congenital malformations in the offspring depend on the type and range from 0.6% to 8%.

Only a few conditions place a patient at a high risk to advise against pregnancy (Table 31–2). High-risk patients with severe cyanotic congenital heart disease, marked decreased functional capacity, or Eisenmenger syndrome should be advised against pregnancy.

Table 31-2. High-Risk Conditions That Warrant Advice against Pregnancy.

	Condition	Maternal Risk	Fetal Risk
1.	Cyanotic congenital heart disease	4–34% MI/stroke/death	12–40% miscarriage
2.	Eisenmenger syndrome	35% MI/stroke/death	30% miscarriage
3.	Severe pulmonary hypertension (> 75% of systemic blood pressure)	30–40% death	10% fetal loss
4.	NYHA class III/IV symptoms	10–56% death	30% fetal loss
5.	Severe symptomatic obstructive valvular lesions	56–78% CHF or pulmonary edema	11% death 33–66% preterm delivery
6.	Marfan syndrome with thoracic aorta > 4.0 cm	11–50% risk of dissection	50% risk of inheriting the syndrome 4–20% risk of fetal/neonatal death
7.	Loeys-Dietz syndrome	9% death in non-pregnant with aorta < 4.5 cm	50% risk of inheriting the syndrome

Data from Crawford MH. Cardiology. 2001; Drenthen W. J Am Coll Cardiol. 2007;49:2303-2311; Hameed A. J Am Coll Cardiol. 2001;37:893-899; Silversides CK. Am J Cardiol. 2003;91:1382-1389; Elkayam U. J Am Coll Cardiol. 2005;46:223-230; Lind J. Eur J Obstet Gynecol Reprod Biol. 2001;98:28-35; Elkayam U. Ann Intern Med. 1995;123:117-122; Sliwa K. Lancet. 2006;368:687-693; Williams JA. Ann Thorac Surg. 2007;83:757-763.

1. Acyanotic heart disease

A. ATRIAL SEPTAL DEFECT—Secundum atrial septal defect is the most common congenital cardiac abnormality encountered during pregnancy. Patients with uncomplicated atrial septal defects usually tolerate pregnancy with little problem. Patients may not be able to tolerate the acute blood loss that can occur at the time of delivery because of increased shunting from left to right caused by systemic vasoconstriction associated with hypotension. The incidence of supraventricular arrhythmias may increase in older pregnant patients, which may result in right ventricular failure and venous stasis leading to paradoxical emboli. Low-dose aspirin, once daily after the first trimester until delivery may help prevent clot formation. Pulmonary hypertension from an atrial septal defect usually occurs late in life, past the childbearing years. Bacterial endocarditis prophylaxis is not recommended. Vaginal delivery is preferred over cesarean section. Risk of occurrence in the offspring is about 2.5%.

B. VENTRICULAR SEPTAL DEFECT—Most isolated ventricular septal defects have closed by adulthood. Women with ventricular septal defects generally fare well in pregnancy if the defect is small and pulmonary artery pressure is normal. Congestive heart failure and arrhythmia are reported only in patients with decreased left ventricular systolic function prior to pregnancy. Endocarditis prophylaxis during delivery is not recommended.

C. CONGENITAL AORTIC STENOSIS—This is most commonly caused by a congenital bicuspid aortic valve. The prevalence in the general population is 1–2% but may be as high as 9–21% in some families, where the condition appears to be autosomal dominant with reduced penetrance. The condition is usually more common in men (2:1 ratio). In patients with congenital aortic stenosis, the outcome during pregnancy depends on the severity of the obstruction. Pregnancy is usually well tolerated in mild-to-moderate aortic stenosis (aortic valve area [AVA] 1.0–2.0 cm^2). Patients with severe aortic stenosis with a valve area of < 1.0 cm^2 and mean transvalvular gradients greater than 50 mm Hg may experience an increased risk of complications (from 10% to 44%) and fetal morbidity is increased. The increased cardiac output and decreased systemic vascular resistance of pregnancy creates an additional hemodynamic burden in these patients. Syncope, cerebral symptoms, dyspnea, angina pectoris, and even heart failure may occur for the first time during pregnancy. The rate at which valve replacement is necessary after pregnancy is markedly increased. Ideally, balloon valvuloplasty or valve replacement should be performed before pregnancy in symptomatic patients with severe aortic stenosis. Valvuloplasty, if needed, is preferred over surgery during pregnancy. Hemodynamic monitoring during labor and delivery should be performed in patients with moderate to severe aortic stenosis. Endocarditis prophylaxis is not recommended for vaginal delivery. As part of the bicuspid aortic valve syndrome, the aortic root often will be dilated, evidence that the condition is not only a disease of the valve but of the connective tissue as well. When the aortic root is dilated there is an increased risk of aortic dissection during pregnancy, and such events have been reported when the aorta is greater than 40 mm, although the true incidence is unknown. Obtaining serial echocardiograms at least every 3 months to monitor progression of root dilatation appears prudent. The risk for the condition in the offspring is variable but at least 4%.

D. PULMONIC STENOSIS—The natural history of pulmonic stenosis favors survival into adulthood even with severe obstruction to right ventricular outflow. Mild-to-moderate pulmonic stenosis (peak gradient < 50 mm Hg) usually presents no increased risk during pregnancy. Patients with severe pulmonic stenosis may occasionally tolerate pregnancy without the development of congestive heart failure. Vaginal delivery is tolerated well. Ideal treatment consisting of balloon valvuloplasty should be performed before conception but may be performed safely during pregnancy if necessary. The risk in the offspring is about 3.5%.

E. Coarctation of the aorta—In uncomplicated coarctation of the aorta, pregnancy is usually safe for the mother but may be associated with fetal underdevelopment because of the diminished uterine blood flow. The blood pressure may decrease slightly, as during normal pregnancy, but still remains elevated. Maternal deaths in these patients are usually the result of aortic rupture or cerebral hemorrhage from an associated berry aneurysm of the circle of Willis. Patients with the greatest risk during pregnancy are those with severe hypertension or associated cardiac abnormalities, such as bicuspid aortic valves. Treatment consists of limitation of physical activity and maintenance of systolic blood pressure around 140 mm Hg for fetal circulation; β-blockers are preferred and should be continued through delivery. Patients with severe uncorrected coarctation and poorly controlled hypertension should undergo cesarean section. Surgical treatment should be reserved for patients in whom complications develop, eg, aortic dissection, uncontrollable hypertension, and refractory heart failure.

F. Patent ductus arteriosus—Most patients with a patent ductus arteriosus undergo repair in childhood. A normal pregnancy can be expected in patients with small-to-moderate shunts and no evidence of pulmonary hypertension. Patients with a large patent ductus arteriosus, elevated pulmonary vascular resistance, and a reversed shunt are at greatest risk for complications during pregnancy. The decreased systemic vascular resistance associated with pregnancy increases the right-to-left shunt and may cause intrauterine oxygen desaturation. Patients in whom heart failure develops are treated with digoxin and diuretics. Closure of the patent ductus arteriosus may be done safely during pregnancy using a percutaneous ductal occluder device. The preferred mode of delivery is vaginal in most patients, with hemodynamic monitoring considered at the time of delivery. The risk of patent ductus arteriosus occurring in an offspring is about 4%.

2. Cyanotic heart disease

A. Tetralogy of Fallot—This is the most common cyanotic congenital heart disease found in pregnant patients. The syndrome consists of pulmonary stenosis, right ventricular hypertrophy, an overriding aorta, and a ventricular septal defect. The decrease in systemic vascular resistance, the increased cardiac output, and the increased venous return to the right heart augment the amount of right-to-left shunt and further decrease the systemic arterial saturation. Acute blood loss during postpartum hemorrhage is particularly dangerous because venous return to the right heart is impaired. The labile hemodynamics during labor and the peripartum period may precipitate cyanosis, syncope, and even death in surgically untreated women. Patients with uncorrected or partially corrected tetralogy of Fallot are advised against becoming pregnant because they have a high rate of miscarriages (12–40%) as well as a high risk of heart failure (15–25%); arrhythmias (5%) and stroke, myocardial infarction (MI), or death (4–34%). Patients who have had good surgical repair may anticipate successful pregnancies, although the risk of arrhythmias may be increased. Antibiotic prophylaxis is recommended for patients with uncorrected tetralogy of Fallot and those in whom prosthetic material has been placed within 6 months. The risk in the offspring is approximately 4%.

B. Eisenmenger syndrome—This syndrome may occur due to several types of congenital heart disease and is characterized by systemic level pulmonary hypertension with right-to-left or bidirectional shunt with deoxygenation. The risk of maternal and fetal morbidity and mortality is so high that patients are advised against becoming pregnant. There is a 35% chance of MI, stroke, or death in the mother and almost 30% offspring mortality.

3. Surgically corrected congenital heart disease—The obstetric care of patients who have had surgical correction of a congenital heart disease requires an understanding of the type of surgical procedure, the sequelae, and the hemodynamic consequences. Although atrial flutter may occasionally develop following surgical closure, the successful closure of an uncomplicated atrial septal defect results in no increased maternal risk during pregnancy. Surgical closure of a patent ductus arteriosus that is not associated with pulmonary hypertension is also not associated with maternal complications during pregnancy. In pulmonary hypertension that develops before surgical closure, the decrease in the pulmonary vascular resistance may not be complete, and complications during pregnancy will depend on its severity. Correction of congenital pulmonary stenosis with either surgery or balloon dilatation that leaves little or no transvalvular gradient presents no difficulty to pregnant patients. Surgical correction of coarctation of the aorta with complete relief of the obstruction decreases the development of associated hypertension and the risk of aortic rupture during pregnancy. Successful repair of tetralogy of Fallot with little residual gradient across the pulmonary outflow tract and relief of the cyanosis should result, with careful management, in a normal pregnancy. Pregnancy after repair of complex congenital heart disease is increasingly encountered. In such patients, the outcome depends on the mother's functional status, the type of repair, the sequelae, and the cardiovascular response to an increase in stress.

Drenthen W et al. Outcome of pregnancy in women with congenital heart disease: a literature review. J Am Coll Cardiol. 2007 Jun 19;49(24):2303–11. [PMID: 17572244]

Elkayam U et al. Valvular heart disease and pregnancy: part I: native valves. J Am Coll Cardiol. 2005 Jul 19;46(2):223–30. [PMID: 16022946]

B. Valvular Heart Disease

No randomized controlled trial data are available to guide decision making for pregnant women with valvular heart disease. However, many patients with valvular heart disease can be treated successfully through their pregnancy with conservative medical treatment, focusing on optimization of intravascular volume and systemic load. Ideally, symptomatic patients should be treated before conception. Drugs, in general, should be avoided whenever possible. Antibiotics for infective endocarditis prophylaxis for uncomplicated vaginal delivery are not indicated, unless a prosthetic valve was placed within 6 months. Although there is little supportive data, antibiotic prophylaxis is often given for complicated vaginal deliveries.

1. Mitral valve disease

A. MITRAL STENOSIS—Mitral stenosis is the most commonly encountered acquired valvular lesion in pregnancy and is almost always caused by rheumatic heart disease. Mitral stenosis may be first diagnosed during pregnancy and is the valvular disorder most likely to develop serious complications during pregnancy. Increased left atrial pressure and even pulmonary edema due to a decrease in diastolic filling time during the tachycardia of pregnancy may develop in women who were previously asymptomatic. In critical mitral stenosis, due to a large diastolic gradient (even at rest), any demand of increased cardiac output results in a significant elevation in the left atrial pressure and pulmonary edema. The most common symptoms include dyspnea, fatigue, orthopnea, and dizziness or syncope. Signs and symptoms of mitral stenosis may develop for the first time during pregnancy. The greatest danger is in late pregnancy and labor due to increased heart rate and cardiac output, blood volume expansion, and intensified oxygen demand. Mild-to-moderate mitral stenosis (mean diastolic pressure gradient less than 10 mm Hg) may be managed safely with the use of diuretics to relieve pulmonary and systemic congestion and β-blockers to prevent tachycardia to optimize diastolic filling. Diuretics, β-blockers, digoxin, or DC cardioversion for atrial fibrillation should be instituted in cases of hemodynamic compromise, taking into consideration maternal safety. Refractory cases and patients with severe mitral stenosis with heart failure prompt mechanical relief, either by percutaneous balloon valvuloplasty or surgery, preferably before conception if the valve is anatomically suitable. Patients with a history of acute rheumatic fever and carditis should continue receiving penicillin prophylaxis.

B. MITRAL REGURGITATION—Mitral regurgitation (most commonly due to mitral valve prolapse) in the absence of NYHA class III or IV heart failure symptoms is generally tolerated well during pregnancy, even if severe. The decrease in systemic blood pressure in pregnancy may reduce the amount of mitral regurgitation. Left ventricular dysfunction, if severe, may precipitate heart failure. Medical management includes use of diuretics; in rare instances, surgical management is necessary, preferably mitral valve repair, which is indicated for severe, acute regurgitation or ruptured chordae and uncontrollable heart failure symptoms. In the future, percutaneous mitral valve repair may be an option for severe, symptomatic mitral regurgitation during pregnancy.

C. MITRAL VALVE PROLAPSE—Mitral valve prolapse is the most common heart disease encountered in pregnancy. Patients without comorbidity, such as a connective tissue, skeletal, or other cardiovascular disorders, tolerate pregnancy. The click and murmur become less prominent during pregnancy. No special precautions for isolated mitral valve prolapse are required. Antibiotic prophylaxis is not recommended. The incidence of complications of the mitral valve prolapse (3%) is similar in pregnant and nonpregnant patients.

2. Aortic valve disease

A. AORTIC STENOSIS—Aortic stenosis in pregnancy is most commonly caused by a congenital bicuspid aortic valve (see previous section).

B. AORTIC REGURGITATION—Isolated chronic aortic regurgitation without left ventricular dysfunction is usually tolerated well. Even if patients are symptomatic, they can often be treated medically with salt restriction, diuretics, and vasodilators. The most common causes are rheumatic disease, bicuspid aortic valve, endocarditis, and a dilated aortic root. Surgery is only indicated for patients with refractory (NYHA class III or IV) symptoms. Acute aortic regurgitation is not well tolerated and should be regarded as a surgical emergency.

3. Pulmonic and tricuspid valve disease

A. PULMONIC VALVE REGURGITATION—Pulmonic valve regurgitation may occur in isolation or in combination with other heart lesions. Isolated pulmonic regurgitation can be managed conservatively.

B. TRICUSPID VALVE DISEASE—Tricuspid valve disease may be congenital or acquired. Isolated tricuspid valve disease can be managed successfully with diuretics. Special care should be given to diuretic-induced hypoperfusion.

4. Prosthetic heart valves—Females with a prosthetic heart valve can usually tolerate the hemodynamic burden of pregnancy without difficulty. The function of the prosthesis can be evaluated and monitored throughout the pregnancy with noninvasive Doppler echocardiography. Two types of

heart valves are available with their own distinct risks and advantages: tissue valves and mechanical prostheses. The main differences between the types are durability, risk of thromboembolism, valve hemodynamics, and effect on fetal outcome.

Tissue valves (bioprostheses) may be selected for a pregnant patient to avoid anticoagulation and risk of thromboembolism and should be considered in women of childbearing age who desire a pregnancy if there are no other indications for anticoagulation, and if the patient accepts the eventual need for replacement of the prosthesis. Bioprostheses in young women are associated with an increased risk of structural valve deterioration, which in some reports appear further accelerated in pregnancy. The risk of failure is estimated to be at least 50% in 10 years and higher if in the mitral position. Therefore, most women of childbearing age will need reoperation and the risk of a second open heart surgery should be considered when discussing the risk with the patient. The newer pericardial bioprostheses may offer better durability, but not enough data are available at the moment to make an estimate of the risk. Homografts appear to have a very low risk of failure even in younger patients and also offer superior hemodynamic profiles over other valves and should therefore be considered when possible.

Mechanical valves are indicated in pregnant patients with other coexisting heart disorders requiring anticoagulation, eg, atrial fibrillation, apical thrombus, or history of thromboembolism. Maternal thromboembolism complicates 4–14% of pregnancies in women with mechanical valves despite a therapeutic international normalized ratio (INR). This complication is more likely in patients with the older generation valves (caged-ball, tilting disk) in the mitral

position but is also reported in the newer bileaflet valves. The choice of prosthetic valve and the safe method of anticoagulation are therefore still of concern in pregnant patients and need further study.

Unfortunately, significant maternal and fetal risk of either hemorrhage or thrombosis with the accompanying use of warfarin or heparin remains a major problem. The decision on the choice of anticoagulation should therefore be made with both the patient and the physician after full discussion of potential risks and benefits, and the risk of pregnancy in patients with prosthetic heart valves should be discussed in detail with the patient and the family prior to conception.

The incidence of warfarin embryopathy has been estimated to be 4–10% and occurs after the embryo has been exposed to warfarin during the first trimester. Heparin, which does not cross the placenta, was believed to be safe for use during pregnancy; however, studies have reported the risk of thromboembolism, including fatal valve failure, may be as high as 12–24% in high-risk patients receiving either subcutaneous unfractionated heparin or low-molecular-weight heparin (LMWH). More recently, an 8.6% risk of valve thrombosis in pregnant patients treated with a subcutaneous LMWH was demonstrated. Many of these cases may be attributed to either inadequate dose, lack of monitoring, or subtherapeutic anti-Xa levels. In studies where anti-Xa levels were monitored, the risk of thromboembolism was very low (2%). High-risk cases may benefit from addition of low-dose aspirin. Table 31–3 shows a recommended regimen for anticoagulation in mechanical prosthetic heart valves taking into account the risk of the patient as well as the risk of side effects from the drugs.

Table 31–3. Recommended Approach for Anticoagulation Prophylaxis in Women with Prosthetic Heart Valves during Pregnancy.

	Higher Risk	Lower Risk
Conditions	First-generation prosthetic heart valve (eg, Starr-Edwards, Bjork Shiley) in the mitral position. Atrial fibrillation. History of thromboembolism while receiving anticoagulation therapy.	Second-generation prosthetic heart valve (eg, St. Jude Medical, Medtronic-Hall) in mitral position. Any mechanical prosthetic heart valve in the aortic position.
Treatment	Warfarin (INR 2.5-3.5) to 35th week, then UFH (mid-interval aPTT > 2.5) or LMWH (pre-dose anti-Xa ~0.7) + ASA 80-100 mg per day. OR UFH (aPTT 2.5-3.5) or LMWH (pre-dose anti-Xa ~0.7) for 12 weeks, followed by warfarin (INR 2.5-3.5) to 35th week, then UFH (aPTT > 2.5) or LMWH (pre-dose anti-Xa ~0.7) + aspirin 80-100 mg/day.	Subcutaneous UFH (mid-interval aPTT 2.0-3.0) or LMWH (pre-dose anti-Xa ~0.6) for 12 weeks, followed by warfarin (INR 2.5-3.0) to 35th week, then subcutaneous UFH (mid-interval aPTT 2.0-3.0) or LMWH (pre-dose anti-Xa ~0.6). OR Subcutaneous UFH (mid-interval aPTT 2.0-3.0) or LMWH (pre-dose anti-Xa ~0.6) throughout pregnancy.

aPTT, activated partial prothrombin time; INR, international normalized ratio; LMWH, low-molecular-weight heparin; UFH, unfractionated heparin.
Modified, with permission, from Elkayam U. JACC. 2005;46:403-10.

5. Infective endocarditis—Underlying structural abnormalities of the heart predispose patients to the development of infective endocarditis. The most common cause is rheumatic heart disease, with others being mitral valve prolapse, injecting drug abuse, and iatrogenic procedures. The estimated incidence of infective endocarditis during pregnancy is 0.005–1.0% of all pregnancies. Although it is rare, the development of infective endocarditis during pregnancy can have devastating consequences, with maternal and fetal mortality rates estimated to be 22% and 15%, respectively. The clinical diagnosis and the management of infective endocarditis in pregnancy is the same as for nonpregnant patients (see Chapter 29); however, special consideration must be given to the diagnostic and therapeutic approaches during pregnancy to reduce the risk to the fetus.

6. Rheumatic heart disease—Despite an overall decline in the incidence of rheumatic heart disease in Europe and North America, rheumatic valvular disease remains common in women of childbearing age.

The cardiac involvement in acute rheumatic fever is a pancarditis involving the endocardium, myocardium, and pericardium. It is the involvement of the endocardium, including the valvular and the subvalvular apparatus that gives rise to the acute manifestations as well as causes the development of chronic rheumatic valvular heart disease. The specific valvular conditions are described in previous sections. The mitral valve is most commonly affected, followed by the aortic valve, and less frequently the tricuspid and pulmonic valves.

Mild rheumatic fever may be difficult to diagnose in pregnancy due to tachycardia, functional murmur, and anemia. The management of acute rheumatic fever is similar in pregnant and nonpregnant patients and consists of bed rest, anemia correction, and penicillin. In severe cases, vasodilators, positive inotropes, or even surgery may be required. Echocardiography can be performed safely during pregnancy to delineate myocardial and heart valve function.

American College of Cardiology/American Heart Association Task Force on Practice Guidelines; Society of Cardiovascular Anesthesiologists; Society for Cardiovascular Angiography and Interventions; Society of Thoracic Surgeons, Bonow RO et al. ACC/AHA 2006 guidelines for the management of patients with valvular heart disease: a report of the American College of Cardiology/American Heart Association Task Force on Practice Guidelines (writing committee to revise the 1998 Guidelines for the Management of Patients With Valvular Heart Disease): developed in collaboration with the Society of Cardiovascular Anesthesiologists: endorsed by the Society for Cardiovascular Angiography and Interventions and the Society of Thoracic Surgeons. Circulation. 2006 Aug 1;114(5):e84–231. [PMID: 16880336]

Campuzano K et al. Bacterial endocarditis complicating pregnancy: case report and systematic review of the literature. Arch Gynecol Obstet. 2003 Oct;268(4):251–5. [PMID: 12728325]

Elkayam U et al. Valvular heart disease and pregnancy: part I: native valves. J Am Coll Cardiol. 2005 Jul 19;46(2):223–30. [PMID: 16022946]

Elkayam U et al. Valvular heart disease and pregnancy: part II: prosthetic valves. J Am Coll Cardiol. 2005 Aug 2;46(3):403–10. [PMID: 16053950]

Reimhold SC et al. Clinical practice. Valvular heart disease in pregnancy. N Engl J Med. 2003 Jul 3;349(1):52–9. [PMID: 12840093]

Stout KK et al. Pregnancy in women with valvular heart disease. Heart. 2007 May 5;93(5):552–8. [PMID: 16905631]

C. Myocarditis

This inflammatory process is either focal or diffuse and involves the heart musculature. Of all the infectious and noninfectious causes, viral infection with **coxsackie B virus** is the most common, accounting for nearly 50% of cases. Acute rheumatic fever is discussed in the previous section. Other important causes include **AIDS** and **Chagas disease** due to *Trypanosoma cruzi*, which is the most common cause in South and Central America. Only a few cases of myocarditis have been reported in pregnancy. Clinical manifestations range from incidental finding of silent myocarditis to overt heart failure with hemodynamic collapse. In the acute stage, the electrocardiogram (ECG) is almost always abnormal, showing Q waves with ST and T wave changes, which may mimic acute MI. The erythrocyte sedimentation rate (ESR) and cardiac enzymes are usually elevated. Viral cultures may or may not be helpful. Noninvasive imaging studies may reveal regional wall motion abnormalities. Although endomyocardial biopsy is the gold standard for the diagnosis of myocarditis, a negative result does not rule it out and rarely does the biopsy aid in diagnosing the etiology or guide management. Therefore, endomyocardial biopsy is not routinely recommended. All pregnant women in whom myocarditis is suspected should be hospitalized. Therapy is supportive, with bed rest; avoidance of strenuous activity; and treatment of heart failure with digoxin, diuretics, and vasodilators. Angiotensin-converting enzyme (ACE) inhibitors should be avoided because of the risk of fetal anomalies. Administration of corticosteroids and immunosuppressive therapy has been controversial and has demonstrated no proven benefit. Potential complications of myocarditis include arrhythmia, heart blocks, and cardiogenic shock. Anticoagulation should be seriously considered, especially for patients with severe left ventricular dysfunction.

D. Cardiomyopathy

1. Peripartum cardiomyopathy—This rare but distinct form of heart failure with left ventricular dysfunction occurs during pregnancy or postpartum. Classically, it is described as occuring between the last month of pregnancy and 5 months postpartum, but cases that do not appear different have been reported from week 17 of pregnancy to 6 months postpartum. Peripartum cardiomyopathy remains a diagnosis of exclusion. The prevalence appears to be increasing, but this is most likely due to increased diagnosis with the common use of echocardiography. Its estimated incidence in the United States is 1 in 4000 and may be higher in other countries. Its cause is unknown but is probably multifactorial. Histopathology reveals a dilated heart with pale myocardium, but myocardial biopsy is of little value. Because signs and symptoms of normal pregnancy resemble heart failure, peripartum cardiomyopathy is easily missed or diagnosed late in the course. Peripartum cardiomyopathy usually presents with dyspnea, cough, orthopnea, paroxysmal nocturnal dyspnea, fatigue, palpitations, and chest pain. Echocardiography is central to diagnosis. The echocardiogram demonstrates dilated left ventricle with marked overall impairment of systolic function. Pulmonary artery catheter placement should be considered for optimized treatment of these patients. Medical therapy is essentially supportive and similar to that for other forms of heart failure and includes salt restriction, diuretics, digoxin, and afterload reduction with hydralazine (the drug of choice). Angiotensin-converting enzyme inhibitors are contraindicated during pregnancy because of associated fetal central nervous system anomalies but can be used after delivery. Heparin should seriously be considered for treating possible thromboembolic phenomena in pregnant patients with very low left ventricular ejection fraction (< 35%). In cases refractory to medical therapy, use of an intra-aortic balloon pump for temporary stabilization and left ventricular assist device as a bridge to transplant are indicated. Most patients recover partially or even completely. However, mortality rates of 10–56% have been reported. Nevertheless, women with a history of peripartum cardiomyopathy have a significant risk of deleterious fetal and maternal outcome in subsequent pregnancies, even if their left ventricular function has returned to normal. Patients who have had fulminant courses and whose left ventricular function has remained depressed should be advised against becoming pregnant again. Recovery of left ventricular function may continue beyond 6 months, and repeat echocardiograms are recommended.

2. Hypertrophic cardiomyopathy—This primary myocardial disease shows a characteristic hypertrophy of the left or right ventricular myocardium. The hypertrophy is asymmetric and most commonly involves the intraventricular septum (asymmetric septal hypertrophy). Pathophysiologic mechanisms include presence of a hyperdynamic left ventricle, obstruction of left ventricular outflow tract, mitral regurgitation, and myocardial ischemia. Prevalence in the young population (aged 23–35 years) is 2 per 1000. A large number of patients are asymptomatic. Severe illness is manifested by poor functional capacity, heart failure, and sudden death.

Dyspnea is the most common symptom, with others being chest pain (which may be postprandial), dizziness, syncope, and palpitations. In younger patients, sudden death may be the first manifestation, with an annual incidence in the population being 6%. Physical examination varies from normal to characteristic findings in patients with high gradi-

ents. The auscultatory hallmark is a diamond-shaped, grade 3–4/6 systolic murmur, heard best at apex radiating to the left sternal border. The murmur increases in intensity during the strain phase of the Valsalva maneuver. Electrocardiogram shows ventricular hypertrophy, ST and T changes, and Q waves in inferolateral leads. Ventricular arrhythmias are commonly seen on Holter monitoring. Echocardiography diagnostically demonstrates asymmetric septal hypertrophy (with a ratio of septum to posterior wall thickening exceeding 1.5) and decreased septal motion.

Most patients do well during pregnancy. High-risk pregnant patients with a higher likelihood of worsening symptoms during pregnancy include those who were symptomatic prior to pregnancy and asymptomatic patients with left ventricular dysfunction. Increased incidence of supraventricular as well as ventricular arrhythmia in pregnancy has been reported. Maternal hypertrophic cardiomyopathy does not influence fetal outcome, although in about half of the patients it is familial with autosomal-dominant inheritance and confers a 50% risk for affection of the child. Genetic counseling is therefore recommended and a detailed discussion regarding risks and a thorough evaluation of the patient is required prior to conception.

In asymptomatic patients, outcome is usually good, but close monitoring is recommended. Therapy needs to be individualized in symptomatic patients. β-Blockers have been used most frequently and relatively safely in symptomatic patients but are not recommended for routine use. Of the calcium channel blockers, verapamil has been used sporadically in pregnant patients. Dual-chamber pacing for arrhythmia has been shown beneficial but is reserved for severely symptomatic cases refractory to medical therapy. Surgical myectomy has not yet been reported in pregnancy. Atrial fibrillation occurs in 10% of the patients, leading to an increased risk of systemic emboli and hemodynamic worsening. Sotalol, procainamide, and DC cardioversion have all been used to treat pregnant patients. Prophylactic placement of an implantable cardioverter-defibrillator should be considered in patients with high-risk features similar to nonpregnant patients. Alcohol septal ablation may reduce symptoms but does not alter prognosis. Hemodynamic monitoring with a pulmonary catheter is recommended for clinical deterioration encountered during labor and delivery and should be considered even in asymptomatic patients. Fortunately, the strain of vaginal delivery is well tolerated in women with hypertrophic cardiomyopathy. Cesarean section is reserved for obstetric indications. Epidural anesthesia should be avoided. Magnesium should be used for tocolysis if needed.

Autore C et al. Risk associated with pregnancy in hypertrophic cardiomyopathy. J Am Coll Cardiol. 2002 Nov 20;40(10):1864–9. [PMID: 12446072]

Elkayam U et al. Maternal and fetal outcomes of subsequent pregnancies in women with peripartum cardiomyopathy. N Engl J Med. 2001 May 24;344(21):1567–71. [PMID: 11372007]

Pearson GD et al. Peripartum cardiomyopathy: National Heart, Lung, and Blood Institute and Office of Rare Diseases (National Institutes of Health) workshop recommendations and review. JAMA. 2000 Mar 1;283(9):1183–8. [PMID: 10703781]

Sliwa K et al. Peripartum cardiomyopathy. Lancet. 2006 Aug 19;368(9536):687–93. [PMID: 16920474]

E. Coronary Artery Disease

Coronary artery disease is a leading cause of death in women in the United States. Coronary artery disease kills more women than the next 16 leading causes of death combined. The incidence of MI during pregnancy and postpartum is estimated to be 3–7 in 100,000 and predominantly antepartum or intrapartum. Because of a trend toward older childbearing age, the incidence of coronary artery disease may be increasing. Earlier studies reported a mortality rate of 37–50% due to MI during pregnancy. However, recent data suggest the rate is much lower at 5–8%, possibly due to improved diagnosis and treatment. The risk of MI in pregnancy is increased threefold to fourfold in comparison with the nonpregnant state. Risk factors include age (30-fold increased if older than 40 years compared with younger than 20 years), hypertension, diabetes mellitus, smoking, and thrombophilia (Table 31–4). The causes of MI in pregnancy include atherosclerosis, congenital lesions (anomalous origin of coronary artery), inflammatory diseases of coronary arteries (Kawasaki disease), connective tissue or vasospastic disorders, and spontaneous coronary artery dissection, which may account for up to 20% of cases. Up to 30% of the women who undergo coronary angiography will have normal or nonobstructive coronary arteries indicating that vasospasm and spontaneous lysis of thrombus play a role in the process.

Most MIs that occur during pregnancy are anterior and transmural, involving the left anterior descending artery. Successful treatment of acute MI during pregnancy with thrombolytic therapy has been reported, but given the risk of placental and fetal bleeding, percutaneous coronary intervention is the preferred treatment for acute ST-elevation MI in pregnancy. β-Blockers are the mainstay of medical therapy. Efforts should be made to limit myocardial oxygen consumption, particularly during late pregnancy and delivery, in women with known coronary artery disease.

Table 31–4. Risk Factors for Pregnancy-Related Acute Myocardial Infarction.

Risk Factor	Univariate Risk Odds Ratio	P Value	Multivariate Risk Odds Ratio	P Value
Age, years				
< 20 (Ref)	1		1	
20–24	2.4	NS	1.9	NS
25–29	4.3	0.02	3.3	NS
30–34	9.5	< 0.01	6.7	< 0.01
35–39	20.5	< 0.01	16.0	< 0.01
≥ 40	31.6	< 0.01	15.2	< 0.01
Race				
White (Ref)	1		1	
Black	1.4	NS	1.4	NS
Hispanic	0.5	0.02	0.8	NS
Condition				
Hypertension	11.7	< 0.01	21.7	< 0.01
Diabetes	3.2	< 0.01	3.6	< 0.01
Smoking	6.2	< 0.01	8.4	< 0.01
Anemia	2.0	< 0.01	1.6	NS
Thrombophilia	22.3	< 0.01	25.6	< 0.01
Preeclampsia	1.6	0.03	0.1	< 0.01
Postpartum bleeding	2.1	0.02	1.8	NS
Transfusion	7.4	< 0.01	5.1	< 0.01
Postpartum infection	2.5	0.04	3.2	0.02

Modified, with permission, from James AH. Circulation. 2006;113:1564–1571.

The most common presentation is angina pectoris. Patients with high index of suspicion should undergo a stress test for risk stratification. Left ventricular function needs to be assessed to determine the choice of therapy and predict likelihood of survival. The normal physiologic changes of pregnancy may precipitate myocardial ischemia and heart failure in women with left ventricular impairment caused by an infarct. Troponin I remains the most useful marker for monitoring pregnant women for a myocardial injury because it is undetectable during normal labor and delivery. Lipid-lowering drugs of the statin-type are contraindicated during pregnancy due to reported teratogenicity, and the risk clearly outweighs the potential benefit.

Ladner HE et al. Acute myocardial infarction in pregnancy and the puerperium: a population-based study. Obstet Gynecol. 2005 Mar;105(3):480–4. [PMID: 15738011]

James AH et al. Acute myocardial infarction in pregnancy: a United States population-based study. Circulation. 2006 Mar 28;113(12):1564–71. [PMID: 16534011]

F. Arrhythmias

Most arrhythmias occurring during pregnancy are benign. Sinus tachycardia, sinus arrhythmia, sinus bradycardia, atrial premature beats, and ventricular premature beats are relatively common during pregnancy. These arrhythmias are hemodynamically insignificant and require no treatment, and the patient can be reassured of their innocence. The occurrence of more complex arrhythmias should, however, raise the suspicion of underlying cardiac disease. Symptomatic arrhythmias, which are rare during pregnancy, may develop during an otherwise uncomplicated pregnancy or in association with underlying cardiac disease. In fact, cardiac arrhythmias may be the first manifestation of cardiac disease during pregnancy.

1. Supraventricular arrhythmias

A. PAROXYSMAL SUPRAVENTRICULAR TACHYCARDIA—The most common arrhythmia encountered during pregnancy is paroxysmal supraventricular tachycardia (PSVT); it has been estimated to occur in approximately 3% of pregnant patients. In patients with a previous history of PSVT, the frequency and severity of the episodes may increase during pregnancy. The symptoms of PSVT are dyspnea, lightheadedness, and anxiety in patients without underlying cardiac disease. In patients with underlying cardiac abnormalities, angina, heart failure, and syncope may occur as a result of myocardial ischemia and decreased cardiac output. Although there is concern about the effects of hypotension on the fetus during these episodes, women with PSVT do not have an increase in perinatal complications.

B. ATRIAL FLUTTER AND ATRIAL FIBRILLATION—Atrial flutter, which is uncommon during pregnancy, and atrial fibrillation are usually found in patients with underlying cardiac disease. The hemodynamic consequences and the associated symptoms depend on the underlying cardiac status. During pregnancy, atrial fibrillation is most commonly found in association with mitral stenosis. The development of this arrhythmia in these patients may precipitate congestive heart failure and embolic events. Consideration should be given to anticoagulation therapy if persistent. β–Blockers and digoxin are preferred for rate control.

C. ATRIOVENTRICULAR NODAL REENTRANT TACHYCARDIA— This arrhythmia may present the first time during pregnancy. Structural heart disease needs to be excluded with an echocardiogram. Adenosine can be safely given and usually terminates the arrhythmia. In recurrent cases, a β-blocker can be given, but drugs should be avoided if possible. The patients should be instructed in the Valsalva maneuver, which may terminate the tachycardia.

D. WOLFF-PARKINSON-WHITE SYNDROME—This preexcitation syndrome usually occurs in patients without underlying cardiac disease. Patients with Wolff-Parkinson-White (WPW) syndrome may have recurrent arrhythmias—most commonly, atrioventricular (AV) reentry tachycardia, atrial fibrillation, or atrial flutter. The hemodynamic effects of the associated arrhythmias are related to the type of arrhythmia and the ventricular rate. Many patients with WPW syndrome are asymptomatic, but pregnancy is associated with an increased incidence of arrhythmias in women with this syndrome.

2. Ventricular arrhythmias

A. PREMATURE VENTRICULAR COMPLEXES—Premature ventricular complexes (PVCs) are relatively common in pregnant women and are associated with complaints of palpitations. Pregnant women with PVCs and no underlying cardiac disease have an excellent prognosis and require no treatment. Reassurance to the patient is frequently all that is required, along with avoidance of such aggravating factors as smoking and stimulants.

B. VENTRICULAR TACHYCARDIA—Defined as the occurrence of three or more consecutive ventricular complexes, ventricular tachycardia is a serious cardiac arrhythmia that, if sustained, can lead to death. Ventricular tachycardia is rare during pregnancy, but when it occurs, it is usually associated with underlying cardiac disease. The most common cardiac abnormalities associated with ventricular tachycardia are mitral valve prolapse, valvular disease, and cardiomyopathy. The prognosis for patients with nonsustained ventricular tachycardia (less than 30 seconds in duration) and no underlying cardiac disease is excellent. In such patients, the ventricular tachycardia is catecholamine-sensitive, and extreme exercise should be avoided. In some patients, therapy with β-adrenergic blocking drugs may be indicated. Sustained ventricular tachycardia (more than 30 seconds in duration) or hemodynamically significant ventricular tachycardia is usually associated with underlying cardiac disease, and therapy with antiarrhythmics is usually indicated. Such patients should also undergo evaluation for such precipitating factors as myocardial ischemia, electrolyte imbalance, congestive heart failure, digitalis intoxication, stimulants, and hypoxia. Drugs that can be used are procainamide, lidocaine, or sotalol. Amiodarone should be avoided. In hemodynamically unstable patients, immediate DC cardioversion should be performed. Patients with aborted sudden death, syncopal ventricular tachycardia, ventricular fibrillation or flutter should have an implantable cardioverter-defibrillator implanted, preferably under echocardiographic guidance.

3. Heart blocks—First-degree heart block is evident as PR prolongation on the ECG and results from an increased time of conduction through the AV junction. First-degree heart block is primarily associated with rheumatic heart disease or digitalis therapy and does not usually require therapy. Second-degree heart block can may be divided into two types: Mobitz type I (Wenckebach) and Mobitz type II. Mobitz type I is characterized by progressive lengthening of the PR interval until an impulse is blocked. It is a relatively benign disorder and occurs when vagal tone is increased. Treatment is seldom indicated. Mobitz type II is a sudden block of conduction without previous prolongation of the PR interval. It often precedes the development of complete heart block. It is rare during pregnancy but may occur in association with rheumatic heart disease or infections. If the ventricular rate is slow and the patient is symptomatic, treatment with permanent pacing is indicated.

Complete heart block can be congenital or acquired. Its onset is usually prior to the pregnancy, and it rarely progresses. Approximately half the cases of complete heart block occurring during pregnancy have an associated ventricular septal defect. Other causes include ischemic heart disease, myocarditis, and rheumatic heart disease. The need for pacemaker therapy depends on the ventricular escape rate. Symptoms are rare at a rate of 50–60 beats/min; if the rate suddenly slows, however, syncope may develop. Permanent pacing is indicated in such patients.

Trappe HJ. Acute therapy of maternal and fetal arrhythmias during pregnancy. J Intensive Care Med. 2006 Sep–Oct;21(5):305–15. [PMID: 16946446]

G. Pericardial Diseases

Pericarditis is usually a mild, self-limited disease. Its incidence, diagnosis, and treatment are similar in pregnant and nonpregnant patients. Most pregnancies, even the complicated ones, may safely reach full term. Idiopathic pericarditis is the most common cause of pericardial disease, others being trauma, infections (viral, bacterial, fungal, tuberculosis), radiation, and collagen vascular diseases.

Sharp, stabbing chest pain that is exacerbated in the supine position and relieved by leaning forward is the most common complaint. Pathognomonic finding of pericardial friction rub is best heard with the diaphragm of the stethoscope over the second and fourth intercostal spaces in midclavicular line or the left sternal border, with the patient leaning forward and inspiring deeply. Characteristic ST-segment elevations with upward concavity and upright T waves have been reported in 80% of patients with acute pericarditis. Echocardiography is an important diagnostic modality and may reveal thickened pericardium, pericardial effusion and, most importantly, cardiac tamponade.

Pregnant patients in whom pericarditis is suspected should be hospitalized for complete bed rest. Nonsteroidal antiinflammatory drugs (NSAIDs), aspirin, and indomethacin are effective analgesics. Corticosteroids should be avoided in tuberculosis. Pericardiectomy is reserved for severe, relapsing pericarditis, refractory to medical treatment. Symptoms of a complicating pericardial effusion with cardiac tamponade mimics the symptoms of pregnancy and includes shortness of breath, dyspnea on exertion, and fatigue. Echocardiogram will quickly establish the diagnosis. Treatment for symptomatic cardiac tamponade is percutaneous drainage with surgical pericardial window reserved for refractory cases.

Asymptomatic pericardial effusion is frequently encountered in all trimesters, most commonly in the third, but resolves postpartum. Pericardial constriction has been rarely reported in pregnancy, although it could occur as a pericarditis sequel. Most patients have dyspnea, marked edema, and ascites in the latter half of pregnancy. Diuretics, corticosteroids, and pericardiectomy (reserved for refractory cases, and associated with reasonable maternal and fetal risk) have all been used to treat pericardial constriction in pregnant patients. Preterm delivery and fetal death have been reported.

H. Pulmonary Hypertension

1. Primary pulmonary hypertension—This uncommon although distinct entity is defined as *mean* pulmonary artery pressure by right heart catheter of more than 30 mm Hg at rest, or more than 40 mm Hg during exercise, without a demonstrable cause. Primary pulmonary hypertension poses a significant risk to pregnant women, with mortality approaching 40%, warranting prevention of pregnancy or early therapeutic abortion. The most common presenting symptoms are dyspnea, fatigue, chest pain, palpitations, syncope or near syncope, and Raynaud phenomenon. Characteristic physical findings are a result of markedly increased pulmonary pressures, leading to right ventricular hypertrophy and failure with decreased cardiac output. The echocardiogram reveals elevated pulmonary artery pressures, right atrial enlargement, right ventricular hypertrophy, and tricuspid regurgitation. A new onset or worsening of symptoms is commonly seen in the second and third trimesters.

Treatment with prostacyclin infusion for short periods to lower pulmonary artery pressure in pregnancy has been reported to be safe and effective. Incidents of premature labor and delivery are high. Patients should lie in the left lateral decubitus position to improve cardiac output.

Planned vaginal delivery seems to be safe in stable patients. Epidural anesthesia has been used in most reported cases. Patients should be monitored for 7–10 days postpartum prior to discharge to ensure stability. Due to its grave prognosis and a high incidence of maternal and fetal morbidity and mortality, pregnancy is contraindicated in patients with primary pulmonary hypertension (see Table 31–2). Therapeutic abortion is indicated as soon as possible if pregnancy occurs. Adequate counseling should be provided to all patients regarding sterilization.

Stewart R et al. Pregnancy and primary pulmonary hypertension: successful outcome with epoprostenol therapy. Chest. 2001 Mar;119(3):973–5. [PMID: 11243988]

2. Thromboembolic disease—Venous thromboembolic disease is a leading cause of morbidity and mortality during pregnancy and postpartum. Venous thromboembolism affects pregnant women five times more frequently than nonpregnant women. It is estimated to complicate 2 in 1000 pregnancies. The diagnosis is complicated by symptoms similar to usual pregnancy symptoms such as shortness of breath, tachycardia, and leg swelling. As many as up to 33% of deep venous thrombosis may occur in the first trimester, although the risk is highest postpartum (five times higher than during the pregnancy). The immediate postpartum period risk for pulmonary embolism is 15 times greater than during the pregnancy. Risk factors for venous thromboembolism includes age > 35 years, weight > 165 lbs, a family or personal history of deep venous thrombosis or pulmonary embolism, varicose veins, smoking, or any known hypercoagulable state as well as multiple previous pregnancies. Pulmonary embolism will occur in 15–24% of patients with untreated deep venous thrombosis and may be fatal in 15%. Diagnosis of deep venous thrombosis should be made with compression ultrasound or impedance plethysmography. Magnetic resonance imaging (MRI) can be performed to diagnose iliac thrombosis. The diagnosis of pulmonary embolism is complicated by the need to avoid radiation in the pregnant patient. However, ventilation-perfusion scannning is considered safe throughout pregnancy and should be the first step in the diagnosis of a pulmonary embolism. To further decrease radiation, consideration should be given to performing perfusion scan alone. If there is no defect, then pulmonary embolism would be very unlikely. The gold standard for pulmonary embolism is pulmonary angiogram. Except in the first trimester, pulmonary angiogram exposes the fetus to less radiation than a helical CT scan. An echocardiogram may support the diagnosis of acute embolus by demonstrating right heart enlargement without hypertrophy and elevated pulmonary artery pressure. Hypokinesis with relative sparing of the right ventricular apex may be seen. The main treatment for deep venous thrombosis during pregnancy consists of heparin, although warfarin can be given after the first trimester until 35 gestation weeks. If unfractionated heparin is used, a target activated partial prothrombin time level should be

2.0–2.5. If an LMWH is used, the patient should be monitored with anti-Xa levels. Pulmonary embolism, if stable, should be treated with intravenous heparin for at least 5 days. Oral anticoagulation should be continued for 6 months thereafter. In unstable pulmonary embolism, consideration to thrombolysis and embolectomy should be given. An inferior vena caval filter may also be needed.

Heit JA et al. Trends in the incidence of venous thromboembolism during pregnancy or postpartum: a 30-year population-based study. Ann Intern Med. 2005 Nov 15;143(10):697–706. [PMID: 16287790]
Stone SE et al. Pulmonary embolism during and after pregnancy. Crit Care Med. 2005 Oct;33(10 Suppl):S294–300. [PMID: 16215350]

I. Diseases of the Aorta

1. Marfan syndrome—Marfan syndrome is an inheritable autosomal-dominant connective tissue disorder of the fibrillin gene on chromosome 15 with a prevalence of 1 in 3000–5000 individuals. It involves the ocular, skeletal, and cardiovascular systems. Patients are predisposed to aortic dissection or actual rupture of the aorta most commonly originating in the ascending portion during pregnancy, most likely in the third trimester. High-risk patients have significant associated cardiac abnormalities, such as mitral valve prolapse, mitral and aortic regurgitation, and an aortic root greater than 4.0 cm in diameter. All women with Marfan syndrome planning to become pregnant should undergo a screening transthoracic echocardiogram. High-risk patients (aortic root > 4.0 mm or rapidly progressive dilatation) should have elective surgery before conception, preferably with valve-sparing surgery if no significant aortic regurgitation is present. If the diagnosis is made during pregnancy, β-blockers are strongly recommended, with some authorities advocating prompt termination of pregnancy with aortic repair. Close follow-up with echocardiography should be performed. Women at increased risk for complications during pregnancy should be advised against attempting a pregnancy that may be associated with a 50% maternal mortality rate (Table 31–2). Patients with no dissection or aortic root enlargement can deliver vaginally with epidural anesthesia and facilitated stage 2 of labor. However, if there is aortic root enlargement, aortic regurgitation, or rapid progression of the aorta size, caesarean delivery is recommended. The risk of the offspring inheriting the disorder is 50%.

2. Loeys-Dietz syndrome—This is a recently recognized syndrome caused by genetic mutation in transforming growth factor (TGF)-β with autosomal dominant inheritance with variable clinical expression. The most common manifestations are aortic aneurysms with a high risk of dissection, hypertelorism, bifid uvula or cleft palate, generalized arterial tortuosity, and aneurysms throughout the arterial tree. Loeys-Dietz syndrome may be misdiagnosed as Marfan syndrome, but patients with Loeys-Dietz syndrome will have normal fibrillin gene. Women with this syndrome should be advised against pregnancy due to the risk of aortic dissection with normal aortic diameter and a risk for uterine rupture during pregnancy.

Immer FF et al. Aortic dissection in pregnancy: analysis of risk factors and outcome. Ann Thorac Surg. 2003 Jul;76(1):309–14. [PMID: 12842575]

Milewicz DM et al. Treatment of aortic disease in patients with Marfan syndrome. Circulation. 2005 Mar 22;111(11):e150–57. [PMID: 15781745]

Williams JA et al. Early surgical experience with Loeys-Dietz: a new syndrome of aggressive thoracic aortic aneurysm disease. Ann Thorac Surg. 2007 Feb;83(2):S757–63. [PMID: 17257922]

J. Hypertension

Hypertension affects 12% of pregnancies and is responsible for 18% of maternal deaths in the United States. Hypertension in pregnancy is defined as an increase in systolic blood pressure of 30 mm Hg or more or in diastolic pressure of 15 mm Hg or more. The hypertension may be chronic (> 135/85 mm Hg before pregnancy or before 20 weeks gestation and persistent more than 6 weeks postpartum), transient, or part of preeclampsia or eclampsia (hypertension after 20 gestation weeks with new proteinuria > 300 mg over 24 hours and edema). The drug treatment of choice for mild hypertension is methyldopa. For severe hypertension drugs such as hydralazine, labetalol, and nifedipine can be used. Target diastolic blood pressure is just below 100 mm Hg for severe cases and lower to 85 mm Hg for nonemergencies.

Vidaeff AC et al. Acute hypertensive emergencies in pregnancy. Crit Care Med. 2005 Oct;33(10 Suppl):S307–12. [PMID: 16215352]

▶ Clinical Findings

A. History

The evaluation of heart disease in pregnancy is difficult due to the normal anatomic and physiologic changes of pregnancy. A careful history taking therefore is very important and should include a history of rheumatic fever, valvular disorder, arrhythmia, congenital heart disease, coronary risk factors or established coronary artery disease, and cardiac surgery.

B. Symptoms and Signs

Reduced exercise tolerance and fatigue are the most common symptoms reported in pregnant women, probably due to increased body weight and anemia. Dizziness, light-headedness, or even syncopal episodes may occur during the latter part of pregnancy because mechanical compression of the uterus on the inferior vena cava decreases venous return, and thus the cardiac output. Palpitations are also a frequent complaint but usually are not associated with a significant arrhythmia. Dyspnea and orthopnea, probably due to hyperventilation, are also reported.

C. Physical Examination

The physical examination of pregnant patients with normal cardiovascular systems changes because of the increased hemodynamic burden. The evaluation of patients with suspected heart disease during pregnancy requires a thorough knowledge of the normal physiologic changes (see Table 31–1).

A normal pregnant patient has a slightly fast resting heart rate, large pulse, slightly widened pulse pressure, and warm extremities. Jugular venous distention is seen starting at the twentieth week. Edema of the ankles and legs is commonly encountered in late pregnancy. A prominent but unsustained left ventricular impulse may be palpated in late pregnancy and may simulate the volume overload seen in aortic or mitral regurgitation. The auscultatory findings of normal pregnancy begin late in the first trimester and usually disappear 2–4 weeks after delivery. During cardiac auscultation, the first heart sound is loud and exhibits an exaggerated splitting. The second heart sound during late pregnancy is often increased and may exhibit persistent expiratory splitting, especially with the patient in the left lateral position. A third heart sound has been reported to be frequent in late pregnancy. However, because of its association with heart failure, the presence of a third heart sound should lead to further investigation of underlying heart disease, especially in women with symptoms and other signs suggestive of heart disease. A fourth heart sound is rarely heard during a normal pregnancy.

Systolic murmurs are common during pregnancy and result from the increased blood volume and hyperkinetic state. Most frequently they are innocent early systolic murmurs, grade 1–2/6, that are best heard at the lower left sternal border and over the pulmonary area, radiating to the suprasternal notch or to the left of the neck. They usually represent vibrations created by ejection of blood into the pulmonary trunk. A cervical venous hum or mammary souffle heard best in the right supraclavicular area in a supine position is a benign systolic, or a continuous, murmur occurring in late pregnancy (Table 31–5). Diastolic heart murmurs are unusual and usually represent valvular abnormalities.

D. Diagnostic Difficulties

Although systolic murmurs are common, the finding of a diastolic murmur is rare during a normal pregnancy and should warrant further diagnostic evaluation. Both systolic and diastolic murmurs associated with cardiac disease can increase or decrease in intensity during pregnancy. Innocent flow murmurs and benign vascular murmurs usually decrease in the sitting position. The systolic murmurs of aortic or pulmonic stenosis usually increase in intensity because of the increased cardiac output and blood volume. The diastolic murmur of mitral stenosis is also increased and may even be first detected during pregnancy. The augmented blood volume and the increased heart rate of pregnancy shorten the diastolic filling period and increase the rate of blood flow across the mitral valve. In contrast, murmurs of

Table 31–5. Cardiovascular Signs and Symptoms in Normal Pregnancy.

Symptoms
Fatigue
Orthopnea
Dyspnea
Decreased functional capacity
Dizziness
Syncope
Physical signs
Jugular venous distention
Displaced left ventricular apical impulse
Right ventricular heave
Palpable pulmonary impulse
Increased intensity of the first heart sound
Persistent splitting of the second heart sound
Systolic ejection murmur at the left lower sternal border or pulmonary area with radiation to the neck
Cervical venous hum, mammary souffle

mitral or aortic regurgitation may soften or even disappear during pregnancy as a result of the decrease in peripheral vascular resistance. The circulatory changes of pregnancy also affect the auscultatory findings in cardiac abnormalities, such as mitral valve prolapse and hypertrophic cardiomyopathy, which are dependent on volume. The increase in left ventricular volume during pregnancy may attenuate or abolish the click and late systolic murmur typical of mitral valve prolapse. The systolic murmur of hypertrophic obstructive cardiomyopathy may also decrease or disappear as the left ventricular volume increases during pregnancy.

E. Diagnostic Studies

1. Electrocardiography—The ECG is an important diagnostic technique that can indicate the presence of underlying cardiac abnormalities. Cardiac chamber hypertrophy, myocardial ischemia and infarction, pericarditis, myocarditis, conduction abnormalities, and the presence of atrial and ventricular arrhythmias may be detected by electrocardiography. In patients with suspected cardiac arrhythmias, ambulatory Holter monitoring may be indicated. During normal pregnancy, sinus tachycardia, a shift of the axis to the left or right may be observed, and transient ST abnormalities are common.

2. Echocardiography—Transthoracic echocardiography is an important diagnostic noninvasive study, which can be performed safely in pregnancy. The intracardiac structures can be evaluated for abnormalities of the great vessels, cardiac chambers, and heart valves. Chamber sizes and ventricular function can also be measured.

During the echocardiographic examination, the normal physiologic changes that occur with pregnancy should be kept in mind. When the patient is evaluated in the left lateral position, an increase in the diastolic dimensions of the right and left ventricles is common because of volume increases that occur with a normal pregnancy. Because of the increase in the left ventricular dimensions, mitral valve prolapse may improve or disappear during pregnancy. Right and left atrial dimensions may also increase slightly; these changes increase as the pregnancy progresses. Small pericardial effusions have been noted in late pregnancy in healthy women.

Doppler echocardiography provides reliable quantitative and qualitative information regarding the presence and severity of valvular stenosis and regurgitation. Doppler echocardiography can measure the valve area and gradients across stenotic valves. Small degrees of pulmonary, tricuspid, and mitral regurgitation have frequently been found in normal individuals, whether pregnant or not. In patients with congenital heart disease (corrected or uncorrected) Doppler echocardiography can detect the presence of intracardiac shunts and estimate the shunt ratios by determining the right and left cardiac outputs. It can measure pulmonary artery systolic pressure to assess the effects of the valvular lesions and intracardiac shunts on the pulmonary circulation.

Transesophageal echocardiography (TEE) provides superior images of the intracardiac structures and great vessels, providing the same detailed analysis of cardiac structure, function, and hemodynamic assessment possible with transthoracic echocardiography. Transesophageal echocardiography can be used for patients in whom the transthoracic examination is technically suboptimal and for those with suspected prosthetic or native valve dysfunction, infective endocarditis, congenital heart disease, or aortic dissection. Although experience with TEE during pregnancy has been limited, the procedure should be considered in pregnant patients for whom the risks are less than the possible benefit. The procedure should be performed by an experienced echocardiographer, and fetal monitoring, in addition to the routine monitoring of the patient, should be available (Table 31–6).

Table 31–6. Normal Diagnostic Test Findings in Pregnancy.

Electrocardiogram
Sinus tachycardia
Increased incidence of arrhythmias
QRS axis deviation
Increased amplitude of R wave in lead V_2
ST segment and T wave changes
Small Q waves
Echocardiogram
Mildly increased biatrial size
Increased biventricular dimensions
Mildly increased left ventricular systolic function
Small pericardial effusion
Increased tricuspid valve diameter
Mild tricuspid, pulmonic, and mitral regurgitation
Chest roentgenogram
Increased lung markings
Horizontal positioning of the heart
Straightened left upper cardiac border

3. Exercise tolerance test—Little is known about the safety of an exercise test to establish ischemic heart disease in pregnancy. Fetal bradycardia, marked hypoxia, acidosis, and severe hypothermia at peak exercise have been reported. In light of these facts, the use of a submaximal stress test (approximately 70% of the maximal predicted heart rate) with close fetal monitoring is recommended, until more information regarding its safety is available. Maximal oxygen consumption, unchanged in pregnancy, could be used for the assessment of the functional status in cardiac patients during pregnancy.

4. Chest radiography—The usefulness of chest films during pregnancy is limited because of the potential hazard to the fetus from radiation exposure. Whenever a chest film is believed necessary, the abdominopelvic area should be shielded with lead to minimize exposure. The normal cardiac changes of pregnancy, such as chamber enlargement and the horizontal position of the heart because of the elevation of the diaphragm, should not be misinterpreted as cardiac disease. Newer and more accurate techniques such as Doppler echocardiography have largely replaced chest films in the evaluation of cardiac structure and function.

5. Radionuclide studies—Myocardial perfusion scans and radionuclide ventriculography should be avoided, if possible, especially in the first trimester of pregnancy because of the risk of rare but possible fetal malformations. Also, in women of childbearing age, the incidence of coronary heart disease is low and other noninvasive techniques, such as exercise echocardiography, can be used to assess coronary artery disease. In cases of suspected pulmonary embolism, a limited ventilation-perfusion scan (only performing the perfusion phase) may be performed weighing out the risks and the benefits.

6. Magnetic resonance imaging—Magnetic resonance imaging provides multiplanar images of the body with excellent soft-tissue contrast without the use of ionizing radiation. Magnetic resonance imaging is in general regarded safe in pregnancy. However, safety data are limited. Therefore, MRI should be limited to cases where ultrasonography are inconclusive and where patient care depends on further imaging. Gadolinium contrast appears to be safe. However, the safety is not very well proven in the fetus, and therefore, should be reserved for cases where this type of study is important for the health of the mother.

7. Pulmonary artery catheterization—Bedside hemodynamic monitoring can be performed with a balloon-tipped pulmonary artery catheter. In most patients, inflating the balloon permits flotation of the catheter through the right heart without the need for fluoroscopy. With the catheter in the pulmonary artery, the balloon is inflated until it occludes a small vessel; the pulmonary artery wedge pressure obtained reflects the left ventricular end-diastolic pressure. Pulmonary artery pressures and cardiac output can also be mea-

sured. The placement of a balloon flotation catheter should be considered during the early stages of labor in any patient with cardiac disease who has been symptomatic during the pregnancy. Furthermore, because of postpartum hemodynamic changes, hemodynamic monitoring should be continued for up to 48 hours following delivery.

8. Cardiac catheterization—In some patients with cardiac disease who decompensate during pregnancy, complete diagnostic information cannot be obtained by noninvasive methods alone. This is particularly important when surgical intervention is contemplated. Cardiac catheterization in these patients may need to be performed during pregnancy. Because the radiation required for the performance of this technique has potentially adverse effects on the fetus, cardiac catheterization should be performed only if the needed information cannot be obtained by any other means. Whenever possible, cardiac catheterization should be performed after major organogenesis has occurred (more than 12 weeks after the last menses). The brachial approach is the preferred method to minimize the risk of radiation exposure to the abdomen, which should be lead shielded. The exposure to x-rays should be reduced to a minimum; catheter position can be guided in some cases by Doppler and contrast echocardiography.

▶ Treatment

A. Pharmacologic Treatment

Treatment of the pregnant patient with cardiac disease requires the collaborative consultation of the obstetrician and cardiologist at regular intervals during gestation and careful planning for delivery with the anesthesiologist. All cardiovascular drugs during pregnancy should be avoided, if possible, especially in the first trimester. Most cardiovascular drugs cross the placenta and are secreted into the breast milk, mandating a detailed evaluation of risk-to-benefit ratio (Table 31–7).

1. Heart failure—Treatment of heart failure is more challenging in pregnant patients than in nonpregnant women. Salt restriction and activity limitation are extremely important. In patients with pulmonary congestion, medical therapy should begin with digoxin. Although digoxin has been safely used during pregnancy for many years, blood levels should be monitored to avoid toxicity. Diuretics, although not teratogenic may cause impaired uterine blood flow and placental perfusion, and hence should only be used in severely symptomatic patients. Thiazide diuretics have been associated with neonatal thrombocytopenia, jaundice, hyponatremia, and bradycardia.

Afterload is already reduced during pregnancy, hence further reduction in afterload may only be beneficial in selected cases. Hydralazine, the most frequently used afterload-reducing agent during pregnancy, is a direct arteriolar dilator and has not been associated with adverse fetal effects. Angiotensin-converting enzyme inhibitors are contraindi-

Table 31–7. Alphabetical List of the Commonly Used Cardiovascular Medications, Their Potential Fetal Side Effects, and Overall Safety.

Drugs	Potential Side Effects	Safety
ACE-I	IUGR, prematurity, low birth weight, neonatal renal failure, bony malformations, limb contractures, patent ductus arteriosus, death	Contraindicated
Adenosine	Limited data (in first trimester only)	Safe
Amiodarone	IUGR, prematurity, hypothyroidism, prolonged QT in the newborn	Unsafe
ARB	Same as ACE-I	Contraindicated
β-Blockers	Fetal bradycardia, hypoglycemia and apnea at birth, IUGR, uterine contraction initiation	Safe
Calcium channel blocker	Maternal hypotension leading to fetal distress, birth defects	Verapamil safe
Digoxin	Low birth weight	Safe
Disopyramide	Uterine contraction initiation	Safe
Diuretics	Hyponatremia, bradycardia, jaundice, low platelets, impaired uterine blood flow	Potentially unsafe
Heparin	None reported	Probably safe
Hydralazine	None reported	Safe
Lidocaine	CNS depression due to fetal acidosis with high blood levels	Safe
Mexiletine	IUGR, fetal bradycardia, neonatal hypoglycemia, and hypothyroidism	Safe
Nitrates	Fetal bradycardia	Probably safe
Nitroprusside	Thiocyanate toxicity	Potentially unsafe
Procainamide	None reported	Safe
Quinidine	Premature labor, fetal VIII cranial nerve damage with high blood levels	Safe
Sotalol	Limited data; bradycardia, reports of death	Probably safe
Warfarin	Embryopathy, in utero fetal hemorrhage, CNS abnormalities	Unsafe

ACE-I, angiotension-converting enzyme inhibitor; ARB, angiotensin receptor blockers; CNS, central nervous system; IUGR, intrauterine growth retardation.

cated in pregnancy due to their associated increased risk of premature delivery, low birth weight, fetal hypotension, renal failure, bony malformations, persistent patent ductus arteriosus, respiratory distress syndrome, and even death. Angiotensin II receptor blockers have similar adverse reactions and are thus rendered unsafe. Data on nitrates are limited and require further evaluation. β-Blockers may be used safely.

2. Arrhythmias—During pregnancy, any precipitating factors of arrhythmia should be avoided or corrected. In general, conservative treatment of cardiac arrhythmias is indicated. DC cardioversion is the treatment of choice in patients with hemodynamic compromise due to arrhythmia. Although no antiarrhythmic is completely safe during pregnancy, most are tolerated well and are relatively safe. Drugs with the longest record of safety should be used as first-line therapy. Digoxin, although one of the safest drugs for treating arrhythmia during gestation, may cause increased risk of prematurity and intrauterine growth retardation. Adenosine has been reported safe and successful in terminating supraventricular tachycardias during pregnancy.

Quinidine, with minimal fetal risk, has the longest record of being used safely and effectively in the treatment of both atrial and ventricular tachycardia during pregnancy. When quinidine is indicated during pregnancy, blood levels should be closely monitored because of drug interactions with warfarin may develop excessively prolonged prothrombin time, with the potential for hemorrhage. Procainamide has also been used safely and is the drug of choice in the treatment of wide-complex tachycardias.

Amiodarone is associated with fetal hypothyroidism, smaller size at birth for date of gestation, and prematurity, and is also secreted in breast milk. Amiodarone is thus reserved only for treating life-threatening arrhythmias or those refractory to other medical therapy. Verapamil, although used during pregnancy, should be discontinued at the onset of labor to avoid dysfunctional labor and postpartum hemorrhage.

β-Adrenergic blocking agents are relatively safe and have frequently been used in pregnant patients to treat arrhythmia, hypertrophic cardiomyopathy, and hyperthyroidism. Propranolol is a nonselective β-blocker that has been used frequently during pregnancy. Fetal and newborn heart rate, blood glucose levels, and respiratory status should be monitored closely.

Lidocaine may be used for ventricular tachycardia, especially in the setting of an acute MI, but it requires close monitoring of blood levels.

3. Thrombosis and thromboembolism—Even though increased concentrations of clotting factors and platelet adhesiveness, and decreased fibrinolysis in pregnancy result in an overall increased risk of thrombosis and embolism, the actual incidence of venous thromboembolism during pregnancy is lower than previously reported. The gestational age at presentation appears to be equally distributed. Pulmonary embolism cases are reported to occur most commonly in the postpartum period and are strongly associated with a cesarean section. About 40% of asymptomatic patients with deep venous thrombosis may indeed have a pulmonary embolism.

The major indications for anticoagulants during pregnancy include the presence of mechanical heart valves and prophylaxis for recurrent pulmonary thromboembolism. Some patients with rheumatic heart disease with atrial fibrillation and cardiomyopathies may also be candidates for anticoagulation during pregnancy. The best method of anticoagulation in a pregnant patient is still controversial. A recommended regimen is suggested in Table 31–3.

Warfarin has been associated with fetal wastage due to spontaneous abortion and stillbirths, optic nerve atrophy and blindness, microcephaly, mental retardation, and even death due to intracranial hemorrhage. Its use in the first trimester is associated with warfarin embryopathy in 4–10% of newborns, a syndrome comprising nasal bone hypoplasia and epiphyseal stippling. Warfarin poses significant risks to both the mother and the fetus during labor and delivery; however, breast-feeding women can be prescribed warfarin because it is not secreted in the breast milk. In the second trimester, warfarin is the treatment of choice, with INR monitoring. Therefore, warfarin should be given only after the 12th gestational week and should be stopped before delivery around 35th week.

Heparin is generally the drug of choice for anticoagulation in pregnant patients, unless there is a very high risk for thromboembolism (see section on prosthetic heart valves). As soon as pregnancy is diagnosed, oral anticoagulants should be discontinued and subcutaneous heparin, with a goal partial thromboplastin time (PTT) of 2–2.5 times normal, should be initiated. If LMWH is used, anti-Xa levels should be monitored. Complications of heparin administration include abdominal wall hematoma or abscess, thrombocytopenia, alopecia, and osteoporosis. At the 36th week of gestation, subcutaneous heparin should be switched to intravenous route. To avoid the risk of bleeding during labor and delivery, heparin should be discontinued 24 hours prior. Anticoagulation should then be resumed 4 hours after delivery.

Low-dose aspirin has been safely used in pregnancy. Dipyridamole should not be used in a pregnant patient. Thrombolytic therapy has been used safely and effectively but should be avoided whenever possible.

4. Endocarditis prophylaxis—The American Heart Association does not recommend prophylaxis for infective endocarditis in pregnant patients expected to have an uncomplicated course of pregnancy and labor and delivery. However, because of the unpredictability of labor and delivery, many clinicians opt to treat. Women undergoing urinary catheter placement in established urinary tract infection, and vaginal delivery in vaginal infection should receive intramuscular or intravenous antibiotics. The conservative approach is to administer endocarditis prophylaxis in pregnant patients with mechanical prosthetic heart valves, a history of infective endocarditis, those with most congenital heart disorders, obstructive hypertrophic cardiomyopathy, and those with mitral valve prolapse with mitral regurgitation who are undergoing interventions likely to cause septicemia.

Joglar JA et al. Antiarrhythmic drugs in pregnancy. Curr Opin Cardiol. 2001 Jan;16(1):40–5. [PMID: 11124717]

B. Surgical Treatment

Ideally, most cardiac diseases requiring surgical correction are diagnosed and treated before the patient becomes pregnant, so the data are anecdotal. In general, cardiac surgery in pregnant patients is not associated with significant maternal risk but may cause fetal wastage. Fetal risk has been reported to be as high as 33%. Pregnant women requiring cardiac surgery need utmost care, adequate valve selection, and anticoagulation to ensure a good outcome.

Surgery should be reserved for severely symptomatic patients and those who are refractory to medical therapy, and it should be avoided in the first trimester, if possible. Procedures not involving cardiopulmonary bypass are preferred because of associated risks of fetal bradycardia and hypoperfusion.

C. Labor and Delivery

Labor and delivery are periods of maximal hemodynamic stress during pregnancy. Pain, anxiety, and uterine contractions all contribute to altered hemodynamics. Oxygen consumption is higher, and cardiac output is increased up to 50%. Both systolic and diastolic pressures are increased significantly during uterine contractions, especially in the second stage. Anesthesia and analgesia during labor and delivery may affect oxygen consumption, but they do not reduce increased cardiac output secondary to uterine contractions.

Acute decompensation may develop in patients with preexisting cardiac disease. This increase in preload and cardiac output can be devastating in a patient with limited cardiac reserve or an obstructive valvular lesion. Patients at greatest risk for complications during labor and delivery include those with significant pulmonary hypertension and those in NYHA functional class III or IV.

The preferred method of delivery is vaginal, with careful attention paid to pain control by regional anesthesia to avoid tachycardia. Postpartum hemorrhage and excessive fluid intake should be prevented. Invasive hemodynamic monitoring may be needed in some cases to guide treatment rapidly during labor and delivery. In these patients, the monitoring should be continued for at least 24–48 hours after delivery or until hemodynamic stability is ensured. Cesarean section, with few exceptions, should be performed only for obstetric indications because it can also create blood loss and fluid shifts. Regardless of the delivery method, however, effective pain control is absolutely essential. Antibiotic prophylaxis should be administered when indicated.

▶ **Prognosis**

Maternal mortality and morbidity rates during pregnancy depend on the underlying cardiac lesion and the functional status of the patient (see Table 31–2). The greatest risk of maternal mortality (25–50%) is for patients with pulmonary hypertension, Eisenmenger syndrome, NYHA class III and IV, and Marfan syndrome with a dilated aorta. Pulmonary vascular disease prevents the adaptive mechanisms of normal pregnancy and makes labor, delivery, and the early postpartum period particularly problematic. Moderate-to-severe mitral stenosis, aortic stenosis, the presence of mechanical prosthetic valves, uncomplicated coarctation of the aorta, uncorrected congenital heart diseases (without Eisenmenger syndrome), and Marfan syndrome with a normal aorta are associated with a 5–10% mortality rate. Left-to-right shunts, pulmonary valve disease, corrected congenital heart disease, bioprosthetic valves, and mild-to-moderate mitral stenosis have a mortality rate of less than 1%.

The functional status of a patient should be classified according to the NYHA classification system. Patients in class I or II can be expected to undergo pregnancy with a less than 0.5% risk of death.

Mauri L et al. Valvular heart disease in the pregnant patient. Curr Treat Options Cardiovasc Med. 2001 Feb;3(1):7–14. [PMID: 11139785]

Sadler L et al. Pregnancy outcomes and cardiac complications in women with mechanical bioprosthetic, and homograft valves. BJOG. 2000 Feb;107(2):245–53. [PMID: 10688509]

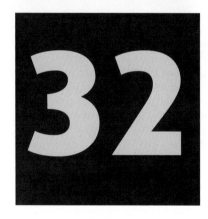

Endocrinology & the Heart

B. Sylvia Vela, MD & Michael H. Crawford, MD

Endocrinology involves the study of glands that secrete hormones into the circulation for effects at distant target sites. At present, more than 100 hormones are known to be released into the circulation, with more than 200 types of receptors on target cells in the human body. Many of these cells contain literally thousands of receptors on their surfaces. Because these hormone receptors are so ubiquitous throughout the body, the presence or absence of a single hormone can have multiple effects on one or more organ systems, including the cardiovascular system. This chapter considers most of the common and some uncommon endocrinopathies that can affect the heart, addressing specifically how they can be recognized and treated to best restore cardiovascular health.

THYROID & THE HEART

Thyroid hormone has profound effects on the cardiovascular system, regulating vascular tone and contractility and the metabolic demands of the body. Thyroid disease often presents solely with cardiovascular manifestations, necessitating a thorough search for this potentially reversible cause of heart disease.

Thyroid hormone regulates oxidative and metabolic processes throughout the body by directing cellular protein synthesis at the nuclear level. Both overproduction or underproduction of thyroid hormone can disrupt normal metabolic function. Under the control of pituitary release of thyroid-stimulating hormone (TSH), the thyroid gland secretes tetraiodothyronine (T_4) and triiodothyronine (T_3), mostly bound to plasma proteins. The free, or unbound, fraction of hormone negatively feeds back at the level of the hypothalamus and pituitary to suppress further release of thyroid-releasing hormone (TRH) and TSH. One step necessary in the production of thyroid hormone is the trapping of iodine by the gland.

1. Hyperthyroidism

ESSENTIALS OF DIAGNOSIS

▶ Suppressed TSH below the lower normal limits.

▶ High free T_4, total T_4, and free thyroxine index, or high free T_3 or total T_3 radioimmunoassay in T_3 toxicosis.

▶ High 24-hour radioactive iodine uptake in Graves disease or toxic multinodular goiter; low uptake in thyroiditis or exogenous cause.

▶ Symmetric goiter (often with bruit) and exophthalmos in Graves disease.

▶ General Considerations

In hyperthyroidism, increased levels of thyroid hormone result in a hyperdynamic cardiovascular system. The enhanced diastolic and systolic performance is due to the effect of T_3 on the regulation of specific cardiac genes. These genes promote the expression of structural proteins of the contractile apparatus of the cardiac myocyte. In addition, thyroid hormone increases calcium-activated adenosine triphosphatase (ATPase), which increases intracellular calcium concentration and inotropism.

In general, the hyperdynamic activity of the hyperthyroid cardiovascular system is similar to that of other conditions in which the sympathetic nervous system is activated with the release of catecholamines. There is enhanced cardiac output, increased stroke volume, enhanced left ventricular contractility, decreased systemic vascular resistance, tachycardia with a wide pulse pressure, a hyperdynamic precordium, increased myocardial oxygen consumption, and increased coronary flow. Although systolic contraction and diastolic relaxation are augmented, the heart is functioning near capacity, with little cardiac reserve.

Surprisingly, catecholamine levels are low or normal in hyperthyroidism, and these catecholamine-like effects are believed to be due in part to a demonstrable increase in the responsiveness of β-catecholamine receptors. The causes of hyperthyroidism are listed in Table 32–1.

▶ Clinical Findings

A. Symptoms and Signs

1. Systemic symptoms and signs—Patients with hyperthyroidism often complain of weight loss despite an increased appetite; this helps distinguish this condition from other wasting conditions such as cancer or AIDS. Occasionally, the appetite may be so great as to result in weight gain. A fine resting tremor of the hands is noticed, along with nervousness, anxiety, insomnia, mood swings, and irritability. Heat intolerance and sweaty skin are seen. Proximal muscle weakness and muscle wasting may be prominent. An increased number of bowel movements or diarrhea is due to decreased transit time in the gut. Diplopia on lateral gaze is seen in Graves ophthalmopathy as a result of extraocular muscle hypertrophy.

2. Cardiovascular symptoms and signs—Frequently, the patient has cardiovascular symptoms, including palpitations, dyspnea, and atypical chest pain. Cardiac arrhythmias are common, especially atrial premature contractions and atrial fibrillation. In the elderly, atrial fibrillation may be the only manifestation of thyrotoxicosis, a condition known as **apathetic hyperthyroidism.** Approximately 10–20% of patients with atrial fibrillation are thyrotoxic, and 10–20% of thyrotoxic patients have atrial fibrillation. The risk of arterial thromboembolism is increased in thyrotoxic patients with atrial fibrillation, as it is in other patients with atrial fibrillation. Other atrial dysrhythmias, such as paroxysmal atrial tachycardia and atrial flutter, are unusual. Ventricular arrhythmias usually indicate underlying cardiac disease.

Exercise intolerance and dyspnea on exertion can occur with or without left-sided heart failure. Heart failure is usually precipitated by atrial fibrillation, in which the rapid ventricular rate and the loss of the atrial kick impair diastolic filling. Most patients with heart failure have underlying cardiac disease that predisposes them to the development of ventricular dysfunction. High-output heart failure can also occur, but it is rare.

Often, thyrotoxicosis precipitates exacerbation of angina when the increased demands placed on the heart by the

Table 32–1. Causes of Hyperthyroidism.

Etiology	Comments
Graves disease	Symmetric smooth goiter, ophthalmopathy, elevated/^{131}I uptake, homogeneous uptake on thyroid scan, TSH-receptor antibodies
Toxic multinodular goiter	Nodular goiter, nonhomogeneous uptake on thyroid scan
Autonomous thyroid nodule	Single large "hot" nodule on thyroid scan, suppressing rest of thyroid tissue
Thyroiditis	
Subacute	Tender firm goiter, low ^{131}I uptake, transient high ESR
Radiation	Tender goiter, low ^{131}I uptake, high ESR; occurs after ^{131}I therapy
Painless (silent)	Nontender goiter, low ^{131}I uptake, normal ESR
Postpartum	Nontender goiter, low ^{131}I uptake, antithyroid antibodies, transient; tends to recur with each pregnancy
Exogenous	
Amiodarone	Low or normal ^{131}I uptake
Iatrogenic	Absent goiter, low serum thyroglobulin, low ^{131}I uptake
Factitious	Absent goiter, low serum thyroglobulin, low ^{131}I uptake
Iodine induced	Low ^{131}I uptake, high 24-h urinary iodide excretion; history of iodine ingestion or exposure (contrast agents)
Rare causes	
Struma ovarii	Low ^{131}I uptake; may have palpable ovary
Trophoblastic tumor	Very high HCG
Metastatic follicular carcinoma	Usually obvious metastases on ^{131}I scan
TSH-producing adenoma	TSH not suppressed, tumor on CT or MRI of pituitary; consider if gland regrows post thyroidectomy or ^{131}I treatment

CT, computed tomography; ESR, erythrocyte sedimentation rate; HCG, human chorionic gonadotropin; ^{131}I, radioactive iodine; MRI, magnetic resonance imaging; TSH, thyroid-stimulating hormone.

thyrotoxic state are accompanied by the underlying fixed atherosclerotic lesions of coronary artery disease. The angina improves once the thyrotoxicosis is treated, and frank myocardial infarction precipitated by thyrotoxicosis is rare.

B. Physical Examination

Stare, lid retraction, and lid lag are usually present because of the high catecholamine-like state. Exophthalmos, proptosis, and diplopia are only seen in Graves disease and are caused by hypertrophy of the extraocular muscles. In most conditions a goiter is present. Absence of a goiter, especially in a young person, should raise the suspicion of factitious hyperthyroidism; elderly patients, however, may not have a palpable goiter in the presence of disease.

The precordium is hyperdynamic, with loud heart sounds reflecting accelerated atrioventricular flow. Systolic ejection murmurs may be heard, reflecting increased flow across the aortic and pulmonic valves. The pulse is rapid and bounding. The skin has an unusually soft and velvety texture and is often sweaty. There is proximal muscle weakness, with patients often having difficulty rising from a squatting position. Deep tendon reflexes are hyperreflexic, and a resting tremor is present. Dermopathy or localized edema may be present on the shins (pretibial myxedema). In younger patients, especially young women, Graves disease is the most common cause of thyrotoxicosis. Graves disease is an autoimmune disease in which antibodies to the TSH receptor stimulate both excessive thyroid growth and thyroid hormone production. These patients typically have a symmetric goiter (often with a bruit) with or without exophthalmos. In the elderly, especially those with apathetic hyperthyroidism, symptoms and signs may be absent. Toxic multinodular goiter is a more common diagnosis in patients over the age of 40. Usually these goiters are very large and nodular (as the name suggests). Iatrogenic or factitious thyrotoxicosis should always be considered; these patients typically have no goiter, and the thyroglobulin level is suppressed. Clinicians should suspect hyperthyroidism in patients with persistent sinus tachycardia and atrial fibrillation, unexplained congestive heart failure, or unstable angina.

C. Diagnostic Studies

1. Electrocardiography and echocardiography—Sinus tachycardia is usually present, although any supraventricular tachycardia can be seen. Atrial fibrillation occurs in 10–20% of hyperthyroid patients; its prevalence in the population at large is 0.4%. On echocardiography, a hypercontractile state is seen with rapid filling of a highly compliant ventricle. Increased left ventricular mass and cardiac hypertrophy can also be seen.

2. Laboratory findings—Diagnosis is made by measurement of thyroid function tests (Table 32–2). Thyroid-stimulating hormone should be suppressed below the lower limit of detection, and the free T_4 or free thyroxine index (FTI) should be elevated, confirming the diagnosis. If the free T_4 or FTI is normal, measurement of total or free T_3 is recommended to rule out a condition known as T_3 toxicosis, in which the serum T_4 level is normal, but the total or free T_3 is elevated. If the only abnormality is a suppressed TSH level, subclinical hyperthyroidism versus a systemic nonthyroidal illness must be considered. Thyroid function tests should be repeated after any period of illness to determine whether the abnormal thyroid function tests have resolved and were due to nonthyroidal illness.

Other tests that may be helpful include measurement of antithyroid antibodies (antimicrosomal or thyroidperoxidase antibodies) or TSH receptor antibody, which are elevated in patients with Graves disease. Thyroglobulin levels will be suppressed in patients with factitious or iatrogenic thyrotoxicosis. Before treatment with radioactive iodine, all suspected hyperthyroid patients should have a radioactive iodine uptake (RAIU) test to ensure that hyperthyroid patients with thyroiditis or exogenous hyperthyroidism are not mistakenly

Table 32–2. Tests in Hyperthyroidism.

Condition	T_4	T_3	TSH	^{131}I Uptake
Graves disease	↑, N	↑	↓	↑↑↑
Multinodular goiter	↑, N	↑	↓	↑↑
Solitary nodule	↑, N	↑	↓	↑ or nl
Early subacute and silent thyroiditis	↑	↑	↓	↓
Exogenous T_4	↑	↑	↓	↓
Exogenous T_3	↓	↑	↓	↓
Iodine-induced	↑	↑	↓	↓
Ectopic	↑, N	↑	↓	↓
TSH-producing pituitary tumor	↑, N	↑	↑, N	↑

^{131}I, radioactive iodine; T_4, tetraiodothyronine; T_3, triiodothyronine; TSH, thyroid-stimulating hormone.

treated for these transient, reversible conditions. Elevated RAIU is seen in Graves disease, toxic multinodular goiter, and occasionally in an autonomously functioning thyroid nodule. In contrast, a decreased RAIU is seen in thyroiditis and exogenous hyperthyroidism. Thyroid scans rarely add any useful information to a good physical examination in patients with diffusely enlarged thyroid glands. In Graves disease, the scan typically shows an enlarged symmetric gland with homogeneous uptake. Thyroid scans are occasionally helpful in identifying an adenoma or multinodular gland, in which one or more cold spots are seen.

► Treatment

Treatment is directed at rapidly improving symptoms and reducing demands on the heart. The mainstay of treatment is accomplished by preventing thyroid hormone synthesis and release with antithyroid drugs, followed by radioactive iodine thyroid ablation (Table 32–3). β-Blockers are most commonly used to improve symptoms. If the tachycardia is considered to be significantly deleterious in patients with heart failure, esmolol, which has a rapid onset of action and short half-life, may be given intravenously; it should be stopped—with rapid reversal—if heart failure worsens. Tremor and tachycardia will improve almost immediately with β-blocker therapy although systolic and diastolic con-tractile performance will not change due to direct effects of thyroid hormone on cardiac muscle. Of the oral β-blockers, propranolol is preferred because it also prevents the periph-eral conversion of T_4 to T_3. The dose should be titrated to the patient's pulse and is usually 20–80 mg four times daily. Occasionally, high doses (80–320 mg four times daily) of propranolol are required in thyroid storm.

Thionamides are used to prevent thyroid hormone release and synthesis, by blocking iodine oxidation, organifi-cation, and iodotyrosine coupling. Propylthiouracil (PTU) and methimazole are the thionamides used in the United States. Because they deplete intrathyroidal stores of thyroid hormone, they circumvent the precipitation of thyroid storm that can result from radiation thyroiditis after radio-active iodine ablation. Doses typically begin at 50–100 mg three times daily of PTU and 10–30 mg daily of methima-zole. Methimazole may be preferred because of its once-a-day dosing and lower incidence of side effects. These drugs are typically withdrawn 3–5 days prior to radioactive iodine ablation and restarted 3–5 days after ablation. Thionamides are known to cause nausea and rash and, of most concern, agranulocytosis in 10% of patients.

Other drugs, including lithium, iodides, and corticoster-oids, are usually reserved for the prevention of life-threaten-ing conditions such as thyroid storm; occasionally, they are used for patients with severe congestive heart failure or

Table 32–3. Agents Used to Treat Hyperthyroidism.

Agent	Dose	Mechanism of Action
Thionamides		
Propylthiouracil	50–300 mg, PO three times daily	Inhibits thyroid hormone synthesis
		Inhibits T_4 conversion to T_3
Methimazole	10–60 mg, PO once daily	Inhibits thyroid hormone synthesis
β-Blockers		
Propranolol	10–80 mg, PO q6–8h	Decreases β-adrenergic activity; inhibits T_4 conversion to T_3
Atenolol	50–100 mg/day PO	Decreases β-adrenergic activity
Nadolol	80–160 mg/day PO	Decreases β-adrenergic activity
Metoprolol	100–200 mg/day PO	Decreases β-adrenergic activity
Iodides		
SSKI	5 drops PO q6–8h	Prevents thyroid hormone release
Lugol	5 drops PO q6–8h	Prevents thyroid hormone release
Ipodate	3 g PO q2–3 days or 0.5 g/day	Prevents thyroid hormone release
Radioactive iodine	Calculated dose	Destroys overfunctioning thyroid
Other agents		
Lithium	300 mg PO three times daily (monitor blood levels)	Prevents thyroid hormone release
Hydrocortisone	50–100 mg IV q6–8h	Decreases peripheral conversion of T_4 to T_3; prevents thyroid hormone release

SSKI, saturated solution of potassium iodide; T_4, tetraiodothyronine; T_3, triiodothyronine.

unstable angina secondary to thyrotoxicosis. Lithium prevents thyroid hormone release, and the dosage is determined by monitoring therapeutic serum levels. Iodides abruptly prevent the release of thyroid hormone. They **must** be used in conjunction with thionamides because rebound or escape occurs commonly. Doses are usually 3–5 drops of a supersaturated potassium iodide solution or Lugol solution (50 mg of iodide per drop) every 6–8 hours.

Parenteral corticosteroids are usually given in stress doses for thyroid storm. Corticosteroids inhibit thyroid hormone secretion and prevent peripheral conversion of T_4 to T_3. Doses are usually 50–100 mg of hydrocortisone every 6–8 hours.

Radioactive iodine (^{131}I) is the preferred and definitive treatment for thyrotoxicosis in patients with a high RAIU. Because thyroid tissue is the only tissue that requires iodine (for thyroid hormone synthesis), ^{131}I is used for thyroid gland destruction. The advantages of radioactive iodine include the fact that usually only a single treatment is needed and that it is relatively safe and inexpensive. Because the treatment usually requires 3–6 months to resolve the hyperthyroidism, most patients will require interim therapy with thionamides during that time. The patient is usually rendered hypothyroid as a result of the treatment and is then treated with long-term thyroid hormone replacement.

Patients with multinodular goiters, who have lower RAIU (than do patients with Graves disease), often have an inadequate response to ^{131}I, and may require re-treatment or surgery. Pregnant patients should not receive ^{131}I and should therefore be treated with PTU, with or without β-blockers, or with subtotal thyroidectomy in the second trimester.

Aspirin, nonsteroidal antiinflammatory drugs, and—rarely—corticosteroids are used if painful thyroiditis is present. Thyroiditis is reversible and requires short-term therapy only. β-Blockers can be used temporarily to improve thyrotoxic symptoms.

Treatment of congestive heart failure and atrial fibrillation are essentially the same as for a euthyroid individual. Treatment should include use of a nonselective β-blocker (eg, propranolol) or a selective $β_1$-blocker (eg, metoprolol) to normalize the heart rate. The physician should be aware, however, that treatment of atrial fibrillation is limited to control of the ventricular rate because cardioversion will not be successful as long as the thyrotoxicosis is present. In addition, patients may be relatively resistant to digoxin. Usually, sinus rhythm returns within 6 weeks with resolution of the thyrotoxic state. Older patients with underlying cardiac disease may not spontaneously revert and may require cardioversion. Anticoagulation should be considered until the patient is euthyroid and in sinus rhythm.

Once the patient becomes euthyroid, the hyperdynamic cardiovascular manifestations disappear. Atrial fibrillation should convert to normal sinus rhythm in more than 60% of patients, and angina should improve because of decreased demands on the heart.

▶ Prognosis

The prognosis is generally excellent for most hyperthyroid conditions. Graves disease and autonomously functioning thyroid nodules usually respond well to ^{131}I and do not recur. As noted previously, multinodular goiters may be relatively resistant to ^{131}I and may ultimately require subtotal thyroidectomy. Despite surgical treatment, multinodular goiters frequently recur.

Frost L et al. Hyperthyroidism and risk of atrial fibrillation or flutter: a population-based study. Arch Intern Med. 2004 Aug 9–23;164(15):1675–8. [PMID: 15302638]
Klein I et al. Thyroid hormone and the cardiovascular system. N Engl J Med. 2001 Feb 15;344(7):501–9. [PMID: 11172193]
Shimizu T et al. Hyperthyroidism and the management of atrial fibrillation. Thyroid. 2002 Jun;12(6):489–93. [PMID: 12165111]

2. Hypothyroidism

 ESSENTIALS OF DIAGNOSIS

▶ Thyroid-stimulating hormone levels above the range of normal (primary hypothyroidism).

▶ Low free T_4 or low FTI.

▶ General Considerations

Hypothyroidism is the term given to any degree of thyroid hormone deficiency. The term **myxedema** is reserved for patients with thyroid hormone deficiency of such severity that profound hypothermia, hypoventilation, hypotension, and central nervous system signs are evident on physical examination. It is estimated that anywhere from 0.5% to 5.0% of the adult population of the United States has underlying hypothyroidism.

Hypothyroidism is associated with accelerated atherosclerosis, likely from the accompanying hyperlipidemia. The atherosclerosis is especially pronounced in the presence of hypertension; however, angina is uncommon and the incidence of myocardial infarction is not increased. This is probably due to the decreased metabolic demands placed on the heart in the hypothyroid state. More commonly, angina is precipitated or worsened by rapid thyroid hormone replacement.

▶ Clinical Findings

A. Symptoms and Signs

1. Systemic symptoms and signs—Hypothyroidism is an insidious disease and may be subtle in its progression and presentation. Patients typically complain of weight gain (although morbid obesity does not occur), weakness, lethargy, fatigue, depression, muscle cramps, constipation, cold intolerance, dry skin, and coarse hair. Women often have menstrual disorders (most commonly amenorrhea), and men may have impotence or decreased libido.

2. Cardiovascular symptoms and signs—Cardiovascular findings are the opposite of those found in hyperthyroidism. There is a decrease in cardiac output because of a reduction in stroke volume and heart rate, reflecting the loss of inotropism and chronotropism characteristic of thyroid hormone. Congestive heart failure rarely occurs because the decrease in cardiac output is usually matched by a decrease in metabolic demand. Myocardial oxygen consumption appears to be decreased below levels expected by the reduced workload to an extent that the hypothyroid heart can be thought of as being more efficient. Systemic vascular resistance is increased and blood volume is reduced, causing prolongation of circulation time and a decrease in blood flow to the periphery. In most tissues, this decrease in tissue perfusion is accompanied by decreased oxygen consumption, so that the mixed arteriovenous oxygen difference remains normal. The hemodynamic alterations resemble those of congestive heart failure except that pulmonary congestion does not occur, and pulmonary artery and right ventricle pressures are often normal. In addition, cardiac output and systemic vascular resistance increase normally in response to exercise, unlike heart failure from other causes.

Marked hypothyroidism must be present for several months before cardiovascular manifestations occur. Common complaints of hypothyroid patients are exertional dyspnea, decreased exercise tolerance, and easy fatigability. As the hypothyroidism worsens, congestive heart failure and pleural and pericardial effusions become prominent. Myxedematous heart failure can be distinguished from other causes in that it responds to exercise with an increased heart rate; improves with thyroid hormone replacement, but not digitalis and diuretics; rarely results in pulmonary congestion; and exhibits high protein content effusions.

B. Physical Examination

Hypothermia, bradycardia with weak arterial pulses, and mild hypertension are characteristic vital signs. The hypertension may be due to increased peripheral resistance. Thyroid hormone replacement will normalize blood pressure in approximately one-third of these patients. The patient may appear pale, with periorbital edema and facial puffiness. Hair and skin are usually coarse and dry. Goiter is present in patients with Hashimoto thyroiditis, congenital enzyme deficiencies, iodine deficiency, and thyroid hormone resistance; it is also present in patients taking amiodarone and antithyroid drug therapy such as thionamides and lithium.

Percussion of the chest may reveal pleural effusions from increased capillary permeability and the leakage of proteins into the interstitial space. Distant heart sounds are present,

especially if a pericardial effusion is present. Reflexes are characteristically delayed in the return phase. Nonpitting edema may be present as a result of the deposition of mucopolysaccharides. Severe hypothyroidism can progress to myxedema coma, and anasarca may be present. In the presence of congestive heart failure, pitting edema may be superimposed on the nonpitting edema.

C. Diagnostic Studies

1. Electrocardiography and echocardiography—Electrocardiographic (ECG) changes include sinus bradycardia, prolonged PR and QT intervals, low voltage complexes, and flattened or inverted T waves. Atrial, ventricular, and intraventricular conduction delays are three times as likely in patients with myxedema as in the general population. Pericardial effusion is probably partly responsible for these ECG changes.

Pericardial effusions occur in as many as 30% of all hypothyroid patients. Cardiac tamponade is unusual because of the slow accumulation of fluid, which does not increase pericardial pressure excessively. Echocardiographic studies have revealed asymmetric septal hypertrophy and obstruction of the left ventricular outflow tract in some patients. These findings disappear when the hypothyroidism is treated.

2. Laboratory findings—Asymptomatic hypothyroid individuals—such as the elderly—frequently go unrecognized. Therefore, all elderly patients and patients with premature atherosclerosis should be screened for primary hypothyroidism with a TSH test. Although the most common cause of hypothyroidism is Hashimoto thyroiditis, there are other causes of hypothyroidism (Table 32–4).

In primary hypothyroidism, TSH level is elevated, and T_4 level, free T_4 level, and FTI are reduced. The absence of an elevated TSH level indicates either nonthyroidal illness or hypothalamic-pituitary dysfunction. Severely ill patients are unlikely to have panhypopituitarism in the absence of other hormone deficiencies.

Occasionally, TSH level is mildly elevated in the face of a normal T_4 level. Subclinical hypothyroidism, as opposed to recovery from a nonthyroidal illness, must be considered. These patients are typically asymptomatic but are at intermediate risk for cardiovascular disease when compared with euthyroid or frankly hypothyroid individuals.

Antithyroid antibodies (antimicrosomal or thyroid peroxidase antibodies) are elevated in Hashimoto thyroiditis. Creatine kinase isoenzymes are increased in hypothyroidism, although the isoenzyme pattern is usually MM and not MB. Hypothyroidism is a common cause of hyperlipidemia; 95% of hypothyroid individuals will have an elevated cholesterol, and 70% will have elevation in both cholesterol and triglycerides. Anemia of chronic disease may be seen, as may hyponatremia from impaired free-water clearance.

Table 32-4. Causes of Hypothyroidism.

Causes	Comments
Destructive	
Radioactive iodine ablation	No palpable thyroid tissue
Thyroid surgery	Scar evident
External radiation to neck	History of malignancy
Infiltrative diseases	Diagnose by fine-needle aspirate
Autoimmune	
Hashimoto thyroiditis	Goiter, antithyroid antibodies
Following Graves disease	History of Graves; may have ophthalmopathy
Hereditary or congenital	
Congenital dyshormonogenesis	Goiter, usually diagnosed in childhood
Thyroid hormone resistance	Rare, familial
Iodine deficiency	Cretin if untreated; unusual in United States
Drug-induced	
Lithium	Goiter, on lithium, usually with underlying predisposition to thyroid disease
Thionamides	History of hyperthyroidism
Iodines	Wolff-Chaikoff effect
Pituitary/hypothalamic failure	Other hormone deficiencies usually apparent

► Treatment

Thyroxine therapy reverses all of the cardiovascular manifestations associated with hypothyroidism. The most important consideration with thyroid hormone replacement therapy is the speed of rendering the patient euthyroid. Young patients without evidence of cardiac disease can be replaced with full doses of thyroxine. Patients over the age of 55 or patients with evidence or suspicion of cardiac disease require slow and judicious use of thyroid hormone replacement to prevent exacerbation of angina or precipitation of myocardial infarction. The typical regimen would begin with 25 mcg (0.025 mg/day) or one-fourth of a normal replacement dose, gradually increased over several months to normal replacement doses of approximately 100–150 mcg (0.1–0.15 mg/day). Because the half-life of T_4 is 1 week, patients will notice alleviation of their symptoms in 1–2 months after reaching a typical replacement dose.

Patients with unstable angina and hypothyroidism are more difficult to treat because of the risk of exacerbating the angina. Very small doses of hormone should be used, and the dosage increments must be made slowly over a longer-than-usual time. If necessary, angioplasty or coronary artery bypass grafting (CABG) should be recommended, after which—if revascularization is complete—thyroid hormone replacement can occur at the usual dosage and rate. Angioplasty and CABG surgery can safely be done in a hypothyroid individual without significantly increasing morbidity and mortality. Adjustments in anesthesia and drug doses should be made because their decreased metabolic clearance makes hypothyroid patients very sensitive to these agents.

Treatment of myxedema coma is controversial. Many authors recommend high initial doses of intravenous T_4 (400 mcg) to saturate receptors and replenish diminished stores, followed by 100 mcg/day. Others prefer a more conservative approach of 50–100 mcg/day intravenously. Stress doses of hydrocortisone should also be administered (100 mg intravenously every 6–8 hours) because hypothyroidism and adrenal insufficiency frequently coexist, and thyroid hormone replacement may precipitate adrenal crisis.

► Prognosis

In the absence of coexisting heart disease, treatment with thyroid hormone and restoration of a euthyroid status correct the hemodynamic, ECG, and serum enzyme alterations and restores heart size to normal. Therapy is lifelong, and relapses occur if the patient is noncompliant or taken off therapy for any reason.

Flynn RW et al. Mortality and vascular outcomes in patients treated for thyroid dysfunction. J Clin Endocrinol Metab. 2006 Jun;91(6):2159–64. [PMID: 16537678]

Hak AE et al. Subclinical hypothyroidism is an independent risk factor for atherosclerosis and myocardial infarction in elderly women: The Rotterdam Study. Ann Intern Med. 2000 Feb 15;132(4):270–8. [PMID: 10681281]

Monzani F et al. Effect of levothyroxine on cardiac function and structure in subclinical hypothyroidism: a double blind, placebo-controlled study. J Clin Endocrinol Metab. 2001 Mar; 86(3):1110–5. [PMID: 11238494]

Tielens ET et al. Changes in cardiac function at rest before and after treatment in primary hypothyroidism. Am J Cardiol. 2000 Feb 1;85(3):376–80. [PMID: 11078310]

Toft AD et al. Thyroid disease and the heart. Heart. 2000 Oct; 84(4):455–60. [PMID: 10995425]

3. Effect of Heart Disease on Thyroid Function

Acute or chronic illness, such as occurs with myocardial infarction, congestive heart failure, and during the postoperative period of cardiopulmonary bypass, can make the interpretation of thyroid function tests difficult. Levels of T_3 and T_4 can drop as much as 20–40%, the so-called nonthyroidal illness. Thyroid-stimulating hormone is inhibited centrally and can be suppressed further by use of drugs, such as dopamine or corticosteroids, to undetectable levels. As recovery from the underlying illness occurs, the TSH level may rise above normal into the hypothyroid range. Consequently, patients with significant cardiovascular disease in a coronary care unit are likely to have abnormal thyroid function tests. In general, thyroid function testing should not be requested unless suspicion of thyroid disease is great because of such symptoms as goiter, ophthalmopathy, or unexplained atrial fibrillation.

4. Cardiovascular Drugs & the Thyroid

Normally, the thyroid gland secretes approximately 20% of the T_3 that is in the peripheral circulation. The remaining 80% is produced from monodeiodination of T_4 by the enzyme 5'-deiodinase. Propranolol and amiodarone inhibit the deiodinase enzyme and prevent peripheral conversion of T_4 to T_3 (the more potent thyroid hormone). This leads to low T_3 levels, which stimulates transient TSH release from the pituitary and consequent T_4 release from the thyroid. The overall result is a transiently elevated TSH for the first 1–3 months, a slightly elevated T_4 with a low-normal T_3. Typically, the patient remains euthyroid. Iodine is a major component of amiodarone; constituting 37% of the compound by weight. Maintenance doses of amiodarone (200–600 mg) provide 75–225 mg of iodine daily. Because the normal optimal daily intake of iodine is considered to be 150–200 mcg, amiodarone provides a massively expanded iodine pool. Normally, the thyroid gland adjusts to the increased iodine substrate; however, in some individuals thyroid dysfunction, that is, thyrotoxicosis and hypothyroidism may occur. Because the elimination half-life of amiodarone is so long (22–55 days) and due to tissue storage of the drug and its slow release, thyroid dysfunction has been reported to occur even after discontinuation of the medication.

Overall incidence of thyroid dysfunction in patients receiving amiodarone is estimated to be between 2% and 24%. Amiodarone-induced thyrotoxicosis (AIT) is more common in countries with low iodine uptake, and amiodarone-induced hypothyroidism in areas that are iodine replete.

Amiodarone-induced thyrotoxicosis may occur at any time during or even after amiodarone treatment, particularly in patients with an underlying predisposition to thyroid disease, who have a goiter. Presenting symptoms and signs include weight loss, weakness, tremor, or new or recurrent atrial tachyarrhythmias. Classic symptoms may be masked by the antiadrenergic effects of amiodarone. Biochemical diagnosis is straightforward if the T_3 or free T_3 level is elevated and the TSH level is suppressed to undetectable levels.

Pathogenesis is complex and can involve excessive thyroid hormone synthesis from the iodine load (so called type I AIT), or destructive thyroiditis (type II AIT). Features of both types of AIT can be seen in Table 32–5.

Table 32–5. Features of Amiodarone-Induced Thyrotoxicosis.

	Type I	Type II
Pathogenesis	Excess hormone synthesis due to excess iodine	Excess hormone release due to thyroid destruction
Goiter	Often present; multinodular or diffuse	Occasionally present; small diffuse, firm, may be tender
Autoantibodies	May be present	Usually absent
IL-6	Normal/elevated	Markedly elevated
Radioactive iodine uptake	Low or normal	Low or suppressed
Color-flow doppler	Normal or increased flow	Decreased flow
Thyroid ultrasound	Nodular, hypoechoic, large	Normal
Therapy	Methimazole or PTU, perchlorate may be necessary, thyroidectomy may be necessary	Steroids
Subsequent hypothyroidism	No, unless thyroidectomy performed	Possible

Il-6, interleukin-6; PTU, propylthiouracil.

Therapy for AIT is difficult and requires knowledge of the underlying pathogenesis. In type I AIT, thionamides should be used to block further organification of iodine and synthesis of hormones. Larger than usual doses are often required (methimazole 40–60 mg/day or propylthiouracil 600–800 mg/day) because the iodine-rich gland is resistant to thionamide therapy. Potassium perchlorate (800–1000 mg/day for 15–45 days), a drug that inhibits iodine uptake into the gland, can also be used although with caution because agranulocytosis, aplastic anemia, and nephrotic syndrome have occurred at doses > 1.5 g. Discontinuation of amiodarone, although often difficult, may be recommended and necessary in some cases. Thyroidectomy can be undertaken in severe cases unresponsive to medical therapy.

Type II AIT can be treated with high-dose corticosteroids (prednisone 30–40 mg/day or equivalent) for 3 months with a gradual slow taper to minimize recurrence. Discontinuation of amiodarone is usually not necessary because the thyroiditis resolves within several weeks to months and rarely recurs. If the two types of AIT cannot be distinguished, therapy with both corticosteroids and antithyroid drugs should be started.

Radioactive iodine therapy is not helpful because the high iodine concentration in the plasma and thyroid gland prevents the uptake of ^{131}I. In patients with a history of AIT who require restarting amiodarone, consideration of ^{131}I ablation prior to reinstitution of the drug should be strongly considered.

Like amiodarone, radiologic contrast material containing iodine such as that used in cardiac catheterizations, has the potential for causing transient thyrotoxicosis and for potentially causing decompensation in a patient with coronary artery disease.

Amiodarone-induced hypothyroidism occurs more frequently in the United States than AIT due to iodine sufficiency of the population. Patients typically are older and frequently have an underlying predisposition to thyroid disease as evidenced by the presence of antithyroid antibodies. Diagnosis is confirmed by an elevated TSH level in conjunction with a low T_4 or free T_4 level.

The proposed pathogenesis is continual inhibition of thyroid hormone synthesis from excess iodine; the so called Wolff-Chaikoff effect. Treatment is much simpler than that for AIT because thyroid hormone replacement can easily be given along with amiodarone therapy. The goal of therapy is to bring the TSH and T_4 or free T_4 levels to the upper range of normal or slightly above normal. This target mimics the range of thyroid function seen in euthyroid individuals who take amiodarone.

Daniels GH. Amiodarone induced thyrotoxicosis. J Clin Endocrinol Metab. 2001 Jan;86(1):3–8. [PMID: 11231968]

Martino E et al. The effects of amiodarone on the thyroid. Endocr Rev. 2001 Apr;22(2):240–54. [PMID: 11294826]

PARATHYROID & THE HEART

Parathyroid hormone (PTH) is responsible for calcium, phosphate, and magnesium homeostasis throughout the body. Although PTH itself has few effects on the heart, an excess or deficiency of this hormone can affect the cardiovascular system indirectly through its regulation of calcium.

1. Hyperparathyroidism

 ESSENTIALS OF DIAGNOSIS

▶ Inappropriately normal or elevated PTH levels.

▶ Serum calcium level more than 10 mg/dL when corrected for serum albumin, or ionized calcium level higher than upper limit of normal range.

▶ Increased 24-hour urine calcium (more than 200 mg).

▶ Elevated alkaline phosphatase.

▶ Decreased phosphate.

▶ General Considerations

Primary hyperparathyroidism is most commonly due to overproduction of PTH from a parathyroid adenoma. Rare causes include parathyroid hyperplasia in familial cases, often in the setting of a multiple endocrine neoplasia (MEN) syndrome. Secondary hyperparathyroidism occurs in hypocalcemic states in which the lack of negative feedback of calcium to the parathyroid glands results in overproduction of PTH and is usually seen in the setting of chronic hypocalcemia, vitamin D deficiency, or renal failure. Tertiary hyperparathyroidism can occur when chronic overstimulation of the parathyroid gland (as in renal failure) causes the autonomous release of PTH.

When the disorder is detected in an outpatient setting, the most common diagnosis is primary hyperparathyroidism from a parathyroid adenoma. Although parathyroid hyperplasia is rare, it is usually found in the setting of MEN, a rare hereditary condition of multiple endocrine neoplasias. Multiple endocrine neoplasia type I comprises hyperparathyroidism, pituitary adenoma, and pancreatic islet-cell tumor; MEN II consists of hyperparathyroidism, medullary thyroid carcinoma, and pheochromocytoma. Granulomatous disease, such as tuberculosis or histoplasmosis, can cause hypercalcemia by increased 1-α-hydroxylase activity, which converts the inactive 25-hydroxy vitamin D to the active 1,25-dihydroxy vitamin D. All patients with hypercalcemia should be queried regarding calcium (including over-the-counter calcium carbonate antacids) and vitamin intake to rule out milk-alkali syndrome and vitamin D and A toxicity. Thyrotoxicosis can cause hypercalcemia because of increased bone turnover. Adrenal insufficiency is another cause of hypercalcemia.

When detected in an inpatient setting, hypercalcemia is usually the harbinger of malignancy and portends a poor prognosis. Malignancies associated with hypercalcemia include bone metastases; multiple myeloma; lymphoma; leukemia; and squamous cell cancers, primarily of the head and neck, which secrete PTH-related peptide. This can bind to PTH receptors and cause PTH-like effects.

The hyperparathyroid state, by altering serum calcium and PTH, has the potential to adversely effect the cardiovascular system. Hypertension; left ventricular hypertrophy (LVH); hypercontractility; arrhythmias; calcific deposits in the myocardium, aortic and mitral valves, and coronary arteries have all been described. Some but not all studies have demonstrated an increased incidence of cardiovascular death that seems to correlate with the degree and duration of disease.

▶ Clinical Findings

A. Symptoms and Signs

1. Systemic symptoms and signs—Most patients with chronic hyperparathyroidism are asymptomatic and are detected through routine laboratory testing. Others complain of nonspecific symptoms such as fatigue and vague aches and pains.

2. Cardiovascular symptoms and signs—Arrhythmias are uncommon, but acute hypercalcemia can cause bradycardia and first-degree heart block. Acute elevation of calcium may cause hypertension, although this may be due to renal damage from nephrocalcinosis and elevated peripheral vascular resistance—a direct effect of calcium on the vascular smooth muscle cells. Left ventricular hypertrophy is noted in as many as 80% of patients referred for parathyroidectomy and can be reversible particularly in normotensive individuals. Valvular sclerosis, on the other hand, does not appear to improve after parathyroidectomy but also does not appear to progress. However, the mortality rate associated with cardiovascular disease in patients with primary hyperparathyroidism does not seem to be increased.

B. Physical Examination

Calcium deposition in the cornea, or band keratopathy, may be noted. In hyperparathyroidism secondary to renal failure, calcium and phosphate may precipitate in the soft tissues and in and around joints. These precipitants are usually readily seen on radiograph, palpated on physical examination and, if severe, can limit mobility of the joints.

C. Diagnostic Studies

1. Electrocardiography and echocardiography—Hypercalcemia decreases the plateau phase of the cardiac action potential, reflected by a shortened ST segment and a reduced QT interval. The QT interval corrected for heart rate is probably the most reliable ECG index of hypercalcemia.

With severe hypercalcemia (calcium level > 16 mg/dL, or 4 mmol/L), the T wave widens, tending to increase the QT interval.

Echocardiography reveals a high incidence of LVH and calcification of aortic and mitral valves as well as the coronary tree and myocardium. Several studies have shown improvement after successful parathyroidectomy in subjects with symptomatic hyperparathyroidism.

2. Laboratory findings—Typically, both serum calcium and ionized calcium are elevated, with an inappropriately normal or elevated PTH. Other causes of hypercalcemia are accompanied by a suppressed or low normal PTH. The 24-hour urine calcium level is usually more than 200 mg. Phosphate levels are usually low or low normal because PTH has a phosphaturic effect on the kidney, and a hyperchloremic metabolic acidosis is present because of the bicarbonaturic effect of PTH. Alkaline phosphatase levels may be elevated, especially in the setting of hyperparathyroid bone disease.

▶ Treatment & Prognosis

Parathyroidectomy is the definitive treatment for hyperparathyroidism and is indicated in all patients with symptoms as well as patients believed to be at high risk for progressive disease.

Successful parathyroidectomy normalizes calcium, phosphate, PTH, and alkaline phosphatase levels while improving bone density, slowing the progression of renal insufficiency, diminishing LVH, and improving symptoms. Hypertension may persist or progress in a percentage of patients, most likely the result of nephrocalcinosis and irreversible renal impairment. Postoperative hypocalcemia is common and may be transient or permanent. If it is permanent, the patient will require lifelong calcium and vitamin D replacement.

Medical treatment is less preferable than surgery unless the patient has a contraindication to the latter. Current medical treatment is limited and includes administration of the bisphosphonates, pamidronate or risedronate, and estrogen in postmenopausal women.

Andersson P et al. Primary hyperparathyroidism and heart disease—a review. Eur Heart J. 2004 Oct;25(20):1176–87. [PMID: 15474692]

Bilezikian JP. Primary hyperparathyroidism when to operate and when to observe. Endocrinol Metab Clin N Am. 2000 Sep;29(3):465–78. [PMID: 11033756]

Strewler GJ. Medical approaches to primary hyperparathyroidism. Endocrinol Metab Clin North Am. 2000 Sep;29(3):523–39. [PMID: 11033759]

2. Hypoparathyroidism

Hypoparathyroidism usually occurs in the postoperative setting after neck or thyroid surgery; it also occurs idiopathically. A functional hypoparathyroidism can occur in patients with magnesium deficiency because magnesium is a cofactor for PTH action on bone. Symptoms include tingling around the mouth and in the hands and feet. Cardiovascular manifestations are rare. The physical examination reveals positive Chvostek and Trousseau signs. Laboratory evaluation reveals a low serum calcium or ionized calcium with a low or inappropriately low normal PTH level. Hypoparathyroidism is associated with a prolonged QT interval on the ECG because of ST-segment lengthening; the T wave is usually normal. Impaired left ventricular function has been reported. Restoration of eucalcemia may improve cardiac function.

Lehmann G et al. ECG changes in a 25-year-old woman with hypocalcemia due to hypoparathyroidism. Chest. 2000 Jul;118(1): 260–2. [PMID: 10893393]

ADRENAL & THE HEART

1. Pheochromocytoma

ESSENTIALS OF DIAGNOSIS

▶ Biochemical evidence of excess catecholamines.

▶ Adrenal tumor or tumor along the sympathetic chain (paraganglioma).

▶ Headache, palpitations, sweating in conjunction with either hypertension (may be paroxysmal) or orthostatic hypotension.

▶ Pressor response to anesthesia induction or to antihypertensive or sympathomimetic drugs.

▶ General Considerations

Catecholamine-secreting neoplasms, or pheochromocytomas, can be life-threatening and cause hypertension, arrhythmia, and hyperglycemia. One case per 2 million persons is diagnosed annually in this country, accounting for less than 0.1% of underlying primary causes of hypertension. Despite the rarity of this condition, its importance cannot be overstated because correct diagnosis and treatment leads to cure, and a missed diagnosis can be fatal. Ninety percent of pheochromocytomas are located in the adrenals; 10% arise from extra-adrenal chromaffin tissue along the sympathetic chain and are known as paragangliomas. Cardiac pheochromocytoma arising from the visceral autonomic paraganglia (atrium or interatrial septum) or branchiomeric paraganglia (branchial arch) are extremely rare. Approximately 10% are malignant, and recurrences can be seen in 6–23% of cases.

Most pheochromocytomas secrete predominantly norepinephrine; about 15% secrete mainly epinephrine. The majority of pheochromocytomas occur sporadically; occasionally (about 10% of cases), they are seen as part of a familial syndrome such as MEN IIa (hyperparathyroidism, medullary thyroid cancer, pheochromocytoma), MEN IIb (pheochromocytoma, medullary thyroid carcinoma, mucosal neuromas, marfanoid habitus), or von Hippel-Lindau disease (cerebelloretinal hemangioblastomas, pheochromocytoma, pancreatic islet cell tumors, renal cell cysts, testicular cysts). Affected family members may have only one manifestation of these syndromes. All members of the family should be screened for pheochromocytomas up until the age of 40 because of the potentially life-threatening nature of these tumors.

▶ Clinical Findings

A. Symptoms and Signs

1. Systemic symptoms and signs—The release of catecholamines from the tumor is unpredictable and usually causes paroxysmal attacks of headache, palpitations, and sweating. Together with hypertension, these three symptoms when present have a diagnostic specificity of 94% and sensitivity of 91%. When this triad of symptoms is absent, pheochromocytoma can be excluded with 99.9% certainty. Patients may also complain of increased nervousness, irritability, and an impending sense of doom. Mild abdominal pain and constipation are relatively common. Pallor and hyperventilation may be noted on examination. The clinician should suspect a pheochromocytoma in any patient in whom a sudden elevation of blood pressure develops during anesthesia induction.

2. Cardiovascular symptoms and signs—The effects of catecholamines on the heart are mediated by β_1-receptors and include increased heart rate, enhanced contractility, and augmented conduction velocity—all of which contribute to an increase in cardiac output. Eighty-five percent of patients will have hypertension, which can be either sustained, labile (with hypotension and hypertension) or paroxysmal. Patients without hypertension most likely secrete dopa or dopamine, which can be vasodilating. Orthostatic hypotension is often noted, and the combination of severe hypertension and orthostasis should suggest the possibility of pheochromocytoma. Light-headedness and syncope occur rarely.

Both dilated and hypertrophic cardiomyopathies and myocarditis have been described with pheochromocytoma, and exposure to high levels of catecholamines can cause contraction-band necrosis and fibrosis. The cardiomyopathy is reversible if the excessive catecholamine stimulus is removed early, before extensive replacement fibrosis takes place. Chest pain, angina, and acute myocardial infarction may occur in the absence of coronary artery occlusive disease. Catecholamine-induced increases in myocardial oxygen consumption, myocarditis, and coronary artery spasm likely contribute to the infarction. Cardiac arrhythmias such as atrial and ventricular fibrillation occur, especially in the setting of surgical resection of the tumor. Sudden death is not an uncommon presentation for patients with pheochromocytoma. Pulmonary edema and shock may also be presentations of such patients; shock may be associated with myocarditis or infarction, or it may follow a hypertensive crisis.

B. Physical Examination

Sustained or paroxysmal hypertension is common. Orthostasis is also often seen, and noncardiogenic pulmonary edema of obscure origin has also been described. Retinal hemorrhage or papilledema is a rare occurrence.

C. Diagnostic Studies

1. Electrocardiography and imaging—Electrocardiographic changes are common; nonspecific ST-T wave changes and prominent U waves may be seen. Sinus tachycardia, sinus bradycardia, and atrial and ventricular tachyarrhythmias have all been noted and may be associated with palpitations. Conduction disturbances, including right and left bundle branch block and signs of left ventricular hypertrophy sometimes occur.

Clinically significant cardiomyopathy and increased left ventricular mass have been noted on echocardiography. Computed tomography or magnetic resonance imaging are useful for localizing the tumors. Occasionally, radionuclide imaging with ^{123}I-metaiodobenzylguanidine is used to detect small tumors, but its sensitivity can be affected by drugs such as labetolol.

2. Laboratory findings—Elevations in plasma catecholamines or their metabolites are necessary for the diagnosis in addition to localization-imaging studies. The most useful tests are 24-hour collections of urinary metanephrines, and free catecholamines. Most clinicians favor urinary or plasma metanephrines as the initial screening test. In general, if the results are equivocal, plasma catecholamines should be measured. Plasma catecholamines must be collected after placement of an intravenous catheter for 30 minutes, with the patient resting supine, preferably in a quiet room to avoid release of catecholamines from pain or emotional arousal. False-positive results should be minimized by avoiding drugs, foods, and conditions that affect the tests (Table 32–6).

Occasionally, suppressive pharmacologic testing may be needed, if all prior testing is equivocal and clinical suspicion is high. The clonidine-suppression test is the most widely used. The test is performed by measuring plasma catecholamines at rest and 3 hours after oral administration of 0.3 mg of clonidine. In patients with pheochromocytoma, catecholamines remain unchanged because tumor secretion is unaffected by the centrally acting clonidine. Patients with essential hypertension, on the other hand, will decrease their catecholamine levels to less than 500 pg/mL.

▶ Treatment

Treatment involves the prevention of cardiovascular complications such as myocardial infarction, heart failure,

Table 32–6. Drugs, Foods, and Conditions That Artificially Increase or Decrease Tests for Pheochromocytoma.

Test	Increase	Decrease
Metanephrines, VMA	Sympathomimetics: amphetamines, ephedrine, nasal decongestants, bronchodilators	Large doses of ganglionic blockers: guanethidine, reserpine
Catecholamines	Levodopa	Fenfluramine
	Rapid clonidine withdrawal	Renal insufficiency
	Excess banana ingestion	Malnutrition, dysautonomia, quadriplegia
	Nitroprusside, nitroglycerin	
	Theophylline, aminophylline	
	Severe stress	
	Diseases: intracranial lesions, psychosis, Guillain-Barré, lead poisoning, eclampsia, hypoglycemia, carcinoid, acute porphyria, acrodynia, quadriplegia, amyotrophic lateral sclerosis	
	Fluorescent substances: quinidine, chloral hydrate, tetracyclines, niacin, erythromycin, quinine, bretylium, methenamine, methocarbamine	
Catecholamines	Ethanol, isoproterenol, methylidopa, MAO inhibitors, phenothiazines, α-methyl p-tyrosine, methenamine, bilirubin, labetalol	
Metanephrines	Ethanol, methyldopa, MAO inhibitors, benzodiazepines, phenothiazines	Radiopaque media: renografin, Hypaque-M, Renovist, Cardiografin, Urografin, conray
VMA	Lithium, nalidixic acid, methocarbamol, glycerol guaiacolate, p-aminosalicylic acid, salicylates, mephenesin, sulfonamides, chocolate, citrus, tea, vanilla, coffee	Ethanol, MAO inhibitors, disulfiram, clofibrate, mandelamine, salicylates

MAO, monoamine oxidase; VMA, vanillylmandelic acid.

hypertensive crisis and stroke, arrhythmias, and sudden death; it also involves surgical removal of the tumor. Recent advances in localizing imaging studies and the emergence of laparoscopic adrenalectomy along with proper preoperative medical preparation have reduced morbidity and mortality significantly. Preoperative α- and β-blockade is used to reverse the effects of excessive catecholamines and prevent crisis. Because most pheochromocytomas secrete norepinephrine, α-blockade should be given first to prevent aggravation of hypertension and precipitation of coronary spasm or pulmonary edema from unopposed α-receptor stimulation. The most frequently used combination of drugs is phenoxybenzamine, started at 20 mg/day and increasing to 80–100 mg/day, as tolerated, and propranolol or labetalol to control hypertension and arrhythmias. Phenoxybenzamine causes orthostasis and should be titrated according to the severity of the orthostasis before the β-blocker is added. Blood pressure control should be attempted for 2 weeks before surgery. Metyrosine is a drug that inhibits the rate-limiting step in catecholamine synthesis by 40–80%. It can be used in patients with inoperable pheochromocytoma, or it can be used preoperatively if the hypertension is difficult to control. Doses are 250 mg three times daily, increased by increments of 250–500 mg to a maximum of 4 g/day.

▶ Prognosis

Nonmalignant surgically treated pheochromocytoma has a 5-year survival rate of 95%. In malignant disease, the 5-year survival is less than 50%. If a surgical cure is achieved before the cardiovascular system has been irreparably damaged, cardiovascular health will be completely restored. In 25% of patients, hypertension persists due to underlying essential hypertension or irreversible vascular or renal damage but is usually well-controlled with standard antihypertensive agents. However, in this instance, a search for a second or residual tumor should be considered.

Duh QY. Evolving surgical management for patients with pheochromocytoma. J Clin Endocrinol Metab. 2001 Apr;86(4):1477–9. [PMID: 11297570]

Klingler HC et al. Pheochromocytoma. Urology. 2001 Jun;57(6):1025–32. [PMID: 11377298]

Liao WB et al. Cardiovascular manifestations of pheochromocytoma. Am J Emerg Med. 2000 Sep;18(5):622–5. [PMID: 10999582]

Neumann HP et al; Freiburg-Warsaw-Columbus Pheochromocytoma Study Group. Germ-line mutations in nonsyndromic pheochromocytoma. N Engl J Med. 2002 May 9;346(19):1459–66. [PMID: 12000816]

Pacak K et al. Pheochromocytoma: recommendations for clinical practice from the First International Symposium. October 2005. Nat Clin Pract Endocrinol Metab. 2007 Feb;3(2):92–102. [PMID: 17237836]

Plouin PF et al. Factors associated with perioperative morbidity and mortality in patients with pheochromocytoma: analysis of 165 operations at a single center. J Clin Endocrinol Metab. 2001 Apr;86(4):1480–6. [PMID: 11297571]

2. Adrenal Insufficiency

 ESSENTIALS OF DIAGNOSIS

▶ Inability to increase cortisol to more than 20 mg/dL in response to synthetic adrenocorticotrophic hormone (ACTH) during rapid ACTH stimulation testing.

▶ Orthostatic hypotension, salt wasting, hyperkalemia in primary adrenal insufficiency (Addison disease).

▶ Hyponatremia in both primary and secondary (pituitary) adrenal insufficiency.

▶ Elevated ACTH in Addison disease.

▶ Hypovolemic shock, hypoglycemia, fever in adrenal crisis.

▶ General Considerations

Deficient production of glucocorticoids, mineralocorticoids, or both results in adrenal insufficiency. This is classified into two types: primary adrenal insufficiency, or Addison disease, in which the adrenal cortex is destroyed; and secondary adrenal insufficiency, in which ACTH hyposecretion leads to decreased production of adrenal glucocorticoids.

Today, the most common cause of Addison disease is autoimmune destruction of the adrenal cortex. Adrenal hemorrhage, metastasis, AIDS, and granulomatous diseases (such as tuberculosis and histoplasmosis) are other etiologic considerations. Adrenal hemorrhage usually occurs in the setting of anticoagulation. The most common cause of secondary adrenal insufficiency is withdrawal of corticosteroids, which suppresses the hypothalamic pituitary adrenal axis and therefore causes glucocorticoid deficiency. Adrenal insufficiency is rare in the general population, with an incidence of < 0.01%. However, the overall risk of adrenal insufficiency is increased in critically ill patients, especially those over the age of 55 who are hypotensive and require pressors. Estimates are that in this setting adrenal insufficiency is present in 30–40%.

▶ Clinical Findings

A. Symptoms and Signs

1. Systemic symptoms and signs—Glucocorticoid deficiency causes fatigue, anorexia, nausea, vomiting (and therefore weight loss), hypotension, and hypoglycemia. Mineralocorticoid or aldosterone deficiency causes renal sodium and bicarbonate wasting, resulting in hyponatremia, hyperkalemia, acidosis, and profound dehydration. Acute adrenal insufficiency or crisis occurs when the patient is exposed to stresses such as infection, trauma, and surgery, and cannot compensate adequately with augmented glucocorticoid release.

2. Cardiovascular symptoms and signs—Hypotension, often orthostatic, is present in 90% of patients and may cause syncope. Chronic adrenal insufficiency is characterized by decreased systemic vascular resistance and decreased myocardial contractility. On the other hand, acute adrenal insufficiency can have variable cardiac function with low, normal, or high systemic vascular resistance, cardiac output, and capillary wedge pressure. Thus, in acute adrenal insufficiency—which can be superimposed on a setting of chronic adrenal insufficiency—the patient may be in hypovolemic shock, accompanied by fever, volume depletion, depressed mentation, nausea, vomiting, abdominal pain, and hypoglycemia. Patients often seem as though they have an acute abdominal emergency and can mistakenly be taken for exploratory surgery—which can be lethal in this setting. Shock and coma can rapidly progress to death, if untreated. Adrenal crisis should be considered in any patient with unexplained hypovolemic shock.

B. Physical Examination

The classic physical examination finding for chronic primary adrenal insufficiency is hyperpigmentation of the skin and mucous membranes, especially over pressure points such as the knuckles, toes, elbows, and knees and also in scars, palmar creases, nail beds, areolae, and the perianal and perivaginal areas. The hyperpigmentation is caused by increased levels of ACTH, which are released along with melanocyte-stimulating hormone and stimulate the melanocyte receptor. Vitiligo is a clue that the adrenal insufficiency is autoimmune in nature. Calcification of the pinna and the loss of pubic and axillary hair from decreased production of adrenal androgens may also be seen. In secondary adrenal insufficiency, patients lack the hyperpigmentation; the presence of cushingoid features suggests glucocorticoid withdrawal.

C. Diagnostic Studies

1. Electrocardiography and echocardiography—Electrocardiographic findings include sinus bradycardia, sinus tachycardia, nonspecific T wave changes, peaked T waves if hyperkalemia is prominent, and low voltage and a shortened QT interval if hypercalcemia is present. Echocardiography reveals small cardiac chambers with normal function.

2. Laboratory findings—Hyponatremia, hyperkalemia, hypercalcemia, hypoglycemia, and acidosis are seen in Addison disease. Patients with secondary adrenal insufficiency will not have hyperkalemia because their renin and angiotensin system is able to stimulate aldosterone production. A normocytic, normochromic anemia with lymphocytosis and eosinophilia is seen on the blood smear.

The rapid ACTH stimulation test is used to diagnose adrenal insufficiency. Administration of synthetic ACTH (cosyntropin) causes an elevation of cortisol within 30–60 minutes. Failure to increase cortisol to 20 mg/dL confirms the insufficiency. An ACTH level can help distinguish primary from secondary causes; hypersecretion is characteristic of primary adrenal insufficiency only.

In the setting of critical illness, the diagnosis of adrenal insufficiency is more problematic. Although it is well known that stress such as that seen with hypotension, inflammation, sepsis, or surgery results in elevated cortisol levels, the definition of adrenal insufficiency in this setting is less clear. Most authors believe that a stress cortisol level in critically ill patients should be > 25 mcg/dL. When the level of stress is uncertain, the low-dose corticotropin stimulation test (1 mcg) can be used. Failure to increase stimulated cortisol to > 25 mcg/dL indicates the need for treatment with corticosteroids.

▶ Treatment

The treatment of adrenal crisis is lifesaving. If the patient is in serious shock, delay of treatment to make the diagnosis of adrenal crisis is both unwise and dangerous. Patients should receive stress doses of corticosteroids, such as 100 mg of hydrocortisone intravenously every 6–8 hours, starting immediately. Saline volume resuscitation along with glucose infusion is necessary to correct volume and electrolyte abnormalities. A search for the underlying precipitant, such as infection, should be undertaken and treated as necessary. Once the patient is safely over the crisis, corticosteroids can be slowly withdrawn, and the diagnosis of adrenal insufficiency confirmed. An alternative approach would be to use dexamethasone, 2–4 mg intravenously initially, which does not interfere with the cortisol assay; perform the rapid ACTH stimulation test; and then switch to hydrocortisone. The treatment of chronic Addison disease involves both glucocorticoid and mineralcorticoid replacement.

Rivers EP et al. Adrenal insufficiency in high-risk surgical ICU patients. Chest. 2001 Mar;119(3):889–96. [PMID: 11243973]
Zaloga GP et al. Hypothalamic-pituitary-adrenal insufficiency. Crit Care Clin. 2001 Jan;17(1):25–41. [PMID: 11219233]

3. Cushing Syndrome
▶ General Considerations

The term **Cushing syndrome** refers to excess cortisol in the circulation. **Cushing disease** is that state of hypercortisolemia caused by an ACTH-producing pituitary adenoma. Other causes of Cushing syndrome are ectopic ACTH production from tumors, such as small cell carcinoma of the bronchus; primary adrenal disease, such as glucocorticoid-secreting adrenal tumors; or the exogenous use of corticosteroids. **Pseudo-Cushing syndrome** refers to patients who, on screening, appear to have hypercortisolemia but have relatively few physical signs. These patients typically are alcoholic or obese or have psychiatric conditions. Confirmatory testing for Cushing syndrome is normal in pseudo-Cushing.

Patients with Cushing syndrome typically have central obesity, hypertension, hyperlipidemia, and hyperglycemia; it is not surprising that they are at risk for coronary artery disease. The longer the duration of the hypercortisolemia, the greater the risk of coronary disease and congestive heart failure.

▶ Diagnostic Considerations

Diagnosis requires three steps: screening, confirmation, and determination of the cause. Screening tests are a 24-hour urine collection for free cortisol, or a 1-mg overnight dexamethasone-suppression test. Patients with Cushing or pseudo-Cushing syndrome will have an elevated urinary free cortisol level, and 1 mg of dexamethasone will not suppress their cortisol to less than 5 mg/dL. Confirmation requires a low-dose (2 mg/day) dexamethasone-suppression test, with or without corticotropin-releasing factor testing. True Cushing syndrome will not suppress with low-dose testing. To determine cause, an ACTH level should be performed. Elevated ACTH indicates a pituitary tumor or ectopic production of ACTH. Low ACTH levels indicate adrenal disease. High-dose (8 mg) dexamethasone suppression testing and the cortisol-releasing hormone stimulation test are the main tests used to differentiate pituitary from ectopic sources of ACTH. Inferior petrosal sinus sampling should be reserved for patients with confusing hormonal testing who have a pituitary adenoma on imaging studies or in patients in whom an ectopic source of ACTH is suspected. Imaging should be done after the biochemical workup is completed to localize the tumor.

▶ Treatment

Treatment involves surgical removal of the pituitary tumor, with or without radiation, in Cushing disease; removal of the adrenal tumor; or removal of the ectopic source of ACTH production. If these procedures are not feasible, medical treatment can be done, using adrenolytic therapy such as mitotane, or adrenocortical-blocking drugs such as aminoglutethimide, metyrapone, or ketoconazole.

Boscaro M et al. The diagnosis of Cushing's syndrome: atypical presentations and laboratory shortcomings. Arch Intern Med. 2000 Nov 13;160(20):3045–53. [PMID: 11074733]

Newell-Price J et al. Cushing's syndrome. Lancet. 2006 May 13;367(9522):1605–17. [PMID: 16698415]

4. Primary Hyperaldosteronism
▶ General Considerations

The increased and autonomous production of aldosterone by the adrenal gland is known as primary hyperaldosteronism. Consequences of excessive aldosterone production include sodium retention, with plasma volume expansion and hypertension; renal loss of potassium and bicarbonate, causing hypokalemia and alkalosis; and suppression of renin and angiotensin. Hyperaldosteronism is the most common secondary cause of hypertension. As many as 12–20% of cases referred to hypertension clinics have primary hyperaldosteronism.

Patients usually come to medical attention because of hypertension and hypokalemia. The hypertension may be moderately severe, requiring several antihypertensives; malignant hypertension, however, is rare. Despite the sodium retention, edema is not a feature of hyperaldosteronism; the kidney can presumably compensate for the excess sodium. The heart is usually only modestly enlarged and heart failure is rarely seen. Electrocardiographic changes are those of mild LVH and hypokalemia.

▶ Diagnostic Considerations

The diagnosis should be considered in any hypertensive patient with spontaneous hypokalemia, resistant hypertension, adrenal incidentaloma, or in patients in whom secondary hypertension is suspected. Basal plasma renin activity should be suppressed, with elevated plasma aldosterone and an elevated aldosterone/renin ratio. If this is the case, the diagnosis can be confirmed by demonstrating failure of the elevated aldosterone to suppress normally with salt or saline loading. The patient must discontinue any antihypertensives that affect the renin-angiotensin-aldosterone axis for 3–6 weeks before salt suppression testing; α-adrenergic blockers can be used to control blood pressure. The patient is typically placed on a high-salt diet (> 120 mEq/day) with sodium chloride supplementation for 3–4 days to suppress aldosterone; on the last day of the high-salt diet, a 24-hour urine is collected to test for aldosterone, sodium, and creatinine. If urinary Na is > 200 mEq and aldosterone is > 12 mcg, unsuppressibility of aldosterone is documented. After confirmation of hyperaldosteronism, imaging of the adrenals should be performed with computed tomography to look for hyperplasia versus adenoma. In equivocal cases, adrenal vein sampling for aldosterone can be performed.

▶ Treatment

Treatment for adenoma involves surgical resection. In as many as 70% of patients, this cures the hypertension and hypokalemia. The blood pressure, however, may require several months following surgery to return to normal. Medical therapy for patients who are not surgical candidates or those with hyperplasia includes the aldosterone-antagonists spironolactone (100–200 mg/day) or eplerenone (25–100 mg/day), the diuretic amiloride (10–40 mg/day), and calcium channel blockers.

Young WF Jr. Minireview: primary aldosteronism–changing concepts in diagnosis and treatment. Endocrinology. 2003 Jun;144(6):2208–13. [PMID: 12746276]

ACROMEGALY & THE HEART

ESSENTIALS OF DIAGNOSIS

▶ Elevated somatomedin C.

▶ Inability to suppress growth hormone to less than 2 ng/mL during glucose tolerance test.

▶ Pituitary adenoma found on magnetic resonance imaging.

▶ General Considerations

Acromegaly is caused by the excessive secretion of growth hormone (GH) by a pituitary adenoma in an adult; gigantism occurs in children. It is characterized by bony overgrowth, organomegaly, and premature death, often due to cardiovascular, cerebrovascular, and respiratory dysfunction. In rare cases, carcinoid, small-cell, islet cell, and other tumors can secrete GH-releasing hormone ectopically and cause acromegaly. The effects of GH are mediated through the insulin-like growth factor 1 (IGF-1 or somatomedin C) in the liver and the periphery.

▶ Clinical Findings

A. Symptoms and Signs

1. Systemic symptoms and signs—Excessive GH causes bony, soft tissue, and visceral overgrowth. Patients may also complain of symptoms related to the local expanse of the tumor such as headache or bitemporal hemianopsia. Impotence, galactorrhea, and amenorrhea may result from cosecretion of prolactin or the destruction of normal gonadotrophs by the tumor. Other symptoms include excessive sweating, hoarseness, carpal tunnel syndrome, polyuria, and polydipsia.

2. Cardiovascular symptoms and signs—Cardiac dysfunction and heart failure are a major cause of death in acromegalics. The older the patient and the longer the duration of disease, the more likely acromegalic cardiomyopathy will develop. The most striking clinical feature is concentric biventricular hypertrophy with inadequate filling leading to both systolic and diastolic dysfunction. Histologic findings include interstitial fibrosis, collagen deposition, myofibrillar derangement, lymphomononuclear infiltration, and myocyte apoptosis resembling myocarditis.

Other factors can potentially contribute to the cardiac dysfunction. The coexistence of hypertension, diabetes, or both in this condition can accelerate the cardiac hypertrophy. Hypertension, the most common cardiovascular finding in acromegalics, is usually mild in nature and easily treated with antihypertensives. The mechanism of the hypertension may be due to increased sodium, extracellular fluid, and plasma volume.

Because of the role of GH as a counterregulatory hormone for hypoglycemia, most acromegalics have either glucose intolerance or frank diabetes, which may explain their increased incidence of premature coronary artery disease. Untreated acromegaly is associated with hypertriglyceridemia and elevated levels of apoprotein A-1, apoprotein E, fibrinogen, and plasminogen activator inhibitor-1 activity.

A rare disorder known as **Carney syndrome** involves any three of the following: GH-secreting pituitary tumors, cardiac or cutaneous myxoma, Sertoli cell tumors, cutaneous hyperpigmentation, and pigmented nodular adrenocortical disease. The myxomas seen in Carney syndrome are usually multiple and may involve more than one chamber. Family members should be screened with echocardiography.

B. Physical Examination

Because acromegaly is such an insidious disease, changes in the body occur gradually and usually go unnoticed until complications develop. Bitemporal hemianopsia may be detected on gross confrontation, indicating optic chiasm compression from the tumor. Thickened, oily skin, particularly of the face, and other facial changes, including thick lips, macroglossia, bulbous nose, frontal bossing, prominent cheek bones, hollow temporal fossa, and malocclusion with protrusion of the lower jaw, are usually seen. Synovial and periarticular swelling may be noted, and dorsal kyphosis, barrel chest, and spade-like hands with sausage-like digits are seen. The chest examination is most remarkable for galactorrhea. Abdominal examination may reveal generalized organomegaly.

C. Diagnostic Studies

1. Electrocardiography and echocardiography—Cardiomegaly is present, even in the absence of hypertension, suggesting a direct effect of GH on the myocyte. Both symmetric and asymmetric cardiac hypertrophy have been seen on echocardiography. In early disease, both ventricular dimension and wall thickness are increased; therefore, relative wall thickness remains unchanged. In later stages, impaired diastolic filling and cardiac dilatation occur, leading to congestive heart failure.

Electrocardiographic abnormalities include ST depression and nonspecific T wave changes, LVH, and intraventricular conduction defects. Cardiac arrhythmias often occur, with ventricular ectopics and atrial fibrillation or flutter being the most frequent.

2. Laboratory findings—Diagnostic tests includes random and glucose-suppressed GH levels, along with somatomedin C or IGF-1 levels. Because GH secretion is episodic, a random level alone is rarely helpful. Normally, GH is suppressed to less than 2 ng/mL in response to glucose infusion. Other findings often associated with acromegaly include hyperglycemia, hyperphosphatemia, and hypertriglyceridemia.

▶ Treatment

The goal in treating acromegaly is to normalize GH and somatomedin C concentrations in order to prevent early cardiovascular mortality. Treatment includes surgical removal of the pituitary adenoma with postoperative radiation therapy, or medical therapy with octreotide (200–500 mcg/day subcutaneously) or bromocriptine (5–30 mg/day). Many authors have suggested that once control of the disease occurs, defined as a GH level of < 2 ng/mL and a normal age-adjusted IGF-1 level, the progression of cardiac disease can be arrested and cardiovascular mortality reduced. The hypertension, heart failure, and arrhythmias are treated conventionally.

AACE Acromegaly Guidelines Task Force. AACE Medical Guidelines for Clinical Practice for the diagnosis and treatment of acromegaly. Endocr Pract. 2004 May–Jun;10(3):213–25. [PMID: 15382339]

Colao A et al. Growth hormone and the heart. Clin Endocrinol(Oxf). 2001 Feb;54(2):137–54. [PMID: 11207626]

Fazio S et al. Cardiovascular effects of short-term growth hormone hypersecretion. J Clin Endocrinol Metab. 2000 Jan;85(1):179–82. [PMID: 10634384]

Melmed S. Medical progress: Acromegaly. N Engl J Med. 2006 Dec 14;335(24):2558–73. [PMID: 17167139]

Vitale G et al. Cardiovascular complications in acromegaly. Minverva Endocrinol. 2004 Sep;29(3):77–88. [PMID: 15282442]

GROWTH HORMONE DEFICIENCY

Unlike acromegaly, in which cardiac involvement has been appreciated for many decades, the cardiac abnormalities associated with adult growth hormone deficiency (GHD) have only recently been recognized. Growth hormone deficiency is associated with abnormal body composition with increased fat mass, abnormal lipid metabolism, impaired capacity for exercise, decreased bone mineral density, decreased quality of life and a risk of increased mortality from cardiovascular disease that is approximately twice that found in the normal population. Myocardial infarction, cardiac failure, and cerebrovascular accidents are the main causes of death.

The precise mechanisms responsible for the increase in cardiovascular disease are unknown, but a characteristic hypokinetic syndrome has been described. In this syndrome, a decrease in left ventricular and septal wall thickness is noted on echocardiography along with low heart rate and blood pressure. One study using radionuclide angiography has noted decreased left ventricular ejection fraction (LVEF) compared with that in controls.

Most commonly, adult GHD results from childhood onset of GHD that continues throughout life. Thus, the patient with a history of pituitary or hypothalamic disease, childhood-onset GHD, cranial irradiation or trauma is a candidate for GHD testing. Testing consists of provocative stimulation with an insulin tolerance test. A biochemical diagnosis of adult GHD is determined by a subnormal response, for example, a peak level of GH < 5 ng/mL. Testing should not be performed in patients with ischemic heart disease or seizure disorder. Treatment is initiated with a daily subcutaneous injection of 2–5 mcg/kg/day of GH and can be titrated to 10–12 mcg/kg/day. Side effects are dose-dependent and consist of fluid retention and carpal tunnel syndrome.

Growth hormone therapy has been implicated in the health of the endothelium and increases nitric oxide production in in vitro studies. In humans with GHD, short-term treatment has been shown in various studies to increase cardiac mass, decrease carotid intimal medial thickness, reverse early atherosclerotic changes in major arteries, and possibly improve the vasodilatory function of the endothelium. However, the hypertrophic effect of long-term replacement with GH appears to subside over time. It remains to be seen if GH replacement therapy will reduce the prevalence of cardiovascular disease in this population.

Colao A et al. Growth hormone and the heart. Clin Endocrinol (Oxf). 2001 Feb;54(2):137–54. [PMID: 11207626]

CARCINOID TUMORS & THE HEART

▶ General Considerations

Carcinoid tumors are neuroendocrine tumors containing vasoactive secretagogues and are found in the gastrointestinal tract, urogenital tract, or the pulmonary bronchioles. Although these tumors can secrete a number of hormones, including ACTH and GH-releasing hormone, they most commonly secrete serotonin and serotonin metabolites. The presentation of the patient depends on the location of the carcinoid. Symptoms include flushing of the head and neck, with liver metastases, and bronchospasm with pulmonary carcinoid.

A unique endocrine effect of carcinoid tumors is fibrotic plaque-like thickenings on the endocardium of the tricuspid and pulmonic valves, atria, and ventricles. Deposition may also be seen on the superior and inferior venae cavae, pulmonary artery, and coronary sinus. The right side of the heart is affected predominantly, and although left-sided heart disease may occur, it is of lesser significance. Thickening of the valves results in tricuspid regurgitation and pulmonic stenosis. If the tricuspid regurgitation is severe, right-sided heart failure and cardiomegaly result. Nearly half of patients who die of carcinoid die of congestive heart failure.

Elaboration of serotonin by the tumor is believed to mediate the fibrosis; however, lowering serotonin levels does not cause regression of the plaques. Diagnosis is made by documenting more than 30 mg of 5-hydroxy indole acetic acid (a serotonin metabolite) in a 24-hour urine collection. Normal individuals secrete less than 10 mg in 24 hours, and values between 10 and 30 mg are equivocal. Testing must be done while the patient has been on a diet free of serotonin-rich foods for several days. Localization should be attempted with bowel series, computed tomography, somatostatin receptor scintigraphy, or positron emission tomography. All patients with carcinoid should have echocardiography to look for heart involvement.

▶ Treatment

Treatment is surgical removal of the tumor if it has not metastasized. Synthetic somatostatin (octreotide) has been shown to shrink tumor metastases in addition to decreasing serotonin levels. Unfortunately, the heart disease does not improve with reduction of serotonin levels, and some patients will require valve replacement.

Ganim RB et al. Recent advances in carcinoid pathogenesis, diagnosis and management. Surg Oncol. 2000 Dec;9(4):173–9. [PMID: 11476988]

Kulke MH. Clinical presentation and management of carcinoid tumors. Hematol Oncol Clin North Am. 2007 Jun;21(3):433–55. [PMID: 17548033]

Moller JE et al. Prognosis of carcinoid heart disease: analysis of 200 cases over two decades. Circulation. 2005 Nov 22;112(21):3320–7. [PMID: 16286584]

DIABETES MELLITUS & THE HEART

▶ General Considerations

The incidence of coronary artery disease in persons with diabetes is two to four times that for persons without diabetes, with cardiovascular disease reigning as the number one cause of death. Two types of vascular disease are seen: macrovascular disease, causing atherosclerosis and arteriosclerosis; and microvascular disease, producing retinopathy, nephropathy, neuropathy, and possibly small artery occlusion in the heart as well. Macrovascular disease develops prematurely in diabetic patients and is usually severe, with a striking predominance in diabetic women. Diabetics with no history of coronary heart disease (CHD) have identical risk of cardiovascular death as do patients with myocardial infarction. Consequently, the Adult Treatment Panel III has designated diabetes as a CHD risk equivalent.

A large body of evidence now links endothelial dysfunction to microangiopathy and atherosclerosis in diabetes. The evidence is particularly striking in persons with type 1 diabetes with microalbuminuria and proteinuria; however, endothelial dysfunction also occurs in patients with type 2 diabetes and normal urinary albumin excretion as well as in patients with insulin resistance who are normoglycemic. Once established, endothelial dysfunction induces changes in vascular tone, reactivity, and function that contribute to the progression of vascular disease. Insulin sensitizers, hypolipidemic therapy, and angiotensin-converting enzyme inhibitors have all been shown to improve endothelial function.

Hyperinsulinemia and insulin resistance have been postulated to relate directly to both hypertension and CHD in type 2 diabetes. The so-called metabolic syndrome is a constellation of metabolic risk factors that includes obesity, insulin resistance, elevated triglycerides, low high-density lipoprotein, hypertension, and fasting hyperglycemia. It enhances the risk for CHD at any given low-density lipoprotein level. To achieve maximum benefit from risk factor modification, the underlying insulin resistant state must be a primary target of therapy.

▶ Clinical Findings

Angina and myocardial infarction in persons with diabetes are often manifested by atypical symptoms. Painless myocardial infarction may occur, and unusual pain patterns may delay diagnosis. Diabetic patients have a high mortality rate from myocardial infarction; recurrence is frequent, and the long-term prognosis is poor, with a higher incidence of congestive heart failure and ventricular rupture. Diabetic men have a 2.4-fold increase in heart failure, but diabetic women have a particularly high incidence: 5.1 times that of persons without diabetes. Diabetic cardiomyopathy occurs even in the absence of epicardial vessel disease, causing some investigators to hypothesize a preponderance of small-vessel disease. Autonomic neuropathy frequently occurs and results in sympathetic denervation manifested by a fixed tachycardia with subsequent parasympathetic damage that results in lowering of the heart rate. Complete autonomic cardiac denervation finally occurs, resulting in a heart rate that is no longer responsive to such physiologic stimuli as standing.

Echocardiographic studies show abnormal systolic and diastolic function, with impaired diastolic filling as one of the earliest manifestations of diabetic cardiomyopathy. Various studies have shown diabetic patients to have a delayed opening of the mitral valve, a longer preejection period, and a shorter left ventricular ejection time, resulting in decreased filling and contractility. Other studies have shown an increase in contractility in patients with diabetes of recent onset. The cause of the left ventricular dysfunction is probably multifactorial, reflecting the effects of both hypertension and coronary atherosclerosis.

▶ Treatment

Diet, oral hypoglycemics, insulin sensitizers, and insulin remain the mainstay of therapy for hyperglycemia. Recent studies have illustrated that tight glucose control decreases the progression and development of diabetic microvascular complications. Few trials examining tight glucose control have shown a substantial reduction in macrovascular disease and whether tight glucose control influences CHD risk is still unclear. To prevent microvascular disease, target hemoglobin A_1C levels should be less than 7%, which corresponds with mean glucose levels of 150 mg/dL.

Current trial evidence suggests that aggressive treatment of hypertension and hyperlipidemia results in large and statistically significant reductions in cardiac event rates for patients with type 2 diabetes. Most studies have shown that cardiovascular benefits begin to accrue 2–4 years from the onset of treatment. Early and vigorous antihypertensive therapy with angiotensin-converting enzyme inhibitors or angiotensin receptor blockers should be first-line therapy. β-Blockers, calcium antagonists, and diuretics in low dose are second-line therapy, with the goal being a systolic and diastolic blood pressure of less than 130/80 mm Hg. Diabetic patients require more antihypertensive therapy to reach this goal; the majority needing two to three drugs concomitantly, but these patients also reap more benefit in terms of reduction in cardiovascular mortality rate per millimeter of mercury reduction of blood pressure compared with hypertensive patients without diabetes.

The benefits of aggressive lipid-lowering therapy in patients with type 2 diabetes and CHD has been demonstrated in several major secondary prevention trials with statin drugs. A few primary prevention trials have shown a decreased risk of CHD in the small number of diabetic persons studied. Target lipid levels are similar to those for patients with established CHD and include an low-density lipoprotein of < 100 mg/dL, triglycerides < 150 mg/dL, high-density lipoprotein > 45 mg/dL in women and > 55 mg/dL in men. Statin therapy is preferred as first-line therapy unless triglycerides are markedly elevated above 500 mg/dL, necessitating use of fibrates as first-line therapy.

Treatment of CHD for diabetic patients is similar to that for nondiabetic persons with some important caveats. Endothelial dysfunction and the platelet and coagulation disturbances characteristic of type 2 diabetes have been postulated to affect morbidity and mortality in the setting of unstable angina, non–ST-segment elevation myocardial infarction, and after percutaneous transluminal coronary angioplasty (PTCA), stenting, and CABG. Diabetic patients have higher rates of adverse outcomes and restenosis in these settings.

Given the known hemostatic disturbances associated with type 2 diabetes, current evidence supports aggressive antiplatelet therapy. The optimal therapeutic modality of diabetic patients with multivessel disease is controversial. Some studies have shown that diabetic patients with multivessel disease treated with bypass surgery have a marked decrease in cardiovascular mortality rates when compared with patients who receive percutaneous interventions. Superiority has been demonstrated for internal mammary artery grafts when bypass surgery is performed compared with saphenous vein grafts.

Overall, persons with diabetes who have multivessel disease appear to do better with CABG using the internal mammary artery than with percutaneous coronary intervention, but there are still many unanswered questions. Until future trial results become available and new technologies and medical therapies emerge, aggressive secondary prevention and ongoing management of CHD in the setting of diabetes will continue to pose a challenge.

Bhatt DL et al. Abciximab reduces mortality in diabetics following percutaneous coronary intervention. J Am Coll Cardiol. 2000 Mar 15;35(4):922–8. [PMID: 10732889]

Booth GL et al. Relation between age and cardiovascular disease in men and women with diabetes compared with non-diabetic people: a population-based retrospective cohort study. Lancet. 2006 Jul 1;368(9529):29–36. [PMID: 16815377]

Brooks RC et al. Clinical trials of revascularization therapy in diabetics. Curr Opin Cardiol. 2000 Jul;15(4):287–92. [PMID: 11139093]

Calles-Escandon J et al. Diabetes and endothelial dysfunction: a clinical perspective. Endocr Rev. 2001 Feb;22(1):36–52. [PMID: 11159815]

Hu G et al. The effect of diabetes and stroke at baseline and during follow-up on stroke mortality. Diabetologia. 2006 Oct;49(10):2309–16. [PMID: 16896934]

Gæde P et al. Multifactorial intervention and cardiovascular disease in patients with type 2 diabetes. N Engl J Med. 2003 Jan 30;348(5):383–93. [PMID: 12556541]

Goldberg IJ. Clinical review 124: Diabetic dyslipidemia: causes and consequences. J Clin Endocrinol Metab. 2001 Mar;86(3):965–71. [PMID: 11238470]

Hammoud T et al. Management of coronary artery disease: therapeutic options in patients with diabetes. J Am Coll Cardiol. 2000 Aug;36(2):355–65. [PMID: 10933343]

Huang ES et al. The effect of interventions to prevent cardiovascular disease in patients with type 2 diabetes mellitus. Am J Med. 2001 Dec 1;111(8):633–42. [PMID: 11755507]

McFarlane SI et al. Insulin resistance and cardiovascular disease. J Clin Endocrinol Metab. 2001 Feb;86(2):713–8. [PMID: 11158035]

Expert Panel on Detection, Evaluation and Treatment of High Blood Cholesterol in Adults. Executive Summary of the Third Report of the National Cholesterol Education Program (NCEP) Expert Panel on Detection, Evaluation and Treatment of High Blood Cholesterol in Adults (Adult Treatment Panel III). JAMA. 2001 May 16;285(19):2486–97. [PMID: 11368702]

Roffi M et al. Platelet glycoprotein IIb/IIIa inhibitors reduce mortality in diabetic patients with non-ST-segment-elevation acute coronary syndromes. Circulation. 2001 Dec 4;104(23):2767–71. [PMID: 11733392]

Stratton IM et al. Association of glycaemia with macrovascular and microvascular complications of type 2 diabetes (UKPDS 35): prospective observational study. BMJ. 2000 Aug 12;321(7258):405–12. [PMID: 10938048]

Vega GL. Results of Expert Meetings: Obesity and Cardiovascular Disease. Obesity, the metabolic syndrome, and cardiovascular disease. Am Heart J. 2001 Dec;142(6):1108–16. [PMID: 11717620]

ESTROGENS & THE HEART

1. Hormone Replacement Therapy

A great deal of interest has recently focused on estrogens and coronary artery disease. There is a strong link between menopause and increased CHD in women. Postmenopausal status or premature menopause without hormone replacement therapy (HRT) was previously considered a risk factor of coronary artery disease by the Adult Treatment Panel II based on several observational studies, such as the Nurses' Health Study, which suggested that current users of HRT had a 40% lower risk for CHD. This observation was supported by mechanistic studies of cellular and molecular actions of estrogen on lipids, hemostasis, endothelial function, and vascular reactivity.

The Adult Treatment Panel III deleted postmenopausal status without HRT as a CHD risk factor after unexpected results from the Heart and Estrogen/progestin Replacement Study (HERS), the first prospective, blind, placebo-controlled, randomized trial of HRT in secondary prevention of CHD. The investigators found no benefit from 4 years of treatment with HRT in women with prior CHD.

Importantly, HERS demonstrated a 52% increased risk of major coronary events within the first year of the trial. During the second year, risk was equal in the two groups, and by years 4–5 risk was higher in the placebo group. The early increase in risk suggests that HRT may predispose to thrombosis, arrhythmia, or ischemia.

The Estrogen Replacement on the Progression of Coronary Artery Atherosclerosis (ERA) trial demonstrated that postmenopausal HRT is not beneficial in the short term (3 years) in preventing progression or inducing regression of coronary atherosclerosis in women with established CHD who undergo angiography.

It should be noted that both HERS and ERA were designed to examine the role of HRT in secondary prevention. The Women's Health Initiative is the first trial examining the effect of HRT in primary prevention and was terminated in early 2002 due to increased risk of invasive breast cancer. Rates of CHD, stroke, deep venous thrombosis, and pulmonary embolism were higher in women receiving HRT. Therefore, postmenopausal HRT cannot be recommended solely for prevention of CHD.

Herrington DM et al. Effects of estrogen replacement on progression of coronary artery atherosclerosis. N Engl J Med. 2000 Aug 24;343(8):522–9. [PMID: 10954759]

Hulley S et al. Randomized trial of estrogen plus progestin for secondary prevention of coronary heart disease in postmenopausal women. Heart and Estrogen/progestin Replacement Study (HERS) Research Group. JAMA. 1998 Aug 19;280(7):605–13. [PMID: 9718051]

Tolbert T et al. Cardiovascular effects of estrogen. Am J Hyperten. 2001 Jun;14(6 Pt 2):186S–193S. [PMID: 11411755]

Rossouw JE, et al; Writing Group for the Women's Health Initiative Investigators. Risks and benefits of estrogen plus progestin in healthy postmenopausal women: principal results from the Women's Health Initiative randomized controlled trial. JAMA. 2002 Jul 17;288(3):321–33. [PMID: 12117397]

2. Oral Contraceptives

Oral contraceptives have long been touted as risks for deep venous thrombosis, myocardial infarction, and stroke. The high risk reported in early studies was increased among women who were cigarette smokers. Women who had stopped taking oral contraceptives did not appear to be at increased risk, suggesting a coagulation rather than a progressive atherosclerotic effect of these agents. Most of these studies used high-dose estrogen preparations. Current day oral contraceptives are low-dose estrogen ($\leq$ 50 mg) and some are progestin only; they are generally safe. Otherwise healthy women who are not diabetic or hypertensive and do not smoke have no excess risk.

Rosondaal FR et al. Female hormones and thrombosis. Arterioscler Thromb Vasc Biol. 2002 Feb 1;22(2):201–10. [PMID: 11834517]

Tanis BC et al. Oral contraceptives and the risk of myocardial infarction. N Engl J Med. 2001 Dec 20;345(25):1787–93. [PMID: 11752354]

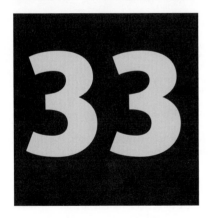

33

Connective Tissue Diseases & the Heart

Carlos A. Roldan, MD

The connective tissue diseases are immune-mediated inflammatory diseases, primarily of the musculoskeletal system; however, they frequently also involve the cardiovascular system. The most important of these diseases are systemic lupus erythematosus, rheumatoid arthritis, scleroderma, ankylosing spondylitis, polymyositis/dermatomyositis, and mixed connective tissue disease. They affect the valve leaflets, coronary arteries, pericardium, myocardium, conduction system, and great vessels with different rates of prevalence and degrees of severity. Although heart involvement in patients with connective tissue diseases contributes significantly to their morbidity and mortality rates, there is a large discrepancy between clinically recognized heart disease and postmortem series. Furthermore, the pathogenesis, natural history, and effects of therapy are incompletely understood. Increased awareness and better understanding of the cardiovascular disease associated with connective tissue diseases may lead to earlier recognition, treatment and, perhaps, increased longevity.

SYSTEMIC LUPUS ERYTHEMATOSUS

ESSENTIALS OF DIAGNOSIS

▶ Musculoskeletal and mucocutaneous manifestations of systemic lupus erythematosus (SLE).

▶ Libman-Sacks vegetations, atrioventricular (AV) valve regurgitation, myocarditis, vascular thrombotic disease, and SLE.

▶ Cardioembolism and SLE.

▶ Acute pericarditis with antinuclear antibodies detected in the pericardial fluid.

▶ General Considerations

Systemic lupus erythematosus is a multisystem chronically recurrent inflammatory disease that affects the musculoskel-

etal, mucocutaneous, visceral, and central nervous systems. Symptoms include fatigue, myalgias, arthralgias or arthritis, photosensitivity, and serositis. The prevalence of SLE varies widely, from 4 to 250 cases per 100,000 persons. It is more frequent in a patient's relatives than in the general population. Systemic lupus erythematosus is predominantly seen in females, with a female-to-male ratio of 10:1. The pathophysiology of the disease is related to the multiorgan deposition of circulating antigen-antibody complexes and activation of the complement system, leading to humoral- and cellular-mediated inflammation.

Although SLE affects the cardiovascular system with varied frequency and degrees of severity, cardiovascular disease is the third most important cause of death in SLE patients (after infectious, renal, and central nervous system diseases). The most significant SLE-associated heart diseases are valvular heart disease, arterial or venous thrombosis and systemic thromboembolism, coronary artery disease (CAD), and pericarditis. Myocarditis or cardiomyopathy and cardiac arrhythmias or conduction disturbances are less common.

The pathogenesis of SLE-associated cardiovascular disease is believed, as it is for the primary disease, that the immune complex deposition and complement activation lead to an acute, chronic, or recurrent inflammation of the valve leaflets, endocardium, vascular endothelium, pericardium, myocardium, or conduction system. The presence in these tissues of immune complexes, complement, antinuclear antibodies, lupus erythematosus cells, mononuclear inflammatory cells, necrosis, hematoxylin bodies, and deposits of fibrin and platelet thrombi support this theory. Many studies suggest that antiphospholipid antibodies (aPL) (IgA, IgG, or IgM anticardiolipin antibodies [aCL], lupus-anticoagulant [LA], or antibodies to plasma phospholipid-binding protein β_2-glycoprotein I) cause cardiovascular injury. These antibodies, present in as many as half of SLE patients, are directed against negatively charged phospholipids present in the membrane of endothelial cells causing endothelial dysfunction, vascular injury, and increased arterial or venous thrombogenesis.

1. Valvular Heart Disease

▶ General Considerations

Valvular heart disease is the clinically most important and frequent of the SLE-associated cardiovascular manifestations. Valvular heart disease is associated with an increased morbidity and mortality of SLE patients. It has been categorized as vegetations (Libman-Sacks endocarditis), leaflet thickening, valve regurgitation and, infrequently, valve stenosis. The actual prevalence of clinically recognized valve disease is unknown. Although not consistently demonstrated, rates of valve disease are probably higher in patients who have had SLE for more than 5 years, in those treated with corticosteroids, in those with higher disease damage scores, in those with moderate to high levels of aPL, and in those older than 50 years of age.

The pathogenesis of SLE valve disease include (1) an immune-complex mediated inflammation with subendothelial deposition of immunoglobulins and complement leading to an increased expression of $\alpha_3\beta_1$-integrin on the endothelial cells; (2) increased amount of collagen IV, laminin, and fibronectin; (3) proliferation of blood vessels; (4) inflammation and fibrosis; and finally, (5) commonly associated increased local or systemic thrombogenesis.

The proposed mechanisms of valve damage by aPL include (1) binding of aPL, which induces activation of endothelial cells and up regulation of the expression of adhesion molecules, secretion of cytokines, and abnormal metabolism of prostacyclins; (2) increased oxidized low-density lipoprotein (LDL taken up by macrophages leads to macrophage activation and further damage to endothelial cells); (3) aPL interference with the regulatory functions of prothrombin and with the production of prostacyclin and endothelial relaxing factor, protein C, protein S, and tissue factor; and (4) a heparin-like–induced thrombocytopenia. All these factors lead to increased vasoconstriction, platelet aggregation, and thrombus formation.

A. Valve Vegetations, or Libman-Sacks Endocarditis

Considered pathognomonic of SLE-associated valve disease, noninfective valve vegetations are almost exclusively seen on the mitral and aortic valves. Most vegetations are located on the coaptation portions of the leaflets, on the atrial side for the mitral valve, and the aortic vessel or ventricular side for the aortic valve. The valve vegetations are usually less than 1 cm^2 in size, have irregular borders and heterogeneous echodensity, and have no independent motion (Figures 33–1 and 33–2). Most valves with vegetations have associated thickening or regurgitation. Although valve vegetations have been seen more commonly in younger persons (younger than 40 years), their temporal association with SLE activity, severity, duration, and therapy has been variable.

Pathologic examination reveals that active Libman-Sacks vegetations have central fibrinoid necrosis with fibroblastic proliferation and fibrosis, surrounded by mononuclear and polymorphonuclear cellular infiltration, small hemorrhages, and platelet thrombus. Healed vegetations have central fibrosis, minimal or no inflammatory cell deposition, and no or hyalinized and endothelialized thrombus. Active, healed, and mixed vegetations can be seen in the same valve.

B. Valve Thickening

Leaflet thickening with or without abnormal mobility results from replacement of the normal spongiosum and endothelial layers by postinflammatory fibrous tissue and infrequently by calcification. Valve thickening may be seen in up to half of patients; it is generally diffuse, with greater involvement of the middle and tip portions (Figures 33–1 and 33–2). When leaflet thickening is localized, the basal, middle, and tip portions are equally affected. Valve thickening predominantly affects the mitral and aortic valves and is commonly associated with valve regurgitation, valve vegetations, or both. In young patients with no atherogenic risk factors, associated valve calcification is uncommon (< 5%). However, in middle age patients with traditional atherogenic risk factors, mitral annular and aortic valve calcification are common (20%).

C. Valve Regurgitation

This most frequent abnormality is predominantly mild in severity and therefore usually clinically silent. Although the prevalence of regurgitation is similar for the mitral, tricuspid, and pulmonic valves (about 50–75%) and the lowest for the aortic valve (25%), the mitral and aortic valves are those most commonly associated with complications. Mitral or aortic valve stenosis associated with respective valve regurgitation is uncommon.

▶ Clinical Findings

A. Symptoms and Signs

Unless it is severe, valve disease is generally asymptomatic or overshadowed by the musculoskeletal and systemic inflammatory symptoms. However, subclinical valve disease is commonly first manifested with cardioembolism. Recent studies report that valve disease detected by transesophageal echocardiography (TEE), especially mitral valve vegetations, are two to four times more common in patients with focal ischemic brain injury on magnetic resonance imaging (MRI), in those with stroke or transient ischemic attack (TIA), and in those with nonfocal neuropsychiatric manifestations of cognitive dysfunction, acute confusional state, seizures, or psychosis (Figure 33–1). In these series, valve vegetations were strong independent predictor of brain injury and focal or nonfocal neuropsychiatric manifestations. These data suggest that valve disease in lupus patients is a source of fibrin or platelet macro- or microembolism to the brain. Also, severe valve regurgitation resulting from recurrent or acute native and

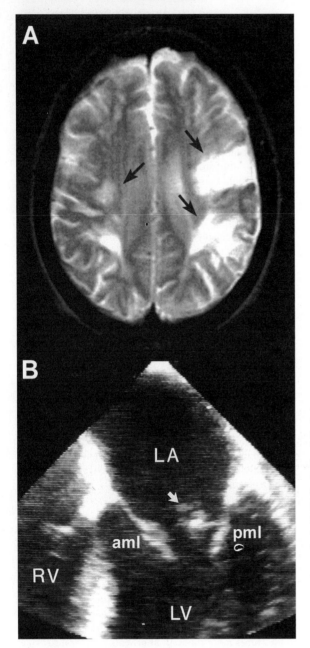

▲ **Figure 33–1.** Recurrent strokes and mitral valve thickening with a large Libman-Sacks vegetation in a 47-year-old woman with systemic lupus erythematosus. **A:** This T_2-weighted magnetic resonance imaging of the brain demonstrates generalized cortical atrophy, multiple areas of old cerebral infarcts characterized by loss of both gray and white matter (*arrows*) in a cortical and subcortical pattern. Also, multiple areas of deep white matter abnormality consistent with widespread ischemic cerebrovascular disease is noted. **B:** This transesophageal four-chamber echocardiographic view shows diffuse thickening predominantly of the middle and tip portions of the anterior (aml) and posterior (pml) mitral leaflets. A large vegetation with heterogeneous echoreflectance and irregular borders is noted on the atrial side of the posterior mitral leaflet (*arrow*). Moderate mitral regurgitation was present. LA, left atrium; LV, left ventricle; RV, right ventricle.

bioprosthetic valvulitis, noninfective mitral valve chordal rupture, or infective endocarditis occur in at least 20% of patients. Infective endocarditis can mimic, accompany, or trigger a flare of SLE and lead to severe valvular dysfunction, heart failure, and death from septicemia. Similarly, a flare of SLE can mimic infective endocarditis (pseudo-infective endocarditis). A low white count, elevated aPL and anti-DNA antibodies, depressed complements, and negative or low C-reactive protein support the diagnosis of active SLE with pseudo-infective endocarditis.

B. Physical Examination

The physical findings of musculoskeletal and mucocutaneous disease generally predominate in SLE patients, even in those with cardiovascular disease. If moderate-to-severe

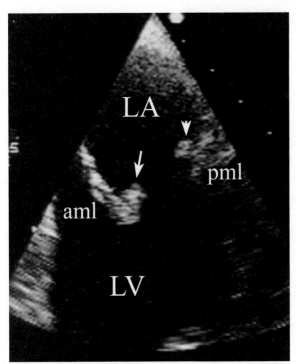

▲ Figure 33–2. Mitral valve Libman-Sacks vegetations in a 37-year-old woman with systemic lupus erythematosus and a stroke. This transesophageal echocardiogram demonstrates a Libman-Sacks vegetation on the atrial side and tip of the anterior mitral leaflet (aml) (*arrow*) and a second vegetation on the midportion of the posterior leaflet (pml) (*arrowhead*). Associated diffuse thickening of both mitral leaflets is also noted. Moderate mitral regurgitation was demonstrated by color-Doppler.

mitral or aortic regurgitation or stenosis is present, the auscultatory findings found on physical examination will be typical. Less significant degrees of regurgitation (these are the majority) may not be clinically detected or may be mistaken for functional murmurs related to fever, anemia, hypertension, or volume overload.

C. Diagnostic Studies

1. Electrocardiography—Results of electrocardiographic (ECG) studies are nonspecific. Left atrial abnormality and left ventricular (LV) hypertrophy can be seen in patients with chronic and severe aortic or mitral regurgitation.

2. Chest radiography—Cardiomegaly with LV and left atrial enlargement may be seen in the presence of significant mitral or aortic regurgitation.

3. Echocardiography—Transthoracic color-flow Doppler echocardiography (TTE) is the most commonly applied tech-

nique for the diagnosis of SLE-associated valve disease. This technique accurately determines the presence and severity of valve regurgitation or stenosis and abnormal leaflet thickening, but not of vegetations. The prevalence of Libman-Sacks vegetations by TTE is less than 10%. This technique will also detect associated increased wall thickness, chamber enlargement, ventricular diastolic or systolic dysfunction, and associated left atrial and pulmonary hypertension. Transesophageal echocardiography is superior to TTE in detecting and characterizing SLE-associated valve masses and leaflet thickening. Transesophageal echocardiography detects valve vegetations in up to 35% of patients. By serial TEE, Libman-Sacks vegetations resolve, appear de novo, or change their morphology over time and are not temporally related to SLE activity, severity, duration, or therapy. Therefore, TEE is indicated to exclude sources of cardioembolism in patients with a focal neurologic defect or in patients with a nonfocal neurologic deficit (moderate or worse cognitive dysfunction, seizures, acute confusional state, or psychosis) and cerebral infarcts on MRI, and in patients with suspected complicating infective endocarditis.

▶ Treatment

A. Specific Antiinflammatory Therapy

Currently, prospective data are limited regarding whether corticosteroids, disease modifying antirheumatic drugs (DMARDs), or immunosuppressive therapy are beneficial in treating SLE-associated valve disease. In general, treatment focuses on managing active SLE disease with antiinflammatory or immunosuppressive agents rather than on managing valve disease specifically.

B. Long-Term Anticoagulation

Long-term anticoagulation is beneficial in patients with Libman-Sacks vegetations and previous systemic embolism independently of aPL.

C. Other Therapy

Diuretics, vasodilators, or high-risk prosthetic valve replacement is indicated in severe symptomatic valve disease, including those cases complicated by infective endocarditis. The mortality rate associated with valve replacement in SLE patients is twice that for patients without SLE.

2. Pericarditis
▶ General Considerations

Pericarditis, with or without effusion or pericardial thickening, is common in postmortem series. Also, about half of lupus patients suffer at least one episode of symptomatic pericarditis. Most episodes are acute and are frequently associated with active SLE and valvulitis, myocarditis, pleuritis, or nephritis. Cardiac tamponade or constrictive pericarditis rarely occurs (< 2%).

▶ Clinical Findings

A. Symptoms and Signs

The diagnosis of pericarditis is based on clinical manifestations rather on the echocardiogram, because an effusion or pericardial thickening are frequently absent. Symptomatic pericarditis is generally acute and uncomplicated and is most commonly seen during flare-ups of the disease. Asymptomatic pericardial disease may be present in some patients. It is manifested by incidentally detected small effusions in most cases and far less frequently by pericardial thickening found on echocardiography. Asymptomatic pericardial disease is generally seen in patients with stable disease that is either mildly active or in remission. Occasionally, acute pericarditis, cardiac tamponade, or both may be the initial manifestation of SLE. Chronic constrictive pericarditis is rare. Infectious pericarditis is rare but catastrophic and most commonly caused by *Staphylococcus aureus*. Finally, a pericardial effusion in SLE patients may also be secondary to severe uremia or nephrotic syndrome.

Because it is frequently symptomatic, acute pericarditis is the SLE-related cardiovascular disease most often detected clinically. It may present with fever, tachycardia, pleuritic chest pain and, on auscultation, the presence of a pericardial rub. If a large effusion is present, decreased heart sounds, jugular venous distention, and pulsus paradoxus may be noted.

B. Laboratory Findings

Pericarditis typically yields serofibrinous, fibrinous or, rarely, serosanguineous exudative fluid containing low complement level and antinuclear antibodies. By immunofluorescence, the pericardium shows granular deposition of immunoglobulins and C3.

C. Diagnostic Studies

1. Electrocardiography—The ECG most frequently shows no abnormalities or nonspecific ST segment and T wave changes. The characteristic diffuse ST-segment elevation with upward concavity and PR segment depression of acute pericarditis are common. Low voltage or electrical alternans may also be seen if a large pericardial effusion is present.

2. Chest radiography—The chest radiography is generally of little diagnostic value because most patients with acute pericarditis have no—or only small—pericardial effusions. If a large pericardial effusion is present, cardiomegaly with a characteristic water-bottle shape may be seen.

3. Echocardiography—Since pericardial chest pain can be masked by musculoskeletal or pleural pain, echocardiography has complementary diagnostic value. Echocardiography may demonstrate small pericardial effusions, or none. Small, asymptomatic pericardial effusions have also been found in up to 20% of SLE patients hospitalized with active disease. However, the absence of an effusion on echocardiography

does not exclude a clinically suspected pericarditis. In cases of pericarditis with large pericardial effusion and clinically suspected cardiac tamponade, echocardiography may demonstrate right atrial or ventricular diastolic collapse and significant respiratory variability of the mitral or tricuspid Doppler inflows, indicating the need for therapeutic pericardiocentesis. Also, echocardiographically guided pericardiocentesis has been successfully performed in lupus patients with hemodynamically significant pericardial effusions. Also, serial follow-up echocardiography after pericardiocentesis or after antiinflammatory therapy is helpful to guide the need of future interventions. Echocardiography is less useful in detecting pericardial thickening or calcification in cases of suspected chronic pericardial constriction.

4. Computed tomography and magnetic resonance imaging—These techniques are preferred methods for assessing pericardial thickening when the echocardiogram suggests constriction.

▶ Treatment

A. Medical Therapy

Most rheumatologists use low-dose prednisone (10–20 mg/day for 7–14 days) rather than nonsteroidal antiinflammatory drugs (NSAIDs) for symptomatic pericarditis. The use of NSAIDs is limited by associated renal disease, thrombocytopenia, or anticoagulation. Chronically recurrent pericarditis is treated with hydroxychloroquine or immunosuppressive agents.

B. Surgical Therapy

Pericardiocentesis should be performed when large effusions are unresponsive to medical therapy and when cardiac tamponade or complicating infectious pericarditis with effusion are suspected.

Pericardiectomy has been performed in isolated cases of SLE-associated chronic pericardial constriction.

3. Myocarditis or Cardiomyopathy
▶ General Considerations

Myocarditis can be seen in autopsy series in up to 80% of patients with SLE; by contrast, only 20% of cases can be clinically detected. Myocardial disease in SLE patients has four principal causes. First, a primary acute, chronic, or recurrent myocarditis is the most common. Primary myocarditis with LV diastolic and, rarely, global or regional systolic dysfunction occur in at least 10% of patients. Rarely, acute myocarditis complicated with heart failure may be the initial manifestation of active SLE. An association of cellular antigen Ro (SS-A) and La (SS-B) antibodies and this type of myocarditis has been established, but their primary pathogenic role is still undefined. The second most common cause of myocardial diastolic and uncommonly systolic dysfunction results from endothelial dysfunction–mediated microvascular CAD. Small vessel vasculitis or epicardial coronary arteritis is rare. The third cause is myocardial dysfunction resulting from severe mitral or aortic regurgitation. Finally, a potentially reversible chloroquine sulfate–induced dilated or restrictive cardiomyopathy has been reported.

Clinical Findings

A. Symptoms and Signs

Acute myocarditis typically manifests with fever, tachycardia, chest pain and, rarely, with symptoms of heart failure, arrhythmias, or conduction disturbances. The myocarditis is generally mild and usually does not cause LV systolic dysfunction. However, up to one-third of young patients with active SLE have asymptomatic diastolic dysfunction. Occasionally, severe dilated cardiomyopathy is seen. Characteristic manifestations of an acute coronary syndrome will be present in those patients with myocardial dysfunction secondary to coronary arteritis, coronary atherosclerosis, small-vessel vasculitis, acute coronary thrombosis without underlying atherosclerosis, or coronary embolism from aortic or mitral valve masses.

If diastolic or systolic dysfunction is present, tachycardia, fourth and third heart sounds, pulmonary rales, and edema may be found.

B. Diagnostic Studies

1. Electrocardiography—Nonspecific ST segment and T wave abnormalities and atrial or ventricular ectopic complexes are common. Rarely, atrial or ventricular tachyarrhythmias can be detected.

2. Chest radiography—Cardiomegaly may be present if dilated cardiomyopathy has developed.

3. Echocardiography—Generally, no abnormalities are detected in acute myocarditis. When the myocarditis is severe, diffuse or regional wall motion abnormalities may be observed. Doppler echocardiography series, including tissue Doppler in asymptomatic young patients without systemic or pulmonary hypertension and normal LV systolic function, have demonstrated up to one-third of LV and right ventricular (RV) diastolic dysfunction, predominantly of impaired relaxation. Diastolic dysfunction occurs three to four times more frequently in patients with active SLE. In unselected patients, the prevalence of LV systolic dysfunction is low.

4. Radionuclide studies—Either first-transit or gated-acquisition radionuclide angiography also can be used to assess ventricular systolic and diastolic dysfunction, wall motion abnormalities, and chamber enlargement. In up to one-third of SLE patients, this technique has shown an abnormal ventricular function response to exercise, as evidenced by a fall or subnormal rise in ejection fraction and the appearance of new or worsened wall motion abnormalities indicative of myocarditis or CAD. Reversible, fixed, or mixed myocardial perfusion defects can be seen in patients with normal epicardial coronary arteries indicative of active or past myocarditis or small vessel disease.

5. Endomyocardial biopsy—Tissue samples may demonstrate SLE-associated myocarditis or cardiomyopathy when a clinical or serologic diagnosis cannot be made.

6. Cardiac biomarkers—Mild elevation of troponin I will be more common than elevation of creatine phosphokinase (CPK).

Treatment

A. Specific Antiinflammatory Therapy

In outpatients, acute myocarditis is treated with high-dose oral prednisone; in hospitalized patients with acute myocarditis, intravenous methylprednisolone (1–2 mg/kg/day) is given. A course of 7–14 days is generally recommended, but the dose and duration can be titrated based on the clinical response. Long-term immunosuppression with intravenous cyclophosphamide or oral mycophenolate may be required.

B. Other Therapy

Symptomatic therapy with NSAIDs or other analgesics, bed rest, and ECG monitoring for detection of arrhythmias are indicated. If symptomatic dilated cardiomyopathy is present, diuretics, vasodilators, and digoxin therapy are used.

4. Thrombotic Diseases

General Considerations

Deep venous thrombosis, pulmonary embolism, and peripheral or cerebral arterial thrombosis are common in SLE patients. Acute coronary thrombosis in the absence of angiographic CAD has also been reported. Both arterial and venous thrombotic events have been associated with aPL. Patients with SLE are subject to intracardiac thrombosis and cerebral or systemic thromboembolism independently of or exacerbated by aPL. Current data support that SLE cerebrovascular disease is commonly associated and likely causally related to cardioembolism from Libman-Sacks endocarditis. In recent series, mitral or aortic valve vegetations were two to four times more common and strong independent predictors of focal ischemic brain injury on MRI; stroke or TIA; and nonfocal neurologic dysfunction, such as cognitive dysfunction, acute confusional state, or seizures. In fact, microembolic events during transcranial Doppler echocardiography are common in patients with cerebral ischemic events.

Clinical Findings

A. Symptoms and Signs

Although acute pleuritic chest pain and tachycardia could be related to the presence of pericarditis, pleuritis, or pneumonitis, they should prompt the suspicion of pulmonary embolism and

DVT. Focal and nonfocal transient or permanent neurologic deficits are commonly due to cardioembolism from valvular or myocardial disease and rarely due to vasculitis or cerebritis.

B. Laboratory Findings

Antiphospolipid antibodies are highly associated with venous or arterial thrombotic events. However, these antibodies can be present in SLE patients without thrombosis and infrequently in patients who do not have SLE. Therefore, routine measurement of aPL to identify patients at high thrombotic risk and as a basis for prophylactic anticoagulant therapy is still undefined.

C. Diagnostic Studies

1. Transesophageal echocardiography—Transesophageal echocardiography should be considered in SLE patients with focal neurologic deficits, in those with nonfocal neurologic deficits and focal brain injury on brain MRI, and in those with peripheral arterial thrombosis to exclude cardioembolism as the cause.

2. Doppler echocardiography, plethysmography, scintigraphy, or venogram—These imaging methods of the lower extremities should be performed if DVT is suspected.

3. High resolution computed tomography of the chest or pulmonary ventilation-perfusion scan—These methods should be considered if pulmonary embolism is clinically suspected.

▶ Treatment
A. Specific Antiinflammatory Therapy

Corticosteroids or immunosuppressive agents may be beneficial in patients with active SLE and noninfective vegetations with or without thrombosis or thromboembolism.

B. Other Therapy

Anticoagulation with warfarin is the therapy of choice in patients with DVT, pulmonary embolism, and in those with noninfective valve vegetations and stroke or TIA or cerebral infarcts on MRI.

5. Coronary Artery Disease
▶ General Considerations

Postmortem studies in SLE patients have demonstrated up to a 25% prevalence of CAD, but clinically evident disease or arteritis is uncommon. Functional or small vessel CAD is more frequent than epicardial coronary disease in clinical and postmortem series.

After controlling for traditional risk factors for CAD, the risk of functional (abnormal vasodilation or microvascular disease) or subclinical atherosclerotic epicardial CAD in lupus patients is four to eight times higher than matched controls. Risk factors for CAD in SLE patients are a longer mean duration of the disease, a longer mean duration and dose of prednisone therapy, a high disease damage score, and SLE-induced dyslipidemia (high levels of oxidative LDL, low levels of HDL, or high levels of pro-inflammatory HDL). However, a high Framingham risk score is also an important predictor.

The proposed pathogenetic mechanisms for CAD include (1) activation of cellular and humoral immunity (including aPL) with activation of macrophages, CD4+CD28–T cells and dendritic cells. The cytotoxicity of these cells to the endothelium and vascular wall result in decreased production of prostacyclin and prostaglandin I and consequently in increased vasoconstriction. Also, vascular wall cytotoxicity result in an increased thrombosis via release of platelet-derived growth factor and thromboxane A_2. Cytotoxic cells also produce interferon-γ, which destabilizes atherosclerotic plaques by suppressing synthesis of collagen, increase proliferation of smooth muscle cells, and activation of macrophages to release free radicals and matrix metalloproteinases; (2) increased oxidation of LDL; (3) increased production of inflammatory cytokines and chemokines such as heat shock proteins, C-reactive protein, rheumatoid factor, tumor necrosis factor-α, and interleukins. These cytokines are expressed on the endothelium of coronary arteries, recruit inflammatory cells, promote abnormal vascular smooth cell proliferation, induce oxidative stress, endothelial apoptosis, and further up-regulation of adhesion molecules and chemokines; and (4) exacerbation of dyslipidemia (high levels of very low density lipoproteins and triglycerides and low levels of high-density lipoproteins), homocysteinemia, and insulin resistance. Uncommon pathogenetic factors include coronary arteritis, in situ coronary thrombosis, or embolization from a Libman-Sacks vegetation.

▶ Clinical Findings
A. Symptoms and Signs

The presentation of CAD in SLE patients is not unique and involves stable or exertional angina, unstable angina, acute ST or non-ST elevation MI or, rarely, heart failure from ischemic LV dysfunction. In addition, fatal MI can occur in SLE patients, and some data suggest an increased risk of myocardial rupture after MI in SLE patients treated with corticosteroids. Coronary arteritis should be suspected in a young patient with an acute ischemic syndrome, active SLE, and evidence of vasculitis affecting other organs. Also, coronary embolism or in situ thrombosis warrant consideration when MI occurs in the presence of a cardioembolic substrate (valve vegetations) or moderate to high levels of aPL.

B. Diagnostic Studies

Electrocardiography, exercise testing with or without perfusion scanning, and echocardiography, can be used in SLE patients in whom CAD is suspected. However, the diagnostic value of these techniques is inferior to that in the general population due to their young age, female predominance, and lower prevalence of obstructive epicardial CAD. Electron beam computed tomography has demonstrated a high prevalence (30–45%) of coronary calcification in asymptomatic patients. None of these techniques, including angiography, can reliably differentiate coronary arteritis from common coronary atherosclerosis. Suspected epicardial CAD may warrant coronary angiography because of the confounding clinical, echocardiographic, and myocardial perfusion features of functional or small vessel CAD or lupus myocarditis.

▶ Treatment

A. Specific Antiinflammatory Therapy

If coronary arteritis is suspected, high-dose corticosteroids (1–2 mg/kg/day) are used initially, and followed by intravenous cyclophosphamide or oral mycophenolate. The duration of therapy is usually based on clinical response. Corticosteroids may have some additional danger in patients with recent transmural MI.

B. Other Therapy

Except for the use of immunosuppressive agents in suspected arteritis, the treatment of epicardial CAD is not different from that in the general population. Both percutaneous coronary intervention (PCI) and bypass surgery have been successfully performed in SLE patients.

6. Cardiac Arrhythmias & Conduction Disturbances

▶ General Considerations

The prevalence of these abnormalities is unknown. Although they are common with myocarditis and highly associated with the presence of anti-Ro antibodies, no primary pathogenetic role of these antibodies has been demonstrated. Atrial fibrillation or flutter may be seen during episodes of acute pericarditis. Rarely, ventricular arrhythmias or conduction disturbances may be associated with acute myocarditis. Chronic conduction disturbances may be due to the inflammation and fibrosis of the conduction system frequently found at autopsy. Electrocardiography is the most valuable technique for detecting arrhythmias and conduction disturbances.

▶ Treatment

A. Specific Antiinflammatory Therapy

Although experience is limited, acute high-degree AV blocks may resolve with the use of high-dose corticosteroids.

B. Other Therapy

Temporary pacing is an alternative treatment for acute AV blocks. Permanent pacemakers should be used in cases of symptomatic high-grade AV blocks that are unresponsive to corticosteroids.

▶ Prognosis

The overall survival rate of SLE patients is about 75% over 10 years. If the heart, lung, kidney, or central nervous system is clinically involved, the prognosis is worse. Cardiovascular disease is the third major cause of mortality in SLE patients, after infectious and renal diseases. Valvular, myocardial, or CAD are known to decrease the survival of SLE patients.

Chung CP et al. Cardiovascular risk scores and the presence of subclinical coronary artery atherosclerosis in women with systemic lupus erythematosus. Lupus. 2006;15:562–9. [PMID: 17080910]

Costedoat-Chalumeau N et al. Cardiomyopathy related to antimalarial therapy with illustrative case report. Cardiology. 2007; 107(2):73–80. [PMID: 16804295]

Doria A et al. Cardiac involvement in systemic lupus erythematosus. Lupus. 2005;14(9):683–6. [PMID: 16218467]

Farzaneh-Far A et al. Relationship of antiphospholipid antibodies to cardiovascular manifestations of systemic lupus erythematosus. Arthritis Rheum. 2006 Dec;54(12):3918–25. [PMID: 17133599]

Galie N et al. Pulmonary arterial hypertension associated to connective tissue diseases. Lupus. 2005;14(9):713–7. [PMID: 16218473]

Law WG et al. Acute lupus myocarditis: clinical features and outcome of an oriental case series. Lupus. 2005;14(10):827–31. [PMID: 16302678]

Locht H et al. IgG and IgM isotypes of anti-cardiolipin and anti-beta2-glycoprotein antibodies reflect different forms of recent thrombo-embolic events. Clin Rheumatol. 2006 Mar;25(2): 246–50. [PMID: 16177835]

Molad Y et al. Heart valve calcification in young patients with systemic lupus erythematosus: a window to premature atherosclerotic vascular morbidity and a risk factor for all-cause mortality. Atherosclerosis. 2006 Apr;185(2):406–12. [PMID: 16046220]

Perez-Villa F et al. Severe valvular regurgitation and antiphospholipid antibodies in systemic lupus erythematosus: a prospective, long-term, followup study. Arthritis Rheum. 2005 Jun 15;53(3):460–7. [PMID: 15934103]

Roldan CA et al. Transthoracic echocardiography versus transesophageal echocardiography for the detection of Libman-Sacks endocarditis: a randomized controlled study. J Rheumatol. 2008 Feb;35(2):224–9. [PMID: 18085739]

Roldan CA et al. Valvular heart disease as a cause of cerebrovascular disease in patients with systemic lupus erythematosus. Am J Cardiol. 2005 Jun 15;95(12):1441–7. [PMID: 15950567]

Roldan CA et al. Valvular heart disease is associated with nonfocal neuropsychiatric systemic lupus erythematosus. J Clin Rheumatol. 2006 Feb;12(1):3–10. [PMID: 16484873]

Weich HS et al. Large pericardial effusions due to systemic lupus erythematosus: a report of eight cases. Lupus. 2005;14(6):450–7. [PMID: 16038109]

RHEUMATOID ARTHRITIS

ESSENTIALS OF DIAGNOSIS

▶ Clinical evidence of rheumatoid arthritis.

▶ Granulomatous valve disease, predominantly of the mitral and aortic valves.

▶ Pericarditis and myocarditis with granuloma on biopsy.

▶ General Considerations

Rheumatoid arthritis is an immune-mediated chronic inflammatory disease characterized by morning stiffness, arthralgias, or arthritis, predominantly of the metacarpophalangeal or proximal interphalangeal joints; rheumatoid nodules; serum IgM or IgG rheumatoid factor; and articular erosions seen on a radiograph. The disease prevalence is about 1%, and it affects females more than males with a ratio of 2–4:1. The natural history of the disease is such that the median life expectancy is reduced by 7 years in men and 3 years in women. The most common causes of death are articular and extra-articular complications such as atlantoaxial subluxation, cricoarytenoid synovitis, sepsis, cardiopulmonary complications, and diffuse vasculitis. Rheumatoid arthritis patients with the worst prognosis are those with positive rheumatoid factor, nodular disease, and male gender.

Rheumatoid cardiovascular disease is produced by a nonspecific immune-complex mediated inflammation, vasculitis, or granulomatous deposition on the pericardium, myocardium, heart valves, coronary arteries, aorta, or the conduction system. Clinically apparent rheumatoid heart disease occurs in one-third of patients, compared with up to 80% in autopsy series. Rheumatoid heart disease may appear as pericarditis, myocarditis, valvular heart disease, conduction disturbances, coronary arteritis, aortitis, or cor pulmonale.

Predictors for clinically apparent cardiovascular disease vary among reported series and include male sex, advanced age at the onset of the disease, hypertension, corticosteroid therapy early in the disease, long-standing disease; active extra-articular, erosive polyarticular, and nodular disease; systemic vasculitis; and high serum titers of rheumatoid factor, higher erythrocyte sedimentation rates (ESR), and higher levels of haptoglobin, von Willebrand factor, and plasminogen activator inhibitor. These findings suggest an inflammatory and prothrombotic processes leading to cardiovascular disease. Heart disease is the third leading cause of death in patients with rheumatoid arthritis and accounts for nearly 40% of their mortality.

1. Rheumatoid Pericarditis

The prevalence of pericarditis is higher in hospitalized patients with active disease. Pericarditis generally follows the diagnosis of rheumatoid arthritis. There is a high association between pericarditis and IgG or IgM rheumatoid-factor positivity, rheumatoid nodular disease, and ESR of > 55 mm/h. Rheumatoid pericarditis occurs by three mechanisms: a nonspecific immune-complex inflammatory process, vasculitis and, less frequently, granulomatous or nodular disease.

▶ Clinical Findings

A. Symptoms and Signs

Rheumatoid pericarditis is generally uncomplicated and most commonly is evidenced by typical pleuritic pain. About one-third of patients are asymptomatic. On physical examination most will have a pericardial rub. Rarely, complicating cardiac tamponade or constrictive pericarditis may occur, generally in adult patients with active and severe disease of a longer duration and in those with extra-articular involvement. Dyspnea and orthopnea, edema, jugular venous distention, rales, pulsus paradoxus, Kussmaul sign, and hepatojugular venous distention are common when cardiac compression is present.

B. Laboratory Findings

Findings commonly associated with rheumatoid pericarditis include an ESR > 55 mm/h and high titers of rheumatoid factor. Pericardial fluid is exudative and serosanguineous, with a high protein content and high lactate dehydrogenase (LDH) but a characteristically low glucose level, and may contain rheumatoid factor. The cellular content is usually more than 2000 cells/mcL, predominantly neutrophils. On pericardial biopsy (by immunofluorescence), granular deposits of IgG, IgM, C3, and C1q are seen in the interstitium and blood vessel walls of the pericardium.

C. Diagnostic Studies

1. Electrocardiography—An electrocardiogram commonly shows nonspecific ST segment and T wave changes; a classic diffuse ST segment elevation and PR depression can be seen. Low voltage or electrical alternans may be seen with large pericardial effusions.

2. Chest radiography—The chest radiography is generally normal. Cardiomegaly is seen in patients with large pericardial effusions. Pericardial calcifications are rarely seen.

3. Echocardiography—This is the most important diagnostic technique for rheumatoid pericardial disease. The most common findings are pericardial effusion and pericardial thickening. Right atrial or ventricular diastolic compression may be seen with large pericardial effusions and may indicate tamponade hemodynamics. The presence of pericardial thickening and calcification without significant effusion, and the presence of symptoms or signs of cardiac compression, suggest constrictive pericarditis, which can be confirmed by cardiac catheterization. However, absence of pericardial abnormalities on echocardiography does not exclude the presence of pericarditis in a patient with typical symptoms or a pericardial rub. Finally, echocardiography is commonly used to guide pericardiocentesis.

4. Computed tomography or magnetic resonance imaging—These imaging methods are superior to echocardiography in detecting pericardial thickening and calcification in patients with suspected constrictive pericarditis.

▶ Treatment

Corticosteroids are frequently successful in treating most cases. If large pericardial effusions or tamponade are present, pericardiocentesis is indicated. For chronic constrictive pericarditis, high-risk pericardiectomy has been performed. The use of intrapericardial corticosteroids at the time of pericardiocentesis is controversial.

▶ Prognosis

The prognosis of rheumatoid arthritis in the presence of pericardial disease is unaltered when the pericardial involvement is mild. Large pericardial effusions with tamponade or chronic constrictive pericarditis, however, increases the morbidity and mortality rates among rheumatoid patients.

2. Rheumatoid Valvular Heart Disease
▶ General Considerations

Rheumatoid valvular heart disease is produced by a nonspecific acute, chronic, or recurrent immune-complex inflammatory process, vasculitis, or deposition of granulomata on the valve leaflets. The inflammatory process consists of infiltration with plasma cells, histiocytes, lymphocytes, and eosinophils that lead to leaflet fibrosis, thickening, and retraction. The valve granulomata, which resemble rheumatoid nodules, are present inside any portion of the four valves, valve rings, papillary muscle tips, and atrial or ventricular endocardium. The aortic and mitral valves are most often affected. The granulomata are most commonly located at the basal or mid portion of the valves; usually focal, and generally produce none or mild valve dysfunction.

Rheumatoid valvular heart disease is more commonly subclinical and can manifest in 4 forms: (1) healed valvulitis with residual leaflet fibrosis and regurgitation and rarely stenosis; (2) valve nodules; (3) acute or chronic valvulitis with variable degrees of regurgitation and with Libman-Sacks–like vegetations; and rarely, (4) aortitis with aortic root dilatation and aortic regurgitation. Acute and chronic valvulitis with resulting leaflet thickening and fibrosis is indistinguishable from that seen in SLE. In contrast, valve nodules appear to be unique to rheumatoid arthritis.

In previous series using TTE, rheumatoid valve disease has been reported in patients with long-standing rheumatoid disease and severe cases with erosive polyarticular and nod-

ular disease, systemic vasculitis, and high levels of rheumatoid factor. In a recent TEE series, no correlation was found between valve disease and the duration, activity, severity, pattern of onset and course, extra-articular disease, serology, or therapy of rheumatoid arthritis. Therefore, a clinical or laboratory predictor or marker of rheumatoid valve disease is still undefined.

▶ Clinical Findings
A. Physical Examination

The physical examination in rheumatoid valve disease may not be revealing because in most cases the degree of valve dysfunction is mild. In the rare cases of acute mitral or aortic valvulitis resulting in severe valve regurgitation or acute severe valve regurgitation from "rupture" of a nodule or a large nodule affecting leaflets coaptation, classic auscultatory findings and associated signs of left or biventricular failure may be present. Uncommonly, a clinical syndrome of systemic embolism can result from a thrombus or a valve strand over imposed on a valve nodule or valve thickening or from Libman-Sacks–like vegetations complicating acute valvulitis.

B. Diagnostic Studies

1. Electrocardiography and chest radiography—The ECG and chest radiography have limited diagnostic value. Both techniques may show chamber enlargement in cases of severe valve disease.

2. Color-flow Doppler echocardiography—Transthoracic echocardiography is the most used test for detecting and assessing the severity of rheumatoid valve disease. In a recent series using TEE in 34 patients with rheumatoid arthritis, 20 (59%) patients had mainly left-sided valve disease (valve nodules in 11 [32%], valve thickening in 18 [53%], at least moderate mitral or mild aortic regurgitation in 7 [21%], and valve stenosis in 1 [3%]). *Valve nodules* were generally single and small (4–12 mm), of homogenous echoreflectance and of oval-shape with regular borders, typically located at the leaflets' basal or mid portions, and equally affected the aortic and mitral valves. In one patient, mitral and aortic valve thickening was associated with mitral valve Libman-Sacks–like vegetations. *Valve thickening* was equally diffuse or localized. When the thickening was localized, it affected any leaflet portion, was usually mild, involved the mitral and aortic valves similarly, and rarely involved the annulus and subvalvular apparatus (Figure 33–3).

▶ Treatment

No specific antiinflammatory therapy for rheumatoid valve disease has been established. The use of corticosteroids, other immunosuppressive agents, or tumor necrosis factor-α receptor inhibitors in cases of acute severe valvulitis has

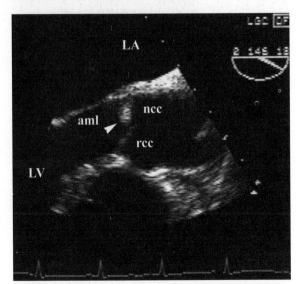

▲ **Figure 33–3.** Rheumatoid aortic valve nodule in a 48-year-old woman with rheumatoid arthritis. This transesophageal echocardiographic view longitudinal of the left ventricular outflow tract demonstrates a well defined nodule with oval shape and homogeneous soft tissue echoreflectance within the midportion of the aortic noncoronary cusp (ncc) (*arrowhead*). In contrast, the right coronary cusp (rcc) is normal. Aortic valve regurgitation was not demonstrated. aml, anterior mitral leaflet; LA, left atrium; LV, left ventricle.

resulted in significant improvement. Also, in patients with Libman-Sacks–like vegetations, anticoagulation and antiinflammatory therapy has resulted in improvement of valve masses and prevention of recurrent embolic events. Although no prospective trial is available, prophylactic antiplatelet therapy may prevent cardioembolism in patients with valve nodules or thickening. Although the morbidity and mortality rates associated with valve surgery are higher in patients with rheumatoid arthritis than in those without rheumatoid arthritis, mitral or aortic valve replacement or homograft root-and-valve replacement has been successfully performed in acute or chronic severe valve regurgitation.

3. Rheumatoid Myocarditis
▶ General Considerations

Rheumatoid myocarditis is observed in as much as 30% of patients in postmortem series but is rare in clinical and echocardiographic reports. Rheumatoid myocarditis is more common in patients with active and extra-articular disease, highly positive rheumatoid factor, and in those with systemic vasculitis. Rheumatoid myocarditis may result from autoimmunity, vasculitis, or granulomata deposition; rarely, it is

due to amyloid infiltration. Recently, a dilated or restrictive cardiomyopathy due to chloroquine therapy and characterized by myocyte enlargement due to perinuclear vacuolization and abundant myelinoid figures within myocytes has been reported. Unless granulomata are present, rheumatoid myocarditis is difficult to differentiate on histopathology from other types of myocarditis.

▶ Clinical Findings

The clinical presentation of rheumatoid myocarditis is similar to that for myocarditis from other causes. Most commonly it is mild, asymptomatic, and clinically unrecognized. When it is symptomatic, nonspecific symptoms of fatigue, dyspnea, palpitations, and chest pain may be present. The chest pain is usually pleuritic and probably reflects the presence of myopericarditis. Rarely, severe acute myocarditis with LV dysfunction may present as congestive heart failure or symptomatic atrial or ventricular arrhythmias.

A. Physical Examination

Fever and sinus tachycardia are common. First and second heart sounds are normal; a third or fourth heart sound may rarely be present. Functional systolic murmurs are common. If myopericarditis is present, a pericardial rub may be detected.

B. Laboratory Findings

Myocarditis has been associated with the presence of anti-SS-A/anti-SS-B autoantibodies. In some cases, elevation of myocardial isoenzymes, such as troponin I and CPK-MB may be seen.

C. Diagnostic Studies

1. Electrocardiography—An ECG generally shows nonspecific ST segment and T wave abnormalities. Atrioventricular conduction disturbances and atrial or ventricular ectopy can be detected. As a result of residual interstitial myocardial fibrosis, patients have higher dispersion of repolarization as manifested by prolongation of the uncorrected and corrected QT intervals.

2. Echocardiography—Recent series using pulse and tissue Doppler, transmitral color flow propagation velocity, and myocardial performance index in young asymptomatic and nonhypertensive patients have demonstrated a high prevalence of diastolic dysfunction, predominantly of impaired relaxation. Also, longitudinal series have demonstrated a high incidence (40%) of clinical diastolic heart failure independent of traditional cardiovascular risk factors for diastolic dysfunction. Less commonly, echocardiography may show segmental wall motion abnormalities or diffuse LV contractile dysfunction and chamber dilatation in cases of severe myocarditis. The echocardiographic features of amyloidosis due to rheumatoid arthritis are nonspecific but may coexist or mimic rheumatoid constrictive pericarditis.

3. Radionuclide scanning—Scanning with indium-111, gallium-67, or technetium-99 may show focal patchy or diffuse myocardial uptake indicative of myocardial inflammation, necrosis, or both.

Treatment & Prognosis

Few data are available about the treatment of rheumatoid myocarditis. Few patients have shown benefit with high oral or intravenous doses of corticosteroids in severe cases. Also, the incidence of heart failure decreases with tumor necrosis factor-α blocker therapy. The value of cytotoxics is undefined. Nonspecific therapy includes bed rest, analgesics, and cardiac monitoring for at least 48–72 hours. The natural history and prognosis of rheumatoid myocarditis are unknown.

4. Rheumatoid Coronary Artery Disease

General Considerations

After controlling for traditional atherogenic risk factors, patients with rheumatoid arthritis have two to three times more common epicardial and small vessel CAD than matched controls. Except for aPL, the pathogenetic factors for these two types of CAD in rheumatoid patients is similar to those described for patients with SLE. Obstructive epicardial CAD is probably as common as abnormal coronary artery vasodilation or microvascular disease. Patients older than 50 years are more prone to epicardial atherosclerotic CAD. About 66% of asymptomatic patients with established rheumatoid arthritis have coronary artery calcification on electron-beam CT, compared with 40% in those with recent onset of the disease. Patients with parameters of active and chronic inflammation have reduced small and large arteries elasticity and have a twofold independent risk of MI, heart failure, stroke, and cardiovascular mortality compared with matched controls. Also, rheumatoid patients with acute coronary syndromes have two times higher recurrence rate of events and mortality than matched controls. Coronary arteritis is rare and occur in patients with rheumatoid nodules, overt vasculitis, rapidly progressive rheumatoid disease, and high titers of rheumatoid factor.

Clinical Findings

A. Symptoms and Signs

Most patients with rheumatoid arthritis who have CAD are asymptomatic. Atherosclerotic CAD will manifest as chronic stable angina, unstable angina, or acute MI, whereas coronary arteritis is more commonly seen as unstable angina or acute MI.

Tachycardia, third or fourth heart sounds, and pulmonary rales, if LV failure is present, are seen during acute ischemic syndromes.

B. Diagnostic Studies

1. Electrocardiography—An ECG will show diagnostic Q waves indicative of previous MI, ST elevation or depression suggestive of epicardial or subendocardial ischemic injury, or T wave inversion suggestive of ischemia.

2. Echocardiography—Resting and stress echocardiography are useful in the detection of wall motion abnormalities in those with obstructive CAD, but have decreased sensitivity for microvascular disease. Transthoracic echocardiography has also been used to assess coronary flow reserve in those with microvascular disease. During severe ischemia, echocardiography may show segmental wall motion abnormalities or myocardial scars if previous infarction has occurred. This technique will also determine the presence (or absence) of LV dysfunction and its severity.

3. Other tests—Patients with high ESR (≥ 60 mm/h), C-reactive protein, serum amyloid, soluble vascular adhesion molecule-1, and interferon-γ have abnormal small and large arteries vasodilatory response and are at increased risk for cardiovascular events and mortality. Electron-beam CT detects subclinical coronary artery calcification in patients with established disease.

Myocardial isoenzymes, such as troponin I, CPK-MB or LDH_1, may be elevated if myocardial necrosis has occurred. Exercise treadmill testing, with or without radionuclide scanning or echocardiography, can be used to detect suspected CAD. Coronary angiography should be considered when there is a high suspicion of CAD, an abnormal exercise treadmill test, or incapacitating symptoms. The diagnosis of coronary arteritis can be suspected if multiple stenotic lesions and aneurysmal lesions are found in the epicardial coronary arteries.

Treatment

Although experience in this area is limited, suspected severe and symptomatic coronary arteritis can initially be treated with high doses of corticosteroids and intravenous cyclophosphamide or oral mycophenylate in conjunction with heparin, aspirin, nitrates, and calcium channel or β-blockers. No data are available about PCIs in coronary arteritis. Symptomatic atherosclerotic CAD should be treated medically or with coronary revascularization as appropriate. Amelioration of inflammation with low-dose corticosteroids, tumor necrosis factor-α blockers, or statins may decrease the effects of vascular inflammation and dysfunction and consequently of coronary events. Furthermore, cyclooxygenase-2 selective inhibitors, which inhibit prostaglandin I-2 (a vasodilator and inhibitor of platelet aggregation) and NSAIDs increase the risk of acute coronary syndromes in rheumatoid patients.

5. Conduction Disturbances

General Considerations

The prevalence of AV or intraventricular conduction disturbances in patients with rheumatoid arthritis may not be different from that in age-matched controls in the general population. Possible mechanisms include acute inflammation of the

AV node or His bundle (related to pancarditis), vasculitis of the arterioles supplying the conduction pathway, granulomata deposition in the conduction system, and amyloid infiltration.

Clinical Findings

The mean age of patients with conduction disturbances is generally more than 60 years, and most of these patients have severe forms of rheumatoid arthritis with nodular disease, requiring corticosteroid therapy. The conduction disturbances are generally mild, asymptomatic, and incidentally diagnosed by ECG.

A. Symptoms and Signs

In extremely rare cases, high-degree AV block may be evidenced with tiredness, dizziness, presyncope, or syncope. Although it is uncommon, complete AV block may be asymptomatic because the joint disease severely limits the patient's activity. Rarely, AV block is transient and can be reversed with antiinflammatory therapy.

B. Diagnostic Studies

The best diagnostic methods are routine ECG, 24-hour or longer ECG monitoring, or both.

Treatment

The treatment of severe and symptomatic high-degree AV or intraventricular blocks associated with acute myocarditis or valvulitis consists of temporary pacing and high-dose corticosteroids. Patients who are unresponsive to this therapy should receive permanent pacemakers.

6. Rheumatoid Pulmonary Hypertension

General Considerations

The causes of pulmonary hypertension with normal pulmonary venous pressure include serum hyperviscosity, interstitial fibrosis, obliterative bronchiolitis, and pulmonary vasculitis. The prevalence of these diseases is uncertain, but low. Since the mortality rate is high within 1 year of diagnosis, prompt diagnosis is vital. Lung biopsy or bronchoalveolar lavage may confirm pulmonary vasculitis and bronchiolitis obliterans, both of which are responsive to immunosuppressive therapy.

Severe pulmonary hypertension may lead to RV hypertrophy, enlargement, and dysfunction (cor pulmonale) and produce the symptoms and signs of right-sided heart failure.

Clinical Findings

A. Symptoms and Signs

Dyspnea is a common manifestation of pulmonary hypertension and cor pulmonale. However, moderate pulmonary hypertension not associated with cor pulmonale can be asymptomatic.

Findings on physical examination include a parasternal heave, split second heart sound with loud pulmonic component, tricuspid regurgitation, right-sided S_3 gallop and, rarely, hepatomegaly and edema.

B. Diagnostic Studies

1. Electrocardiography—An ECG may show right atrial and ventricular enlargement and right bundle branch block.

2. Color-flow Doppler echocardiography—This technique may show right atrial and ventricular enlargement, hypertrophy or dysfunction, tricuspid regurgitation, and evidence of high pulmonary artery systolic pressure. Pulmonary hypertension may not be accompanied by echocardiographic evidence of cor pulmonale, especially if the pulmonary artery pressure is less than 50 mm Hg. In controlled series of asymptomatic patients, the prevalence of pulmonary hypertension on echocardiography is five times higher in rheumatoid patients than in controls (21% versus 4%). Echocardiography can rule out left-sided heart disease as a cause of pulmonary hypertension. Echocardiography can also assess response to therapy.

3. Open-lung biopsy and bronchoalveolar lavage—These methods should be done if severe pulmonary vasculitis or bronchiolitis obliterans is suspected as the cause of pulmonary hypertension.

Treatment & Prognosis

The treatment of pulmonary hypertension from pulmonary vasculitis is immunosuppressive agents or corticosteroids, but the prognosis is poor, and most patients die within 1 year of diagnosis.

Arslan S et al. Diastolic function abnormalities in active rheumatoid arthritis evaluation by conventional Doppler and tissue Doppler: relation with duration of disease. Clin Rheumatol. 2006 May;25(3):294–9. [PMID: 16222411]

Cauduro SA et al. Echocardiographically guided pericardiocentesis for treatment of clinically significant pericardial effusion in rheumatoid arthritis. J Rheumatol. 2006 Nov;33(11):2173–7. [PMID: 17086604]

Chung CP et al. Increased coronary-artery atherosclerosis in rheumatoid arthritis: relationship to disease duration and cardiovascular risk factors. Arthritis Rheum. 2005 Oct;52(10):3045–53. [PMID: 16200609]

Douglas KM et al. Excess recurrent cardiac events in rheumatoid arthritis patients with acute coronary syndrome. Ann Rheum Dis. 2006 Mar;65(3):348–53. [PMID: 16079169]

Gerli R et al. Cardiovascular involvement in rheumatoid arthritis. Lupus. 2005;14(9):679–82. [PMID: 16218466]

Nicola PJ et al. Contribution of congestive heart failure and ischemic heart disease to excess mortality in rheumatoid arthritis. Arthritis Rheum. 2006 Jan;54(1):60–7. [PMID: 16385496]

Roldan CA et al. Characterization of valvular heart disease in rheumatoid arthritis by transesophageal echocardiography and clinical correlates. Am J Cardiol. 2007 Aug 1;100(3):496–502. [PMID: 17659935]

Young A et al; Early Rheumatoid Arthritis Study (ERAS) group. Mortality in rheumatoid arthritis. Increased in the early course of disease, in ischaemic heart disease and in pulmonary fibrosis. Rheumatology (Oxford). 2007 Feb;46(2):350–7. [PMID: 16908509]

SCLERODERMA

ESSENTIALS OF DIAGNOSIS

▶ Sclerotic skin, esophageal dysfunction, Raynaud phenomenon.

▶ Functional or structural small vessel CAD.

▶ Multisegmental myocardial perfusion abnormalities.

▶ Diastolic heart failure.

▶ Pulmonary hypertension and cor pulmonale.

▶ General Considerations

Scleroderma, or systemic sclerosis, is a generalized disorder characterized by excessive accumulation of connective tissue; fibrosis; and degenerative changes of the skin, skeletal muscles, synovium, blood vessels, gastrointestinal tract, kidney, lung, and heart. Raynaud phenomenon, esophageal dysfunction, and sclerotic skin characterize the disease and are present in more than 90% of patients. The two major clinical variants are diffuse cutaneous (20% of cases) and limited cutaneous disease (80%). The less common diffuse type is characterized by skin thickening of the distal and proximal extremities and the trunk, with frequent involvement of the kidney, lung, or heart. In the more common limited type, which includes the CREST syndrome (calcinosis, Raynaud phenomenon, esophageal dysfunction, sclerodactyly, and telangiectasia), the skin changes are limited to the face, fingers, and distal portions of the extremities. A third, uncommon variant is the overlap syndrome that includes scleroderma in association with other connective tissue disease.

The incidence of scleroderma is 10–20 per million population per year. The disease affects all races, is three times more common in women than in men, and usually occurs between the ages of 30 and 50 years. The diffuse cutaneous type has a poorer prognosis than does the limited type. The overall cumulative survival rates after 3, 6, and 9 years are 86%, 76%, and 61%, respectively. The prognosis is worst for males who are older than 50 years with kidney, lung, or heart disease. Pulmonary disease, including pulmonary hypertension, and renal diseases are the major causes of death; these are followed by heart disease, with a cumulative survival of only 20% at 7 years. The major causes of cardiac death are structural and functional microvascular ischemic heart disease, followed by refractory heart failure, sudden death, and pericarditis. Scleroderma cardiac disease manifests predominantly as microvascular CAD, myocarditis, and pulmonary

hypertension with or without cor pulmonale. Pericarditis, conduction disturbances, and arrhythmias are less common. Clinically overt scleroderma heart disease is reported in less than one-fourth of patients; the rate rises to as high as 80% in autopsy series. Scleroderma heart disease is generally less common and less severe in the limited type than in the diffuse type.

1. Coronary Artery Disease
▶ Pathophysiology

In scleroderma, the intramyocardial coronary arteries and arterioles are affected by abnormally increased small vessel vasoconstriction due to an immune-mediated endothelial cell injury and increased production of platelet-derived growth factor impairing the endothelial response to vasodilation. The intramyocardial coronary arteries and arterioles are also affected by mast cell degranulation of histamine, prostaglandin D_2, and leukotrienes C_4 and D_4, leading to coronary vasoconstriction. Also, obstructive microvascular disease occurs due to immune-complex mediated intimal inflammation, fibrinoid necrosis, stimulation of fibroblasts, collagen deposition, and ultimately vessel thrombosis. In contrast, the prevalence of epicardial atherosclerotic disease in patients with scleroderma is probably similar to that of a general population. The common finding on autopsy of myocardial contraction-band necrosis (necrotic myocardial cells with dense eosinophilic bands) is likely related to intermittent intramyocardial coronary spasm or intramyocardial Raynaud phenomenon. Furthermore, almost all patients with evidence of intramyocardial CAD have peripheral Raynaud phenomenon.

▶ Clinical Findings
A. Symptoms and Signs

Chest pain is uncommon; when present, it is related more commonly to pericarditis or esophageal reflux than to myocardial ischemia. Most patients, even with resting or stress-induced myocardial perfusion imaging defects or wall motion abnormalities, are asymptomatic. Although intramyocardial coronary vasospasm is the rule, severe vasospasm of the epicardial coronary arteries leading to transmural MI has rarely been reported.

B. Diagnostic Studies

1. Electrocardiographic exercise testing—This method has limited sensitivity because the prevalence of epicardial CAD in patients with scleroderma is low.

2. Radionuclide studies—Resting or exercise-induced multisegmental perfusion abnormalities are common; they are frequently reversed or improved with nifedipine or dipyridamole, which suggests recurrent vasospastic episodes leading to myocardial ischemia or fibrosis. Cold-induced reversible or partially reversible myocardial perfusion defects, further support coronary vasospasm. On myocardial perfusion, most patients show fixed defects and some show reversible defects or both fixed and reversible defects (Figure 33–4). Most patients have normal LV function at rest despite the high frequency of perfusion defects, but almost half have an abnormal LV response (a failure to increase the ejection fraction more than 5% from baseline) during exercise radionuclide ventriculography.

3. Echocardiography—Due to the predominant involvement of the intramyocardial coronary arteries, echocardiographic findings typical of transmural MI are uncommon. Using contrast-enhanced pulse wave Doppler TTE in a series of 27 patients without clinical evidence of ischemic heart disease, reduction in coronary flow reserve (≤ 2.5) in the left anterior descending coronary artery during adenosine infusion was detected in 52% of patients, compared with 4% of matched controls. Reduction in coronary flow reserve is more common in the diffuse form of scleroderma and is related to the duration and severity of the disease. As a result of functional and later on of obliterative microvascular disease, LV and RV diastolic and uncommonly systolic dysfunction can occur. Occasionally, a transmural MI due to epicardial coronary vasospasm can occur, and its echocardiographic diagnosis relies on the same findings as those of atherosclerotic disease. The cold pressor test with simultaneous echocardiography demonstrates transient wall motion abnormalities in patients with angiographically normal or mild epicardial CAD.

4. Coronary angiography—This diagnostic study usually shows normal epicardial coronary arteries, a slow dye flow indicative of increased intramyocardial coronary resistance, and impaired coronary sinus blood flow indicative of abnormal coronary flow reserve.

▶ Treatment

Nifedipine and nicardipine have demonstrated short-term improvement in the number and severity of perfusion defects, but their long-term benefit is unknown. Captopril has shown similar beneficial effects.

2. Myocarditis
▶ General Considerations

Two types of scleroderma myocardial disease are described. The most common is due to recurrent intramyocardial ischemia leading to fibrosis; the second and less common, an acute inflammatory myocarditis. Patients with scleroderma who have skeletal myopathy have twice the prevalence of myocardial disease, compared with those patients without peripheral myopathy. Myocardial disease is also more common and severe in patients with diffuse cutaneous disease, anti-Scl70 antibodies, and older than 60 years.

Clinically apparent myocarditis is rare, but postmortem series report a high prevalence. Focal or diffuse myocardial fibrosis and contraction-band necrosis are common. Contraction-band necrosis typical of transient coronary occlusion and reperfusion is common but not pathognomonic.

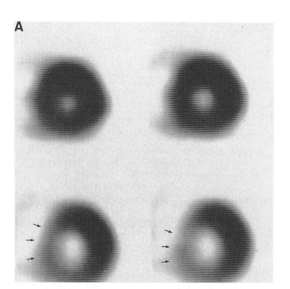
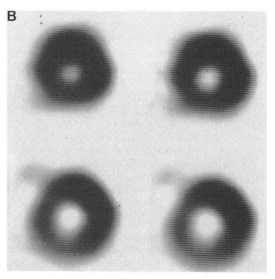

▲ **Figure 33–4.** Intramural coronary artery disease in a patient with scleroderma. **A:** This short-axis postexercise perfusion scan of the left ventricle shows septal and inferoseptal wall ischemia (*small arrows*) that resolve on the resting images. **B:** This patient had normal epicardial coronary arteries.

These pathologic findings differ from atherosclerotic myocardial disease by their lack of relation to coronary arteries and frequent involvement of the RV and subendocardium.

Clinical Findings

A. Symptoms and Signs

Focal or diffuse myocardial fibrotic disease may result in significant LV diastolic or systolic dysfunction, arrhythmias, and conduction disturbances. Patients with skeletal myopathy and those with myocarditis more commonly have clinical heart failure. Insidious symptoms are most common and the physical findings of heart failure are similar to those of other conditions. Acute symptoms of heart failure and sudden death rarely occur.

B. Diagnostic Studies

If clinical or laboratory evidence of myositis is present, diagnostic screening for asymptomatic cardiac involvement is warranted.

1. Electrocardiography—A septal infarction pattern is seen in some patients, correlating with septal or anteroseptal thallium perfusion abnormalities, despite the presence of normal epicardial coronary arteries. This may represent septal fibrosis.

2. Echocardiography—Left ventricular systolic dysfunction is uncommon in asymptomatic patients, but when associated with heart failure portends an 80% mortality rate at 1 year. In contrast, a high prevalence (30–50%) of LV diastolic dysfunction is seen in patients with either diffuse or limited cutaneous disease, compared with < 10% in controls. Similarly, a high prevalence (40%) of RV diastolic dysfunction independently of pulmonary hypertension has been reported. Left ventricular diastolic dysfunction correlates with high levels of soluble vascular cell adhesion molecules-1 and ESR as well as the duration and severity of Raynaud phenomenon. Also, RV dysfunction in patients with normal pulmonary artery pressure improves with nicardipine therapy. These data support functional microvascular CAD as the cause of diastolic dysfunction. However, a decreased and heterogeneous integrated backscatter in the subendocardium by ultrasonic videodensitometry in young, nonhypertensive patients supports interstitial collagen deposition and fibrosis as another cause of myocardial dysfunction.

3. Radionuclide studies—Radionuclide angiography demonstrates abnormal resting ejection fraction in 15% of patients. Myocardial perfusion scanning is a sensitive method for diagnosis and follow-up of the myocardial disease and for assessing therapeutic responses.

4. Endomyocardial biopsy—This technique has been used occasionally to diagnose scleroderma myocardial disease; however, the heterogenous and nonspecific pattern of involvement limit the sensitivity and specificity of this technique.

Treatment

Calcium channel blockers may abolish or decrease the frequency and severity of episodes of ischemia and thereby of myocardial fibrosis, but this hypothesis has not been longitudinally tested. The use of intravenous methylprednisolone in acute inflammatory myocarditis is controversial. Otherwise, symptomatic LV systolic or diastolic dysfunction is treated with current standard therapy.

Prognosis

The presence of an S_3 gallop is indicative of LV systolic dysfunction and increases the risk of death by more than 500%. Patients with heart failure have a 100% mortality rate at 7 years, with the highest number (80%) occurring during the first year after diagnosis.

3. Conduction Disturbances & Arrhythmias

General Considerations

Conduction defects occur in up to 20% of patients with scleroderma; the highest prevalence is seen in those patients with demonstrated myocarditis or myocardial perfusion defects. Fibrous replacement of the sinoatrial and AV nodes, bundle branches, and surrounding myocardium is seen on postmortem series of patients with conduction disturbances.

Clinical Findings

A. Symptoms and Signs

Arrhythmias are common and frequently associated with active myocarditis. Atrial or ventricular premature contractions, supraventricular tachycardias, and nonsustained ventricular tachycardia are also common. Ventricular and supraventricular arrhythmias are more common in patients with diffuse cutaneous disease than in those with the limited type. Palpitations occur in 50% of patients. Syncope (Stokes-Adams attacks) can occur and are related to either high-degree AV block or ventricular arrhythmias; it may occasionally be the primary manifestation of scleroderma. Syncope can also occur in patients with severe pulmonary hypertension. Forty percent to 60% of cardiac deaths in patients with scleroderma who have active myocarditis may be sudden and related to ventricular arrhythmias.

B. Diagnostic Studies

1. Electrocardiography—Most patients have a normal ECG, which is highly predictive of normal LV function. The presence of left or right bundle branch block or bifascicular block generally correlates with resting or exercise-induced LV systolic dysfunction. Also, LV potentials on signal-averaged ECG, complex atrial and ventricular arrhythmias, or conduction abnormalities on ECG are common and correlate with LV dysfunction or myocardial perfusion defects.

2. Electrophysiologic studies—These studies show a high prevalence of abnormal sinoatrial and AV nodes and His-Purkinje function and conduction. However, electrophysiologic studies are recommended only for patients with syncope of undefined origin, for those with sustained ventricular tachycardia, or for survivors of sudden cardiac death.

Treatment

A pacemaker is indicated for symptomatic high-grade conduction disturbances, and antiarrhythmic or implantable cardioverter-defibrillator therapy is appropriate for symptomatic arrhythmias.

Prognosis

The presence on ambulatory ECG of frequent ventricular and supraventricular arrhythmias predicts a mortality risk two to six times higher than that of patients without arrhythmias. Because these arrhythmias are strong independent predictors of sudden cardiac death, 24-hour ambulatory ECG monitoring should be considered in patients with scleroderma to identify patients at high risk for sudden cardiac death. Cardiac conduction defects on the resting ECG also indicate a poor prognosis with a mortality rate of 50% by 6 years following diagnosis.

4. Pericarditis
General Considerations

The pathogenesis of scleroderma pericardial disease is unknown and is usually clinically silent. A low clinical prevalence of pericardial disease contrast with that of postmortem and echocardiographic series (~50%). Fibrinous pericarditis, chronic fibrous pericarditis, pericardial adhesions, and pericardial effusion are the pathologic types described.

Clinical Findings
A. Symptoms and Signs

Pericardial disease is rarely the initial manifestation of scleroderma. Symptomatic pericardial disease occurs in less than 20% of patients. The most common clinical presentation is a chronic pericardial effusion with dyspnea, orthopnea, and edema; it is less frequently seen as an acute pericarditis with fever, pleuritic chest pain, dyspnea, and pericardial rub. Cardiac tamponade or pericardial constriction is rare. Symptomatic pericardial disease is two to four times more common in patients with the diffuse form of scleroderma than in those with the limited cutaneous form of the disease.

B. Diagnostic Studies

1. Echocardiography—Echocardiography commonly shows asymptomatic small pericardial effusions and uncommonly pericardial thickening. It can also confirm clinically suspected cardiac tamponade.

2. Computed tomography and magnetic resonance imaging—These imaging studies are important diagnostic adjuncts to echocardiography. They aid in the assessment of pericardial thickening or calcification in patients with suspected chronic constriction (Figure 33–5).

3. Other tests—Pericardial fluid aspirates are usually exudative without autoantibodies, immune complexes, or complement depletion. Antiphospholipid antibodies may be associated with pericardial disease.

Treatment

Symptomatic pericarditis or significant pericardial effusions can be treated with NSAIDs. If tamponade is suspected, pericardiocentesis is usually successful. Corticosteroids alone are not effective in patients with large, chronic pericardial effusions.

Prognosis

Patients with pericarditis and moderate pericardial effusion have a cumulative survival of only 25% after 6–7 years, with the highest mortality rates the first year after diagnosis. This high mortality rate is believed to be related to complicating or accompanying progressive renal failure in patients with chronic pericardial effusions and to sudden death in those with associated acute myopericarditis or myocarditis.

5. Valvular Heart Disease

The true prevalence of valvular heart disease in patients with scleroderma is unknown, but it is rarely recognized clinically. Postmortem series report a prevalence of up to 18%. Systemic embolism in association with echocardiographically defined noninfective mitral valve vegetations, similar to those of SLE, has been described. One echocardiographic series reported a 67% frequency of mitral regurgitation in scleroderma patients, compared with only 15% in controls. Nonspecific thickening of the mitral or aortic valves without significant regurgitation also can be seen. In addition, a disproportionately high clinical and echocardiographic prevalence of mitral valve prolapse has been described in patients with either diffuse or limited scleroderma.

6. Secondary Scleroderma Heart Disease

Secondary causes of scleroderma heart disease are related to pulmonary and systemic hypertension. Pulmonary fibrosis can occur in up to 80% and pulmonary hypertension with cor pulmonale in up to 40–50% of patients. Pulmonary hypertension secondary to inflammatory vasculopathy or pulmonary vasospasm is less common and more commonly associated with the limited cutaneous type and overlap syndrome. Abnormal pulmonary function tests, abnormal lung uptake of gallium and technetium-99m sestamibi, and radiographic abnormalities often precede cor pulmonale on echocardiography. In patients with pulmonary hypertension, a higher

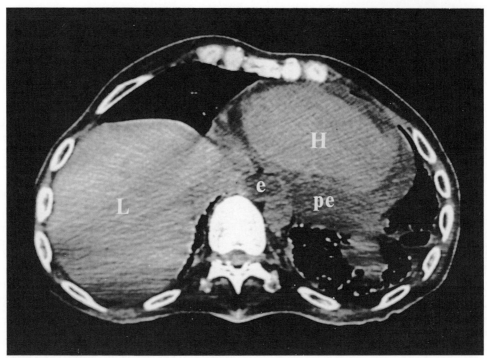

▲ **Figure 33–5.** This CT scan of the chest shows a large pericardial effusion (pe) predominantly posteriorly located in a patient with scleroderma and pericarditis. No pericardial thickening or calcification was detected. Esophageal (e) dilatation is noted. H, heart; L, liver.

prevalence and severity of RV diastolic dysfunction independently of age and LV mass has been reported. An RV tissue Doppler E velocity of < 0.11 m/sec select patients with pulmonary artery pressure > 35 mm Hg. Patients with pulmonary hypertension have a decreased survival of 81%, 63%, and 56% at 1, 2, and 3 years, respectively, from the diagnosis.

Oxygen, calcium channel blockers, and angiotensin-converting enzyme inhibitors have provided long-term benefits. Selected patients with severe scleroderma–related lung disease can undergo lung transplantation with similar morbidity and mortality to that of patients without scleroderma.

Hypertension and hypertensive heart disease are generally related to renovascular disease. The prognosis is related to the severity of the heart disease.

Ferri C et al. Heart involvement in systemic sclerosis. Lupus. 2005;14(9):702–7. [PMID: 16218471]

Maione S et al. Echocardiographic alterations in systemic sclerosis: a longitudinal study. Semin Arthritis Rheum. 2005;34(5):721–7. [PMID: 15846587]

Meune C et al. Myocardial contractility is early affected in systemic sclerosis: a tissue Doppler echocardiography study. Eur J Echocardiogr. 2005 Oct;6(5):351–7. [PMID: 16153555]

Tarek el-G et al. Coronary angiographic findings in asymptomatic systemic sclerosis. Clin Rheumatol. 2006 Jul;25(4):487–90. [PMID: 16440131]

Vacca A et al. Absence of epicardial coronary stenosis in patients with systemic sclerosis with severe impairment of coronary flow reserve. Ann Rheum Dis. 2006 Feb;65(2):274–5. [PMID: 16410537]

ANKYLOSING SPONDYLITIS

 ESSENTIALS OF DIAGNOSIS

▶ Characteristic lumbar spine and sacroiliac arthritis.

▶ Positive HLA-B27 assay.

▶ Aortic root sclerosis and dilation, leaflet thickening, and subaortic bump on echocardiography.

▶ Aortic regurgitation.

▶ General Considerations

Ankylosing spondylitis, also known as Marie-Strümpell, or Bekhterev disease, is an inflammatory disorder that affects predominantly the vertebral and sacroiliac joints. It manifests itself as chronic low back pain and limitation of back motion and chest expansion. Less frequently, it affects the peripheral joints and extra-articular organs such as the heart. The disease is estimated to affect 1 in 2000 of the general population, predominantly white men less than 40 years old; the male-to-female ratio is 3–12:1. More than 90% of patients are positive for the histocompatibility antigen HLA-B27. Although the manifestations of the cardiovascular disease generally follow the arthritic syndrome by 10–20 years, they sometimes precede it. The most important cardiovascular manifestations of the disease are aortitis, with or without aortic regurgitation; conduction disturbances; mitral regurgitation; myocardial dysfunction; and pericardial disease. The clinical prevalence of cardiovascular disease in ankylosing spondylitis varies widely. The rates are higher in patients with more than 20 years of disease duration, in those who are older than age 50, and in those with peripheral articular involvement.

1. Aortitis & Aortic Regurgitation

▶ **General Considerations**

The pathogenesis of aortitis is still undefined. Increased platelet-aggregating activity and platelet-derived growth factor are believed to be pathogenetic factors in the characteristic proliferative endarteritis of aortic root disease. The inflammatory process also is mediated by plasma cells and lymphocytes. It occurs in the intima, media, and adventitia of the proximal aortic wall and sinus of Valsalva and results in a marked fibroblastic reparative response, fibrous thickening, and calcification, especially of the adventitia and intima. This process extends proximally to the aortic annulus, valve cusps, and adjacent commissures. The consequent dilatation and thickening of the aortic root and annulus and the thickening or retraction of the aortic valve cusps cause aortic regurgitation generally of mild to moderate degree. Severe aortic regurgitation is rare. The mitral valve is frequently involved by downward extension of the aortic root fibrosis into the intervalvular fibrosa and base of the anterior mitral leaflet. This often results in localized fibrotic thickening at the base of the anterior mitral leaflet forming the characteristic "subaortic bump."

▶ **Clinical Findings**

The most common and characteristic manifestation of ankylosing spondylitis–associated heart disease is proximal aortitis, with or without aortic regurgitation. Associated mitral valve disease is also common. Aortitis and aortic regurgitation are generally mild to moderate, clinically silent, and chronic. In rare cases, severe aortic regurgitation from severe acute or chronic aortitis or valvulitis or complicating infective endocarditis occurs. Clinically silent aortic root or valve disease, with or without aortic regurgitation, can be present in one-third of patients before the joint disease manifests itself. Although it happens rarely, severe aortic regurgitation may present with mild or no articular disease.

A. Physical Examination

The most common and salient clinical findings in patients with ankylosing spondylitis will be those of the articular disease because cardiac disease when present is generally mild to moderate and asymptomatic.

B. Diagnostic Studies

1. Chest radiography—The appearance of the cardiac silhouette and great vessels is usually normal. If severe aortic root disease or aortic regurgitation is present, the ascending aorta may appear dilatated or elongated, and LV and atrial enlargement may be noted.

2. Color-flow Doppler echocardiography—By TEE, aortic root thickening, increased stiffness, and dilatation is seen in 60%, 60%, and 25% of patients, respectively. Aortic valve thickening detected in 40% of patients is manifested mainly as nodularities of the aortic cusps. Mitral valve thickening seen in 30% of patients manifests predominantly as basal thickening of the anterior mitral leaflet, forming the characteristic "subaortic bump" (Figure 33–6). Valve regurgitation seen in almost 50% of patients is moderate in one-third of them. Aortic root disease and valve disease is related to the duration of ankylosing spondylitis but not to its activity, severity or therapy. Associated LV enlargement, hypertrophy, and systolic or diastolic function can also be assessed.

3. Radionuclide ventriculography—This method can assess LV systolic or diastolic function and LV enlargement.

▶ **Treatment**

A. Medical Therapy

1. Specific antiinflammatory therapy—No data are available regarding the role of corticosteroids in the aortic root and valve disease associated with ankylosing spondylitis.

2. Other therapy—Vasodilators can be used in patients with significant aortic regurgitation.

B. Surgical Therapy

Aortic valve replacement has been successfully performed in patients with severe and symptomatic aortic regurgitation.

2. Conduction Disturbances

Conduction disturbances are the second most common associated heart disease, although their pathogenesis is unknown. Although the prevalence of HLA-B27 is increased in patients with ankylosing spondylitis who have implanted pacemakers for heart block, it may be absent in these patients. Furthermore, because HLA-B27 may be present in 6% of normal patients, it cannot be implicated as a primary pathogenetic factor in ankylosing spondylitis–associated conduction disturbances. Conduction disturbances can be

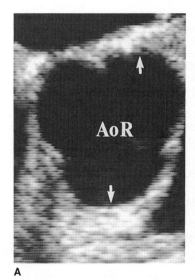

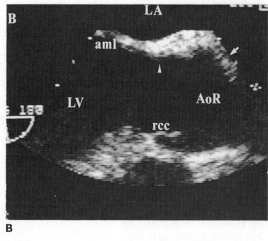

▲ **Figure 33–6.** Aortic root and valve disease in a patient with ankylosing spondylitis. **A:** This transesophageal basilar short-axis view shows marked aortic root thickening, predominantly of the posterolateral and anteromedial walls (*arrows*). Mild aortic root dilation is present. **B:** Transesophageal basilar longitudinal close-up view of the aortic root also shows the marked thickening of the posterior wall (*arrow*) extending to the basilar portion of the anterior mitral leaflet (subaortic bump; *arrowhead*). Mild localized thickening of the right coronary cusp tip is noted. Moderately severe aortic regurgitation was detected on color-flow mapping. The distance between the dots at the edge of the image is 1 cm. aml, anterior mitral leaflet; AoR, aortic root; LA, left atrium; LV, left ventricle; rcc, right coronary cusp.

the result of the subaortic fibrotic process extending to the basilar septum, leading to destruction or dysfunction of the AV node, the proximal portion of the bundle of His, bundle branches, and fascicles. In fact, echocardiographic studies have demonstrated an association of conduction disturbances with aortic root thickening and subaortic bump.

▶ **Clinical Findings**

The prevalence of conduction disturbances varies greatly, but is at least 20%. Atrioventricular blocks (first, second and, rarely, third degree) are most frequent, followed by sinus node dysfunction (sinus arrhythmias, sinoatrial block, sinus arrest, and sick sinus syndrome) and bundle branch or fascicular block.

Patients with conduction disturbances are generally asymptomatic and can be detected before clinically manifested in less than one-fifth of patients. The conduction disturbances can occasionally be transient, and symptomatic patients can be treated with temporary pacing. The prevalence of aortic root disease and valve regurgitation is high in the presence of conduction disturbances, in contrast to the small number of cases of aortic regurgitation in patients without conduction disturbances. Occasionally, severe conduction disturbances associated with symptoms requiring cardiac pacing may precede the diagnosis of ankylosing spondylitis. Therefore, unrecognized ankylosing spondylitis should be considered in patients with unexplained conduction disturbances or aortic regurgitation.

A. Physical Examination

Severe bradyarrhythmias will be clinically detected if patients are symptomatic; otherwise, conduction disturbances are generally incidentally detected with ECG.

B. Diagnostic Studies

Electrocardiography, including 24-hour ambulatory and event monitoring, can detect the described conduction disturbances.

▶ **Treatment**

A. Specific Antiinflammatory Therapy

Antiinflammatory therapy has not proved beneficial in patients with conduction disturbances.

B. Other Therapy

Permanent pacing has been successfully performed. The most common indications for pacing are complete heart block and sick sinus syndrome.

3. Mitral Valve Disease

The prevalence of mitral valve disease is about 30%, but it is generally not significant and therefore frequently unrecognized. Mitral valve disease is generally asymptomatic and frequently incidentally detected by echocardiography. The pathogenesis of mitral valve disease is related to the extension of the aortic root fibrosis into the subaortic basilar portion of the anterior mitral leaflet, producing the characteristic subaortic bump. Mitral regurgitation results from either the decreased anterior leaflet mobility caused by the basilar subaortic bump or, less frequently, from LV dilatation caused by aortic regurgitation. Only a few cases of mitral regurgitation severe enough to require valve replacement have been reported.

4. Myocardial Disease, Pericardial Disease, & Bacterial Endocarditis

Primary myocardial disease is rare. Although its pathogenesis is unknown, it is caused by a diffuse increase in the myocardial interstitial connective tissue and reticulum fibers. It may manifest as LV systolic dysfunction and dilatation in up to one-fifth of patients. Doppler echocardiography series in patients younger than 50 years old with no clinical heart disease have uncommonly reported LV systolic dysfunction. In contrast, about one-third of patients have diastolic dysfunction, predominantly impaired relaxation. Diastolic dysfunction is unrelated to age, disease duration, or disease activity. Rarely, cardiac amyloidosis with diastolic heart failure has been reported. Rarely, secondary myocardial dysfunction relates to chronic volume overload of aortic or mitral regurgitation. If significant LV systolic or diastolic dysfunction is present, third or fourth heart sounds and pulmonary rales may be present. Echocardiography is the best diagnostic method to show primary or secondary LV dysfunction. No specific therapy is available for primary myocardial disease.

Although the true prevalence of **pericardial disease** is unknown, it is rare in ankylosing spondylitis, and its pathogenesis is also undefined. It is generally asymptomatic and usually incidentally detected by echocardiography as pericardial thickening or small pericardial effusions. No specific therapy is available.

▶ Prognosis

The overall prognosis of patients with ankylosing spondylitis is good and almost comparable to that of a general population. In the past, the presence of severe cardiovascular disease significantly decreased the survival of these patients. Currently, improved diagnostic and therapeutic technologies have allowed early diagnosis, appropriate follow-up, and proper timing of valve replacement or pacemaker implantation in patients with cardiovascular disease. These factors have made the prognosis of ankylosing spondylitis with cardiovascular disease more benign.

Brunner F et al. Ankylosing spondylitis and heart abnormalities: do cardiac conduction disorders, valve regurgitation and diastolic dysfunction occur more often in male patients with diagnosed ankylosing spondylitis for over 15 years than in the normal population? Clin Rheumatol. 2006 Feb;25(1):24–9. [PMID: 16247583]

Divecha H et al. Cardiovascular risk parameters in men with ankylosing spondylitis in comparison with non-inflammatory control subjects: relevance of systemic inflammation. Clin Sci (Lond). 2005 Aug;109(2):171–6. [PMID: 15801904]

Han C et al. Cardiovascular disease and risk factors in patients with rheumatoid arthritis, psoriatic arthritis, and ankylosing spondylitis. J Rheumatol. 2006 Nov;33(11):2167–72. [PMID: 16981296]

POLYMYOSITIS/DERMATOMYOSITIS

 ESSENTIALS OF DIAGNOSIS

▶ Muscle weakness, characteristic skin lesions.

▶ Myocarditis and arrhythmias or conduction disturbances.

▶ Pericarditis, coronary arteritis, valve disease.

▶ General Considerations

Polymyositis or dermatomyositis is an acquired, chronic, inflammatory myopathy that presents clinically as symmetric proximal muscle weakness of the extremities, trunk, and neck. Dermatomyositis differs from polymyositis by the presence of a rash on the face, neck, chest and extremities, most commonly over the extensor surfaces, especially the dorsum of the hands and fingers. The incidence of polymyositis and dermatomyositis is estimated to be one to five new cases per million population per year in the United States. Overlap syndrome is the association of polymyositis/dermatomyositis with other connective tissue diseases, such as scleroderma, SLE, and rheumatoid arthritis. Rarely, polymyositis or dermatomyositis can be associated with the aPL syndrome. Adults in the fourth to sixth decades are most commonly affected. Both childhood polymyositis/dermatomyositis and that with malignancy are less common. Females, especially black females, are predominantly affected. A cumulative survival rate of 50–75% after 6–8 years has been reported. The major causes of death (in descending order) are malignancy, sepsis, and cardiovascular disease. Poor prognostic indicators of the disease include an age older than 45 years, cardiopulmonary disease, and cutaneous necrotic lesions.

▶ Clinical Findings

Polymyositis/dermatomyositis–associated heart disease is not uncommon and is manifested predominantly as myocarditis and arrhythmias or conduction disturbances. Dilated cardiomyopathy, pericarditis, coronary vasculitis, pulmonary hypertension with cor pulmonale, mitral valve prolapse, and hyperkinetic heart syndrome have also been reported. Clinically overt heart disease is less common than that found in postmortem series. Clinical heart disease is more common in polymyositis and overlap syndrome than in dermatomyositis or in malignant and childhood polymyositis/dermatomyositis. The presence of heart disease does not correlate with age, disease activity, severity, or duration and does not differ between men and women.

1. Myocarditis

Myocarditis is characterized at postmortem by diffuse interstitial and perivascular lymphocytic infiltration, contraction-band necrosis, and fibrosis. In one postmortem series, myocarditis was seen in half the patients, manifested equally as active myocarditis or focal myocardial fibrosis. Approximately 10–20% of them have dilated cardiomyopathy. Acute myocarditis as the principal manifestation of polymyositis has been reported in only two cases, one case mimicking acute MI, and the second case leading to fatal cardiac arrhythmias. A high correlation has been demonstrated between myocarditis and active myositis. About half of patients with peripheral myositis, as indicated by uptake of technetium-99m pyrophosphate, also have myocardial uptake. Increased myocardial uptake is also frequently associated with depressed ejection fraction and abnormal wall motion (shown by radionuclide ventriculography), which is further supportive of myocardial inflammation. Myocarditis may manifest itself clinically as congestive heart failure or as dilated cardiomyopathy.

2. Arrhythmias & Conduction Disturbances

Right bundle branch block, left anterior fascicular block, bifascicular block, nonspecific intraventricular conduction block, left bundle branch block, and AV block can occur. Occasionally, conduction disturbances can progress to more severe forms, despite remission of the disease, and permanent pacing has been required in a few cases.

The prevalence of arrhythmias varies. The most common arrhythmias are premature ventricular and atrial beats. Supraventricular tachyarrhythmias and ventricular tachycardia are rare. Sudden cardiac death may occur in a small number of patients. Active myocarditis or residual myocardial degeneration and fibrosis extending to the sinoatrial, AV nodal, and bundle branches explain the arrhythmias and conduction abnormalities.

3. Coronary Arteritis

The clinical prevalence is unknown. One postmortem series demonstrated the presence of coronary arteritis in 30% of patients, manifested as active vasculitis with intimal proliferation or as medial necrosis with calcification.

4. Valvular Heart Disease

Except for a higher prevalence of mitral valve prolapse, no other specific valve disease has been reported. The cause of mitral prolapse has not been determined.

5. Pericarditis

Acute uncomplicated pericarditis with small-to-moderate pericardial effusions has been described; acute pericarditis with cardiac tamponade and chronic constrictive pericarditis are rare. Pericarditis affects less than 20% of adults and slightly more than that in children. Echocardiography, however, shows a prevalence of pericardial effusion, usually small, in up to 25% in adults and up to 50% in children. One large series reported a higher prevalence of pericarditis in overlap syndrome than in isolated polymyositis or dermatomyositis. Only rarely does pericarditis form part of the initial clinical presentation of polymyositis/dermatomyositis.

6. Pulmonary Hypertension, Cor Pulmonale, & Hyperkinetic Heart Syndrome

Both pulmonary hypertension secondary to interstitial lung disease and primary pulmonary vasculopathy leading to cor pulmonale have been found. In hyperkinetic heart syndrome, abnormally increased LV performance has been demonstrated in up to one-third of patients with polymyositis. The cause of this asymptomatic abnormality is unknown.

▶ Treatment & Prognosis

The benefit of corticosteroid therapy in patients with conduction disturbances, myocarditis, or pericarditis is uncertain. Available data are limited about the natural history, effect of therapy, and prognosis in polymyositis/dermatomyositis–associated heart disease.

Finsterer J et al. Restrictive cardiomyopathy in dermatomyositis. Scand J Rheumatol. 2006 May–Jun;35(3):229–32. [PMID: 16766371]
Allanore Y et al. Effects of corticosteroids and immunosuppressors on idiopathic inflammatory myopathy related myocarditis evaluated by magnetic resonance imaging. Ann Rheum Dis. 2006 Feb;65(2):249–52. [PMID: 16410529]
Lundberg IE. Cardiac involvement in autoimmune myositis and mixed connective tissue disease. Lupus. 2005;14(9):708–12. [PMID: 16218472]

MIXED CONNECTIVE TISSUE DISEASE

ESSENTIALS OF DIAGNOSIS

▶ Raynaud phenomenon, sclerodactyly.

▶ Myopathy.

▶ Pericarditis, pulmonary hypertension.

▶ High ribonucleoprotein antibody titers.

General Considerations

Patients with mixed connective tissue disease are those with clinical findings of SLE, rheumatoid arthritis, scleroderma, and polymyositis. Characteristically, these patients have high titers of antibodies to nuclear ribonucleoprotein (RNP) and speckled antinuclear antibodies. Rheumatoid agglutinins also occur in more than half of patients. The disease occurs at all ages, affecting predominantly females (80%). Its prevalence is similar to that of scleroderma, more common than polymyositis, but less than SLE. This disease has no particular racial or ethnic predominance. Primary cardiac involvement in mixed connective tissue disease is infrequent and less common than in other connective tissue diseases.

Clinical Findings

A. Symptoms and Signs

Pericardial disease manifested as pericarditis, small pericardial effusions, or pericardial thickening is the most common. Pericarditis is more common in children, affecting almost half of patients. In rare cases, pericarditis is the initial presentation of the disease. Mitral valve prolapse has also been reported in this disease, with an unusually high prevalence (30%). Verrucous thickening of the mitral valve and regurgitation have been infrequently detected and are indistinguishable from those of SLE. Infrequently, supraventricular or ventricular arrhythmias and conduction disturbances have been reported. Functional or microvascular disease is the most common type of associated CAD. Acute coronary syndromes may also result from coronary vasospasm, in situ thrombosis, coronary embolism form a valve vegetation, and rarely arteritis. Myocarditis is characterized on histology by interstitial lymphocytic infiltrates and variable degrees of myocardial fibers necrosis and when acute can be reversible with corticosteroids and intravenous pulse cyclophosphamide. On echocardiography, the spectrum of the disease ranges from diastolic dysfunction to global or regional LV systolic dysfunction and heart failure. Acute myocarditis may mimic a myocardial infarction, can be complicated by congestive heart failure and death. Because of the high frequency of pulmonary disease (80%) in patients with mixed connective tissue disease, pulmonary hypertension associated with pulmonary fibrosis or proliferative pulmonary vasculopathy of the small and medium-sized pulmonary arteries can occur, especially in patients with features of scleroderma. Pulmonary thromboembolism is rare.

The clinical manifestations of primary cardiac disease, pulmonary hypertension, and cor pulmonale associated with mixed connective tissue disease do not differ from the other connective tissue diseases.

B. Diagnostic Studies

The methods used to diagnose cardiac disease associated with mixed connective tissue disease are the same used for other connective tissue diseases.

Treatment

Little data are available about the treatment of heart disease associated with mixed connective tissue disease. Pericarditis generally responds well to corticosteroids. Nifedipine has demonstrated both acute and sustained reduction in pulmonary vascular resistance in patients with pulmonary hypertension.

Prognosis

The overall mortality rate of patients with mixed connective tissue disease is 13% at 6–12 years. The prognostic implications of cardiac disease associated with mixed connective tissue disease are unknown.

Bezerra MC et al. Cardiac tamponade due to massive pericardial effusion in mixed connective tissue disease: reversal with steroid therapy. Lupus. 2004;13(8):618–20. [PMID: 15470773]

Jang JJ et al. A teenager with mixed connective tissue disease presenting with acute coronary syndrome. Vasc Med. 2004 Feb;9(1):31–4. [PMID: 15230486]

The Athlete's Heart

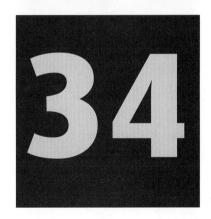

Cedela Abdulla, MD & J. V. (Ian) Nixon, MD, FACC, FAHA

ESSENTIALS OF DIAGNOSIS

► History of athletic training and performance.

► Enhanced exercise ability ($\dot{V}o_{2max}$ > 40 mL/kg/min).

► Resting bradycardia.

► Increased left ventricular mass by echocardiography.

► General Considerations

The concept of the athlete's heart is one that has been postulated for almost 100 years, promulgating the idea that myocardial hypertrophy could be a purely physiologic phenomenon. Media attention to the sudden deaths of widely known athletes has helped focus attention on the important distinction between pathologic cardiac hypertrophy and physiologic hypertrophy and the upper limits of the latter.

The adaptations of the human body to physical training involve (but are not confined to) the cardiovascular system. The exercise-related changes in other organ systems influence the cardiovascular response to exercise. It is important for the physician to be familiar with the physiologic responses to physical training in order to distinguish them from similar changes that can occur with cardiovascular disease.

Different forms of exercise produce a number of physiologic responses. Also, cardiovascular responses to short-term training and prolonged training differ. Exercise generally takes two basic physiologic forms—dynamic and static, or isometric, exercise—although most athletic activities are a variable combination of both forms of exercise. Dynamic exercise constitutes an alteration in the length of skeletal muscle with comparatively little change in muscle tension. Static exercise is essentially the reverse—that is, a marked alteration in skeletal muscle tension with little or no change in muscle length. Distance running is a classic example of dynamic exercise; weight lifting is a classic example of static exercise.

The morphologic and physiologic consequences of dynamic and isometric exercise are significant and may simulate changes associated with cardiac disease. The normal limits of changes that are due to athletic conditioning require careful identification. Awareness of these limits improves the physician's ability to determine the end points at which normal anatomy and physiology become clinical disease.

Maron BJ et al. The heart of trained athletes: cardiac remodeling and the risks of sports, including sudden death. Circulation. 2006 Oct 10;114(15):1633–44. [PMID: 17030703]

► Physiology of Exercise Training

The acute cardiovascular responses to exercise are specific and vary with different forms of exercise (Figure 34–1). There are also specific adaptive responses to exercise, particularly to dynamic exercise. In particular, the adaptive change in heart rate from an alteration in vagal parasympathetic tone defines the normal physiologic range; as noted earlier, this may be initially misinterpreted as representative of cardiovascular disease.

A. Acute Responses to Exercise

1. Dynamic exercise—Several acute cardiovascular responses to dynamic exercise are typical (Figure 34–1). As would be anticipated in meeting the demands of aerobic exercise, oxygen consumption increases because of an increase in both cardiac output and the arteriovenous oxygen difference. The increase in arteriovenous oxygen difference results from an increase in the oxygen extraction, or demand, by the exercising skeletal muscle and the increase in muscular capillary blood flow. Oxygen consumption is linearly related to the workload achieved during dynamic exercise. Maximal oxygen consumption ($\dot{V}o_{2max}$) is a highly reproducible measure of total aerobic capacity and thus dynamic exercise performance. Aerobic capacity varies with

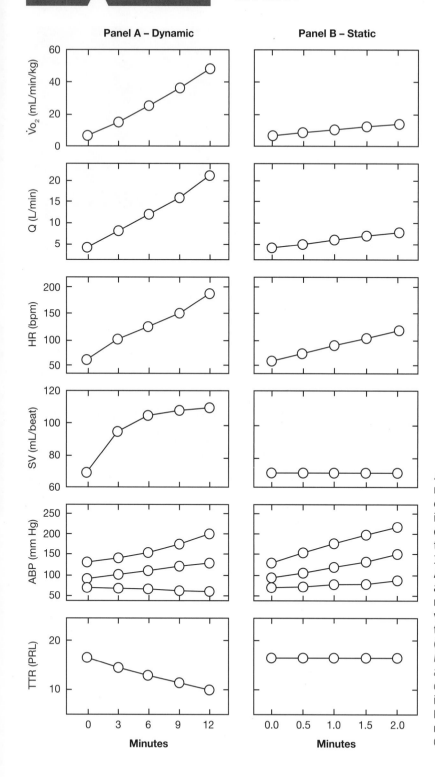

▲ **Figure 34–1.** Cardiovascular response to exercise. **A:** Response to dynamic exercise progressively increasing workload to maximal oxygen consumption. **B:** Response to static handgrip contraction at 30% maximal voluntary contraction. ABP, systolic, mean and diastolic arterial blood pressures; HR, heart rate; Q, cardiac output; SV, stroke volume; TPR, total peripheral resistance; $\dot{V}o_2$, oxygen consumption. (Reprinted with permission from Mitchell JH, Raven PB. Cardiovascular adaption to physical activity. In: Bouchard C et al, editors. Physical Activity, Fitness and Health: International Proceedings and Consensus statement. Human Kinetics Publishers: Champain IL; 1994.)

training, lean body mass, age, and gender and is significantly influenced by the individual's genetic characteristics. In children, gender differences are seen only after puberty, when the aerobic capacity of girls and young women tends to be approximately 30% less than that of boys and young men of the same age. Although incompletely explained, these differences are believed to be multifactorial; females, for example, have a lower lean body mass and a lower hemoglobin level. Maximal oxygen consumption diminishes with increasing age, as a result of such factors as the gradual detraining effect of age, an alteration in cardiac stiffness, and a reduction in β-adrenergic responsiveness that produces an attenuated heart rate response to exercise. Although it may be improved by dynamic training in older individuals, this improvement may well be due to an increased arteriovenous oxygen difference as much as to an increase in cardiac output and stroke volume. Furthermore, the improvement in $\dot{V}O_{2max}$ is relative when the overall decline in fitness is taken into account.

Oxygen consumption is also linearly related to cardiac output during dynamic exercise. The increase in cardiac output results principally from an increase in heart rate. Some increase in stroke volume takes place, resulting from the increase in venous return produced by the increasing skeletal muscle activity. The increase in left ventricular stroke volume during dynamic exercise is larger in an upright than in a supine position, but the absolute stroke volume at peak exercise is greatest in the supine position. Other hemodynamic responses contribute to the increased stroke volume. Intrathoracic pressure is reduced, left ventricular filling pressure rises, the mitral valve orifice enlarges, and the left ventricular end-diastolic volume increases. The net effect of these changes is activation of the Frank-Starling mechanism during the early initial and lower levels of dynamic exercise. Subsequently, at higher levels of exercise, sympathetic activation augments the Frank-Starling response in increasing stroke volume by increasing myocardial contractility and reducing end-systolic volume.

Resting heart rate is determined by vagal tone coupled with the level of sympathetic reflex activation. In the upright (versus supine) position, for example, resting heart rate is higher because of a mildly increased level of sympathetic activation. The initial increase in heart rate during exercise is due to a reduction in vagal tone, a central nervous system response mediated by stimulation of mechanoreceptors in the activated skeletal muscles. The heart rate increase is subsequently maintained by sympathetic activity and increased circulating catecholamines.

Systolic blood pressure increases during dynamic exercise, with a minimal increase in either diastolic or mean arterial pressure. The magnitude of the response is determined by the size of the activated muscle mass. Thus, the response during large muscle or leg exercise is greater than during small muscle or arm exercise. There is a greater increase in pulmonary arterial pressure than in systemic pressure during exercise because the change in vascular resistance is less in the pulmonary vasculature. This relative increase in pulmonary pressures is believed to augment pulmonary oxygen transport during exercise.

2. Static exercise—In static exercise, intramuscular pressure increases dramatically, with a resultant reduction or obliteration of exercising skeletal muscle blood flow (Figure 34–1). Static exercise is sustained by anaerobic mechanisms, and the consequent increases in oxygen consumption and cardiac output are much less than during dynamic exercise. Furthermore, oxygen consumption and cardiac output increase after static exercise, presumably because of an immediate increase in blood flow to the involved muscles to rectify the oxygen debt acquired by anaerobic mechanisms during the static exercise.

The increase in cardiac output during static exercise is due mainly to the increase in heart rate; stroke volume remains almost unchanged. Systolic blood pressure increases significantly during static exercise. Because stroke volumes and systemic vascular resistance change only minimally, this increased arterial pressure is due to the effects of increased muscle contraction on arterial pressure waves. Although arteriovenous oxygen difference remains unchanged during static exercise, an increase does take place immediately following release as a result of increased blood flow to the muscle bed.

B. Effects of Systematic Exercise Training

As previously stated, $\dot{V}O_{2max}$ is an accurate and reproducible measure of aerobic capacity and thus becomes an objective measure of dynamic fitness. In normal men, $\dot{V}O_{2max}$ ranges from 25 mL/kg/min to 40 mL/kg/min, with the lower values occurring in the older individuals. More than 50 mL/kg/min is considered representative of an elite level of fitness (the level may go as high as 80 mL/kg/min), reflecting an increase in maximal cardiac output and arteriovenous oxygen difference.

1. Dynamic exercise training—This type of training decreases resting heart rate because of an adaptive increase in vagal tone; it also decreases the heart rate response at any level of exercise. The heart rate response to maximal exercise, however, is identical in both the trained and untrained individual. Therefore, the increase in maximum cardiac output associated with dynamic training is due to increased stroke volume. It should also be noted that these physiologic adaptive changes to dynamic training occur in association with morphologic and physiologic changes in the heart.

2. Static exercise training—This type of training does not produce the same degree of $\dot{V}O_{2max}$ as does dynamic training. It is probable that the use of anaerobic rather than aerobic mechanisms to generate muscle energy requires a lower increase in cardiac output. Although morphologic changes do occur, the hemodynamic response to static exercise is similar in trained and untrained individuals.

3. Cross training—Dynamic training improves the response to static exercise in that the increased stroke volume at a lower heart rate allows the subject to sustain a greater cardiac pressure load and thus improve isometric performance. Static exercise training does not improve dynamic performance, however, except in areas or activities where greater strength or power is required (eg, pole vaulting).

4. Cardiovascular response—The frequency, intensity, and duration of exercise all affect the cardiovascular response. To obtain a significant training effect requires 30 minutes of dynamic exercise at 60–80% of maximal $\dot{V}O_2$ three times per week. Little effect is seen unless rates of more than 130 bpm are achieved for prolonged periods. Although lower levels and less frequent episodes of training may create a training effect, cessation of exercise produces a rapid detraining effect—which is complete within 3 weeks.

Measurement of the heart rate provides a good index of training. As discussed earlier, the alteration in resting heart rate is said to be due to an increase in vagal parasympathetic tone rather than a decrease in sympathetic tone or lower circulating catecholamine levels. In trained athletes, circulating levels of both epinephrine and norepinephrine are lower during dynamic and static exercise, with a lower heart rate response to the relative intensity of both forms of exercise.

Systematic training has some effects on other organ systems. Total blood and plasma volumes increase with dynamic training; these changes are thought to be related to increases in renin activity and serum albumin levels. Higher hemoglobin levels lead to an increase in both maximal oxygen consumption and endurance. Well-trained athletes use oxygen more efficiently, and the vascular conductance of skeletal muscle changes, resulting in a greater arteriovenous oxygen difference during dynamic exercise. Dynamic exercise training also increases high-density lipoprotein levels and decreases low-density lipoprotein and very-low-density lipoprotein levels, as well as body weight.

C. Morphologic Responses to Training

Physiologic hypertrophy is a prominent feature of the athlete's heart. The morphologic adaptations to the increased stroke volume induced by exercise conform to the principles of Laplace law, which relates the wall tension to intracavitary size and pressure. The increase in wall thickness in the setting of volume and pressure overload tends to normalize wall stress in both dynamic and isometric exercise (Figure 34–2).

The availability of two-dimensional and Doppler echocardiography and radionuclide ventriculography has allowed for the assessment of the mechanics of systolic and diastolic function in the trained athlete. The value of these technologies, although substantial, is limited by the inability to directly measure changes in intracardiac pressures, making absolute conclusions regarding detailed adaptive changes

more difficult. Nevertheless, when compared with matched controls (age, gender, and body surface area), any relative changes in parameters of systolic or diastolic function are valid. It is also evident that the functional changes are consequences of the adaptive morphologic changes of the dynamically and isometrically trained athlete. Noninvasive parameters of systolic function in trained athletes usually fall within accepted normal limits. The occasional abnormal findings may be satisfactorily explained as secondary to the adaptive morphologic changes associated with the different types of training. Similarly, noninvasive parameters of diastolic function usually fall within a normal range of values at rest, irrespective of the type of training.

Echocardiography allows cardiac anatomy to be detailed in a noninvasive serial manner; it is particularly useful in finding and documenting changes in cardiac morphology in athletes. Changes in cavity sizes, left ventricular wall thickness, and left ventricular mass have been documented in a number of studies of athletes undergoing both dynamic and static exercise training (Figure 34–2).

1. Left ventricular cavity—A consistent finding in dynamically trained athletes is an increased left ventricular end-diastolic dimension, which is present irrespective of body surface area, height, or gender. Compared with sedentary control subjects, the left ventricular end-diastolic dimension is increased by approximately 10% in the trained athlete, which represents an increase in end-diastolic volume of approximately 33%. Most dynamically trained athletes have an end-diastolic dimension of 60 mm or less. In contrast, left ventricular end-diastolic dimension is not altered with static exercise training, whether expressed in absolute values, or normalized by body surface area, weight, or lean body mass. This difference is believed to reflect the pressure, rather than volume load, on the left ventricle that is created by isometric training. The end-systolic dimension and volume remain within normal limits in the endurance athlete, producing the increase in stroke dimension and volume associated with dynamic exercise training.

2. Left ventricular wall thickness—Concomitant with the increase in left ventricular cavity size in the dynamically trained athlete, left ventricular posterior wall and interventricular septal thickness increase. The increase (compared with sedentary controls) in left ventricular posterior wall thickness is as high as 19%; in the same study, 98% had a left ventricular posterior wall thickness of 12 mm or less. Isometric exercise produces septal wall thicknesses of up to 16 mm. These increased values fall within an acceptable range when normalized for body surface area, weight, or lean body mass.

Although septal hypertrophy is a characteristic of hypertrophic cardiomyopathy, the increase in septal thickness in athletes is rarely above 16 mm and the septal-posterior wall thickness ratio does not increase above 1.2:1. Furthermore, there is no evidence in the literature that primary hypertrophic cardiomyopathy may develop with training.

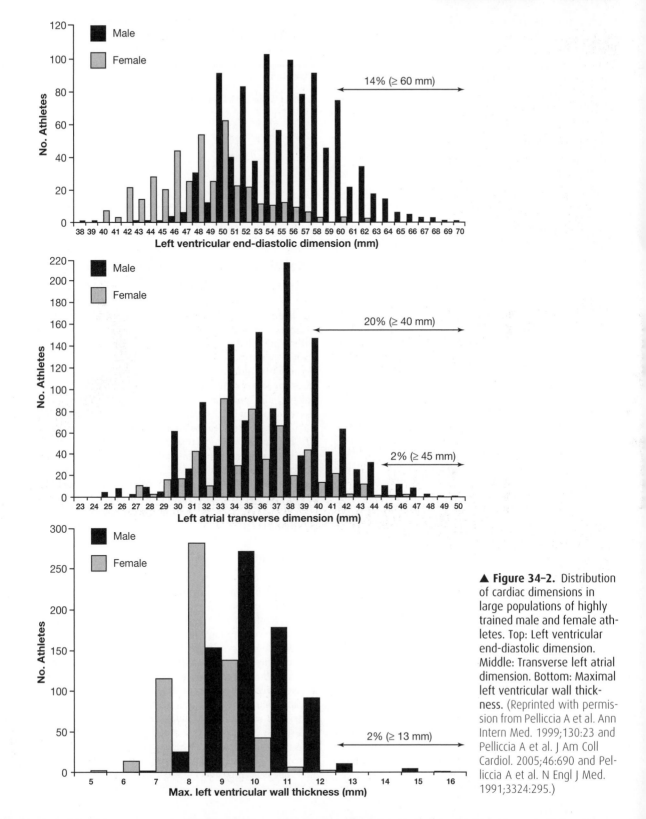

▲ **Figure 34–2.** Distribution of cardiac dimensions in large populations of highly trained male and female athletes. Top: Left ventricular end-diastolic dimension. Middle: Transverse left atrial dimension. Bottom: Maximal left ventricular wall thickness. (Reprinted with permission from Pelliccia A et al. Ann Intern Med. 1999;130:23 and Pelliccia A et al. J Am Coll Cardiol. 2005;46:690 and Pelliccia A et al. N Engl J Med. 1991;3324:295.)

3. Left ventricular mass—Estimates of left ventricular mass incorporate measurements of intraventricular septum and posterior wall thickness, both of which increase significantly in trained athletes. It is therefore reasonable to expect a significant increase in left ventricular mass in both dynamically and isometrically trained athletes. An increase of as much as 45% is found, even after normalization for body surface area.

4. Right ventricular cavity—Increases of up to 24% in right ventricular cavity dimensions may be seen in trained athletes.

5. Left atrial cavity—Increases in left atrial cavity size are also found in trained athletes and appear to be related to both the intensity and duration of the exercise.

D. Electrocardiography

Any type of athletic training in any form can alter the electrocardiogram (ECG) (Table 34–1). In a recent survey of 1005 trained athletes, 40% of ECGs were abnormal. It is important to know the effects of normal training on the ECG as well as the ECG abnormalities that warrant further investigation. Alterations on the ECG also depend on the nature, intensity, and level of training. The ECG reflects the morphologic adaptive changes of the heart—sinus bradycardia and voltage criteria for left ventricular hypertrophy (LVH)—that are due to the nature of the training. In the dynamically trained athlete in particular, the sinus bradycardia, which can be profound, reflects the adaptive increase in left ventricular cavity size that delivers large stroke volumes at rest and during exercise. Sinus bradycardia is usually due to high vagal tone, which may also be associated with sinus arrhythmia, sinoatrial block, multifocal atrial rhythms, junction rhythms, first-degree atrioventricular block, and Mobitz I second-degree atrioventricular block. All these abnormalities disappear during exercise. The P wave of the ECG may be notched and increased in amplitude. Interventricular conduction abnormalities are common in athletes. The ST segment may be elevated and the T wave increased in amplitude. Occasionally in trained athletes, the ST segment may be depressed and the T wave biphasic or inverted, all of which correct during exercise. These latter findings at rest are characteristic of ischemic heart disease, however, and their existence in the athlete warrants further investigation.

Distinguishing between physiologic and pathologic LVH by ECG may not be possible, particularly in a young athlete. The adaptive development of LVH and sinus bradycardia is characteristic of the trained athlete, as is the loss of these adaptive characteristics as a detraining effect. In the older athlete, where the prevalence of ischemic heart disease is much higher, voltage criteria for LVH, ST- and T-wave abnormalities, and repolarization abnormalities of the QRS complex are more common. The threshold for pursuing further investigation of abnormal ECG findings should be much lower in these older athletes.

Table 34–1. Effects of Dynamic and Isometric Exercise and Training on the Electrocardiogram.

Notched P waves
Voltage criteria for LVH
Interventricular conduction abnormalities
Symmetric peaked T waves
Sinus bradycardia
Sinus arrhythmia
Sinoatrial block
Multifocal atrial rhythm
Junctional rhythm
First-degree AV block
Mobitz I second-degree AV block

AV, atrioventricular; LVH, left ventricular hypertrophy.

E. Racial Differences in Response to Training

No detailed studies addressing the adaptive responses to training in the black athlete have yet been completed. Circumstantial evidence, however, would suggest that these responses may differ in black athletes. It is known that LVH is more prevalent in a black hypertensive population than in a white population, given similar levels of blood pressure elevation. Because a racial difference appears to exist in the blood pressure response to both dynamic and isometric exercise, the potential for an increased prevalence and greater degree of LVH appears to exist among black athletes. A study of black collegiate athletes showed that more than 30% had an interventricular septal thickness of more than 13 mm; a separate study of white athletes found only 3% with similar increases in thickness. These factors, coupled with the occurrence of sudden death in athletes—including black athletes—clearly indicate the need for studies of trained black athletes as well as comparative studies of black and white athletes.

F. Detraining

The adaptive responses to both dynamic and isometric exercise training persist only if the training continues with sufficient duration and intensity. Cessation of the training activity results in a temporal regression of these adaptive changes: the detraining effect. Although this effect is consistent despite age, gender, or the overall duration or type of training, the time course appears to be influenced by these factors. Following cessation of training, a regression of physiologic hypertrophy of up to 60% takes place within 7 days, so-called left ventricular remodeling. Both posterior left ventricular wall thickness and interventricular septal thickness regress equally, and the septal-posterior wall thickness ratio remains unchanged. The left ventricular end-diastolic dimension decreases within 7 days, with little change thereafter. The detraining effect is also associated with a reduction in $\dot{V}O_{2max}$. After 12 weeks of inactivity (cessation of training),

$\dot{V}O_{2max}$ decreases up to 16%, with half of this loss occurring in the first 3 weeks. Maximal cardiac output during exercise is also reduced by up to 8% in the first 3 weeks of detraining.

Germann CA et al. Sudden cardiac death in athletes: a guide for emergency physicians. Am J Emerg Med. 2005 Jul;23(4):504–9. [PMID: 16032621]

Pellicia A et al. Clinical significance of abnormal electrocardiographic patterns in trained athletes. Circulation. 2000 Jul 18;102(3):278–84. [PMID: 10899089]

Pelliccia A et al. Remodeling of left ventricular hypertrophy in elite athletes after long-term deconditioning. Circulation. 2002 Feb 26;105(8):944–9. [PMID: 11864923]

Sharma S et al. Physiologic limits of left ventricular hypertrophy in elite junior athletes: relevant to differential diagnosis of athlete's heart and hypertrophic cardiomyopathy. J Am Coll Cardiol. 2002 Oct 16;40(8):1431–6. [PMID: 12392833]

► Sudden Death in Athletes

The publicity attached to the sudden deaths of high-profile collegiate and professional athletes has raised the general awareness of sudden death in young athletes and led to a reappraisal of the validity and extent of a preparticipatory medical examination. It should be noted, however, that despite the publicity, the incidence of sudden death in athletes is very low, irrespective of age. In young athletes, it is rare. The incidence increases with age and an increased prevalence of coronary atherosclerosis; however, it remains very low. Little data exist on the incidence of sudden death in female athletes. Further studies have shown that while sports activities may be associated with sudden death, the individual sports were the trigger rather than the cause in athletes with cardiovascular disease.

The causes of sudden death in athletes appear to be related to age and the nature of the trained athlete population. Athletes younger than 35 years are likely to die of hypertrophic cardiomyopathy (about 50%) or coronary artery anomalies (Table 34–2). In hypertrophic cardiomyopathy, sudden deaths occur during exercise rather than at rest and are thought to be due to ventricular arrhythmias, particularly in individuals with ventricular arrhythmias documented prior to death. One study has shown exercise-induced ischemia as a prodromal feature of sudden death in hypertrophic cardiomyopathy, although a direct cause-and-effect relationship has not been established. It should be noted, however, that the prevalence of hypertrophic cardiomyopathy in young athletes is very low and has been shown not to warrant routine Doppler echocardiographic surveys. The prevalence increases in individuals with symptoms of exertional or postexertional syncope or arrhythmias, or with a family history of similar symptoms or sudden death. Furthermore, the magnitude of LVH appears to be directly related to the risk of sudden death. A variant of hypertrophic cardiomyopathy as a cause of sudden death is idiopathic LVH. These individuals have normal myocardial histology and LVH and thus have changes consistent with the training activity of the individual.

Table 34–2. Causes of Sudden Death in Athletes under 35 Years.

Hypertrophic cardiomyopathy
Aberrant coronary arteries
Premature atherosclerosis
Arrhythmogenic right ventricular dysplasia
Marfan syndrome
Idiopathic left ventricular hypertrophy
Mitral valve prolapse syndrome
Wolff-Parkinson-White syndrome
Prolonged QT syndrome
Myocarditis
Coronary artery vasospasm
Blunt chest trauma
Kawasaki disease
Heat stroke

Among athletes older than 35 years, the most common cause of sudden death is coronary atherosclerosis (Figure 34–3 and Table 34–3). Furthermore, older athletes tend to jog rather than engage in group sports activities. Risk factors for cardiovascular disease are usually present in those older than 35 years who have exercise-related sudden death; they also may show prodromal features of angina or unusual fatigue. Retrospective reviews of these individuals often show a history of hypertension, cigarette smoking, and hyperlipidemia, and a family history of ischemic heart disease.

The second most common cause of sudden death in athletes younger than 35 years is a coronary artery anomaly, which invariably precipitates death during exercise (all coronary anomalies may predispose to sudden death). Both angina and syncope have retrospectively been identified as prodromal features of this condition; these symptoms should prompt an immediate evaluation of a young athlete. Right ventricular dysplasia and Uhl anomaly are rare causes of sudden death in young athletes, who may have a history of syncope, palpitations, or ventricular tachycardia.

There is a paucity of literature of sudden death following anabolic steroid use, usually in weight lifters. Accelerated atherosclerosis in young subjects has been reported at autopsy in these individuals.

Corrado D et al. Does sports activity enhance the risk of sudden death in adolescents and young adults? J Am Coll Cardiol. 2003 Dec 3;42(11):1959–63. [PMID: 14662259]

Germann CA et al. Sudden cardiac death in athletes: a guide for emergency physicians. Am J Emerg Med. 2005 Jul;23(4):504–9. [PMID: 16032621]

► The Preparticipation Physical Examination

The identification of sudden death in athletes by the media has stressed the importance of establishing guidelines and internationally accepted levels of practice to evaluate any type of

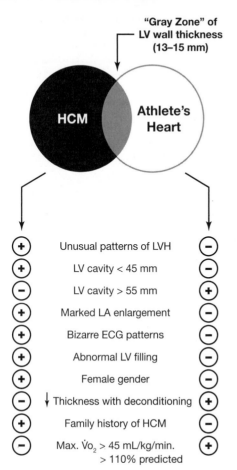

▲ Figure 34–3. Distinction between hypertrophic cardiomyopathy (HCM) and the athlete's heart, when there is a "gray zone" of morphologic overlap. LVH, left ventricular hypertrophy; LA, left atrial; ECG, electrocardiogram; $\dot{V}o_2$, oxygen consumption. (Reprinted with permission from Maron BJ et al. Circulation. 1995;91:1596.)

cope at rest or during exercise, dyspnea, angina or its equivalents, and palpitations need to be recorded. In older athletes, close attention should be paid to the existence of cardiovascular risk factors as well as the symptoms and manifestations of coronary artery disease.

Physical examinations should exclude Marfan syndrome. Arterial blood pressure should be measured accurately. Auscultation of the heart should be comprehensive, keeping in mind that both S_3 and S_4 sounds are common in athletes, as are pulmonary arterial flow murmurs in young athletes and aortic valve flow murmurs in older athletes. The cardiac examination should include the upright position to lessen innocent murmurs and intensify the murmur from hypertrophic cardiomyopathy. Because of the significance of hypertrophic cardiomyopathy, when a systolic murmur is auscultated, its features during squatting and during and after the Valsalva maneuver should be characterized.

Further testing is not routinely required, unless warranted by an abnormal feature of the history or physical examination. Furthermore, should a cardiovascular test be carried out, the limitations of the procedure as well as the altered normal ranges of parameters evaluated by the procedure must be kept in mind. The extent of any evaluation beyond the history and physical examination depends on any abnormality that emerges. The routine use of electrocardiography, exercise testing, and echocardiography is precluded on a cost-benefit basis as a population-based screening tool because of the very low prevalence of sudden death in the trained athlete population. It is possible that the threshold for a diagnostic echocardiogram may be lower for an older or masters athlete, again emphasizing its indication is provided by any potential abnormality emerging from the detailed history and physical examination, and previously substantiated cardiovascular risk factors.

There are other relevant reasons for forgoing expensive cardiovascular tests. The morphologic changes produced by the various forms of athletic training often produce changes in certain tests (particularly the echocardiogram) that would

athlete prior to their partication in their athletic endeavor. Although standard levels of care have not yet been substantiated by evidence-based measures, many reputed societies have begun to introduce certain expected predictors of cardiovascular disease and sudden death for further evaluation. All athletes of any age should undergo a preparticipation cardiac examination and subsequent regular periodic examinations. These should be done in a closed setting, providing time for a detailed history and physical examination, rather than in an assembly-line atmosphere. Knowledge of the subject and the subject's family history are essential. The history should detail any information regarding congenital heart disease in the subject or family members as well as sudden death of any family members. Symptoms such as exercise intolerance, syn-

Table 34–3. Causes of Sudden Death in Athletes over 35 Years.

Coronary atherosclerosis
Hypertrophic cardiomyopathy
Aberrant coronary arteries
Premature atherosclerosis
Right ventricular dysplasia
Marfan syndrome
Idiopathic left ventricular hypertrophy
Mitral valve prolapse syndrome
Wolff-Parkinson-White syndrome
Prolonged QT syndrome
Myocarditis
Coronary artery vasospasm

be abnormal in a normal, sedentary, age-matched population. It must be remembered that the normal range of values for athletes varies considerably from the accepted normal ranges of left ventricular cavity size, posterior wall and interventricular septal thickness, and left ventricular wall mass. The same applies to routine ECGs in this population, in that abnormal ECG findings may be normal variants in a group of trained athletes. In addition, the incidence of false-positive exercise stress tests appears to be higher in a population of trained athletes. Although these observations do not completely preclude the use of cardiovascular tests, they reinforce the conclusion that they need not be done routinely.

Corrado D et al. Does sports activity enhance the risk of sudden death in adolescents and young adults? J Am Coll Cardiol. 2003 Dec 3;42(11):1959–63. [PMID: 14662259]

Corrado D et al; Study Group of Sport Cardiology of the Working Group of Cardiac Rehabilitation and Exercise Physiology and the Working Group of Myocardial and Pericardial Diseases of the European Society of Cardiology. Cardiovascular pre-participation screening of young competitive athletes for prevention of sudden death: proposal for a common European protocol. Consensus statement of the Study Group of Sport Cardiology of the Working Group of Cardiac Rehabilitation and Exercise Physiology and the Working Group of Myocardial and Pericardial Diseases of the European Society of Cardiology. Eur Heart J. 2005 Mar;26(5):516–24. [PMID: 15689345]

Maron BJ et al. 36th Bethesda Conference. Introduction: eligibility recommendations for competitive athletes with cardiovascular abnormalities—general considerations. J Am Coll Cardiol. 2005 Apr 19;45(8):1318–21. [PMID: 15837280]

Pelliccia A et al; Study Group of Sports Cardiology of the Working Group of Cardiac Rehabilitation and Exercise Physiology and the Working Group of Myocardial and Pericardial Diseases of the European Society of Cardiology. Recommendations for competitive sports participation in athletes with cardiovascular disease: a consensus document for the Study Group of Sports Cardiology of the Working Group of Cardiac Rehabilitation and Exercise Physiology and the Working Group of Myocardial and Pericardial Diseases of the European Society of Cardiology. Eur Heart J. 2005 Jul;26(14):1422–45. [PMID: 15923204]

Pfister GC et al. Preparticipation cardiovascular screening for US collegiate student-athletes. JAMA. 2000 Mar 22–29;283(12):1597–9. [PMID: 10735397]

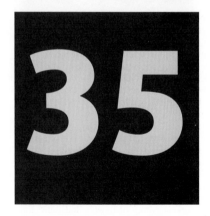

35

Thoracic Aortic Aneurysms & Dissections

John A. Elefteriades, MD

ANEURYSMS

ESSENTIALS OF DIAGNOSIS

▶ Ascending aortic diameter > 4 cm on imaging study.
▶ Descending aortic diameter > 3.5 cm on imaging study.

▶ General Considerations

In the ascending aorta, aneurysms tend to take on three common patterns, as indicated in Figure 35–1. These include the supracoronary aortic aneurysm, annuloaortic ectasia (marfanoid), and tubular diffuse enlargement.

The most common pattern is that of supracoronary dilatation of the ascending aorta. In this pattern of disease, the short segment of aorta between the aortic annulus and the coronary arteries remains normal in size. Sinuses are "preserved," meaning that the aorta indents normally, forming a "waist," near the level of the coronary arteries. For this type of aneurysm, a supracoronary tube graft suffices.

In the second type, annuloaortic ectasia, the aortic annulus itself becomes dilated, giving a shape to the aorta like an Erlenmeyer chemistry flask. In this type of disease, the segment of aorta between the annulus and the coronary arteries is diseased, dilated, and thinned. Sinuses are "effaced," meaning that the normal indentation, or waist, is lost. When surgery is required, the entire aortic root must be replaced.

In the third type of ascending aortic disease, the configuration is midway between the previous two patterns, that is, there is some dilatation of the annulus and root and some effacement of the sinuses, but these elements are not dramatic. The overall appearance is that of a large tube, rather than a flask. For such aortas, either supracoronary tube grafting or aortic root replacement may be appropriate.

The Crawford classification (Figure 35–2) is used to categorize the appearance of an aneurysm in the descending aorta and thoracoabdominal aorta. This classification is based on the longitudinal location and extent of aortic involvement and has implications for surgical strategy and affects the risk of perioperative complications.

Type I aneurysms involve most of the thoracic aorta and the upper abdominal aorta. Type II aneurysms, the most extensive and most dangerous to repair, involve the entire descending and abdominal aortas. Type III aneurysms involve the lower thoracic and abdominal aortas. Type IV aneurysms are predominantly abdominal but involve thoracoabdominal exposure because of the proximity of the upper border to the diaphragm.

▶ Etiology

The genetics of Marfan disease, a well-known cause of aneurysms of the thoracic aorta, have been well delineated, with over 85 mutations identified at one locus on the fibrillin gene.

Increasingly, it is being appreciated that patients who do not have Marfan disease also manifest familial clustering of thoracic aortic aneurysms and dissections. Patients with aneurysms often answer one or both of the following questions affirmatively: "Do you have any family members with aneurysms anywhere in their bodies? Did any of your relatives die suddenly or unexpectedly of apparent cardiac causes?" Detailed construction of family trees on over 500 patients with thoracic aneurysm have indicated that 21% of aneurysm probands have a first-degree relative with a known or likely aortic aneurysm. The true number is certainly much higher, as these estimates are based only on family interview and not on head-to-toe imaging of relatives. Figure 35–3 shows the 21 positive family trees of the first 100 families analyzed. The most likely pattern of inheritance appears to be autosomal-dominant with incomplete penetrance. A most recent analysis has shown that the location of the proband's aneurysm largely influences the location of the aneurysms in the family members. If the proband has an ascending aneurysm, the likelihood is that the family mem-

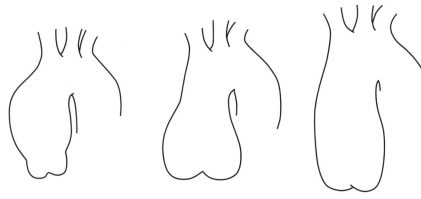

Supracoronary
aneurysm

Annuloaortic ectasia
(marfanoid)

Tubular diffuse
enlargement

▲ **Figure 35–1.** The three common patterns of ascending aortic aneurysm.

bers have ascending aneurysms. If, however, the proband has a descending aneurysm, it is likely that the family members have abdominal aortic aneurysms. These proband-family member observations are in keeping with the general con-

cept that aneurysm disease divides at the ligamentum arteriosum: Ascending and arch aneurysms represent one disease, largely nonarteriosclerotic, while descending and abdominal aneurysms represent another disease, largely arteriosclerotic.

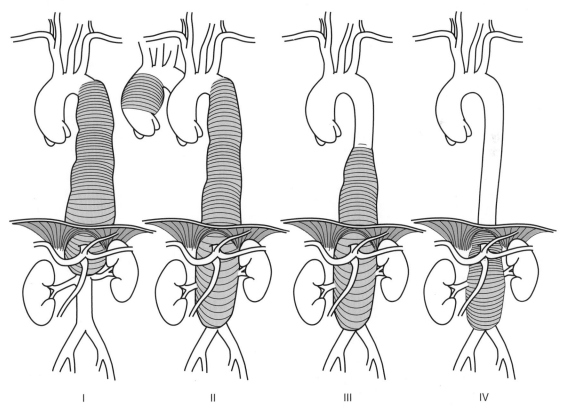

I   II   III   IV

▲ **Figure 35–2.** The Crawford classification of descending and thoracoabdominal aneurysms. See text for description of each type. (Reprinted, with permission, from Edmunds LH Jr, ed. Cardiac Surgery in the Adult. New York: McGraw-Hill, 1997.)

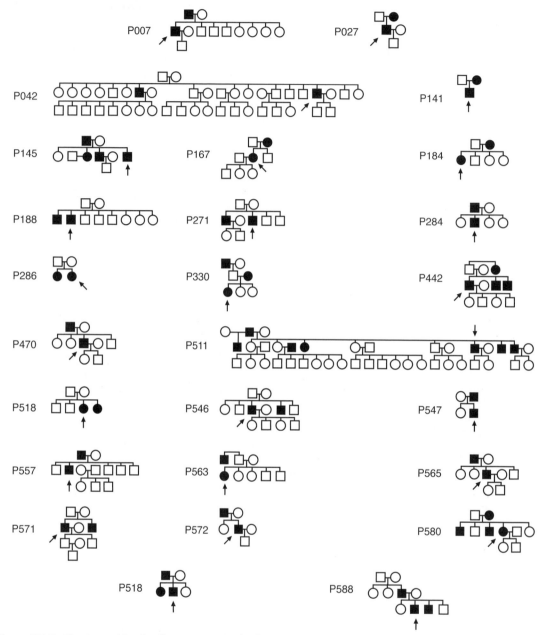

▲ **Figure 35–3.** The 21 positive family trees among the first 100 families assessed for genetic patterns of thoracic aortic disease.

Application of modern molecular genetic techniques is successfully making progress toward determining the specific genetic aberrations responsible for these family clusterings and for thoracic aneurysms in general. Specific sites of genetic mutations that underlie many of the instances of familial inheritance, including the so-called TAAD1 (Tho-

racic Aortic Aneurysm and Dissection 1) locus, has been uncovered. Examination of single nucleotide polymorphisms (SNPs) in the blood of hundreds of patients with thoracic aortic aneurysms via genome-wide surveys using large (> 30,000) SNP libraries has been examined. An "RNA signature" in the blood of patients with thoracic aortic aneurysm was found, which can predict with about 85% accuracy from a blood test alone whether the patient harbors a thoracic aortic aneurysm. This "signature" is composed of specific RNAs that are either markedly up-regulated or markedly down-regulated in aneurysm patients, compared with healthy controls. These RNA profiles reflect alterations in RNA expression brought about by the aneurysm disease. The corresponding analyses of DNA polymorphisms, which would reflect the underlying mutations in the genome, is nearing fruition.

Patients who have a genetic predisposition for aneurysm development, specifically those patients with annuloaortic ectasia or ascending dissection, are significantly protected from arteriosclerosis (Figure 35–4). It appears likely that the same mutations that promote lysis of the aortic wall also prevent plaque build-up.

Accepting that most patients with aneurysms have an underlying genetic predisposition to the condition, how does this genetic programming lead to the development of an aneurysm? Rapid progress is being made in elucidating these mechanisms. Aneurysm formation is currently thought to involve the following processes (Figure 35–5): extracellular matrix proteolysis, chronic inflammation, cytokine activity, and smooth muscle cell loss. The identification of these mechanisms raises the intriguing possibility of interfering pharmacologically with this pathophysiology, so aneurysm formation or progression can be stopped. The importance of the transforming growth factor-β (TGF-β) pathway in aneu-

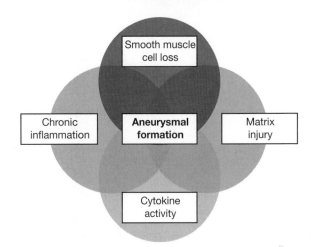

▲ **Figure 35–5.** Diagram illustrating the overlapping cellular and molecular processes that contribute to aortic aneurysm formation.

rysm formation has been demonstrated; the ability of angiotensin receptor blocking medications (eg, losartan) to interfere with this pathophysiologic mechanism is being tested, and experimental results are promising. At this time, however, it may be said that no specific pharmacologic strategy exists for delaying aneurysm progression. Results of trials of proteolytic antagonists and β-blockers have been underwhelming. The potential roles of statin medications, antiinflammatory agents (cyclooxygenase [COX]-2 inhibitors), immunosuppressants (sirolimus), and antibiotics (doxycycline), are being investigated.

The proteolytic enzymes called matrix metalloproteinases (MMPs) are receiving extensive attention in aneurysm pathophysiology. These powerful enzymes are found in excess in thoracic aortic aneurysms (Figure 35–6) and are thought to play a major role in destroying the substance of the aortic wall, leading to decreases wall strength and, ultimately, dilatation and rupture.

The biologic changes in the aortic wall discussed above are vitally important, but hemodynamic forces need to be considered as well. As the ascending aorta reaches a diameter of 6 cm, the distensibility vanishes, so that the aorta becomes essentially a rigid tube (Figure 35–7). Because of this rigidity, the force of systole can no longer be beneficially dissipated by elastic expansion of the aorta, and this translates into increased wall stress. Especially at high blood pressures, this wall stress becomes excessive, setting the stage for disruption of the aortic wall via rupture or dissection. It is instructive to note how closely this mechanical data dove-tails with the clinical behavior of the aorta: The mechanical properties deteriorate at 6 cm diameter, and that is precisely the hinge point for clinically manifest rupture and dissection.

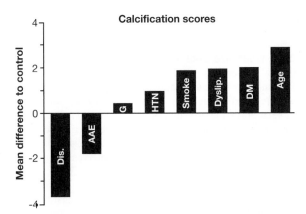

▲ **Figure 35–4.** Difference in overall calcification scores relative to the control group for all risk factors analyzed. Note that patients with ascending aortic dissection or annuloaortic ectasia are significantly "protected" from arteriosclerosis, manifesting lower calcification scores. Dis, ascending aortic dissection; AAE, annuloaortic ectasia; G, male gender; HTN, hypertension; Smoke, smoking history; Dyslip, dyslipidemia; DM, diabetes mellitus; Age, age (in 10-year intervals).

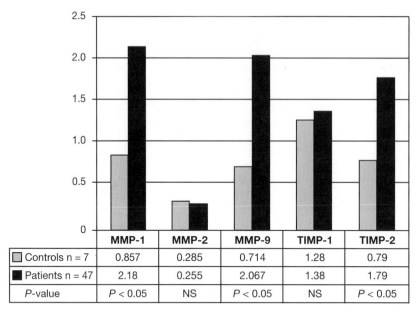

	MMP-1	MMP-2	MMP-9	TIMP-1	TIMP-2
Controls n = 7	0.857	0.285	0.714	1.28	0.79
Patients n = 47	2.18	0.255	2.067	1.38	1.79
P-value	*P* < 0.05	NS	*P* < 0.05	NS	*P* < 0.05

▲ **Figure 35-6.** Note overabundance of matrix metalloproteinase (MMP)-1 and MMP-9 in aortas of patients with thoracic aortic aneurysm, compared with controls. This information suggests an important role for MMP enzymes in the pathophysiology of aneurysm disease.

▶ Clinical Findings

A. Natural History

The Yale computerized database now contains information on nearly 3000 patients with thoracic aortic aneurysm, including some 9000 tabulated serial imaging studies and 9000 patient-years of follow-up. This database and these methods of analysis have permitted assessment of multiple fundamental topics and questions regarding the natural behavior of the thoracic aorta and have shed light on appropriate criteria for surgical intervention.

1. How fast does the thoracic aorta grow?—Calculation of growth rate of the aorta is more complicated than simply subtracting the original size of the aorta from the current size and dividing by the length of follow-up. Different modalities (echocardiography, computed tomographic [CT] scan, and magnetic resonance imaging [MRI]) may give different values. In addition, some interobserver variability may occur in size assessment. And, most importantly, some scans may show smaller size than original measurements. (This does not imply that the aorta gets smaller, but rather that variability in measurement can happen, especially in huge samples of data.) If these negative changes are truncated, falsely high growth rates result. Via specifically developed statistical methods designed to account for these potential sources of error, the annual growth rate of an aneurysmal thoracic aorta has been determined to be 0.12 cm on average. The descending aorta grows faster than the ascending aorta, at 0.19 cm/year compared with 0.07 cm/year. Also, the larger the aorta becomes, the faster it grows.

2. At what size does the aorta dissect or rupture?—Critical to decision-making in aortic surgery is an understanding of when complications occur in the natural history of unrepaired thoracic aortic aneurysms. In the case of the thoracic aorta, the two complications that are vitally important are rupture and dissection. Knowing when these complications are likely would permit rational decision-making regarding elective, preemptive surgical intervention to prevent them.

Size criteria apply *only* to asymptomatic aneurysms. Symptomatic aneurysms should be resected regardless of size. The usual symptom produced by an aortic aneurysm is pain. For ascending aneurysms, this pain is usually felt anteriorly, under the breastbone. For descending thoracic aneurysms, the pain is usually felt in the interscapular region of the upper back. For thoracoabdominal aneurysms, the pain is usually felt lower in the back and in the left flank. Other symptoms may occasionally be produced by thoracic aortic aneurysms, including bronchial obstruction, esophageal obstruction, and phrenic nerve dysfunction, and also constitute indications for surgical intervention.

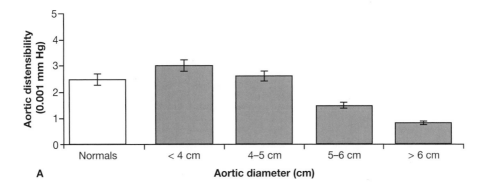

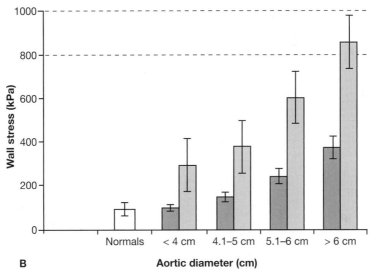

▲ **Figure 35–7. A:** Distensibility values in normal aortas and aortic aneurysms of different diameters. Distensibility of ascending aortic aneurysms decreases rapidly as diameter increases, to very low values at dimensions > 6 cm. At 6 cm, the aorta is essentially a rigid tube, unable to dissipate the force of systole by expanding phasically during the cardiac cycle. **B:** Exponential relationship between wall stress and aneurysm size in ascending aortic aneurysms. The dark columns represent a blood pressure of 100 mm Hg, and the light columns represent a blood pressure of 200 mm Hg. The lines at 800–1000 kPa represent the range of maximum tensile strength of the human aorta. Note that a patient with a 6-cm aneurysm and a blood pressure of 200 mm Hg (as during stress or extreme exertion) "flirts" with the limits of the ultimate strength of his or her aorta wall.

Initial statistical analysis revealed sharp "hinge points" (Figure 35–8) in aortic size at which rupture or dissection occurred. For the ascending thoracic aorta, the hinge point occurs at 6.0 cm. By the time aortas reach this size, 31% have ruptured or dissected. For the descending aorta, the hinge point is located at 7.0 cm. By the time descending aortas reach this size, 43% have ruptured or dissected.

If a surgeon were to wait for the aorta to achieve the median size at time of complications in order to intervene, by definition rupture or dissection would have occurred in half of the patients (Figure 35–9). Accordingly, it is important to intervene before the median value is attained. The following recommendations take this factor into account, permitting preemptive surgical extirpation before rupture or dissection in most patients.

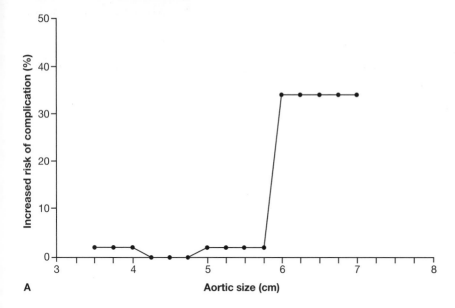

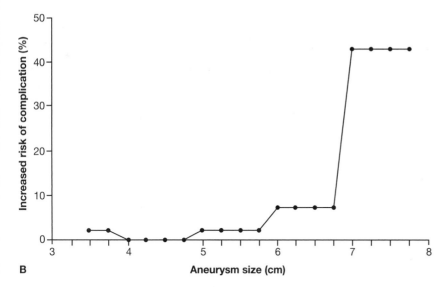

▲ **Figure 35-8.** The "hinge-points" (*arrows*) in the cumulative, life-time incidence of complications (rupture or dissection) of thoracic aortic aneurysms, based on size. By the time the aorta reaches the dimensions on the x-axis, the percentage of patients shown on the y-axis has already incurred rupture or dissection. **A:** Curve for the ascending aorta. **B:** Curve for the descending aorta.

Current recommendations are listed in Table 35–1 and are based on the hinge points noted in Figure 35–8. Specifically, prophylactic extirpation of the aneurysmal ascending aorta is recommended when the aneurysm measures 5.5 cm; for the descending aorta, which does not rupture until a larger size, surgical intervention is recommended when the aneurysm measures 6.5 cm. Application of these criteria will prevent most ruptures and dissections, without prematurely exposing the patient to the risks and inconveniences of surgery.

It is well-known that patients with Marfan disease are prone to unpredictable dissection at an early size. For this reason, earlier intervention is recommended for patients with Marfan disease as indicated in Table 35–1.

For patients with a positive family history, but without Marfan disease, the same criteria is applied as for Marfan disease because the data indicate malignant behavior of the aneurysm in these patients as well.

If the patient has a positive family history, or if an afflicted family member has suffered rupture, dissection, or

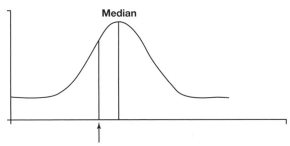

Median

▲ **Figure 35–9.** A schematic representation of the importance of selecting a criterion for intervention before complications (rupture or dissection) commonly occur. Utilization of the median as the criterion level would allow half the population to realize a devastating complication before preemptive intervention. Accordingly, a criterion below the median is selected (*arrow*), to allow preemptive intervention before a large proportion of patients have suffered a complication.

death, preemptive surgical extirpation is carried out earlier than otherwise.

Studies of aortic anatomy increasingly recognize that patients with a bicuspid aortic valve also have inherently deficient aortas. Therefore, lower intervention dimensions are used for patients with bicuspid aortic valve as well. Table 35–2 indicates that a bicuspid aortic valve is actually a more common cause of aortic dissection than Marfan disease. Table 35–2 compares the general incidence of Marfan disease with that of bicuspid aortic valve. Although the incidence of dissection is 5% for bicuspid valve disease, compared with 40% for patients with Marfan disease, bicuspid valve disease is so much more common that it causes more total cases of dissection than Marfan disease. This factor must be taken into account in planning surgical repair of the ascending aorta of the patient with a bicuspid aortic valve when the aorta is still in the aneurysmal stage, and not yet a dissection.

3. What is the yearly rate of rupture or dissection for thoracic aortic aneurysms?—The preceding data indicate the cumulative *lifetime* rates of dissection or rupture by the time the aorta reaches a certain size. Determining the *yearly* risk of complications from the natural history of thoracic aortic aneurysm is more challenging because it requires extremely robust data. Such data must produce enough hard end points to permit analysis within a year's time for differ-

Table 35–1. Size Criteria for Surgical Intervention for Asymptomatic Thoracic Aortic Aneurysm.

	Marfan's	Non-Marfan's
Ascending	5.0 cm	5.5 cm
Descending	6.0 cm	6.5 cm

ent size strata. The following equation calculates the yearly rate of rupture:

$$\ln \lambda = -21.055 + 0.0093 \, (\text{age}) + 0.842 \, (\text{pain}) + 1.282 \, (\text{COPD}) + 0.643 \, (\text{diameter of descending aorta}) + 0.405 \, (\text{diameter of abdominal aorta})$$

Calculations of yearly rates of rupture or other complications based on size of the aorta have also been produced. These yearly rates are expressed based simply on the size of the aorta (Figure 35–10).

These data all point to a diameter of 6 cm as a very dangerous size threshold. At or above this size, the yearly risk for rupture is about 4%, the yearly risk of dissection is about 4%, and the risk of death is about 11%. (Death is often directly related to catastrophic complications from the aneurysm.) The chance of any one of these phenomena occurring—rupture, dissection, or death—is 14%/year. As a mnemonic point of reference, a 6-cm aneurysm can be equated to about the diameter of a soft-drink can. When a thoracic aortic aneurysm reaches the diameter of a soda can, it has certainly attained the point where it poses a major risk to the patient.

These analyses should permit accurate decision making when seeing a patient during an office visit and considering preemptive surgical extirpation of thoracic aneurysms. These data allow the physician to form a reasonable estimate of the individual patient's risk of dissection, rupture, or death for each future year of life, if the aorta is not resected. The risk of rupture, dissection, or death based on aortic size is presented graphically in Figure 35–10.

The question arises whether the same surgical intervention criteria should apply for a small woman as for a large man. It is true that a larger individual can be "allowed" a larger aorta, generally speaking. Conversely, even a moderate-sized aneurysm can be quite threatening in an individual of small stature. For this reason, adverse event rates (rupture or dissection) based on aortic size corrected for body surface area (BSA) have been analyzed. By plotting the aneurysm

Table 35–2. Aortic Manifestation of Connective Tissue Disease.

	Incidence in General Population	Rate of Dissection (per affected individual)	Number of Dissections Caused (per 10,000 population)
Marfan syndrome	0.01% (1 in 10,000)	40%	0.4 persons
Bicuspid aortic disease	1–2% (100–200 in 10,000)	5%	5–10 persons

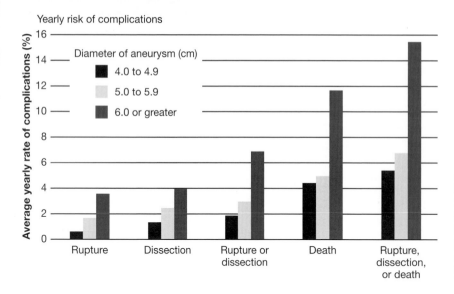

Yearly risk of complications

▲ **Figure 35–10.** Probabilities that rupture, dissection, or death will occur have been calculated for aortic aneurysms in the chest. The likelihood of these events jumps sharply for aneurysms that reach 6 cm or higher.

size along the horizontal scale and the BSA along the vertical scale, each particular patient can be classified into low-, medium-, or high-risk categories—thus taking account of the aneurysm size in relation to the patient's physical size.

B. Symptoms and Signs

Most thoracic aortic aneurysms are asymptomatic and are detected fortuitously during imaging of other thoracic structures. When they are symptomatic, deep visceral pain in the upper anterior chest or interscapular back can occur. This pain differs from angina pectoris because it is not necessarily precipitated by exertion nor relieved by rest or nitroglycerin. Often, it is rather constant and not influenced by body motion or position. All patients with chest pain should have a screening chest radiograph. Rupture of a thoracic aneurysm usually causes excruciating pain, accompanied by profound dyspnea as the chest fills with blood, and quickly results in shock. A large ascending aortic aneurysm occasionally may result in dysphagia or stridor due to esophageal or large airway obstruction. Rarely, a large aneurysm may cause bone pain due to pressure against thoracic skeletal structures.

C. Physical Examination

Physical examination is usually unremarkable. The presence of a murmur of aortic regurgitation should raise the suspicion of ascending aortic aneurysm, as should features suggestive of Marfan syndrome or related conditions. Rarely, an abnormal pulsation will be felt due to a large aneurysm contacting the chest wall.

D. Diagnostic Studies

The remarkable strides made in recent decades in three-dimensional body imaging have dramatically advanced the

diagnosis and treatment of thoracic aortic aneurysm. Echocardiography (especially transesophageal) and CT and MRI scans all yield images that clarify the presence, location, size, and extent of aneurysmal disease. An example of the precise imaging afforded by MRI is indicated for a specific, very extensive aneurysm in Figure 35–11.

In this era of specialized three-dimensional imaging, it is important not to forget the chest radiograph, which can often yield significant information about the thoracic aorta.

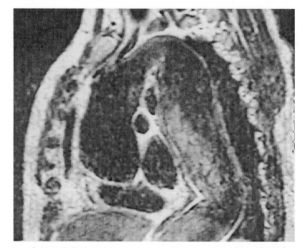

▲ **Figure 35–11.** Magnetic resonance scan of massively dilated aorta, which extends from the aortic valve to the iliac bifurcation. Note that the heart is compressed to a small shadow crushed between the elongated aorta and the diaphragm. This aneurysm was successfully resected in two stages.

An example is provided in Figure 35–12. Ascending aortic aneurysm presents as a bulge beyond the right hilar border. Arch aneurysm produces enlargement of the aortic knob. Descending thoracic aneurysm is often easily seen as a deviation of the stripe of the descending aorta, which normally runs parallel to and just left of the vertebral column.

▶ Treatment

A. Risks of Aortic Surgery

It is certainly helpful to know numerically and statistically the cumulative and yearly rates of rupture, dissection, and death imposed by an aortic aneurysm of a specific size. On the other hand, the equation is incomplete without consideration of the risks inherent in elective, prophylactic surgical extirpation of the thoracic aorta. Certainly these are major operations, and the surgical risks most feared include death, stroke, and paraplegia. However, these operations have become safer, reflecting increased surgical experience, improved perfusion techniques, improved (non-porous) grafts, effective anti-fibrinolytic agents for perioperative use, improved methods of spinal cord preservation, and the advent of centers specializing in aortic care and surgery. A recently published report emphasizes the "safety of thoracic aortic surgery in the present era." Mortality rates and rates of other complications after aortic surgery are quite low, especially for operations performed electively on stable patients, in whom the safety of ascending aortic and aortic arch surgery is as high as 98%. Table 35–3 shows the pertinent rates of morbidity and mortality.

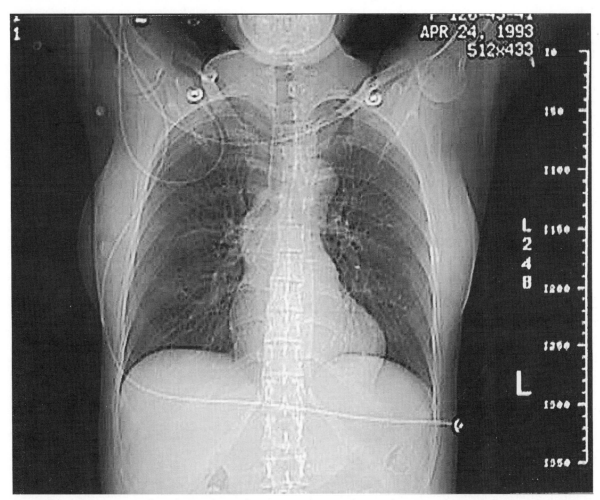

▲ **Figure 35–12.** An exemplary chest radiograph indicating that significant information about the aorta can be gleaned from this simple test. Note the bulge of the ascending aorta to the right of the upper mediastinal border. This young patient with Marfan disease suffered dissection at an ascending aortic dimension of 4.8 cm.

Table 35–3. Current Risks of Thoracic Aortic Surgery.

	Mortality (%)	Stroke (%)	Paraplegia (%)
Ascending/arch	2.9	3.0	0.5
Descending/ thoracoabdominal	2.9	4.2	5.3

Data are for elective procedures, which is the category to whom surgical decision criteria are applied. Data from Achneck H, Rizzo JA, Tranquilli M, Elefteriades JA. Safety of thoracic aortic surgery in the present era. Ann Thorac Surg. In press.

These rates are typical of those at other centers with a focused interest and a specific program in thoracic aortic diseases. It should be noted that stroke can complicate not only ascending and arch operations, but also descending aortic operations.

B. Indications and Contraindications

By considering the rates of natural rupture, dissection, and death from the thoracic aneurysm itself versus the risks of operation, the physician can make an informed recommendations about elective, preemptive surgery. Once patients and their families are provided the natural history and surgical risk data, they often have strong opinions of their own. Some patients are reluctant to undergo major surgery, with its significant attendant risks, for an asymptomatic problem. Most patients, however, seem to feel they will never be comfortable until the threatening aneurysm is resected.

One more very important general point needs to be considered. Once the aorta has dissected, the prognosis is thereafter adversely affected (Figure 35–13). Patients who required emergency surgery not only had a higher rate of early mortality, but their survival curve was dramatically poorer. The patients who elected for surgery showed a survival rate very similar to that of a normal population. The poor long-term outlook for patients who required emergency surgery is due largely to the fact that, even after surgical replacement of portions of the aorta, the remainder of this vital organ will forever remain dissected. Because the aortic wall was deficient to start with, at half-thickness, after dissection, it is rendered even more vulnerable to subsequent enlargement and rupture.

C. Surgical Techniques

As discussed, the type of operation for the ascending aorta is based on the pattern of aneurysmal pathology. For many

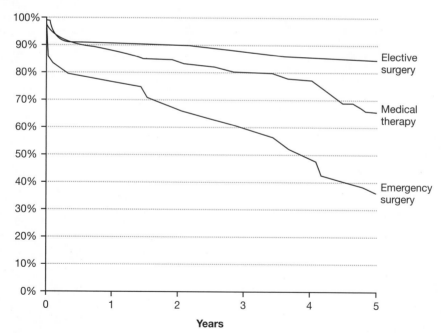

▲ **Figure 35–13.** Long-term survival rates based on treatment. Medically treated patients had, of course, smaller and less symptomatic aneurysms. Note particularly that patients having emergent surgery not only manifested a higher likelihood of perioperative mortality, but also had a poorer long-term outlook. On the other hand, patients who received elective surgery, showed excellent survival rates, comparable to an age and sex-matched normal population. This data argues for elective, prophylactic extirpation of the aneurysmal aorta, before rupture or dissection can occur.

patients, a supracoronary tube graft suffices (Figure 35–14A). For others, a composite graft, including both a valve and a graft, with obligate coronary artery reimplantation, is appropriate (Figure 35–14B). New valve-sparing aortic replacement procedures have been developed. The appropriate application of these procedures will become clearer as more patients are monitored into the medium term and as more centers accumulate experience with these innovative techniques.

The main debate regarding the procedure for ascending aortic operations and those on the aortic arch concerns the optimal means of protecting brain function during the time that anastomoses in the vicinity of the aortic arch are performed. Deep hypothermic circulatory arrest—a state of suspended animation, which is generally safe for 30–45 minutes or longer—is preferred by many surgeons, for its simplicity and effectiveness. In a study on 400 patients, the effectiveness of this remarkable technique as a sole means of

brain preservation was confirmed. Retrograde cerebral perfusion—via the superior vena cava—has its advocates, although the actual amount of effective brain perfusion achieved by this means has been questioned. Direct perfusion of the head vessels—usually via a cannula in the innominate artery or cannulas in both the innominate and the left carotid artery—also has its supporters, despite its added complexity. Direct perfusion is gaining in popularity, and it does provide a margin of protection, especially for very complex arch reconstructions or for surgical teams relatively inexperienced with arch replacement. No technique has been demonstrated conclusively superior over the others. Some recent attempts have been made to develop a solution and technique for "cerebroplegia," which takes a cue from the paralyzing cardioplegia used to protect the heart, without success.

For descending and thoracoabdominal operations, the technique of left atrial to femoral artery bypass has become

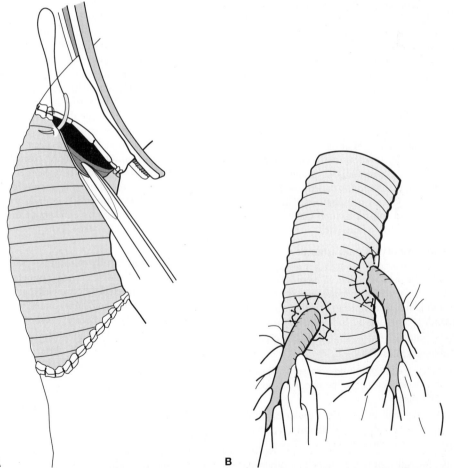

A **B**

▲ **Figure 35–14. A:** Supracoronary tube graft replacement and **B:** composite graft replacement. (A: Reprinted, with permission, from Cooley DA, Wukasch DC. Techniques in Vascular Surgery. Philadelphia: WB Saunders, 1979.)

extremely popular. This method takes strain off the heart by diverting blood away from the left ventricle. This approach mitigates the effect of high aortic cross-clamping on cardiac afterload. It also perfuses the lower body, especially the extremely vulnerable spinal cord. Despite decades of concerted attention, paraplegia from descending and thoracoabdominal aortic replacement continues to be a major clinical problem. The cause is multifactorial, with clamp time, air and particulate embolism, and disconnection of critical intercostal branches all playing a role. Besides the benefits of left atrial to femoral artery perfusion, most authorities feel that routine spinal fluid drainage and deliberate maintenance of a strong postoperative blood pressure (to encourage collateral blood flow) are also effective adjuncts against the complication of postoperative paraplegia.

D. Specific Clinical Scenarios and Issues

1. Patient with pain, but aneurysm smaller than criteria

The answer to whether such an aorta should be replaced is a resounding yes. The dimensional criteria are specifically intended for asymptomatic patients. Any and all symptomatic aneurysms need to be resected because symptoms are a precursor to rupture. Aneurysm pain represents stretching or irritation of the aortic adventitia, the adjacent chest wall, the mediastinal pleura, or some other structure impinged on by the expanding aneurysm. Even an aorta smaller than the criterion can rupture or dissect. Such a patient is of extreme concern, and preemptive resection is needed. In one case, a patient complained of typical pain of an ascending aortic aneurysm. The aorta was 5.0 cm. Because the medical team thought this was too small for resection, they underestimated the symptoms at presentation. The aorta subsequently ruptured and the patient died within 48 hours. This point cannot be overemphasized: The size criteria are explicitly intended only for asymptomatic patients; *all symptomatic aneurysms need to be resected.*

2. Differentiating aneurysm pain from musculoskeletal pain

This very important point is not always easy to determine, even in the most experienced hands. The patient usually has a good sense of whether the pain is originating from muscles and joints. The clinician usually gets an additional understanding by asking the following questions:

   a. Is the pain influenced by motion or position? (If so, it is probably musculoskeletal.)

   b. Do you have a history of lumbosacral spine disease or chronic low back pain? (If so, the symptoms may not be aortic in origin.)

   c. Do you feel the pain in the interscapular back? (An affirmative answer indicates an almost certain relationship to thoracic aortic aneurysm.)

Presume that the pain is aortic in origin if no other cause can be conclusively established. This is the only approach that can prevent rupture.

3. Appropriate interval for serial aortic imaging

Patients with a thoracic aortic aneurysm should be monitored indefinitely. Stable, asymptomatic patients can undergo imaging about once every 2 years, remembering that the aneurysmal aorta grows at a relatively slow 1 mm/year. In case of new onset of symptoms, imaging should be done promptly, regardless of the interval from the prior scan. For new patients, for whom only one size data point is available, imaging should be done at short intervals until the behavior of aorta is understood. Imaging may be done every 3–6 months for new patients with moderately large aortas. Remember to compare the present scan with the patient's *first* scan, not with the last prior scan. That is the way to detect growth. Many a patient has suffered because scans were only compared with the last prior scan, and major growth went undetected.

4. Choice of imaging modality for serial follow-up

Three quality imaging techniques are currently available: echocardiography, CT scan, and MRI. If echocardiography is chosen, it is important to remember that a standard transthoracic echocardiogram cannot see the distal ascending aorta, the aortic arch, or the descending aorta with conclusive accuracy because of intervening air-containing lung tissue. Supplement such studies with a periodic CT scan or MRI, which can visualize the entire aorta. The choice between CT and MRI may depend on ease of availability and radiologic expertise in a particular environment. Both modalities can image the entire aorta extremely well. Elevated creatinine or contrast allergy may contraindicate CT and instead favor MRI. The need to evaluate complex aortic lesions in multiple imaging planes would also favor MRI (although very recently concerns have been raised about the risk to the kidneys of gadolinium contrast agents used for MRI scanning). Of course, indwelling metallic foreign objects, such as pacemakers or metal artifacts from previous surgery, may make CT the necessary choice instead of MRI.

5. Evaluation of family members

The data on familial inheritance has become strong enough that the treating physician is obligated to recommend that family members be evaluated. Physicians of family members should be made aware that aneurysm disease has been diagnosed in the family. A CT scan is recommended for adult males and for females beyond childbearing age. For children and for females of childbearing age, echocardiography of the ascending aorta and abdominal aorta is recommended. Investigators hope to identify humoral markers or genetic aberrations that can be used for familial screening of the aneurysm trait soon.

6. Activity restrictions

Continuation of any and all aerobic activities, including running, swimming, and bicycling is recommended. Serious weight lifters, at peaks of exertion, can elevate systolic arterial pressure to 300 mm Hg. This type of instantaneous hypertension is, of course, not prudent for aneurysm patients. Weight lifters should limit themselves to one-half their body weight. The evidence for effort-induced aortic dissection is mounting. Participation in contact sports or those that might produce an abrupt physical impact, such as tackle football, snow skiing, water skiing, and horseback riding, is proscribed.

7. Role of stent grafting—A word of caution is appropriate concerning stent grafts. Multiple thoracic stent products previously in clinical trials have been recalled by the US Food and Drug Administration. Owing to the very high need for subsequent conventional surgery after abdominal aneurysm stent placement, the recent large, multicenter Eurostar study questioned the very efficacy and advisability of stent grafting. Endoleak, stent dislodgement, and aneurysm expansion or rupture were disturbingly widespread in medium-term follow-up. It should be remembered that stents were designed to keep tissue from encroaching on the vessel lumen, not to keep the vessel from expanding. One noted authority believes that the aneurysmal aorta essentially "ignores" the stent graft, dilating regardless of the stent, at its own pace. (Personal communication, Dr. L. Svennson.) Also remember that the natural history of the thoracic aorta is that they grow slowly, and that hard end points (rupture, dissection, and death) take years to be realized. For this reason, short-term stent studies are nearly meaningless. Long-term studies are needed. This new modality should be approached with enthusiasm tempered by caution. Its advent should not at this point influence overall intervention strategy.

Achneck HE et al. Safety of thoracic aortic surgery in the present era. Ann Thorac Surg. 2007 Oct;84(4):1180–5. [PMID: 17888967]

Coselli JS et al. Cerebrospinal fluid drainage reduces paraplegia after thoracoabdominal aortic aneurysm repair: results of a randomized clinical trial. J Vasc Surg. 2002 Apr;35(4):631–9. [PMID: 11932655]

David TE. Aortic valve-sparing operations for aortic root aneurysm. Semin Thorac Cardiovasc Surg. 2001 Jul;13(3):291–6. [PMID: 11568875]

Davies RR et al. Yearly rupture or dissection rates for thoracic aortic aneurysms: simple prediction based on size. Ann Thorac Surg. 2002 Jan;73(1):17–27. [PMID: 11834007]

Davies RR et al. Novel measurement of relative aortic size predicts rupture of thoracic aortic aneurysms. Ann Thorac Surg. 2006 Jan;81(1):169–77. [PMID: 16368358]

Elefteriades JA. Beating a sudden killer. Sci Am. 2005 Aug;293(2):64–71. [PMID: 16053139]

Elefteriades JA et al. Endovascular stenting for descending aneurysms: wave of the future or the emperor's new clothes? J Thorac Cardiovasc Surg. 2007 Feb;133(2):285–8. [PMID: 17258546]

Elefteriades JA et al. Litigation in nontraumatic aortic diseases—a tempest in the malpractice maelstrom. Cardiology. 2008;109(4):263–72. [PMID: 17873491]

Goldstein LJ et al. Stroke in surgery of the thoracic aorta: incidence, impact, etiology, and prevention. J Thorac Cardiovasc Surg. 2001 Nov;122(5):935–45. [PMID: 11689799]

Habashi JP et al. Losartan, an AT1 antagonist, prevents aortic aneurysm in a mouse model of Marfan syndrome. Science. 2006 Apr 7;312(5770):117–21. [PMID: 16601194]

Hasham SN et al. Mapping a locus for familial thoracic aortic aneurysms and dissections (TAAD2) to 3p24-25. Circulation. 2003 Jul 1;107(25):3184–90. [PMID: 16847387]

Koullias GJ et al. Increased tissue microarray matrix metalloproteinase expression favors proteolysis in thoracic aortic aneurysms and dissections. Ann Thorac Surg. 2004 Dec;78(6):2106–10. [PMID: 15561045]

Laheij RJ et al. Need for secondary interventions after endovascular repair of abdominal aortic aneurysms. Intermediate-term follow-up results of a European collaborative registry (EUROSTAR). Br J Surg. 2000 Dec;87(12):1666–73. [PMID: 11122182]

Svensson LG et al. Prospective randomized neurocognitive and S-100 study of hypothermic circulatory arrest, retrograde brain perfusion, and antegrade brain perfusion for aortic arch operations. Ann Thorac Surg. 2001 Jun;71(6):1905–12. [PMID: 11426767]

AORTIC DISSECTION

ESSENTIALS OF DIAGNOSIS

▶ Usually middle-aged or elderly hypertensive men; occasionally, young patients with history of Marfan syndrome, other connective tissue disorder. Rarely, young women in late pregnancy or labor.

▶ Acute chest pain, frequently with hemodynamic instability.

▶ Possible appearance of shock but normal or elevated blood pressure.

▶ Various neurologic symptoms, such as Horner syndrome, paraplegia, and stroke.

▶ Absent or unequal peripheral pulses.

▶ Aortic regurgitation.

▶ Widened mediastinum on chest radiograph.

▶ Confirmatory aortic imaging study.

▶ General Considerations

A. Terminology

Aortic dissection refers to a splitting of the layers of the aortic wall (within the media) permitting longitudinal propagation of a blood-filled space within the aortic wall. Aortic dissection is thought to be the most common cause of death related to the human aorta (Figure 35–15).

Three related but distinct entities—acute aortic transection, rupture of aortic aneurysm, and aortic dissection—are commonly confused, both in substance and in terminology (Figure 35–16). **Acute aortic transection** is a traumatic phenomenon, with disruption of the wall of the aorta, without a propagating dissection. The aortic wall is intrinsically normal and resistant to the dissection process. **Rupture** of aortic aneurysm is self-explanatory; however, confusion in terminology may arise if an acute aortic transection or an

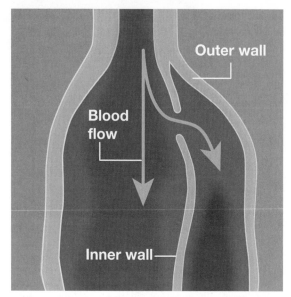

▲ **Figure 35–15.** Schematic depiction of aortic dissection.

acute aortic dissection happens to rupture—a common eventuality. **Acute aortic dissection** refers to the very specific process of separation of layers of the aortic wall discussed fully in this chapter. For dissection to occur, the aortic wall must nearly always be affected by structural disease of the media.

Recent years have brought recognition of two important variants of aortic dissection: intramural hematoma (IMH) and penetrating aortic ulcer (PAU) (Figure 35–17).

Intramural hematoma of the aorta differs from typical dissection in that there is no flap defining a true and a false lumen, and the hematoma is located circumferentially around the aortic lumen, rather than obliquely oriented across the aortic lumen. Whether the IMH arises from a small intimal tear (not detected radiographically) or from a rupture of a vasa vasorum within the aortic wall remains controversial. The clinical course is variable; the hematoma may persist, reabsorb (returning the aorta to a normal appearance), lead to aneurysm with the possibility of rupture, or convert to dissection. Penetrating aortic ulcer involves a local penetration deep into the wall of the aorta, resembling a penetrating ulcer of the stomach. This lesion disrupts the internal elastic lamina and erodes into the media, which in some cases may mimic or initiate aortic dissection, pseudoaneurysm formation, IMH, or rupture. Extensive arteriosclerosis is a common accompaniment of PAU (Figure 35–17).

It is important to recognize that IMH and PAU are diseases of advanced age. In addition, it is important point to mention that although branch vessel occlusion is part and parcel of typical aortic dissection, the variants of aortic dissection PAU and IMH never occlude branch vessels.

The general management of these lesions is still a matter of debate. Most authorities believe that descending aortic IMH and PAU can be managed medically, with "anti-impulse" therapy (see Treatment section). However, early (but not immediate) surgical intervention is preferred in suitable operative candidates to preempt rupture due to a high incidence of death from rupture. Some of the discrepancy in recommendations also has to do with regional differences: in Japan, IMH behaves in a more benign fashion than in the Western world, perhaps reflecting fundamental genetic differences in the aortic wall, or differences in body size and aortic dimension.

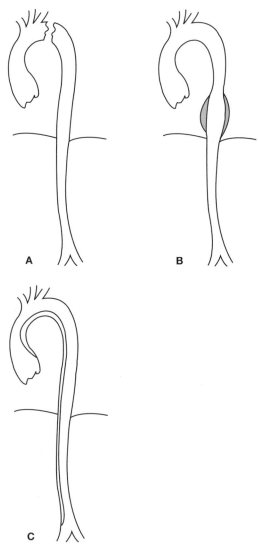

▲ **Figure 35–16.** Frequently confused terminology. See text for a description of the very different disorders of acute aortic transection **(A)**, ruptured aortic aneurysm **(B)**, and acute aortic dissection **(C)**.

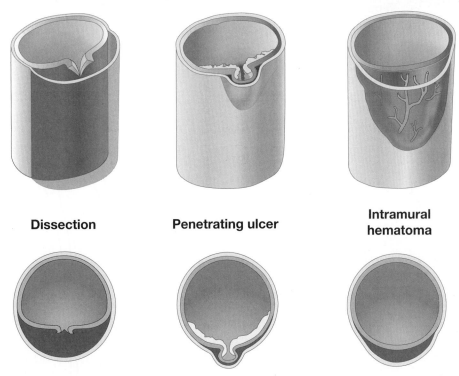

Dissection   **Penetrating ulcer**   **Intramural hematoma**

▲ **Figure 35–17.** Schematic of variant forms of aortic dissection: typical dissection, penetrating ulcer, and intramural hematoma. A true dissection has to have a flap.

For ascending variant dissections IMH and PAU, most authorities agree on aggressive immediate surgical intervention, although one recent paper from Japan challenges the need for routine surgery, even in this anatomic location.

B. Anatomic Classification

Aortic dissections may be ascending (type A) or descending (type B). The two patterns are determined by the location of the inciting intimal tear. Tears occur in two very specific locations: (1) in the ascending aorta, 2–3 cm above the coronary arteries and (2) in the descending aorta, 1–2 cm beyond the left subclavian artery. The first type of tear produces ascending dissection and the second, descending dissection. Please note that ascending dissections usually go around the aortic arch to involve the descending and abdominal portions of the aorta (Figure 35–18).

▶ Clinical Findings

A. Symptoms and Signs

Aortic dissection produces intense, severe pain, often described as tearing or shearing in quality. This pain is sudden in onset (a differentiating feature from the pain of

myocardial infarction) and very severe in intensity. Most patients describe this as the most intense pain of their lives, more intense even than childbirth or a kidney stone. The pain of ascending dissection is felt in the anterior chest, substernally, and that of a descending dissection is felt posteriorly, between the scapulae. The "tearing," "shearing," "knife-like" quality of the pain is quite consistent with the pathophysiology. The pain can migrate downward, into the flank or pelvis, as the dissection process propagates distally. Impending aortic rupture should be considered when pain subsides and later recurs. On occasion, painless dissection does occur, perhaps as often as 15% of patients; this is usually picked up later, on a routine imaging study done for another reason.

B. Diagnostic Studies

1. Chest radiography—Chest radiography is a useful screening test. Many, if not most, aortic dissections occur in the background of a chronic aortic aneurysm. To the astute observer, chronic thoracic aneurysms can be visualized on a chest radiograph. The enlarged ascending aorta will protrude to the right of the upper mediastinal border, an arch aneurysm will show as an exaggerated aortic knob, and a descend-

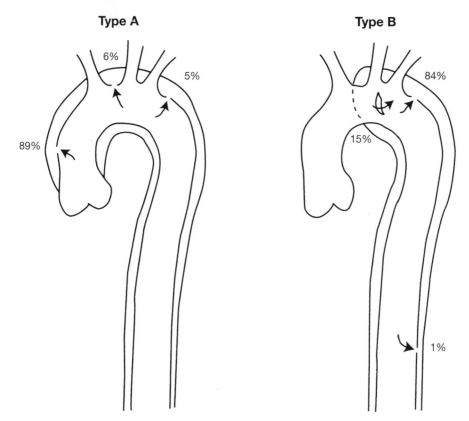

▲ **Figure 35–18.** Stanford classification system. (Reprinted, with permission, from Daily PO et al. Ann Thorac Surg. 1970;10:244.)

ing aortic aneurysm will be visible as a left-deviated stripe of the descending aorta. In case of aortic dissection, chest radiography will usually provide additional clues: most commonly, widening of the mediastinal shadow, pleural effusion, or inward displacement of aortic medial calcification.

2. Three-dimensional imaging methods—Multiple types of three-dimensional imaging modalities are pertinent in aneurysm disease and aortic dissection and all have excellent sensitivity and specificity: transesophageal echocardiography (TEE), CT scanning, and MRI. Many patients undergo a TEE and either a CT or an MRI. The CT or MRI shows the three-dimensional structure of the entire aorta. The TEE, while partially blinded to the aortic arch and abdominal aorta, provides information about pericardial effusion and tamponade, valve function, and left ventricular function. Transesophageal echocardiography images both ascending and descending aortas well.

The primary diagnostic criterion for aortic dissection by CT or MRI is demonstration of two contrast-filled lumens separated by an intimal flap. Sensitivity and specificity of CT and MRI for diagnosis of aortic dissection are approaching 100%. Transesophageal echocardiography does not lag far behind in accuracy. Contrast aortography, once the gold standard, has fallen by the wayside for diagnosis of aortic dissection, being more invasive and not offering nearly the amount of three-dimensional anatomic information afforded by CT, MRI, and TEE.

▶ **Differential Diagnosis**

The imaging studies discussed above provide specific information that rules in or out the presence of aneurysm or dissection. The main diagnostic issue involves (1) maintaining a high index of suspicion for aneurysm disease and (2) being aware of the protean presentations of aneurysm disease. In particular, aortic dissection has been called "the great masquerader" because it can produce symptoms related to virtually any organ. A high index of suspicion is required to establish the diagnosis promptly, since the presentations of aortic dissection are so myriad and mimic a wide array of other diseases. Specifically, all patients admitted with chest pain without obvious cause should have their thoracic aorta imaged. Patients with a ruptured or dissected thoracic aorta often "masquerade" as heart attacks. It is especially important to rule out aortic dissection in patients about to be treated for myocardial infarction, as administration of thrombolytic drugs in patients with acute aortic dissection is associated with a high mortality rate.

Among conditions for which aortic dissection can be confused are myocardial infarction, musculoskeletal chest pain, pericarditis, pleuritis, pneumothorax, pulmonary embolism, cholecystitis, ureteral colic, appendicitis, mesenteric ischemia, pyelonephritis, stroke, transient ischemic attack, and primary limb ischemia. Especially troublesome to clinicians in emergency departments are patients with abdominal symptoms and signs without apparent abdominal cause; aortic dissection must be considered in such patients.

Given the extensive differential diagnosis, aggressive, objective diagnostic testing is necessary when the possibility of aortic dissection is considered. The diagnosis is most strongly suggested when migratory chest and back pain of less than 24 hours duration arises in a patient with a history of hypertension. The following recommendations are made for the physicians who are the first to evaluate such patients: (1) Keep aortic dissection (and ruptured thoracic or abdominal aneurysm) in the differential diagnosis. (2) Image freely and liberally to rule out aortic pathology. A CT scan can exclude all three major chest diagnoses likely to result in death: coronary artery disease, pulmonary embolism, and aortic aneurysm or dissection. The modern 64-slice scanners are ideal for this purpose. (3) Remember the D-dimer test. A negative D-dimer, which is most commonly applied to rule-out pulmonary embolism, also rules out aortic dissection. The clot that forms in the false lumen of an aortic dissection liberates D-dimer quite strikingly. This simple blood test is nearly 100% sensitive in picking up aortic dissection. (4) Remember to look at the aorta, even if the CT scan is ordered for other, especially abdominal, examination.

Attention to these recommendations will also serve to discourage litigation for failure to diagnose aortic dissection.

▶ Treatment

A. Pharmacotherapy

Most patients will require intensive medical therapy for acute aortic dissection, either as sole treatment or as a stabilizing measure until appropriate surgical therapy is undertaken.

It has been recognized that aortic dissection propagates more vigorously when either blood pressure or force of cardiac contraction are excessive. Accordingly, blood pressure needs to be controlled in patients with acute aortic dissection or other acute aortic syndromes, including aortic rupture or impending rupture. Nitroglycerin or nitroprusside are usually used for this purpose, because of their effectiveness, their rapid onset of action, and their quick cessation of action upon discontinuation. Blood pressure should be reduced as low as possible without producing neurologic dysfunction or oliguria. Usually, the severity of

general occlusive vascular disease determines how low the blood pressure can safely be taken. The blood pressure may be lowered to 90–100 mm Hg initially, until the patient's response can be evaluated. For older patients with extensive end-organ vascular disease, lowering the blood pressure pharmacologically to 120–130 mm Hg may need to be satisfactory.

However, to lower blood pressure by afterload reduction alone would actually increase the sheer stress on the aortic wall. It is crucial to decrease the force of cardiac contraction (Figure 35–19). The morphology of the arterial pulse wave must be blunted by decreasing the force of cardiac contraction. The dp/dt, reflected in the upslope of the initial portion of the aortic pulse wave, must be decreased, usually by administering a short-acting β-blocker, such as esmolol. Another approach is administration of the α- and β-adrenergic antagonist labetalol by intravenous infusion. When β-blocking drugs are contraindicated, calcium channel blockers are a reasonable substitute.

Together, the afterload reduction and the β-blockade are referred to as "anti-impulse" therapy for acute aortic dissection. Regardless of whether the dissection is ascending or descending, or whether or not the patient will be taken emergently to the operating room, such therapy must be instituted—to discourage rupture or extension of the dissection. Anti-impulse therapy is the appropriate initial response

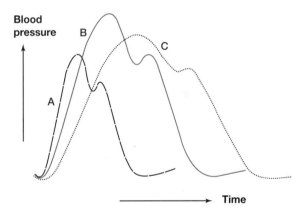

▲ **Figure 35–19.** Diagram of aortic pressure curves under various conditions. The continuous line **(B)** represents the baseline state. Administration of a vasodilator agent such as nitroprusside is represented by the dashed curve **(A)**. There is significant decrease in pressure levels and acceleration in heart rate, but this is accompanied by a steepest slope of the ascending portion of the curve (increased dp/dt_{max}). β-Blockade administration is represented by the dotted line **(C)**. Although the degree of pressure lowering is usually smaller, the drug negative inotropic and chronotropic effects result in decreased impulse and dp/dt_{max}.

once the diagnosis of any type of acute aortic dissection or related process is made. Often, such therapy is undertaken while imaging studies are being performed to confirm the diagnosis of aortic dissection and define the anatomic type, location, and extent of the process. Definitive therapeutic decisions and treatments will follow.

B. Surgical Treatment

For acute aortic dissection, the following guidelines regarding definitive therapy apply.

Ascending aortic aneurysms require urgent surgery because death from intrapericardial rupture, aortic regurgitation, or myocardial infarction from coronary artery involvement usually occurs in patients who do not undergo surgery. The dissection layers are reapproximated as a "sandwich" between layers of Teflon felt (Figure 35–20). Overall survival at experienced centers is about 85% for patients with acute type A aortic dissection. The exact surgical procedure performed, vis-à-vis the proximal aortic root and the coronary arteries varies depending on the circumstances. For patients in whom dissection occurs in the setting of Marfan disease or other cause of annuloaortic ectasia (proximal root enlargement), the aortic valve, aortic root, and ascending aorta are replaced with a prefabricated "composite graft" including both a valve and a graft (see Figure 35–15B).

Descending dissections, in the absence of specific vascular complications, do well with medical management (short- and long-term "anti-impulse" therapy with β-blockers and afterload-reducing medication). If a specific complication occurs, this is addressed directly by surgery ("complication-specific" approach to descending aortic dissection). Ninety-one percent of patients survived the initial hospitalization (type B aortic dissection is "milder" than type A dissection) and about 66% had a completely uncomplicated course while receiving anti-impulse medical therapy alone. The majority of complications were related to vascular malperfusion of specific organs.

The subacute and chronic stages of aortic dissection are managed differently. Once the patient with type A dissection has been brought safely through surgery, or the type B patient has been stabilized with anti-impulse therapy, they are observed closely for the first month, with repeat aortic imaging. After that point, it is uncommon for the dissection to extend, cause symptoms, or rupture in the short-term to mid-term. The patients are then monitored the same as those with chronic aneurysm. Over years, enlargement of the dissected aorta will develop in some patients and require resection. The same dimensional criteria for surgical intervention can be applied as for non-dissected aneurysms. It is usually the most proximal portion of the descending aorta, just beyond the subclavian artery, that dilates first and requires surgical replacement.

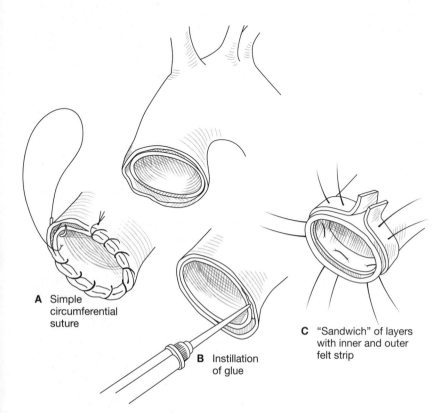

A Simple circumferential suture

B Instillation of glue

C "Sandwich" of layers with inner and outer felt strip

▲ **Figure 35–20.** Alternate methods of dealing with the dissection prior to anastomosis.

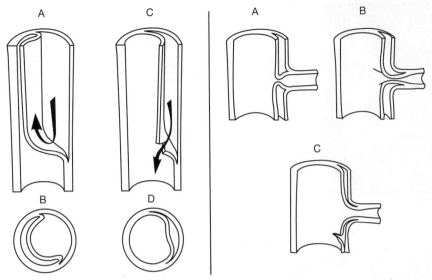

▲ Figure 35–21. Depiction of means by which the dissected lumen can compromise the true lumen, seen in various planes. The figures on the left look at the aorta itself. Note the relief of impingement when the flap fenestrates (images left, C and D and right, C).

▶ Prognosis

Aortic dissection is often fatal without early diagnosis and aggressive treatment. The presenting symptoms and signs are so myriad and nonspecific (see above) that dissection may be overlooked initially in up to 40% of cases; in fact, the diagnosis is not made until postmortem examination in a disturbingly large fraction of patients. This can be a frequent cause of litigation, and guidelines have recently been outlined so litigation can be avoided. Few other conditions demand such prompt diagnosis and treatment, since the mortality rate of untreated dissection approaches 1–2% per hour during the first 48 hours, 89% at 14 days, and 90% at 3 months.

Aortic dissection can result in death in four ways: (1) intrapericardial rupture (of an ascending dissection), (2) acute aortic regurgitation (from an ascending aortic dissection), (3) free rupture into the pleural space (of a descending dissection), and (4) occlusion of any branch of the aorta (with consequent organ ischemia).

Branch vessel occlusion comes about via impingement on the true lumen of any branch vessel (coronaries to iliacs) by the distended false lumen (Figure 35–21). The acute aortic regurgitation of an ascending dissection may be very poorly tolerated, compared with chronic aortic regurgitation, because the sudden nature allows no time for cardiac adaptation. Cardiogenic shock may result.

Elefteriades JA. What operation for acute Type A dissection? J Thorac Cardiovasc Surg. 2002 Feb;123(2):201–3. [PMID: 11828276]

Hatzaras IS et al. Role of exertion or emotion as inciting events for acute aortic dissection. Am J Cardiol. 2007 Nov 1;100(9):1470–2. [PMID: 17950810]

Hatzaras I et al. Weight lifting and aortic dissection: more evidence for a connection. Cardiology. 2007;107(2):103–6. [PMID: 12821554]

Tittle SL et al. Midterm follow-up penetrating ulcer and intramural hematoma of the aorta. J Thorac Cardiovasc Surg. 2002 Jun;123(6):1051–9. [PMID: 12063450]

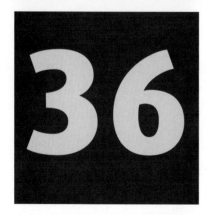

Evaluation & Treatment of the Perioperative Patient

Sanjiv J. Shah, MD

The prevalence of cardiovascular disease and the death rate associated with it rises sharply after age 45, an age when the incidence of noncardiac surgeries is also increasing, and approximately one-third of the 25 million surgical procedures done annually are performed in patients with cardiovascular diseases. Cardiac deaths and nonfatal myocardial infarction (MI) occur in about 0.2% of all cases of general anesthesia and surgery (about 500,000 events annually). Cardiac deaths account for approximately 40% of all perioperative mortality, the same proportion as sepsis, although in many cases the cause of death is multisystem organ failure. These figures underestimate the total effect of cardiovascular diseases because another 500,000 persons a year suffer nonfatal MI, unstable angina, or congestive heart failure (CHF) perioperatively, prolonging both their time in the intensive care unit and the total hospital stay.

Although there is great potential to reduce perioperative cardiovascular risk, it is also impractical, unnecessary, and potentially harmful to perform cardiovascular testing in all patients prior to noncardiac surgery. Therefore, it is important to determine perioperative risk, decide whether cardiac testing is appropriate, and to provide prophylactic treatment to reduce risk.

▶ Preoperative Risk Assessment

An individual patient's preoperative risk profile depends on three main factors: the patient's history, current medical and functional status, and the type of surgery. Preoperative electrocardiography can detect arrhythmia and prior silent MI, but it rarely changes management.

Table 36–1 lists cardiac risk based on type of noncardiac surgery. In the evaluation of perioperative patients, understanding the nature of the surgery is of prime importance. Is this an emergency surgery? If yes, the clinician should advise to proceed with the surgery and evaluate the patient's cardiac risk postoperatively. On the other hand, if the patient is young, without systemic disease, and undergoing a minor surgery or procedure, the clinician should advise to proceed with surgery without further cardiac workup. However,

most patients who require perioperative cardiac consultation are not so straightforward. In these patients, there are three algorithms that can help identify perioperative risk and the need for further cardiac testing.

A. Algorithms

1. Revised Cardiac Risk Index (RCRI)—This algorithm is simple to use, and it helps identify patients who require β-blockers perioperatively. *However, the RCRI may have less accuracy in patients undergoing major vascular surgery.* Use the RCRI as follows:

  a. Assign 1 point to each of the following risk factors if present:
    • High-risk surgery (intraperitoneal, intrathoracic, suprainguinal vascular).
    • Ischemic heart disease (history of MI or current angina, use of sublingual nitroglycerin, recent abnormal stress test, Q waves on electrocardiogram [ECG], or history of coronary revascularization with ongoing chest pain).
    • History of heart failure.
    • History of cerebrovascular disease (stroke, transient ischemic attack).
    • Diabetes mellitus requiring insulin.
    • Preoperative creatinine > 2.0 mg/dL.

  b. Assign a risk class to determine cardiac complication rate to help counsel the patient and also the surgeon:
    • Class I: zero risk factors, 0.4%
    • Class II: one risk factor, 0.9%
    • Class III: two risk factors, 6.6%
    • Class IV: three or more risk factors, 11.0%

  c. Patients who are categorized as having risk class III or IV will require additional cardiac testing for risk stratification and more aggressive perioperative medical management to reduce the risk of complications.

Table 36–1. Cardiac Risk Stratification for Noncardiac Surgical Procedures According to ACC Guidelines.

High (Reported cardiac risk often greater than 5%)
  Emergent major operations, particularly in the elderly
  Aortic and other major vascular surgery
  Peripheral vascular surgery
  Anticipated prolonged surgical procedures associated with large
    fluid shifts and/or blood loss
Intermediate (Reported cardiac risk generally less than 5%)
  Carotid endarterectomy surgery
  Head and neck surgery
  Intraperitoneal and intrathoracic surgery
  Orthopedic surgery
  Prostate surgery
Low (Reported cardiac risk generally less than 1%)
  Endoscopic procedures
  Superficial procedure
  Cataract surgery
  Breast surgery

ACC, American College of Cardiology.
Reproduced with permission from Eagle KA, et al. Circulation. 2002;105:1251.

2. American College of Cardiology/American Heart Association (ACC/AHA) Guidelines—These guidelines are somewhat cumbersome (Figure 36–1). In simplified terms, the ACC/AHA guidelines recommend noninvasive cardiac stress testing in patients with two or more of the following risk factors:

- Intermediate clinical predictors: mild angina, prior MI, compensated or prior heart failure, diabetes mellitus, or renal insufficiency.
- Poor functional capacity (< 4 metabolic equivalents): cannot walk more than one or two blocks on level ground; cannot do light housework, such as washing dishes or dusting; cannot climb a flight of stairs or walk up a hill.
- High-risk surgery: vascular surgery, prolonged procedure, or anticipated large fluid shifts or blood loss.

3. American College of Physicians (ACP) Guidelines—In general, the ACP guidelines advocate less perioperative cardiac testing while the ACC/AHA guidelines lean toward more perioperative cardiac testing. The ACP approach, which is also quite lengthy, is as follows:

a. Is the patient young, without systemic disease and undergoing a minor surgery? If yes, no further evaluation required. If no, proceed with further evaluation.

b. Is this an emergency surgery? If yes, no further evaluation required and recommend proceeding with the operation. If not, proceed with further evaluation.

c. Apply the Modified Cardiac Risk Index (assign points for each risk factor):

- Coronary artery disease: MI < 6 months ago? 10 points; MI > 6 months ago? 5 points; angina walking one or two blocks or climbing one flight of stairs? 10 points; angina with any physical activity? 20 points.
- Alveolar pulmonary edema: in last week? 10 points; ever? 5 points.
- Suspected critical aortic stenosis? 10 points.
- Arrhythmias: rhythm other than sinus? 5 points; more than five premature ventricular contractions/minute? 5 points.
- Poor medical status? Any one of the following (P_{O_2} < 60 mm Hg, P_{CO_2} > 50 mm Hg, potassium < 3 mmol/L, creatinine > 3 mg/dL, blood urea nitrogen > 50 mg/dL, or bedridden): 5 points.
- Age > 70 years: 5 points.
- Emergency surgery: 10 points.

d. Add up points for above risk factors:

- Score < 15: proceed to next step.
- Score > 20: the patient is at high risk for cardiac complications. Optimize medical management and consider angiography or revascularization based on same criteria for nonsurgical patient.

e. Collect cardiac variables and assign risk:

- Age over 70 years, angina, ECG evidence of ST-segment depression or of history of MI or Q waves ventricular arrhythmia, diabetes mellitus, hypertension with left ventricular hypertrophy, history of heart failure.
- If the patient has fewer than two of the above variables, he or she is at low risk for cardiac complications and no further testing is needed.
- If the patient has two or more of the above variables, he or she is at intermediate risk for cardiac complications; proceed to next step.

f. Is the patient undergoing vascular surgery? If the answer is no, additional testing is not necessary. If the answer is yes, proceed to next step (noninvasive cardiac stress testing).

g. Perform noninvasive cardiac stress testing. If the test results are normal, no further testing is needed. If the results are abnormal, consider angiography or revascularization based on the same criteria as for the nonsurgical patient.

B. Intermediate Risk Patients

While perioperative management of low-risk and high-risk patients is relatively straightforward, the management of patients who fall into the intermediate risk is more challenging. Low-risk patients can proceed to surgery without further cardiac evaluation. For high-risk patients, management should include one or more of the following: postpone or cancel surgery until high-risk features improve or resolve, start

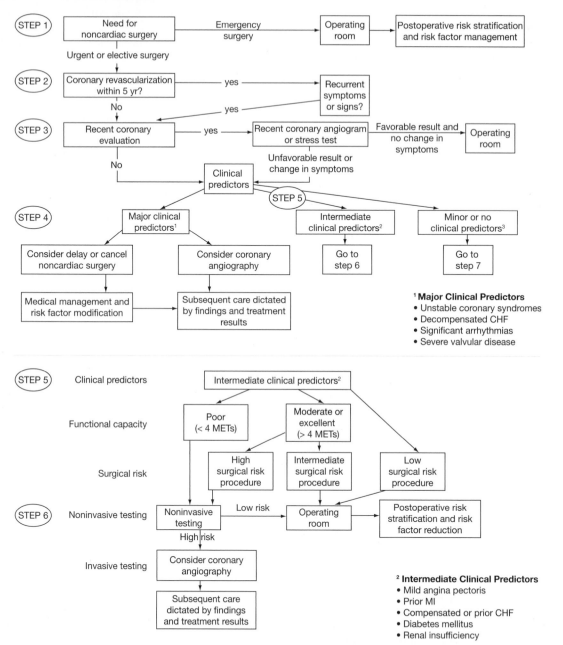

▲ Figure 36–1. American Heart Association/American College of Cardiology guidelines for preoperative evaluation prior to noncardiac surgery. CHF, congestive heart failure; ECG, electrocardiogram; METs, metabolic equivalents; MI, myocardial infarction. (Reproduced, with permission, from Fleisher LA et al. J Am Coll Cardiol. 2007;50:1707.) (continued)

treatment of the underlying high-risk features, or proceed to invasive testing. In high-risk patients with a high pretest probability of disease, noninvasive tests are not helpful, because a negative result will most likely be a false negative.

Intermediate-risk patients derive the most benefit from perioperative medical management or stress testing, or both.

For most patients in the intermediate risk category, it is important to obtain imaging with the stress test because ECG

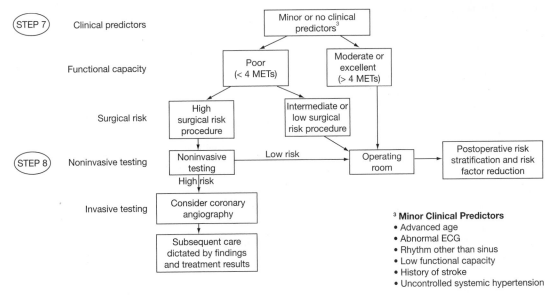

▲ Figure 36-1. (*Continued*)

alone is unlikely to move the posttest probability beyond the threshold for treatment or no treatment.

1. Exercise versus pharmacologic stress testing—The choice between exercise and pharmacologic stress testing follows the same guidelines as those for routine, nonperioperative stress testing. Exercise testing can provide valuable information on functional capacity, but patients may not be able to reach 85% of maximal predicted heart rate due to deconditioning or β-blocker use. Since β-blockers are important in the perioperative period, withholding them is not ideal.

Dipyridamole or adenosine is preferred in cases where arrhythmia (eg, rapid atrial fibrillation) or frequent premature atrial or ventricular beats are present. These agents are relatively contraindicated in patients with significant bronchospasm, in whom dobutamine is the agent of choice.

2. Type of imaging technique—When choosing either echocardiography or nuclear imaging (the two most commonly available stress imaging modalities), it is most important to determine which modality has better reliability and expertise at the clinician's hospital or clinic. In published studies, both imaging techniques have good negative predictive value (> 90%) but poor positive predictive value (< 25%). Echocardiography with contrast (to assist in endocardial border definition) may be more helpful in obese patients (who may have more attenuation defects on nuclear imaging). Nuclear imaging may be more useful in patients with left bundle branch block and when atrial fibrillation is present. Newer modalities include rubidium positron emission tomography (PET) scanning, which provides better resolution images. However, patients must be cooperative and must

be able to hold still for longer periods of time. Cardiac computed tomography provides anatomic assessment of the coronary arteries but does not provide data on ischemic burden, and has not been adequately evaluated in the perioperative setting.

C. Understanding Cardiac Complications

Despite the risks during general anesthesia, including myocardial depression, transient hypotension, and tachycardia, very few cardiac events occur during the surgery itself. The incidence of perioperative cardiac complications actually peaks between 2 and 5 days postoperatively. These data imply that factors activated during or following surgery, and not only the surgery itself, are crucial in determining adverse outcomes.

Pneumonitis and microatelectasis produce ventilation-perfusion mismatch, and sedation or analgesia may cause respiratory depression and interfere with coughing, all of which contribute to arterial hypoxemia. Thrombocytosis and a generalized hypercoagulable state, caused by increased fibrinogen and activators from the damaged tissue, favor thrombosis. At the same time, sympathetically mediated increases in heart rate, blood pressure, and contractility increase myocardial oxygen consumption, whereas thrombotic tendencies, anemia, and arterial desaturation impede oxygen delivery to the myocardium. In a patient with underlying coronary artery disease, this situation may lead to myocardial ischemia or infarction. The imbalance may be further exaggerated because antihypertensive or anginal medications are often withheld. By the third or fourth postoperative day, the patient is hypermetabolic, with negative nitrogen and potassium balances. A natriuresis follows, which can produce hypovolemia and further activate the sympathetic nervous system.

All of these factors provide the exact setting in which a perioperative MI may occur. Perioperative MI carries a high mortality and presents atypically (usually without chest pain). Clues such as hypotension, pulmonary edema, altered mental status, and arrhythmia may be the only signs alerting the clinician to the possibility of a perioperative MI. Therefore, those caring for perioperative patients must have a high level of suspicion in order to detect perioperative MI.

Fleisher LA et al. ACC/AHA 2007 Guidelines on Perioperative Cardiovascular Evaluation and Care for Noncardiac Surgery: Executive Summary: A Report of the American College of Cardiology/American Heart Association Task Force on Practice Guidelines (Writing Committee to Revise the 2002 Guidelines on Perioperative Cardiovascular Evaluation for Noncardiac Surgery). J Am Coll Cardiol. 2007;50:1707–32. [PMID: 17950159]

Guidelines for assessing and managing the perioperative risk from coronary artery disease associated with major noncardiac surgery. American College of Physicians. Ann Intern Med. 1997;127(4):309–12. [PMID: 9265433]

▶ Treatment to Reduce Perioperative Risk

Knowledge of how new therapies can reduce cardiac risk has progressed rapidly in recent years. Perioperative medicine now provides "risk management" (through medicine such as β-blocker) in addition to the standard risk prediction. In general, the higher the patient's risk, the greater benefit derived from the use of therapies such as β-blockers and statins. Therefore, healthcare providers should use the Revised Cardiac Risk Index (see above) to stratify patients, and then use this to determine whether or not to treat.

A. β-Blockers

These agents are first-line therapy to reduce perioperative morbidity and mortality in high-risk patients. Current guidelines have advocated β-blockers in almost all intermediate- or high-risk patients undergoing noncardiac surgery. However, two recent studies in vascular surgery patients did not show a benefit, and a meta-analysis of seven randomized controlled trials did not conclusively show a benefit with β-blockers. Another recent retrospective review of 600,000 patients showed that β-blocker benefit was greater in higher-risk patients. Therefore, the decision to use β-blockers should be individualized. If the patient is already taking a β-blocker for other reasons (eg, coronary artery disease), β-blockers should be continued in the perioperative setting. Patients with an RCRI score (see above) of ≥ three benefit from β-blockers, while those with an RCRI score of zero are harmed by β-blockers.

In patients deemed to benefit from β-blockers in the perioperative setting, oral metoprolol is started on the day of the perioperative visit. For patients who were taking β-blockers before the surgery, the dose is titrated to a heart rate of 60 bpm. Postoperatively, metoprolol is started at 5–10 mg intravenously every 4–6 hours as needed to keep the heart rate 60–70 bpm until the patient can take oral medications. Oral β-blockers are then continued for 30 days postoperatively and indefinitely in patients who were previously taking these medications.

B. Statins

One small randomized controlled trial and several observational studies have found a benefit to statin use, with greater benefit in higher risk patients. Therefore, if there are no major contraindications, intermediate- and high-risk patients should be taking a statin prior to major noncardiac surgery.

C. Clonidine

There is evidence that clonidine (an α_2-adrenergic agonist) reduces MI and mortality in high-risk vascular surgery patients. Clonidine's transdermal delivery system works well in the perioperative setting, but clonidine is not ideal for outpatient management and carries the risk of rebound hypertension. For these reasons, clonidine should not be used routinely but can be a good choice for in-hospital control of hypertension in the perioperative patient who cannot take oral medications.

D. Calcium Channel Blockers

Verapamil and diltiazem (centrally acting calcium channel blockers) are second-line therapy for reducing perioperative ischemia or arrhythmia, or both. Use in high-risk patients who have a contraindication to β-blockers.

E. Maintanence of Normothermia

Maintaining normal body temperature is easy to perform, low risk, and has been shown to significantly reduce perioperative cardiac events in high-risk patients undergoing major abdominal or vascular surgery.

F. Deep Venous Thrombosis Prophylaxis

Although not a routine part of perioperative cardiac risk assessment and treatment, it is important to check for appropriate perioperative deep venous thrombosis (DVT) prophylaxis since DVT (with resultant pulmonary embolism) can cause significant cardiac instability and death. Low-molecular-weight-heparins are being used increasingly in place of unfractionated heparin and appear equivalent or, in some cases, superior.

G. Endocarditis Prophylaxis

Recommendations for management of endocarditis prophylaxis have changed dramatically with the publication of the new AHA guidelines. In general, the new AHA guidelines advocate less use of antibiotic prophyalxis because of the lack of evidence of benefit in humans, and the fact that transient bacteremia occurs frequently, and there is no evidence that dental and other procedures increase rates of bacteremia more than activities of daily living alone. The AHA guidelines state that only patients at the highest risk for endocarditis should receive antibiotic prophylaxis. These high-risk patients include those with prosthetic cardiac valve, previous infective endocarditis, unrepaired cyanotic congenital heart disease (including palliative shunts and conduits), completely repaired congenital heart defect with prosthetic material or device during the first 6 months post-procedure, repaired congenital heart defects with residual defects at site of prosthetic material which prevent endothelialization, and patients who have undergone heart transplantation in whom significant valvular heart disease develops.

Prophylaxis for dental procedures in the aforementioned patients is only recommended if the procedure involves manipulation of gingival tissue, manipulation of periapical region of teeth, or perforation of the oral mucosa.

Endocarditis prophylaxis is no longer recommended for genitourinary or gastrointestinal procedures.

H. Perioperative Medication Management

Management of outpatient medications in the perioperative period is underappreciated but extremely important for ensuring an optimal patient outcome. Many times, essential medications are discontinued and not restarted before the patient is discharged from the hospital, leading to potentially disastrous outcomes. Other times, the conversion of oral to intravenous (and back to oral) dosing of medications causes under- or over-treatment.

1. Anticoagulation management—Nowhere is perioperative medication management more important than in anticoagulation, since use of anticoagulants can cause increased bleeding intra- and post-operatively. Alternatively, too little anticoagulation can lead to severe morbidity (eg, stroke, MI, and stent thrombosis) and even death.

A. WARFARIN—One of the most common reasons for cardiac consultation (besided assessing perioperative risk) is to manage warfarin perioperatively. Although the risks of discontinuing warfarin therapy 4 days prior to surgery are low, in the few patients in whom thromboembolism develops, the results (stroke, pulmonary embolism, MI, or death) can be devastating. Therefore, in high-risk patients, bridging with unfractionated or intravenous heparin is important and can reduce perioperative risk of thromboembolism. However, use of heparins can increase bleeding. Therefore, it is important to carefully select patients who will need bridging with heparin. The keys to optimal warfarin management is to identify the indication for warfarin, and assess the patient's risk for thromboembolism. Bridging with heparin is advised in the following situations: (1) atrial fibrilla-

tion and rheumatic heart disease, history of thromboembolism, or mechanical heart valve; (2) older mechanical heart valve in mitral position (single-disk or caged-ball), or recently placed mechanical valve (< 3 months); or (3) hypercoagulable state, venous or arterial thromboembolism in prior 3 months, acute intracardiac thrombus visualized on echocardiogram.

Bridging is advised on a case-by-case basis (weighing risks and benefits) in patients with significant (recurrent) cerebrovascular disease, newer model mechanical valve (ie, bileaflet tilting disk) in mitral position, older mechanical valve in aortic position, atrial fibrillation with multiple risk factors for cardiac embolism, and history of venous thromboembolism (> 3 months ago). Bridging is not advised in patients with a newer-model mechanical valve in the aortic position, atrial fibrillation without multiple risk factors for cardiac embolism, or in patients with a history of one remote (> 6 months ago) venous thromboembolism.

Warfarin should be stopped 4 days prior to surgery if preoperative INR is 2.0–3.0 (with modification of timing if INR is < 2.0 or > 3.0). In patients who require bridging with a heparin, there is evidence that low-molecular-weight heparin (eg, enoxaparin) is just as effective and safe (if not more so) than unfractionated heparin. Enoxaparin (1 mg/kg twice daily), if not contraindicated, is started 36 hours after the last dose of warfarin and is discontinued 24 hours prior to surgery. On postoperative day 1, warfarin is restarted at the preoperative outpatient dose. At 24 hours postoperatively, the patient is evaluated and enoxaparin is restarted if hemostasis has been achieved. Once INR is in the therapeutic range, enoxaparin can be discontinued.

B. ASPIRIN AND CLOPIDOGREL—Controversy exists regarding the optimal management of antiplatelet therapy in patients undergoing noncardiac surgery, especially in patients with drug-eluting stents. It appears that decreased endothelialization of drug-eluting stents predisposes these patients to stent thrombosis for quite some time after stent placement.

In patients who do not have a coronary stent and who are at low risk for perioperative cardiac events, aspirin and clopidogrel should be discontinued 7–10 days prior to noncardiac surgery.

In patients with coronary stents, especially drug-eluting stents, the risk of stent thrombosis greatly increases when aspirin and clopidogrel are stopped prematurely. Recent AHA/ACC guidelines state that aspirin and clopidogrel should not be discontinued for at least 1 month after bare metal stent and for at least 12 months after the placement of a drug-eluting stent. If surgery cannot be deferred, aspirin should be continued in the perioperative period, and in extremely high-risk patients, intravenous glycoprotein IIb–IIIa inhibitors (which have a shorter half-life than clopidogrel) can be used to try to prevent stent thrombosis (although the increased risk of significant bleeding must also be taken into consideration).

It is now clear that cardiologists must discuss with their patients the need for prolonged dual antiplatelet therapy prior to percutaneous coronary intervention, so that if noncardiac surgery is possible in the near future, drug-eluting stents should be avoided.

2. Antiarrhythmics—These medications should be continued up to the day of surgery, and if necessary in the immediate postoperative period (in an intravenous form).

Amiodarone is a common oral antiarrhythmic that needs to be converted to an intravenous format in the perioperative period. Since intravenous bolus of amiodarone can cause hypotension, it is more ideal to add up the total daily oral dose of amiodarone and convert that dose to a prolonged or continuous infusion (eg, instead of giving 200 mg intravenously as a bolus once daily, give 0.15 mg/min intravenously continuously over 24 hours, or give the 200 mg intravenously over a 4–6 hours).

Digoxin dose should generally be reduced slightly in the perioperative period, especially in elderly patients or those in whom worsening renal function is to be expected.

3. Nonsteroidal antiinflammatory drugs (NSAIDs)—These medications can predispose elderly and other high-risk patients to perioperative renal failure, especially with perioperative dehydration and hypotension. Therefore, NSAIDs should be discontinued at least 3 days prior to surgery and restarted if necessary upon discharge from the hospital.

I. Prophylactic Coronary Revascularization

For patients who are intermediate or high-risk, and who eventually undergo coronary angiography, there are three possibilities: no significant coronary artery disease, left main or triple-vessel coronary artery disease, and single- or two-vessel coronary artery disease.

1. No significant coronary artery disease—Noncardiac surgery can proceed without further testing, although perioperative risk reduction with β-blockers and other agents will be important.

2. Left main or triple-vessel coronary artery disease—These patients, who are on the opposite extreme, are very high-risk and should undergo prophylactic coronary artery bypass grafting. Alternatively, in institutions with expertise, percutaneous coronary intervention is another possibility.

3. Single- or two-vessel coronary artery disease—In these patients, the decision for prophylactic revascularization is more difficult. The Coronary Artery Revascularization Prophylaxis (CARP) trial showed that in patients with single- or two-vessel coronary artery disease (> 70% stenosis) undergoing noncardiac vascular surgery, prophylactic revascularization was no better than medical management for the prevention of short- and long-term perioperative cardiac

events. It is important to note that all patients underwent coronary angiography and those with triple-vessel or left main coronary artery disease were excluded from the trial. Therefore, in patients found to have single- or two-vessel coronary disease, medical management in the perioperative period, even before high-risk vascular surgery, is just as safe as prophylactic revascularization and does not delay noncardiac surgery. If patients must undergo percutaneous coronary intervention preoperatively, balloon angioplasty alone avoids the necessity to continue dual antiplatelet therapy. If stents are placed, it is extremely important to follow recommendations for perioperative management of aspirin and clopidogrel (see section on Perioperative Medication Management above).

Auerbach AD et al. Beta-blockers and reduction of cardiac events in noncardiac surgery: scientific review. JAMA. 2002 Mar 20;287(11):1435–44. [PMID: 11903031]

Auerbach AD. Perioperative cardiac risk reduction: doing it right. Cleve Clin J Med. 2006 Mar;73 Suppl 1:S25–9. [PMID: 16570544]

Devereaux PJ et al. How strong is the evidence for the use of perioperative beta blockers in non-cardiac surgery? Systematic review and meta-analysis of randomized controlled trials. BMJ. 2005 Aug 6;331(7512):313–21. [PMID: 15996966]

Durazzo AE et al. Reduction in cardiovascular events after vascular surgery with atorvastatin: a randomized trial. J Vas Surg. 2004 May;39(5):967–75. [PMID: 15111846]

Grines CL et al; American Heart Association; American College of Cardiology; Society for Cardiovascular Angiography and Interventions; American College of Surgeons; American Dental Association; American College of Physicians. Prevention of premature discontinuation of dual antiplatelet therapy in patients with coronary artery stents: a science advisory from the American Heart Association, American College of Cardiology, Society for Cardiovascular Angiography and Interventions, American College of Surgeons, and American Dental Association, with representation from the American College of Physicians. Circulation. 2007 Feb 13;115(6):813–8. [PMID: 17224480]

Jaffer AK. Anticoagulation management strategies for patients on warfarin who need surgery. Cleve Clin J Med. 2006 Mar;73 Suppl 1:S100–5. [PMID: 16570558]

Lindenauer PK et al. Lipid-lowering therapy and in-hospital mortality following major noncardiac surgery. JAMA. 2004 May 5;291(17):2092–9. [PMID: 15126437]

Lindenauer PK et al. Perioperative beta-blocker therapy and mortality after major noncardiac vascular surgery. N Engl J Med. 2005 Jul 28;353(4):349–61. [PMID: 16049209]

McFalls EO et al. Coronary-artery revascularization before elective major vascular surgery. N Engl J Med. 2004 Dec 30;351(27):2795–804. [PMID: 15625331]

Poldermans D et al. Statins are associated with a reduced incidence of perioperative mortality in patients undergoing major noncardiac vascular surgery. Circulation. 2003 Apr 15;107(14):1848–51. [PMID: 12695283]

Wijeysundera DN et al. Alpha-2 adrenergic agonists to prevent perioperative cardiovascular complications: a meta analysis. Am J Med. 2003 Jun 15;114(9):742–52. [PMID: 12829201]

Wijeysundera DN et al. Calcium channel blockers for reducing cardiac morbidity after noncardiac surgery: a meta-analysis. Anesth Analg. 2003 Sep;97(3):634–41. [PMID: 12933374]

Wilson W et al; American Heart Association Rheumatic Fever, Endocarditis, and Kawasaki Disease Committee; American Heart Association Council on Cardiovascular Disease in the Young; American Heart Association Council on Clinical Cardiology; American Heart Association Council on Cardiovascular Surgery and Anesthesia; Quality of Care and Outcomes Research Interdisciplinary Working Group. Prevention of infective endocarditis: guidelines from the American Heart Association: a guideline from the American Heart Association Rheumatic Fever, Endocarditis, and Kawasaki Disease Committee, Council on Cardiovascular Disease in the Young, and the Council on Clinical Cardiology, Council on Cardiovascular Surgery and Anesthesia, and the Quality of Care and Outcomes Research Interdisciplinary Working Group. Circulation. 2007 Oct 9;116(15):1736–54. [PMID: 17446442]

► Special Populations

A. Vascular Surgery

Of all noncardiac surgeries, intra-abdominal and intrapelvic vascular surgeries are perhaps the highest risk because of the nature of the surgery and the nature of the patients who have peripheral vascular disease, since many of these patients have significant coronary risk factors and coronary artery disease.

For patients undergoing elective high-risk vascular surgery, the ACC/AHA guidelines are useful for determining whether these patients need further risk stratification with noninvasive cardiac testing. Kertai and colleagues have published a more detailed risk prediction model, customized for type of vascular surgery, which may be useful in cases where level of risk is not obvious, or for surgeons, patients, or families who want a more detailed risk assessment.

In patients who require coronary angiography because they are high-risk, or because they are intermediate risk with an abnormal stress test, the results of the CARP trial (see above under Prophylactic Coronary Revascularization) help clinicians better understand which patients can be adequately treated with medical therapy alone.

B. Aortic Stenosis

In patients with severe or critical aortic stenosis, risks of a perioperative cardiac complication are very high. The risk correlates with aortic valve mean gradient, as measured by echocardiography. Even moderate aortic stenosis (mean gradient of > 25 mm Hg) has been associated with an adjusted relative risk of 5.2 for perioperative cardiac complications.

Noninvasive stress testing is unnecessary and potentially dangerous in these patients. If the patient has symptomatic aortic stenosis, postpone the noncardiac surgery until after the patient undergoes coronary angiography, aortic valve replacement, and coronary artery bypass grafting (if the patient is found to have significant coronary artery disease). In asymptomatic patients with severe aortic stenosis, preoperative aortic valve replacement (prior to elective noncardiac surgery) is usually the best option because of the very high-risk nature of these patients. If aortic valve replacement is not an option, percutaneous aortic valvuloplasty can be considered, though it carries a significant risk of thromboembolism and aortic stenosis recurrence. These risks must be weighed against the risk of cancelling surgery or operating with significant aortic stenosis.

C. Heart Failure

Patients with a history of hospitalization for heart failure, and especially those with current signs and symptoms of heart failure, are at high risk for perioperative cardiac events. In these patients, heart failure should be treated and volume status optimized prior to surgery, since the risks of heart failure outweigh the need for surgery in most cases. As the number of patients with heart failure increases along with the aging population, more patients who undergo noncardiac surgery will have a history of heart failure. Even though heart failure is a greater risk of perioperative cardiac events than coronary artery disease, there are few studies on the optimal perioperative treatment of patients with heart failure, especially those with preserved ejection fraction.

D. Pulmonary Hypertension

In patients with significant pulmonary hypertension, the risks of general anesthesia are extraordinarily high. Pulmonary hypertension can be thought of as a fixed obstruction to cardiopulmonary blood flow, and therefore prevents increase in cardiac output necessary in the perioperative state. It is therefore very similar to critical aortic stenosis in this aspect. In these cases, a pulmonary hypertension specialist should be consulted. Elective surgeries should be postponed indefinitely until the patient is treated with vasodilators to reduce the perioperative risk. If surgery is absolutely necessary, it is advisable that these patients undergo continuous monitoring with pulmonary artery catheter intraoperatively. Intraoperative inhaled nitric oxide can be used to decrease pulmonary artery pressures.

E. Pacemakers and Defibrillators

There is a small risk that prolonged electrocautery could trigger, reprogram, or inadvertently offset an implantable cardioverter defibrillator (ICD). Electrocautery may also interfere with pacemaker output and anesthetic agents may interfere with pacing thresholds. Some manufacturers have recommended that the device be inactivated during surgery. Supraventricular tachycardias, which are fairly common in the postoperative period, may exceed the rate threshold of the ICD and can cause inappropriate shocks to be delivered. Implantable cardioverter defibrillators should be interrogated before surgery to assess underlying rhythm and frequency of discharges. In pacemaker-dependent patients, the rate response feature should be tuned off. The ICD defibrillation capacity should be disengaged just prior to surgery and resumed immediately after surgery, and an external defibrillating device with personnel able to handle it should be close to the patient at all times during the period that the ICD is off. Of note, an anteroposterior lead placement of the external pacer paddles away from the device pocket is required in the event of external cardioversion or defibrillation.

Christ M et al. Preoperative and perioperative care for patients with suspected or established aortic stenosis facing noncardiac surgery. Chest. 2005 Oct;128(4):2944–53. [PMID: 16236971]

Kertai MD et al. Aortic stenosis: an underestimated risk factor for perioperative complications in patients undergoing noncardiac surgery. Am J Med. 2004 Jan 1;116(1):8–13. [PMID: 14706659]

Kertai MD et al. Optimizing the prediction of perioperative mortality in vascular surgery by using a customized probability model. Arch Intern Med. 2005 Apr 25;165(8):898–904. [PMID: 15851641]

Index

Note: Page numbers followed by *t* indicate tables; those followed by *f* indicate figures.